D1416582

MANUAL OF

Critical Care Nursing

Nursing Interventions and
Collaborative Management

MANUAL OF
Critical Care Nursing
Nursing Interventions and Collaborative Management

Edited by

Marianne Saunorus Baird, RN, MN
Clinical Nurse Specialist
Saint Joseph's Hospital of Atlanta
Atlanta, Georgia

Janet Hicks Keen, RN, MSN, CIC, CCRN
Director, Emergency Department
Saint Joseph's Hospital of Atlanta
Atlanta, Georgia

Pamela L. Swearingen, RN
Special Project Editor

FIFTH EDITION

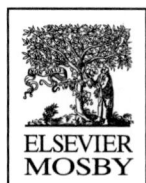

ELSEVIER
MOSBY

ELSEVIER
MOSBY

11830 Westline Industrial Drive
St. Louis, Missouri 63146

MANUAL OF CRITICAL CARE NURSING
Copyright © 2005, 2001, 1995, 1991, 1998 by Mosby, Inc. All rights reserved.

NOTICE

Nursing is an ever-changing field. Standard safety precautions must be followed, but as new research and clinical experience broaden our knowledge, changes in treatment and drug therapy may become necessary or appropriate. Readers are advised to check the most current product information provided by the manufacturer of each drug to be administered to verify the recommended dose, the method and duration of administration, and contraindications. It is the responsibility of the licensed prescriber, relying on experience and knowledge of the patient, to determine dosages and the best treatment for each individual patient. Neither the publisher nor the author assumes any liability for any injury and/or damage to persons or property arising from this publication.

The Publisher

ISBN-13: 978-0-323-02657-4
ISBN-10: 0-323-02657-5

Executive Publisher: Barbara Nelson Cullen
Developmental Editor: Julie Vitale
Publishing Services Manager: Deborah Vogel
Project Manager: Mary Drone
Design Manager: Gail Hudson

Printed in the United States of America

Last digit is the print number: 9 8 7 6 5 4 3 2

Working together to grow
libraries in developing countries
www.elsevier.com | www.bookaid.org | www.sabre.org

ELSEVIER   BOOK AID International   Sabre Foundation

Contributors

JENNI JORDAN ABEL, RN, BA, CME
Staff Nurse, Surgical Intensive Care Unit
University of Colorado Hospital
Denver, Colorado

PATRICE C. AL-SADEN, RN, CCRC
Clinical Research Associate on Staff
The Feinberg School of Medicine
Northwestern University
Northwestern Memorial Hospital
Chicago, Illinois

LINDA S. BAAS, RN, PHD, ACNP, CCNS
Associate Professor, College of Nursing
University of Cincinnati
Acute Care Nurse Practitioner, Heart Failure Program, University Hospital
Cincinnati, Ohio

MARIANNE SAUNORUS BAIRD, RN, MN
Clinical Nurse Specialist
Saint Joseph's Hospital of Atlanta
Atlanta, Georgia

CAROL A. BARCH, MN, CCNS, FNP, ANCC
Department of Neurology Clinical Administrator
UPMC Stroke Institute Program Administrator
University of Pittsburgh Medical Center
Pittsburgh, Pennsylvania

SUSAN BETHEL, RN, MS, CNRN
Director of Nursing
Clinical Programs & Research
Greenville Hospital System
Greenville, South Carolina

CHERYL L. BITTEL, RN, MSN, CCRN
Clinical Nurse Specialist
Saint Joseph's Hospital of Atlanta
Atlanta, Georgia

MIMI CALLANAN, RN, MSN
Epilepsy Clinical Nurse Specialist
Department of Neurology
Stanford University Medical Center
Stanford, California

GRETCHEN J. CARROUGHER, RN, MN
Clinical Faculty, School of Nursing
University of Washington
Research Nurse Supervisor, Department of Surgery
Department of Rehabilitation Medicine, University of Washington
Seattle, Washington

ALICE E. DAVIS, PHD, RN, CNRN, GNP
Assistant Professor
University of Michigan
Ann Arbor, Michigan

BEVERLY GEORGE-GAY, RN, MSN, CCRN
Nurse Educator
Critical Care Programs
Virginia Commonwealth University Medical Center
Richmond, Virginia

KAREN GOFF, RN, BSN
Data Integration Analyst
Saint Joseph's Hospital of Atlanta
Atlanta, Georgia

SHARI HONARI, RN, BSN
Burn Research Supervisor
University of Washington Burn Center at Harborview Medical Center
Seattle, Washington

MARGUERITE MCMILLAN JACKSON, RN, PHD, FAAN, CIC
Associate Clinical Professor of Family & Preventive Medicine
Director, Administrative Unit
National Tuberculosis Curriculum Consortium (NTCC)
Division of Pulmonary & Critical Care Medicine
School of Medicine
University of California, San Diego
San Diego, California

DAN KIDWELL, AS, RRTE, RCP
Network Clinical Practice Specialist
The Community Health Network
Indianapolis, Indiana

CATHERINE OSIKA LANDRETH, BSN, MS, CCRN, CEN
Trauma Program Coordinator
Clinical Nurse Specialist
Greenville Hospital System
Greenville, South Carolina

LYNDA LILES, RN, BS, MBA, CCRN
Performance Improvement Specialist
Staff Nurse
Coronary Care Unit
Saint Joseph's Hospital of Atlanta
Atlanta, Georgia

ANDREA LIPSMEYER, RN, BSN
Staff Nurse
Labor and Delivery
North Carolina Women's Hospital
Chapel Hill, North Carolina

CHARLOTTE HARRISON MACKEY, RN, MSN, EDD
Assistant Professor of Nursing
West Chester University
West Chester, Pennsylvania

CHERYL MCKAY, RN, MSN, CCNS
Clinical Nurse Specialist
HCA Healthcare
Edmond, Oklahoma

BARBARA MCLEAN, RN, MN, CCRN, CCNP, CCNS, FCCM
Nurse Intensivist
Atlanta Medical Center
Atlanta, Georgia

THERESA MURRAY, RN, MSN, CCRN
Clinical Nurse Specialist for Critical Care
The Community Health Network
Indianapolis, Indiana

MARGUERITE J. MURPHY, RN, MSN
Assistant Professor
School of Nursing
Medical College of Georgia
Augusta, Georgia

PAUL SCHMIDT, RPH, BCPS
Adjunct Faculty
Mercer University
Atlanta, Georgia
University of Georgia
Athens, Georgia
Pharmaceutical Care Pharmacist
Saint Joseph's Hospital of Atlanta
Atlanta, Georgia

NANCY STOTTS, RN EDD, FAAN
Professor
University of California, San Francisco
San Francisco, California

THOMAS K. WEICHART, RN, MSN, MSA, CCRN
Captain, U.S. Army
Emergency Department
Womack Army Medical Center
Fort Bragg, North Carolina

PATRICIA D. WEISKITTEL, MSN, CNN, CS
Renal Transplant Clinical Nurse Specialist
University Hospital
Cincinnati, Ohio

LAURA D. WILLIAMS, BSN, MBA, CCRN, NCBF
Palliative Care Coordinator
Saint Joseph's Hospital of Atlanta
Atlanta, Georgia

Reviewers

JENNIFER BASLER, RN, MSN, CCRN
Clinical Nurse Specialist for Cardiovascular Services
Appleton Medical Center
Appleton, Wisconsin

LOUISE M. DIEHL-OPLINGER, RN, MSN, CCRN, APRN, BC, CLNC
Staff Development Instructor
Warren Hospital
Phillipsburg, New Jersey

KAREN HEMPSTEAD, RN, MSN
Director of Education, Mountain View Regional Medical Center
Associate Professor of Nursing
Department of Nursing
New Mexico State University
Las Cruces, New Mexico

ANN M. PRICE, MSC, BSC, PGCE, RN
Senior Lecturer in Critical Care, Adult Nursing Department
Canterbury Christ Church University College
Canterbury, Kent, England

LESLIE TONEY, RN, BSN
Practical Nursing Instructor
Wes Watkins Technology Center
Wetumka, Oklahoma

Preface

Manual of Critical Care Nursing: Nursing Interventions and Collaborative Management, fifth edition, is a clinically focused reference designed to assist nurses with various levels of expertise in the evaluation and management of the human responses to potentially life-threatening conditions. Consideration is given to the physical, emotional, mental, and spiritual impact of critical illness on both the patient and his or her support system. Assessment, planning, and implementation of care, with subsequent evaluation parameters, are presented. Desired nursing outcomes are specific, positive statements that facilitate measurable evaluation of care. Suggested time frames for outcome criteria are included with each outcome statement. Time frames provided are guidelines, since each patient's response time to both illness and interventions is unique.

Each chapter provides a brief review of pathophysiology, physical assessment, diagnostic testing, collaborative management, NANDA-approved nursing diagnoses and nursing interventions, patient-support system teaching, and discharge planning information specific to each disorder or management strategy. Overall content is a balance of information needed to manage the technology of the critical care environment along with the challenges of patient care related to each illness. Cross references to the appropriate labels derived by the Nursing Interventions Classification (NIC) are included to provide a platform for reference if additional details of care are desired.

More generic information is included in Chapter 1: General Concepts in Caring for the Critically Ill, in which assessment and management strategies for nutritional support, mechanical ventilation, hemodynamic monitoring, sedating and paralyzing agents, alterations in consciousness, wound and skin care, pain, prolonged immobility, psychosocial support for the patient, family and support system and the ethical considerations in critical care are presented. Research boxes containing pertinent clinical data are located in each chapter, along with elder icons located in the margin, which emphasize content pertinent to older adults.

For clarity and consistency throughout the book, normal values are given for hemodynamic monitoring and other measurements. All values should be individualized to each patient's baseline health status. To best assess improvement or deterioration in status, knowledge of the patient's condition before critical illness is essential. Although the book offers many interventions for each disorder, not all interventions are appropriate for every patient. Our intent is to offer a thorough list of interventions that can be chosen as needed in planning care for individual patients.

New to the Fifth Edition

- Critical care content throughout the manual, including appendices, has been thoroughly **revised and updated** by clinical experts.
- Sections on **Emerging Infections, Bioterrorism, High-Risk Obstetrics Patients,** and **Thyroid Disease** have been added.
- Content regarding **intensive insulin therapy to manage blood glucose** and emerging strategies for **managing systemic inflammatory response syndrome to preserve the vascular endothelium** are expanded.
- **New medications used to manage anticoagulation, fibrinolysis,** and recent data regarding evaluation of **alternatives to blood transfusions for anemia** are included.
- New **implantable cardiac support devices** and guidelines medications used for management of **heart failure, blood pressure, and dysrhythmias,** including **neurohormonal, antihypertensive and diuretic therapies,** are detailed.
- Recent changes in guidelines used in the **management of burn and trauma** patients are included.

- New and upcoming **strategies used in mechanical ventilation, including noninvasive positive pressure ventilation (NPPV)** and **prevention of ventilator associated pneumonia,** are reviewed.
- Current medications and other **strategies used to manage organ transplantation** are detailed.
- Care plans have been **redesigned to emphasize key actions** and lengthy paragraphs have been formatted into easily scanned lists for quicker, easier reading when possible.
- Principles of management of **delirium, restlessness, pain, and agitation** are presented.

Readers who desire more information on disorders traditionally seen in the medical-surgical nursing environment (e.g., chronic obstructive pulmonary disease, chronic renal failure, diverticulosis and cancer) are encouraged to read the *Manual of Medical-Surgical Nursing Care: Nursing Interventions,* fifth edition, edited by Pamela L. Swearingen.

Manual of Critical Care Nursing was written to supplement critical care textbooks and assumes that the reader has a basic background in critical care pathophysiology and assessment parameters. The book can serve as a resource not only for clinicians, but for academicians and students as well. The textual information and numerous tables will stimulate the clinician's recall of previously learned concepts. Academicians can use the book in teaching students to apply theoretical concepts to clinical practice. Students will find the book to be an excellent tool in helping them assess the patient systematically, as well as in setting priorities in nursing interventions. Nursing diagnoses are presented in order of priority.

Our primary goal is to provide the staff and students in critical care a wealth of knowledge in a quick and easy-to-use format. We welcome feedback from nurses who use the book on a daily basis so we can enhance its usefulness in future editions.

Marianne Saunorus Baird
Janet Hicks Keen
Pamela L. Swearingen

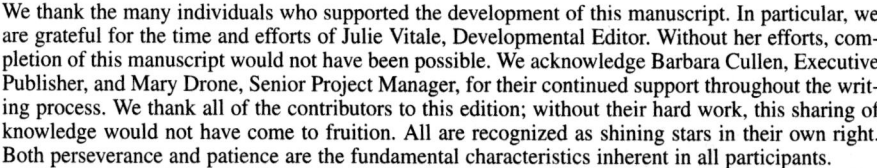

Acknowledgments

We thank the many individuals who supported the development of this manuscript. In particular, we are grateful for the time and efforts of Julie Vitale, Developmental Editor. Without her efforts, completion of this manuscript would not have been possible. We acknowledge Barbara Cullen, Executive Publisher, and Mary Drone, Senior Project Manager, for their continued support throughout the writing process. We thank all of the contributors to this edition; without their hard work, this sharing of knowledge would not have come to fruition. All are recognized as shining stars in their own right. Both perseverance and patience are the fundamental characteristics inherent in all participants.

We extend special recognition to Susan Bethel, RN, MS, CNRN; Catherine Osika-Landreth, BSN, MS, CCRN, CEN, and Thomas K. Weichart, RN, MSN, MSA, CCRN, for "going the extra mile" with their contributions to the manuscript.

MSB
JHK
PLS

I acknowledge the support of my husband Thom; my daughter Rachel; my colleagues, Polly Willis, Susan Axelrod, Debra Bonser, and Terry Hackworth; my parents, John and Irene Saunorus; and the divine inspiration and strength that helped me when I was most in need.

MSB

Contents

CHAPTER 1

General Concepts in Caring for the Critically Ill

Nutritional Support

The goal of nutritional support therapy is to identify preexisting malnutrition, prevent further protein-calorie deficiencies, optimize the patient's current state, and reduce further morbidity. Outcomes for patients with protein-calorie malnutrition demonstrate increased mortality and morbidity, including weakness, compromised immunity, decreased wound healing, infection, and organ failure. When protein-calorie malnutrition, marasmus, is complicated with stressors, such as burns, trauma, surgery, or sepsis, the neuroendocrine response results in hypermetabolism, hypercatabolism, insulin resistance with hyperglycemia, and depletion of lean body mass. The body adapts to starvation through a series of hormonal changes that compensate for the decreased intake of nutrients. If starvation is prolonged, the body uses its own substrate to optimize survival, with a resulting loss of skeletal muscle and adipose tissue.

NUTRITIONAL ASSESSMENT

Multiple sources of information are used, including medical and nutritional history, anthropometric data (body measurements), biochemical analysis of blood and urine, and duration of the disease process. With a critically ill individual, this history may be obtained from significant others.

Medical/nutritional history: A nutritional history identifies individuals who are or may be at risk for malnutrition. Medical history is included to assess diseases or conditions affecting nutritional status. Describe the adequacy of both usual and recent food intake. Focus on factors which may have impaired adequate selection, preparation, ingestion, digestion, absorption, and excretion of nutrients. Include the following:

- Comprehensive review of usual dietary intake, including food allergies, food aversions, use of nutritional supplements including vitamins and alternative/complementary therapies
- Recent weight loss or gain—planned or unplanned
- Chewing or swallowing difficulties
- Nausea, vomiting, or pain with eating
- Altered pattern of elimination (e.g., constipation, diarrhea)
- Diseases/conditions increasing energy needs (e.g., burns, extensive wounds, decubitus ulcers, sepsis, surgery, trauma)
- Chronic disease affecting utilization of nutrients (e.g., malabsorption, pancreatitis, diabetes mellitus)

- Use of medications (e.g., laxatives, antacids, antibiotics, antineoplastic drugs)
- Who obtains food and prepares meals
- Cultural preferences restricting specific nutrient intake or causing excessive intake
- Alcohol or drug use
- Recent fad or vegetarian diets

Physical assessment: Most physical findings are not conclusive for particular nutritional deficiencies. Compare current assessment findings with past assessments, especially related to the following:
- Loss of muscle and adipose tissue
- Work and muscle endurance, neuromuscular function
- Changes in hair, presence of skin lesions

Anthropometric data: Anthropometrics is the measurement of the body or its parts. Pounds and inches are converted to metric measurements using the following formulas:

Divide pounds by 2.2 to convert to kilograms (kg).

Multiply inches by 2.54 to convert to centimeters (cm).

- *Height:* Used to determine ideal weight and body mass index; if unavailable, obtain estimate from family or significant others.
- *Weight:* A readily available and practical indicator of nutritional status that can be compared with previous weight and ideal weight or used to calculate body mass index. Large changes may reflect fluid retention (edema, third spacing), diuresis, dehydration, surgical resections, traumatic amputations, or weight of dressings or equipment. Remember 1 liter (L) of fluid equals approximately 2 pounds (lb). Use actual body weight to avoid overfeeding in starved patients and ideal body weight in patients who weigh >120% of ideal body weight (Table 1-1).
- *Body mass index (BMI):* Used to evaluate adult weight. One calculation and one set of standards apply to both men and women:

T A B L E 1 - 1   Height and Weight Guidelines for Men and Women

Height	Men (weight in lb)			Women (weight in lb)		
	Small frame	Medium frame	Large frame	Small frame	Medium frame	Large frame
4 ft 10 in	—	—	—	102-111	109-121	118-131
4 ft 11 in	—	—	—	103-113	111-123	120-134
5 ft	—	—	—	104-115	113-126	122-137
5 ft 1 in	—	—	—	106-118	115-129	125-140
5 ft 2 in	128-134	131-141	138-150	108-121	118-132	128-143
5 ft 3 in	130-136	133-143	140-153	111-124	121-135	131-147
5 ft 4 in	132-138	135-145	142-156	114-127	124-138	134-151
5 ft 5 in	134-140	137-148	144-160	117-130	127-141	137-155
5 ft 6 in	136-142	139-151	146-164	120-133	130-144	140-159
5 ft 7 in	138-145	142-154	149-168	123-136	133-147	143-163
5 ft 8 in	140-148	145-157	152-172	126-139	136-150	146-167
5 ft 9 in	142-151	148-160	155-176	129-142	139-153	149-170
5 ft 10 in	144-154	151-163	158-180	132-145	142-156	152-173
5 ft 11 in	146-157	154-166	161-184	135-148	145-159	155-176
6 ft	149-160	157-170	164-188	138-151	148-162	158-179
6 ft 1 in	152-164	160-174	168-192	—	—	—
6 ft 2 in	155-168	164-178	172-197	—	—	—
6 ft 3 in	158-172	167-182	176-202	—	—	—
6 ft 4 in	162-176	171-187	181-207	—	—	—

$$BMI \ (kg/m^2) = \frac{Weight \ (kg)}{Height \ (m) \times Height \ (m)}$$

BMI values of 20-25 are optimal; values >25 indicate obesity; and values <20 indicate underweight status and significant increase in morbidity, and are associated with longer intensive care unit stay, increased postoperative complications, and higher readmission rates.

- *Midarm muscle circumference (MAMC):* measures muscle mass of mid upper arm using a formula.
- *Triceps skinfold thickness (TSF):* Measured at the midpoint of the upper arm by taking half the distance between the olecranon and the acromion process and grasping the skin and subcutaneous tissue at the back of the arm approximately 1 cm from the midpoint. Surgical calipers are used to measure the skinfold. A TSF measurement of <3 mm signals severely depleted fat stores.

Specially trained clinicians and dietitians should perform this assessment for more accurate and consistent results. The skill level and technique used varies among clinicians.

DIAGNOSTIC TESTS

No laboratory test specifically measures nutritional status. Status can be estimated, however, using the following guidelines.

Visceral protein status: Normal values may vary with different laboratory procedures and standards. If hydration status is normal and anemia is absent, albumin and transferrin levels may be the initial parameters used.

- **Serum albumin** (3.5-5.5 g/dl): associated with increased morbidity in critical illness if <3.5 g/dl. Has a long half-life (19 days) and changes slowly in response to nutritional support when protein-calorie malnutrition is present.
- **Prealbumin** (20-30 mg/dl): reliable indicator of response to nutritional therapy. Has a short half-life (24-48 hr). May not be as reliable if patient is severely stressed or ill.
- **Retinal binding protein** (4-5 mg/dl): indicator with shortest half-life (10 h), used to assess the response to nutritional therapy. Not as reliable if patient is severely stressed or ill.
- **Transferrin** (180-260 mg/dl): indicator with a longer half-life (9 days), used as a baseline indicator of protein intake and synthesis.

Nitrogen balance: Used to discern if the patient is anabolic (building body stores or healing) or catabolic (breaking down body stores, deteriorating). If more nitrogen is received than excreted, nitrogen is said to be positive and an anabolic state exists. When nitrogen excretion is higher than intake, a negative balance or catabolic state exists. Most nitrogen loss occurs through the urine, with a small, constant amount lost via skin and feces. Nitrogen balance studies should be performed by specialists, because accurate measurement of 24-hr food intake and urine output is required. Heavy losses of protein in the presence of ascites, large wounds, and excessive chest tube drainage are difficult to measure but should be considered.

ESTIMATING NUTRITIONAL REQUIREMENTS

Energy needs: The primary goal of nutritional support is to meet the energy needs for body temperature, metabolic processes, and tissue repair. The nutritional plan should avoid overfeeding and the complications associated with excessive caloric intake. Energy needs can be estimated using the following options:

Indirect calorimetry: Specialized personnel and access to a metabolic cart are required to provide accurate results. It measures oxygen consumption and carbon dioxide production as a by product of metabolism and gives the basal energy expenditure (BEE).

Harris Benedict equations: Most common method to determine BEE. It is calculated using the following equations developed by Harris and Benedict:

$$BEE \ (male) = 66 + (13.7 \times W) + (5 \times H) - (6.8 \times A)$$

$$BEE \ (female) = 655 + (9.6 \times W) \ (1.7 \times H) - (4.7 \times A)$$

when:

$$W = weight \ (kg); \ H = height \ (cm); \ A = age \ (yr)$$

The BEE is multiplied by a stress factor that is estimated from the degree of stress and the need for weight maintenance or repletion. Multiplying the BEE by 1.2-2.5 provides a range appropriate for most patients. The lower factor is appropriate for patients without significant stress, whereas the higher factor is appropriate for patients with higher levels of stress, such as occurs with major trauma, sepsis, or burns.

Protein needs: Protein requirements for maintenance therapy are 0.8 g/kg/day. Critically ill patients may need an estimated 1.5-2 g/kg/day. Fever, infection, and wounds increase needs to the same range. Severe stress or burns may increase this requirement to 3 gm/kg/day.

Provision of energy and protein:

- *Carbohydrate (CHO):* Glucose administration of 5 mg/kg/min is a suitable amount. Carbohydrates provided in excess of this amount are not well utilized and may lead to hyperglycemia, excessive CO_2 production, hypophosphatemia, fat deposits in the liver, transient elevated liver enzymes, and fluid overload.
- *Protein:* Approximate ratio of g CHO to g nitrogen is 150:1. 1 g nitrogen = 6.25 g protein.
- *Fat requirements:* If protein and glucose are supplied as outlined, the remainder of needed calories can be supplied as fat. Fat can be administered in minimal quantities to satisfy needs for essential fatty acids, or it can be provided in larger quantities, as tolerated, to meet energy needs.
- *Abnormal elevations in liver enzymes:* Often occur in patients maintained on total parenteral nutrition (TPN) longer than 3 weeks. Usually the enzymes return to normal upon cessation of TPN. Giving cyclic TPN, in which the patient receives TPN for 12-16 hr out of 24 hr, may prevent enzyme elevation.
- *Including protein in caloric count:* Although controversy still exists as to whether to count protein calories (4 cal/g) in parenteral nutrition, many clinicians do include them based on the rationale that they are included when calculating enteral and oral caloric intake. Also, it is impossible to prevent some protein from being used for energy once it is administered.

Vitamin and essential trace mineral requirements: In general, follow the Recommended Dietary Allowances (RDAs) to provide minimum quantities of vitamins, minerals, and essential fatty acids. For specific patients, supplements of specific vitamins or minerals are needed in increased amounts for existing disease states (e.g., zinc and vitamins A and C for burns; thiamine, folate, and vitamin B_{12} for chronic alcohol ingestion).

Fluid requirements: Many factors affect fluid balance. All sources of intake (oral, enteral, intravenous, and medications), as well as output (urine, stool, drainage, emesis, fluid shifts, and respiratory and evaporative losses), must be considered. Fluid intake is closely associated to energy provided. Approximately 1 ml fluid per calorie is the standard method to calculate fluid requirements. Fever increases fluid needs, and fluid intake should be closely monitored in renal and cardiac dysfunction.

Special diets for organ-specific pathology: Costly, and the metabolic advantages of some products remain unproven.

- *Hepatic failure:* Branched-chain amino acids in combination with reduced aromatic amino acid concentrations may help alleviate encephalopathy associated with hepatic failure.
- *Renal disease:* High percentages of essential amino acids are used to improve nitrogen use and decrease urea formation.
- *Respiratory disease:* A low-protein and low-carbohydrate diet decreases CO_2 production and, consequently, the work of breathing.
- *Diabetes:* Reduced carbohydrates and higher fiber content used for glucose intolerance. Fat consists of higher monounsaturated fatty acids to stay within guidelines for prevention of coronary artery disease.

NUTRITIONAL SUPPORT MODALITIES

Studies indicate enteral feedings prevent passage of bacteria from the gastrointestinal (GI) tract into the lymphatic system (bacterial translocation) and other organs, reducing a major source of sepsis and possible organ failure. Cost, safety, and convenience considerations have been the rationale for using enteral over parenteral nutritional support, but the potential physiologic benefits are a more compelling argument. Enteral feedings foster wound healing and immunocompetence and preserve gut function.

Enteral formulas: Composed of a wide variety of standard and modular formulas. See also Table 1-2.

- *Standard:* Consist of intact proteins and a caloric source; most are lactose-free; all are sterile, and suitable for small-bore feeding tubes and have a fixed nutrient composition. Vitamins and trace elements and minerals are included.
- *Modular:* Consist of a single nutrient that may be combined with other modules (nutrients) for a formula tailor-made for an individual's specific deficits (e.g., carbohydrate, fat, protein, vitamin modules).

TABLE 1-2 Types of Enteral Formulations

Enteral formula	Description
Blenderized diet	
Compleat, Compleat Modified, Vitaneed	Nutritionally complete, requiring complete digestive capabilities; composed of natural foods, including meat, vegetables, milk, and fruit
Milk-based formula	
Meritene, Sustagen, Carnation Instant (if mixed with milk)	Nutritionally adequate diet for general nutritional support
Lactose-free formula	
Ensure, Entrition 1, Isocal, Osmolite	Nutritionally adequate, liquid preparation; used for general nutritional support; isoosmolar or hypoosmolar; all except Osmolite are low residue
Elemental or chemically defined	
Criticare HN	Low-Na+, lactose-free, high-N diet; 40% protein supplied as small peptides; nutritionally adequate; used for general nutritional support
Travasorb NH	Nutritionally adequate; used for general nutritional support; contains additional hydrolyzed protein that is readily digested and absorbed
Specialty formulas **Hepatic failure**	
Hepatic Travasorb	Nutritionally complete; has a greater ratio of branched chain to aromatic amino acids while restricting total amino acid concentrations and adding nonprotein calories
Hepatic-Aid II	Nutritionally incomplete powder diet with essential nutrients in easily digestible form; high in branched chain amino acids; low in aromatic amino acids and methionines
Renal failure	
Renal Travasorb	Electrolyte, lactose, fat-soluble, vitamin-free; high in calories; contains mostly essential amino acids; restricted total protein content may reduce or postpone need for dialysis
Amin-Aid	Nutritionally incomplete supplement with essential nutrients in readily digestible form with minimal electrolytes
Respiratory insufficiency	
Pulmocare	Nutritionally complete; contains a higher proportion of fat to carbohydrates; reduces CO_2 production
Hypermetabolic and trauma states	
Trauma-Aid HB	High in branched-chain amino acids; readily digestible essential nutrients
Trauma Cal	Nutritionally adequate with high proportions of protein and calories in a limited volume
Modular formulas	Offer highly flexible tailoring of nutrients (e.g., fat [Lipomul], protein [Pro Mod], and carbohydrates [Moducal]) for specific patient needs

Continued

T A B L E 1 - 2   Types of Enteral Formulations—cont'd

Enteral formula	Description
Fiber enhanced	
Ultracal, Boost with Fiber, Compleat, FiberSource, Ensure Fiber, Jevity, Nutren with Fiber	Nutritionally complete; require intact GI function and absorption; hypertonic; milk, soy, or sodium and calcium caseinate protein source; some brands come in standard and high-calorie or high-nitrogen concentrations
Standard formula Osmolite, Isocal, Boost, Ensure, IsoSource, Nutren, ReSource	Nutritionally complete; typically 1 or 1.06 calorie/ml, low-residue liquid formula used for standard tube feedings; some come in closed system to minimize contamination
Calorically dense Novasource 2.0, Resource 2.0, TwoCal HN, Nutren 2.0, NuBasics, 2.0, Deliver 2.0	Calorie content is 2 calories/ml to provide adequate nutrients in lower volume for volume-restricted patients; some standard products also come in 1.5 calorie/ml concentration
Elemental or semi-elemental	
Impact, Peptinex, Tolerex, Vivonex, AlitraQ, Criticare HN, Crucial, Optimental, Peptamen, Peritive, Reabilan, Subdue	Designed for easy absorption for patient who has poor absorption or atrophied intestine; protein source is free amino acids or protein hydrolysates (peptides) or both; fat source are oils easily absorbed: MCT, soybean, canola, safflower; no fiber; some have flavor packets for oral use
Disease specific	
Liver failure: Hepatic-Aid II, NutriHep	Branched-chain amino acids, no fiber, minimal-to-no vitamin or minerals
Renal failure: Nepro, Renalcal, Amin-Aid, Suplena, NutriRenal Diet, Magnacal Renal	Essential amino acids, designed to minimize protein load and reduce need for dialysis. minimal or no vitamins or minerals
Glucose intolerance: glytrol, choice DM, DiabetiSource, Glucerna	Reduced carbohydrate, higher fiber content, nutritionally complete for glucose intolerance from diabetes or stress
Pulmonary failure: NutriVent, Oxepa, Pulmocare, Respalor, NovaSource Pulmonary	Moderate fat content with less saturated fats
Other specialty products	Lower carbohydrate, calorically dense designed to decrease CO_2 production
Impact, Promote, ProtainXL, Peritive	Fortified with protein, vitamins, and minerals that enhance wound healing and immune function (i.e., zinc, vitamin C, arginine); many are higher in fiber

Modified from Webber KS. In Swearingen PL, Ross DG, editors: *Manual of medical-surgical nursing care: nursing interventions and collaborative management,* ed 4, St Louis, 1999, Mosby.

- **Specialty:** Enteral formulas that are disease-specific as described in previous section on special diets for organ-specific pathology.
Nutritional composition:
- **Carbohydrates:** The most easily digested and absorbed component in enteral formulas; 80% of all carbohydrates are broken down and absorbed as simple glucose in the normal intestine. Nearly all enteral formulas are lactose-free to avoid problems in individuals with lactase deficiencies.
- **Fiber:** Included in many commercial preparations because it is claimed to be helpful in controlling blood glucose, reducing hyperlipidemia, and controlling bowel disorders, such as diverticula. High-

fiber products are highly viscous and require a large-bore feeding tube, such as a 10 French (10 Fr), or an infusion pump. Begin the infusion slowly to reduce transient symptoms of gas and abdominal distention.

- **Protein:** Three forms commonly used:
  - ❏ *Polymeric:* Protein found in complete and original form (e.g., commercial and blenderized whole food diets that require normal levels of pancreatic enzyme).
  - ❏ *Semielemental:* Protein that has been broken down into smaller forms to assist absorption. It is better absorbed in short bowel syndrome or pancreatic insufficiency.
  - ❏ *Elemental:* Protein that requires no further digestion and is ready for absorption. Is most useful in severe malabsorption.
- **Fat:** Two forms are the primary sources:
  - ❏ *Long-chain triglycerides (LCT):* A major source of essential fatty acids, fat-soluble vitamins, and calories.
  - ❏ *Medium-chain triglycerides (MCT):* Foster the absorption of fat but have lower incidence of nausea and vomiting, abdominal distention, and diarrhea.

Types of feeding tubes and sites:
- **Stomach:** Easiest site for tube placement; simulates normal GI function; may be used for intermittent or continuous feedings. The stomach is the site reserved for patients who are alert, with intact gag and cough reflexes. Entry site is nasal, oral, or percutaneous.
  - ❏ *Small-bore:* Soft polyurethane or silicone with or without weighted tip; designed for long-term use; size 6-12 Fr; length 36-45 in. Some nasoenteric feeding tubes have a Y port added, allowing irrigation and medication administration without disconnecting the administration set.
  - ❏ *Large-bore:* Stiff, polyvinyl chloride; size 10-18 Fr; used for short-term (<1 week) feeding after gastric suction is no longer needed.
  - ❏ *Surgical gastrostomy:* A soft tube inserted directly into the stomach. Complications may include infections, leakage, catheter occlusion and expulsion. Placed in operating room at time of other GI surgery or when percutaneous gastrostomy unable to be done for technical reasons.
  - ❏ *Percutaneous endoscopic gastrostomy (PEG):* Soft tube inserted into the stomach via the esophagus and then drawn through the abdominal skin using a stab incision.
- **Small bowel (postpyloric feeding):** Used for patients with diminished protective pharyngeal reflexes; the small bowel is less affected by postoperative ileus than the stomach and colon. Tube placement is more difficult. Continuous feedings are tolerated better, inasmuch as the continuous drip approximates normal gastric delivery to the small bowel. Entry sites are nasal, oral, duodenal, and jejunal. Nurses and other health care professionals can be taught to insert postpyloric feeding tubes using oral or nasal entry sites.
  - ❏ *Dual tubes:* Placed either via gastrostomy or nasally. Have one port for feeding into the jejunum and a second port that allows for aspiration and decompression of the stomach.
  - ❏ *Duodenum/jejunum:* Minimizes risk of vomiting and aspiration compared with gastric feedings. Small-bore feeding tubes can be inserted nasally or orally and pushed past the ligament of Trietz into the jejunum (postpyloric feeding). A jejunostomy tube is soft, small-bore feeding tube inserted directly into the jejunum, via percutaneous endoscopic (PEJ) or open surgical approach. These tubes are not easily dislodged.

Infusion rates: See Table 1-3.

Management of complications: See Table 1-4.

Parenteral nutrition (PN): The post-injury metabolic stress response is said to peak at 3-4 days. Initiating nutritional support within 48 hr by supplying nutrients to prevent catabolism of skeletal and visceral protein stores can decrease morbidity in a previously well-nourished person who is critically ill. Use of parenteral nutrition in a well-nourished surgical patient may not improve outcome when used for less than 7 days.

Parenteral nutrition provides some or all nutrients using either a peripheral venous catheter (IV) or central venous catheter (CVC). IV nutrition can meet total nutritional needs in patients who cannot be given enteral support safely or whose GI tract cannot be accessed. Parenteral nutrition is also used when the GI tract is unable to function, such as in the case of motility disorders.

- **Parenteral solutions:** These solutions are derived from combinations of dextrose, amino acids, fat, electrolytes, water, vitamins, and trace elements. Total nutrient admixtures (TNA) are formulated by combining dextrose, fat, and amino acids in one container; or, less commonly, dextrose and amino acids are combined and a separate delivery device is used for fat. A 0.22 micron in-line filter cannot be used with TNA because it traps lipid molecules.
  - ❏ *Carbohydrates:* Dextrose solutions are used to meet part of the patient's energy needs. With excess CHO intake, insulin demand, CO_2 generation, and O_2 consumption are increased, leading to respiratory distress and hypermetabolism.

TABLE 1-3   Methods and Rates of Administration for Enteral Products

Type	Typical rate of administration	Comments
Bolus	250-400 ml 4-6 x/day	May cause cramping, bloating, nausea, diarrhea, aspiration; not recommended for critically ill patients
Intermittent	120 ml isotonic formula with 30-50 ml H_2O; flush over 30-60 min *Advancement:* Increase formula q8-12h by 60 ml if residual <1/2 volume of previous feeding	Starting regimen Should not exceed 30 ml/min; may cause cramping, nausea, bloating, diarrhea, aspiration
Continuous	40-50 ml/hr, full strength, isotonic formula *Advancement:* If serum albumin levels <2.5 g/dl or initial loose stools, dilute formula to 150 mOsm	Starting regimen Allows more time for absorption of nutrients

Modified from Webber KS: Providing nutritional support. In Swearingen PL, Ross DG, editors: *Manual of medical-surgical nursing care,* ed 4, St Louis, 1999, Mosby.

TABLE 1-4   Management of Complications in the Tube-Fed Patient

Complication/possible causes	Suggested management strategy
Nausea and vomiting	
Fast rate	Decrease rate.
Fat intolerance	Fat should compose no more than 30%-40% of total intake.
Lactose intolerance	As prescribed, change to lactose-free product
Delayed gastric emptying	See **Risk for aspiration**, p. 12.
Product odor	Mask with flavoring.
Blocked tube	
Viscous formula/medications; inadequate flushing	Flush tube with 50-150 ml water after each feeding/medication administration. Flush q4h with 30 ml water.
Instillation of crushed medications	Do not instill crushed medications in small-bore tubes. Substitute liquid preparations after consulting a pharmacist and prescriber. Some medications may be crushed into a fine powder and dissolved. Check with pharmacist, since crushing can alter medication characteristics. Never crush time-released medications. Incompatibilities between drugs and feeding formulas are possible.

❏ *Protein:* Essential and nonessential amino acid formulations are available in concentrations of 3% to 15%. Special amino acid formulations for specific disorders are available (see "Estimating Nutritional Requirements," p. 3).

❏ *Fat:* Lipids are an isotonic solution providing essential fatty acids and a source of concentrated calories. For best use and tolerance, lipids should be infused with carbohydrates and protein over no less than 8 h. Symptoms of an adverse reaction include febrile response, chills and shivering, and pain in the chest and back. A second type of adverse reaction occurs with prolonged use of IV fat emulsions and may result in a transient increase in liver enzyme levels, kernicterus, eosinophilia, and thrombophlebitis. Maintain the infusion rate at 1 ml/min for the first 15-30 min as a test dose. Subsequent infusions are given over 12-24 hr. Patients receiving Diprivan, which is lipid-based, should not also receive fat emulsion.

Selection of feeding site:
- *Central Venous IV Catheter (CVC):* Used for infusion of large amounts of nutrients or electrolytes with smaller fluid volumes (hypertonic solutions) than those in peripheral parenteral nutrition. The solution usually is delivered through a large-diameter vein (e.g., superior vena cava via the subclavian vein). The volume of blood flow rapidly dilutes the hypertonic solutions and decreases irritation of vein walls. However, there are more complications with CVC than with the peripheral route (Table 1-5).
- *Peripheral venous (IV): Generally not as effective as central venous administration.* The need for low osmolality of solutions (<800 milliosmole [mOsm]/L) reduces efficacy of treatment. Combining solutions of dextrose, amino acids, and lipids with lower osmolality can provide a concentrated energy source which can be delivered through a peripheral vein, usually of the hand or forearm. Reserved for individuals who need partial or total nutritional support for short periods when CVC access is unavailable or not warranted.

Types of catheters: See Table 1-6.

Monitoring infusion rates: PN is given at a constant rate using an infusion pump. When initiated, the infusion rate is gradually increased to avoid hyperglycemia and fluid overload. For example, 1 L is infused the first day. Volume is increased to 2 L on the second day while monitoring tolerance of

TABLE 1-5   Catheters Used in Parenteral Nutrition

Catheter	Description
Subclavian/jugular	
Single lumen	Inserted at bedside. Multiple uses for specimen retrieval, feeding, and medication administration increase the risk of infection, especially in compromised patients.
Multilumen	Inserted at bedside. Dedication of one lumen in this catheter is common practice, enabling other lumen(s) to be used for medication administration and laboratory monitoring.
Right atrial (e.g., Hickman, Broviac)	Composed of silicone rubber with plastic external segment, which is implanted in OR. Its safety enables use by home care patients.
Implantable (e.g., Infuse-a-Port, Port-a-Cath)	Implanted in OR. Designed for repeated access, making the need for repeated venipuncture unnecessary.

Modified from Webber KS. In Swearingen PL, Ross DG, editors: *Manual of medical-surgical nursing care,* ed 4, St Louis, 1999, Mosby.

TABLE 1-6   Management of Complications in Patients Receiving Parenteral Nutrition

Potential complications	Management strategy
Pneumothorax	Ensure that x-ray is done immediately after insertion. To determine placement of catheter before initiating feeding. Monitor for diminished or unequal breath sounds, tachypnea, dyspnea, and labored breathing.
Subclavian artery injury	If pulsatile, bright red blood returns into the syringe, assist with immediate removal of the needle and apply pressure for 10 min anteriorly and posteriorly at the point of penetration.
Catheter occlusion	If solution is infusing sluggishly, flush line with heparinized saline. Check to see if line or tubing is kinked. If line is occluded, try to aspirate clot and contact health care provider, who may prescribe a thrombolytic agent.

fluid and dextrose intake. If a higher rate is needed, it is achieved by day 3. Discontinuation of PN is accomplished by reducing the rate by half for 12 hours then by half again for 12 h. Once the rate is at 40 ml or below, it can be discontinued.

Managing complications: See Table 1-5.

Electrolyte imbalances occurring in both enteral and parenteral nutrition: See Table 1-7.

T A B L E 1 - 7   Possible Electrolyte Imbalances Occurring in Enteral and Parenteral Nutrition

Sodium: Daily requirement is 60-150 mEq. Sodium is the primary extracellular cation in maintaining concentration and volume of extracellular fluid.

Complication	Pathophysiology/strategy
Hypernatremia	In PCM, patients have increased sodium because of extravascular volume expansion and intravascular volume depletion. Monitor sodium levels as depletion resolves, edema decreases, and diuresis occurs. Hypernatremia also occurs in patients receiving hypertonic tube feedings without adequate water supplements. **Sources:** Amino acid solutions contain varying amounts of sodium (up to 70 mEq/L): some antibiotics (e.g., sodium penicillin) also have a high sodium content (31-200 mEq/dl). Corticosteroids may cause sodium retention, and blood products can contain increased levels (130-160 mEq/L).
Hyponatremia	Can be a problem in patients with gastric suctioning and in those receiving diuretic agents or those with SIADH. **Replacement:** TPN solutions can replace sodium by using acetate, phosphate, or chloride salt form, depending on underlying disease state. The phosphate form should not be used in patients with renal failure. In academia, the acetate form is preferred to correct the imbalance.

Potassium: Daily requirement is 50-100 mEq. Potassium is the major intracellular cation required for neurotransmission, protein synthesis, cardiac and renal function, and carbohydrate metabolism.

Complication	Pathophysiology/strategy
Hyperkalemia	May be caused by excessive parenteral or enteral potassium supplementation or increased tissue catabolism, especially in renal insufficiency. **Sources:** Amino acid solutions contain potassium. Elevated potassium levels occur in patients receiving ACE inhibitors, heparin, cyclosporine, and potassium-sparing diuretics.
Hypokalemia	May occur during anabolism (tissue synthesis) in patients being refed. Potassium shifts into intracellular space, and patients require supplementation. It also may occur in patients with high GI losses or increased loss from diuretics. Potassium levels in patients with acid-base disorders may be misleading: potassium decreases by 0.4-1.5 mEq/L for every 0.1 increase in pH. **Replacement:** In daily TPN solutions, 80-120 mEq may be given to patients with no renal problems. Potassium can be replaced using acetate, phosphate, and chloride forms, depending on the underlying disease state, but it should be titrated separately to avoid wasting TPN solutions. Infusion rates >0.5 mEq/kg/h are associated with cardiac irregularities.

Phosphorus: Daily requirement is 2.5-4.5 mg/dl. Phosphorus is required for release of oxygen from hemoglobin in the form of 2,3-diphosphoglycerate and for bone deposition, calcium regulation, and synthesis of carbohydrates, fats, and protein.

T A B L E 1 - 7 **Possible Electrolyte Imbalances Occurring in Enteral and Parenteral Nutrition—cont'd**

Complication	Pathophysiology/strategy
Hyperphosphatemia	Occurs in catabolic stress, renal failure, and hypocalcemia. Treatment involves ingestion of aluminum antacids, which bind phosphate in the intestine. **Sources:** Phosphorus-rich solutions, antacids, diuretic agents, and steroids.
Hypophosphatemia	A complication with a high mortality, often found in malnourished patients on refeeding. As the patient receives fluids containing dextrose, phosphorus shifts rapidly into the intracellular space, causing hypophosphatemia. **Replacement:** Phosphate-rich TPN solutions.

Magnesium: Daily requirement is 18-30 mEq. Magnesium is required for carbohydrate and protein metabolism and enzymatic reactions.

Complication	Pathophysiology/strategy
Hypermagnesemia	Transient elevations can occur with use of diuretics or extracellular volume depletion. **Source:** Magnesium-containing antacids
Hypomagnesemia	Low levels commonly occur in patients with severe malnutrition or lower GI losses and in those given insulin for hyperglycemia. For anabolism to occur, the body requires 2 mEq of magnesium per gram of nitrogen. **Replacement:** Parenteral magnesium

Calcium: Daily requirement is 1000-1500 mg. Calcium is a necessary ingredient of the cells that play a major role in neurotransmission and bone formation.

Complication	Pathophysiology/strategy
Hypercalcemia	Occurs in thiazide diuretic use, prolonged immobilization, and decreased excretion. **Source:** Side effect of diuretic use.
Hypocalcemia	May occur from reduced total body calcium or reduced ionized calcium. It also occurs with hyperphosphatemia. A deficit can be misleading, inasmuch as serum calcium is bound to protein and varies with changing albumin levels. Also, in acidosis, a lower pH results in release of more calcium from protein, which elevates serum calcium levels. The opposite is true as pH rises. **Replacement:** Calcium-rich parenteral solutions.

TRANSITIONAL FEEDING

A period of adjustment is needed before discontinuing nutritional support. Taper enteral and parenteral nutrition as oral intake increases. Patients receiving parenteral nutrition may have some mucosal atrophy of the bowel and need a period of adjustment before the bowel can fully resume its normal function.

NURSING DIAGNOSES AND INTERVENTIONS

For patients receiving enteral and parenteral nutrition
Altered nutrition: Less than body requirements, related to inability to ingest, digest, or absorb nutrients
Desired outcome: Within 7 days of initiating parenteral/enteral nutrition, patient has improving nutritional status, evidenced by level weight or steady weight gain of ¼-½ lb/day; improved or normal measures of protein stores (serum albumin, transferrin, thyroxine-binding prealbumin, and retinol-binding protein); positive nitrogen balance as measured by nitrogen balance studies; presence of wound granulation; and absence of infection (see "Risk for infection," p. 13).
• Ensure nutritional screening and assessment of patient within 72hr of admission; document. See "Nutritional Assessment," p. 1. Reassess weekly.

- Monitor electrolytes, blood urea nitrogen (BUN), and blood sugar daily until stabilized. Ensure that serum albumin, transferrin, or prealbumin and trace elements are monitored weekly. Document.
- Weigh patient daily.
- Record intake and output (I&O) carefully, tracking fluid balance trends.
- Check volume infused and rate of infusion hourly.
- Ensure that patient receives the prescribed amount of nutrients.

Risk for aspiration: related to GI bleeding; delayed gastric emptying; site of feeding tube
Desired outcome: Patient is free of aspiration problems as evidenced by auscultation of clear breath sounds; vital signs (VS) within patient's baseline; and absence of signs of respiratory distress.

- Check x-ray film for position of feeding tube before feeding. Mark and secure tubing for future reference. Insufflation with air and aspiration of stomach contents are commonly used to confirm position thereafter but do not guarantee correct position.
- Assess respiratory status q4h, observing respiratory rate and effort, and presence of adventitious breath sounds.
- Monitor temperature q4h.
- Auscultate for bowel sounds, percuss abdomen, and assess abdominal contour and girth q8h. Consult physician if bowel sounds are absent, the abdomen becomes distended, or nausea and vomiting occur.
- Elevate head of bed (HOB) ≥30 degrees during and for 1hr after feeding. If this is not possible or comfortable for patient, turn patient into a slightly elevated, right side-lying position to enhance gravity flow from the stomach to the pylorus.
- Consult physician if gastric residual is >2 times the hourly rate. Hold feeding for 1 hr, and recheck residual.
- Stop tube feeding ½-1hr before chest physical therapy, suctioning, or placing patient supine.
- Discuss with physician the possibility of placing feeding tube beyond the pylorus.
- As prescribed, administer metoclopramide HCl or other agents that promote gastric motility.

Diarrhea (or risk for same): related to bolus feeding; lactose intolerance; bacterial contamination; osmolality intolerance; medications; low fiber content
Desired outcome: Patient has formed stools within 24-48 hr of intervention.

General
- Assess abdomen and GI status, including bowel sounds, distention, consistency and frequency of bowel movements, cramping, skin turgor, and other indicators of hydration.
- Monitor I&O status carefully.

Specific problems
- Bolus feeding: Switch to intermittent or continuous feeding method.
- Avoid lactose containing products.
- Bacterial contamination:
  - ❏ Obtain stool sample for culture and sensitivity, *Clostridium difficile* as ordered.
  - ❏ Use clean technique in handling feeding tube, enteral products, and feeding sets.
  - ❏ Change all equipment q24h.
  - ❏ Refrigerate all opened products but discard after 24 hr.
  - ❏ Discard feedings hanging for >8 hr.
- Osmolality intolerance
  - ❏ Determine osmolality of feeding formula. Most are isotonic (plasma osmolality 300 mOsm). If hypertonic, reduce rate. If problem continues, dilute to ½ formula and ½ water but maintain rate.
- Medications
  - ❏ Monitor use of antibiotics, antacids, potassium chloride, and sorbitol in liquid medications. Dilute liquid medications with water.
  - ❏ As prescribed, administer *Lactobacillus acidophilus* to restore GI flora or use tincture of opium to decrease GI motility.
  - ❏ Low fiber content: Add bulk-forming agents (psyllium or fiber-enriched enteral formula).

Impaired tissue integrity (or risk for same): related to mechanical irritant (presence of enteral tube)
Desired outcome: At time of discharge from critical care, patient's tissue is intact with absence of erosion around orifices, excoriation, skin rash, or mucous membrane breakdown.

Nasoenteric tube/ postpyloric feeding tube
- Assess nares for irritation or tenderness q8h and alter position to avoid pressure. Use hypoallergenic tape to anchor tube.
- Use a small-bore tube if possible.

- If long-term support is needed, discuss using gastrostomy or jejunostomy tube with physician.
- Give ice chips, chewing gum, or hard candies prn if permitted.
- Apply petroleum jelly to lips q2h.
- Brush teeth and tongue q8h.

Gastrostomy tube/PEG
- Assess site for erythema, drainage, tenderness, and odor q4h.
- Monitor placement of tube q8h.
- Secure tube so there is no tension on patient's tissue and skin.
- For first three days after insertion, clean skin with 1:1 solution of water and H_2O_2. Wipe with gauze. After day 3 wash skin with soap and water daily; pat dry.

Jejunostomy tube/PEJ
- Assess site for erythema, drainage, tenderness, and odor q4h.
- Secure tube to avoid tension. Coil tube on top of dressing if necessary.
- Skin care is same as for gastrostomy tube.

Risk for infection: related to central line or malnutrition

Desired outcome: Patient is free of infection as evidenced by temperature and VS within normal limits; total lymphocytes 25%-40% (1500-4500 µl); white blood cell (WBC) count ≤11,000/mm^3; and absence of clinical signs of sepsis, including erythema and swelling at insertion site, chills, fever, and glucose intolerance.
- Ensure adequate nutritional support, based on individual needs. See "Nutritional Assessment," p. 1.
- Twice weekly and prn, monitor total lymphocyte count, WBC count, and differential for values outside normal range.
- Check blood glucose q6h for values outside normal range.
- Examine catheter insertion site(s) q8h for erythema, swelling, or purulent drainage.
- Use meticulous sterile technique when changing central line dressing, containers, or lines.
- Avoid using nutritional support catheter for blood drawing, pressure monitoring, or administration of medications or other fluids.
- Change all administration sets and rotate insertion site within the time frame per policy.
- Do not allow solutions to hang longer than 24 hr.
- If sepsis is suspected, take blood specimens for culture and administer antibiotics as prescribed. Remove catheter and culture as prescribed.

Altered cardiopulmonary tissue perfusion (or risk for same): related to interruption of arterial flow (air embolus)

Desired outcome: Patient has adequate cardiopulmonary tissue perfusion as evidenced by VS, arterial blood gas (ABG) values, and arterial oximetry within normal limits; and absence of dyspnea, tachypnea, cyanosis, chest pain, tachycardia, and hypotension.
- Check chest x-ray film to determine catheter position.
- Use Trendelenburg position when changing tubing or when central vein catheters are inserted or removed.
- Teach patient Valsalva maneuver (if possible) for implementation during tubing changes.
- Use Luer-Lok connectors on all connections.
- Use occlusive dressing over insertion site for 24 hr after catheter is removed to prevent air entry via catheter-sinus tract.
- Monitor patient for chest pain, tachycardia, tachypnea, cyanosis, and hypotension.
- If air embolus is suspected, clamp the catheter and turn patient to left side-lying Trendelenburg position to trap air in the right ventricle. Administer high-flow oxygen and contact physician immediately.

Risk for fluid volume deficit: related to failure of regulatory mechanisms; hyperglycemia; hyperglycemic hyperosmolar nonketotic syndrome (HHNS)

Desired outcome: Patient's hydration status is adequate as evidenced by baseline VS; glucose <300 mg/dl; balanced I&O; urine specific gravity 1.010-1.025; and electrolytes within normal limits.
- Weigh patient daily; monitor I&O hourly.
- Consult physician for urine output <1 ml/kg/h.
- Check urine specific gravity; consult physician for value >1.035.
- Monitor serum osmolality and electrolytes daily and prn; consult physician for abnormalities.
- Monitor for circulatory overload during fluid replacement.
- Monitor for indicators of hyperglycemia. Perform finger stick q6h prn until blood glucose is stable. Administer insulin as prescribed to keep blood glucose levels <180 mg/dl.

Research Brief 1-1   To evaluate the potential for using pH and bilirubin measurements in determining feeding tube placement, 437 gastrointestinal samples for pH and bilirubin were taken from acutely ill adults who had newly inserted small-bore feeding tubes placed. One sample was inadvertently taken from a tube placed in the right, mainstem bronchus. Seeing the pH difference, 149 additional respiratory tract samples were taken. Patients' enteric pH-altering medications or tube feedings were excluded. A pH of >5 with bilirubin <5mg/dl indicated a respiratory aspirate, whereas pH >5 with bilirubin ≥5 indicated intestinal tube placement. Gastric tube placement reflected pH <5 with bilirubin ≥5. Use of pH monitoring may enable reducing the number of x-ray films needed for enteric tube placement.

From Metheny NA et al: pH and concentration of bilirubin in feeding tube aspirates as predictors of tube placement, *Nurs Res* 48(4):189-197, 1999.

• Assess rate and volume of nutritional support hourly. For HHNS discontinue infusion until blood glucose and fluid balance is normalized. Reset to prescribed rate as indicated.
• Provide 1 ml water for each calorie of enteral formula provided (or 30-50 ml/kg body weight).

ADDITIONAL NURSING DIAGNOSES

For other nursing diagnoses and interventions, see "Fluid and Electrolyte Disturbances," p. 538, which includes discussion of the electrolyte abnormalities listed in Table 1-7.

Mechanical Ventilation

To ensure optimal care of the patient who requires mechanical ventilation, the practitioner must have adequate knowledge of the equipment and processes involved in mechanical ventilation. An in-depth discussion of the entire process is beyond the scope of this book; therefore it is assumed that the reader has basic knowledge on which to build.

TYPES OF VENTILATORS

Three categories of ventilators are used to deliver oxygen and artificial respiration.
Positive pressure: Most widely used ventilator type. It is designed to deliver a preset volume of gas (tidal volume) which creates positive pressure during inspiration. The machine attempts to deliver the predetermined tidal volume independent of normal changes in airway resistance or lung compliance. To prevent acute lung injury, the ventilator is equipped with safety mechanisms that are set to terminate inspiration when peak inspiratory pressures are excessive. Generally these pressure limits are set 10-20 cm H_2O above the patient's normal delivery pressure. The ventilator automatically terminates inspiration once a preset pressure is reached, at which time the patient exhales passively. When airway resistance increases because of mucus secretions or bronchospasm, the inspiratory cycle may terminate before adequate tidal volume is delivered.
Negative pressure: Intrapleural pressure ranges from -2 to -10 cm H_2O. The positive pressure ventilators already discussed can generate 5-120 cm H_2O pressure to deliver a breath. Negative pressure ventilators generate subatmospheric pressure to the thorax and trunk to initiate respiration and do not require intubation for use. The iron lung, chest cuirass shell, and poncho chest shell are examples. Since these devices are noninvasive, there has been a resurgence of interest in their use for long-term home therapy.
High-frequency: Jet ventilation and high-frequency oscillation are alternative types of ventilators in which small tidal volumes are delivered at high rates. The resulting lower airway and intrathoracic pressures may reduce the risk of ventilator-induced lung injury. Barotrauma and circulatory depression are associated with the high peak airway pressures of conventional ventilation. Tidal volume is low and minute ventilation is high, making this ideal ventilation for patients with major airway disruption. High-frequency ventilation requires the use of a specially designed endotracheal (ET) tube. The three basic mechanisms that are used are discussed in Table 1-8.

MODES OF POSITIVE PRESSURE MECHANICAL VENTILATION

Most patients require ET intubation or a tracheostomy in place prior to initiating mechanical ventilation. Continuous positive airway pressure (CPAP) and bilevel positive airway pressure (BiPAP) can be delivered by face mask.

TABLE 1-8 High-Frequency Jet Ventilation

Mode	Rate	Tidal volume	Mechanism
High-frequency positive pressure ventilation (HFPPV)	60-100 cpm	3-6 ml/kg	Pneumatically controlled valve connected to high-pressure gas source; pulses gas into airway while additional gases are entrained into the airway via a humidification circuit
High-frequency jet ventilation (HFJV)	100-200 cpm	50-400 ml	Gas under pressure is propelled through a narrow cannula (inserted in ET tube) while additional gases are entrained through a humidifier
High-frequency oscillations (HFO)	>200 cpm (800-3000 vibrations/ min)	50-80 ml	Gas is oscillated through ET tube via a piston; gas flows over the connection, and PEEP is created via resistant tubing on the outflow port; gas exchange occurs primarily by diffusion

cpm, Cycles per minute; *ET,* endotracheal; *PEEP,* positive end-expiratory pressure.

Controlled mandatory ventilation (CMV): Delivers a preset tidal volume at a preset rate, ignoring the patient's own ventilatory drive (the patient cannot trigger this machine). Use is generally restricted to patients with central nervous system (CNS) dysfunction, drug-induced paralysis or sedation, or severe chest trauma for whom negative pressure-driven respiratory effort is undesirable. This is the simplest but least frequently used mode.

Assist-control ventilation (A/C or ACV): Delivers a preset tidal volume when the patient initiates a negative pressure respiratory effort (inspiration) or independently of the patient's effort if the preset time limit is reached. With adequate tidal volume delivery, work of breathing is decreased and alveolar ventilation improves. Although machine sensitivity can be adjusted to prevent hyperventilation in patients whose respiratory rate increases because of mild anxiety or neurologic factors, use of sedatives should be used to facilitate control of the respiratory rate. If hyperventilation cannot be controlled, the patient may need to be changed to synchronized intermittent mandatory ventilation.

Synchronized intermittent mandatory ventilation (SIMV): Delivers a preset tidal volume at a preset rate. Patient can also breathe spontaneously (at his or her own rate and tidal volume) between ventilator breaths. The ventilator is synchronized to deliver a mandatory breath when the patient initiates inspiration. This is the most frequently used mode of ventilation.

Positive end-expiratory pressure (PEEP): Delivers a constant set pressure at the end of expiration. This pressure counteracts small airway collapse and keeps alveoli open to optimize gas exchange across the alveolar-capillary membrane, thereby decreasing shunting. Frequently used in conjunction with mechanical ventilation to improve ventilatory function, reflected by increased partial pressure of oxygen in arterial blood (Pao_2). PEEP increases functional residual capacity (FRC) and compliance while decreasing dead space ventilation and shunt fraction. Very effective for atelectatic alveoli, as well as for alveoli that are filled with fluid. Does not improve lung function due to poor perfusion. Generally, PEEP pressures range from 2.5-20 cm H_2O. Higher pressures (>35 cm H_2O) may be used if the patient can tolerate the increase and if the condition is warranted. Application of PEEP increases intrathoracic pressure and can compromise the patient's hemodynamic status by compressing the heart and great vessels. Increased intrathoracic pressure decreases venous return, right ventricular filling pressures, and cardiac output, which may cause or potentiate hypotension and shock. Patients with intravascular volume depletion are at higher risk. High levels of PEEP can cause pneumothorax, particularly if lung compliance is diminished.

Note: Continuous positive airway pressure functions in the same manner as PEEP but is a mode used independently of mechanically delivered breaths and is continuous throughout the spontaneous respiratory cycle. Can be delivered to patients using a specially designed, tight-fitting face mask, or through an ET tube or tracheostomy.

Bilevel positive airway pressure (BiPAP): A mode of ventilatory support that uses alternating inspiratory positive pressures (IPAP) and expiratory positive pressures (EPAP) to enhance variable spontaneous tidal volumes. The resistance and compliance of the airways will determine the IPAP "driving pressure" necessary to produce a desired tidal volume. The level of EPAP needed is based on the oxygenation status of the patient. The physician determines a tidal volume goal (usually 8-12 ml/kg) and an oxygenation goal the clinician will use to determine the titration range for IPAP, EPAP, and Fio_2. Bilevel mode can be found on many conventional ventilators and on freestanding units used for noninvasive positive pressure ventilation (NPPV). In this mode, BiPAP is most often delivered using a specially designed, tight-fitting face mask, or on patients with a tracheostomy tube in place.

Pressure support ventilation (PSV): Augments or supports a patient's spontaneous inspiration with a preselected pressure level. Pressure is applied at the initiation of inspiration and ends when a minimum inspiratory flow rate is reached. The patient retains control over inspiratory time and flow rate, expiratory time, frequency, tidal volume, and spontaneous minute ventilation. PSV creates less dyssynchrony (patient's breathing is not in harmony with ventilator-delivered breaths) than assist-control or SIMV alone. Inspiratory work is decreased by compensating for resistance created by the demand valve or ET tube size. PSV may be combined with SIMV to improve patient tolerance of mechanical ventilation and to decrease the work of breathing through the ET tube. PSV is often used to facilitate weaning from mechanical ventilation.

Pressure control ventilation (PCV): Ventilation designed to control inspiratory pressure. A tidal volume goal (usually 4-12 ml/kg) is ordered by the physician. The respiratory care clinician selects the inspiratory pressure (IP), usually 10-40 cm H_2O, and the breath is delivered at a rapid flow rate. The compliance and resistance of the airways determine the tidal volume achieved from the inspiratory cycle. Both inspiratory and expiratory times can be set. PCV mode is frequently used for patients with high peak inspiratory pressures (PIP) due to acute lung injury (ALI) or Acute Respiratory Distress Syndrome (ARDS). The set respiratory rate must be increased to facilitate adequate minute ventilation. This mode is usually accompanied by PEEP therapy.

Inverse ratio ventilation (IRV): Technique in which the inspiratory phase is prolonged and the expiratory phase is shortened. Normal inspiration/expiration (I/E) ratio is 1:2. During IRV, the I/E ratio is increased to >1:1 (e.g., 2:1), thereby promoting alveolar recruitment, which improves oxygenation at lower levels of PEEP. The patient will require administration of a paralyzing agent and sedation to minimize the discomfort and anxiety associated with this unusual breathing pattern.

ADDITIONAL MODES AND ADJUNCTS OF MECHANICAL VENTILATION

The following list is a small sample of current and experimental ventilator modes and adjuncts that work in conjunction with ventilator modes:

Airway pressure release ventilation (APRV): This mode is similar to CPAP. Patients are allowed to breathe spontaneously by combining two separate levels of CPAP. Periodically, the pressure is reduced to the lower of the two levels to reduce mean airway pressure during spontaneous exhalation. The drop in pressure facilitates a more effective exhalation.

Proportional assist ventilation (PAV): In this mode of ventilation, the ventilator automatically adjusts airway pressure in response to the patient's ventilatory patterns. The ventilator frequently adjusts needed support based on the patient's inspiratory flow rate, exhaled tidal volume, compliance, and resistance.

ADJUNCTS TO MECHANICAL VENTILATION

AutoFlow: A new advance in volume-controlled modes of mechanical ventilation. The ventilator automatically regulates inspiratory flow. This autoregulation works in conjunction with the set tidal volume and the patient's lung compliance.

Extracorporeal membrane oxygenation (ECMO): Technically not a mode of mechanical ventilation, ECMO is very expensive and limitedly available. It is used to support oxygenation and ventilation for patients with severe respiratory failure who are unable to be managed with other modes of ventilation. ECMO requires that the patient's blood be directed from the body into external membranes for oxygenation and removal of carbon dioxide. ECMO is used primarily in the pediatric population.

Mandatory minute ventilation or minimum minute ventilation (MMV): Provides a predetermined minute ventilation to augment the patient's spontaneous minute ventilation (breathing efforts). Used to prevent hypoventilation and respiratory acidosis during ventilator weaning when SIMV is supporting the patient.

Partial liquid ventilation (PLV): Still considered experimental, partial liquid ventilation uses perfluorocarbon liquids to augment diffusion. Liquid perfluorocarbon is instilled into the lungs until the level approximates FRC. Standard mechanical ventilation is then superimposed.

Tracheal gas insufflation (TGI): Used to reduce the amount of dead space in the patient-ventilator system. Still considered experimental, caregivers introduce a small-caliber catheter through an angled, side-arm adapter into a specially designed ET tube to inject a secondary flow of gas just above the carina, which helps remove ("washes out") CO_2 during expiration.

COMPLICATIONS RELATED TO MECHANICAL VENTILATION

Barotrauma and pneumothorax: Barotrauma can occur when ventilatory pressures increase intrathoracic and intrapleural pressures, causing damage to the lungs, the major vessels, and possibly all organs in the thorax, with referred damage to the abdomen. If severe, barotrauma can lead to pneumothorax; a partially or totally collapsed lung. Symptoms vary depending on the amount of lung collapsed.

Tension pneumothorax: Develops when pressurized air escapes from the lungs, enters and collects in the thoracic cavity, causing one or both lungs to collapse. High pressure from mechanical positive pressure ventilation may tear diseased or fragile lung tissue, leading to this life-threatening complication. Symptoms include respiratory distress, fluctuations in blood pressure (BP), shifting of the trachea toward the unaffected side, and sudden and sustained increases in peak inspiratory pressure.

Caution: If tension pneumothorax is suspected, the patient should be disconnected from the ventilator immediately and ventilated using a bag/valve/tube device ("Ambu Bag"). The nurse should prepare the patient for immediate chest tube insertion/placement.

Gastrointestinal complications: Peptic ulcers with profound hemorrhage may develop as a result of physiologic pressures and stress. Histamine H_2-receptor antagonists (e.g., cimetidine), and/or sucralfate (Carafate) may be administered to prevent these ulcers from developing. In addition, gastric dilation can occur as a result of the large amounts of air swallowed in the presence of an artificial airway. If gastric dilation is left untreated, paralytic ileus, vomiting, and aspiration may develop. Extreme dilation can compromise respiratory effort because of the restriction of diaphragmatic movement. Treatment includes insertion of a gastric tube orally or nasally (oral placement may be preferred) connected to low intermittent suction to remove air from the GI tract.

Hypotension with decreased cardiac output: Develops as a result of decreased venous return secondary to increased intrathoracic pressure caused by positive pressure ventilation. Unless associated with tension pneumothorax, this phenomenon is transient and is seen immediately after the patient has been placed on mechanical ventilation. PEEP, especially at levels >20 cm H_2O, may increase the incidence and severity of this phenomenon because of the compression of the heart and large blood vessels from the increased intrathoracic pressure. IV fluid therapy is used with PEEP to maintain adequate intravascular volume for sufficient cardiac output to perfuse vital organs. Heart rate (HR) and BP should be monitored frequently if the patient is unstable. Cardiac output may be monitored via flow-directed pulmonary artery (Swan-Ganz) catheter. See "Hemodynamic Monitoring," p. 23, for details regarding cardiac output.

Increased intracranial pressure: Occurs as a result of decreased venous return to the heart due to compression of intrathoracic blood vessels, causing blood to pool or accumulate in the head. See "Traumatic Brain Injury," p. 98, for additional information.

Research Brief 1-2   A total of 813 patients who received prolonged (>48 hours) mechanical ventilation were studied to determine the relationship between age and hospital costs. Severity of illness, comorbidities, length of stay, hospital costs and mortality were measured. The association between age and hospital cost was evaluated independently using linear regression analysis. Mean age was 60.4 ± 18.8 years. Hospital mortality was 36%. Median total hospital costs were $56,056 and daily costs were $2,655. Older age was associated with lower hospital costs for all cost departments examined, except for respiratory care and intensive care unit room costs. Decreased hospital resource use in older patients may be related to a preference for less aggressive care by older patients, their families and/or health care providers.

From Lakshmipathi C et al: Hospital costs in patients receiving prolonged mechanical ventilation: does age have an impact? *Crit Care Med* 31(6):1746-1751, 2003.

Fluid imbalance: Increased production of antidiuretic hormone (ADH) occurs as a result of increased pressure on baroreceptors in the thoracic aorta, which causes the system to react as if the body were volume-depleted. ADH stimulates the renal system to retain water. Patients may need diuretics if signs of hypervolemia are present. Be alert to new symptoms of dependent edema or adventitious breath sounds.

Ventilator-acquired pneumonia: Studies indicate that 70%-90% of mechanically ventilated patients have been colonized by hospital-acquired bacteria in the oropharynx, trachea, or digestive tract. Aspiration of bacteria from the oropharynx is a leading cause of ventilator-acquired pneumonia. The onset of infection may have several mechanisms:

- Presence of an ET/tracheostomy tube creates a bypass of upper respiratory tract defense mechanisms of cough and mucociliary clearance action.
- Contaminated secretions pool above the ET/tracheostomy tube cuff and leak into the lower respiratory tract.
- Supine positioning, the presence of a nasogastric tube, or reflux of bacteria from the stomach contribute to oropharyngeal colonization. The medications that mechanically ventilated patients may receive to prevent gastrointestinal bleeding alter the gastric pH. Use of sucralfate, which does not increase gastric pH, decreases the incidence of pneumonia when compared with antacids alone or in combination with hydrogen ion antagonists.
- Use of contaminated equipment/supplies, inadequate hand washing, or poor infection control practices may directly inoculate the tracheobronchial tree with pathogens. Consult with your infection control practitioner for additional practice guidelines.

Anxiety: Many individuals experience anxiety related to the discomfort associated with loss of control over their ventilatory process and the perception that their health status is threatened. Hypoxemia and air hunger, if present, contribute to anxiety and prompt rapid, shallow, and often irregular respiratory efforts. Coordinated and effective ventilation may not be possible with severe anxiety and agitation. Diligent administration of anxiety-relieving drugs and analgesics, along with close monitoring of the patient's response to potent medications, may be necessary to reduce the work of breathing and facilitate effective mechanical ventilation. The use of an approved sedation scale is also recommended. (See "Sedating and Paralytic Agents," p. 32.) In extreme cases, if a patient is unable to tolerate the ventilator mode most appropriate for his or her condition and cannot be managed using high-dose antianxiety agents, sedatives, and analgesics, the physician may consider use of neuromuscular blockade to facilitate more effective ventilation. Neuromuscular blockade should be reserved for only the most extreme situations, wherein the patient's life is threatened by the overall energy expenditure related to fear, anxiety, or inability to attain control over his or her breathing pattern despite other efforts. (See "Neuromuscular Blockade," p. 33.)

WEANING THE PATIENT FROM MECHANICAL VENTILATION

Successful weaning depends more on the patient's overall condition than on the technique used. Physiologic factors (cardiovascular status, fluids and electrolyte balance, acid-base balance, nutritional status, comfort, and sleep pattern) and emotional factors (fear, anxiety, coping skills, general emotional state, ability to cooperate) are important and must be evaluated both before and during the weaning process. Adequate pulmonary function parameters must be attained before the weaning process is begun (Table 1-9). Goals for the weaning process are listed in Table 1-10. Traditionally, three methods are employed for weaning the patient from mechanical ventilation.

Intermittent mandatory ventilation (IMV): Ventilator-generated breaths are decreased gradually while the patient builds muscle strength and endurance. This is the most widely accepted method for patients receiving long-term ventilatory support.

Pressure support ventilation (PSV): Assists the patient's normal breathing pattern with positive airway pressure (1-20 cm H_2O pressure) applied during inspiration. Pressure support is added to SIMV (see p. 15), to decrease the work of breathing through the demand flow system, to overcome resistance of the ET tube, and to enhance spontaneous tidal volumes. Patients control their ventilatory rate, inspiratory time, tidal volume, and inspiratory flow rate. When the patient stops inhaling, the positive pressure stops. The amount of pressure support is gradually decreased as the patient is weaned from the ventilator.

T-piece method: A T-shape adapter is placed at the end of the ET tube. Patient is taken off the ventilator and initiates spontaneous respiratory effort for increasingly longer periods. The T-piece method may be used starting with 1-2 min off the ventilator, followed by 58-59 min on, with a gradual reversal of this ratio until the patient breathes independently. In this manner the patient builds strength and endurance for independent respiratory effort. The T-piece method does not allow for

TABLE 1-9 Pulmonary Function Parameters for the Patient Being Weaned From Mechanical Ventilation

Pulmonary function	Optimal parameters	Definition
Minute ventilation	≤10 L/min	Tidal volume × respiratory rate; if adequate, means patient is breathing at a stable rate with adequate tidal volume
Negative inspiratory force	≥ − 20 cm H_2O	Measures respiratory muscle strength; maximum negative pressure that patient is able to generate to initiate spontaneous respirations; indicative of patient's ability to initiate inspiration independently
Maximum voluntary ventilation	≥2 × resting minute ventilation	Measures respiratory muscle endurance; indicates patient's ability to sustain maximal respiratory effort
Tidal volume	5-10 ml/kg	Indicates patient's ability to ventilate lungs adequately
Arterial blood gases	Pao_2 ≥ 60 mm Hg Pao_2 ≤ 45 mm Hg pH 7.35-7.45 or patient's baseline	
Fractional concentration of inspired oxygen (Fio_2)	≤ 0.40	

TABLE 1-10 Goals for Weaning

RR	<25 breaths/min
Tidal volume (V_T)	At least 3-5 ml/kg
HR/BP	Within 15% of baseline
Arterial pH	≥7.25
Pao_2	≥60 mm Hg and stable
Pao_2	≤45 mm Hg and stable
O_2 saturation	≥90%
Cardiac dysrhythmias	None
Use of accessory muscles of respiration	None

BP, Blood pressure; *HR,* heart rate; *RR,* respiratory rate.

mandatory mechanical ventilatory assistance or mandatory minute ventilation (MMV) in the event of patient apnea and must be used in conjunction with monitoring devices.

TROUBLESHOOTING MECHANICAL VENTILATOR PROBLEMS

The most important assessment factor in troubleshooting a mechanical ventilator is the effect on the patient. Regardless of which alarm sounds, always assess the patient first to evaluate his or her physiologic response to the problem. (See Tables 1-11 and 1-12 for processes that contribute to high-pressure and low-pressure alarm situations.) If at any time the patient is not receiving the proper volumes, or the nurse is unable to properly assess and manage the alarm situation, take the patient off the ventilator and contact the respiratory therapist immediately.

T A B L E　1 - 11　　**Processes Contributing to High-Pressure Alarm Situations**

Increased airway resistance	Decreased lung compliance
Patient requires suctioning	Pneumothorax
Kinks in ventilator circuitry	Pulmonary edema
Water or expectorated secretions in circuitry	Atelectasis
Patient coughs or exhales against ventilatory breaths	Worsening of underlying disease process
Patient biting ET tube	ARDS
Bronchospasm	
Herniation of airway cuff over end of artificial airway	
Change in patient position that restricts chest wall movement	
Breath stacking	

ARDS, Acute respiratory distress syndrome; *ET*, endotracheal.

T A B L E　1 - 12　　**Processes Contributing to Low-Pressure Alarm Situations**

Patient disconnected from machine
Leak in airway cuff
　Insufficient air in cuff
　Hole or tear in cuff
　Leak in one-way valve of inflation port
Leak in circuitry
　Poor fittings on water reservoirs
　Dislodged temperature-sensing device
　Hole or tear in tubing
　Poor seal in circuitry connections
Displacement of airway above vocal cords
Loss of compressed air source

NURSING DIAGNOSES AND INTERVENTIONS

Impaired gas exchange (or risk for same): related to altered oxygen supply secondary to non-physiologic tidal volume distribution associated with mechanical ventilation
Desired outcome: Patient has adequate gas exchange as evidenced by Pao_2 >60 mm Hg; $Paco_2$ 35-45 mm Hg; Spo_2 >92%; Svo_2 >60%; and respiratory rate (RR) 12-20 breaths/min
- Observe for, document, and report any changes in patient's condition consistent with increasing respiratory distress. (See "Clinical Presentation" in "Acute Respiratory Failure," p. 202.)
- Position patient to allow for maximal alveolar ventilation and comfort. Remember that in normal situations the dependent lung receives more ventilation and more blood flow than the nondependent lung; however, during mechanical ventilation the dependent portion of the lung receives less distribution of tidal volume than do the nondependent areas.
　❏ Analyze Spo_2, Svo_2, and ABG results with patient in different positions to determine adequacy of ventilation.
　❏ Use postural drainage principles where appropriate.
　❏ In unilateral lung disease, position patient with healthy lung down.
　❏ In bilateral lung disease, position patient in right lateral decubitus position, inasmuch as the right lung has more surface area. If ABG results show that the patient tolerates left lateral decubitus

position, alternate between the two positions. Rotational therapy (rotating patient and/or use of a chest percussion bed) may be effective.
- Turn patient q2h or more frequently if signs of deteriorating pulmonary status occur.
- Auscultate over artificial airway to assess for leaks.
- Assess ventilator for proper functioning and parameter settings, including Fio_2, tidal volume, rate, mode, peak inspiratory pressure, and temperature of inspired gases. In addition, ensure that circuits are tight and alarms are set. Policy and procedure guidelines should at a minimum require thorough ventilator checks every 2 hr. These should be systematically documented in the medical record, most likely the respiratory care practitioner. Assessing the ventilator for proper function and the patient's response to this therapy is a collaborative effort in most situations between nursing and respiratory care personnel.
- Keep ventilator circuitry free of condensed water and expectorated secretions. Fluids may obstruct the flow of gases to and from the patient. The water is a warm, moist environment that is ideal for the growth of microorganisms. Gloves should be worn any time the ventilator circuit is manipulated.
- Monitor serial ABG results. Be alert for hypoxemia (decreases in Pao_2) or hypercapnia (increases in $Paco_2$) with concomitant decrease in pH (<7.35), which can signal hypoventilation and/or inadequate oxygenation. Also observe for decreased $Paco_2$ (<35 mm Hg) with increased pH (>7.45), which may signal mechanical hyperventilation. Notify physician of dysrhythmias, which can occur even with modest alkalosis if the patient has heart disease or is receiving inotropic medications (see Appendix 7). Arrange for ABG analysis when change in patient's condition warrants.
- Keep manual resuscitator at bedside for ventilation in case of malfunctioning equipment.

Ineffective airway clearance (or risk for same): related to altered anatomic structure secondary to presence of ET or tracheostomy tube
Desired outcome: Patient maintains a patent airway as evidenced by absence of adventitious breath sounds or signs of respiratory distress, such as restlessness and anxiety.
- Assess and document breath sounds in all lung fields at least q2h. Note quality and presence or absence of adventitious sounds.
- Monitor patient for restlessness and anxiety, which can signal early airway obstruction.
- Using sterile technique, suction patient's secretions when needed, based on assessment findings, to maintain a patent airway. Avoid routine or scheduled suctioning. Document amount, color, and consistency of tracheobronchial secretions and the patient's tolerance of the procedure. Collaborate with the respiratory care practitioner and report significant changes (e.g., increase in production of secretions, tenacious secretions, bloody sputum) to physician. Maintain artificial airway in a secure and proper alignment.
- Maintain correct temperature ($32°$-$36°$ C [$89.6°$-$96.8°$ F]) of inspired gas. Cold air irritates airways, and hot air may burn fragile lung tissue.
- Maintain humidification of inspired gas to prevent drying of tracheal mucosa. Without humidification, tracheobronchial secretions may become thick and tenacious, creating mucous plugs that place patient at risk for development of atelectasis and infection.

Ineffective breathing pattern (or risk for same): related to anxiety secondary to use of mechanical ventilation
Desired outcomes: Patient exhibits stable RR of 12-20 breaths/min (synchronized with ventilator) and absence of restlessness, anxiety, lethargy, and/or sounding of high-pressure alarm.
- Monitor for evidence that patient is fighting ventilator: frequent sounding of high-pressure alarm when patient breathes against mechanical inspiration or mismatch of patient's respiratory rate and ventilatory cycle.
- Monitor respiratory rate and quality, and monitor for signs of respiratory distress (e.g., tachypnea, hyperventilation, anxiety, restlessness, lethargy, and cyanosis, which is a late sign).
- Teach patient technique for progressive muscle relaxation (see "Health-Seeking Behavior," p. 259). Stay with patient until the respirations are under control. Reassure patient that he or she will be able to synchronize respirations with the ventilator once he or she relaxes.
- Administer prescribed pain or sedation medication for restlessness; restlessness increases O_2 demand and consumption, thus interfering with adequate ventilation.

Risk for infection: related to increased environmental exposure (contaminated respiratory equipment); tissue destruction (during intubation or suctioning); invasive procedures (intubation, suctioning, presence of ET tube) and presence of critical illness.
Desired outcome: Patient is free of infection as evidenced by normothermia; WBC count $\leq11,000/mm^3$; clear sputum; and negative sputum culture results.
- Assess patient for signs and symptoms of infection, including temperature $>38°$ C ($100.4°$ F), tachycardia (HR >100 beats/min, erythema of tracheostomy, and foul-smelling sputum. Document all significant findings.

- To minimize the risk of cross-contamination, wash hands before and after contact with the respiratory secretions of any patient (even though gloves were worn) and before and after contact with patient who is undergoing intubation.
- Maintain appropriate seal on artificial airway cuff to prevent aspiration of oral secretions.
- Keep cuff sealed and, unless contraindicated, HOB elevated 30-45 degrees, especially for patients receiving continuous gastric feedings. Monitor patient for reflux of feedings, as well as for signs of intolerance to feedings (absence of bowel sounds, abdominal distention, residual feedings >100 ml), which can precipitate vomiting and result in pulmonary aspiration of gastric contents. Consider use of a postpyloric feeding tube if patient is at high risk for aspiration or is intolerant of conventional feeding strategies.
- Recognize that bacteria and spores can be introduced easily during suctioning. Follow standard techniques:
  - ❑ Use aseptic technique during suctioning process, including use of sterile catheter and gloves. Use of lavage solutions is not recommended.
  - ❑ Suction tracheobronchial tree before suctioning the oropharynx to avoid introducing oral pathogens into tracheobronchial tree.
  - ❑ Never store or reuse a single-use suction catheter. Consider use of closed system for suctioning.
  - ❑ Change suction canisters and tubing within the time frame established by agency and/or always when filled. Change canisters and tubing between patients.
- To reduce the risk of infection caused by trauma or cross-contamination, suction on an as-needed basis rather than routinely.
- Wash hands and use sterile gloves when performing tracheostomy care to prevent colonization of stoma with bacteria from practitioner's hands.
- Provide oral hygiene at least q2-4h to prevent overgrowth of normal flora and aerobic gram-negative bacilli. Suction oropharynx and posterior pharynx to prevent pooling of secretions. Products are available to provide continuous suctioning of the posterior pharynx. Oral rinse products with chlorhexidine have been used to help control bacteria.
- Manage water reservoirs and ventilator equipment to reduce potential sources of contamination by following these precautions:
  - ❑ Use sterile fluids in all humidifiers and nebulizers.
  - ❑ Change the entire ventilator circuit (ventilator tubing) within the time frame established by policy, or sooner if soiled with secretions or blood.
  - ❑ Empty condensed water or expectorated secretions in tubes into attached traps. Avoid disconnecting tubing, and do not allow secretions to drain back into patient.
  - ❑ Empty water traps on tubing during each ventilator check.
  - ❑ When disconnecting patient from ventilatory circuits, keep ends of connectors clean. Avoid unnecessary disconnection.
  - ❑ Keep connectors on manual resuscitator bags clean and free of secretions between use. Although no data suggest that disposable bags be changed with any frequency, reusable bags should not be used between patients without sterilization.
- Be aware of special risk factors for patients with tracheostomy tubes, and intervene accordingly:
  - ❑ Maintain tracheostomy tube in a secure and proper alignment to avoid irritation of stoma from too much movement.
  - ❑ Change tracheostomy ties q24h, or more frequently if heavily soiled with secretions or wound exudate.
  - ❑ Perform stoma care at least q8h, using aseptic technique until stoma is completely healed. Keep area around stoma dry at all times to prevent maceration and infection. Change stoma dressing as needed to keep it dry.
  - ❑ Avoid use of cotton-filled gauze or other material that may shed small fibers. Patient may aspirate fibers, which in turn can lead to infection.
  - ❑ Use aseptic technique (including use of sterile gloves and drapes) when changing tracheostomy tube.
  - ❑ Culture secretions or wound drainage; administer antibiotics as prescribed.

Anxiety: related to actual or perceived threat to health status as a result of need for or presence of mechanical ventilation

Desired outcome: During the interval of mechanical ventilation, patient relates the presence of emotional comfort and exhibits a decrease in irritability, with a HR within patient's normal range.
- Because some in the general public equate ventilator placement with a hopelessly chronic, vegetative state, reassure patient and significant others that ventilatory support may be a temporary measure until the underlying pathophysiologic process has resolved. At that time the patient may be weaned from the ventilator. Set timelines for reevaluation of patient's progress.

* Reassure patient that he or she will not be left alone.
* Explain all procedures before they are initiated to patient and significant others. Inform patient of his or her progress.
* Describe and point out the alarm system, explaining that it will alert staff in the event of an accidental disconnection.
* Provide patient with mechanism for communication (e.g., picture board, erasable marker board, pen and paper). See "Impaired Verbal Communication" in "Psychosocial Support," p. 69.
* If aggressive sedation is used, perform "wake up assessments" at least every 24hrand evaluate whether patient needs analgesics for pain control. Sedatives can mask symptoms of pain.

Impaired gas exchange (or risk for same): related to altered oxygen supply secondary to weaning from mechanical ventilation

Desired outcome: Patient has adequate gas exchange as evidenced by Pao_2 >60 mm Hg; $Paco_2$ <45 mm Hg; Spo_2 ≥92%; Svo_2 ≥60%; and pH 7.35-7.45 (or values within 10% of patient's baseline).

* Maintain patient in a comfortable position to enhance ventilation. Many patients find that semi-Fowler's position promotes effective respirations.
* Observe for indicators of hypoxia, including tachycardia, tachypnea, cardiac dysrhythmias, pain, anxiety, and restlessness.
* Assess and record VS q15min for the first hour of weaning, then hourly if patient is stable. Report significant findings to physician, such as increased respiratory effort, hyperventilation, anxiety, lethargy, and cyanosis.
* Check patient's tidal volume after the first 15 min of weaning and as needed. Optimally, it will be within 5-10 ml/kg.
* Obtain specimen for ABG analysis during weaning as indicated. Monitor Spo_2 continuously and as available, Svo_2 for values outside normal range.

Anxiety related to perceived threat to health status secondary to weaning process

Desired outcome: During the weaning process, patient expresses the attainment of emotional comfort and is free of the signs of harmful anxiety as evidenced by HR ≤100 beats/min; RR ≤20 breaths/min; and BP within patient's normal range.

* Before weaning process is initiated, discuss plans for weaning with patient and significant others. Explain that patient's condition will be assessed at frequent intervals during the weaning procedure. Provide time for questions and answers about the procedure.
* Stay with patient during the initial phase of weaning, keeping patient informed of progress being made. Provide positive feedback for positive efforts.
* Teach patient progressive muscle relaxation technique, which may reduce anxiety and fear and thus relax chest muscles. (See "Health-Seeking Behavior," p. 259.)
* Instruct patient to take deep breaths if he or she is capable of doing so. This may provide the confidence of knowing that he or she can initiate and sustain respirations independently.
* Leave call light within patient's reach before leaving bedside. Reassure patient that help is nearby.

You may also wish to refer to the following interventions from the Nursing Interventions Classification (NIC):

NIC Acid-Base Management; Acid-Base Monitoring; Airway Management; Airway Suctioning; Anxiety Reduction; Aspiration Precautions; Bedside Laboratory Testing; Infection Control; Laboratory Data Interpretation; Mechanical Ventilation; Mechanical Ventilatory Weaning; Oxygen Therapy; Positioning; Respiratory Monitoring; Vital Signs Monitoring

ADDITIONAL NURSING DIAGNOSES

Also see nursing diagnoses and interventions under "Prolonged Immobility," p. 61; "Psychosocial Support," p. 68; and "Psychosocial Support for the Patient's Family and Significant Others," p. 78.

Hemodynamic Monitoring

Hemodynamic monitoring refers to the specialized methods used to evaluate cardiovascular performance. It provides information about cardiac performance, tissue perfusion, blood volume, tissue oxygenation, and vascular tone. Indirect methods of hemodynamic monitoring include measurement of arterial pressure via manual or automated BP cuff or Doppler test, and measurement of cardiac output (CO) with an echo Doppler device. Direct methods of measuring hemodynamic values include those obtained by arterial, central venous, and pulmonary artery catheters.

Many critical care patients have cardiovascular disease or are at risk for cardiovascular complications; therefore it is essential to be able to evaluate cardiac function and related factors. Four major cardiac mechanisms determine CO, which is the amount of blood ejected from the heart over 1 min. These mechanisms are preload, afterload, contractility, and heart rate.

Preload: Starling's law of the heart describes the concept of preload: the greater the stretch of the myocardial muscle at the end of diastole, the greater the force of contraction. However, if the stretch is excessive, contractility will diminish. This mechanism enables the heart to pump varying volumes of blood and to coordinate the output of the two ventricles. The volume of blood present in the ventricles coupled with compliance (ability to stretch) of the ventricles at end of diastole determine preload. Factors that affect ventricular blood volume include venous return, circulating blood volume, condition of the heart valves, and atrial contractility. Ventricular compliance is affected by stiffness and thickness of the cardiac muscle. Any stressor that influences one of these factors will result in a change in preload, with a concomitant change in CO. Clinically, preload is described as ventricular end-diastolic pressure (VEDP), because pressure in the ventricles correlates closely with volume. Right ventricular end-diastolic (filling) pressure (RVEDP) is reflected by the right atrial pressure (RAP) or the central venous pressure (CVP). Left ventricular end-diastolic (filling) pressure (LVEDP) is reflected by the left atrial (LA), pulmonary artery diastolic (PAD), or pulmonary artery wedge (PAW) pressure measurements. Heart disease affects preload. Patients with biventricular heart failure and/or "stiff ventricles" are not able to handle increased intravascular volume. Their preload is always high. The diseased heart is very sensitive and has little ability to compensate for volume changes. Patients with heart disease can develop heart failure, so expert monitoring by the clinician is required.

Afterload: Refers to the pressure generated within the ventricular myocardium during systole. The heart must generate enough pressure within the right and left ventricles to overcome the vascular resistance to ejection. The pressures created by the blood volume and vascular tone within the pulmonary, aortic, and systemic circulation can impede ventricular ejection. Other resistant forces include increased blood viscosity, reduced distensibility of the vascular system, and diseased heart valves. Since vascular resistance plays a major role in determining pressures throughout the heart and lungs, afterload is evaluated by calculating the pulmonary vascular resistance (PVR) for right ventricular afterload and systemic vascular resistance (SVR) for left ventricular afterload. The higher the afterload, the greater the myocardial wall pressure and the greater the work of the heart to overcome resistance to flow. Increased cardiac work requires increased myocardial blood flow to deliver additional oxygen. When blood flowing through the coronary arteries is diminished by atherosclerosis, the demand for increased blood needed for increased afterload may not be met, resulting in myocardial ischemia, injury, and possibly infarction. The clinician should be aware that diseased ventricles are extremely sensitive to abrupt changes in afterload.

Contractility: Refers to the inherent capacity of the myocardium to contract. This mechanism functions independently of variations in preload and afterload. Although contractility cannot be measured directly, a change in contractility can be inferred when CO is decreased and other variables that affect CO (i.e., preload, afterload, heart rate) remain the same. Several factors positively influence contractility: sympathetic stimulation, calcium, positive inotropic agents such as digitalis, dobutamine, milrinone, and beta-(β-) adrenergic drugs. Factors such as acidemia, hypoxia, β-blocker drugs, and antidysrhythmic drugs decrease contractility.

Heart rate: Changes in heart rate (HR) affect myocardial functioning significantly. Slight increases in HR with a constant stroke volume (SV) result in increased CO. Very rapid heart rates are associated with a reduction in CO as diastolic time is shortened, resulting in decreased coronary perfusion and reduced ventricular filling time. Bradycardia often results in decreased CO unless there are increases in SV because of longer ventricular filling times. The heart requires more oxygen with increased heart rates but ironically may actually be receiving less oxygen. A HR of 100-130 beats/min is often required to maintain a cardiac output that matches the oxygen demands of hypermetabolic states in the critically ill. Changes in any of the four components discussed produce significant hemodynamic deterioration and imbalance in myocardial oxygen supply and demand for patients with heart disease.

This section focuses on direct methods of hemodynamic monitoring. Normal hemodynamic values with derived parameters are found in Table 1-13.

DIRECT HEMODYNAMIC MEASUREMENT

Arterial pressure monitoring: Arterial catheters are inserted via the radial artery, because this artery is readily accessible and collateral blood flow is usually adequate. The arterial catheter may also be inserted in the femoral or brachial artery. The arterial pressure waveform is displayed on a bedside monitor for continuous observation of systolic, diastolic, and mean arterial pressures. The

T A B L E 1 - 13   Hemodynamic Formulas

Parameter	Formula	Normal values
Cardiac output (CO)	$\dfrac{O_2 \text{ consumption}}{\text{A-V}o_2}$	4-7 L/min
Cardiac index (CI)	$\dfrac{CO}{\text{Body surface area (BSA)}}$	2.5-4 L/min/m²
Coronary perfusion pressure (CPP)	Diastolic BP – PAWP	50-70 mm Hg
Stroke volume (SV)	$\dfrac{CO}{HR} \times 1000$	55-100 ml/beat
Stroke volume index (SVI)	$\dfrac{SV}{BSA}$	30-60 ml/beat/m²
Arterial oxygen content (Cao_2)	(Hgb × 1.34) × Sao_2	18-20 ml/vol%
Venous oxygen content (Cvo_2)	(Hgb × 1.34) × Svo_2	15.5 ml/vol%
Oxygen delivery (Do_2)	Cao_2 × CO × 10	800-1000 ml/min
Oxygen delivery index (Do_2I)	Cao_2 × CI × 10	500-600 ml/min/m²
Arteriovenous oxygen content difference (C[a-v]o_2	Cao_2 – Cvo_2	4-6 ml/vol%
Oxygen consumption (Vo_2)	CO × 10 × C(a-v)o_2	200-250 ml/min
Oxygen consumption index (Vo_2I)	CI × 10 × C(a-v)o_2	115-165 ml/min/m²
Systemic vascular resistance (SVR)	$\dfrac{\text{MAP-RAP}}{CO} \times 80$	900-1200 dynes/sec/cm^{-5}
Pulmonary vascular resistance (PVR)	$\dfrac{\text{PAM – PAWP}}{CO} \times 80$	60-100 dynes/sec/cm^{-5}
Left ventricular stroke work index (LVSWI)	SVI × (MAP – PAWP) × 0.136	40-75 g/m²/beat
Right ventricular stroke work index (RVSWI)	SVI × (MPAP – RAP) × 0.136	4-8 g/m²/beat
Mean arterial pressure (MAP)	$\dfrac{\text{Systolic BP + 2 (Diastolic BP)}}{3}$	70-105 mm Hg
Mean pulmonary artery pressure (MPAP, PAM)	$\dfrac{\text{PAS + 2(PAD)}}{3}$	10-15 mm Hg
Mixed venous oxygen saturation (Svo_2)	(CO × Cao_2 × 10) – Vo_2	60% -80%
Central venous pressure (CVP)		2-6 mm Hg
Right atrial pressure (RAP)		4-6 mm Hg
Left atrial pressure (LAP)		8-12 mm Hg
Right ventricular pressure (RVP)		25/0-5 mm Hg
Pulmonary artery systolic pressure (PAS)		20-30 mm Hg
Pulmonary artery diastolic pressure (PAD)		8-15 mm Hg
Pulmonary artery wedge pressure (PAWP)		6-12 mm Hg

appearance of the arterial waveform is influenced by variations in BP, dysrhythmias, and mechanical factors. Mechanical factors that influence the waveform include overdamping, catheter whip, and inaccurate calibration/zeroing (Table 1-14). Complications of arterial catheters include arterial thrombosis with ischemia, infection, infiltration, and blood loss caused by disconnection. Continuous observation of the arterial line insertion site for infection and leakage is an essential nursing responsibility. Monitor and document pulses distal to the catheter site every 1-2 hr. It is important to note a patient's baseline BP and to compare left and right cuff blood pressures with arterial blood pressures. *Systolic blood pressure:* Determined by (1) the amount of blood ejected by the ventricle per beat (stroke volume), (2) wall compliance of the arterial system, and (3) peripheral resistance. Elevations in systolic pressure produce large, steep waveforms, often reflective of changes in vascular compliance, such as the hypertension seen in patients with atherosclerosis. A decrease in systolic pressure

TABLE 1-14   Mechanical Problems Affecting Hemodynamic Measurements

Problem	Waveform appearance	Cause
Overdamping*	Smaller than usual with a slow rise; diminished or absent dicrotic notch (arterial and pulmonary artery catheters)	Air bubbles in system Thrombus formation Lodging of catheter against vessel wall Kinking or knotting of catheter or tubing Loose connection in tubing or transducer Incorrect calibration Spontaneous catheter migration into a near-wedged position (PA catheter only)
Catheter whip	Erratic, "noisy" waveform with highly variable and inaccurate pressures	Spurious movement of the catheter tip within the vessel lumen (may require repositioning) Catheter too long for vessel (arterial)
No waveform	Complete absence of waveform	Large leak in the system, usually with blood backing up into the tubing Loose or cracked transducer or air intransducer Stopcock turned to wrong position Catheter tip or lumen totally occluded by clot Inadequate pressure (<300 mm Hg) on pressure bag Defective transducer or amplifier
Inability to obtain a wedged reading (PA catheter only)	Absence of wedge waveform after balloon inflation	Balloon rupture Retrograde catheter slippage

*Whenever the amplitude of an arterial or PA waveform decreases, the patient first should be assessed for hypovolemia or shock.

producing smaller, damped waveforms is seen in connection with heart disorders that result in decreased stroke volume or with the use of arterial vasodilators such as nitroprusside, nitroglycerin, and nifedipine.

Diastolic blood pressure: Determined by (1) volume of blood within the arterial system, (2) compliance of the arterial wall, and (3) peripheral resistance. Coronary artery blood flow occurs during diastole, and a drop in diastolic pressure may result in myocardial ischemia as flow is reduced with lower diastolic pressure. Monitoring of diastolic BP is critical, especially when vasodilating drugs are administered, since diastolic BP generally decreases from the effect of these medications.

Mean arterial pressure: normal value is 70-100 mm Hg: The average pressure within the arterial tree throughout the cardiac cycle.

Mean arterial pressure (MAP) reflects the average force that pushes blood through the systemic circulation to the tissues. MAP is the product of CO × SVR. An increase in CO or SVR will increase MAP. A decrease in either value will decrease MAP. Mean arterial pressure is the most accurate noninvasive measurement of central aortic pressure. The intraaortic balloon pump (IABP) provides the most accurate invasive measurement. MAP can be calculated by the following formula:

$$\text{MAP} = \frac{\text{Systolic BP} + 2\,(\text{Diastolic BP})}{3}$$

Central venous pressure: normal value is 2-6 mm Hg: Central venous pressure (CVP) is the measurement of systemic venous pressure at the level of the right atrium (RA). CVP can be measured by a catheter threaded into the jugular, subclavian, or other large vein or by the proximal port of a pulmonary artery (PA) catheter. Since 60% of total blood volume resides in the venous system, the CVP is valuable in assessing for fluid volume excess or deficit and venous tone. The CVP also provides information regarding right ventricular (RV) function. RV failure, cardiac tamponade, fluid volume overload, pulmonary hypertension, tricuspid valve disease, and chronic left ventricular failure may increase CVP. Decreased CVP is most often caused by hypovolemia. Venodilation caused by sepsis, drugs, or neurogenic dysfunction also may decrease CVP. Complications of central venous catheters include venous air embolism, dysrhythmias, hemorrhage, infection, vascular erosion, perforation of cardiac chambers, pneumothorax, and thromboembolic problems.

Pulmonary artery pressures: multiple values are measured (see Table 1-13): Pulmonary artery (PA) pressure monitoring is used to evaluate heart function and pulmonary vascular status. PA catheters (e.g., Swan-Ganz) provide valuable information used to assess and treat life-threatening illness or injury. Blood volume, heart function, and tissue oxygenation can be assessed using various available pressures. PA catheters are inserted via the jugular, subclavian, or femoral vein and passed through the right side of the heart into the PA, where the tip of the catheter is positioned in the pulmonary capillary bed. Pulmonary artery systolic (PAS), pulmonary artery mean (PAM), and pulmonary artery diastolic (PAD) pressures are monitored continuously by the distal port of the PA catheter after the catheter is passed out of the right heart, through the pulmonary valve, and into the pulmonary artery. Pulmonary artery/capillary wedge pressure (PAWP or PCWP) can be assessed after inflating the balloon on the distal end of the catheter, which allows it to float and "wedge" into a smaller branch of the pulmonary artery. Once the artery is occluded by the balloon, the filling pressures of the left heart can be indirectly measured. If an Svo_2 pulmonary artery catheter is used, mixed venous oxygen saturation levels are also continuously monitored. CO can be measured intermittently using thermodilution or, with some PA/Svo_2 catheters, is measured continuously. A full hemodynamic profile can be calculated for the patient, including SV, stroke work, pulmonary vascular resistance, and systemic vascular resistance (see Table 1-13). All values are helpful in determining how to manage the patient's fluid balance, heart function, and vascular tone, and can be individualized to the patient's body size (index values). Abnormal pulmonary artery pressures are discussed in Table 1-15. Complications of PA catheters include ventricular or atrial dysrhythmias, pulmonary ischemia or infarction, valvular damage (tricuspid, pulmonic), pulmonary artery rupture, infection, emboli (thrombotic, air, balloon) and pneumothorax. Incidence of PA catheter complications is about 3%.

Right atrial pressure: normal mean RAP is 4-6 mm Hg: Measured via the proximal catheter port, is essentially the same as CVP. With the PA catheter, RAP can be monitored continuously and displayed on a bedside screen. In addition, the catheter lumen can be used for fluid or drug administration.

TABLE 1-15 Abnormal Pulmonary Artery Pressures

Hemodynamic pressure	Normal range	Clinical conditions
Pulmonary artery systolic pressure (PAS)	20-30 mm Hg	*Increased:* right ventricular failure, chronic left ventricular failure, constrictive pericarditis, cardiac tamponade, pulmonary hypertension (primary or related to lung disease) *Decreased:* hypovolemia, preload reduction
Pulmonary artery diastolic pressure (PAD)*	8-15 mm Hg	*Increased:* left ventricular failure, mitral stenosis, left-to-right shunts, pulmonary hypertension (primary or related to lung disease) *Decreased:* hypovolemia, preload reduction
Pulmonary artery wedge pressure (PAWP)†	6-12 mm Hg	*Increased:* left ventricular failure, cardiac tamponade, mitral valve regurgitation, acute ventricular septal defect, fluid volume overload *Decreased:* hypovolemia, afterload reduction

*PAD may exceed PAWP by ≥5 mm Hg in patients with pulmonary hypertension, hypoxemia, acidosis, pulmonary emboli, and other lung disease.
†PAWP > PAD signals a mechanical problem (i.e., overwedging or improper identification of PAD).

Right ventricular pressure: normal RVP is 25/0-5 mm Hg: Measured during catheter insertion only, can provide information about the function of the right ventricle and the tricuspid and pulmonic valves. Elevation of RV systolic pressure may be seen in pulmonic stenosis, pulmonary hypertension, or ventricular septal defect (VSD) with left-to-right shunt. Elevation of RV diastolic pressure may occur with RV failure, cardiac tamponade, or constrictive pericarditis. It is important for the nurse to identify the normal RV waveform, because a complication of the PA catheter is redirection of the catheter tip into the right ventricle, causing ventricular ectopy.

PA systolic, diastolic, and mean pressures: normal pulmonary artery pressures are 20-30/8-15 mm Hg (PAS/PAD) with PA mean pressure 12-20 mm Hg (PAM): Used to evaluate heart function and pulmonary vascular disease. In patients with healthy pulmonary vasculature, the PAD pressure corresponds closely to the PAWP and reflects the LVEDP. A significant difference (i.e., >5 mm Hg) between the PAD and PAWP is seen with pulmonary disease or a pulmonary embolus. When this occurs, PA systolic and diastolic pressures are elevated, whereas the PAWP remains normal. Specific disease states that elevate PA pressures include pulmonary hypertension, pulmonary embolism, hypoxia, left ventricular failure because of valve disease, myocardial infarction (MI), cardiomyopathy, and left-to-right intracardiac shunt. Decreased PA pressures are seen with hypovolemia and pharmacologic preload reduction.

Pulmonary artery wedge pressure: normal mean PAWP is 6-12 mm Hg: Reflects the LVEDP and is used to evaluate cardiac performance. An elevated PAWP may be seen with left ventricular failure, acute mitral regurgitation, acute VSD, and acute cardiac tamponade. A decreased PAWP is seen with hypovolemia and afterload reduction. PEEP/CPAP >10 cm H_2O may result in falsely elevated pulmonary artery pressures and PAWP. However, patients should not be disconnected from the ventilator to measure pulmonary artery pressures, because significant hypoxemia and inaccurate measurements can result. Correlation of measured pressures with the respiratory cycle improves the accuracy of these measurements.

Cardiac output: normal value is 4-7 L/min: The volume of blood in liters ejected by the heart each minute and the product of the SV and the HR. *SV is the volume of blood ejected by the heart per beat. Normal SV is 55-100 ml/beat.* The CO is often individualized in relation to body size by taking the CO and dividing by the body surface area (BSA) to obtain the value known as the *cardiac index (CI).* Normal CI is 2.5-4 L/min/m². If continuous CO monitoring is done, an average CO is recorded over 3-min intervals and updated every 30-60 sec. Continuous CO monitoring closely and accurately monitors a patient's hemodynamic profile. Benefits of continuous CO monitoring may improve response to changes in output, resulting in improved outcomes for severely ill patients (e. g., cardiomyopathy, ejection fractions [EFs] less than 20%).

Systemic vascular resistance: normal value for SVR is 900-1200 dynes/sec/cm⁻⁵ The major factor that determines left ventricular afterload or resistance that must be overcome prior to left ventricular ejection. The formula for SVR is the following:

$$SVR = \frac{(MAP - RAP)}{CO} \times 80$$

Any factor that increases SVR will increase the workload of the heart and may reduce cardiac output. Vasodilator therapy is used to reduce SVR to normal limits. A low SVR can indicate systemic vasodilation, commonly seen with septic, anaphylactic, and neurogenic shocks. Vasopressors and IV fluids are administered to manage vasodilation along with medications directed at the cause. Patients with low SVR often have high cardiac outputs due to low resistance to ventricular ejection.

Pulmonary vascular resistance: The normal value is 60-100 dynes/sec/cm⁻⁵: Measures right ventricular afterload or the resistance the right ventricle must overcome to eject into the pulmonary circulation. The formula for PVR is the following:

$$PVR = \frac{(PAM - PAWP)}{CO} \times 80$$

PVR may be elevated as a result of primary pulmonary hypertension, or secondary pulmonary hypertension due to mitral or aortic valve disease, congenital heart disease, long-standing left ventricular heart failure, hypoxia, chronic obstructive pulmonary disease (COPD), or pulmonary embolus. Medications may affect the PVR: norepinephrine, vasopressin and neosynephrine increase it, whereas isoproterenol, nifedipine, prostaglandins, sodium nitroprusside, and acetylcholine decrease it.

Mixed venous oxygen saturation (Svo$_2$): normal range for Svo$_2$ is 60%-80%: Can be measured intermittently using mixed venous blood samples from the distal port of the PA catheter or continuously using a fiberoptic Svo$_2$ pulmonary artery catheter. Svo$_2$ is the average percentage of Hgb bound with oxygen in the venous blood and is reflective of the patient's ability to balance oxygen supply and demand at the tissue level. Very low levels (<30%) indicate poor perfusion and are often associated with lactic acidosis. Svo$_2$ monitoring can be used to evaluate the effects of medical and nursing interventions on tissue oxygen use. If the Svo$_2$ value changes by more than 10% for more than 10 min, the nurse should evaluate arterial oxygen saturation (Sao$_2$), CO, Hgb, and oxygen consumption (vo$_2$). By examining the variables involved in tissue oxygenation, the nurse can help determine what is affecting Svo$_2$ (Table 1-16).

Left atrial pressure: the normal value for LAP is 8-12 mm Hg: Left atrial pressure (LAP) is the most direct measure of the volume within the left ventricle at the end of diastole (LVEDP). A small, rigid catheter is inserted into the left atrium during cardiac surgery and brought through the chest wall or epigastric area. Continuous monitoring of LVEDP may be indicated for the cardiac surgery patient with significant pulmonary hypertension. PAWP is no longer reflective of left heart function when severe pulmonary hypertension is present. Since the catheter enters directly into the left atrium, the patient is at high risk for air or tissue emboli. An in-line air filter should be added to the flush system to reduce the risk of air emboli. If the waveform pattern dampens, the catheter should be aspirated until blood is seen. If there is no blood return, consult the physician. **It is not advisable to flush the LA catheter because of the risk of embolization.**

T A B L E 1 - 16 Factors Affecting Mixed Venous Oxygen Saturation

Factor	Effect on Svo$_2$	Clinical examples
Arterial oxygen saturation		
↑ Sao$_2$	↑ Svo$_2$	Supplemental oxygen
↓ Sao$_2$	↓ Svo$_2$	Reduced oxygen supply (e.g., ARDS, ET suctioning, removal of supplemental oxygen)
Cardiac output		
↑ CO	↑ Svo$_2$	Administration of inotropes to increase contractility
↓ CO	↓ Svo$_2$	Dysrhythmias, increased SVR, MI
Hemoglobin		
↓ Hgb	↓ Svo$_2$	Hemorrhage, hemolysis, severe anemia in patients with cardiovascular disease
Oxygen consumption		
↑ Vo$_2$	↓ Svo$_2$	States in which metabolic demand exceeds oxygen supply (e.g., shivering, seizures, hyperthermia, hyperdynamic states)
↓ Vo$_2$	↑ Svo$_2$	States in which there is failure of peripheral tissue to extract or use oxygen: • Significant peripheral arteriovenous shunting: cirrhosis, renal failure • Redistribution of blood away from beds where oxygen extraction occurs: sepsis, acute pancreatitis, major burns • Blockage of oxygen uptake or utilization: cyanide poisoning (including nitroprusside toxicity), carbon monoxide poisoning
Mechanical problems	↑ Svo$_2$	Wedged PA catheter creates falsely elevated Svo$_2$

ARDS, Acute respiratory distress syndrome; *CO,* cardiac output; *ET,* endotracheal; *Hgb,* hemoglobin; *MI,* myocardial infarction; *PA,* pulmonary artery; *SVR,* systemic vascular resistance.

NURSING DIAGNOSES AND INTERVENTIONS

Knowledge deficit: rationale for hemodynamic monitoring and procedure for catheter insertion
Desired outcome: Within 24 hr of catheter placement, patient verbalizes knowledge of the rationale for hemodynamic monitoring; procedure for insertion of lines; and sensations that are experienced during and after the procedure.

- Assess patient's knowledge about hemodynamic monitoring. As indicated, explain to patient/family that hemodynamic monitoring is useful in guiding therapy and that the PA catheter can measure pressures in and near the heart.
- Teach patient about the insertion procedure, emphasizing that a local anesthetic agent will be used, he or she will not be able to move during the procedure, frequent x-rays films will be taken, and a dressing will be applied to the insertion site. Explain to patient that a drape may be placed over patient's face for central or PA catheter insertion.
- Explain the sensations that may be felt during the procedure: a stick from injection of the local anesthetic, pressure as the catheter advances, coldness from the cleansing solution, burning from the injection of lidocaine, claustrophobia from drapes over the face, dull pushing and pulling sensations in the neck, and coldness from the injection of cardiac output iced solution (if used).
- Instruct patient to report any anxiety or discomfort that occurs during the procedure because medications to comfort the patient may be given.

Risk for infection related to presence of invasive hemodynamic catheters
Desired outcome: Patient is free of infection as evidenced by normothermia; WBC count ≤11,000/mm^3; negative culture results; and absence of erythema, heat, swelling, or purulent drainage at the insertion site.

- On a daily basis, monitor temperature for elevations ≥37.7° C (100° F); WBC count for elevation; and catheter insertion site for erythema, tenderness to the touch, local warmth, and purulent drainage.
- As prescribed, obtain culture of any suspicious drainage and report positive findings.
- Use normal saline rather than D$_5$W for hemodynamic flush solution.
- Change hemodynamic tubing, transducer, and flush solution according to hospital protocol.
- Maintain closed system to transducer and for flush solution. Keep all external openings and stopcocks securely capped at all times.
- Use closed system for cardiac output injection fluid.
- Maintain occlusive, dry sterile dressing over insertion site.
- Change dressing per hospital protocol, using aseptic technique.
- Record date of catheter insertion, and ensure that catheter is changed per agency protocol.
- If infection occurs, send catheter tip for culture and sensitivity test.

Altered cardiopulmonary tissue perfusion (or risk for same) related to interrupted blood flow secondary to migration of PA catheter into a wedged position, "overwedging" of balloon, continuous wedge position, or local vascular thrombosis
Desired outcome: Within 2hrof this diagnosis, patient has adequate pulmonary perfusion as evidenced by normal PA waveform and RR 12-20 breaths/min with normal depth and pattern (eupnea).

- Monitor PA waveform continuously. Report any change in configuration, particularly if the waveform becomes decreased in amplitude and flattened in appearance (see Table 1-14).
- Assess patient for interrupted pulmonary arterial blood flow as evidenced by acute onset of pleuritic chest pain, shortness of breath (SOB), tachypnea, and hemoptysis.
- Evaluate daily, the position of the catheter via chest x-ray. Never push the PA catheter forward in the pulmonary artery to avoid possibility of PA rupture or lodging the catheter in a small vessel.
- Exercise care in taking PAWP measurements. Prolonged and repeated readings can cause trauma to the vessel wall. The catheter can also be "overwedged." Inject enough air to obtain a wedge configuration but no more than the amount recommended by catheter manufacturer. Never pull back on plunger of syringe to remove air; rather, disconnect the syringe and allow passive deflation of the balloon.
- Verify correlation of PAD to PAWP q4-8h. Be aware that PAD may exceed PAWP by ≥5 mm Hg in patients with acidosis, hypoxemia, pulmonary emboli, lung disease, and pulmonary hypertension.
- Consult physician if PA waveform remains in wedged position after balloon deflation.
- Pay special attention to PA waveform when the patient is moved (e.g., when being taken to x-ray department; getting into a chair, when position is changed or bed is made). The monitoring system may not be appropriately leveled with the patient's phlebostatic axis (right atrial level) after the patient has changed position.

Altered peripheral tissue perfusion (involved extremity) related to interrupted blood flow secondary to presence of arterial catheter or thrombosis caused by catheter
Desired outcome: Within 2 hr of this diagnosis, patient has adequate perfusion to affected extremity as evidenced by brisk capillary refill (<2 sec), natural color, warm skin, normal sensation, and the ability to move the fingers.
- Continuously monitor capillary refill, color, temperature, sensation, pulses, and movement. Be alert to indicators of ischemia and teach them to the patient, stressing the importance of notifying staff members promptly if they occur.
- Maintain arterial line on continuous flush at 3 ml/hr with heparinized normal saline (1 U heparin/ml saline or flush solution recommended by agency); ensure that pressure bag remains inflated at 300 mm Hg.
- Ensure tight connections of tubing throughout the system.
- Support patient's wrist or appropriate extremity with armboard or other supportive device to prevent flexion and movement of the catheter.

Risk for injury related to potential for insertion complications secondary to ventricular irritability, patient movement during insertion procedure, or difficult anatomy
Desired outcome: Patient has no complications from PA or CVP catheter insertion as evidenced by normal sinus rhythm on ECG; BP within patient's normal range; HR $\leq$100 beats/min; RR $\leq$20 breaths/min with normal pattern and depth (eupnea); normal breath sounds; and absence of adventitious breath sounds or muffled heart sounds.
- During pre-procedure teaching, caution patient about the importance of remaining still during insertion of catheter. Provide sedation and analgesics as prescribed.

Note: With PA or CVP catheter insertion, the following complications may occur: carotid artery puncture, air embolism, right ventricular perforation, hemorrhage, thoracic duct injury, pneumothorax, and cardiac tamponade. With PA catheter insertion, ventricular dysrhythmias may occur.

- Perform a baseline assessment, monitoring BP, HR, RR, breath sounds, heart sounds, and ECG. Perform a post-procedure assessment, comparing it with baseline findings. Be alert to decreased BP, pulsus paradoxus (see Table 2-8, p. 121), increased HR or RR, diminished or absent breath sounds, and muffled heart sounds, as well as dysrhythmias on ECG. Report significant findings to the physician.
- After the procedure, obtain a chest x-ray as prescribed.
- Keep lidocaine at bedside for immediate IV injection if patient has sustained ventricular dysrhythmias.

Research Brief 1-3 Low peak oxygen consumption (Vo_2) and prolonged QT interval or enhanced QT variability are associated with poor prognosis in patients who have heart failure. In a study that involved 154 transplant candidates, the relation between the QTc interval and other hemodynamic variables was analyzed. Mortality was examined after a mean follow-up of 4.3 $\pm$ 1.8 years. At the end of the study, 47% of patients were dead. An inverse relationship was found between the QTc interval length and peak Vo_2, or peak oxygen consumption. A correlation was not found between QTc interval and LV loading conditions. In summary, a repolarization length measured by the QTc interval is inversely correlated with heart failure severity measured by peak Vo_2 and is independent of LV loading conditions in patients with severe heart failure.

From Boccalandro F et al: Relations among heart failure severity, left ventricular loading conditions and repolarization length in advance heart failure secondary to ischemic or idiopathic dilated cardiomyopathy, *Am J Cardiol* 92(5):544-547, 2003.

Sedating and Paralytic Agents

All critically ill patients experience some degree of anxiety, restlessness, and/or agitation. Severe illness produces anxiety and fear in all but those who are deeply obtunded. Sedative, anxiolytic, and neuromuscular blocking (paralytic) agents are administered to promote comfort and stabilization of the patient. Optimally, potential causes of agitation syndrome can be identified and managed using non-pharmacologic methods. See "Psychosocial Support," p. 68, for nonpharmacologic nursing interventions that should be used along with pharmacotherapy. Anxiety and agitation in critically ill patients are prompted by emotional factors, including fear, loss of physical control, life-threatening illness, inability to communicate (e.g., mechanical ventilation), and feelings of helplessness. Common pathophysiologic factors contributing to agitation syndrome include hypoxemia, impaired cerebral perfusion, infection, alcohol withdrawal, and encephalopathy (Table 1-17).

Inadequate pain control can frequently manifest itself as agitation. Environmental factors such as noise, temperature extremes, and sleep deprivation add to anxiety and agitation. Unrelieved stress,

---

T A B L E 1 - 17   Pathologic Conditions Contributing to Agitation

Addison's crisis
Alzheimer disease
Anxiety disorder
Delirium tremens
Developmental disability
Drug intoxication
Fear
Encephalopathy
  Hepatic
  Metabolic
  Uremic
Hypercarbia
Hyperthyroidism
Hypoglycemia
Hyponatremia
Hypoxemia
Impaired cerebral perfusion
  Cerebral thrombosis
  Subarachnoid hemorrhage
  Intracranial bleeding
  Cerebral vasospasm
  Cerebral edema
Infection
  Meningitis
  Encephalitis
  Brain abscess
  Sepsis syndrome
Opiate withdrawal
Pain, inadequately controlled
Partial drug-induced paralysis
  Antibiotic (e.g., aminoglycosides)
  Electrolyte disorders (e.g., hypophosphatemia)
Sedative withdrawal
Sleep deprivation
Steroid psychosis

---

manifested in the form of anxiety or agitation, retards healing and can increase mortality. The remainder of this section discusses the use of sedatives in situations in which non-pharmacologic interventions are not entirely effective.

The goal of pharmacologic sedation is to reduce anxiety and produce a calm but communicative state. This is best accomplished by administering frequent, incremental doses of sedatives just until the desired effects are achieved. Close monitoring, individualized dosing, and titration to desired effect are essential in avoiding oversedation and toxicity in critically ill patients. Major organ dysfunction, use of multiple medications, tissue catabolism, and other factors render critically ill patients especially vulnerable to the toxic effects of many sedatives. Excessive sedation has been associated with delayed recognition of neurologic events, muscle wasting, and nosocomial complications such as deep vein thrombosis, compression injury, and pneumonia.

Neuromuscular blockade (paralyzing the patient) is used only on mechanically ventilated patients who cannot be stabilized and/or controlled with other sedative, antipsychotic, analgesic, anesthetic, or other adjunctive agents. Paralysis is always done in conjunction with sedation and analgesia, since the patient is unable to breathe and communicate while paralyzed. In the patient who receives paralytics without sedation and analgesia, overwhelming fear and helplessness occurs, as the patient is unable to state needs, cannot move, or take a breath.

ASSESSMENT

Anxiety: Subjective characteristics include increased tension, apprehension, fear, shakiness, uncertainty, distress, difficulty concentrating, and feelings of helplessness. Objective findings include cardiovascular excitation, superficial vasoconstriction, pupil dilation, increased perspiration, restlessness, disturbed sleep patterns, tremors, and facial tension.

Pain: Is what a patient says it is. Use a visual analog scale, numeric scale, and "happy faces" or other coded method to establish baseline and evaluate analgesic effectiveness. Objective findings include autonomic responses such as changes in BP and HR, increased or decreased RR, pupil dilation, increased perspiration, guarding, moaning, crying, restlessness, facial grimace, furrowing of the brow, and rigid muscle tone.

Neuromuscular blockade: The level or depth of paralysis may be quantified using a device called a *peripheral nerve stimulator.* Typically a technique called the *train-of-four (TOF)* is chosen because it imposes the least discomfort. The TOF setting on the peripheral nerve stimulator will deliver four signals along the nerve path. The muscle response is then measured to evaluate how many signals are blocked compared with the number actually delivered. In the absence of neuromuscular blockade, the muscle should move four times equally in response to four signals. As receptors are loaded with neuromuscular blocking agents (NMBAs), fewer muscle contractions are seen (Table 1-18).

COLLABORATIVE MANAGEMENT

A variety of therapeutic options are available to produce sedation in critically ill patients. Assessment and alleviation of pain as a stimulus for anxiety/agitation is essential. Appropriate analgesics must be used and considered for patients in whom pain is a component of agitation.

Opiate analgesics: Reliably relieve pain, are easily titrated, and have significant sedative effects. Morphine is widely used in intermittent bolus dosing and as a continuous infusion. Morphine may be helpful with lung disorders as it dilates the pulmonary bed. Morphine has an active metabolite that accumulates in renal failure and should be reduced by 50% in these patients. Other opiates commonly used include hydromorphone (Dilaudid) and fentanyl citrate (Sublimaze). Demerol is not recommended since it can accumulate with repeated doses, causing an increased risk of neurotoxicity,

---

TABLE 1-18 Nerve Stimulation in Relationship to Percent Blockage

Number of twitches	Percent blockage
4	0-50
3	60-70
2	70-80
1	80-90
None	>90

particularly in patients with renal failure and the elderly. Fentanyl and hydromorphone are more rapidly taken up by the CNS and therefore are more potent than morphine.

Benzodiazepines: Relieve anxiety, promote sleep, and produce sedation by specific depressant effect on gamma-(γ-) aminobutyric acid (GABA) and other nonspecific CNS depressant effects. Benzodiazepines produce muscle relaxation, which has the beneficial effect of reducing dosage requirements when NMBAs are used to induce paralysis. Dose-related effects on mental status range from relief of anxiety to sedation and coma. All benzodiazepines promote amnesia by preventing memory consolidation. This effect is particularly useful in patients undergoing unpleasant procedures. Midazolam (Versed) is reported to be superior to other benzodiazepines in preventing recall. Safety, ease of use, lack of paradoxic agitation, and lack of recall make benzodiazepines attractive choices for sedation in many critical care situations. They are the primary drugs used to alleviate symptoms of acute alcohol withdrawal. Table 1-19 describes specific characteristics of the widely used benzodiazepines.

- *Lorazepam (Ativan):* Most commonly given as an intermittent bolus but sometimes used as a continuous infusion. Lorazepam has no active metabolites; therefore, in patients with advanced age or hepatic failure, drug effects do not seem to accumulate. Lorazepam has the slowest onset and the longest duration of action. Extreme caution should be used when administering lorazepam to the elderly, severely ill, and those with limited pulmonary reserve. If pain is present, an analgesic will need to be prescribed and administered.

- *Diazepam (Valium):* Inexpensive but has a long half-life, which causes prolonged sedation. An active metabolite may result in prolonged sedative effects (up to 200 hr after a given dose). Diazepam should be avoided in patients with liver dysfunction or severe heart failure because of reduced hepatic clearance. Limited solubility in water restricts use of standard formulation to intermittent IV bolus injections. A lipid suspension form of diazepam is now available. This formulation is less irritating to veins and may be used as a continuous IV infusion.

- *Midazolam (Versed):* Short-acting and rapidly metabolized, which makes this drug particularly useful for short procedures such as bronchoscopies and endoscopies. Because of its short half-life, continuous infusions are required to maintain sedation for longer periods. Delayed drug metabolism in some critically ill patients may lead to extended sedation, particularly with sepsis or hepatic impairment. An analgesic is necessary for pain management.

- *Chlordiazepoxide (Librium):* Sometimes used to manage agitation associated with alcohol withdrawal, which commonly contributes to agitation in the critically ill. When physiologically unstable patients are admitted to critical care, it is not always possible to obtain a clear history of alcohol use. The first sign may surface 24-48 hr later, when the patient becomes agitated and restless. However, because of chlordiazepoxide's relatively long half-life and several long-lived active metabolites, it is a poor choice for sedation and delirium tremens prophylaxis, when compared with newer benzodiazepines that are safer and easier to titrate. Lorazepam (Ativan) is generally preferred because of its relatively short duration and simple metabolism.

Anesthetic agents: Although there is no absolute definition of anesthesia, there are four general components: analgesia, amnesia, absence of pathologic reflexes (e.g., vagal response to pain), and lack of purposeful movement. Once restricted to surgical settings, forms of anesthesia are increasingly employed in critical care areas. Anesthesia can be accomplished via use of a single agent or by several combinations of drugs. Many anesthetics are restricted to use by or with the direct supervi-

TABLE 1-19	Benzodiazepine Characteristics			
	Benzodiazepines	**Lorazepam (Ativan)**	**Diazepam (Valium)**	**Midazolam (Versed)**
Dosage	**Intermittent**	0.5-1 mg q1-2h	2.5-5 mg, q3-4h	0.15-0.35 mg/kg, q1-2h
	Continuous	0.25-2 mg/hr 4-35 mcg/min	N/A	0.03-0.22 mg/kg/hr 0.5-4 mcg/kg/min
Pharmacokinetics	**Metabolism**	Hepatic	Hepatic	Hepatic
	Active metabolites	One	Yes	Yes
	Excretion	Renal	Renal	Renal

sion of an anesthesiologist; however, one anesthetic, propofol (Diprivan), has been approved for sedation in mechanically ventilated patients. Propofol is often used in intensive care units (ICUs) for short-term sedation (several hours to 5 days).

- **Propofol (Diprivan):** A lipid suspension that is administered as a titratable, continuous infusion to provide a desired level of sedation to mechanically ventilated patients (Table 1-20). Patients usually awaken readily with prompt return to baseline mental function after sedation with propofol. Recovery time after prolonged infusion is not increased, in contrast to some benzodiazepines. Hemodynamic changes (e.g., vasodilation, decreased MAP) can be minimized by adequate hydration and slow increases in the infusion rate. This agent is particularly useful for patients with neurologic impairment, since the short action allows daily awakening to evaluate the underlying mental status. Propofol is not an analgesic, so pain medication should be dually prescribed and patients should be assessed for pain during daily awakening. Scheduled analgesics or continuous infusion of morphine works well for pain control in patients receiving Diprivan. It is a lipid-base emulsion and is considered a caloric supplement. This should be taken into account when patients are receiving TPN in addition to propofol. Propofol accumulates more readily in obese patients; therefore dosing should be based on ideal body weight in the obese patient.

Antipsychotics: Have been used to reduce agitation in disoriented and agitated patients. Patients should be well hydrated to avoid hypotension associated with parenteral use of these drugs.

- **Haloperidol lactate (Haldol):** A butyrophenone antipsychotic that is especially helpful in managing psychosis and during withdrawal of sedatives. Incremental bolus doses or continuous infusions are used. IV route is considered investigational but has been widely used in critically ill patients because onset of action is rapid and extrapyramidal side effects occur less frequently than with the intramuscular (IM) route. Haldol should be given cautiously to patients with severe cardiovascular disorders because of the possibility of transient hypotension and QT prolongation.

- **Chlorpromazine (Thorazine):** A phenothiazine sometimes used as a sedative, particularly if the patient also displays evidence of psychosis. Chlorpromazine produces alpha-(α-) receptor blockade, and hypotension is likely. For this reason and because it generally is less potent than haloperidol, chlorpromazine is not used frequently in critically ill patients.

Neuromuscular blocking agents: Used when longer periods of complete paralysis are necessary in mechanically ventilated patients. All possible causes of agitation (e.g., pain, fear, suctioning, hypoxemia) must be investigated thoroughly before neuromuscular blockade is initiated. Seek alternative means of management if feasible. NMBAs generally are used in the following situations: (1) to decrease oxygen consumption in patients who otherwise cannot obtain satisfactory oxygen saturation; (2) to alleviate specific medical conditions (e.g., status asthmaticus, tetanus, malignant hyperthermia, status epilepticus, acute respiratory distress syndrome [ARDS]); (3) to immobilize patients for surgical and invasive procedures; and (4) to manage increased intracranial pressure.

- **Depolarizing NMBAs:** Succinylcholine (Anectine) is the only depolarizing NMBA with widespread clinical use. It is used to produce rapid, brief paralysis, most often during emergent intubation. Long-term blockade is not practical because of rapid tachyphylaxis and desensitization of receptors to blocking effects.

- **Nondepolarizing NMBAs:** The class of NMBAs most commonly used in the critically ill patient. The most common agents used are pancuronium (Pavulon), vecuronium (Norcuron), and cisatracurium (Nimbex) (Table 1-21). Many drugs and certain physiologic states can augment or antagonize neuromuscular blockage in the critically ill patient (Table 1-22). These states should be assessed continuously throughout the course of therapy.

T A B L E 1 - 20   Propofol (Diprivan) Characteristics

*Dosage**		1-3 mg/kg/hr
		5-50 mcg/kg/min
Pharmacokinetics	**Metabolism**	Hepatic
	Metabolites	None
	Excretion	Renal
	Half-life	1.5-2hr
Cardiovascular effects		Minimal: 15% ↓BP and MAP (short lived = 15 min)
		(cause: ↓SVR and [–] inotrope)

*Propofol is a sedative-hypnotic at the above recommended dosages but is classified chemically as an anesthetic.

TABLE 1-21   Neuromuscular Blocking Agent Characteristics

	Neuromuscular blocking agents	Pancuronium (Pavulon)	Vecuronium (Norcuron)	Cisatracurium (Nimbex)
Dosage	**Intermittent**	0.04-0.1 mg/kg/q1h prn	0.01-0.015 mg/kg q15min	0.03 m/kg q15min
	Continuous	1-1.6 mcg/kg/min	0.8-1.2 mcg/kg/min	0.5-10 mcg/kg/min
Pharmacokinetics	**Metabolism** **Excretion**	Renal > Hepatic Renal	Hepatic > Renal Renal Renal (15%) Biliary (30%-50%)	Hoffman (organ independent) Elimination
	Metabolites (active or toxic)	Yes	Yes	No
	Half-life (elimination)	132-257 min (2-4 hr)	80-97 min	22-29 min
Cardiovascular effects		Moderate ↑HR, ↓BP, ↑CO	Minimal <1% ↑HR, ↓BP	None on HR and MAP

Important comments:
1. Pancuronium is by far the most cost-effective paralytic agent, followed by vecuronium.
2. Norcuron is 24× as expensive as Pavulon. Nimbex is 53× as expensive as Pavulon.
3. Nimbex is preferred in patients with hepatic or renal dysfunction.

TABLE 1-22   Drugs and Physiologic Conditions That Affect NMBAs

Drugs that augment neuromuscular blockade

Aminoglycoside antibiotics	Lidocaine
Bretylium	Procainamide
Calcium channel blockers	Propranolol
Clindamycin	Quinidine
Cyclosporine	Vancomycin

Drugs that antagonize neuromuscular blockade

Anticholinesterase agents	Phenytoin
Azathioprine	Ranitidine
Carbamazepine	Theophylline
Corticosteroids	

Physiologic conditions that increase neuromuscular blockade

Acidosis	Hypokalemia
Dehydration	Hyponatremia
Hypercalcemia	Hypothermia
Hypermagnesemia	Myasthenia gravis
Hypocalcemia	

Physiologic conditions that decrease neuromuscular blockade

Alkalosis	Hypernatremia
Hyperkalemia	Decreased peripheral perfusion

Clinicians should determine a therapeutic endpoint or goal for paralysis and titrate neuromuscular blockade to achieve that goal. Examples of such therapeutic endpoints are decreases in peak inspiratory pressure, decreases in oxygen consumption, and inability to move. Monitoring the degree of neuromuscular blockade is essential. This can be done by using a peripheral nerve stimulator (see "Assessment," p. 33). Another commonly used method is providing a "drug holiday," to enable return of neuromuscular function to assess muscle strength. NMBAs provide no analgesia or anxiolysis. All patients receiving NMBAs must also have therapy with continuously dosed opiates and anxiolytics.

NURSING DIAGNOSES AND INTERVENTIONS

Anxiety related to actual or perceived threat of death; change in health status; threat to self-concept or role; unfamiliar people or environment; the unknown

Desired outcome: Within 4-6 hr of initiating therapy, patient's anxiety is diminished as evidenced by verbalization of same; HR $\leq$100 beats/min; RR $\leq$20 breaths/min; and decrease in restlessness and extraneous motor movement.

- Carefully assess for and correct factors contributing to anxiety (see Table 1-17).
- Evaluate adequacy of pain control. Administer opiate or other analgesics in appropriate doses on a schedule or through a continuous infusion.
- Initiate non-pharmacologic measures to reduce anxiety (see Table 1-35).
- Administer short-acting benzodiazepine in small doses at frequent intervals. Monitor carefully for excessive sedation and respiratory depression. Have flumazenil (Romazicon) immediately available for reversal of drug effects.
- If anxiety is profound and associated with sensory/perceptual alterations (e.g., hallucinations), consider use of antipsychotic agent. Ensure adequate hydration before use, and monitor closely for hypotension.

Impaired gas exchange (or risk for same) related to decreased oxygen supply secondary to decreased ventilatory drive occurring with sedative use and CNS depression or secondary to decreased chest wall movement occurring with residual neuromuscular blockade

Desired outcome: Within 1 hr of intervention, patient has adequate gas exchange as evidenced by orientation to time, place, and person; Pao_2 $\geq$80 mm Hg; $Paco_2$ 24-30 mm Hg; Spo_2 $\geq$90; and RR 12-20 breaths/min with normal depth and pattern (eupnea).

- Assess patient's respiratory rate, depth, and rhythm at least hourly when heavily sedated. Fully sedated patients require continuous direct monitoring until VS are stable and protective reflexes (e.g., gag reflexes) are present.
- If NMBAs are used, assess depth of paralysis using peripheral nerve stimulator. Titrate dose to maintain desired level of paralysis (see Table 1-18).
- Continuously monitor Spo_2 via pulse oximetry. Alternatively, monitor chest wall movement via apnea monitor. Have appropriate antidote (e.g., naloxone for opiates, flumazenil for benzodiazepines, and pyridostigmine and atropine for NMBAs) and airway management equipment immediately available.
- Position patient to promote full lung expansion, and turn patient to mobilize sputum. Encourage deep breathing at frequent intervals.

Knowledge deficit: lack of recall, related to interrupted memory consolidation secondary to benzodiazepine use

---

Research Brief 1-4   Intensive care units are beginning to use bayesian programs to help determine appropriate levels of sedation in critically ill patients. A study was performed to determine the effectiveness of a bayesian program (PKS system, Abbott) in predicting Versed concentrations and pharmacokinetic parameters in critical care patients. Versed infusions were administered to 42 patients for 2 hr or for several days. The bayesian program was used to predict plasma Versed levels after feedback of 1, 2, or 3 concentrations. There was a high correlation between observed and estimated concentrations. In fact, from 2 or 3 feedback concentrations, Versed pharmacokinetic parameters estimated by PKS were statistically comparable to rich pharmacokinetic parameters. This software appears to be quite helpful to clinicians for dosage adjustment for Versed based on Versed concentrations and clinical sedation.

From Bolon M et al.: Evaluation of the estimation of midazolam concentrations and pharmacokinetic parameters in intensive care patients using a bayesian pharmacokinetic software (PKS) according to a sparse sampling approach, *J Pharm Pharmacol* 55(6):765-771, 2003.

Desired outcome: Within 12 hr of cessation of benzodiazepine therapy, patient recalls information essential to self-protection and self-care.

- Remind patient and family that recall of unpleasant procedures (e.g., cardioversion, endoscopy) will be diminished and that this is a desired effect of the medication.
- Reinforce necessary information (e.g., NPO instructions, need to call for assistance when changing positions, need for deep breathing) with patient and family at frequent intervals until comprehension is demonstrated.
- Review outcome or findings of procedure with patient as necessary until patient expresses satisfactory understanding.

Alterations in Consciousness

Consciousness is a state of awareness of the self and environment composed of three aspects: arousal (ability to awaken), ability to perceive internal and external stimuli, and the ability to perform goal-directed behavior. Alterations in these aspects of consciousness result in a broad spectrum of syndromes including coma, delirium, and agitation. Factors precipitating various alterations in consciousness are listed in Table 1-23. Impaired consciousness results in complications in hospitalized patients, is associated with safety issues and often causes longer hospital stays with higher morbidity and mortality.

T A B L E   1 - 23   Factors Precipitating Alterations in Consciousness

Delirium
　Age
　Aggressive and dominant personality
　Anesthesia time
　Cardiac dysrhythmia
　Body temperature
　Cerebral disorders
　Fluid and electrolyte imbalances
　Drugs
　Metabolic disturbances
　Pulmonary disorders
　Sleep deprivation
　Toxins
　Electrolyte imbalances
　End-stage disease (renal, liver)
　Pulmonary disorders
　Impaired communication
　Withdrawal syndromes
　Neuropsychiatric disorders

Stupor
　Diffuse organic cerebral dysfunction
　Confused with the catatonic behavior of schizophrenia or severe depressive reaction

Coma
　Central nervous system dysfunction
　　Cerebral structural changes (brain injury)
　　Cerebrovascular impairment (hemorrhage, ischemia, or edema)
　Metabolic conditions

Vegetative state (coma vigil)
　Coma related to cerebral or metabolic disorders

Locked-in syndrome
　Supranuclear motor deefferentation related to brainstem injury

---

ASSESSMENT
History and risk factors:
- *Age:* Elders more prone to alterations in consciousness especially with changes in environment or for those who have sundowner's syndrome.
- *Brain injury:* Lesions of the cortex, subcortex, and brainstem caused by global or focal ischemia, stroke, or traumatic brain injury.
- *Cerebral disorders:* Deteriorating brain condition, such as an expanding lesion.
- *Cardiovascular status:* Disorders that lower cardiac output, procedures that cause postcardiotomy delirium, intraaortic balloon pump sequelae, states of lowered perfusion (lowered MAP), and dysrhythmias.
- *Pulmonary disorders:* Those causing hypoxia and hypoxemia.
- *Drug therapy:* Sedation, analgesia, drug toxicity, drug interactions, and drug sensitivity.
- *Surgical factors:* Nature and extent of surgery and anesthesia time.
- *Perceptual/sensory factors:* Sleep deprivation, sensory overload, sensory deprivation, impaired sensation (hypesthesia, decreased hearing or vision), impaired perception (inability to identify environmental stimuli), and impaired integration (inability to integrate environmental stimuli).
- *Metabolic factors:* Changes in glucose level, hypermetabolism, hypometabolism, and endocrine crises.
- *Fluid and electrolyte disturbances:* Sodium and potassium imbalances, hypovolemia.

Clinical presentation:
- *Delirium/acute confusional state:* A state of disordered attention which reflects an underlying acute or subacute process. Usually a transient condition (may be prolonged) that develops along a continuum including of clouding of consciousness, attention deficit, global cognitive impairment, and psychosis. Symptoms include disorientation to time, place, and person; disorganized thinking; fear; irritability; misinterpretation of sensory stimuli (e.g., pulling at tubes and dressings); appears distracted; altered psychomotor activity; altered sleep-wake cycles; memory impairment; hallucinations; inappropriate communication (e.g., yelling, swearing, nonsensical speech); and dreamlike delusions. Lucid intervals alternate with episodes of delirium. Patients may have difficulty following commands. Daytime drowsiness is contrasted with nighttime agitation. Clinical variants of delirium include the quiet form, hyperactive-hyperalert form, hypoactive-hypoalert form, and a combination form that includes lethargy and agitation (Figure 1-1).

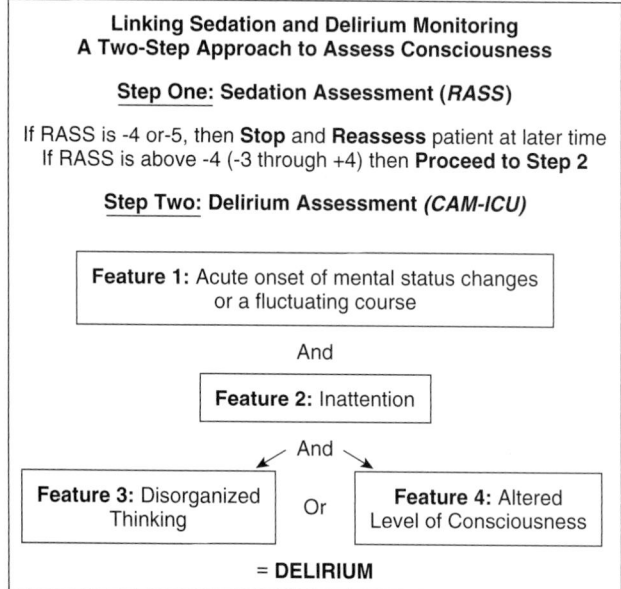

Figure 1-1:   Linking sedation and delirium monitoring: a two-step approach to assess consciousness. Copyright E. Wesley Ely, MD, MPH, and Vanderbilt University, 2002.

- *Stupor:* A deep sleep with responsiveness only to vigorous and repeated stimuli with return to unresponsiveness when the stimulus is removed. Stupor usually is related to diffuse organic cerebral dysfunction but may be confused with the catatonic behavior of schizophrenia or the behavior associated with a severe depressive reaction.
- *Coma:* An alteration in arousal and diminished awareness of self and environment. No understandable response to external stimuli or inner need is elicited. No language is spoken. There are no covert or overt attempts at communication nor eye opening. Spontaneous purposeful movement and/or localizing movements are absent. Motor responses to noxious stimuli are reflexive and do not result in recognizable defensive movements. Sleep-wake cycles are absent on the electroencephalogram (EEG). The extent of coma is difficult to quantify because limits of consciousness are difficult to define. Self-awareness can only be inferred from appearance and actions. Coma occurs when normal CNS function is disrupted by alteration in the cerebral structure (brain injury), cerebrovascular impairment (hemorrhage, ischemia, or edema), or metabolic conditions (hepatic encephalopathy). If coma persists for longer than 4 weeks, it is defined as transitioning to a vegetative state.
- *Minimally conscious state (MCS):* Describes patients who demonstrate inconsistent but reproducible behavior indicating awareness of self and environment. Generally they cannot reliably follow commands or communicate but show visual fixation and tracking, and have emotional and/or behavioral responses to external stimuli. Once the patient consistently follows commands, can reliably communicate, and uses objects in a functional way, the minimal conscious state ends. Although the etiology is uncertain, MCS seems to be related to diffuse, bilateral, subcortical, and hemispheric damage.
- *Akinetic mutism (AM):* A subcategory of MCS in which a decrease in spontaneity and initiation of actions, thoughts, speech, or emotion is present. Sensory motor function is normal. Visual tracking and eye movements are intact, and there is occasional speech and movement to commands. However, internally guided behavior is absent because cortical activation is inadequate. AM is associated with orbito-mesial frontal cortex, limbic system, and reticular formation lesions.
- *Vegetative state (VS):* Vegetative state is a subacute or chronic condition that may follow the coma of brain injury or occur independently of coma (e.g., dementia). Transition from coma to VS occurs if coma persists for longer than 4 weeks. Onset of VS is signaled by a return of wakefulness (eyes are open and sleep patterns may be observed) with return of spontaneous control of autonomic function but without observable signs of cognitive function. The patient cannot follow commands, offers no comprehensible sounds, and displays no localization to stimuli. There is complete loss of meaningful interaction with the environment. The vegetative state may exist for many years because the autonomic and vegetative functions necessary for life have been preserved.
- *Locked-in syndrome (LIS):* Characterized by paralysis of all four extremities and the lower cranial nerves but with preservation of cognition. Associated with deefferentation (disruption of the pathways of the brainstem motor neurons), this condition prevents the patient from communicating with a full range of language and body movement. Generally, consciousness, vertical eye movement, and eyelid blinking are intact and provide a mechanism for communication. LIS is classified by the degree of voluntary speech and motor function preservation. In complete LIS there is total immobility and anarthria (inability to speak). In incomplete LIS there is vertical eye movement and blinking function. LIS can be distinguished from a vegetative state because patients give appropriate signs of being aware of themselves and their environment. Often, sleep patterns are disrupted.

Physical assessment: Requires a thorough evaluation of mental/emotional status, cranial nerve function, motor function, sensory function, and reflex activity. Baseline neurologic findings elicited from each component of the examination must be documented. When alterations in consciousness are manifested, the mental/emotional component of the examination is of particular importance. In patients who are unconscious or demonstrate low-level function, assessment techniques are used that do not require patient participation, such as coma and cognitive functioning scales. The purpose of assessment is to determine the extent of wakefulness and cognition through observed responses, such as eye opening, movement of the head and body, verbalization, and ability to follow commands. These observations alone will not fully discriminate the subtle differences in altered states of arousal. Assessment should be accompanied by an in-depth history focusing on the possible etiology of the change in cognition. Extensive cognitive testing including attention, concentration, memory, and learning assessments is performed when the patient is arousable and aware.

- *Mental status testing:* A subjective assessment requiring patient cooperation for best results (Table 1-24).

T A B L E 1 - 24   Mental Status Component of the Neurologic Examination

1. General appearance
2. Behavior (with and without stimulation)
3. Language and speech characteristics (organization, coherence, and relevance)
4. Mood and affect
5. Judgment
6. Abstract thinking
7. Orientation (time, place, person)
8. Attention and concentration
9. Memory (recent, remote)
10. Cognition (following commands, fund of knowledge, interpretation of information, problem solving)

T A B L E 1 - 25   Mini Mental Status Examination

1. What is the year, season, date, day, month (5 points)
2. Where are we: state, county, town, hospital, room (5 points)
3. Name three objects (3)
4. Count backward by sevens (e.g., 100, 93, 86, 79, 72) (5 points)
5. Repeat same three objects from number 3 above (3 points)
6. Name a pencil and watch (2 points)
7. Follow a three-step command (3 points)
8. Write a sentence (1 point)
9. Follow the command "close your eyes" (1 point)
10. Copy a design (e.g., two hexagons) (1 point)

- *Mini-mental status examination:* Objective neuropsychologic tool used to measure orientation, recall, attention, calculation, and language. Scores less than 23 (total 25) indicate cognitive dysfunction. Patient participation is necessary for this examination (Table 1-25).
- *Glasgow Coma Scale:* Quantitative, three-part scale that assesses the patient's ability to open his or her eyes, to move, and to speak/communicate. Scores range from 3 to 15, with 3 being unresponsive to all stimuli and 15 being awake, alert, and oriented. Patients who are unable to cooperate can be evaluated using this scale. See Appendix 3.
- *Coma recovery scale:* Quantitative 35-item scale used to assess brain function at four levels (generalized, localized, emergent, cognitively mediated). Seven responses are evaluated: arousal and attention, auditory perception, visual perception, motor function, oromotor ability, communication, and initiative. Patients who are unable to cooperate can be evaluated using this scale.
- *Confusion assessment method:* A four-part scale used to evaluate confusion. Onset and course, inattention, disorganized thinking, and level of consciousness are assessed.
- *Rancho Los Amigos (RLA) cognitive functioning scale:* An eight-level scale that describes levels of cognitive functioning. Levels range from unresponsive to sensory stimuli to purposeful/appropriate actions. Patients who cannot cooperate can be evaluated using this scale. See Table 1-26.

DIAGNOSTIC TESTS

Neurodiagnostic testing: See "Traumatic Brain Injury," p. 98.

Neuropsychologic testing: Although not a routine part of critical care, neuropsychologic testing should be planned and implemented for patients with brain injury or altered consciousness when they enter the recovery phase. This testing provides a comprehensive baseline for rehabilitation by evaluating higher cortical functions, such as memory, learning, and language.

T A B L E 1 - 26   Cognitive Rehabilitation Goals

Level	Response	Goal/intervention
I II III	None Generalized Localized	*Goal:* Provide sensory input to elicit responses of increased quality, frequency, duration, and variety. *Intervention:* Give brief but frequent stimulation sessions, and present stimuli in an organized manner, focusing on one sensory channel at a time; for example: *Visual:* Intermittent television, family pictures, bright objects *Auditory:* Tape recordings of family or favorite song, talking to patient, intermittent TV or radio *Olfactory:* Favorite perfume, shaving lotion, coffee, lemon, orange *Cutaneous:* Touch or rub skin with different textures such as velvet, ice bag, warm cloth *Movement:* Turn, ROM exercises, up in chair *Oral:* Oral care, lemon swabs, ice, sugar on tongue, peppermint, chocolate
IV	Confused, agitated	*Goal:* Decrease agitation, and increase awareness of environment. This stage usually lasts 2-4 wk. *Intervention:* Remove offending devices (e.g., NG tube, restraints), if possible. Do not demand patient follow-through with task. Provide human contact unless this increases agitation. Provide a quiet, controlled environment. Use a calm, soft voice and manner around patient.
V VI	Confused, inappropriate Confused, appropriate	*Goal:* Decrease confusion and incorporate improved cognitive abilities into functional activity. *Intervention:* Begin each interaction with introduction, orientation, and interaction purpose. List and number daily activity in the sequence in which it will be done throughout the day. Maintain a consistent environment. Provide memory aids (e.g., calendar, clock). Use gentle repetition, which aids learning. Provide supervision and structure. Reorient as needed.
VII	Automatic, appropriate	*Goal:* Integrate increased cognitive function into functional community activities with minimal structuring. *Intervention:* Enable practicing of activities. Reduce supervision and environmental structure. Help patient plan adaptation of ADLs and home living skills to home environment.

Modified from Rancho Los Amigos Hospital, Inc, Levels of Cognitive Functioning (scale based on behavioral descriptions or responses to stimuli). From Swift CM: Neurologic disorders. In Swearingen PL, editor: *Manual of medical-surgical nursing care,* ed 4, St Louis, 1999, Mosby.
ADLs, Activities of daily living; *NG,* nasogastric; *ROM,* range of motion.

COLLABORATIVE MANAGEMENT

For delirium:
• Determine and correct physiologic imbalances and drug interactions.
• Correct sensory/perceptual deficits (e.g., provide hearing aid, eyeglasses).
• Reorient patient to the self and environment.
• Perform neuropsychologic testing.
• Implement appropriate medications to help control behavior.
• See "Sedating and Paralytic Agents," p. 32).

For coma:
• Assess cognitive function using the RLA score or coma recovery scale.
• Initiate a sensory stimulation program for patients with low level cognition.
• Minimize stimulation for confused or agitated patients.
• Consult with rehabilitation services including physical, occupational, and speech therapy.
• Plan care to prevent or minimize problems related to the injury (e.g., spasticity, swallowing disorders) and complications of immobility (e.g., disuse syndrome, contractures, pressure ulcers).

For locked-in syndrome:
• Establish a communication system/pattern.
• Consult a mental health professional to assess the psychologic impact of this syndrome.
• Consult with rehabilitation (see preceding section on Coma).
• Provide a normal day/night routine to help minimize sleep-wake cycle disturbances.

For vegetative state:
• Perform neurodiagnostic and neuropsychologic testing to confirm the diagnosis.
• Provide essential supportive care to minimize complications such as pressure ulcers and aspiration.
• Initiate a sensory stimulation program for low-level cognitive function, including visual, auditory, tactile, gustatory and vestibular stimuli (see Box below).

SENSORY STIMULATION (SS) PROGRAMS AS AN INTERVENTION TECHNIQUE IN THE CRITICALLY ILL

STRONG EVIDENCE	INSUFFICIENT EVIDENCE	RECOMMENDATIONS
SS programs appear to be safe to administer.	There is still no clear evidence that increased arousal is brain injury recovery or SS program enhanced recovery.	SS programs can be initiated as an adjustment therapy.
SS programs do not increase ICP or CPP and do not affect HR or BP.	It is unclear how the time when SS was started (early or late) influences outcome.	SS program can be incorporated into daily nursing routine.
A positive trajectory of recovery has been documented in all studies.	It is unclear how the type of program (multimodal or unimodal) influences outcome.	Use rest periods between sessions to diminish fatigue.
	It is unclear what type of stimulation is most useful for increasing arousal (e.g., novel, familiar music, voices).	Stop intervention if an unstable medical status develops, and resume when patient is stable.
	It is unclear how long daily stimulation should last (concentrated or multiple short sessions).	Include family in intervention program.

From Kater K: Response of head-injured patients to sensory stimulation, *West J Nurs Res* 11(1):20-33, 1989; Lewinn E, Dimancescu M: Environmental deprivation and enrichment in coma, *Lancet* 2:156-157, 1978; Mackay L et al: Early intervention in severe head injury: long-term benefits of a formalized program, *Arch Phys Med Rehabil* 73:635-641, 1992; Mitchell S et al: Coma arousal procedure: a therapeutic intervention in the treatment of head injury, *Brain Inj* 4:273-279, 1990; Schinner K et al: Effects of auditory stimuli on intracranial pressure and cerebral perfusion pressure in traumatic brain injury, *J Neurosci Nurs* 27(6):336-341, 1994; Wilson S et al: Vegetative state and response to sensory stimulation: an analysis of 24 cases, *Brain Inj* 10(11):807-818, 1996.
BP, blood pressure; CPP, cerebral perfusion pressure; HR, heart rate; ICP, intracranial pressure.

NURSING DIAGNOSES AND INTERVENTIONS

Sensory/perceptual alterations related to physiologic changes; psychologic changes; environmental changes; sensory deprivation; sensory overload; drug interactions

Desired outcomes: If cause of alteration in consciousness is an extracerebral event, within 72 hr of this diagnosis, patient's level of arousal and cognition improve and patient responds consistently and appropriately to stimuli. If cause is cerebral, increased arousal and improvements in cognition may take days to weeks.

NIC Cognitive Ability: Ability To Execute Complex Mental Processes; Cognitive Orientation: Ability to Identify Person, Place, and Time; Information Processing: Ability to Acquire, Organize, and Use Information

- Eliminate environmental causes of sensory/perceptual deficit.
  - ❑ Assess patient for potential causes of sensory/perceptual deficits. For the hearing- or vision-impaired patient, wearing eyeglasses or hearing aids will decrease misinterpretation of visual and auditory stimuli.
  - ❑ Assess environment for potential causes of disorientation and confusion. Maintain day/night environment as much as possible. Keep clocks and calendars within patient's field of vision.
- Develop a plan of care consistent with sensory/perceptual deficit.
- Assess patient for sensory deprivation and sensory overload. Decrease or increase stimulation based on RLA assessment (see Box, p. 43) and patient's needs. For example, agitated and confused individuals require structure and reorientation interventions, whereas those who are comatose or stuporous require stimulation techniques.
  - ❑ Orient patient to time, place, and person during all interactions. Explain procedures in terms patient can understand.
  - ❑ Teach significant others reorientation and sensory stimulation strategies, and provide liberal visitation to facilitate their assistance.
  - ❑ Assess underlying cause of confusion or delirium before using sedation, anxiolytic, analgesic, or antipsychotic drug therapy (see "Sedating and Paralytic Agents," p. 32). Also see "Psychosocial Support," p. 68, for this nursing diagnosis.

NIC Cognitive Restructuring; Cognitive Stimulation; Environmental Management; Reality Orientation; Dementia Management; Electrolyte Management; Delirium Management

Impaired verbal communication related to neurologic deficits

Desired outcome: If cause of alteration in consciousness is an extracerebral event, within 72 hr of this diagnosis, patient communicates needs and feelings and exhibits decreased frustration and fear related to communication barriers. If cause is cerebral, improvement in communication may take days to weeks.

NIC Communication ability: Ability to receive, interpret, and express spoken, written, and nonverbal messages

- Determine underlying cause of impaired communication, including physiologic (cortical, brainstem, or cranial nerve injury) or psychologic (depression, fear, or anger).
- When communicating with these patients, use their name, face them, use eye contact if they are awake, speak clearly, and use a normal tone of voice.
- Be alert to nonverbal messages, especially eye movement, blinking, facial expressions, and head and hand movements. Attempt to validate these signals with the patient.
- Assure patient that you are attempting to find methods that promote communication if patient's needs cannot always be understood.
- For the patient who does not respond to or acknowledge verbal stimulation, continue communication attempts.
- Teach significant others methods of communication, and encourage them to continue attempts at communication.
- Brainstem-evoked potentials and audiometry (hearing test) can provide useful information related to a patient's ability to receive and process auditory stimuli. Detection and treatment of otitis media in patients who have ET tubes will improve hearing.
- Obtain a speech therapy consultation to assess nature and severity of communication impairment and assist in developing a communication plan. Special attention is required for individuals with locked-in syndrome.
- Obtain a mental health consultation to assist with patient who is angry, frustrated, and fearful because of the communication impairment.

NIC Communication Enhancement: Speech Deficit; Support System Enhancement

Impaired physical mobility related to perceptual or cognitive impairment; imposed restrictions of movement

Desired outcome: By the time of discharge from the critical care unit, patient demonstrates range of motion (ROM) and muscle strength within 10% of baseline parameters.

- Assess muscle strength and tone to determine type of interventions required. Consult physical therapy and occupational therapy for evaluation and treatment plan.
- Manage decreased muscle tone (flaccidity):
  ❑ Maintain body alignment and positioning.
  ❑ Perform passive ROM and stretching exercises.
  ❑ Avoid prolonged periods of limb flexion.
  ❑ Apply splints and other adaptive devices to maintain functional position of the extremities.
  ❑ Turn patient q2h.
  ❑ Consider chair sitting as the patient stabilizes.
- Manage increased muscle tone (spasticity):
  ❑ Avoid supine position; use side-lying, semiprone, prone, and high Fowler's positions.
  ❑ Position limbs opposite flexion posture.
  ❑ Use skeletal muscle relaxant, such as baclofen (Lioresal), as prescribed for decreasing tone.
- Monitor calcium and alkaline phosphatase levels. Increased levels can lead to the development of heterogenous ossification, which often is seen with states of impaired mobility, such as spinal cord injury. See "Fluid and Electrolyte Disturbances," p. 538.
- Maintain patient's skin integrity. See "Wound and Skin Care" in the following section.
- Prevent pulmonary complications in the following ways:
  ❑ Encourage coughing and deep breathing if patient is able, or suction as needed.
  ❑ Assess swallowing ability before initiating oral feedings. Obtain dysphagia consultation (usually from a speech therapist) if swallowing reflexes are impaired.
  ❑ Initiate enteral feeding protocol for patients with feeding tubes to prevent aspiration. See "Nutritional Support," p. 1.

NIC Bed Rest Care; Positioning; Exercise Promotion; Self-Care Assistance

ADDITIONAL NURSING DIAGNOSES

Also see nursing diagnoses and interventions under "Nutritional Support," p. 1; "Sedating and Paralytic Agents," p. 32; "Prolonged Immobility," p 61; and **Risk for disuse syndrome,** in "Traumatic Brain Injury," p. 109.

Wound and Skin Care

A wound is a disruption of tissue integrity caused by trauma, surgery, or an underlying medical disorder. Wound management is designed to promote healing, prevent infection and/or reduce deterioration in wound status.

WOUNDS CLOSED BY PRIMARY INTENTION

Clean surgical or traumatic wounds whose edges are closed with sutures, clips, sterile tape strips, or wound glue are referred to as wounds closed by *primary intention*. Impairment of healing most frequently manifests as dehiscence, evisceration, infection, or delayed healing. Individuals at high risk for disruption of wound healing include those who are obese, diabetic, elderly, malnourished, receiving steroids, immunosuppressed, undergoing chemotherapy or radiation therapy, or receiving vasopressors. Coexistent infections at another body site and colonization with microorganisms such as methicillin-resistant *Staphylococcus aureus* (MRSA) are factors that may contribute to the development of infection.

ASSESSMENT

Optimal healing: Immediately after injury, the incision line is warm, reddened, indurated, and tender. Inflammation normally subsides in 3 to 5 days. A healing ridge, a palpable accumulation of scar tissue, forms by day 7 to 9 after injury. In patients who undergo cosmetic surgery, a healing ridge is purposely avoided to minimize scar formation (Table 1-27).

Impaired healing: Lack of an adequate inflammatory response; continued drainage from the incision line 2 days after injury (when no drain is present); absence of a healing ridge by day 9 after injury; presence of purulent drainage. See Table 1-27.

DIAGNOSTIC TESTS

Complete blood count (CBC) with white blood cell (WBC) differential: To assess for anemia and presence of infection. Low hemoglobin (Hb) indicates anemia and decreased ability to carry oxygen to the tissues. For optimal healing, the Hb should be within a normal range. Increased WBC count signals infection. The production of more immature WBCs (shift to the left) occurs with infection but will be less pronounced if patient is immunosuppressed.

Gram stain of wound fluid or tissue: If infection is suspected, to identify the presence of pathogenic organism, and aid in initial antimicrobial therapy.

Culture and sensitivity: To determine optimal antibiotic. Infection is said to be present when 10^5 organisms per gram of tissue are present, or fever and drainage are present.

COLLABORATIVE MANAGEMENT

Application of a sterile dressing in surgery or at the time of injury: To protect wound from external contamination or trauma or provide pressure. Usually, surgeon or advanced practice nurse changes the initial dressing.

Nutrition (oral diet, enteral nutrition, parenteral nutrition): To provide sufficient nutrients for wound healing.

Multivitamins (all but especially C) and minerals (especially zinc and iron): To correct any deficits and support healing.

Pain control: To maximize subcutaneous blood flow to the wound to support healing.

Insulin: As needed to control glucose levels in individuals with diabetes mellitus (DM) or hyperglycemia from other causes (e.g., steroid therapy, TPN, enteral nutrition). Hyperglycemia may delay healing. Critically ill patients often develop insulin resistance, resulting in hyperglycemia.

Local or systemic antibiotics: Given when infection is present and sometimes used prophylactically.

Incision and drainage: To drain pus when infection is present and localized. Healing occurs by secondary intention. The wound may be irrigated to flush out organisms.

NURSING DIAGNOSES AND INTERVENTIONS

Impaired tissue integrity: Wound, related to altered circulation; metabolic disorders (e.g., DM); alterations in fluid volume and nutrition; medical therapy (chemotherapy, radiation therapy, steroid administration)

Desired outcome: Patient exhibits the following signs of wound healing: well-approximated wound edges; good initial postinjury inflammatory response (erythema, warmth, induration, pain); no inflammatory response after the fifth day after injury; no drainage (without drain present) 48 hr after closure; healing ridge present by postoperative day 7 to 9. Tissue integrity is restored.

- Assess wound for indications of impaired healing, including absence of a healing ridge, presence of drainage or purulent exudate, and delayed or prolonged inflammatory response. Monitor VS and lab work for signs of infection, including elevated temperature, HR, and WBC. Document findings.

TABLE 1-27   Assessment of Healing of Wounds Closed by Primary Intention

Expected findings	Abnormal findings
Edges well approximated	Edges not well approximated
Good inflammatory response (redness, warmth, induration, pain) lasting 3-5 days	Decreased inflammatory response or inflammatory response that lasts more than 5 days after injury
No drainage (without drain present) 2 days after closure	Drainage continues more than 2 days after injury
Healing ridge present by postinjury day 7-9	No healing ridge present by day 9
	Hypertrophic scar or keloid present

- Use standard (universal) precautions and follow proper infection-control techniques when changing dressings. If a drain is present, keep it sterile, maintain patency, and handle it gently to prevent it from becoming dislodged. If wound care will be necessary after hospital discharge, teach the dressing change procedure to the patient and significant others.
- For persons with hyperglycemia, perform serial monitoring of blood glucose and administer insulin to keep glucose level in a normal range.
- Explain to patient that deep breathing promotes oxygenation, which enhances wound healing. Stress the importance of position changes and activity as tolerated to promote ventilation. Splint incision as needed.
- Monitor volume status by checking BP, HR, and capillary refill time in the tissue adjacent to incision, moisture of mucous membranes, skin turgor, and I&O.
- For nonrestricted patients, ensure a fluid intake of at least 2-3 L/day.
- To provide nutrients for healing, provide a diet with adequate protein, calories, vitamins and minerals. Encourage between-meal supplements and give frequent small feedings as needed.

SURGICAL OR TRAUMATIC WOUNDS HEALING BY SECONDARY INTENTION

Wounds healing by *secondary intention* are those with tissue loss or heavy contamination that form granulation tissue and contract in order to heal. Most often, impairment of healing is caused by increased contamination and impairment of perfusion, oxygenation, and nutrition, which results in a delay in the healing process. Individuals at risk for impaired healing include those who are obese, diabetic, malnourished, elderly, receiving steroids, immunosuppressed, undergoing radiation therapy or chemotherapy, or receiving vasopressors.

ASSESSMENT

Optimal healing: Initially the wound edges are inflamed, indurated, and tender. Pale granulation tissue on the floor and walls progresses to a deeper pink and then to a beefy red; it should be moist. Epithelial cells from the tissue surrounding the wound gradually migrate across the granulation tissue. As healing occurs, the wound edges become pink and wound contraction occurs. When present, a tract or sinus gradually decreases in size as healing occurs. The time frame for healing depends on the size and location of the wound, as well as on the patient's physical and psychologic status (Table 1-28).

Impaired healing: Exudate, slough, and necrotic material appear on the floor and walls of the wound and do not abate as healing progresses. Note their distribution, color, odor, volume, and adherence. The periwound skin is assessed for signs of tissue damage, including disruption, discoloration, and increasing pain. When a drain is in place, the volume, color, and odor of the drainage are evaluated. See Table 1-28.

DIAGNOSTIC TESTS

CBC with WBC differential; Gram stain, tissue biopsy or culture and sensitivity of drainage: See discussion, "Wound Closed by Primary Intention," p. 45.

T A B L E 1 - 28   Assessment of Healing of Wounds Closing by Secondary Intention

Expected findings	Abnormal findings
Granulation tissue initially pale and moist and then becomes pink and beefy red over time	Granulation tissue remains pale or is excessively dry or moist
No odor	Abnormal odor
No slough or necrotic tissue	Slough or necrotic tissue
No tunneling or undermining	Tunneling or undermining
	Pain
	Wound breakdown

COLLABORATIVE MANAGEMENT

Débride slough and necrotic tissue: To remove dead tissue. Use surgical or sharp débridement for rapid removal and enzymatic (e.g., Accuzyme) or autolytic (e.g., hydrocolloid dressing) for slower removal.

Dressings: To keep healthy wound tissue moist, provide antiseptic agent to decrease wound surface bacterial counts, or débride the wound (Table 1-29).

Warming dressing: To assist with controlling the ambient environment around the wound to enhance closure.

Wound cleansing: To remove waste products and dislodge and remove bacteria, necrotic tissue, foreign bodies, and exudate.

Fluids (oral/IV): To ensure adequate intravascular volume to support healing.

Topical or systemic vitamin A: As needed to reverse adverse effects of steroids on healing. Use is limited to 7 to 10 days.

Drain(s): To remove excess tissue fluid or purulent drainage.

Vacuum-assisted closure: To draw the edges of the wound together, reduce edema, increase blood flow, and stimulate granulation tissue formation.

Skin graft/cultured keratinocytes/cultured skin substitute: To provide coverage of wound if necessary.

TABLE 1-29   Dressings Used for Wound Care

Dressing	Advantages	Disadvantages
Transparent dressing (e.g., Op-Site, Tegaderm, Bioclusive)	Transparent so can view wound; prevents loss of wound fluid; protects from external contamination; protects from friction and shear.	Nonabsorptive, may result in maceration of periwound tissue.
Hydrocolloid (e.g., Duoderm, Restore, Cutinova)	Maintains moist wound surface while minimizing pooling; facilitates autolytic débridement; easy to apply, reduces pain.	Cannot be used with heavily draining wounds; opaque; exudates present on removal may be confused with infection; some roll.
Hydrogel (e.g., Curasol, Nu-gel, Vigilon)	Nonadherent; rehydrates wound; minimizes pain; can be used with infected wounds.	Cannot be used with heavily draining wounds; may macerate periwound skin.
Foam (e.g., Allevyn, Hydrosorb, Lyofoam)	Absorptive; nontraumatic; easy to apply and remove.	Not intended for dry wounds; may require tape or secondary dressing to secure.
Alginates (e.g., Kaltostat, Sorbsan)	Highly absorbent; can use on infected wounds; remove without trauma to wound.	Cannot be used for dry wounds; requires secondary dressing; may have foul odor when removed.
Gauze (e.g., 2 x 2, 4 x 4, roller gauze)	Inexpensive; easy to use; ideal for packing wound.	May result in tissue maceration if inserted too moist; may result in tissue disruption if allowed to dry out.
Composites (e.g., Alldress, Telfa Plus)	Use for partial to full-thickness wounds.	Adhesive borders may disrupt surrounding skin.

Tissue flap: To fill tissue defect and provide wound closure with its own blood supply.
Growth factors: Naturally occurring proteins that stimulate new cell formation (e.g., platelet-derived growth factor, insulin).
Hyperbaric oxygen: Used with difficult wounds to support oxidative processes in healing.
Regular diet, multivitamins and minerals, insulin, pain control, supplemental oxygen, antibiotics, and incision and drainage: See discussion, "Wounds Closed by Primary Intention," p. 45.

NURSING DIAGNOSES AND INTERVENTIONS

Impaired tissue integrity: Wound, related to presence of contaminants; metabolic disorders (e.g., DM); medical therapy (e.g., chemotherapy, radiation therapy); altered perfusion; immunosuppression; malnutrition
Desired outcomes: Patient's wound exhibits the following signs of healing: initially, postinjury wound edges are inflamed, indurated, and tender; with epithelialization, edges become pink within 1 wk of injury; granulation tissue develops (identified by pink tissue that becomes beefy red) within 1 wk of injury; and there is no odor, exudate, or necrotic tissue. Patient or significant other successfully demonstrates wound care procedure before hospital discharge, if appropriate.

- Monitor for the following signs of impaired healing: initially postinjury, decreased inflammatory response or inflammatory response that lasts >5 days; epithelialization slowed or mechanically disrupted and noncontinuous around the wound; granulation tissue remains pale or excessively dry or moist; presence of odor, exudate, necrotic tissue, pain, and/or wound breakdown.
- Apply prescribed dressings (see Table 1-29). Insert dressing into all tracts to promote gradual closure of those areas. Ensure good hand washing before and after dressing changes, and dispose of contaminated dressings appropriately.
- When a drain is used, maintain its patency, prevent kinking of the tubing, and secure the tubing to prevent the drain from becoming dislodged.
- To help prevent contamination, cleanse the skin surrounding the wound with soap and water. Use minimal friction with cleansing if tissue is friable.
- If cleansing is used, apply high-pressure irrigation using a 35-ml syringe with an 18-gauge angiocath. If the tissue is friable or the wound is over a major organ or blood vessel, use extreme caution with the irrigation pressure. To remove contaminants effectively, use a large volume of irrigant (e.g., 100-150 ml).
- When topical enzymes are prescribed, follow package directions carefully. Be aware that some agents, such as povidone-iodine, deactivate the enzymes. Protect undamaged skin with zinc oxide, aluminum hydroxide paste, or skin sealant.
- Teach patient or significant other the prescribed wound care procedure, if indicated.

PRESSURE ULCERS

Pressure ulcers are a disruption in tissue integrity and are caused by excessive tissue pressure or shearing of blood vessels. High-risk patients include the elderly and those who have decreased mobility, decreased level of consciousness (LOC), impaired sensation, debilitation, incontinence, sepsis/elevated temperature, malnutrition, or are receiving vasopressors or treatment with invasive devices that restrict mobility.

ASSESSMENT

High-risk individuals should be identified upon admission assessment, with daily assessments during hospitalization, using a standard assessment tool. When pressure ulcers are present, their severity can be staged on a scale of I to IV.
Stage I: Nonblanchable erythema of intact skin. In dark-skinned individuals, discoloration of the skin, warmth, edema, induration, and hardness may be the only indication of a Stage I pressure ulcer.
Stage II: Partial-thickness skin loss that involves epidermis and/or dermis; seen as an abrasion, blister, or shallow crater.
Stage III: Full-thickness skin loss that involves subcutaneous tissue but does not extend through fascia.
Stage IV: Full-thickness injury that involves muscle, bone, or supporting structures. See "Surgical or Traumatic Wounds Healing by Secondary Intention," p. 47, for other assessment data.

DIAGNOSTIC TESTS

See "Diagnostic Tests" p. 46.

COLLABORATIVE MANAGEMENT

See "Collaborative Management" in "Surgical Wounds Healing by Primary Intention," p. 45, and "Collaborative Management" in "Surgical or Traumatic Wounds Healing by Secondary Intention," p. 47.

NURSING DIAGNOSES AND INTERVENTIONS

Impaired tissue integrity (or risk for same) related to excessive tissue pressure; shearing forces; altered circulation

Desired outcomes: If patient at risk: patient's tissue remains intact. After interventions/instructions, patient participates in preventive measures and verbalizes understanding of the rationale for these interventions. For those with ulcers, ulcer is clean and decreasing in size. There is no slough tissue, necrotic tissue, or odor present.

- Identify individuals at risk, and systematically assess skin over bony prominences daily; document.
- Establish and post a position-changing schedule.
- Assist patient with turning q1-2h. Use pillows or foam wedges to prevent direct pressure on bony prominences. Patients with a history of previous tissue injury will require pressure relief measures more frequently. Because high Fowler's position results in increased shearing, use low Fowler's position and alternate supine position with prone and 30-degree elevated side-lying positions.
- For immobile patients, float the heels using pillows inserted under the length of the calf.
- Minimize friction on tissue during activity. Lift rather than drag patient during position changes and transferring; use a draw sheet to facilitate patient movement. Do not massage over bony prominences.
- Minimize skin exposure to moisture. Cleanse at the time of soiling and at routine intervals. Use moisture barriers and disposable briefs as needed.
- Use a mattress that reduces pressure, such as foam, alternating air, gel, or water.

Impaired tissue integrity: Presence of pressure ulcer with increased risk for further breakdown, related to altered circulation; presence of contaminants or irritants (chemical, thermal, mechanical)

Research Brief 1-5   The purpose of the study was to determine whether the addition of the anabolic steroid, oxandrolone, to standard aggressive surgical management (débridement and diet) would control the catabolism of acute necrotizing fasciitis. Patients (n = 21) were randomly assigned to the standard care or the standard care plus oxandrolone group. Data on weight loss and nitrogen balance showed that patients who received oxandrolone had a significantly lower rate of catabolism and less lean body mass loss than those who received standard care.

From Demling RH, DeSanti L: Effect of the anabolic steroid oxandrolone on the rate of catabolism in acute necrotizing fasciitis. *WOUNDS: Compend Clin Res Pract* 15(5):143-148, 2003.

Desired outcomes: Stages I and II are healed within 7 to 10 days; stages III and IV may require months to heal. After intervention/instructions, patient/caregiver verbalizes causes and preventive measures for pressure ulcers and successfully participates in the plan of care to promote healing and prevent further breakdown.

- Evaluate stage of pressure ulcer. See "Assessment," p. 49.
- Maintain a moist physiologic environment to promote tissue repair and minimize contaminants. Change dressings as prescribed.
- Be sure patient's skin is kept clean with regular bathing, and be especially conscientious about washing urine and feces from the skin. Soap should be used and then thoroughly rinsed from the skin.
- If the patient has excessive perspiration, ensure frequent bathing and change bedding as needed.
- To absorb moisture and prevent shearing when the patient is moved, apply heel and elbow covers as needed.
- Teach patient and significant others the importance of and measures for preventing excess pressure as a means of preventing pressure ulcers.

- Provide wound care as needed (described under "Surgical or Traumatic Wounds Healing by Secondary Intention," p. 47).

ADDITIONAL NURSING DIAGNOSES

Also see **Impaired tissue integrity** under "Surgical or Traumatic Wounds Healing by Secondary Intention," p. 49.

NIC Skin Surveillance; Incision Site Care; Wound Care; Pressure Ulcer Care; Pressure Ulcer Prevention; Wound Irrigation

Pain

PATHOPHYSIOLOGY

Critically ill patients endure substantial pain from pathologic conditions, injury, therapeutic interventions such as surgery, and multiple invasive diagnostic procedures. Even seemingly unconscious patients experience pain. The patient's pain experience is compounded by fear, anxiety, and multiple barriers to communication. In addition, pain control frequently assumes a low priority when juxtaposed against respiratory or hemodynamic instability, either of which is common in critical care areas. The presence of pain is a significant stressor for critically ill patients and contributes to and potentiates other problems such as confusion, inadequate ventilation, immobility, sleep deprivation, depression, and immunosuppression.

The subjective nature of pain adds to its complexity. Pain has been defined by the International Association for the Study of Pain as "an unpleasant sensory and emotional experience associated with actual or potential tissue damage or described in terms of such damage." Pain is a warning signal to which the body responds to prevent further injury. Noxious substances that are released in response to damaged tissue initiate the pain (nociceptive) nerve transmission. Afferent nerve fibers such as A delta (Aδ) and C fibers respond to pain stimuli peripherally and relay this information to the spinal cord entering through the dorsal horn. Aδ fibers are small, myelinated, fast-conducting fibers that transmit pain sensation that is well localized. C fibers are small, unmyelinated, slow-conducting fibers that transmit poorly localized, dull, aching pain sensations.

In the dorsal horn, nociceptive neurotransmitters are released in response to the nociceptive input that activates the second-order dorsal horn neurons. The activation of the second-order neurons results in (1) spinal reflex responses such as vasoconstriction, muscle spasm, and increased sensitization and (2) activation of the ascending tracts, which transmits the nociceptive input to several regions within the brain. This is where several responses to pain occur, including the perception of pain and the emotional and behavioral responses.

Uncontrolled pain: a widespread problem

Characteristic pain patterns develop according to the area affected and the underlying pathophysiologic process. Despite the availability of effective analgesics and new pain-control technologies, many critically ill patients continue to be underassessed and treated inadequately for pain. Patients may report their pain as less than it truly is for fear of addiction or upsetting the nurse.

Professional and patient-related barriers have contributed to poor pain management. These barriers include (1) societal expectations concerning pain (e.g., unrelieved pain is expected and accepted in certain situations such as during surgical or invasive procedures, treatment for malignant conditions, or as a normal part of aging); (2) professionals' knowledge deficits regarding the pharmacokinetics and equianalgesic dosing; (3) patients' lack of knowledge concerning the side effects of unrelieved pain and the lack of knowledge of pain management in general; (4) inadequate pain assessment techniques by health care professionals; (5) inappropriate professional attitudes and beliefs (e.g., certain patients do not have pain [e.g., neonates], pain management is low priority); (6) inappropriate patients' attitudes and beliefs (e.g., pain builds character, pain is a part of procedures; and (7) fear of tolerance, addiction, and analgesic side effects by both professionals and patients.

Uncontrolled pain has multisystem effects. The cardiovascular effects of unrelieved pain are increased HR, BP, SVR; increased myocardial oxygen consumption; altered regional blood flow; and deep vein thrombosis. The pulmonary effects noted of uncontrolled pain are decreased lung volumes, atelectasis, decreased cough effort, increased sputum retention, and hypoxemia. Gastrointestinal and genitourinary effects are decreased gastric and bowel motility and urinary retention. The neuroendocrine response to uncontrolled pain is to release more of the stress hormones such as catecholamines, cortisol, and glucagon. Psychologic effects are anxiety, fear, and sleeplessness. Nurses have an ethical obligation to relieve pain and reduce associated physiologic and psychologic risks of untreated pain.

Pain management must be made a priority and a visible part of daily patient care. Methods which make pain management more visible and a priority include (1) displaying pain assessment tools in patients' rooms; (2) designating pain as the fifth vital sign to signify its importance; and (3) incorporating pain assessment into documentation tools. Continuous assessment and documentation increases awareness and effectiveness of pain intervention.

ASSESSMENT

A thorough baseline assessment, whenever possible, is important in accurately evaluating and managing pain. Frequent, brief assessments are necessary postoperatively and during acute episodes of pain until the pain is well controlled. Health care professionals need to establish a good rapport with patients and use therapeutic communication skills.

History and risk factors: Question patient regarding previous or current pain; usual ways in which pain is described and expressed; previously used pharmacologic and non-pharmacologic methods of pain control; previous history of chemical dependence, including alcohol use; attitudes and beliefs toward pain and use of opioid, anxiolytic, or other medications; typical coping responses for pain or stress; and expectations regarding pain management.

Subjective presentation: Because pain is subjective, the mainstay of pain assessment should be patients' self-report. Patients should be asked to describe the nature of the pain (e.g., location, intensity, quality, the timing of the pain, aggravating/alleviating factors). One or more of several pain assessment tools should be used to assist the patient in rating pain. Comparisons of the patient's ratings before and after a given intervention are useful in guiding therapy.

Numeric rating scale (NRS): Patient ranks pain numerically, usually from 1 to 10.

Visual analog scale (VAS): Patient marks a 10-cm line to indicate pain intensity.

Adjective rating scale (ARS): Patient selects an adjective that best describes the pain intensity.

Objective presentation: Used to supplement self-reports or used exclusively if the patient is unconscious or has other profound communication barriers.

Physiologic: Responses to pain are related to autonomic nervous system stimulation, as seen in increases in HR, BP, and RR, all which are associated with untreated pain. Other physiologic responses associated with autonomic stimulation are listed in Table 1-30.

Behavioral: Social, cultural, ethnic, and environmental factors affect a patient's understanding of and attitudes toward pain. Patients respond according to learned attitudes and beliefs. A number of nonverbal indicators are listed in Table 1-31.

Vital signs and hemodynamics: With untreated pain, usually reflect autonomic stimulation (e.g., elevated HR, RR, BP, SVR). IV opiate analgesics promptly reduce SVR directly as a result of vasodilation and indirectly as a result of pain relief.

COLLABORATIVE MANAGEMENT

Opioid agonists: Centrally-acting analgesics that bind with receptors in the CNS and other tissues, thus blocking pain sensation and causing various other effects, including feelings of well-being, peripheral vasodilation, and possibly respiratory depression. They are used to manage moderate to severe acute pain. For the most effective therapy, titrate in small increments to produce the desired analgesia with minimal side effects. "As needed" dosing provides poor pain management because of

---

T A B L E 1 - 30   Autonomic Indicators of Pain

Diaphoresis, pallor

Vasoconstriction

Increased systolic and diastolic blood pressure

Increased pulse rate (>100 beats/min)

Papillary dilation

Change in respiratory rate (usually increased to >20 breaths/min)

Muscle tension or spasm

Decreased intestinal motility, evidenced by nausea, vomiting, abdominal distention, and possibly ileus

Endocrine imbalance, evidenced by sodium and water retention and mild hyperglycemia

T A B L E 1 - 31 Nonverbal Indicators of Pain	
Skeletal muscle tension	**Psychic reactions**
Facial grimace, tension	Short attention span
Guarding or splinting of the affected part	Irritability
Restlessness	Anxiety
Increase in motor activity	Sleep disturbances
Decrease in motor activity	Anger
	Crying
	Fearfulness
	Withdrawal

delays in administration and fluctuations in the patient's analgesic blood levels. Patient-controlled analgesia (PCA) pumps, continuous peripheral or epidural infusions, and small, frequent IV bolus dosing are effective methods used for patients in critical care areas. Opioid tolerance, physiologic or psychologic dependence, and addiction are unusual when opioids are used to manage acute pain in patients without a history of chemical dependency. Parenteral opioids may cause hypotension in patients with hypovolemia. Restore fluid volume before or concurrently with administration. Some patients are at a greater risk for respiratory depression. Those at greater risk are the opioid naïve, those with compromised pulmonary status or neuromuscular disease, the extremely young (neonates), and the elderly. Opioid-induced respiratory depression can be prevented with careful titration and monitoring.

Elderly people are more sensitive to the therapeutic and toxic effects of analgesics. The distribution of medications is altered by age. With aging, lean body mass decreases and body fat increases. Also, muscle and soft-tissue mass decrease, and body water declines. This results in water-soluble opioid analgesics such as morphine having a lower volume of distribution. This causes an increased speed of onset of action and raises peak concentration, which is associated with increased toxicity. Lipid-soluble opioid analgesics (e.g., fentanyl) may be more widely distributed, resulting in a delayed onset of action and accumulation with repeated doses. Because of age-related changes in metabolism and elimination, the elderly are also at risk for drug-accumulation toxicity. In treating the elderly, it is best to start at lower doses (50%-75% of recommended younger adult doses); increase the interval between doses; use opioids with shorter half-lives (morphine, hydromorphone, oxycodone); and closely observe for signs of toxicity.

With careful assessment, proper dosing and titration, knowledge of analgesic onset and peak times, and careful monitoring, the risk for respiratory depression is low. However, naloxone (Narcan), an opioid antagonist, should be immediately available to reverse respiratory depression. See Table 1-32 for equianalgesic doses of narcotic analgesics and Table 1-33 for uses of opioid and opioid agonist-antagonist analgesia.

- *Morphine:* Most frequently used opioid; considered "first-line" therapy for moderate to severe acute pain. With its vasodilatory effects and little effect on CO and HR, morphine is beneficial for patients with left ventricular failure, pulmonary hypertension, or pulmonary edema. Rapid IV injection may trigger histamine release with related vasodilation, decreased preload, and decreased BP. Continuous opioid infusion minimizes hemodynamic changes that can occur with bolus dosing. Epidural administration may result in reduced responsiveness of the respiratory center in the brainstem to carbon dioxide. This results in gradual decrease in the depth and rate of respiration, increase in $Paco_2$, increase in sedation level, and respiratory acidosis.
- *Hydromorphone (Dilaudid):* Highly effective opioid; substitute analgesic for patient with morphine allergy or intolerance.
- *Meperidine (Demerol):* Indicated for brief courses (i.e., <48 hr) in patients with allergy or intolerance to morphine, hydromorphone, or other opiates. Its toxic metabolite, normeperidine, is a cerebral irritant and may cause seizures, which has decreased its usage in critical care patients, especially the elderly.
- *Fentanyl:* Potent synthetic opioid. IV preparation is especially useful in critical care because of minimal cardiovascular effects, short duration of action, and rapid onset of action. Duration of

action increases with repeated doses. Caution must be taken if large doses of fentanyl are given rapidly. This may cause chest wall muscle rigidity requiring ventilatory support and rapid-acting muscle relaxants.

Caution: A fentanyl patch may be used for continuous analgesia, usually with supplemental doses of morphine or other opiate titrated to produce analgesia for breakthrough pain, but should be used only for patients with opiate tolerance. A fentanyl patch is not recommended for mild pain, acute postoperative pain, or intermittent pain because of its slow onset (12-16 hr) and long duration and because it is difficult to reverse its side effects and adverse effects. Respiratory depression with hypoventilation occurs, as with morphine. Transdermal fentanyl absorption can be increased in patients with elevated temperatures.

Opioid agonist-antagonists: Stimulate and antagonize opiate receptors to varying degrees, depending on agent and dose. They may precipitate withdrawal in patients receiving opiates on a regular basis (Tables 1-32 and 1-33).
• *Pentazocine (Talwin):* Predominately agonist effects but with weak antagonist activity. It may cause increased MAP, LVEDP, and mean PAP, thus increasing myocardial workload.
• *Butorphanol (Stadol):* Adverse effects reported in patients with congestive heart failure (CHF) or acute MI. It may be useful in decreasing side effects associated with epidural morphine.
Nonsteroidal antiinflammatory drugs (NSAIDs): They are used to treat mild to moderate pain and are used as an adjunct with opioids to treat moderate to severe pain. NSAIDs inhibit the synthesis and release of prostaglandins peripherally, rendering afferent receptors less sensitive to bradykinin, histamine, and serotonin, which in turn decreases pain receptor stimulation. Most NSAIDs are given orally (e.g., ibuprofen, aspirin), but injectable NSAIDs such as ketorolac are available. Prostaglandin inhibition leads to decreased renal blood flow and acute renal failure; increased gastric irritation; and decreased platelet adhesiveness, which may result in bleeding complications (Table 1-34).
• *Ketorolac (Toradol):* Effective for short-term use in relieving mild to moderate pain. Effect on ventilation is minimal, and the drug has been effective when given on an alternate schedule with morphine or other opiate analgesic during ventilator weaning of postoperative patients. Renal toxicity is possible, which limits use to patients with normal renal function. Bleeding complications are more likely with high-dose therapy and in older adults.
Other pharmacologic interventions: Sedatives and anxiolytics (e.g., midazolam [Versed]) are often used to reduce anxiety associated with pain and to promote amnesia when painful procedures are planned. Spinal analgesia with a local anesthetic agent may be used with epidural opiates. Intermittent or continuous local neural blockade, such as intercostal nerve block, is used for specific localized pain.
Non-pharmacologic interventions: Include sensory, emotional, and cognitive interventions, such as massage, relaxation, distraction, guided imagery, repositioning, and TENS unit. These interventions are used for mild pain and anxiety and as adjuncts to pharmacologic management of moderate to severe pain (Table 1-35).

NURSING DIAGNOSES AND INTERVENTIONS

Pain: related to biophysical injury secondary to pathology; surgical, diagnostic, or treatment interventions; or related to trauma
Desired outcomes: Within 1 hr of initiating therapy, patient's subjective evaluation of discomfort improves, as documented by a pain scale. Patient does not exhibit nonverbal indicators of pain (see Table 1-31). Autonomic indicators (see Table 1-30) are diminished or absent. Verbal responses, such as crying or moaning, are absent.
• Develop a systematic approach to pain management for each patient. The primary nurse should collaborate with the physician and patient for optimal management of pain. See Figures 1-2 and 1-3 for pain treatment flow charts for preoperative and postoperative patients.
• Monitor patient at frequent intervals for the presence of discomfort. Use a formal, patient-specific method of assessing pain. One method is to have the patient rate discomfort on a scale of 0 (no dis-

T A B L E 1 - 32   Equianalgesic Doses of Narcotic Analgesics

Class/name	Route	Equianalgesic dose (mg)*	Average duration (hr)
Morphine-like agonists			
Codeine	IM, SC	130[†]	3
	PO	180[†]	3
Hydromorphone	IM, SC	1.5	4
(Dilaudid)	PO	6-7.5	4
Levorphanol	IM, SC	2	6
(Levo-Dromoran)	PO	4	6
Morphine	IM, SC	10	4
Oxycodone (Percodan)	PO	30[†]	4
Oxymorphone	IM, SC	1	4
(Numorphan)	Rectal	15-20	4
Meperidine-like agonists			
Fentanyl (Sublimaze)	IV, IM, SC	0.1	3-4[‡]
Meperidine (Demerol)	IM, SC	100	3
Methadone-like agonists			
Methadone	IM, SC	10	6
(Dolophine)	PO	10-20	6
Propoxyphene			
(Darvon)	PO	130-250[†]	4
Mixed agonist-antagonist			
Buprenorphine			
(Buprenex)	IM	0.3-0.4	4
Butorphanol (Stadol)	IM, SC	2	3
Nalbuphine (Nubain)	IM, SC	10	3-4
Pentazocine (Talwin)	IM	150	3
	PO	60	3

Modified from Hazard V, Hopfer DJ: *Davis' drug guide for nurses*, ed 5, Philadelphia, 1997, Davis; Macintyre PE, Ready LBN: *Acute pain management: a practical guide*, London, 1996, Saunders; Salerno E: Pharmacologic approaches. In Salerno E, Willens JS, editors: *Pain management handbook: an interdisciplinary approach*, St Louis, 1996, Mosby.
*Recommended starting dose; actual dose must be titrated to patient response.
[†]Starting doses lower (codeine 30 mg, oxycodone 5 mg, meperidine 50 mg, propoxyphene 65-130 mg, pentazocine 50 mg).
[‡]Respiratory depressant effects persist longer than analgesic effects.
IM, Intramuscular; *IV,* intravenous; *PO,* oral; *SC,* subcutaneous.

comfort) to 10 (worst pain). Other methods may be used, but the method selected should be used consistently and patient's report should be respected.
- Evaluate patients with acute and chronic pain for nonverbal indicators of discomfort (see Table 1-31).
- Evaluate patients with acute pain for autonomic indicators of discomfort (see Table 1-30). Be aware that patients with chronic pain (>6 mo duration) will not exhibit an autonomic response.
- Evaluate health history for evidence of alcohol and drug (prescribed and nonprescribed) use. Individuals with a history of chemical dependence may require a higher dose for effective analgesia. Persons with evidence of chronic or acute hepatic insufficiency require a reduced dose and careful selection of appropriate analgesics. Consult pain control team if available. All care providers must be consistent in setting limits while providing effective pain control through pharmacologic and non-pharmacologic methods. Psychiatric consultation may be warranted. Be aware that some opioid agonist-antagonist analgesics (e.g., butorphanol, buprenorphine, pentazocine) have strong narcotic antagonist activity and may trigger withdrawal symptoms in individuals with opiate dependency.

TABLE 1-33   **Use of Opioid and Opioid Agonist-Antagonist Analgesia**

Route	Commonly prescribed medications	Advantages	Disadvantages
Continuous IV infusion	Morphine, fentanyl (Sublimaze), hydromorphone (Dilaudid)	• Useful for severe, predictable pain • Relieves pain with lower doses than IV bolus • Avoids peaks and valleys of pain present with IV bolus and IM injections	• Requires frequent observation to monitor flow rate • VS must be monitored often, especially respiratory status • Weaning necessary
IV bolus	Morphine, fentanyl, hydromorphone, meperidine (Demerol)	• Useful for severe, intermittent pain (i.e., for procedures, treatments) • Rapid onset of action	• Relatively short duration of pain relief • Fluctuating levels • Possibility of excessive sedation as drug levels peak
Patient-controlled analgesia (PCA); may be delivered IV or SC	Morphine, fentanyl, buprenorphine (Buprenex)	• Useful for moderate to severe pain • Enables titration by patient for effective analgesia without excessive sedation • Relief of pain with lower dosages of medication • Immediate delivery of medication • Patient's sense of self-control lowers anxiety • Less nursing time spent preparing medications	• Pumps necessary to deliver drug are expensive • Patient must have clear mental status • Health care provider resistance to self-administration by patient
Epidural and intrathecal	Morphine, fentanyl, local anesthetics (e.g., bupivacaine)	• Provides greater analgesia with less CNS depression than parenteral narcotics • Enables direct binding of narcotics to opioid receptor sites in the spinal cord, thereby minimizing CNS depression • Directly blocks pain impulse transmission to central cortex when anesthetics are used	• Difficult to assess patency and placement • Significant infection risk

T A B L E 1 - 33 **Use of Opioid and Opioid Agonist-Antagonist Analgesia—cont'd**

Route	Commonly prescribed medications	Advantages	Disadvantages
IM/SC injection	Meperidine, morphine, pentazocine (Talwin), nalbuphine (Nubain), butorphanol (Stadol), buprenorphine	• Useful for moderate to severe pain • Longer duration of action than with IV route • Faster pain relief than with oral medication • SC route useful for patients with poor IV access and little muscle mass	• Variable absorption and fluctuating levels, especially in hypotensive and edematous patients • Possibility of excessive sedation as drug levels peak • Potential delay in administration • Demerol's propensity toward seizures decreases its efficacy

CNS, Central nervous system; *IV,* intravenous; *IM,* intramuscular; *SC,* subcutaneous; *VS,* vital signs.

• Administer opioid and related mixed agonist-antagonist analgesics as prescribed (see Table 1-33). Monitor for side effects, such as respiratory depression, excessive sedation, nausea, vomiting, and constipation. Be aware that meperidine (Demerol) may produce excitation, muscle twitching, and seizures, especially in conjunction with phenothiazines. Do not administer mixed agonist-antagonist analgesics concurrently with morphine or other pure agonists, because reversal of analgesic effects may occur. Meperidine is poorly tolerated by the elderly.
• Assess patients receiving opioid analgesics at frequent intervals for evidence of excessive sedation when awake or respiratory depression (i.e., RR <10 breaths/min or Sao_2 <90%-92%). In the presence of respiratory depression, reduce the amount or frequency of the dose as prescribed. Have naloxone (Narcan) readily available to reverse severe respiratory depression.

Note: Because of respiratory depression and excessive sedation, older adults and individuals with asthma, COPD, and other respiratory disorders should be monitored closely when receiving opiate analgesics.

• If the patient is receiving epidural or intrathecal narcotic, monitor closely for side effects and complications.
• Check patient's analgesia record for the last dose and amount of medication given during surgery and in the postanesthesia care unit. Be careful to coordinate timing and dose of postoperative analgesics with previously administered medication.

T A B L E 1 - 34 **Common Non-narcotic and Nonsteroidal Antiinflammatory Analgesics**

Acetaminophen (Tylenol, Tempra)
Acetylsalicylic acid (aspirin)
Ibuprofen (Motrin, Advil, Nuprin)
Indomethacin (Indocin)
Ketorolac (Toradol)
Naproxen (Naprosyn, Anaprox, Aleve)

T A B L E　1 - 35　Common Non-Pharmacologic Methods of Pain Control

Physical therapies/modalities
- Massage: To relax muscular tension and increase local circulation. Back and foot massage are especially relaxing.
- ROM exercises (passive, assisted, or active): To relax muscles, improve circulation, and prevent pain related to stiffness and immobility.
- Heat/cold applications: To alter pain threshold, reduce muscle spasm, and decrease vascular congestion, particularly in the area of injury. Cold decreases initial tissue injury response. Heat facilitates clearance of tissue toxins and fluids.
- Transcutaneous electrical nerve stimulation (TENS): A battery-operated device used to send weak electric impulse via electrodes placed on the body. The sensation of pain is reduced during and sometimes after treatment.

Emotional interventions
- Prevention and control of anxiety: Limiting anxiety reduces muscle tension and increases the patient's pain tolerance. Anxiety and fear contribute to autonomic stimulation and pain responses. Progressive relaxation exercises and encouraging slow, controlled breathing may be helpful.
- Promoting self-control: Feelings of helplessness and lack of control contribute to anxiety and pain. Techniques such as PCA and promoting self-helping behaviors contribute to feelings of self-control.

Cognitive interventions
- Preparatory information: Preparing the patient by explaining what can be expected, thereby reducing stress and anxiety. Preoperative teaching is an example of this technique.
- Patient education: Teaching methods for preventing or reducing pain. Examples include suggesting comfortable postoperative positions, methods of ambulation, and splinting of incisions when coughing.
- Distraction: Encouraging patient to focus on something unrelated to the pain. Examples include conversing, reading, watching television or videos, listening to music, relaxation techniques (see "Health-seeking behavior," p. 259)
- Humor: Can be an excellent distraction and may help the patient cope with stress.
- Guided imagery: The patient employs a mental process that uses images to alter a physical or emotional state. This technique promotes relaxation and decreases pain sensations.
- Biofeedback: The patient learns conscious control of physiologic processes that normally are controlled unconsciously. Muscle tension and chronic or episodic pain may be reduced.

Many of these techniques may be taught to and implemented by the patient and significant others.
PCA, Patient-controlled analgesia; *ROM,* range of motion.

- Administer non-narcotic and nonsteroidal antiinflammatory agents (see Table 1-34) as prescribed for relief of mild-to-moderate pain or on alternating schedule with opiate analgesics for moderate-to-severe pain. NSAIDs are especially effective when pain is associated with inflammation and soft-tissue injury. Ketorolac (Toradol) may be given IM or IV when oral agents are contraindicated. Monitor for excessive bleeding, gastric irritation, and renal compromise in patients receiving NSAIDs.
- Administer prn analgesics before pain becomes severe. Prolonged stimulation of pain receptors results in increased sensitivity to painful stimuli and will increase the amount of drug required to relieve pain.
- Administer intermittently scheduled or supplemental analgesics before painful procedures (e.g., suctioning, chest tube removal) and ambulation and at bedtime, scheduling them so that their peak effect is achieved at the inception of the activity or procedure.
- Augment analgesic therapy with sedatives and tranquilizers to prolong and enhance analgesia. Avoid substituting sedatives and tranquilizers for analgesics.
- Wean patient from opioid analgesics by decreasing dosage or frequency of the drug. When changing route of administration or medication, be certain to employ equianalgesic doses of the new drug (see Table 1-32).
- Augment action of medication by employing non-pharmacologic methods of pain control (see Table 1-35). Many of these techniques may be taught to and implemented by the patient and significant others.

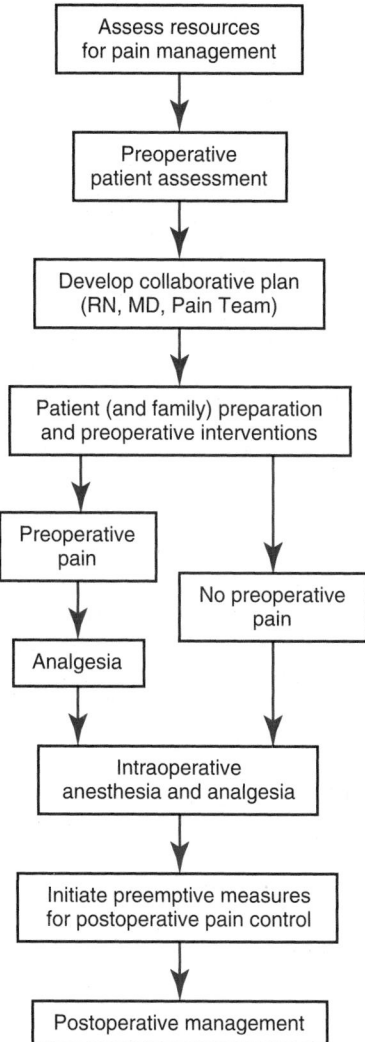

Figure 1-2: Pain treatment flow: preoperative and intraoperative phases.
Acute Pain Management Guideline Panel: *Acute pain management: operative and medical procedures and trauma, clinical practice guideline,* AHCPR Pub No 92-0032, Agency for Health Care Policy and Research, Public Health Service, Rockville, MD, 1992, US Department of Health and Human Services.

- Maintain a quiet environment to promote rest. Plan nursing activities to enable long periods of uninterrupted rest at night.
- Evaluate for and correct nonoperative sources of discomfort (e.g., position, full bladder, infiltrated IV site).
- Position patient comfortably, and reposition at frequent intervals to relieve discomfort caused by pressure and to improve circulation.
- Sudden or unexpected changes in pain intensity can signal complications such as internal bleeding or leakage of visceral contents. Carefully evaluate the patient's report of pain, compare to previous pain reports, and consult the surgeon immediately.
- Document efficacy of analgesics and other pain control interventions, using the pain scale or other formalized method.

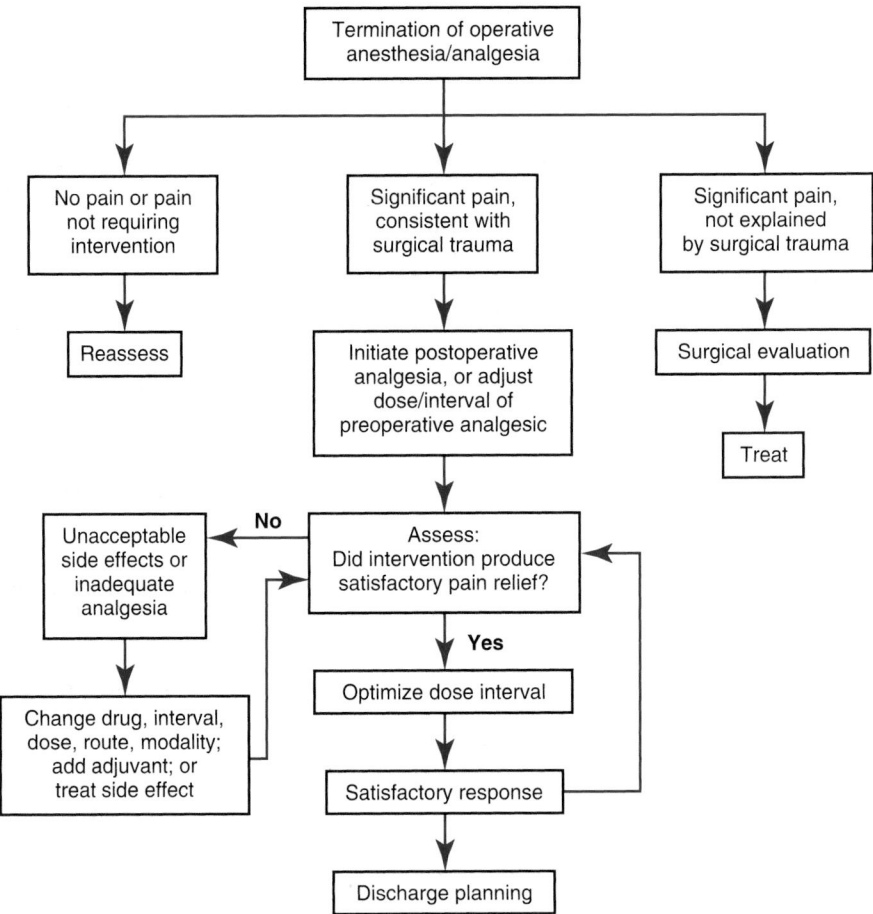

Figure 1-3:   Pain treatment flow chart: postoperative phase.
Acute Pain Management Guideline Panel: *Acute pain management: operative and medical proce-
dures and trauma, clinical practice guideline,* AHCPR Pub No 92-0032, Agency for Health Care
Policy and Research, Public Health Service, Rockville, MD, 1992, US Department of Health and
Human Services.

NIC Analgesic Administration; Pain Management; Analgesic Administration: Intraspinal; Patient-
Controlled Analgesia (PCA) Assistance
Ineffective breathing pattern: related to neuromuscular impairment secondary to central respiratory depression; pain-induced splinting
Desired outcome: Patient exhibits effective ventilation within 30 min of this diagnosis as evidenced
by relaxed breathing; RR 12-20 breaths/min with normal depth and pattern (eupnea); clear breath
sounds; normal color; PaO_2 ≥80 mm Hg; pH 7.35-7.45; $PacO_2$ 35-45 mm Hg; HCO_3^- 22-26 mEq/L;
and SpO_2 ≥92%.
• Assess and document respiratory rate and depth qh. Note signs of respiratory compromise, including RR <10 or >26; shallow or grunting respirations; use of accessory muscles of respiration; prolonged inspiratory/expiratory ratio; pallor or cyanosis; decreased vital capacity; and increased
residual volume. Consult physician for evidence of respiratory compromise.

- Monitor Spo_2 and ABG values. Consult physician for decreased Spo_2 (<90%-92%) or increased $Paco_2$ (>45 mm Hg).
- Assess and document LOC q1-2h.
- Use apnea monitor as indicated.
- Keep naloxone (Narcan) at patient's bedside during and for 24 hr after epidural or intrathecal administration.
- Maintain IV access for immediate administration of naloxone to reverse respiratory depression.
- Respiratory depression may persist for as long as 24 hr after the last dose of epidural morphine. Monitor for respiratory depression during and for 24 hr after patient's receipt of epidural or intrathecal opioids.

NIC Airway Management; Respiratory Monitoring; Oxygen Therapy; Aspiration Precautions

Urinary retention: related to inhibition of reflex arc secondary to opioid action

Desired outcomes: Within 4 hr of this diagnosis, complete bladder emptying is achieved. Overflow incontinence is absent.

- Monitor for symptoms of urinary retention: bladder distention, frequent voiding of small amounts of urine, sensation of bladder fullness, residual urine, dysuria, and overflow incontinence.
- Monitor I&O precisely.
- Catheterize bladder intermittently or insert indwelling catheter as prescribed.
- Administer IV naloxone as prescribed.

NIC Urinary Retention Care; Urinary Catheterization

Risk for impaired skin integrity: related to itching secondary to alteration in sensory modulation from opioid effects

Desired outcome: Patient's skin remains intact.

- Decrease the opioid dose via epidural or PCA infusion.
- Administer diphenhydramine or hydroxyzine as prescribed. Monitor sedation when antihistamine added.
- Maintain comfortably cool environment.
- Apply cool, moist compresses.
- If relief from the above measures is inadequate, administer small amounts of IV naloxone as prescribed.

See also "Prolonged Immobility" in following section.

NIC Skin Surveillance; Positioning; Pressure Ulcer Prevention

Prolonged Immobility

NURSING DIAGNOSES AND INTERVENTIONS

Activity intolerance: related to prolonged bed rest; generalized weakness; an imbalance between oxygen supply and demand

Desired outcome: Within 48 hr of discontinuing bed rest, patient exhibits cardiac tolerance to low-intensity exercise as evidenced by HR ≤20 beats/min over resting HR; systolic BP ≤20 mm Hg over or under resting systolic BP; SaO_2 >90%; Svo_2 ≥60%; RR ≤20 breaths/min; normal sinus rhythm; warm and dry skin; and absence of crackles, murmurs, and chest pain.

- **Perform ROM exercises bid to qid on each extremity**. Individualize the exercise plan on the basis of the following guidelines:
  - ❑ *Mode or type of exercise:* Begin with passive exercises, moving the joints through the motions of abduction, adduction, flexion, and extension. Progress to active-assisted exercises, in which you support the joints while the patient initiates muscle contraction. When the patient is able, supervise him or her in active isotonic exercises, during which the patient contracts a selected muscle group, moves the extremity at a slow pace, and then relaxes the muscle group. Have the patient repeat each exercise 3-10 times.

Caution: Avoid isometric exercises in cardiac patients. Stop any exercise that causes muscular or skeletal pain. Consult with a physical therapist for necessary modifications.

Intensity: Begin with 3-5 repetitions as tolerated by the patient. Assess exercise tolerance by measuring HR and BP at rest, peak exercise, and 5 min after exercise. If HR or systolic BP increases >20 beats/min or >20 mm Hg over the resting level, decrease the number of repetitions. If HR or systolic BP decreases >10 beats/min or >10 mm Hg at peak exercise, this could be a sign of left ventricular failure, denoting that the heart cannot meet this workload. For other adverse signs and symptoms, see "Assessment," which follows.

Duration: Begin with 5 min or less of exercise. Gradually increase the exercise to 15 min as tolerated.

Frequency: Begin exercises bid-qid. As the duration increases, the frequency can be reduced.

Assessment of exercise tolerance: Be alert to signs and symptoms that the cardiovascular and respiratory systems cannot meet the demands of the low-level ROM exercises. Excessive SOB may occur if (1) transient pulmonary congestion occurs secondary to ischemia or left ventricular dysfunction; (2) lung volumes are decreased; (3) oxygen-carrying capacity of the blood is reduced; or (4) there is shunting of blood from the right to the left side of the heart without adequate oxygenation. If CO does not increase to meet the body's needs during modest levels of exercise, systolic BP may fall; the skin may become cool, cyanotic, and diaphoretic; dysrhythmias may be noted; crackles may be auscultated; an S_3 or a systolic murmur of mitral regurgitation may occur. If the patient tolerates the exercise, increase the intensity or number of repetitions each day. See Table 1-36 for physiologic effects of bed rest (deconditioning).

- **Ask patient to rate perceived exertion (RPE)** experienced during exercise, using the following scale developed by Borg (1982):
    0 Nothing at all
    1 Very weak effort
    2 Weak (light) effort
    3 Moderate
    4 Somewhat stronger effort
    5 Strong effort
    6
    7 Very strong effort
    8
    9 Very, very strong effort
    10 Maximal effort
    The patient should not experience an RPE >3 while performing ROM exercises. Reduce the intensity of the exercise and increase the frequency until an RPE of ≤3 is attained.
- **Increase activity as the patient's condition improves.** Progress to sitting in a chair as soon as possible. Assess for orthostatic hypotension, which can occur as a result of decreased plasma volume and difficulty in adjusting immediately to postural change. Prepare the patient by increasing the amount of time spent in high Fowler's position and moving the patient slowly and in stages. (See Table 4-1 on activity progression.)
- **Have patient perform self-care activities** such as eating, mouth care, and bathing as tolerated.
- **Teach and involve significant others** in interventions for preventing deconditioning.
- **Provide emotional support** to help allay fears of failure, pain, or medical setbacks.

▌NIC Exercise Therapy: Ambulation; Energy Management; Cardiac Care: Rehabilitative

---

T A B L E 1 - 36   Physiologic Effects of Bed Rest (Deconditioning)

Increased heart rate and blood pressure for submaximal workload

Decrease in functional capacity

Decrease in circulating volume

Orthostatic hypotension

Reflex tachycardia

Modest decrease in pulmonary function

Increase in thromboemboli

Loss of muscle mass

Loss of muscle contractile strength

Deficient protein state

Negative nitrogen state

Risk for disuse syndrome: related to mechanical or prescribed immobilization; severe pain; altered LOC
Desired outcome: Patient displays full ROM without verbal or nonverbal indicators of pain.

Note: ROM exercises should be performed every day for all immobilized patients with *normal* joints and no surgical- or injury-related contraindication. Modification may be required for patients with flaccidity (e.g., immediately after stroke or spinal cord injury) to prevent subluxation; or for patients with spasticity (e.g., during the recovery period for patients with stroke or spinal cord injury) to prevent an increase in spasticity. Consult with physical therapist or occupational therapist for assistance with modifying the exercise plan for these patients. In addition, be aware that ROM exercises are contraindicated during the inflammatory phase of rheumatologic disease and for dislocated or fractured joints.

- **Prevent joint contractures**. The following areas are at high risk for joint contractures:
  - ❑ *Shoulders*: can become "frozen" to limit abduction and extension;
  - ❑ *Wrists:* can "drop," prohibiting extension;
  - ❑ *Fingers*: can develop flexion contractures that limit extension;
  - ❑ *Hips*: can develop flexion contractures that affect the gait by shortening the limb or can develop external rotation or adduction deformities that affect the gait;
  - ❑ *Knees*: can develop flexion contractures that limit extension and alter the gait;
  - ❑ *Feet:* can "drop" as a result of plantar flexion, which limits dorsiflexion and alters the gait.
- **Change the patient's position at least q2h.** Post a turning schedule at patient's bedside. Position changes will not only maintain correct body alignment, thereby reducing strain on the joints, but will also prevent contractures, minimize pressure on bony prominences, and promote maximal chest expansion.
- **Position to achieve proper standing alignment:** head neutral or slightly flexed on the neck, hips extended, knees extended or minimally flexed, and feet at right angles to the legs. Maintain this position with pillows, towels, or other positioning aids.
  - ❑ *HOB elevated 30 degrees*: extend the patient's shoulders and arms, using pillows to support the position, and allow the fingertips to extend over the edge of the pillows to maintain normal arching of the hands.
  - ❑ *Prevent hip flexion contractures*: ensure that the patient is prone or side-lying with the hips extended for the same amount of time patient spends in the supine position.

Caution: Because elevating the HOB promotes hip flexion, ensure that patient spends equal time with the hips in extension. When patient is in the side-lying position, extend the lower leg from the hip to help prevent hip flexion contracture.

- **Prone Positioning:** When able to place patient in the prone position, use a special prone positioning device or move patient to the end of the bed and allow the feet to rest between the mattress and footboard. This not only will prevent plantar flexion and hip rotation, but also will prevent injury to the heels and toes. Place thin pads under the angles of the axillae and the lateral aspects of the clavicles to prevent internal rotation of the shoulders and maintain anatomic position of the shoulder girdle. Ensure adequate lung expansion and padding to prevent pressure sores on the face. When using prone positioning for treatment of ARDS, be sure to establish a schedule that optimizes use of this position. Often the patient is prone for up to 6 hr, followed by 2 hr on the back.

Note: Guidelines for the optimal use of prone positioning to improve oxygenation for the patient in ARDS are not well established.

- **Maintain the joints in neutral position:** use the following as indicated: pillows, rolled towels, blankets, sandbags, antirotation boots, splints, and orthotics. When using adjunctive devices, monitor the involved skin at frequent intervals for alterations in integrity and implement measures to prevent skin breakdown.

- **Assess for foot drop.** Inspect the feet for plantar flexion and evaluate patient's ability to pull the toes upward toward the nose. Although feet posture naturally in plantar flexion, be particularly alert to the patient's inability to pull the toes up. To prevent foot drop, foam boots or "high top" tennis shoes may be used to support the feet. Document this assessment daily. Teach patient the rationale and procedure for ROM exercises, and have patient return the demonstrations, if able.
- **Ensure that patient does not exceed his or her tolerance.** Provide passive exercises for patients unable to perform active or active-assistive exercises. In addition, incorporate movement patterns into care activities, such as position changes, bed baths, getting the patient on and off the bedpan, or changing the patient's gown. Ensure that joints especially prone to contracture are exercised more stringently.
- **Assess patient's existing muscle mass, strength and joint motion.** Perform and document limb girth measurements, dynamography (hand-grip device that measures muscle strength), ROM, and exercise baseline limits. Explain to patient that muscle atrophy occurs because of disuse or failure to use the joint. Inform patient that disuse may result in a decrease in muscle mass and blood supply and a loss of tissue elasticity surrounding joints, resulting in pain and further difficulty moving.
- **Emphasize the importance of exercise.** Maintaining or increasing muscle strength and tissue elasticity surrounding joints is imperative. If unsure about patient's complicating pathology, consult with physician about the appropriate form of exercise for patient.
- **Promote self-care.** Maximal participation in self-care as tolerated helps to maintain muscle strength and enhances a sense of participation and control.
- **For *non*cardiac patients needing greater help with muscle strength.** Assist with resistive exercises (e.g., moderate weightlifting to increase the size, endurance, and strength of the muscles). For patients in beds with overhead frames, provide the means for resistive exercise using weights and pulleys. First, determine patient's baseline level of performance on a given set of exercises, and then set realistic goals with the patient for repetitions.
- **Use isometric exercises if the joints require rest.** With these exercises, teach patient to contract a muscle group and hold the contraction for a count of 5 or 10. The sequence is repeated for increasing numbers or repetitions until an adequate level of endurance has been achieved. Thereafter, maintenance levels are performed.
- **Reinforce progress.** Provide a chart to show patient's progress combined with large amounts of positive reinforcement. Post the exercise regimen at the bedside to ensure consistency by all health care personnel.
- **Balance rest and activity.** Provide periods of uninterrupted rest between exercises/activities to enable patient to replenish energy stores.
- **Consult rehabilitation services.** Seek a referral to a physical therapist (PT) or occupational therapist (OT) as appropriate.

NIC Positioning; Pressure Management; Exercise Therapy: Joint Mobility; Exercise Therapy: Muscle Control

Altered oral mucous membrane: related to ineffective oral hygiene

Desired outcome: Patient's oral mucosa, lips, and tongue are intact within 24 hr before discharge from intensive care unit.

- **Assess patient's oral mucous membrane,** lips, and tongue at least q4h, noting presence of dryness, exudate, swelling, blisters, and ulcers.
- **Offer sips of water or ice chips to prevent dryness** if patient is alert and able to take oral fluids.
- **Perform mouth care q2-4h,** using a soft-bristle toothbrush to cleanse the teeth and a moistened cloth or sponge-tip applicator to moisten crusty areas or exudate on tongue and oral mucosa. For patients who are intubated, suction mouth continuously during oral hygiene to remove fluid and debris.
- **Apply lip balm q2h and prn** to prevent cracking of lips.
- **Consider using an artificial saliva preparation** to assist in keeping mucous membrane moist.
- **Have patient wear dentures as possible,** to improve communication and enhance comfort.

NIC Oral Health Maintenance

Self-care deficit: related to cognitive, neuromuscular, or musculoskeletal impairment; activity intolerance secondary to prolonged bed rest

Desired outcome: Patient's physical needs are met by patient, nursing staff, or significant others.

- **Assess patient's ability to perform self-care** on the basis of functional status (e.g., comatose state, hemiplegia, sensory or motor deficit, alterations in vision).

- **If patient is comatose**, meet all patient's physical needs, including bathing, oral hygiene, feeding, and elimination. Involve significant others in the plan of care. Explain all procedures to patient and significant others before performing them.
- **For patient who is not comatose**, collaborate with him or her on a plan of care that promotes as much self-care as patient is capable of providing. Schedule care activities around the periods of time patient has the most energy to meet his or her needs. Use assessment criteria for activity tolerance, p. 61, to evaluate patient's tolerance of the activity.
- **If patient is alert**, keep toiletries and other necessary items within reach.
- **Do not rush patient**; allow adequate time for performance of self-care activities.
- **Encourage patient**; reinforce the value of progress that is made.
- **Provide assistive devices.** Consult with occupational therapy department regarding use of devices such as long-handle tools for dressing or picking up objects.
- **If visual impairment exists**, place all objects within patient's field of vision. If diplopia is present, apply an eye patch and alternate it between patient's eyes q2-3h.

NIC Energy Management; Self-Care Assistance

Altered peripheral tissue perfusion: related to interrupted arterial and venous flow secondary to prolonged immobility

Desired outcome: By discharge from the ICU, patient has adequate peripheral circulation as evidenced by normal skin color and temperature and adequate distal pulses (>2+ on a 0-4+ scale) in peripheral extremities.

- **Identify patients at high risk for tissue impairment:** altered LOC, immobility, hypothermia, hyperthermia, cachexia, hypoalbuminemia, inability to perform activities of daily living (ADLs), or advanced age.
- **Identify patients at risk for deep vein thrombosis (DVT):** chronic infection, malignancy, and peripheral vascular disease, those with a history of smoking, and the aged, obese, and anemic.
- **Teach patient the signs of DVT**: pain, redness, swelling, and warmth in the involved area and coolness, unnatural color or pallor, and superficial venous dilation distal to the involved area; and to report signs to a staff member promptly if they occur.
- **Assess lab values and vital signs for risk of DVT.** Note fever, tachycardia, and elevated sedimentation rate (ESR). C-reactive protein is a nonspecific marker of inflammation and may be elevated with DVT. "Hypercoagulable" patients are at higher risk for DVT. In patients prone to DVT, acquire bilateral baseline measurements of the midcalf, knee, and midthigh and record them on patient's initial assessment. Monitor these measurements daily and compare them with the baseline measurements to rule out extremity enlargement caused by DVT.
- **Assess for a positive Homan's sign.** The Homan's sign is not very sensitive or specific for DVT but can be elicited by flexing the knee 30 degrees and dorsiflexing the foot. Pain elicited with the dorsiflexion may indicate DVT, and may warrant further evaluation by a physician.
- **Exercise for DVT prevention.** Teach patient calf-pumping (ankle dorsiflexion-plantar flexion) and ankle-circling exercises. Unless symptomatic, instruct patient to repeat each movement 10 times hourly during extended periods of immobility. Help promote circulation by performing passive ROM or encouraging active ROM exercises. Encourage deep breathing, which increases negative pressure in the lungs and thorax to promote emptying of large veins.
- **Provide mechanical venous compression.** When not contraindicated by peripheral vascular disease, ensure that patient wears antiembolic hose or pneumatic sequential compression stockings. Remove them for 10-20 min q8h, and inspect underlying skin for evidence of irritation or breakdown. Reapply hose after elevating patient's legs at least 10 degrees for 10 min.
- **Position for maximal venous circulation.** Instruct patient not to cross the feet at the ankles or knees while in bed because doing so may cause venous stasis. If patient is at risk for DVT, elevate the foot of the bed 10 degrees to increase venous return.
- **Reduce the potential for thrombus formation and embolization.** Medications such as heparin, low-molecular-weight heparin, aspirin, platelet inhibitors, or sodium warfarin inhibit blood clotting. Administer medication as prescribed, and monitor appropriate laboratory values (e.g., prothrombin time [PT], International Normalized Ratio [INR], and partial thromboplastin time [PTT]). Educate patient to self-monitor for and report bleeding (epistaxis, bleeding gums, hematemesis, hemoptysis, melena, hematuria, and ecchymoses). High-risk patients may have an inferior vena caval (IVC) filter placed to protect against pulmonary embolism.

NIC Embolus Precautions; Circulatory Precautions

Altered cerebral tissue perfusion: (orthostatic hypotension) related to interrupted arterial flow to the brain secondary to prolonged bed rest

Desired outcome: When getting out of bed, patient has adequate cerebral perfusion as evidenced by HR <120 beats/min and BP ≥90/60 mm Hg immediately after position change (or within 20 mm Hg of patient's normal range); dry skin; normal skin color; and denial of vertigo and syncope, with return of HR and BP to resting levels within 3 min of position change.

- **Assess patient for factors that increase the risk of orthostatic hypotension.** Fluid volume changes (e.g., recent diuresis, diaphoresis, change in vasodilator therapy), altered autonomic control (e.g., diabetic cardiac neuropathy, denervation after heart transplant, advanced age), or severe left ventricular dysfunction.
- **Educate the patient.** Explain cause of orthostatic hypotension and measures for prevention.
- **Apply elastic stockings to help prevent orthostatic hypotension.** For patients who continue to have difficulty with orthostatic hypotension, it may be necessary to supplement the hose with elastic wraps to the groin when the patient is out of bed. Ensure that these wraps encompass the entire surface of the legs.
- **Prepare patient for getting out of bed.** Encourage position changes within necessary confines. *Consider using a tilt table* to reacclimate patient to upright positions.
- **Follow these guidelines for mobilization:**
  - ❏ *Closely monitor the BP* of any high-risk patient for whom this will be the first time out of bed.
  - ❏ *Dangle patient's legs at the bedside.* Be alert to indicators of orthostatic hypotension, including diaphoresis, pallor, tachycardia, hypotension, and syncope. Question patient about the presence of lightheadedness or dizziness.
  - ❏ *Check vital signs if indicators of orthostatic hypotension occur.* A drop in systolic BP of 20 mm Hg and an increased pulse rate, combined with symptoms of vertigo and impending syncope, signal the need for return to a supine position.
  - ❏ *Stand at bedside if leg dangling is tolerated.* Have at least two staff members assisting patient. *Progress to ambulation* if no adverse signs or symptoms occur.

▐NIC Energy Management; Surveillance

Constipation: related to less-than-adequate fluid or dietary intake and bulk; immobility; lack of privacy; positional restrictions; use of opioid analgesics

Desired outcomes: Within 24 hr of this diagnosis, patient verbalizes knowledge of measures that promote bowel elimination. Patient relates the return of his or her normal pattern and character of bowel elimination within 3 to 5 days of this diagnosis. The elderly often experience constipation.

- **Assess patient's bowel history.** Determine normal bowel habits and interventions that are used successfully at home.
- **Monitor and document patient's bowel movements, diet, and I&O.** Be alert to the following indications of constipation: fewer than patient's usual number of bowel movements, abdominal discomfort or distention, straining at stool, and patient complaints of rectal pressure or fullness. Fecal impaction may be manifested by oozing of liquid stool and confirmed via digital examination.
- **Auscultate each abdominal quadrant for at least 1 min** to determine the presence of bowel sounds. Normal sounds are clicks or gurgles occurring at a rate of 5-34/min.

Note: Bowel sounds are decreased or absent with paralytic ileus. High-pitched rushing sounds may be heard during abdominal cramping, indicating an intestinal obstruction.

- **Remove rectal fecal impaction.** Use a gloved, lubricated finger to remove stool from the rectum. Digital stimulation alone may prompt a bowel movement. Oil-retention enemas may soften impacted stool.
- **Encourage a high-fiber/high-fluid diet.** Unless contraindicated, a high-roughage diet and a fluid intake of at least 2-3 L/day help to promote regular bowel movements. Individualize fluid intake according to physiologic state for patients with renal, hepatic, or cardiac disorders.
- **Promote bowel regularity.** Offer the bedpan at intervals. Ensure privacy. Time laxatives, enemas, or suppositories to take effect at the time of day the patient normally has a bowel movement. Provide warm fluids before breakfast and encourage toileting to gain advantage of gastrocolic or duodenocolic reflexes.
- **Promote peristalsis.** Encourage as much activity as tolerated.
- **Consult physician for pharmacologic interventions as necessary.** To help prevent rebound constipation, make a priority list of interventions to ensure minimal disruption of patient's normal bowel habits. The following is a suggested hierarchy of interventions:

❑ Bulk-building additives (e.g., psyllium)

❑ Mild laxatives (e.g., apple or prune juice, milk of magnesia)

❑ Stool softeners (e.g., docusate sodium or docusate calcium)

❑ Potent laxatives and cathartics (e.g., bisacodyl, cascara sagrada)

❑ Medicated suppositories

❑ Enemas

- **Discuss the role narcotics and other medications have in constipation.** Consider alternative methods of pain control (see Table 1-35) in an attempt to reduce narcotic dosage.

NIC Constipation/Impaction Management

Diversional activity deficit: related to prolonged illness and hospitalization

Desired outcome: Within 24 hr of intervention, patient engages in diversional activities and relates the absence of boredom.

- **Prevent boredom.** Provide patient with something to read or do. Explore activities patient enjoys. Assess patient's activity tolerance as described on p. 61.
- **Personalize the patient's environment** with favorite objects and photographs. Suggest that significant others bring in a radio or a TV, if not part of the standard room furnishings.
- **Tailor activities to attention span.** Initiate activities that require little concentration, and proceed to more complicated tasks as patient's condition allows. For example, if reading requires more energy or concentration than patient is capable of, suggest that significant others read to patient or bring in audiotapes of books, such as those marketed for the visually impaired.
- **Remember the pleasant past.** Encourage discussion of past activities or reminiscence as a substitute for performing favorite activities during convalescence.
- **Progress activities as patient's endurance improves.** Move from reading to other diversions, such as puzzles, model kits, handicrafts, and computerized games and activities.
- **Encourage visitation by significant others within limits of patient's endurance.** Involve significant others in patient activities, such as playing cards or backgammon. Encourage significant others to stagger their visits throughout the day.
- **Provide social interaction time.** Spend time talking with patient. Arrange for hospital volunteers to visit, play cards, read books, or play board games as appropriate. Consider relocation to a room in an area of high traffic if patient desires more social interaction.
- **Remember the outdoors to promote normalcy.** As patient's condition improves, assist him or her with sitting in a chair near a window. When able, provide opportunities to sit in a solarium so patients can interact together. If the physical condition and weather permit, take patient outside for brief periods. Natural sunlight helps to promote a more normal sleep-wake cycle.
- **Support spiritual, mental, and emotional health.** Request consultation for interventions as appropriate from social services, occupational therapy, pastoral services, and psychiatric nurse.

NIC Energy Management; Activity Therapy; Art Therapy; Recreation Therapy; Self-Responsibility Facilitation; Spiritual Support; Family Support; Emotional Support

Altered sexuality patterns: related to actual or perceived physiologic limitations on sexual performance secondary to disease, therapy, or prolonged hospitalization

Desired outcome: Within 72 hr of this diagnosis, patient relates satisfaction with sexuality and/or understanding of the ability to resume sexual activity.

- **Assess patient's normal sexual function,** including the importance placed on sex in the relationship, frequency of interaction, normal positions used, and the couple's ability to adapt or change to meet requirements of patient's limitations.
- **Identify sexual dysfunction.** Approach patient diplomatically and clarify issues. Indicators of sexual dysfunction can include regression, acting-out with inappropriate behavior such as grabbing or pinching, sexual overtures toward the hospital staff, self-enforced isolation, and other similar behaviors.
- **Encourage acceptable expressions of sexuality.** For example, a woman can wear makeup, jewelry, and her own clothing.
- **Encourage discussion between patient and significant other.** Promote verbalization of feelings and anxieties about sexual abstinence or hurting the patient.
- **Inform patient and significant other if it is possible to have time alone together for intimacy.** Implement a "Do Not Disturb" sign on the door, enforcing privacy by restricting staff and visitors from the room. Encourage intimacy, within the limitations of the environment.

NIC Anxiety Reduction; Body Image Enhancement; Coping Enhancement; Counseling

Altered role performance: dependence versus independence

Desired outcomes: Within 48 hr of this diagnosis, patient collaborates with caregivers in planning realistic goals for independence, participates in own care, and takes responsibility for self-care.

Research Brief 1-6   Understanding the severe consequences of prolonged bed rest and immobility, an interdisciplinary team devised a quality improvement project that would ensure the team would address this need in medical-surgical patients at one institution. An educational program was developed and then chart audits conducted to assess improvements. Because documentation was difficult to assess, the team planned a common language for documentation and this was disseminated throughout the institution. After implementation, there was a significant improvement in order for activity levels. Rates of pneumonia decreased 1.7% and other pulmonary complications decreased 4.3%. These are important outcomes that can reduce hospital stay.

Markey DW, Brown RJ: An interdisciplinary approach to addressing patient activity and mobility in the medical-surgical patient, *J Nurs Care Qual* 16(4):1-12, 2002.

- **Encourage independence.** Ensure that all health care providers are consistent in conveying their expectations of eventual independence within limitations of the endurance, therapy, and pain. Be aware, however, that temporary periods of dependence are appropriate, inasmuch as they enable the person to restore energy reserves needed for recovery.
- **Alert patient to areas of overdependence**, and involve him or her in collaborative goal setting to achieve independence.
- **Do not minimize patient's expressions of feelings of depression.** Allow patient to express emotions, while providing support, understanding, and realistic hope for a positive role change.
- **Provide self-help devices** to increase patient's independence with self-care.
- **Provide positive reinforcement** when patient meets or advances toward goals.

NIC   Normalization Promotion; Role Enhancement

Psychosocial Support

Psychosocial support of patients and their families is an integral component of a patient plan of care. Founded on principles of holistic care, in which body, mind, and spirit operate in tandem, this section addresses psychosocial care within the context of the individual's primary social structure. Considerable overlap will be noted between nursing diagnoses for the patient and those for the family. Nursing interventions should occur simultaneously for both the patient and the family/significant others.

NURSING DIAGNOSES AND INTERVENTIONS

Knowledge deficit: current diet, disease process, health resources, medication, prescribed activity, treatment procedures, treatment regimen

Desired outcome: Before any medical or nursing intervention and within the 24-hr period before discharge from the critical care unit, patient verbalizes understanding of current diet, disease process, health resources, medication, prescribed activity, treatment procedures, and treatment regimen.

- Assess current level of knowledge about diet, disease process, health resources, medication, prescribed activity, treatment procedures, and treatment regimen.
- Assess cognitive and emotional readiness to learn.
- Recognize barriers to learning, such as impaired verbal communication, altered thought processes, confusion, impaired memory, sensory alterations, fear, anxiety, and lack of motivation.
- Assess learning needs, and establish short- and long-term goals.
- Use individualized verbal or written information to promote learning and enhance understanding. Give simple, direct instructions. If indicated, use audiovisual tools to supplement information.
- Encourage significant others to reinforce correct information about diet, disease process, health resources, medication, prescribed activity, treatment procedures, and treatment regimen.
- As appropriate, facilitate referral of neurologically impaired patient to neurologic clinical nurse specialist or other specialist.
- Encourage interest about health care information by involving patient in planning care. Explain rationale for care.
- Interact frequently with patient to evaluate comprehension of information given. Ask patient to repeat what has been explained. Individuals in crisis often need repeated explanations before information can be understood. Also be aware that many individuals may not understand seemingly simple medical terms (e.g., "terminal," "malignant," "constipation").

- As appropriate, assess understanding of informed consent. Assist patient to use information received to make informed health care decisions (e.g., about invasive procedures, surgery, resuscitation).
- Assess understanding of right to self-determination; provide information as indicated. If requested, assist patient with mechanism for executing an advance directive for health care.

NIC Teaching: Disease Process; Teaching: Individual; Patient Rights Protection; Preparatory Sensory Information

Anxiety related to actual or perceived threat of death; change in health status; threat to self-concept or role; unfamiliar people and environment; the unknown

Desired outcomes: Within 1-2 hr of intervention, anxiety is absent or reduced as evidenced by patient's verbalization of same; HR ≤100 beats/min; RR ≤20 breaths/min; and an absence of or decrease in irritability and restlessness.

- Engage in honest communication; empathize. Actively listen, and establish an atmosphere that enables free expression. Express to patient that you care about his or her health.
- Assess level of anxiety. Be alert to verbal and nonverbal cues:
  - ❑ *Mild:* Restless, irritable, asks more questions, focuses on the environment
  - ❑ *Moderate:* Inattentive, expresses concern, narrowed perceptions, disturbed sleep pattern, increased HR
  - ❑ *Severe:* Expresses feelings of doom; rapid speech; tremors; poor eye contact; preoccupation with the past; inability to understand the present; possible presence of tachycardia, palpitations, nausea, and hyperventilation
  - ❑ *Panic:* Cannot concentrate or communicate, distorts reality, increased motor activity, vomiting, tachypnea
- For severe anxiety or panic state, refer to appropriate psychiatric health care team member.
- If hyperventilation occurs, encourage slow, deep breaths by having patient mimic your own breathing pattern.
- Validate the nursing assessment of anxiety with the patient. ("You seem distressed; are you feeling anxious or overwhelmed?")
- After an episode of anxiety, review and discuss the thoughts and feelings that led to the episode.
- Identify coping behaviors currently being used (e.g., denial, anger, repression, withdrawal, daydreaming, drug or alcohol dependence). Review coping behaviors used in the past. Assist in using adaptive coping to manage anxiety.
- Encourage expression of fears, concerns, and questions. ("I know this room looks like a maze of wires and tubes; please let me know when you have any questions.")
- Reduce sensory overload by providing an organized, quiet environment. See "Sensory/Perceptual Alterations," p. 70.
- Introduce self and other health care team members; explain each individual's role as it relates to the plan of care or care map.
- Teach relaxation and imagery techniques. See "Health-Seeking Behavior," p. 259.
- Enable support persons to be in attendance whenever possible.
- Consult palliative care services if available and appropriate.
- Engage in and promote awareness of touch to significant others when appropriate. Kinds of touch are described in Table 1-37.

NIC Anxiety Reduction; Coping Enhancement; Calming Technique

Impaired verbal communication related to neurologic or anatomic deficit (e.g., hearing impairment, visual impairment); psychologic or physical barriers (e.g., tracheostomy, intubation); cultural or developmental differences

Desired outcome: At the time of intervention, patient communicates needs and feelings and relates decrease in or absence of frustration over communication barriers.

- Assess etiology of impaired communication (e.g., tracheostomy, stroke, cerebral tumor, Guillain-Barré syndrome).
- With patient and significant others, assess patient's ability to hear, see, speak, read, write, and comprehend English. If patient speaks a language other than English, collaborate with English-speaking family member or interpreter to establish effective communication.
- When communicating, use eye contact; speak in a clear, normal tone of voice; and face the patient.
- If patient cannot speak because of a physical barrier (e.g., tracheostomy, wired mandibles), provide reassurance and acknowledge frustration. ("I know this is frustrating for you, but please do not give up. I want to understand you.")
- Provide slate, word cards, pencil and paper, alphabet board, pictures, or other communication device to assist patient. Adapt the call system to meet the patient's needs. Document the meaning of the patient's signals in response to questions.

T A B L E 1 - 37   Kinds of Touch

Instrumental touch
- Task or procedure related
- May be negatively perceived but accepted as impersonal

Affective touch
- Expressive, personal
- Caring
- Comforting
- May be positively or negatively perceived
- Influenced by cultural patterns

Therapeutic touch
- A deliberate intervention to accomplish a purpose
- Acupressure
- Use of space around the individual to mobilize energy fields

---

- Explain to significant others the source of the communication impairment; demonstrate effective communication alternatives (see preceding intervention).
- Be alert to nonverbal messages, such as facial expressions, hand movements, and nodding of the head. Validate meanings of nonverbal cues with the patient.
- Recognize that the inability to speak may foster maladaptive behaviors. Encourage patient to communicate needs; reinforce independent behaviors.
- Be honest; do not relate understanding if you cannot interpret patient's communication.
Active Listening; Communication Enhancement: Hearing Deficit, Speech Deficit, Visual Deficit

NIC **Sensory/perceptual alterations:** related to therapeutically or socially restricted environment; psychologic stress; altered sensory reception, transmission, or integration; chemical alteration
Desired outcomes: At the time of intervention, patient verbalizes orientation to time, place, and person; relates the ability to concentrate; and expresses satisfaction with the degree and type of sensory stimulation being received.
- Assess factors contributing to the sensory/perceptual alteration.
  - ❏ *Environmental:* Excessive noise in the environment; constant, monotonous noise; restricted environment (immobility, traction, isolation); social isolation (restricted visitors, impaired communication); therapies.
  - ❏ *Physiologic:* Altered organ function; sleep or rest pattern disturbance; medication; history of altered sensory perception.
- Determine the appropriate sensory stimulation needed; plan care accordingly.
- Control factors that contribute to environmental overload. For example, avoid constant lighting (maintain day/night patterns); reduce noise whenever possible (e.g., decrease alarm volumes, avoid loud talking, keep room door closed, provide ear plugs).
- Provide meaningful sensory stimulation:
  - ❏ Display clocks, large calendars, and meaningful photographs and objects from home.
  - ❏ Depending on patient's preferences, provide a radio, music, reading materials, and tape recordings of family and significant others. Earphones help block out external stimuli.
  - ❏ Position patient toward window when possible.
  - ❏ Discuss current events, time of day, holidays, and topics of interest during patient care activities.
  - ❏ As needed, orient patient to surroundings. Direct patient to reality as necessary.
  - ❏ Establish personal contact by touch to help promote and maintain contact with the real environment.
  - ❏ Encourage significant others to communicate with patient frequently, using a normal tone of voice.
  - ❏ Convey concern and respect. Introduce yourself, and call patient by name.
  - ❏ Stimulate vision with mirrors, colored decorations, and pictures.
  - ❏ Stimulate sense of taste with sweet, salty, and sour substances if appropriate.
  - ❏ Encourage use of appropriate eyeglasses and hearing aids.

- Inform patient before initiating interventions and using equipment.
- Encourage participation in health care planning and decision making whenever possible by asking patient first.
- Provide patients with choices when possible.
- Assess sleep-rest pattern to evaluate its contribution to the sensory/perceptual disorder. Ensure that patient attains at least 90 min of uninterrupted sleep as frequently as possible. For more information, see "Sleep Pattern Disturbance," which follows.

NIC Environmental Management; Cognitive Restructuring; Cognitive Stimulation

Sleep pattern disturbance: related to environmental changes; illness; therapeutic regimen; pain; immobility; psychologic stress

Desired outcomes: After discussion, patient identifies factors that promote sleep. Within 8 hr of intervention, patient attains 90-min periods of uninterrupted sleep and verbalizes satisfaction with ability to rest.

- Assess usual sleeping patterns (e.g., bedtime routine, hours of sleep per night, sleeping position, use of pillows and blankets, napping during the day, nocturia).
- Explore relaxation techniques that promote rest/sleep (e.g., imagining relaxing scenes, listening to soothing music or taped stories, using muscle relaxation exercises).
- Identify causative factors and activities that contribute to sleep pattern disturbance, adversely affect sleep patterns, or awaken patient. Examples include pain, anxiety, depression, hallucinations, medications, underlying illness, sleep apnea, respiratory disorder, caffeine, fear, and medical and nursing interventions.
- Organize procedures and activities to allow for 90-min periods of uninterrupted rest/sleep. Limit visiting during these periods.
- Whenever possible, maintain a quiet environment by providing ear plugs or decreasing alarm levels. The use of "white noise" (e.g., low-pitched, monotonous sounds; electric fan; soft music) may facilitate sleep. Dim the lights for a period of time q24h by drawing the drapes or providing blindfolds.
- If appropriate, limit daytime sleeping. Attempt to establish regularly scheduled daytime activity (e.g., ambulation, sitting in chair, active ROM), which may promote nighttime sleep.
- Investigate and provide non-pharmacologic comfort measures that are known to promote sleep (Table 1-38).

NIC Environmental Management; Environmental Management: Comfort; Sleep Enhancement

Fear: related to separation from support systems; unfamiliarity with environment or therapeutic regimen; loss of sense of control

Desired outcome: After intervention, patient communicates fears and concerns and relates the attainment of increased psychologic and physical comfort.

- Assess perceptions of the environment and health status, and determine contributing factors to feelings of fear. Evaluate verbal and nonverbal responses.
- Acknowledge fears. ("I understand that this equipment frightens you, but it is necessary to help you breathe.")
- Provide opportunities for expression of fears and concerns. ("You seem very concerned about receiving more blood today.") Listen actively. Recognize that anger, denial, occasional withdrawal, and demanding behaviors may be coping responses.
- Encourage asking questions and gathering information about the unknown. Provide ongoing information about equipment, therapies, and routines according to patient's ability to understand.
- To promote an increased sense of control, encourage patient participation in the plan of care whenever possible. Provide continuity of care by establishing a routine and arranging for consistent caregivers whenever possible. Appoint a primary nurse or care manager as appropriate.
- Discuss with health care team members the appropriateness of medication therapy for fear or anxiety that is disabling.
- Explore patient's desire for spiritual, psychologic, or palliative care counseling. Make referrals as appropriate.
- Collaborate with physician about a visit by another individual with the same disorder.
- Allow patient time with significant other if appropriate in reducing patient's fears.

NIC Anxiety Reduction; Counseling; Crisis Intervention; Decision Making Support; Security Enhancement

Ineffective individual coping and ineffective denial related to health crisis; sense of vulnerability; inadequate support systems

Desired outcomes: Within 24 hr of this diagnosis, patient verbalizes feelings, identifies strengths, and begins using positive coping behaviors.

TABLE 1-38   Non-pharmacologic Measures To Promote Sleep

Activity	Example(s)
Mask or eliminate environmental stimuli	Use eyeshields, ear plugs
	Play soothing music
	Dim lights at bedtime
	Mask odors from dressings/drainage; change dressing or drainage container as indicated
Promote muscle relaxation	Encourage ambulation as tolerated throughout the day
	Teach and encourage in-bed exercises and position change
	Perform back massage at bedtime
	If not contraindicated, use a heating pad
Reduce anxiety	Ensure adequate pain control
	Keep patient informed of his or her progress and treatment measures
	Avoid overstimulation by visitors or other activities immediately before bedtime
	Avoid stimulant drugs (e.g., caffeine)
Promote comfort	Encourage patient to use own pillows, bedclothes if not contraindicated
	Adjust bed; rearrange linens
	Regulate room temperature
Promote usual presleep routine	Offer oral hygiene at bedtime
	Provide warm beverage at bedtime
	Encourage reading or other quiet activity
Minimize sleep disruption	Maintain quiet environment throughout the night
	Plan nursing activities to allow long periods (at least 90 min) of undisturbed sleep
	Use dim lights when checking on patient during the night

- Assess patient's perceptions and ability to understand current health status.
- Establish honest communication. ("Please tell me what I can do to help you.") Assist with identifying strengths, stressors, inappropriate behaviors, and personal needs.
- Support positive coping behaviors. ("I see that reading that book seems to help you relax.")
- Provide opportunities for expression of concerns; gather information from nurses and other support systems. Provide explanations about prescribed routine, therapies, and equipment. Acknowledge feelings and assessment of current health status and environment.
- Identify factors that inhibit ability to cope (e.g., unsatisfactory support system, knowledge deficit, grief, fear).
- Recognize defensive and maladaptive coping behaviors (e.g., severe depression, drug or alcohol dependence, hostility, violence, suicidal ideations). Confront these behaviors. ("You seem to be requiring more pain medication. Are you experiencing more physical pain, or does it help you to remove yourself from reality?") Refer patient to case manager, psychiatric liaison, clinical nurse specialist, clergy, or palliative care specialist as appropriate.
- As patient's condition allows, assist with reducing anxiety. See "Anxiety," p. 69.
- Help reduce sensory overload by maintaining an organized, quiet environment. See "Sensory/Perceptual Alterations," p. 44.
- Encourage regular visits by significant others. Encourage them to engage in conversation with patient to help minimize patient's emotional and social isolation.
- Assess significant others' interactions with patient. Attempt to mobilize support systems by involving them in patient care whenever possible.
- As appropriate, explain to significant others that increased dependency, anger, and denial may be adaptive coping behaviors used by patient in early stages of crisis until effective coping behaviors are learned.

NIC Emotional Support; Support System Enhancement

Anticipatory grieving: related to perceived potential loss of physiologic well-being (e.g., expected loss of body function or body part, changes in self-concept or body image, terminal illness)

Desired outcomes: After interventions, patient and significant others/family express grief, participate in decisions about the future, and communicate concerns to health care team members and to one another.

- Assess whether perceived sense of loss is real or unreal to patient.
- Assess factors contributing to anticipated loss.
- Assess and accept patient's behavioral response. Expect reactions such as disbelief, denial, guilt, anger, and depression. Determine stage of grieving as described in Table 1-39.
- Assess spiritual, religious, and sociocultural expectations related to loss. ("Is religion an important part of your life? How do you and your family/significant others deal with serious health problems?") Refer to the clergy or community support groups as appropriate.
- Encourage patient and family/significant others to share their concerns. ("Is there anything you'd like to talk about today?") Also, respect their desire not to speak, and actively listen.
- Demonstrate empathy. ("This must be a very difficult time for you and your family.") Touch when appropriate (see Table 1-37).
- In selected circumstances, provide an explanation of the grieving process. This approach may assist in better understanding and acknowledging feelings.
- Assess grief reactions of patient and family/significant others, and identify a potential for dysfunctional grieving reactions (e.g., absence of emotion, hostility, avoidance). If the potential for dysfunctional grieving is present, refer to case manager, psychiatric clinical nurse specialist, clergy, or palliative care specialist as appropriate.
- When appropriate, assess patient's wishes about tissue donation.

NIC Active Listening; Dying Care; Grief Work Facilitation

Dysfunctional grieving: related to loss of physiologic well-being; fatal illness

Desired outcomes: Within 24 hr of this diagnosis, patient expresses grief, explains the meaning of the loss, and communicates concerns with family/significant others. The patient completes necessary self-care activities.

- Assess grief stage (Table 1-39) and previous coping abilities. Discuss patient's feelings, the meaning of loss, and goals. ("How do you feel about your condition/illness? What do you hope to accomplish in these next few days/weeks?")
- Acknowledge and permit anger; set limits on the expression of anger to discourage destructive behavior. ("I understand that you must feel very angry, but for the safety of others, you may not throw equipment.")

TABLE 1-39 Stages of Grieving

Protest stage	Denial: "No, not me"
	Disbelief: "But I just saw her this morning"
	Anger
	Hostility
	Resentment
	Bargaining to postpone loss
	Appeal for help to recover loss
	Loud complaints
	Altered sleep and appetite
Disorganization	Depression
	Withdrawal
	Social isolation
	Psychomotor retardation
	Silence
Reorganization	Acceptance of loss
	Development of new interests and attachments
	Restructuring of lifestyle
	Return to preloss level of functioning

- Identify suicidal behavior (e.g., severe depression, statements of intent, suicide plan, previous history of suicide attempt). Ensure safety, and refer to case manager, psychiatric clinical nurse specialist, psychiatrist, clergy, or palliative care specialist.
- Encourage patient and family/significant others to participate in ADLs and diversional activities. Identify physiologic problems related to loss (e.g., eating or sleeping disorders), and intervene accordingly.
- Collaborate with physician about a visit by another individual with the same disorder, if appropriate.

Grief Work Facilitation; Anger Control Assistance

■NIC **Powerlessness** related to health care environment; treatment regimen

Desired outcome: Within 24 hr of this diagnosis, patient makes decisions about self-care and therapies and relates an attitude of realistic hope and a sense of self-control.

- Assess personal preferences, needs, values, and attitudes.
- Before providing information, assess patient's understanding of health condition, prognosis, and plan of care.
- Recognize expressions of fear, lack of response to events, and lack of interest in information, any of which may signal a sense of powerlessness.
- Evaluate medical and nursing interventions, and adjust them, as appropriate, to support patient's sense of control. For example, if the patient always bathes in the evening to promote relaxation before bedtime, modify the care plan or map to include an evening bath rather than follow the hospital routine of giving a morning bath.
- Assist patient to identify and demonstrate activities that can be performed independently.
- Whenever possible, offer alternatives related to routine hygiene, diet, diversional activities, visiting hours, or treatment times.
- Ensure privacy and preserve territorial rights whenever possible. For example, when distant relatives and casual acquaintances request information about the patient's status, refer them to the patient or a family member who can provide acceptable amounts of information.
- Discourage patient's dependency on staff. Avoid overprotection and parenting behaviors.
- Assess support systems; enable significant others to be involved in care whenever possible.
- Offer realistic hope for the future. If appropriate, encourage direction of thoughts beyond the present.
- Provide referrals to clergy, palliative care specialists, and other support systems as appropriate.

Emotional Support; Self-Responsibility Facilitation

■NIC **Spiritual distress:** related to separation from spiritual/religious/cultural supports; challenged belief and value system

Desired outcomes: Within 24 hr of this diagnosis, patient verbalizes spiritual or religious beliefs and expresses hope for the future, the attainment of spiritual or religious support, and the availability of what is required to resolve conflicts.

- Assess spiritual or religious beliefs, values, and practices. ("Do you have a religious preference? How important is it to you? Are there any religious or spiritual practices you wish to participate in while in the hospital?")
- Inform patient and family/significant others of the availability of spiritual aids, such as a chapel, religious services, or pastoral care service.
- Present a nonjudgmental attitude toward patient's religious or spiritual beliefs and values. Create an environment that is conducive to free expression and invite patient to share his or her beliefs.
- Identify available support systems that may assist in meeting the patient's religious or spiritual needs (e.g., clergy, patient's fellow church members, support groups).
- Be sensitive to comments related to spiritual concerns or conflicts. ("I don't know why God is doing this to me." "I'm being punished for my sins.")
- Use active listening and open-ended questioning to assist in resolving conflicts related to spiritual issues. ("I understand that you want to be baptized. We can arrange to do that here.")
- Provide privacy and opportunities for religious practices, such as prayer and meditation.
- If spiritual beliefs and therapeutic regimens are in conflict, provide honest, concrete information to encourage informed decision making. ("I understand that your religion discourages receiving blood transfusions. Do you understand that by refusing blood your condition is more difficult to treat?")

Spiritual Support; Hope Instillation; Coping Enhancement

■NIC **Social isolation:** related to altered health status; inability to engage in satisfying personal relationships; altered mental status; altered physical appearance

Desired outcome: Within 24 hr of this diagnosis, patient demonstrates interaction and communication with others.

- Assess factors contributing to social isolation.
  - ❑ Restricted visiting hours
  - ❑ Absence of or inadequate support system
  - ❑ Inability to communicate (e.g., presence of ET tube/tracheostomy)
  - ❑ Physical changes that affect self-concept
  - ❑ Denial or withdrawal
  - ❑ Critical care environment
- Recognize patients at higher risk for social isolation: the older adult, disabled, chronically ill, economically disadvantaged.
- Assist patient with identification of feelings associated with loneliness and isolation. ("You seem very sad when your family leaves the room. Can you tell me more about your feelings?")
- Determine need for socialization, and identify available and potential support systems. Explore methods for increasing social contact (e.g., tapes of loved ones, more frequent visitations/hospital volunteers, scheduled interaction with nurse or support staff).
- Provide positive reinforcement for socialization that lessens feelings of isolation and loneliness. ("Please continue to call me when you need to talk to someone. Talking will help both of us to better understand your feelings.")
- Facilitate patient's ability to communicate with others (see "Impaired Verbal Communication," p. 69).

NIC Socialization Enhancement

Body image disturbance: related to loss of or change in body parts or function; physical trauma

Desired outcomes: Before hospital discharge, patient acknowledges body changes and demonstrates movement toward incorporating changes into self-concept. Maladaptive responses, such as severe depression, are absent.

- Establish open, honest communication. Promote an environment that is conducive to free expression. ("Please feel free to talk to me whenever you have any questions.") Assess indicators suggesting body image disturbance as listed in Table 1-40.
- When planning care, be aware of interventions that may influence body image (e.g., medications, procedures, monitoring).
- Assess knowledge of patient's pathophysiologic process and current health status. Clarify any misconceptions.
- Discuss the loss or change with the patient. Recognize that what may seem to be a small change may be of great significance to the patient (e.g., arm immobilizer, catheter, hair loss, ecchymoses, facial abrasions).
- Explore expressions of concern, fear, and guilt. ("I understand that you are frightened. Your face looks very different now, but you will see changes and it will improve. Gradually you will begin to look more like yourself.")
- Encourage patient and family/significant others to interact with one another. Help family/significant others to support the patient's feelings related to the changed body part or function. ("I know

---

T A B L E 1 - 40   Indicators Suggesting Body Image Disturbance

Nonverbal indicators

Missing body part—internal or external (e.g., splenectomy, amputated extremity)

Change in structure (e.g., open, draining wound)

Change in function (e.g., colostomy)

Avoiding looking at or touching body part

Hiding or exposing body part

Verbal indicators

Expression of negative feelings about body

Expression of feelings of helplessness, hopelessness, or powerlessness

Personalization or depersonalization of missing or mutilated part

Refusal to acknowledge change in structure or function of body part

your son looks very different to you now, but it would help if you speak to him and touch him as you would normally.")

- Encourage gradual participation in self-care activities as the patient becomes physically and emotionally able. Allow for some initial withdrawal and denial behaviors. For example, when changing dressings over traumatized part, explain what you are doing but do not expect the patient to watch or participate initially.
- Discuss the potential for reconstruction of the loss or change (i.e., surgery, prosthesis, grafting, physical therapy, cosmetic therapies, organ transplant).
- Recognize manifestations of severe depression (e.g., sleep disturbances, change in affect, change in communication pattern). As appropriate, refer to case manager, psychiatric clinical nurse specialist, clergy, or support group.
- Help patient attain a sense of autonomy and control by offering choices and alternatives whenever possible. Emphasize strengths, and encourage activities that interest patient.
- Offer realistic hope for the future.

▌NIC Body Image Enhancement; Emotional Support; Grief Work Facilitation

Risk for violence: self-directed or directed at others, related to sensory overload; suicidal behavior; rage reactions; neurologic disease; perceived threats; toxic reaction to medications; substance withdrawal

Desired outcome: Patient does not harm self or others.

- Assess factors that may contribute to or precipitate violent behavior (e.g., medication reactions, inability to cope, suicidal behavior, confusion, hypoxia, substance withdrawal, preictal and postictal states).
- Attempt to eliminate or treat causative factors. For example, provide patient teaching, reorient patient, ensure delivery of prescribed oxygen therapy, and reduce or prevent sensory overload (see "Sensory/Perceptual Alterations," p. 44).
- Assess for history of physical aggression, family violence, and substance abuse as maladaptive coping behaviors.
- Monitor for early signs of increasing anxiety and agitation (e.g., restlessness, verbal aggressiveness, inability to concentrate). Assess for body language that is indicative of violent behavior: clenched fists, rigid posture, increased motor activity.
- Approach patient in a positive manner, and encourage verbalization of feelings and concerns. ("I understand that you are frightened. I will be here from 3 PM to 11 PM to care for you.")
- Offer as much personal and environmental control as the situation allows. ("Let's discuss the care you will need today. What fluids would you like to drink? Would you prefer a bath in the morning or evening?")
- Help patient distinguish reality from altered perceptions. Orient to time, place, and person. Alter the environment to promote reality-based thought processes (e.g., provide clocks, calendars, pictures of loved ones, familiar objects).
- For acute confusion that becomes aggressive, do not attempt to reorient patient and avoid arguing. Instead, provide support by stating, "I believe that you (see, hear) that; however, I do not (see, hear) that." Use nonthreatening mannerisms, facial expressions, and tone of voice.
- Initiate measures that prevent or reduce excessive agitation:
  - ❑ Reduce environmental stimuli (e.g., alarms, loud or unnecessary talking).
  - ❑ Before touching patient, explain interventions, using short, concise statements.
  - ❑ Speak quietly (but firmly, as necessary), and project a caring attitude. ("We are very concerned for your comfort and safety. Can we do anything to help you feel more relaxed?")
  - ❑ Avoid crowding (e.g., of equipment, visitors, health care personnel) in patient's personal environment.
  - ❑ Avoid direct confrontation.
- Explain and discuss patient's behavior with family/significant others. Acknowledge frustration, concerns, fears, and questions. Review safety precautions with family/significant others (Table 1-41).

Hopelessness related to prolonged isolation or activity restriction; failing or deteriorating physiologic condition; long-term stress; loss of faith in God or belief system

Desired outcome: Before hospital discharge, patient verbalizes hopeful aspects of health status and relates that feelings of despair are absent or lessened.

- Develop open, honest communication with the patient. Actively listen, be empathic about patient's fears and doubts, and promote an environment that is conducive to free expression.
- Assess patient's and family's/significant others' understanding of health status and prognosis; clarify any misperceptions.

TABLE 1-41 Safety Precautions in the Event of Violent Behavior

Patient safety
- Remove harmful objects from the environment, such as heavy objects, scissors, tubing
- Apply padding to side rails according to agency protocol.
- If available, use bed alarms.
- Use restraints as necessary and prescribed. Monitor patient's neurovascular status at frequent intervals.
- Set limits on patient's behavior, using clear and simple commands.
- As prescribed, consider chemical sedation when unable to control patient's behavior with other means.
- Explain safety precautions to patient and family/significant others.

Caregiver safety
- Place patient in bed closest to nursing station. Maintain visibility at all times by keeping door open.
- Alert hospital security department when risk of violence is present.
- Do not approach a violent patient without adequate assistance from others.
- Never turn your back on a violent patient.
- Maintain a clam, matter-of-fact tone of voice.
- Monitor security measures at frequent intervals.
- Remain alert.

- Assess for indicators of hopelessness: unwillingness to accept help, pessimism, withdrawal, lack of interest, silence, loss of gratification in roles, previous history of hopeless behavior, hypoactivity, inability to accomplish tasks, expressions of incompetence, closing eyes, and turning away.

Research Brief 1-7 Patients in ICU often experience anxiety, but patients are not always able to respond to current validated measures of anxiety such as the Brief Symptom Inventory. A study was performed to assess the ability of intensive care patients to respond to the Faces Anxiety Scale and to investigate if the scaled yields ordinal and interval data. Forty intensive care patients were asked to respond to the Faces Anxiety Scale, the anxiety subscale of the Brief Symptom Inventory, and a numeric analog anxiety scale; and 100 hospital and university staff and students were asked to place the five faces in rank order. The Faces Anxiety Scale elicited more responses from ICU patients than the numeric analog anxiety scale or the anxiety subscale of the Brief Symptom Inventory. The Faces Anxiety Scale is easy for patients to use, obtains self-report from ICU patients more often than other simple scales, and has evidence of interval scale properties of rank order and equality between the points on the scale.

From McKinley S, Cooke K, Stein-Parbury J: Development and testing of a Faces Scale for the assessment of anxiety in critically ill patients, *J Adv Nurs* 41(1):73-79, 2003.

- Provide opportunities for the patient to feel cared for, needed, and valued by others. For example, emphasize importance of relationships. ("Tell me about your grandchildren." "It seems that your family loves you very much.")
- Support significant others who seem to spark or maintain patient's feelings of hope. ("Your husband's mood seemed to improve after your visit.")
- Recognize factors that promote sense of hope (e.g., discussions about family members, reminiscing about better times).
- Explore patient's coping mechanisms; assist with expanding positive coping behavior (see "Ineffective Individual Coping," p. 71).
- Assess spiritual foundation and needs (see "Spiritual Distress," p. 74).
- Promote anticipation of positive events (e.g., mealtime, grandchildren's visits, bath time, extubation, removal of traction).

- Help patient recognize that although there may be no hope for returning to original lifestyle, there *is* hope for a new but different life.
- Avoid insisting that the patient assume a positive attitude. Encourage hope for the future, even if it is the hope for a peaceful death.
- Set realistic, attainable goals, and reward achievement.

Psychosocial Support for the Patient's Family and Significant Others

NURSING DIAGNOSES AND INTERVENTIONS

Altered family processes related to situational crisis (patient's illness)

Desired outcome: After intervention, family/significant others demonstrate effective adaptation to change/traumatic situation as evidenced by seeking external support when necessary and sharing concerns.

- Assess character of family/significant others: social, environmental, ethnic, and cultural factors; relationships; and role patterns. Identify developmental stage. Be aware that other situational or maturational crises may be ongoing, such as an elderly parent or teenager with a learning disability.
- Assess previous adaptive behaviors. ("How do you react in stressful situations?") Discuss observed conflicts and communication breakdown. ("I noticed that your brother would not visit your mother today. Has there been a problem we should be aware of? Knowing about it may help us better care for your mother.")
- Acknowledge the family's/significant others' involvement in patient care, and promote strengths. ("You were able to encourage your wife to turn and cough. That is very important to her recovery.") Encourage participation in patient care conferences. Promote frequent, regular patient visits.
- Provide information and guidance related to the patient. Discuss the stresses of hospitalization, and encourage discussions of feelings, such as anger, guilt, hostility, depression, fear, or sorrow. ("You seem to be upset since having been told that your husband is not leaving the hospital today.") Refer to clergy, case manager, clinical nurse specialist, social services, or palliative care specialist as appropriate.
- Evaluate interactions among patient and family/significant others. Encourage reorganization of roles and priority setting as appropriate. ("I know your husband is concerned about his insurance policy and seems to expect you to investigate it. I'll ask the financial counselor to talk with you.")
- Encourage family/significant others to schedule periods of rest and activity outside the critical care unit and to seek support when necessary. ("Your neighbor volunteered to stay in the waiting room this afternoon. Would you like to rest at home? I'll call you if *anything* changes.")

NIC Family Integrity Promotion; Family Process Maintenance; Normalization Promotion

Family coping: potential for growth, related to use of support systems and referrals; choosing experiences that optimize wellness

Desired outcomes: At the time of the patient's diagnosis, family/significant others express their intent to use support systems and resources and identify alternative behaviors that promote communication and strengths. Family/significant others express realistic expectations and decrease use of ineffective coping behaviors.

- Assess relationships, interactions, support systems, and individual coping behaviors. Permit movement through stages of adaptation. Encourage further positive coping.
- Acknowledge expressions of hope, future plans, and growth among family members/significant others.
- Encourage development of open, honest communication. Provide opportunities in a private setting for interactions, discussions, and questions. ("I know the waiting room is very crowded. Would you like some private time together?")
- Refer the family/significant others to community or support groups (e.g., ostomy support group, head injury rehabilitation group).
- Encourage exploration of outlets that foster positive feelings, for example, periods of time outside the hospital area, meaningful communication with the patient or support individuals, and relaxing activities (e.g., showering, eating, exercising).

Ineffective family coping: compromised, related to inadequate or incorrect information or misunderstanding; temporary family disorganization and role change; exhausted support systems; unrealistic expectations; fear; anxiety

Desired outcomes: After interventions, family/significant others verbalize feelings, identify ineffective coping patterns, identify strengths and positive coping behaviors, and seek information and support from the nurse or other support systems.

- Establish open, honest communication. Assist in identifying strengths, stressors, inappropriate behaviors, and personal needs. ("I understand your mother was very ill last year. How did you manage the situation?" "I know your loved one is very ill. How can I help you?")
- Assess for ineffective coping (e.g., depression, substance abuse, violence, withdrawal), and identify factors that inhibit effective coping (e.g., inadequate support system, grief, fear of disapproval by others, knowledge deficit). ("You seem to be unable to talk about your husband's illness. Is there anyone with whom you can talk about it?")
- Assess knowledge regarding patient's current health status and therapies. Provide information frequently, and allow sufficient time for questions. Reassess understanding at frequent intervals.
- Provide opportunities in a private setting to talk and share concerns with nurses or other health care providers. If appropriate, refer to psychiatric clinical nurse specialist for therapy.
- Offer realistic hope. Help family/significant others develop realistic expectations for the future and identify support systems that will assist them with planning for the future.
- Reduce anxiety by encouraging diversionary activities (e.g., period of time outside of hospital) and interaction with outside support systems. ("I know you want to be near your son, but if you would like to go home to rest, I will call you if *any* changes occur.")

NIC NIC Family Involvement Promotion; Family Mobilization; Family Support

Ineffective family coping: disabling, related to unexpressed feelings; ambivalent family relationships; disharmonious coping styles among family members/significant others

Desired outcomes: Before hospital discharge, family/significant others verbalize feelings, identify sources of support as well as ineffective coping behaviors that create ambivalence and disharmony, and do not demonstrate destructive behaviors.

- Establish open, honest communication and rapport. ("I am here to care for your mother and to help you, as well.")
- Identify ineffective coping behaviors (e.g., violence, depression, substance abuse, withdrawal). ("You seem to be angry. Would you like to talk to me about your feelings?") Refer to psychiatric clinical nurse specialist, clergy, or support group as appropriate.
- Identify perceived or actual conflicts. ("Are you able to talk freely among yourselves?" "Are your brothers and sisters able to help and support you during this time?")
- Encourage healthy functioning. For example, facilitate open communication and encourage behaviors that support cohesiveness. ("Your mother enjoyed your last visit. Would you like to see her now?")
- Assess knowledge about patient's current health status. Provide opportunities for questions; reassess understanding at frequent intervals.
- Assist with developing realistic goals, plans, and actions. Refer to clergy, case manager, psychiatric nurse, social services, financial counseling, and family therapy as appropriate.
- Encourage family/significant others to spend time outside of the hospital and to interact with support individuals. Respect the need for occasional withdrawal.
- Include the family/significant others in the patient's plan of care. Offer them opportunities to become involved in patient care, for example, ROM exercises, patient hygiene, and comfort measures (e.g., back rub).

NIC NIC Family Support; Family Process Maintenance

Fear: related to patient's life-threatening condition; knowledge deficit

Desired outcome: After intervention, family/significant others relate that fear has been lessened or is manageable.

- Assess fears and understanding related to the patient's clinical situation. Evaluate verbal and nonverbal responses.
- Acknowledge the fears. ("I understand these tubes must frighten you, but they are necessary to help nourish your son.")
- Assess history of coping behavior. ("How do you react to difficult situations?") Determine resources and significant others available for support. ("Who/what usually helps during stressful times?")
- Provide opportunities for expression of fears and concerns. Recognize that anger, denial, withdrawal, and demanding behavior may be adaptive coping responses during initial period of crisis.
- Provide information at frequent intervals about patient's status and the therapies and equipment used. Demonstrate a caring attitude.
- Encourage use of positive coping behaviors by identifying the fear(s), developing goals, identifying supportive resources, facilitating realistic perceptions, and promoting problem solving.

- Recognize anxiety, and encourage family/significant others to describe their feelings. ("You seem very uncomfortable tonight. Can you describe your feelings?")
- Be alert to maladaptive responses to fear: potential for violence, withdrawal, severe depression, hostility, and unrealistic expectations of staff or of patient's recovery. Provide referrals to psychiatric clinical nurse specialist or palliative care specialist as appropriate.
- Offer *realistic* hope, even if it is the hope for the patient's peaceful death.
- Explore desires for spiritual, religious, or psychologic counseling.
- Assess your own feelings about the patient's life-threatening illness. Acknowledge that your attitude and fear may be reflected to the family/significant others.
- For other interventions, see previous nursing diagnoses: "Altered Family Processes," p. 78; "Ineffective Family Coping: Compromised," p. 78; and "Ineffective Family Coping: Disabling," p. 79.

NIC Coping Enhancement; Security Enhancement; Support System Enhancement

Knowledge deficit: patient's current health status; therapies

---

Research Brief 1-8   The long-term effects on patients' families after a prolonged stay in a surgical ICU are unclear. A study was performed to test the hypothesis that illnesses requiring more than 7 days' stay in the surgical ICU would have significant, long-lasting effects on patients' families and would be related to the patients' functional outcome. Maximal dysfunction/impact was compared with patients' functional outcome in 128 ICU patients with 7-day or longer lengths of stay in the ICU. Significant disturbances in the families' lives occurred throughout the 12 months of the study. Nearly 45% of caregivers had to quit work after 1 month, and more than 36% of families lost savings after 1 year. A prolonged stay in the surgical ICU has a profound effect on families that is greatest in the first 3 months and parallels the patient's functional outcome. Systems that provide support to patients and their families should be provided in the hospital and after discharge.

Swoboda S, Lipsett P: Impact of a prolonged critical illness on patients' families, *Am J Crit Care* 11(5):459-466, 2002.

Desired outcome: After intervention, family/significant others verbalize knowledge and understanding about the patient's current diet, disease process, health resources, medication, prescribed activity, treatment procedures, and treatment regimen.

- At frequent intervals, inform the family/significant others about the patient's current health status, therapies, and prognosis. Use individualized verbal, written, and audiovisual strategies to promote understanding.
- Evaluate family/significant others at frequent intervals for understanding of information that has been provided. Adjust teaching as appropriate. Some individuals in crisis need repeated explanations before comprehension can be assured. ("I have explained many things to you today. Would you mind summarizing what I've told you so that I can be sure you understand your husband's status and what we are doing to care for him?")
- Encourage family/significant others to relay correct information to the patient. This also reinforces comprehension for family/significant others and patient.
- Ask if needs for information are being met. ("Do you have any questions about the care your mother is receiving or about her condition?")
- Help family/significant others use the information they receive to guide health care decisions (e.g., regarding patient's surgery, resuscitation, organ donation).
- Promote active participation in patient care when appropriate. Encourage family/significant others to seek information and express feelings, concerns, and questions.

NIC Learning Facilitation; Learning Readiness Enhancement

Ethical Considerations in Critical Care

More controversy surrounds health care decisions made by and for critical care patients than in any other health care area. These decisions have been debated vigorously in the literature, and although some of these issues have been resolved, others continue to be argued. Here we will examine what is currently considered morally acceptable practice.

Health care providers must develop a clear understanding of ethical issues to ensure that the care they provide is morally and legally acceptable. Ethical reasoning enables the health care professional to examine the moral principles involved in decision making and determine what he or she ought to do. There are four predominant principles used in health care ethics for decision making: (1) respect for autonomy (recognizing that each patient has a right to make decisions for himself), (2) nonmaleficence (not harming a patient), (3) beneficence (helping a patient), and (4) justice (treating patients equally). Ethical dilemmas occur when one of these principles conflicts with another. When a patient refuses needed treatment, the principles of autonomy and beneficence are in conflict. Other processes and documents related to decision making are discussed below.

INFORMED CONSENT

Without adequate knowledge, patients and significant others cannot make good decisions. Part of a nurse's obligation is to inform patients and families, in a caring manner, what is to be expected regarding different treatments. Informed consent serves not only to protect the health care provider from liability; its primary purpose is to support the ethical principle of respect for autonomy. Informed consent is instrumental to a patient's right to accept, continue, or reject all or part of health care interventions of any sort. The elements of informed consent should be used as a guide but are not absolutely necessary for all nursing or medical interventions (Table 1-42).

If a patient is unsure, does not understand, or feels pressured about consenting to the treatment plan, nurses are responsible to advocate for the patient and communicate this to the physician and to the hospital administration if necessary.

ADVANCE DIRECTIVES

Advance directives refer to a patient's directions on how to provide care in the event that the patient becomes unable to make decisions. An advance directive can be written or verbal and can be in the form of a living will or a durable power of attorney for health care (DPAHC).

A living will specifies what treatment a patient wants or does not want in the event that the condition is terminal and the patient cannot make health care decisions. A DPAHC appoints a person to make decisions for a patient when the patient cannot make decisions.

A surrogate decision maker is someone named in the DPAHC. When no DPAHC exists, the legal next of kin becomes the surrogate decision maker for the patient. If the patient does not have family or a DPAHC, a court-appointed guardian becomes the surrogate decision maker. This person is obligated to make choices that the patient would make. If those choices are unknown, the surrogate decision maker must try to determine, based on the patient's values, what the patient would want.

Advance directives appeal to the ethical principle of respect for autonomy. When no advance directive is available, we then turn to the ethical principle of beneficence by making decisions in the patient's best interest. Advance directives are supported by the Patient Self-Determination Act, which encourages their use as well as prompts health care providers and institutions to honor them. Interpretation of advance directives can be problematic. Although many patients express a desire for

---

T A B L E 1 - 42   Elements of Informed Consent

Threshold elements (preconditions)
1. Competence (to understand and decide)
2. Voluntaries (in deciding)

Information elements
3. Disclosure (of material information)
4. Recommendation (of a plan)
5. Understanding (of nos. 3 and 4)

Consent elements
6. Decision (in favor of a plan)
7. Authorization (of the chosen plan)

From Beauchamp TL, Childress JF: *Principles of biomedical ethics,* ed 5, pp 80, New York, 2001, Oxford University Press.

no "extraordinary measures," the meaning of this term can vary. For example, a ventilator can be considered "extraordinary," but it is also part of quite common temporary treatments regularly used in critical care. Despite problems with interpretation, caregivers must responsibly deal with their ambiguities and seek to honor their spirit.

CONFIDENTIALITY

Confidentiality in a relationship between a health care provider and a patient means that we do not identify or expose information that is not relevant to care. Also, we do not communicate information gained from a patient except with providers and decision makers identified by the patient. Confidentiality appeals to the ethical principles of respect for autonomy, beneficence, and nonmaleficence. Almost all nursing and medical codes provide for keeping all information about a patient confidential. Any disclosure of patient information should be considered very carefully.

However, there are situations in which we are legally obligated to breach patient confidentiality. These situations include public welfare risks, sexually transmitted diseases, gunshot wounds, and suspected abuse of children, elders, or developmentally disabled individuals. Whereas we are *legally* obligated to report such incidents, we are *morally* obligated to let the patient know that we must report the incident.

QUALITY OF LIFE

Most quality-of-life dilemmas in health care appeal to the ethical principle of justice. A person's quality of life is based on physical, intellectual, emotional, and social components. Although improving quality of life is a primary focus of health care, assessing quality of life is difficult at best. Numerous studies have demonstrated that health care providers consistently rate patients' quality of life lower than the patients do themselves. Studies also reveal that such judgments by health care providers do affect care. Nurses in critical care should be aware they are seeing only a minuscule part of a patient's entire life. Quality-of-life assessments may be based on a patient's medical condition during this time. Patients take into account things such as family, relationships, and finances when assessing their own quality of life.

A patient's assessment of quality of life may be compromised when that patient becomes depressed or newly disabled (e.g., stroke, paraplegia, quadriplegia). Although critical care nurses care for many patients in such situations, it is usually the first time that this patient or family has faced such life-altering circumstances. The stress of the situation makes evaluation of quality of life difficult for them. It is important to provide the patient and family with support and time before making critical decisions.

Studies indicate that health care providers not only base quality of life on the patient's medical condition, but also have social prejudices that affect care. These include prejudices against the elderly, persons with alternative lifestyles, those with alcohol or substance abuse, and patients with criminal activity. Judgments may be passed on to others during nursing reports. This promotes prejudice rather than good care. Our justice system, not our health care system, determines what behaviors to punish and how they should be punished.

WITHHOLDING AND WITHDRAWING TREATMENT

Withholding (not starting) and withdrawing (stopping) treatment are considered to have no moral or legal difference. However, health care providers and patients' family members are misguidedly more comfortable withholding than with withdrawing treatment. Once a treatment has been started and is determined to be of no benefit to the patient, the reasons used to justify withholding treatment can be used when stopping or withdrawing care. The decision can be reinforced by appealing to the principles of nonmaleficence and beneficence along with the knowledge that the treatment has not benefited the patient.

It has been noted that when decisions to withhold resuscitation (do not resuscitate [DNR]) have been made, it seems unclear what other care should be provided. DNR does not mean do not treat. Many patients with DNR orders receive critical care interventions, surgery, and other treatments and then survive to discharge. Once a decision has been made to withhold resuscitation, it is important to clearly define treatments to be withheld or provided.

ASSISTED SUICIDE

Assisted suicide occurs when someone provides a means for a patient to commit suicide (such as deliberately providing enough medicine for an overdose) but the patient actually performs the act that results in death. Although controversy surrounds assisted suicide, the American Nurses Association (ANA), the American Association of Critical Care Nurses (AACN), the American Medical Association (AMA), and the National Hospice Organization (NHO) explicitly oppose it. Most states have laws that make assisted suicide a criminal act. In 1994, Oregon became the first and only state to allow physician-assisted suicide for terminally ill patients. The Oregon law continues to face legal challenges. In the summer of 1997, the U.S. Supreme Court determined that there is no constitutional right to physician-assisted suicide.

EUTHANASIA

Euthanasia refers to one person killing another person without causing pain. Several studies reveal a significant number of nurses believe euthanasia is justifiable and should be legalized. This indicates a serious conflict of interest by health care providers. Euthanasia is illegal, is opposed by nursing and medical codes, and is morally unacceptable. Even if the intent of euthanasia is "compassion" and the patient requests it, if the health care provider intentionally kills a patient, that health care provider is morally and legally responsible for that patient's death.

COMFORT CARE

Patients who are chronically ill, debilitated, or dying are generally isolated from and by society as well as by health care providers. Health care providers now recognize pain and depression may be undertreated in the routine care of patients, and while caring for those who are chronically ill or dying. Concerns center around fears of causing dependence, unresponsiveness, and even death. When faced with a dying patient, it is unreasonable to worry about potential dependence on medication. The benefits of analgesics far outweigh the risks of dependence. Health care providers should try to provide the maximal pain relief possible while preserving responsiveness. When that is not possible, most patients and families choose to accept a decreased responsiveness to ensure that adequate pain relief is provided for the dying patient.

Many health care providers voice concerns that giving potent opioids to a dying patient may actually kill the patient. This concern is magnified when decisions to withdraw and withhold treatments have been made simultaneously. Opioid analgesics afford a broad therapeutic index and have a long history of safe use in medically frail patients. Patients can tolerate increasing doses of opioids without adverse respiratory or cardiovascular effects.

Even though it is very difficult to determine what amount of opioid will cause a person's death, such medicines can still be given by appealing to the principle of double effect. Simplified, this principle explains that giving narcotics to relieve pain is morally acceptable, even while knowing that it may also cause the patient to die sooner. When narcotics and sedatives are given to a patient at the end of life, the intent is to provide comfort until death; the health care provider does not intend to cause the patient to die. If the health care provider gives a medicine with the primary intent of killing a patient, the health care provider is euthanizing that patient and the action is immoral and illegal.

ETHICAL REASONING

When nurses find themselves in a situation in which they think something is "wrong," they should first consider the situation logically and systematically. By doing this, nurses can defend their positions rationally and provide ethically as well as medically sound care.

1. Identify the problem. Is the care provided inappropriate?
2. Determine the relevant facts of the case. These facts include the patient's medical, mental, and emotional condition, as well as the current plan of care.
3. Evaluate personal biases. The nurse must consider his or her personal values and ethical position regarding the situation as it may affect care. Nurses should consider the values and ethical positions of all of the decision makers involved.
4. Check for advance directives. If the patient is incompetent, does he or she have an advance directive?
5. Explore options and their consequences. Explore all plausible options for resolving the dilemma. Consider the consequences of each option.
6. Discuss the relevant ethical principles in the situation. For example, a question asked may be "Will continued aggressive treatment respect the patient's autonomy by following the advance directive?"
7. Rank the acceptable options in order of importance. Develop and implement a plan for choosing options, including timelines for choices.
8. Clarify the expectations and wishes of those involved. Table 1-43 outlines steps used to begin clarifying our understanding of the situation so appropriate decisions can be made.

If direct communication with those involved does not resolve the issue, the bedside nurse should then involve the charge nurse or unit manager. The medical director's involvement may be beneficial also. If assistance is still needed in resolving the dilemma, the Joint Commission on Accreditation of

---

T A B L E   1 - 43   Components of Ethical Reasoning

---

1. Identify the actual problems.
2. Determine the relevant facts of the case.
3. Consider the values and ethical positions of everyone involved.
4. Determine possible options for resolving the dilemma.
5. Consider consequences of each option identified.
6. Apply relevant ethical principles to each option identified.
7. Prioritize acceptable options.
8. Develop and implement a plan to resolve the dilemma.
9. Evaluate the resolution of the dilemma.

Healthcare Organizations (JCAHO) requires that health care providers have access to institutional means for resolving ethical dilemmas (such as an ethics consultant or committee). If a nurse strongly believes that unethical care is being provided and an acceptable resolution to the issue is not found, the nurse should withdraw from caring for that patient. Before withdrawing from that patient, however, the nurse must be replaced by another equally competent nurse who does not oppose the plan of care.

PREVENTIVE ETHICS

Just as it is easier to prevent heart disease than it is to cure it, it is easier to prevent an ethical conflict than it is to resolve one. When evaluating actions taken to resolve a dilemma, nurses should consider how those actions can provide help with future dilemmas. When the bedside nurse first sees signs of a problem, strategies used in previous, similar situations should be employed to prevent this situation from developing into a conflict. Many seemingly ethical problems are actually communication deficits. Such problems may be resolved after gathering information and coordinating a patient care conference involving all relevant persons. All professionals should refrain from speculation or gossip and instead openly communicate with the patient, family, and other members of the care team about the plan of care. The nurse should promote discussions in advance of all possible outcomes. Last and most important, nurses should respect each patient as a person and treat that patient accordingly.

NURSING DIAGNOSES AND INTERVENTIONS

Knowledge deficit: medical/nursing interventions
Desired outcome: Before any medical or nursing intervention, patient/significant others will know, understand, and agree to or refuse the intervention.
• Determine appropriate decision maker
• Assess decision making capacity
• Assess decision maker's understanding of intervention; provide information as indicated
• Determine voluntariness
• Accept patient's/significant others' permission for or refusal of the intervention
▌NIC NIC Teaching: Procedure/Treatment; Teaching: Disease Process; Learning Facilitation
Knowledge deficit: end-of-life decisions
Desired outcome: Patient will know and understand options regarding living wills and DPAHC.
• Provide patient with information regarding living wills and DPAHC.
• Assess understanding of living wills/DPAHC; provide information as indicated.
• Determine who is legally empowered as a surrogate decision maker.
▌NIC NIC Health System Guidance; Patient Rights Protection
Anticipatory grieving related to withholding/withdrawal of treatment; anticipation of loss
Desired outcome: After interventions, patient and significant others communicate feelings and participate in decisions regarding death and dying.
• Assess patient's/significant others' understanding of medical prognosis and planned interventions.
• Provide specific information regarding what to expect, what care/interventions will be given, and what will be withheld/discontinued; answer questions openly.
• Allow for significant others to be with patient during the dying process.
• Provide all comfort measures possible for patient/significant others.

NIC Grief Work Facilitation; Support System Enhancement; Active Listening; Family Support; Environmental Management: Comfort; Spiritual Support; Decision-Making Support

Bibliography

Alanso JA, Kallett RH, Siebal M, et al: *Crit Care Med* 27:A93, 1999.

Alcock NW: Laboratory tests for assessing nutritional status. In Shills ME et al, editors: *Modern nutrition in health and disease,* ed 9, Baltimore, 1999, Williams and Wilkins.

American Association of Cardiovascular and Pulmonary Rehabilitation (AACVPR): *Guidelines for cardiac rehabilitation and secondary prevention programs,* ed 3, Champaign, Ill, 1999, Human Kinetics.

American College of Sports Medicine (ACSM): *Guidelines for exercise testing and prescription,* ed 6, Philadelphia, 2002, Lippincott, Williams & Wilkins.

Anderson J: Management of four arterial blood gas problems in adult mechanical ventilation: decision-making algorithms and rationale for their use, *Crit Care Nurse* 16(3):62-73, 1996.

Apelgren KN et al: Comparison of nutritional indices and outcomes in critically ill patients, *Crit Care Med* 10:305-307, 1982.

Asch DA, DeKay ML: Euthanasia among US critical care nurses: practices, attitudes, and social and professional correlates, *Med Care* 35:890-900, 1997.

Baranoski S: Wound dressings: challenging decisions, *Home Healthcare Nurse* 17(1):19-25, 1999.

Beauchamp TL, Childress JF: *Principles of biomedical ethics,* ed 4, New York, 1994, Oxford University Press.

Bednash G, Ferrell BR: *End-of-life nursing education consortium (ELNEC) faculty guide,* Duarte, Calif, 2002, American Association of Colleges of Nursing and City of Hope National Medical Center.

Benjamin M, Curtis J: *Ethics in nursing,* ed 3, New York, 1992, Oxford University Press.

Benner P. Seeing the person beyond the disease, *Am J Crit Care* 13(1):75-78, 2004.

Borg GV: Psychophysical basis of perceived exertion, *Med Sci Sports Exerc* 14:377-381, 1982.

Bos S: Coma stimulation, *Online J Knowledge Synthesis* 4(1):1997.

Bozeman M: Cultural aspects of pain management. In Salerno E, Willens JS, editors: *Pain management handbook: an interdisciplinary approach,* St Louis, 1996, Mosby.

Branson RD, Campbell RS: Modes of Ventilator Operation. In MacIntyre NR, Branson RD: *Mechanical ventilation,* Philadelphia, 2001, Saunders.

Branson RD, MacIntyre NR: Dual control modes of mechanical ventilation, *Respir Care* 41:294-305, 1996.

Braunwalde E: Valvular Heart Disease. In Braunwald E, editor: *Textbook of cardiovascular disease,* ed 6, Philadelphia, 2001, Saunders.

Brower R et al: Treatment of ARDS: *Chest* 120:1347-1367, 2001.

Byas-Smith M: Management of acute exacerbation of chronic pain syndromes. In Sinatra RS et al, editors: *Acute pain: mechanisms and management,* St Louis, 1992, Mosby.

Case KO, Cuddy PK, McGurk EP: Nutrition support in the critically ill patient. *Crit Care Nurs Q* 22(4):75-89, 2000.

Cassem NH, Lopez GA, Bleck TP: Acute and subacute psychiatric disorders. In Parrillo JE, Dellinger RP: *Critical care medicine: principles of diagnosis and management in the adult,* St Louis, 2002, Mosby.

Celesia G: Persistent vegetative state: clinical and ethical issues, *Theo Med* 18:221-236, 1997.

Chatburn RL, Branson RD: Classification of mechanical ventilators. In MacIntyre NR, Branson RD: *Mechanical ventilation,* Philadelphia, 2001, Saunders.

Clarke EB et.al: Quality indicators for end of life in the intensive care unit. *Crit Care Med* 31(9):2255-2262, 2003.

Conwell Y, Caine ED: Rational suicide and the right to die: reality and myth, *N Engl J Med* 325:1101-1102, 1991.

Curtis JR, Rubenfeld GD: *Managing death in the intensive care unit,* New York, 2001, Oxford University Press.

Davis A, White J: Innovative sensory input for the comatose brain-injured patient, *Crit Care Nurs Clin North Am* 7(2):351-361, 1995.

Davis AJ et al: Nurses' attitudes toward active euthanasia, *Nurs Outlook* 43(4):174-179, 1995.

Darvovic G: *Hemodynamic monitoring, invasive and noninvasive clinical application,* Philadelphia, 2002, Saunders.

Dochterman JM, Bulechek GM, editors: *Nursing interventions classifications (NIC),* ed 4, St Louis, 2004, Mosby.

Duff D, Wells D: Postcomatose unawareness/vegetative state following severe brain injury: a content methodology, *J Neurosci Nurs* 29(5):305-317, 1997.

Evans NJ: The role of total parenteral nutrition in critical illness: guidelines and recommendations, *AACN Clinical Issues* 5:476-484, 1994.

Fahey PJ, Tobin MJ: Weaning from ventilatory support. In Baum GL et al, editors: *Textbook of pulmonary diseases,* ed 6, Philadelphia, 1998, Lippincott-Raven.

Ferrell B, Coyle N: *Textbook of palliative nursing,* New York, 2001, Oxford University Press.

Folstein M, Folstein S, McHugh P: Mini-mental state: a practical method for grading the cognitive state of patients for clinicians, *J Psychiatr Res* 12(5):189-198, 1975.

Frawley M, Habashi N: AACN Clinical Issues, *AACN* 12(2): 234-246, 2001.

Gardner SE, Frantz RA, Doebbeling BN: The validity of the clinical signs and symptoms used to identify localized chronic wound infection, *Wound Repair & Regeneration* 9(3):178-186, 2001.

Gentile MA, Cheifetz IM: Extracorporeal techniques for cardiopulmonary support. In MacIntyre NR, Branson RD: *Mechanical ventilation,* Philadelphia, 2001, WB Saunders.

Giacino J: Disorders of consciousness: differential diagnosis and neuropathologic features, *Semin Neurol* 17(2):105-111, 1997.

Govert JA: Positioning the patient. In MacIntyre NR, Branson RD: *Mechanical ventilation,* Philadelphia, 2001, Saunders.

Hess D: Heliox and inhaled nitric oxide. In MacIntyre NR, Branson RD: *Mechanical ventilation,* Philadelphia, 2001, Saunders.

Heymsfield SB, Baumgartner RN: Nutritional assessment of malnutrition by anthropometric methods. In Shils ME et al, editors: *Modern nutrition in health and disease,* ed 9, Baltimore, 1999, Williams and Wilkins.

Hirschl RB et al: Initial experience with partial liquid ventilation in adult patients with acute respiratory distress syndrome, *JAMA* 275:383-389, 1996.

Howard CA: Mechanical ventilation. In Keen JH, Swearingen PL, editors: *Mosby's critical care nursing consultant,* St Louis, 1997, Mosby.

Inaba-Roland K, Maricle R: Assessing delirium in the acute care setting, *Heart Lung* 21(2):48-55, 1992.

Inouye S et al: Clarifying confusion: the confusion assessment method. A new method for detection of delirium, *Ann Intern Med* 113(12):941-948, 1990.

Jonsen AR et al: *Clinical ethics,* ed 5, New York, 2002, McGraw-Hill.

Kim MJ, McFarland GK, McLane AM: *Pocket guide to nursing diagnoses,* ed 7, St Louis, 1997, Mosby.

Kirby RR, Taylor RW, Civetta JM: Ventilatory support modes. In Kirby RR, editor: *Handbook of critical care,* ed 2, Philadelphia, 1997, Lippincott-Raven.

Knudson NW, Fulkerson WJ: Lung injury from mechanical ventilation. In MacIntyre NR, Branson RD: *Mechanical ventilation,* Philadelphia, 2001, Saunders.

Kress J, O'Connor M: Daily interruption of sedative infusions in critically ill patients undergoing mechanical ventilation, *N Engl J Med* 342:1471-1477, 2000.

Litton K: Delirium in the critical care patient: what the professional staff needs to know, *Crit Care Nurs Q* 26(3):208-213, 2003.

Lode HM et al: Nosocomial pneumonia in the critical care unit, *Crit Care Clin* 14(1):119-133, 1998.

Luer J: Sedation and neuromuscular blockade in patients with acute respiratory failure, *Crit Care Nurse* 22(5):70-75, 2002.

Lynn J, Schuster J, Kabcenell A: *Improving care for the end of life, a sourcebook for health care managers and clinicians,* New York, 2000, Oxford University Press.

MacIntyre NR: Mechanical ventilatory support. In Baum GL et al, editors: *Textbook of pulmonary diseases,* ed 6, Philadelphia, 1998, Lippincott-Raven.

MacIntyre NR: High frequency ventilation. In MacIntyre NR, Branson RD: *Mechanical ventilation,* Philadelphia, 2001, WB Saunders.

MacIntyre NR: Ventilator monitors, displays and alarms. In MacIntyre NR, Branson RD: *Mechanical ventilation,* Philadelphia, 2001, WB Saunders.

MacIntyre NR: Patient-ventilator interactions. In MacIntyre NR, Branson RD: *Mechanical ventilation,* Philadelphia, 2001, WB Saunders.

MacIntyre NR: Weaning mechanical ventilatory support. In MacIntyre NR, Branson RD: *Mechanical ventilation,* Philadelphia, 2001, WB Saunders.

MacIntyre NR: Evidence-based guidelines for weaning and discontinuing ventilatory support, *Chest* 120:375s-396s, 2001.

Mackay L et al: Early intervention in severe head injury: long-term benefits of a formalized program, *Arch Phys Med Rehabil* 73:635-641, 1992.

Malkmus D, Booth B, Kodimer C: *Rehabilitation of the head-injured adult: comprehensive cognitive management,* Downey, Calif, 1980, Professional Staff Association of the Rancho Los Amigos Hospital.

Matzo M, Sherman D: *Palliative care nursing, quality care to the end of life.* New York, 2001, Springer.

McCaffery M: How to calculate a rescue dose, *Am J Nurs* 94(4):65-66, 1996.

McCloskey JC, Bulechek GM, editors: *Nursing interventions classifications (NIC),* ed 3, St Louis, 2000, Mosby.

McConnell, RR Jr: Modifications on conventional ventilation techniques. In MacIntyre NR, Branson RD: *Mechanical ventilation,* Philadelphia, 2001, WB Saunders.

McGee DC, Weinacker AB, Raffin TA: Ethical concerns in managing critically ill patients. In Parrillo JP, Dellinger RP: *Critical care medicine: principles of diagnosis and management in adults,* ed 2, St Louis, 2002, Mosby.

McGinnis C: Parenteral nutrition focus: nutrition assessment and formula composition, *J Infus Nurs* 25:54-64, 2002.

Melltorp G, Nilstun T: The difference between withholding and withdrawing life-sustaining treatment, *Intensive Care Med* 23:1264-1267, 1997.

Milisen K et al: Delirium in the hospitalized elderly: nursing assessment and management, *Nurs Clin North Am* 33(3):417-436, 1998.

Olsen DP: When the patient causes the problem: the effect of patient responsibility on the nurse-patient relationship, *J Adv Nurs* 26:515-522, 1997.

Ozuna J: Persistent vegetative state: important considerations for the neuroscience nurse, *J Neurosci Nurs* 28(3):199-203, 1996.

Plum F, Posner J: *The diagnosis of stupor and coma,* ed 3, Philadelphia, 1980, Davis.

Porta R et al: Mask proportional assist vs pressure support ventilation in patients in clinically stable condition with chronic ventilatory failure. *Chest* 122:479-488, 2002.

Portenoy RK: Morphine infusions at the end of life: the pitfalls in reasoning from anecdote, *J Palliat Care* 12:44-46, 1996.

Prendergast TJ, Puntillo KA: Withdrawal of life support: intensive caring at the end of life, *JAMA* 288(21):2732-2740, 2002.

Punyatavorn W, Bunburaphong S: Validity and reliability of cardiac output by arterial thermodilution and arterial pulse contour analysis compared with pulmonary artery thermodilution in intensive care unit. *J Med Assoc Thailand* 86(Suppl 2):S323-S330, 2003.

Rasanen J: APRV. In Tobin M, editor: *Principles and practice of mechanical ventilation,* Maywood, Ill, 1994, McGraw-Hill.

Reickert C et al: The pulmonary and systemic distribution and elimination of perflubron from adult patients treated with partial liquid ventilation, *Chest* 119:515-522, 2001.

Sanders KM, Stern TA: Management of delirium associated with use of the intra-aortic balloon pump, *Am J Crit Care* 2(5):371-377, 1993.

Schinner K et al: Effects of auditory stimuli on intracranial pressure and cerebral perfusion pressure in traumatic brain injury, *J Neurosci Nurs* 27(6):348-354, 1995.

Shike M: Enteral feeding. In Shils ME et al, editors: *Modern nutrition in health and disease,* ed 9, Baltimore, 1999, Williams & Wilkins.

Shils ME, Brown RO: Parenteral nutrition. In Shils ME et al, editors: *Modern nutrition in health and disease,* ed 9, Baltimore, 1999, Williams and Wilkins.

Siegel MD, Matthay M: Sedatives, analgesics, and paralytic agents in the intensive care unit. In Bone R, editor: *Pulmonary and critical care medicine,* St Louis, 1997, Mosby.

Sosnowski C, Ustik M: Early intervention: coma stimulation in the intensive care unit, *J Neurosci Nurs* 26(6):336-341, 1994.

Stotts NA: Promoting wound healing. In MR Kinney et al, editors: *AACN's clinical reference for critical care nursing,* ed 4, St Louis, 1998, Mosby.

Stotts NA: Impaired healing. In Carrieri V, Lindsey AM, West CM, editors: *Pathophysiological phenomena in nursing: human responses to illness,* ed 3, Philadelphia, 2003, Saunders.

Stotts NA, Hunt TK: Managing bacterial colonization and infection, *Clin Geriatr Med* 13(3):565-574, 1997.

Teasdale G, Jennett B: Assessment of coma and impaired consciousness: a practical scale, *Lancet* 2:81, July 6, 1974.

Tess M: Acute confusional states in critically ill patients: a review, *J Neurosci Nurs* 23(6):398-402, 1991.

Tobin M: Mechanical ventilation: conventional modes and settings. In Fishman AP, editor: *Fishman's pulmonary diseases and disorders,* ed 3, New York, 1998, McGraw-Hill.

Uustal DB: Enhancing your ethical reasoning, *Crit Care Nurs Clin North Am* 2(3):437-442, Sept, 1990.

Velasco B, Richards T, Radovancevic B: Relations among heart failure severity, left ventricular loading conditions, and repolarization length in advanced heart failure secondary to ischemic or idiopathic dilated cardiomyopathy, *Am J Cardiol* 92(5):544-547, 2003.

Wilson S et al: Vegetative state and responses to sensory stimulation: an analysis of 24 cases, *Brain Inj* 10(11):807-818, 1996.

Wunderlink RG, Jennings SG: Noninvasive ventilation. In MacIntyre NR, Branson RD: *Mechanical ventilation,* Philadelphia, 2001, WB Saunders.

Yagan MB: Hospital-acquired pneumonia and its management, *Crit Care Nurs Q* 20(3):43, 1997.

Younces M: Proportional assist ventilation. In Tobin M, editor: *Principles and practice of mechanical ventilation,* Maywood, Ill, 1994, McGraw-Hill.

Multisystem Trauma

Major Trauma

PATHOPHYSIOLOGY

Traumatic injuries are the leading cause of death, lost years of potential life, lifetime disability, lost wages, and expenditure of health care dollars in the United States for persons from 1 to 34 years of age, and the fifth most frequent cause of death for all age-groups. Approximately 60 million people are injured in the United States every year. Of those 30 million require medical care and 3.6 million require hospitalization; nearly 200,000 die following trauma. According to the Center for Injury Research and Policy at Johns Hopkins University, the trauma-related cost for the United States alone exceeds $160 billion annually. Aggressive public education and other prevention measures are needed to reduce the staggering burden. Immediate resuscitation and transport to a designated trauma center must occur promptly to maximize chance of survival, limit comorbidities, and potential permanent disability.

Mechanisms of injury: Injuries can be predicted based on knowledge of the object producing the injury (e.g., motor vehicle, handgun); type of energy released (e.g., kinetic, thermal, chemical); force of energy (e.g., velocity of vehicle or missile); and use of protective devices (e.g., seat belts, air bags, helmets).

Types of injury: *Blunt injuries* occur without interrupting skin integrity. The degree of injury is related to the transfer of energy into the tissues and responsiveness of the anatomic structure involved. The compressible hollow organs (e.g., stomach, bladder) are less likely to rupture than solid organs (e.g., liver, spleen) when force is applied. Common causes of blunt injury are vehicular collisions and falls.

Penetrating injuries are those caused by direct damage from the motion of foreign objects that penetrate tissue. Indirect damage may occur because of tissue deformation associated with energy transference from the penetrating object into the surrounding tissues. A process called *cavitation* occurs when a missile penetrates tissue; the surrounding tissue is briefly displaced, creating a temporary cavity. This process is responsible for the massive tissue damage caused by high-velocity missiles (bullets). Injury inflicted by a stab wound generally follows a more predictable pattern and involves less tissue destruction than does injury from a gunshot wound.

Oxygen delivery and consumption: Massive fluid shifts related to tissue damage and blood loss create a severe fluid volume deficit, which leads to hypovolemic shock unless estimated blood and fluid loss is replaced. Bleeding must be controlled. When the number of red blood cells is reduced from blood loss, cellular oxygen supply is reduced, resulting in end organ hypoxia due to inadequate tissue perfusion. Anaerobic metabolism may ensue if blood and volume replacement is inadequate to maintain blood pressure.

After initial restoration of circulating fluid volume, the body may develop a hyperdynamic circulatory state to help compensate for the cellular oxygen debt incurred. This phase should peak at 48-72 hr and diminish within 7-10 days. The hyperdynamic state is evidenced by an increased cardiac index (CI), oxygen delivery (Do_2), and oxygen consumption (Vo_2). Inability to achieve and maintain a hyperdynamic state is associated with higher mortality and shock-related organ failure.

Neuroendocrine stress response: All body systems require both oxygen and glucose for cellular energy production. Following major injury, the central nervous system (CNS) triggers a series of reactions to increase delivery of oxygen and glucose to the cells. Catecholamines (epinephrine and norepinephrine) and glucocorticoids are released from the adrenal glands to mobilize glycogen stores, increase available glucose and oxygen, suppress pancreatic insulin secretion, and enhance glucose uptake. Hyperglycemia may be noted. Glycogen stores are rapidly depleted (in <24 hr). Without nutrition, energy is generated from the breakdown of the body or catabolism. Breakdown of muscle tissue, fat, and viscera creates a negative nitrogen balance. Subclinical adrenal insufficiency may become clinically apparent after severe injury. Exogenous steroids, insulin, and catecholamines may be administered if shock persists.

The posterior pituitary release of antidiuretic hormone (ADH) promotes water absorption in the distal renal tubules. Intravascular volume increases as urinary output decreases. Blood pressure is increased by the renin-angiotensin-aldosterone system. Aldosterone promotes sodium and water resorption to increase intravascular volume, and renin-angiotensin causes vasoconstriction.

Systemic inflammatory response syndrome: In patients who sustain major trauma, a widespread inflammatory response known as *systemic inflammatory response syndrome* (SIRS) may be triggered by massive tissue injury and the presence of foreign bodies such as road dirt, missiles, and invasive medical devices. Inflammatory mediators activate the coagulation cascade, increased catecholamines stimulate production and release of white blood cells, and endothelial dysfunction ensues. The hemodynamic response and clinical findings are similar to those with sepsis. (See p. 501 for information on SIRS.)

Multiple organ dysfunction syndrome (MODS): The overwhelming inflammation associated with SIRS may lead to *multiple organ dysfunction syndrome* (MODS). MODS is a major cause of late mortality in polytrauma patients, accounting for about 10% of trauma deaths. Inadequate initial resuscitation or inability to achieve and maintain a compensatory hyperdynamic state contributes to the development of organ failure in trauma patients. Presence of endotoxin, tumor necrosis factor (TNF), interleukin-1, and other inflammatory mediators causes vasodilation, leading to hypotension. Capillary dysfunction results in poor cellular circulation and subsequent tissue destruction. Acidosis, pulmonary compromise, and circulatory collapse may result. Clinical trials are underway for therapies to help control inflammatory mediators. Activated protein C (Drotrecogin alfa) is the only approved medication to help control SIRS leading to MODS.

Coagulopathy: Disseminated intravascular coagulopathy (DIC) is a severe acquired bleeding disorder that may be triggered by massive trauma and SIRS. Factors contributing to development of DIC include hypotension, impaired tissue perfusion, capillary dysfunction leading to stasis, hypoxemia, and hypothermia. Massive blood transfusion is associated with abnormal hemostasis. Banked blood >14 days old may be proinflammatory, leading to coagulopathies. Older whole blood may be deficient in coagulation factors and platelets. Replacement of clotting components with fresh-frozen plasma and platelet transfusions may help prevent transfusion-related coagulopathies.

Hypothermia: Multiple factors increase the likelihood of hypothermia in major trauma. Exposed body surface area or viscera may occur at the scene of injury or during the initial resuscitation. Cold blood and room-temperature resuscitation fluids lower the core body temperature. Prolonged exposure to cool temperatures in resuscitation or operative areas is an additional factor. When present, central thermoregulatory failure caused by CNS injury, intoxication, or hypoperfusion contributes to hypothermia. Mild hypothermia can help preserve the function and viability of major organs, particularly when tissue perfusion is diminished as a result of injury, shock, or surgical clamping of arteries. Severe hypothermia creates significant physiologic alterations, including CNS depression, dysrhythmias, acidosis, and significant electrolyte imbalances. Catecholamine infusions are often ineffective until body temperature approaches 93° Fahrenheit.

Psychologic response: Victims of major trauma sustain life-threatening injuries. The patient often is aware of the situation and fears death. Even after the physical condition stabilizes, the patient may have a prolonged and severe psychologic reaction triggered by the trauma called *posttraumatic stress disorder.*

ASSESSMENT

The patient's survival and optimal chance for life without disability depend on a fast, accurate assessment of all major injuries and body systems. Once airway, breathing, circulation, and neurologic status are addressed, a thorough but rapid head-to-toe assessment must follow.

History and risk factors

Mechanism of injury: Knowledge of the events leading to the injury can help predict certain patterns of injury. For example, an unrestrained driver in an automobile collision typically sustains injuries to the cranium, face, cervical vertebrae, torso, and lower extremities. High-velocity gunshot wounds typically result in large, ragged exit wounds with massive internal injury along the missile path.

Intoxicants: Acute alcohol intoxication is a common finding with blunt and penetrating trauma. The presence of alcohol and other intoxicants produces neurologic and pupillary changes that may be incorrectly attributed to CNS injury. In addition, acute alcohol or drug intoxication causes cardiovascular, hematologic, and ventilatory changes that compound injury-related alterations. Finally, intoxicants dull the pain response and may obscure important signs that are useful for accurate diagnosis of injuries.

Preexisting medical conditions: Chronic health conditions such as hypertension, diabetes, chronic obstructive pulmonary disease (COPD), cerebrovascular disorders, renal failure, and immune disorders increase the susceptibility for and impair physiologic responses to injury. Use of prescribed and illicit drugs should be determined. For example, beta-(β-) blocking medications inhibit sympathetic stimulation and limit the patient's ability to compensate for hypovolemia. Individuals with insulin-dependent diabetes may require additional insulin to respond to transient hyperglycemia. Chronic opiate use increases tolerance to opiates, and greater than usual amounts may be necessary for analgesia.

Last meal: Information regarding time, quantity, and type of food or beverage ingested is necessary for planning care to prevent vomiting and reduce the risk of aspiration, especially if surgical intervention is imminent.

Tetanus immunization: Immunization history determines need for tetanus vaccine or immunoglobulin administration (Table 2-1).

Initial subjective presentation: Mild tenderness to severe pain may be present, with the pain either localized to the site of injury or diffuse. Pain may be referred, particularly if abdominal structures are involved. Dyspnea, shortness of breath (SOB), agitation, restlessness, and anxiety are associated with impaired tissue perfusion and oxygenation. Nausea and vomiting may occur, and the conscious patient who has sustained blood loss often complains of thirst, an early sign of hemorrhagic shock. Slurred speech and poor coordination are present with intoxication or CNS impairment caused by decreased cerebral O_2 delivery due to blood loss.

Initial objective presentation (primary survey): Initial objective presentation may vary according to site of injury, blood loss, and involved structures and should be assessed during the primary survey. Primary survey consists of the *ABCD*and*Es*: *A*—airway with cervical spine protection; *B*—breathing: oxygenation and ventilation; *C*—circulation with hemorrhage control; *D*—disability: brief neurologic examination (usually Glasgow Coma Scale [see Appendix 3]); *E*—exposure/envi-

---

T A B L E   2 - 1　**Tetanus Prophylaxis in Routine Wound Management—United States, 1991**

History of absorbed tetanus toxoid (doses)	Clean, minor wounds		All other wounds*	
	Td†	**TIG**	**Td†**	**TIG**
Unknown or <3	Yes	No	Yes	Yes
≥3‡	No§	No	No‖	

Modified from Centers for Disease Control: MMWR 40(RR10):1-28, 1991.

Td, Tetanus and diphtheria (toxoid); *TIG,* tetanus immunoglobulin.

*Such as, but not limited to, wounds resulting from missiles, crushing, burns, and frostbite.

†For children <7 yr: DPT (DT, if pertussis vaccine is contraindicated) is preferred to tetanus toxoid alone. For persons ≥7 yr, Td is preferred to tetanus toxoid alone.

‡If only three doses of fluid toxoid have been received, a fourth dose of toxoid, preferably an absorbed toxoid, should be given.

§Yes, if >10 yr since last dose

‖Yes, if >5 yr since last dose. (More frequent boosters are not needed and can accentuate side effects.)

ronment. For posterior examination, ensure that spinal alignment is maintained while turning patient. General findings are listed below.

Inspection (secondary survey): Abrasions and ecchymoses suggest mechanism of injury and involvement of underlying structures. Ecchymoses may take hours to days to develop, depending on rate of blood loss. Absence of external evidence of injury does not exclude the possibility of serious internal injury. Protrusion of bone fragments and viscera may be present. Entrance and exit wounds (if present) should be determined in the case of penetrating injuries. Protruding instruments should not be removed, because additional harm and renewed bleeding may occur.

Auscultation: Diminished or absent breath sounds, distant heart sounds, diminished or absent bowel sounds.

Palpation: Weak and irregular pulse, cool and clammy skin, subcutaneous emphysema over area of injury, swelling and point tenderness over injured area.

Percussion: Dullness over blood-filled areas or internal hematomas.

Vital signs and hemodynamics

Initial: Widely variable, according to catecholamine response, volume status, and drugs administered. Increased respiratory rate (RR) and compensatory tachycardia are typical. The absence of tachypnea suggests CNS injury or severe intoxication. Patients taking β-blocking medications may not experience tachycardia, and heart rate (HR) may remain within normal limits despite serious blood loss. Blood pressure (BP) may be normal, slightly elevated, or diminished, depending on volume of blood loss. In young adults, compensatory responses maintain a normal BP until major blood loss occurs. If not treated, hypotension with mean arterial pressure (MAP) <70 mm Hg occurs; sometimes very rapidly. Decreased central venous pressure (CVP), pulmonary artery wedge pressure (PAWP), and cardiac output/cardiac index (CO/CI) reflect hypovolemia and should be corrected to maintain euvolemia. Systemic vascular resistance (SVR) is initially elevated as a result of compensatory vasoconstriction.

Hyperdynamic phase: After fluid volume resuscitation, a hyperdynamic circulatory state compensates for the cellular oxygen debt incurred during the initial traumatic injury. Increases in CO/CI are present. Oxygen delivery increases because tissue oxygen needs (Vo_2) increase from factors such as pain, agitation, infection, and tachycardia. Vo_2 may double. Svo_2 usually is elevated (>80%) due to poor cellular oxygen extraction and/or capillary dysfunction. $S\bar{V}R$ is <900 dynes/sec/cm^{-5}, indicative of vasodilation from inflammatory mediators. If there is failure of compensatory mechanisms, MODS may ensue. CO/CI will be decreased and pulmonary artery wedge pressure (PAWP) will be increased. The patient may require vasopressors (e.g., norepinephrine, dopamine) to maintain MAP >70 mm Hg.

DIAGNOSTIC TESTS

Complete blood count (CBC): Serial determination of hematocrit/hemoglobin (Hct/Hgb) reflects the amount of blood lost. If drawn immediately after the injury, Hct/Hgb levels may be normal. Serial Hgb/Hct levels may be markedly decreased during resuscitation and as extravascular fluid mobilizes during the recovery phase. Leukocytosis (elevated white blood cell [WBC] count) is expected initially. Later, an increase in WBCs or a shift to the left may reflect the inflammatory response or may signal infection.

Blood chemistries: Glucose is elevated initially because of catecholamine release and insulin resistance. Ionized calcium levels decline because of metabolic alterations associated with impaired tissue perfusion and binding with citrate from stored blood. Baseline levels of electrolytes, enzymes, and other chemistries are drawn for later comparison and to guide therapy. Venous lactate levels may be elevated if tissue perfusion is inadequate and anaerobic metabolism is present.

Arterial blood gas (ABG) analysis: May show pH <7.35 and HCO_3^- <22 mEq/L because of metabolic acidosis, due to inadequate tissue oxygen delivery leading to anaerobic metabolism and excess lactate production. Decreased Pao_2 is present if ventilation is compromised by pulmonary injury or altered level of consciousness (LOC).

Oximetry (Spo_2 monitoring): Continuous pulse oximetry is used to assess oxygen saturation. Oxygen therapy should be titrated to maintain pulse oximetry reading (Spo_2) of ≥92%, according to individual injuries and preexisting medical conditions.

Type and cross-match: To determine presence of antigens so that recipient and donor blood are compatible. If blood loss requires immediate transfusion, O-negative (without major antigens) blood or type-specific blood is used until a full cross-match can be performed.

Blood alcohol, toxicology screen: Checks for the presence of alcohol or other intoxicant. Positive results are used to guide therapy and prevent acute withdrawal symptoms.

Urinalysis: Done initially to check for the presence of blood caused by urinary tract injury. Later, checks for presence of bacteria caused by urinary tract infection (UTI).

X-ray: Evaluated for presence of fractures, abnormal air or fluids, foreign objects and to determine location of large organs. With polytrauma patients, cervical spine, chest, abdomen, pelvic, and extremity x-ray studies usually are necessary.

Computed tomography (CT): To detect magnitude of soft tissue injury, hematomas, and subtle fractures.

> **Caution:** Because of the risk of rapid deterioration, the patient should be accompanied by an experienced nurse during the CT. Appropriate monitoring and resuscitation equipment must be readily available.

COLLABORATIVE MANAGEMENT

Airway management: A patent airway must be secured when Glasgow Coma Scale (GCS) score <8 or potential for airway compromise is possible. Secure the airway by intubation or cricothyroidotomy, if necessary. If cervical spine injury is suspected, the cervical spine is stabilized during the procedure by maintaining constant in-line positioning with gentle traction. Nasal intubation is preferred to the oral route because there is less manipulation of the cervical spine. The success of any method depends on findings with each patient and the experience of the clinician. Cricothyroidotomy is indicated when other means of intubation are not possible or are contraindicated.

Oxygen: All trauma patients require supplemental oxygen. Blood loss creates reduced oxygen-carrying capacity, and tissue demand for oxygen is greatly increased during the hypermetabolic phase. High-flow oxygen by mask is indicated initially. Oxygen therapy can be titrated according to ABG and pulse oximetry values. Mechanical ventilation may be required.

Fluid management: Underresuscitation as well as overresuscitation of trauma patients during the initial 48-72 hr may lead to shock, MODS, and death. The goal of resuscitation in any trauma patient should be to maintain euvolemia. Two or more large-bore (≥16-gauge) short catheters should be placed to maximize delivery of fluids and blood. Use of intravenous (IV) tubing with an exceptionally large internal diameter (trauma tubing), absence of stopcocks, and use of external pressure are techniques used to promote rapid fluid volume therapy when indicated. When rapid infusion of large amounts of fluid is required, all fluid should be warmed to body temperature to prevent hypothermia. Rapid warmer/infusor devices are available to facilitate rapid administration of blood products. A combination of crystalloids, colloids, and blood products is necessary for most patients with major trauma. Patients with significant craniocerebral trauma have precise fluid requirements (see "Traumatic Brain Injury," p. 103).

Crystalloids: Balanced salt solutions such as 0.9% normal saline (NS), or NaCl, or lactated Ringer's (LR) are commonly used. These solutions are inexpensive and convenient to store, but intravascular retention is poor. Sustained use of normal saline can lead to hyperchloremic metabolic acidosis; therefore LR is generally preferred. NS is used when crystalloids are administered simultaneously through the same IV line as blood products. The ionized calcium in LR can interact with the citrate anticoagulant in banked blood, causing clot formation.

Colloids: The osmotic force generated by the large molecular weight (colloid) substances results in increased plasma osmotic pressure and promotes intravascular fluid retention. Albumin, dextran, and hetastarch are colloid substances in current use. Colloids are generally used as a supplement to crystalloid therapy. To date, resuscitation with crystalloid or colloid remains controversial. Colloids do not readily cross capillary walls or pass between the tissue compartments as easily as crystalloids.

Packed red blood cells (PRBCs): Blood loss is associated with most injuries, and may necessitate massive transfusion. *Massive transfusion* is defined as replacement of one half of the patient's blood volume at one time or complete replacement of the patient's blood volume over 24 hr. If blood loss is very rapid during the initial resuscitation, immediate transfusion with O-negative blood may be required. When bleeding continues, type-specific blood is used until a full cross-match can be performed. The patient must be properly and permanently identified with trauma alias or name, if known, to prevent transfusion errors. Complications of massive transfusion are numerous. Hypocalcemia caused by calcium binding with citrate in stored packed red blood cells (PRBCs) results in depressed myocardial contractility, particularly in hypothermic patients or in those with impaired liver function. One ampule of 10% calcium chloride should be considered for administration after every 4 units of PRBCs. Abnormal hemostasis occurs, since stored PRBCs are deficient in some coagulation factors and platelets. Replacement of clotting components with fresh-frozen plasma and platelet transfusions, as appropriate, will help minimize transfusion-related coagulopathies.

Autotransfusion: Shed blood from the patient can be collected, filtered, and reinfused. Shed blood is captured from chest tube drainage or the operative field and reinfused immediately. Various techniques are used to capture and reinfuse the blood. Advantages of autotransfusion include reduced risk of disease transmission, absence of incompatibility problems, and availability. Disadvantages include risk of blood contamination and presence of naturally occurring factors that promote anticoagulation.

Gastric intubation: Permits gastric decompression, aids in removal of gastric contents, and helps to prevent vomiting or possible aspiration. Contraindicated in patients with basilar skull fractures because of the need to prevent tubes entering the cranial vault via abnormal openings in the fractured skull.

Urinary drainage: An indwelling catheter is inserted to obtain a specimen for urinalysis and to monitor hourly urine output. See "Renal and Lower Urinary Tract Trauma," p. 122, for precautions.

Pharmacotherapy

Antibiotics: Broad-spectrum antibiotics are used initially to prevent infections. More specific antimicrobial agents are used when results from culture and sensitivity tests are available.

Analgesics and anxiolytics: Relief of pain and anxiety are accomplished using intravenous opiates and anxiolytics. All intravenous agents should be carefully titrated to desired effect, while avoiding respiratory depression, masking injury, or disguising changes in physiologic parameters. Use of the World Health Organization (WHO) ladder for pain management and a pain rating scale are essential for the trauma population.

Tetanus prophylaxis: Tetanus immunoglobulin and tetanus-toxoid are considered on the basis of Centers for Disease Control (CDC) recommendations (see Table 2-1).

Nutrition therapy: Infection and sepsis contribute to the negative nitrogen state and increased metabolic needs. Prompt initiation of nutrition therapy is essential for rapid healing and prevention of complications. Parenteral nutrition or postpyloric (jejunal) feedings may be used if postoperative ileus or injury to the gastrointestinal (GI) tract is present. For more information, see "Nutritional Support," p. 1.

Surgery: Need for surgery depends on the type and extent of injuries. The surgical team is coordinated by the trauma surgeon. When several specialty surgeons are required for various injuries, the order of surgeries is coordinated carefully to preserve life and limit the potential for disability.

NURSING DIAGNOSES AND INTERVENTIONS

Fluid volume deficit related to active loss secondary to physical injury or inadequate resuscitation

Desired outcome: Within 12-24 hr of this diagnosis, patient becomes euvolemic as evidenced by MAP $\geq$70 mm Hg; HR 60-100 beats per minute (beats/min); normal sinus rhythm on electrocardiogram (ECG); CVP 2-6 mm Hg; PAWP 6-12 mm Hg; CI $\geq$5 L/min/m^2; SVR 900-1200 dynes/sec/cm^{+5}; urinary output $\geq$0.5 ml/kg/hr; specific gravity 1.010-1.0300; warm extremities; brisk capillary refill (<2 sec); and distal pulses >2+ on a 0-4+ scale.

- Monitor BP q15min, or more frequently in the presence of obvious bleeding or unstable vital signs (VS). Be alert to changes in the MAP of >10 mm Hg. Even a small but sudden decrease in BP may be a signal to consult the physician, especially when the extent of injury is unknown.
- Monitor HR, ECG, and cardiovascular status q15min until volume is restored, with hourly intake and output until VS are stable. Check ECG to note HR elevations and myocardial ischemic changes (i.e., ventricular dysrhythmias, ST segment changes), resulting from dilutional anemia.
- In the patient with volume depletion or active blood loss, administer fluids through several large-caliber ($\geq$16 gauge) catheters or central line. Use short, large-bore IV tubing (trauma tubing) to maximize flow rate. Avoid use of stopcocks, because they slow the infusion rate. Fluids should be warmed to prevent hypothermia.

Caution: Evaluate patency of IV catheters continuously during rapid-volume resuscitation. Hypocalcemia may develop in rapidly transfused patients as a result of stored citrate. Monitor for signs and symptoms such as hyperreflexia or positive Trousseau's or Chvostek's sign.

- Measure pulmonary artery (PA) pressures q1h or more frequently if blood loss is ongoing. Measure CO/CI and calculate SVR and pulmonary vascular resistance (PVR) q4-8h, or more often in unstable patients. Be alert to low or decreasing CVP and PAWP. An elevated HR, along with decreased PAWP, decreased CO/CI, and increased SVR, suggests inadequate fluid resuscitation. During the hyperdynamic phase, calculate Do_2 and Vo_2. Support higher-than-normal values by oxygen and fluid administration, conservation of energy, and other measures according to individual patient. Anticipate higher-than-normal CO/CI and lower-than-normal SVR.

- Measure urinary output q1h. Be alert to output <0.5 ml/kg/hr for 2 consecutive hours. Low urine output usually reflects inadequate intravascular volume in the patient with abdominal trauma.
- Monitor for physical indicators of hypovolemia, including cool extremities, capillary refill >2 sec, and absent or decreased amplitude of distal pulses.
- Estimate ongoing blood loss. Measure all bloody drainage from tubes or catheters, noting drainage color (e.g., coffee-grounds, burgundy, bright red [see Table 2-14]). Note the frequency of dressing changes as a result of saturation with blood to estimate amount of blood loss via wound site.
- Administer oxygen to maximize delivery of oxygen to tissues. Use continuous pulse oximetry to assess for adequate oxygenation. Evaluate ABG values as necessary.

You may also wish to refer to the following interventions from the Nursing Interventions Classification (NIC):

NIC Electrolyte Management; Fluid Management; Fluid Monitoring; Hypovolemia Management; Bleeding Precautions

Pain related to physical injury secondary to trauma or surgery

Desired outcome: Within 2 hr of this diagnosis, patient's subjective or objective (in unconscious, sedated, or paralyzed patient) evaluation of discomfort improves. If patient can give subjective response, document by using pain scale.

- Evaluate patient for presence of preoperative and postoperative pain. Preoperative pain is anticipated and is a vital diagnostic aid. Use a pain scale to rate pain and relief of discomfort. Devise a method to communicate or consider using the Face, Legs, Activity, Cry, Consolability (FLACC) scale for patients with endotracheal (ET) tubes or other barriers to communication.
- Administer opiates and other analgesics as prescribed. Avoid preoperative administration of large doses of opiate analgesics until the patient has been evaluated thoroughly by a trauma surgeon. Tell patient to report unrelieved pain. Postoperatively, administer prescribed analgesics before the pain becomes severe. Analgesics help relieve pain and aid in the recovery process by promoting greater ventilatory excursion. Substance abuse is often involved with injuries. Victims may be drug or alcohol users, with higher-than-average tolerance to narcotics, and may be at risk for alcohol or narcotics withdrawal. Recognize that narcotics decrease GI motility and may delay return to normal bowel functioning. Document the degree of pain relief obtained, using the pain scale or changes in assessment.
- Supplement analgesics with nonpharmacologic maneuvers (e.g., positioning, back rubs, distraction) to aid in pain reduction.
- See p. 51 for additional pain intervention.

NIC Analgesic Administration; Pain Management, Post Anesthesia Care; Positioning

Altered protection related to clotting factor alterations; decreased hemoglobin level

Desired outcomes: Patient is free of symptoms of bleeding as evidenced by absence of bleeding at venipuncture sites, mucous membranes, intravenous catheter insertion sites, incisions, and GI tract. Coagulation profiles return to normal by the time of transfer from intensive care unit (ICU).

- Obtain blood for coagulation and related studies: prothrombin time (PT), thrombin time, partial thromboplastin time (PTT), and Hct, Hgb, and fibrinogen levels, and fibrin degradation products (FDPs).
- Observe for bleeding at venipuncture sites, mucous membranes, urinary catheter insertion sites, incisions, and GI tract. Test GI tract secretions/excretions for occult blood.
- Administer misoprostol (Cytotec), omeprazole (Prilosec), histamine H_2-receptor antagonists, and/or sucralfate (Carafate) as prescribed to reduce gastric acid and prevent erosion of gastric mucosa. Avoid use of cimetidine (Tagamet) because of reduction in hepatic blood flow.
- Avoid intramuscular (IM) injections and venipunctures. Use IV medication administration.
- If DIC is present, see "Disseminated Intravascular Coagulation," p. 489, for treatment.

NIC Infection Control; Infection Protection; Bleeding Precautions

Risk for infection related to inadequate primary defenses secondary to physical trauma or surgery; inadequate secondary defenses as a result of decreased hemoglobin or inadequate immune response; tissue destruction and environmental exposure; multiple invasive procedures

Desired outcome: Patient is free of infection as evidenced by core or rectal temperature <37.7° C (100° F); HR ≤100 beats/min; orientation to time, place, and person; and absence of unusual redness, warmth, or drainage at surgical incisions and drain sites.

- Monitor VS for evidence of infection, noting temperature increases and associated increases in HR and RR. An elevated cardiac output (CO) and a decreased SVR suggest sepsis. Consult surgeon if these are new findings. See Tables 10-1 and 10-2, for hemodynamic profiles of early and late septic shock. Also refer to "Septic Shock," p. 501.
- Evaluate orientation and LOC q2-4h.

- Ensure patency of all surgically placed tubes or drains. Irrigate or attach to low-pressure suction as prescribed. Promptly report unrelieved loss of tube patency.
- Evaluate incisions and wound sites for evidence of infection: unusual redness, warmth, delayed healing, and purulent or unusual drainage.
- Note color, character, and odor of all drainage. Consult physician and culture drainage if it is foul smelling or abnormal.
- Administer parenteral antibiotics in a timely fashion. Reschedule antibiotics if a dosage is delayed for more than 1 hr. Recognize that failure to administer antibiotics on schedule may result in inadequate blood levels and treatment failure.
- Administer tetanus immunoglobulin and tetanus-toxoid as prescribed (see Table 2-1). Ensure that patient receives documentation of tetanus immunization, if given.
- Change dressings as prescribed, using aseptic technique. Prevent cross-contamination from various wounds by changing one dressing at a time.

NIC Infection Control; Infection Protection; Incision Site Care; Vital Signs Monitoring; Tube Care

Impaired tissue integrity related to mechanical factors (including physical injury); related to altered circulation secondary to hemorrhage or direct vascular injury; related to nutritional deficit secondary to hypermetabolic state; and related to impaired physical mobility

Desired outcome: Patient has adequate tissue integrity as evidenced by wound healing within an acceptable time frame according to extent of injury.

- On admission, clean and irrigate all cutaneous injuries with 0.9% NaCl, or use some other procedure according to individual prescription or hospital protocol.
- Assess all wounds, fistulas, and drain sites q4-8h for signs of irritation, infection, and ischemia. Inspect for healing and presence of granulation tissue with each dressing change or assessment.
- Identify infected and devitalized tissue. Aid in the removal of eschar as directed by physician or wound specialist.
- Turn patient q1-2h. Identify need for specialty bed in patients with multiple risk factors for impaired tissue integrity (use individual hospital protocol).
- Promptly change all dressings that become soiled with drainage or blood. Use of a calcium algenate product or the vacuum-assisted closure device (VAC) may be necessary for heavily exudative wounds.
- Protect the skin surrounding tubes, drains, or fistulas, keeping the areas clean and free from drainage. If necessary, apply ointments, skin barriers, or drainage pouches to protect the surrounding skin. Consult wound specialist as necessary.
- Ensure adequate protein and calorie intake for tissue healing (see "Altered Nutrition," p. 97).

NIC • See "Wound and Skin Care," p. 45, for more information.

Wound Care; Incision Site Care

Hypothermia related to exposure at the scene of injury; temporary loss of temperature regulatory mechanisms because of shock or CNS ischemia; surgical exposure of abdominal viscera; administration of large volumes of unwarmed fluid or blood

Desired outcomes: Patient's temperature remains or returns to normal within 24 hr of this diagnosis. Complications of hypothermia are avoided as evidenced by normal sinus rhythm on ECG; patient oriented to time, place, and person; $Pao_2 \geq 80$ mm Hg; and absence of prolonged bleeding from wounds, incisions, and venipuncture sites.

- Warm all fluids administered during the initial resuscitation phase and until the patient approaches normothermia after surgery. Prewarm crystalloids so that they are ready for immediate use. Use rapid-volume infuser for rapid warming of large volumes of blood.
- Keep room temperature as warm as possible in trauma receiving, surgical, and critical care areas. Keep patient dry, and cover head to reduce heat loss.
- Avoid unnecessary exposure. Keep patient covered with warmed or warming blanket.
- Monitor core temperature via rectal or esophageal probe, urinary catheter attachment, or PA catheter until normothermia is attained.
- Be aware that vasodilation during rewarming can result in an intravascular fluid volume deficit and may require vasoactive infusions, along with volume resuscitation.
- Monitor for and promptly report serious dysrhythmias (i.e., atrial fibrillation with rapid ventricular response, ventricular dysrhythmias, atrial ventricular [AV] conduction block), associated with severe or prolonged hypothermia.
- Be aware that hypothermia compromises cortical functioning, and the patient may be confused, disoriented, or somnolent or may have other neurologic derangements. These symptoms may make it difficult to evaluate concurrent head injury.

- Monitor ABG values at frequent intervals for evidence of hypoxemia. Hypothermia causes a shift to the left in the oxyhemoglobin dissociation curve and may impair oxygen unloading to peripheral tissue.
- Because DIC may develop several days after a hypothermic episode, monitor for excessive bleeding from wounds, surgical incisions, and venipuncture sites and promptly report the presence of serious or progressive thrombocytopenia. (See "Disseminated Intravascular Coagulation," p. 489.)

NIC Hypothermia Treatment; Temperature Regulation; Vital Signs Monitoring

Altered nutrition: less than body requirements, related to increased need secondary to hypermetabolic posttrauma state; possible decreased intake secondary to direct injury or surgical disruption of GI tract or ileus

Desired outcome: Within 5 days of this diagnosis, patient has adequate nutrition as evidenced by maintenance of baseline body weight and state of nitrogen balance on nitrogen studies.

- Collaborate with physician, dietitian, and pharmacist to estimate patient's metabolic needs on the basis of type of injury, activity level, and nutritional status before injury.
- Consider patient's specific injuries and preexisting medical condition when planning nutrition.
- Monitor serum markers of nutritional status: prealbumin, transferrin.
- Start enteral feedings as soon as possible (i.e., bowel sounds are present, patient experiences hunger).
- Recognize that opiates decrease GI motility and may cause nausea and vomiting.
- Weigh patient daily to evaluate trend. Be alert to steady decreases in weight, and evaluate loss by assessing and comparing with volume status and fluid shifts.
- Collect 24-hr urine specimen for urea nitrogen value, as prescribed, to evaluate nitrogen balance.
- For additional information, see "Nutritional Support," p. 1.

NIC Nutrition Management; Weight Gain Assistance

Fear related to potentially threatening situation (e.g., serious injuries, hospitalization) and supported by presence of pain, unfamiliarity, and noxious environmental stimuli present in critical care area; communication barrier (e.g., intubation); sensory impairment from direct injuries

Desired outcome: Within 24 hr of this diagnosis, patient exhibits decreased symptoms of fear: apprehension, tension, nervousness, tachycardia, superficial vasoconstriction, aggressiveness, and withdrawal.

- Assess level of fear and understanding of present condition.
- Plan care to provide as restful an environment as possible.
- Provide information regarding nursing care, treatment plan, and progress. It is often necessary to repeat information because injury, stress, and fear can interfere with comprehension.
- Promote visits by family members and significant others.
- Offer to consult hospital chaplain or patient's clergy member as desired by patient.
- Assess and promote patient's usual coping strategies. It may be helpful to interview family members.
- Provide referral to support groups for trauma patients and family members.
- For more information, see this diagnosis in "Psychosocial Support," p. 71.

NIC Anxiety Reduction; Coping Enhancement; Security Enhancement; Support System Enhancement

Risk for injury related to potential for use of alcohol or illicit drugs; propensity for thrill-seeking behaviors

Desired outcomes: The potential for postdischarge use of alcohol or illicit drugs is identified by the time of hospital discharge. The potential for thrill-seeking behaviors is evaluated by the time of hospital discharge.

- Evaluate preinjury status regarding use of intoxicants.
- Assess for preinjury patterns of thrill-seeking behaviors.
- Initiate early referral to social services or discharge planner if need of rehabilitation is anticipated.
- Refer patient and family members or significant others to appropriate rehabilitation program or counseling as indicated. Immediately after serious injury, the patient and family members are very impressionable, making this period an ideal time to begin addressing behaviors that place that patient at risk for additional injury.
- Initiate injury prevention education. Provide instructions on proper seat belt application (across the pelvic girdle rather than across soft tissue of the lower abdomen), firearm safety, injury prevention for infants and children, and other factors suitable for the persons involved.

NIC Impulse Control Training; Risk Identification; Substance Use Prevention; Substance Use Treatment; Vehicle Safety Promotion

Posttrauma syndrome (Posttraumatic stress disorder) related to unanticipated serious physical injury or event resulting in physical trauma

Desired outcomes: By the time of hospital discharge, patient verbalizes that the psychosocial impact of the event has decreased; cooperates with treatment plan; and does not exhibit signs of severe stress reaction, such as display of inconsistent affect, suicidal or homicidal behavior, or extreme agitation or depression.

- Evaluate mental status at systematic intervals during the acute and recovery periods. Be alert to indicators of severe stress reaction such as display of affect inconsistent with statements or behavior, suicidal or homicidal statements or actions, extreme agitation or depression, and failure to cooperate with instructions related to care.
- Anticipate some reexperience of traumatic event. Reassure patient and significant others that this is common.
- Consult with specialist such as psychologist, psychiatric nurse clinician, or pastoral counselor if patient displays signs of severe stress reaction, as described in the first intervention.
- Consider organic causes that may contribute to posttraumatic stress response (e.g., severe pain, alcohol intoxication or withdrawal, electrolyte imbalance, metabolic encephalopathy, impaired cerebral perfusion).
- For other psychosocial interventions, see "Psychosocial Support," p. 68.

NIC Counseling; Support System Enhancement; Support Group

ADDITIONAL NURSING DIAGNOSES

Also see the following as appropriate: "Nutritional Support," p. 1; "Hemodynamic Monitoring," p. 23; "Sedating and Paralytic Agents," p. 32; "Alterations in Consciousness," p. 38; "Wound and Skin Care," p. 45; "Pain," p. 200; "Prolonged Immobility," p. 61; "Psychosocial Support," p. 68; "Psychosocial Support for the Patient's Family and Significant Others," p. 78; other trauma discussions in this chapter; and "SIRS and MODS," pp. 501 and 510.

Traumatic Brain Injury

PATHOPHYSIOLOGY

Trauma to the head from blunt and penetrating forces can result in injury to the brain, support structures, blood vessels, and cranium. Blunt injuries to the head are caused by acceleration, deceleration, and rotational forces (e.g., vehicular collisions, falls, high-impact sports). Penetrating injuries occur from piercing forces that traverse the skull and damage underlying brain tissue and support structures.

The initial impact (force) results in widespread injury due to tissue stresses and strain which activate biomolecular processes within the cells. Injury results from structural and neuronal damage, vascular insufficiency, and inflammation. The cerebral vasculature and skull are often damaged. Tissue stresses result in contusions, diffuse axonal injuries, and compression injuries. Biomolecular processes cause neurexcitation and deafferentation of the neurons. The neurexcitatory injury activates excitatory neurotransmitters (glutamate and aspartate), which depolarize neurons. This neurotransmitter surge causes aberrant cell signaling, leading to long-lasting or permanent neuronal dysfunction. Deafferentation destroys the neurofilament of the axon, and the axon swells and retracts. Reduced blood flow augments cell death.

Outcome after traumatic brain injury can be predicted to some extent based on the type of lesion, severity of injury, and length of coma. Age, preinjury medical status, mechanism of injury, intracranial pressure, and brainstem integrity are important factors influencing outcome.

Changes in intracranial pressure dynamics

Intracranial pressure dynamics (IPD) is based on the volume-pressure relationship within the cranium (Monro-Kellie hypothesis). Three volumes exist within the fixed, rigid cranial vault: the brain, the blood, and the cerebrospinal fluid (CSF). Under normal conditions these volumes exert a pressure that is <15 mm Hg. When any of these volumes increases, pressure increases and compensatory mechanisms (shunting of CSF into the intrathecal space or vasoconstriction to reduce blood volume) are activated to reduce the volume. In addition, the brain requires a constant blood supply to maintain normal function. With brain injury, the intrinsic compensatory mechanisms are damaged or overwhelmed and functions that serve to maintain cerebral perfusion are compromised. Extrinsic measures are necessary to maintain the normal pressure-volume relationship and preserve cerebral perfusion pressure (CPP). Table 6-3 lists indicators of increased intracranial pressure (IICP). Treatment of derangements in IPD is based on the relationship between intracranial pressure (ICP) and CPP and is stated simply:

$$CPP = MAP - ICP$$

MAP is calculated using the following equation:

$$MAP = \frac{\text{Systolic BP} + 2(\text{Diastolic BP})}{3}$$

The goal of treatment is to maintain CPP >70 mm Hg and reduce ICP to <20 mm Hg.

Primary brain injuries

When the skull and brain are subjected to mechanical forces, a host of injuries in the cerebral cortex, brainstem or cerebellum may change cerebral perfusion pressure. Severity of brain injuries is classified using the Glasgow Coma Scale (GCS): mild (GCS score = 13-15), moderate (GCS score = 9-12), and severe (GCS score = ≤8). Specific injuries arising from the mechanical forces are as follows:

Contusion: Bruising that occurs as a result of mechanical forces to the head. Surface (scalp) contusions are focal bruises, lacerations, and capillary hemorrhages found with contact forces. Contusions are associated with fractures. *Coup* (brain injury is directly beneath the site of impact) or *contrecoup* (brain injury is opposite the site of impact) injuries, herniation contusions (parahippocampal structures and cerebellar tonsils forced against the tentorium), and gliding contusions (from rotational forces in the parasagittal areas) can result in focal hemorrhage of the cortex and adjacent white matter.

Diffuse axonal injuries (DAI): Mild to severe injuries which occur when diffuse areas of white matter have been torn or sheared. Injury evolves over time. *Initial* CT scan may not demonstrate a pathologic condition.

Concussion: Neurexcitatory injury sometimes associated with diffuse, axonal brain injuries. Classified as mild (no loss of consciousness, possible brief episodes of confusion or disorientation); moderate (brief loss of consciousness, transient focal neurologic deficits); or severe (prolonged loss of consciousness with sustained neurologic deficits lasting <24 hr).

Secondary brain injuries

Secondary injuries such as inflammation, edema and changes in blood flow occur after the primary processes and further contribute to brain damage. They may be intrinsic or extrinsic.

Intrinsic: Injuries that result from primary brain injury including intracranial hypertension, impaired autoregulation (causes reduced cerebral blood flow), reperfusion injury, brain edema, hemorrhage, herniation, cerebral vasospasm, inflammation, and hyperthermia.

Extrinsic: Injuries unrelated to primary brain injury resulting from inadequate resuscitation, poor oxygenation, extreme hyperventilation, substance abuse, or nosocomial factors such as infections (meningitis) or anesthetic agents used for surgical repair of injuries. (See "Meningitis," p. 384).

Associated skull fractures

Skull fractures occur as a result of blunt or penetrating impact force. Primary and secondary brain injuries are usually present.

Linear skull fractures: Nondisplaced, associated with low-velocity impact.

Basilar skull fractures: Linear, involving the base of the cranium's anterior, middle, and posterior fossae.

Depressed skull fractures: Depression of the skull over the point of impact; may be comminuted (usually closed without direct brain penetration), compressed, or compound (open).

Vascular injuries

Vascular injuries are intrinsic brain injuries resulting from impact force that causes bleeding of cerebral arteries or veins. These injuries usually accompany moderate and severe primary injuries.

Epidural hematomas: Commonly occur after a temporal linear skull fracture that lacerates the middle meningeal artery below it or from fractures of the sagittal and transverse sinuses. The hematoma develops rapidly in the space between the skull and dura.

Subdural hematomas: Bleeding from veins between the dura and the arachnoid spaces; may be acute, subacute, or chronic.

Subarachnoid hemorrhage: Bleeding in the subarachnoid space seen over convexities of the brain or in the basal cisterns.

Intracranial hematomas: Blood collection from injury to the small arteries and veins within the subcortical white matter of the temporal and frontal lobes; usually associated with petechiae, contusions, and edema.

Neurologic complications

Herniation syndromes: Displacement of a portion of the brain through openings within the intracranial cavity that result from increased intracranial pressure. Herniation occurs when there is a pressure difference between the supratentorial and infratentorial compartments within the skull. When herniation occurs, significant portions of the cerebral vasculature is compressed, destroyed, or lacerated, resulting in ischemia, necrosis, and ultimately death.

- *Cingulate herniation:* Occurs because of an increase in ICP in one brain hemisphere. The affected high pressure side shifts towards the low pressure side causing compression of the anterior cerebral artery and internal cerebral vein. Reduced blood flow results in development of cerebral ischemia, edema, and (IICP). Neurologic deficits include decreased LOC, with unilateral or bilateral lower extremity weakness or paralysis.
- *Uncal herniation:* Life-threatening, emergent situation that occurs when an expanding lesion (blood, edema, tumor) of the middle or temporal fossa forces the tip (uncus) of the temporal lobe toward the midline. The uncus protrudes over the edge of the tentorium cerebelli and compresses the oculomotor (third cranial) nerve and posterior cerebral artery. The uncus may be lacerated in the process and the midbrain is compressed against the tentorial edge. The patient manifests a fixed and dilated pupil on the side of herniation, a change in respiratory pattern, marked deterioration in LOC and further elevation in ICP.
- *Central (transtentorial) herniation:* Life-threatening, emergent situation that occurs with expanding lesions of the frontal, parietal, or occipital lobes or with severe, generalized cerebral edema. Often, cingulate and uncal herniation precede this life-threatening process. Table 2-2 describes the clinical features of uncal and central herniation syndromes. Subcortical structures, including the basal ganglia and diencephalon (thalamus and hypothalamus), herniate through the tentorium cerebelli, causing compression of the midbrain and posterior cerebral arteries bilaterally. Symptoms of increased ICP often occur too rapidly to be observed. Changes in respiratory patterns may not be seen in critically ill patients who are mechanically ventilated, depending on mode of ventilation.
- *Transcranial (extracranial) herniation:* Occurs when intracranial contents under pressure are forced through an open wound, surgical site, or cranial vault fracture. Although the resultant loss of brain volume lowers ICP and may prevent intracranial herniation, this is an ominous sign and the patient is at risk for infection, further brain injury, and death.

ASSESSMENT

Baseline physical examination data should include assessment of mental status, cranial nerves, motor status, sensory status, and reflexes. Thereafter, continuous neurologic assessment should be based on the clinical status of the patient. Ideally, a complete neurologic assessment should be performed. However, many components of the examination require patients to follow commands. For patients unable to follow commands, the neurologic assessment should be tailored individually to the patient's abilities and redesigned as necessary. The Glasgow Coma Scale (Appendix 3) and the Rancho Los Amigos cognitive functioning scale (see "Cognitive Rehabilitation Goals," Table 1-26) should be part of the neurologic assessment. Record specific patient responses to stimuli and the type of stimuli required to produce the response. The following are assessment findings related to specific injuries.

Epidural hematoma/linear skull fracture: Scalp lacerations, swelling, tenderness, and ecchymosis. Classic epidural signs are loss of consciousness, followed by a lucid interval and then rapid deterioration. Ipsilateral pupil dilation and contralateral weakness, followed by brainstem compression, occur if treatment is not initiated emergently.

Basilar skull fracture: Dural tears resulting in rhinorrhea and otorrhea are common. Anterior fossa injuries are associated with periorbital ecchymosis (raccoon eyes), epistaxis, damage to cranial nerves I and II, and meningitis. Middle and posterior fossa injuries may damage cranial nerves VII and VIII and are associated with tinnitus, hemotympanum, and destruction of the cochlear vestibular apparatus. Ecchymosis of the mastoid process (Battle's sign) is common.

Compound depressed skull fracture: Neurologic changes are based on the extent of brain injury, but changes in LOC, pupillary changes, headache, cerebral edema, and IICP often accompany these injuries. Physical and diagnostic examination findings may include CSF leaks if the dura has been torn; tympanum rupture; and bruised, lacerated, or contused brain tissue.

TABLE 2-2 Assessment of Central and Uncal Herniations

Criteria	Diencephalic		Midbrain/upper pons	Lower pons/upper medulla
	Early	Late		
Central herniation				
Respiratory pattern	Deep sighs, yawning	Cheyne-Stokes	Hyperventilation that is sustained and regular	Shallow, rapid, irregular
Pupils: size/reaction	Small; react to bright light; small range of contraction	Small; react to bright light; small range of contraction	Midpositioned; irregularly shaped; fixed reaction to light	Midpositioned; fixed
Oculocephalic/oculovestibular responses (doll's eyes phenomenon/ice water caloric)	Full conjugate or slightly roving eye movements; full conjugate lateral; ipsilateral response to ice water ear irrigation	Same as early; nystagmus absent	Impaired; may be dysconjugate	No response
Motor responses				
At rest	Contralateral paresis, which may worsen	Motionlessness	Abnormal extension posturing	Flaccidity
To stimulus	Bilateral Babinski	Abnormal flexion posturing	Rigidity	Bilateral Babinski
		Early third nerve	Late third nerve	
Uncal herniation				
Respiratory pattern	Normal		Hyperventilation that is regular and sustained	
Pupils: size/reaction	Moderate dilation; ipsilateral to primary lesion; sluggish constriction; brisk contralateral papillary reaction		Widely dilated and fixed ipsilateral pupil	
Oculocephalic/oculovestibular responses (doll's eyes phenomenon/ice water caloric)		Present or dysconjugate, full conjugate, slow ipsilateral eye movement or dysconjugate caused by contralateral eye not moving medially	Impaired or absent; Full lateral movement with contralateral eye; absence of medial movement with ipsilateral eye	
Motor response to stimulus		Contralateral extensor plantar reflex	Ipsilateral hemiplegia; abnormal posturing; absence of all responses	

Modified from Plum F, Posner J: *Diagnostic of stupor and coma*, ed 3, Philadelphia, 1980, Davis.

Concussion: Headache, dizziness, vomiting, memory loss, and decreased attention and concentration skills. Moderate and severe injuries require close observation because cerebral edema and IICP can develop.

Contusion: Loss of consciousness is common. Neurologic deficits may be generalized or focal, depending on the site and severity of injury. Cerebral edema and unstable intracranial pressure dynamics may often complicate the primary injury.

Diffuse axonal injury: May occur with other injuries and is characterized by an immediate loss of consciousness. Ischemia is often a secondary complication. Edema and unstable intracranial pressure dynamics are common. Duration of coma varies, depending on the severity of the injury, but often, coma is prolonged and recovery of function is minimal to moderate.

Subdural hematoma: With acute subdural hematoma, neurologic deterioration is seen within 24-72 hr (or earlier) and is manifested by a changing LOC, ipsilateral dilated pupil, and contralateral extremity weakness. Subacute hematoma may present within 48 hr to weeks after injury and manifests initially as a headache. Characteristically there is no clinical sign of improvement. LOC begins to deteriorate, and focal neurologic deficits ensue. Neurologic signs associated with a chronic subdural hematoma may occur weeks or months after injury. The progression of elusive, fluctuating deficits, such as personality changes, memory loss, headache, extremity weakness, and incontinence, may signal chronic subdural hematoma, especially in high-risk groups such as older adults or chronic alcohol users.

Subarachnoid hemorrhage (SAH): Highly associated with headache, changes in LOC, and meningeal signs such as nuchal rigidity, elevated temperature, and positive Kernig's sign (loss of ability to extend leg when thigh is flexed on abdomen).

Intracranial hematoma: Neurologic deficits are based on the site and severity of injury.

Other physical assessment data: Baseline cardiovascular, pulmonary, gastrointestinal, genitourinary, and integumentary data should be completed, with reassessment on an ongoing basis.

NON-NEUROLOGIC COMPLICATIONS

Cardiac dysrhythmias: Commonly seen in brain-injured patients and probably related to autonomic (sympathetic and parasympathetic) derangement or compression of midbrain and brainstem structures. ECG changes seen with elevated ICP are prominent U waves, ST segment changes, notched T waves, and prolongation of the QT interval. Bradycardic, supraventricular, tachycardic, and ventricular dysrhythmias are seen, as well. Cushing's syndrome, characterized by bradycardia, elevated systolic blood pressure (SBP), and a widening pulse pressure, is a late sign indicating mechanical compression or severe metabolic dysfunction of the brainstem.

Aspiration pneumonia: Prevalent complication after brain injury. Aspiration may occur at the time of injury or as an iatrogenic complication of intubation, enteral feedings, or prolonged use of artificial airways. Early detection reduces associated morbidity and mortality and should be incorporated into the plan of care. Tracheobronchial secretions should be checked for glucose (a sign that tube feedings have been aspirated), enteral feeding protocols initiated, and swallowing assessments done. See "Nutritional Support" for "Risk for Aspiration," p. 12, and Table 1-4, which discusses complications in the tube-fed patient.

Other complications: The patient with brain injury is predisposed to numerous complications related to injury of the central and autonomic nervous systems, concurrent injuries, hypoperfusion, and iatrogenic complications. Also see the following as appropriate: "Acute Respiratory Distress Syndrome," p. 189; "Pulmonary Edema," p. 220; "Meningitis," p. 384; "Diabetes Insipidus," p. 400; "Syndrome of Inappropriate Antidiuretic Hormone," p. 404; "Gastrointestinal Bleeding," p. 459; "Anemia," p. 473; and "Disseminated Intravascular Coagulation," p. 489.

DIAGNOSTIC TESTS

Skull x-ray: Detects structural deficits such as skull fractures, facial bone destruction, air-fluid level in sinuses, unusual intracranial calcification, pineal gland location (normally midline), and radiopaque foreign bodies.

Cervical spine x-ray: Demonstrates structural deficits of the spine. Used to rule out cervical spine injuries, including fractures, dislocations, and subluxations. Cervical spine immobilization is mandated in all trauma patients until the cervical spine (C1 through T1) is visualized completely and fractures are ruled out.

Computed tomography (CT): The most important diagnostic tool used to evaluate for primary and secondary brain injuries. Gray and white matter, blood, and CSF are identified by their different radiologic densities. CT is used to diagnose cerebral hemorrhage, infarction, hydrocephalus, cerebral edema, and structural shifts.

Magnetic resonance imaging (MRI): Identifies type, location, and extent of injury. It provides spatial resolution, can follow metabolic processes, and detects structural changes.

Cerebral angiography: Invasive radiographic procedure using dye injected into peripheral vessels to examine the cerebral vasculature. Used as an adjunct study in diagnosing brain injury or if CT is unavailable.

Electroencephalography (EEG): Measures spontaneous brain electrical activity via surface electrodes. Useful in detecting areas of abnormal brain activity (irritability) associated with seizures and generalized brain activity related to drug overdose, coma, or suspected brain death. Drug therapy, especially with anticonvulsants, alters brain activity. Use of these drugs should be documented if the drug cannot be withheld 24-48 hr before performing EEG.

Evoked responses: Evaluates the electrical potentials (responses) of the brain to an external stimulus (i.e., auditory, visual, somatosensory). Provides information related to lesions of the cortex or ascending pathways of the spinal cord, brainstem, or thalamus. Evoked potentials are used to determine the extent of injury in uncooperative, confused, or comatose patients. Should be used when planning rehabilitation activities.

CSF analysis: Used to evaluate for infection in the brain-injured patient. Analysis of CSF should include color, turbidity/cloudiness, red blood cell (RBC) and WBC counts, protein, glucose, electrolytes, gram stain, culture, and sensitivity. *Cerebral microdialysis* is a promising new method of CSF analysis, wherein levels of neurotransmitters and electrolytes are calculated. Abnormal levels can be treated.

Serum laboratory studies: To identify complications associated with injury. WBCs, Hgb, Hct, electrolytes, osmolality, albumin, and transferrin are monitored at least daily, and more frequently during the acute phase.

COLLABORATIVE MANAGEMENT

Management focuses on treating the emergent pathologic condition, controlling ICP, preventing complications, and initiating rehabilitation.

Surgical intervention: Performed to evacuate mass lesions (epidural, subdural, and intracranial hematomas), place an ICP monitoring system, elevate depressed skull fractures, débride open wounds and brain tissue, and repair dural tears or scalp lacerations. Frontal lobectomies may be necessary to control severe increases in ICP.

Management of intracranial pressure dynamics: ICP monitoring is performed by a variety of techniques (Table 2-3). All monitoring systems provide a digital display of ICP, but CPP must be calculated (see p. 99). The goal is to maintain CPP >70 mm Hg.

Reduction of ICP by CSF drainage: Performed using intraventricular or ventriculostomy systems. To prevent herniation when draining CSF, drainage collection bags must be maintained at the level of the tragus of the ear or higher, thereby preventing excessive CSF flow caused by a higher-to-lower pressure gradient.

Hyperventilation via mechanical ventilation: Hyperventilation is no longer recommended as a first-line treatment to reduce ICP. Recent evidence reveals hyperventilation may cause neurologic dysfunction as a result of decreased cerebral perfusion. Maintaining $Paco_2$ at 35 ± 2 mm Hg is now considered optimal ventilation.

Monitoring jugular venous oxygen saturation (Sjo₂): Used to measure cerebral oxygenation by determining oxygen content of cerebral venous blood. Three types of blood flow can be discriminated: normal (Sjo_2 = 55%-70%), oligemic (Sjo_2 <55%), and hyperemia (Sjo_2 >70%). Treatment should be aimed at maintaining normal range.

Diuresis therapy: Reduces cerebral brain volume by removing fluid from the brain's intracellular compartment. Mannitol 20%, an osmotic diuretic, and furosemide (Lasix), a loop diuretic, are generally used. Mannitol may be given in 25-50 g doses as needed to reduce ICP or may be given q4-6h. Furosemide 20-40 mg may be given in conjunction with mannitol. Dehydration is a major complication with continued use of diuretics. Serum electrolyte and osmolality values should be closely monitored. Fluid balance is maintained with fluid therapy (75-100 ml/hr). Replacement of urine losses may be prescribed based on the volume of urine collected 1 hr after giving diuretics. Given either ml for ml or 0.5 ml for ml over a 3- to 4-hr period.

Maintenance of blood pressure to maintain cerebral perfusion pressure: Hypotension and hypertension can contribute to cerebral edema, which compresses blood vessels. Hypotension can result in decreased oxygen delivery to brain cells. The pH is reduced by elevated $Paco_2$, causing cerebral vessels to vasodilate. Hypotension reduces MAP and thus CPP. Dopamine HCl (Intropin), used at doses between 3-5 mcg/kg/min, can effectively increase MAP and raise CPP.

T A B L E 2 - 3 Types of Intracranial Monitoring

System	Type	Placement	Advantages/uses	Disadvantages
Fluid-filled or fiberoptic	Intraventricular cannula	Lateral ventricle in nondominant hemisphere through burr hole	CSF measurement CSF drainage Drug administration Volume-pressure response testing	Rapid CSF drainage can result in collapsed ventricles or subdural hematoma Cannula tip may catch on ventricular wall Risk of intracerebral bleeding and infection May become plugged with debris Possible difficult insertion because of shifting or collapse of ventricle
Fluid-filled	Subarachnoid screw	Subarachnoid space through twist drill hole	Pressure monitoring Less risk of infection than with cannula Useful with small ventricles Does not penetrate brain	Compliance testing maybe unreliable No CSF drainage Some risk of infection Risk of hemorrhage or hematoma during insertion Brain may herniated into bolt, making recording unreliable
Electrical sensor	Epidural sensor	Epidural space Burr hole Fiberoptic sensor	Lowest risk of infection Easy to insert Dura not penetrated	No direct measurement of CSF No CSF drainage Inability to recalibrate to zero Cannot measure volume-pressure response
Fiberoptic	Intraparenchymal	Intraparenchymal via twist drill Fiberoptic sensor	Easy to insert Direct pressure Compliance testing One-time zero and calibration before insertion	Risk of intracerebral bleeding and infection No CSF drainage

CSF, Cerebrospinal fluid.

The effects of hypertension (elevated CPP and increased cerebral edema) are unclear, but increased capillary permeability and petechial hemorrhage are seen. Antihypertensive medications, such as labetalol HCl (Normodyne) or nitroprusside sodium (Nipride), may be required.

Reduction of metabolic demand: Important strategy when treating ICP problems, because cerebral blood supply must match demand to maintain cerebral function.

- *Sedating agents:* Use of individual or combined continuous infusions of sedatives, analgesics, and paralytic drugs to reduce metabolic demand. Midazolam HCl (Versed), opiate analgesics such as fentanyl citrate (Sublimaze) or morphine sulfate, and anesthetic agents such as propofol (Diprivan) are used. Nondepolarizing neuromuscular blocking agents, including vecuronium bromide (Norcuron) or atracurium, are used. See "Sedating and Paralytic Agents," p. 32.
- *Seizure control:* Seizures may occur with focal brain injuries such as depressed, comminuted, or compound skull fractures, contusions, and lacerations. Seizure activity increases the metabolic demand of the brain. Seizure prophylaxis with anticonvulsant agents such as phenytoin sodium (Dilantin) or phenobarbital is often prescribed. When using phenytoin, a 500-1000 mg IV loading dose is given slowly at 50 mg/min, followed by a daily dose of 100 mg tid. Phenytoin cannot be administered with a dextrose solution. Therapeutic levels should be maintained between 10-20 µg/ml. Dosing should be patient-specific (higher levels may be necessary to prevent breakthrough seizures, whereas lower levels may be acceptable if seizures are controlled).
- *Barbiturate coma:* A less often used method of reducing metabolic demand. High doses of barbiturates should not be used without continuous ICP and hemodynamic monitoring and controlled mechanical ventilation. Barbiturates may induce profound cardiac and cerebral depression. Pentobarbital sodium (Nembutal) is the drug of choice. A loading dose between 5-10 mg/kg is given (discontinue if MAP falls <70 mm Hg), followed by a maintenance dose of 1-3 mg/kg/hr to sustain a level of 3-5 mg/dl. Barbiturates are withdrawn gradually as the patient improves. Patients with barbiturate coma require intensive physical care and physiologic monitoring. Assessment of brain death criteria, if appropriate, cannot be initiated until barbiturate levels return to zero.
- *Maintaining body temperature:* For every 1° C in temperature elevation, there is a 10%-13% increase in metabolic rate. Body temperature should be normal to control metabolic demand. Normal temperatures range from 35.8°-37.5° C (96.4°-99.5° F) with a diurnal variation of 1° C. Rectal temperatures are 0.2°-0.6° C higher than oral and can be 0.8° C higher than right atrial, esophageal, and oral temperatures. Evaluation of the etiology of fever is important with brain injury, as it influences treatment choice. Fever may be caused by brain injury *(central fever)*, an infectious process *(peripheral fever)*, or drugs *(drug fever)*. *Central fever* reflects disturbance in the hypothalamic thermoregulatory mechanism. It is characterized by lack of sweating, no diurnal variation, plateaulike elevation patterns, elevations up to 41° C (105.8° F), absence of tachycardia, persistence for days or weeks, and temperature reduction with external cooling rather than with antipyretic agents. *Peripheral fever* is associated with wound infections, meningitis, sepsis, pneumonia, and other bacterial invasion. Sweating, diurnal variation, response to antipyretic agents, and tachycardia are present. *Drug fever* occurs in response to certain medications including antibiotics. External cooling with a hypothermia blanket may cause shivering, the body's mechanism to increase heat production. Shivering increases metabolic demand and may increase ICP. Shivering may be controlled by wrapping distal extremities in bath towels before initiating hypothermia or using chlorpromazine (Thorazine) which, however, must be used with caution because it may cause hypotension. Research on use of hypothermia in treatment of acute brain injury is evolving. If used, follow a strict hypothermia protocol.

Modifying nursing care activities that raise ICP: Transient brief and rapid elevations in ICP are commonly seen during position changes or other nursing care activities, which cannot always be avoided. Generally, the ICP returns to resting baseline within a few minutes. All nursing care activities that increase ICP should be spaced to enable a return of ICP to baseline and maximizing of CPP. Clustering nursing care such as bathing, turning, and suctioning creates a stair-step rise in ICP. Sustained increases (>5 min) should be avoided.

- *Suctioning:* Causes a significant rise in ICP. To minimize adverse effects associated with suctioning, implement the guidelines found in Table 2-4.
- *Neck positioning:* Flexion, extension, and lateral movements of the neck can significantly raise ICP. Maintaining the neck in a neutral position at all times is important. In patients with poor neck control, stabilize the neck with towel rolls or sandbags.
- *Elevating head of bed (HOB):* Although HOB elevation at 30 degrees is believed to improve venous drainage and contribute to ICP reduction, ICP may be improved at higher or lower elevations. Adjust HOB elevation to optimize the patient's CPP and minimize ICP.

T A B L E 2 - 4   Guidelines for Suctioning Patients at Risk for Increased Intracranial Pressure

- Suction only if the clinical status of the patient warrants.
- Precede suctioning with preoxygenation using 100% oxygen.
- Limit each suctioning pass to ≤10 sec.
- Limit suction passes to 2.
- Follow each pass with 60 sec of hyperventilation using 100% oxygen.
- Use negative suction pressure <120 mm Hg.
- Keep patient's head in a neutral position.
- Use a suction catheter with an outer-to-inner diameter ratio of 2:1.

- *Turning:* Turning the patient with IICP is not contraindicated but should be based on the patient's response to turning. Initially, turning from side to side will elevate pressure, but ICP should return to resting baseline after a few minutes. If the ICP does not return to resting baseline within 5 min, CPP may be compromised and the patient should be returned to a position that reduces ICP and maximizes CPP.
- *Bathing:* Although bathing itself has not been documented as raising ICP, the rapid turning from side to side associated with linen changes raises ICP. These "turn procedures" are actually clustered activities because the length of the procedure does not allow sufficient time for the ICP to return to baseline. Evaluation of the patient's response may necessitate performing the linen change in stages or allowing adequate time for ICP to return to resting baseline.
- *Sensory stimulation:* A sensory stimulation program may be implemented safely in comatose patients early after injury when ICP is stable. This rehabilitative technique may be an important adjunct to traditional care (Table 2-5).

Nutritional support: Enteral nutrition helps to maintain the integrity of the gut mucosa and should be initiated as early as possible after injury. When postpyloric (duodenum or jejunum) feeding tubes are used, enteral feedings can be initiated before bowel sounds return to normal. In some cases, gastric tubes for decompression are used simultaneously with the postpyloric tubes. See "Nutritional Support," p. 1, for documentation of proper placement and checking of residual volumes. If enteral feedings are contraindicated or not tolerated by the patient, parenteral feedings are started.

Rehabilitation: Brain injury often results in physical (paralysis, spasticity, and contractures) and cognitive impairments. Consult with physical, occupational, and speech therapists early to minimize deficits and prepare the patient for an acute rehabilitative program. National Institutes of Health (NIH) Consensus Development Conference Recommendations on Rehabilitation of Persons with Brain Injury are available. Support also is available through the Brain Injury Association of America (URL: www.biausa.org).

NURSING DIAGNOSES AND INTERVENTIONS

Impaired gas exchange related to decreased oxygen supply and increased carbon dioxide production secondary to decreased ventilatory drive occurring with pressure on respiratory center, imposed inactivity, and possible neurologic pulmonary edema

Desired outcomes: $Paco_2$ values remain between 35 ± 2 mm Hg. By the time of discharge from ICU or transfer to rehabilitation unit, patient has adequate gas exchange as evidenced by orientation to time, place, and person; Pao_2 ≥80 mm Hg; RR 12-20 breaths/min with normal depth and pattern (eupnea); and absence of adventitious breath sounds.

- Assess patient's respiratory rate, depth, and rhythm. Auscultate lung fields for breath sounds q1-2h and prn. Monitor for respiratory patterns described in Table 2-2. Be alert to IICP (see Table 6-3).
- Assess patient for signs of hypoxia, including confusion, agitation, restlessness, and irritability. Remember that cyanosis is a late indicator of hypoxia.
- Ensure a patent airway via proper positioning of neck and frequent assessment of the need for suctioning. Ensure hyperoxygenation of patient before and after each suction attempt to prevent dangerous, suction-induced hypoxia.
- Monitor ABG values; consult physician for significant findings or changes. Be alert to levels indicative of hypoxemia (Pao_2 <80 mm Hg) and to $Paco_2$ ≥35 ± 2 mm Hg, inasmuch as levels higher than this range may increase cerebral blood flow and thus ICP.
- Ensure that oxygen is delivered within prescribed limits.

TABLE 2-5   Management of Severe Brain Injury

Treatment	Level of evidence*	Recommendation
Blood pressure and oxygenation	Guideline	Avoid early postinjury episodes of hypotension <90 mm Hg or hypoxia <60 mm Hg.
ICP treatment threshold	Guideline	Treatment to lower ICP should be initiated at 20-25 mm Hg.
CPP treatment	Option	CPP should be maintained at >70 mm Hg. Maintain MAP >90 mm Hg.
Hyperventilation	Guideline	Avoid prophylactic hyperventilation (<35 mm Hg) the first 24 hours postinjury. May use hyperventilation for refractory IICP.
Mannitol	Guideline	Use intermittent boluses of 0.25 – 1 mg/kg
Barbiturates	Guideline	May be considered in hemodynamically stable patients refractory to other methods to reduce ICP.
Glucocorticoids	Standard	Use is not recommended.
Nutrition	Guideline	Replace 140% of resting metabolic expenditure in unparalyzed patients and 100% in paralyzed patients using parenteral or enteral methods. By day 7, feedings should contain at least 15% protein.
Seizure prophylaxis	Guideline	Anticonvulsants can be considered an option for high-risk patients early after injury.
	Standard	Not recommended for preventing late posttraumatic seizures.

Modified from Brain Trauma Foundation: Guidelines for the management of severe head injury, *J Neurotrauma* 13:639-734, 1996.

Standard = high level of certainty; *Guideline* = moderate clinical certainty; *Option* = unclear clinical certainty. Level of evidence is based on scientific literature where the highest degree of certainty is drawn from prospective randomized clinical trials.

*Level of evidence denotes the degree that the recommendation represents clinical certainty.

- Assist with turning q2h, within limits of patient's injury, to promote lung drainage and expansion and alveolar perfusion. Unless contraindicated, raise HOB 30 degrees to enhance gas exchange.
- Encourage deep breathing at frequent intervals to promote oxygenation. Avoid coughing exercises for patients at risk for IICP.
- Evaluate the need for an artificial airway in patients unable to maintain airway patency or adequate ventilatory effort.

NIC Airway Management; Oxygen Therapy; Respiratory Monitoring

Risk for infection: CNS, related to inadequate primary defenses secondary to direct access to the brain in the presence of skull fracture, penetrating wounds, craniotomy, intracranial monitoring, or bacterial invasion caused by pneumonia or iatrogenic causes

Desired outcome: Patient is free of infection as evidenced by normothermia; WBC count ≤11,000 /µl; negative culture results; HR ≤100 beats/min; BP within patient's normal range; and absence of agitation, purulent drainage, and other clinical indicators of infection.

- Assess VS at frequent intervals for indicators of CNS infection. Be alert to elevated temperature and increased HR and BP.
- Monitor patient for signs of systemic infection, including discomfort, malaise, agitation, and restlessness.

- Inspect cranial wounds for the presence of erythema, tenderness, swelling, and purulent drainage. Obtain prescription for culture as indicated.
- Apply a loose sterile dressing (sling) to collect CSF drainage. Do not pack. Record amount, color, and character of drainage.
- Caution patient against coughing, sneezing, nose blowing, or Valsalva's or similar maneuvers, because these activities can damage the dura further. Use orogastric tubes if basilar skull fractures or severe frontal sinus fractures are present.
- Ensure timely administration of prescribed antibiotics.
  - ❑ Apply basic principles for care of any invasive device used with ICP monitoring:
  - ❑ Use good hand-washing technique before caring for patient.
  - ❑ If patient is not comatose, encourage him or her not to touch device; apply restraints *only* if necessary to keep patient from harm. Restraints can increase ICP by causing straining.
  - ❑ Maintain aseptic technique during care of device, following agency protocol.

NIC Infection Control; Infection Protection

Decreased adaptive capacity: intracranial, related to decreased cerebral perfusion pressure or infections that can occur with secondary head injury

Desired outcomes: Within 12-24 hr of treatment/interventions, patient has adequate intracranial adaptive capacity as evidenced by equal and normoreactive pupils; RR 12-20 breaths/min with normal depth and pattern (eupnea); HR 60-100 beats/min; ICP 0-15 mm Hg; CPP 60-80 mm Hg; and absence of headache, vomiting, and other clinical indicators of IICP. Optimally, by the time of discharge from ICU or transfer to rehabilitation unit, patient is oriented to time, place, and person and has bilaterally equal strength and tone in the extremities.

- Assess neurologic status at least hourly. Monitor pupils, LOC, and motor activity; also perform cranial nerve assessments (see Appendix 4). A decrease in LOC is an early indicator of IICP and impending herniation. Changes in the size and reaction of the pupils, a decrease in motor function (e.g., hemiplegia, abnormal flexion posturing), and cranial nerve palsies all indicate impending herniation.
- Monitor VS at frequent intervals. Be alert to changes in respiratory pattern, fluctuations in BP and pulse, widening pulse pressure, and slow HR.
- Monitor patient for indicators of IICP (see Table 6-3).
- Monitor hemodynamic status to evaluate CPP and ensure that it is 60-80 mm Hg. Be alert to decrease in mean systolic arterial blood pressure (<80 mm Hg) or increase in MAP. Perform ongoing assessment of ICP and CPP, recording pressures at least hourly until stable. Consult physician if pressure changes significantly (e.g., >15 mm Hg or other preestablished range). Perform ongoing calibration and zeroing of transducer to ensure accuracy of readings.
- Maintain a patent airway, and ensure precise delivery of oxygen to promote optimal cerebral perfusion.
- Facilitate cerebral venous drainage by maintaining neck in neutral position.
- To help prevent fluid volume excess, which could add to cerebral edema, ensure precise delivery of IV fluids at consistent rates.
- Ensure timely administration of medications that are prescribed for the prevention of sudden increase or decrease in BP, HR, RR.
- Treat elevations in ICP immediately (Table 2-6).

NIC Cerebral Edema Management; Cerebral Perfusion Management; Intracranial Pressure (ICP) Monitoring; Neurologic Monitoring

Ineffective thermoregulation related to trauma associated with injury to or pressure on the hypothalamus

---

T A B L E 2 - 6   Nursing Interventions for Patients With Increased Intracranial Pressure

- Maintain HOB elevation at level that keeps ICP <20 mm Hg and CPP >70 mm Hg.
- Loosen constrictive objects around neck to facilitate venous blood flow from the head.
- With position changes, ensure ICP and CPP return to baseline or stay within acceptable parameters within 5 minutes of turn.
- Maintain head in neutral position.
- Correct factors that may increase ICP such as hypoxia, pain, anxiety, fear, and abdominal or bladder distention.
- Evaluate activities that increase ICP (e.g., suctioning, bathing, dressing changes) and reorganize care to minimize elevations.

ICP, Intracranial pressure; *CPP,* cerebral perfusion pressure.

Desired outcome: Patient becomes normothermic within 24 hr of this diagnosis.
* Monitor for signs of hyperthermia: temperature >38.3° C (101° F), pallor, absence of perspiration, torso that is warm to the touch.
* As prescribed, obtain blood, urine, and sputum specimens for culture to rule out underlying infection.
* Be alert to signs of meningitis: fever, chills, nuchal rigidity, Kernig's sign, Brudzinski's sign (see "Meningitis," p. 384).
* Assess wounds for evidence of infection, including erythema, tenderness, and purulent drainage.
* If patient has hyperthermia, remove excess clothing and administer tepid baths, hypothermic blanket, or ice bags to axilla or groin.
* As prescribed, administer antipyretics such as acetaminophen.
* As prescribed, administer chlorpromazine to treat or prevent shivering, which can cause further increases in ICP.
* Keep environmental temperature at optimal range.
* Assess for possible drug fever reaction, which can occur with antimicrobial therapy.

NIC **Temperature Regulation; Fever Treatment**

Risk for disuse syndrome related to immobilization and prolonged inactivity secondary to brain injury, spasticity, or altered LOC

Desired outcome: Patient has baseline/optimal ROM without verbal or nonverbal indicators of pain.
* Begin performing passive range-of-motion (ROM) exercises q4h on all extremities as soon as patient's acute condition stabilizes. Monitor ICP during exercise, being alert to dangerous elevations outside of the established parameters. Consult with physical therapist accordingly.
* Teach passive ROM exercises to significant others. Encourage their participation in patient exercise as often as they are able.
* Reposition patient q2h within restrictions of the head and other injuries, using log-rolling technique as indicated.
* Ensure proper anatomic position and alignment. Support alignment with pillows, trochanter rolls, wrapped sandbags.
* For patient with spasticity, use foot cradles to keep linens off the feet. To maintain dorsiflexion, provide patient with shoes that are cut off at the toes, with the shoes ending just proximal to the head of the patient's metatarsal joints. Because there is no contact of the balls of the feet with a hard surface, the risk of spasticity will be minimized. Consult occupational therapist for use of splints or other supportive device.
* For patient without spasticity, use foot supports to prevent plantar flexion and external hip rotation.
* To maintain anatomic position of the hands, provide spastic patient with a splint or a cone that is secured with an elastic band. Either device will limit spasticity by pressing on the muscles, while the elastic band will stimulate the extensor muscles, thereby promoting finger extension.

NIC **Exercise Therapy: Joint Mobility; Positioning**

Impaired corneal tissue integrity (or risk for same) related to irritation associated with corneal drying and reduced lacrimal production secondary to altered consciousness or cranial nerve damage

Desired outcome: Patient's corneas are moist and intact.
* Assess for indicators of corneal irritation: red and itching eyes, ocular pain, sensation of a foreign object in the eye, scleral edema, and blurred vision.
* Avoid exposing patient's eyes to irritants such as baby powder or talc.
* Lubricate patient's eyes q2h with isotonic eye drops or ointment.
* Facilitate an ophthalmic consultation as indicated.

NIC **Medication Administration: Eye**

ADDITIONAL NURSING DIAGNOSES

Also see "Decreased adaptive capacity: intracranial" in "Cerebral Aneurysm and Subarachnoid Hemorrhage," p. 363. As appropriate, see nursing diagnoses and interventions under "Alterations in Consciousness," p. 44; "Care of the Patient After Intracranial Surgery," p. 365; and "Meningitis," p. 384. See "Risk for Trauma" in "Status Epilepticus," p. 372. Also see nursing diagnoses and interventions under "Nutritional Support" (particularly "Risk for Aspiration," p. 12); "Mechanical Ventilation," p. 14; "Hemodynamic Monitoring," p. 23; "Prolonged Immobility," p. 61; "Psychosocial Support," p. 68; and "Psychosocial Support for the Patient's Family and Significant Others," p. 78. The patient with craniocerebral trauma is at risk for diabetes insipidus and syndrome of inappropriate antidiuretic hormone. See "Fluid Volume Deficit" in "Diabetes Insipidus," p. 403; and "Risk For Injury" in "Syndrome of Inappropriate Antidiuretic Hormone," p. 405.

Chest Trauma

PATHOPHYSIOLOGY

Chest trauma is a complex, multidimensional problem categorized by cause. Thoracic trauma can be severe enough to cause pulmonary or cardiac contusion, airway rupture, or tracheobronchial injury and can interfere with heart and lung function. In-depth physical assessment is critical after the patient's injury.

Blunt injury: Chest injury resulting from forceful, direct contact of an object or extremity with the chest, such as a steering wheel in vehicular collision, a beating, a fall, or a crush injury. Usually the chest wall remains closed (no communication of the chest cavity with outside atmospheric pressure). Rib fractures are the most common blunt injury. Both blunt and penetrating chest wounds can lead to pneumothorax.

Penetrating injury: An open chest injury resulting from stab or missile wounds to the thorax. The chest cavity is open and affected by the outside atmospheric pressure. Pneumothorax is likely. Gunshot wounds are the most common missile-type penetrating injuries, and knife wounds the most common stabbing chest injuries.

ASSESSMENT

Subtle signs, symptoms and changes in the patient's condition can indicate serious problems. Treat the patient as if a spinal cord injury is present until ruled out. Small changes in mental status may signal a central nervous system insult or hypoxemia.

Blunt injury: Dyspnea, SOB, agitation, restlessness, anxiety, and severe chest pain during respirations that the patient can localize.

Potential injuries: Pneumothorax, hemothorax, rib fractures, flail chest, pulmonary contusion, blunt cardiac injury.

Inspection: RR >20 breaths/min; hyperpnea; ventilatory distress; use of accessory muscles of respiration; nasal flaring; stridor; decreased tidal volume; hemoptysis; asymmetric chest wall motion; paradoxical chest wall motion; inability to clear tracheobronchial secretions; splinting; jugular venous distention; cyanosis or pallor of the skin, lips, and nail beds; and ecchymosis, which can signal injury to underlying organs.

Palpation: Tracheal deviation; subcutaneous emphysema of the neck and upper portion of the chest; tenderness at fracture points; bony crepitus; weak pulse; cool, clammy skin; protrusion of bony fragments.

Percussion: Dullness over lung fields, which can signal hemothorax or atelectasis; hyperresonance over lung fields signaling pneumothorax.

Auscultation: Diminished or absent breath sounds, bony crepitus over fracture sites, muffled heart tones, decreased BP, pericardial friction rub, pulsus paradoxus, apical tachycardia. Bowel sounds may be heard in the thorax as a result of rupture or tear of the diaphragm, allowing herniation of abdominal contents into the thorax.

Penetrating injury: Dyspnea, SOB, moderate chest pain, restlessness, anxiety.

Potential injuries: Hemothorax, pneumothorax, tension pneumothorax, hemorrhage, shock, and infection.

Note: Perform a complete and rapid assessment with the patient's clothing removed. Entry sites may be deceptive. The skin has an elastic quality, tends to close behind the penetrating object, and may mask size and extent of injury. Log-roll the patient to assess for posterior wound(s).

Inspection: RR >20 breaths/min; hyperpnea; respiratory distress; use of accessory muscles of respiration; nasal flaring; decreased tidal volume; asymmetric chest wall movement; inability to clear tracheobronchial secretions; splinting; and cyanosis or pallor of the skin, lips, and nail beds. During inspection, estimate blood loss on clothing and locate both entry and exit sites. Be alert to presence or severity of other wounds or to presence of ecchymosis, which can signal injury to underlying internal organs. Assess for presence or absence of pulsations of the penetrating object, which may be imbedded in a major organ or blood vessel. Do not remove any penetrating object. The object may have a sealing or tamponade effect. Removing it could result in uncontrollable bleeding from the organ or penetrated blood vessels.

Palpation: Tracheal deviation, subcutaneous emphysema, weak or irregular pulse, cool and clammy skin.

Percussion: Dullness over lung fields from hemothorax or atelectasis; hyperresonance results from pneumothorax.

Auscultation: Assess for sucking sound during inspiration over entry wounds; diminished breath sounds; respiratory stridor; muffled heart tones; apical tachycardia or bradycardia from shock, bowel sounds in thorax.

Flail chest: Occurs when two or more adjacent ribs are fractured in two or more places (or the sternum is fractured, along with ribs adjacent to the sternal fracture). Paradoxic chest wall motion, the hallmark symptom, results when the fracture segment is free of the bony thorax and moves independently in response to intrathoracic pressure. Normally the chest expands on inspiration, creating a negative intrathoracic pressure; the chest wall retracts during expiration in response to positive pressure inside the chest. Since the flail chest segment is no longer attached to the bony thorax, it follows the pressure and retracts on inspiration (negative pressure is a pulling pressure) and bulges on expiration (positive pressure is a pushing pressure). Flail chest injury are associated with pulmonary contusions.

DIAGNOSTIC TESTS

Chest x-ray: Confirms presence of air or fluid in the pleural space; may determine extent of hemothorax or pneumothorax; confirms presence or absence of fractures of the bony thorax, and mediastinal shift.

ABG analysis: Evaluates oxygenation and acid-base balance. May reflect hypoxemia (Pao_2 <80 mm Hg) and hypercapnia ($Paco_2$ >45 mm Hg) with concomitant respiratory acidosis (pH <7.35). Pulse oximetry should be used for continuous monitoring of oxygen saturation (see, p. 176).

ECG monitoring: Reveals presence or absence of life-threatening dysrhythmias. An analysis of the heart's electrical activity is provided by 12-lead ECG. Althouh dysrhythmias are a common complication after chest trauma, this important test often is overlooked. Continuous ECG monitoring should be continued if serious dysrhythmias occur or patient complains of cardiac-related chest pain.

Echocardiogram: Assesses damage to the structures of the heart and estimates CO.

Hgb/Hct values: Levels determine the need for blood transfusion or fluid volume replacement.

COLLABORATIVE MANAGEMENT

Interventions are directed toward managing acute respiratory compromise while correcting the underlying injuries that may cause deterioration in the patient's condition.

Oxygen therapy: Device is determined by patient's response to therapy and range from nasal cannula to 100% nonrebreathing mask, depending on extent of hypoxemia.

Intubation: Maintains patent airway, decreases airway resistance and respiratory effort, provides route for easy removal of airway secretions, and allows for manual or mechanical ventilation, as necessary.

Mechanical ventilation: For cases of extreme respiratory distress or ventilatory collapse (see p. 14).

Blood replacement: A high priority in the trauma victim. Blood loss is replaced with packed RBCs or whole fresh blood, if available. Blood replacement via autotransfusion is widely accepted. Use of colloid versus crystalloid fluids for volume replacement remains controversial. Volume is more often replaced with crystalloid fluids (e.g., normal saline, lactated Ringer's solution) rather than colloidal IV fluids (e.g., plasma, albumin). Colloids increase the risk of developing acute respiratory distress syndrome (ARDS) and acute renal failure (ARF) and are more expensive; furthermore, research has failed to demonstrate significant benefit.

Chest tubes: Chest tubes are used to remove fluid or trapped air from the chest cavity. A thoracic catheter is inserted, usually through the second intercostal space, the midclavicular line, or the fifth lateral intercostal space, midaxillary line. Placement depends on the location and extent of the hemothorax, effusion, or pneumothorax. The catheter can be connected to a one-way flutter valve (for air evacuation only) or to a closed chest drainage system. Tension pneumothorax is a life-threatening emergency requiring pleural decompression.

Analgesia: Manages pain to minimize splinting and improve breathing. Opioid analgesics are used cautiously to avoid respiratory depression. An epidural patient-controlled analgesia (PCA) pump or an intercostal nerve block may help to relieve local rib pain.

Pleural decompression for tension pneumothorax: Relieves life-threatening tension pneumothorax. A 14-gauge needle or IV catheter is inserted into the second intercostal space at the midclavicular line to relieve the pressure in the chest cavity.

Stabilization and fixation of flail chest: Most flail chest injuries stabilize within 10-14 days without surgical intervention. Stabilization of fractures is achieved using a volume-cycled ventilator.

During surgery, a flail segment can be externally fixated by wiring or otherwise attaching the segment to the intact bony structures.

Thoracotomy: Consider following stabilization if a massive air leak is noted in the chest drainage system, and for continued or increased bleeding from chest tubes, refractory hypotension, acute deterioration, and cardiac tamponade.

NURSING DIAGNOSES AND INTERVENTIONS

Risk for fluid volume deficit related to active loss secondary to excessive bleeding occurring with chest trauma

Desired outcome: Patient is normovolemic as evidenced by BP and HR within patient's normal limits; stable weight; urine output ≥0.5 ml/kg/hr; chest drainage ≤100 ml/hr; and RR ≤20 breaths/min with normal depth and pattern (eupnea).

- Note condition of dressings at frequent intervals. Check linens beneath patient. Report excessive drainage or bleeding (e.g., if dressings are saturated in less than 4 hr during the first 24-48 hr). Bleeding should subside in less than 48 hr. Dressing changes should be required bid, for serosanguinous or serous drainage. Any bright red bleeding should be reported promptly.
- Monitor drainage in closed chest-drainage system. Report significant increase in bright red blood or other drainage. Amounts >100 ml/hr are usually considered excessive.
- Monitor autotransfusion equipment. Collaborate with physician for additional transfusion/fluid requirements based on the amount and rate of bleeding. Record accurate I&O status.
- Assess VS frequently until stable. Hypotension, tachycardia, and tachypnea may signal shock.
- Assess for adequate hydration. Monitor daily weight, fluid intake, and urinary output.
- Monitor Hgb to assess hemostasis. Decreased hemoglobin may reflect bleeding.

NIC Airway Management; Analgesic Administration; Bleeding Reduction; Blood Products Administration; Fluid/Electrolyte Management; Fluid Management; Fluid Monitoring; Hypovolemia Management; Oxygen Therapy; Pain Management; Respiratory Monitoring; Shock Management; Shock Management: Volume

ADDITIONAL NURSING DIAGNOSES

Also see "Posttrauma Response" in "Major Trauma," p. 97; and "Impaired Gas Exchange," p. 200, and "Pain," p. 200, in "Pneumothorax." For other nursing diagnoses and interventions, see "Psychosocial Support," p. 68, and "Psychosocial Support for the Patient's Family and Significant Others," p. 78.

Near Drowning

PATHOPHYSIOLOGY

Drowning is death by asphyxia caused by submersion in fluid; a common cause of traumatic death among young people, especially boys. *Near drowning* is survival of more than 24 hr following a drowning. Many drownings or near drownings are preceded by alcohol or drug ingestion, diving injuries, or medical catastrophies such as seizures or myocardial infarctions. Hypoxia, hypotension, pulmonary edema, and respiratory and metabolic acidosis may occur after near drowning. Potential complications include neurologic deficits from cerebral anoxia, acute renal failure secondary to acute tubular necrosis, and DIC. Near drowning can be categorized in two ways:

Near drowning with aspiration (wet): Aspiration of the submersion fluid or gastric contents occurs in 85%-90% of victims of near drowning. Hypoxia can result from laryngospasm, bronchospasm, airway obstruction from aspirated contaminants, or pulmonary edema. *Freshwater (hypotonic) aspiration* results in loss of surfactant, caused by the presence of hypotonic solution in the lungs. Without surfactant, atelectasis ensues because surface tension of the lung tissue increases, causing alveoli to collapse. Lung compliance decreases. The atelectasis and pulmonary edema lead to a ventilation-perfusion mismatch, adding to the hypoxia and acidosis. *Saltwater (hypertonic) aspiration* results in a rapid shift of water and plasma proteins from the circulation into the alveoli. The fluid-filled alveoli are not ventilated, while continued perfusion leads to ventilation-perfusion mismatch and hypoxia. The aspirated volume of either freshwater or saltwater is usually small, so there is little effect on total blood volume. The intravascular depletion often results from increased capillary permeability (from anoxia) and loss of protein in the pulmonary edema fluid. Any aspirated contaminants (e.g., algae, chemicals, sand) may cause or contribute to obstruction and lead to asphyxiation. Bacterial pneumonia can develop, depending on the type of contaminant in the aspirant, and chemical pneumonitis can occur if gastric contents were aspirated.

Near drowning without aspiration (dry): Death may result from asphyxiation secondary to laryngospasm. Laryngospasm may be stimulated by irritation of the trachea due to aspiration of fluid, or from pain. Represents 10%-15% of cases.

Many deaths attributed to near drowning may actually result from one of two separate phenomena leading to aspiration: (1) *immersion syndrome:* sudden immersion in cold water, resulting in hyperventilation, which increases the risk of swallowing or inhaling large amounts of cold water; cold water may stimulate vagally mediated bradycardia that results in loss of consciousness or asystolic cardiac arrest; and (2) *hyperventilation syndrome:* occurs when divers hyperventilate to increase the duration of breath-holding under water. The normal impetus to breathe (increased $PaCO_2$) is not present following hyperventilation. With exercise, oxygen stores continue to be used. Since breath-holding may not be terminated before the patient's oxygen content has reached dangerously low levels, dysrhythmias, seizures, or death from hypoxia can occur.

Hypothermia may occur with a near drowning. Defined as a drop in core temperature to 33° C (91.4° F) or below, its progression can cause muscle activity and vital functions to cease, resulting in ventricular fibrillation (happens at about 28° C [82.4° F]). Hypothermia may protect the brain from permanent anoxic damage by decreasing cerebral metabolism by as much as 50%. Resuscitation should be continued until the victim is rewarmed to at least 32° C (89.6° F), since the heart may start beating at that temperature. Resuscitation remains possible after 30 min of submersion. Resuscitation efforts frequently should be continued for at least 1 hr. All near drowning victims should receive aggressive initial resuscitation.

ASSESSMENT

Clinical presentation: Depending on severity and duration of hypoxia, symptoms may include unconsciousness, seizures, nonspecific alterations in mental status (e.g., confusion, irritability, lethargy), neurologic deficits (motor, speech, visual), mild coughing, pink and frothy sputum, vomiting, substernal chest pain, mottled and cold skin, cyanosis, fixed and dilated pupils, and abdominal distention.

Physical assessment: Pulmonary edema may cause resonance over lung fields and tactile fremitus. Lung auscultation may reveal apnea, tachypnea, shallow or gasping respirations, crackles, rhonchi, wheezes, supraventricular dysrhythmias, bradycardia, tachycardia, and ventricular fibrillation.

DIAGNOSTIC TESTS

ABG values: Initially may be normal or reflect hypoxemia (PaO_2 <80 mm Hg), hypercapnia ($PaCO_2$ >45 mm Hg), and metabolic and respiratory acidosis (pH <7.35, serum bicarbonate <22 mEq/L). Often $PaCO_2$ returns to normal while hypoxemia persists. Continuous pulse oximetry should be used to monitor oxygen saturation.

> **Note:** Since respiratory status can deteriorate quickly, serial ABG monitoring should be performed.

CBC: Determines a baseline hematologic status, which may reflect the presence of infection.

Serum electrolyte levels: Life-threatening changes in electrolyte levels are unusual after near drowning. Electrolyte disturbances are related to the quantity and tonicity of the water aspirated.

Blood urea nitrogen (BUN) and creatinine levels: Reflect the effects of hypoxia on renal tubular function. Creatinine is the most sensitive indicator of renal dysfunction, whereas uremia causes malaise. Acute tubular necrosis is a potential complication.

Chest x-ray: Serial x-ray studies should be done to determine presence of infiltrates, atelectasis, and pulmonary edema. The alveolar filling pattern of noncardiogenic pulmonary edema is evidenced by a soft, fluffy appearance with poorly demarcated lesions, often referred to as a *ground-glass* appearance.

Skull and spine x-ray: Obtaining cervical and complete spinal x-ray films must be done to rule out brain/spinal trauma from head, neck, or back injury. Until x-ray study results are known, the patient's neck and spine must be immobilized.

COLLABORATIVE MANAGEMENT

Oxygen therapy: Oxygen (100%) is initiated immediately to treat hypoxia and is continued. All patients, including those who are alert with spontaneous ventilation, are at risk for hypoxia and acidosis. Warmed oxygen 40°-43° C (104°-109.4° F) may be used as part of the rewarming process for patients with hypothermia.

Endotracheal (ET) intubation and mechanical ventilation: Intubation provides a patent airway for patients who are unable to manage secretions. Mechanical ventilation is used to manage respiratory failure due to reduced lung compliance, or if for any reason the patient is unable to maintain effective respiratory effort. Patients with freshwater aspiration require 1.5-2 times normal tidal volume at slower rates to allow optimal lung expansion and ventilation of alveoli.

Positive end-expiratory pressure (PEEP): If the patient is unresponsive to high levels of oxygen ($FiO_2 \geq 0.50$ to maintain a $PaO_2 \geq 60$ mm Hg), PEEP improves oxygenation by preventing the collapse of alveoli during expiration. PEEP is especially useful after freshwater aspiration, since surfactant is reduced and alveoli are more prone to collapse. The pressure keeps alveoli open despite inadequate surfactant. PEEP should be removed cautiously, since levels of surfactant can remain low for 48-72 hr after freshwater aspiration.

Bronchoscopy: To remove aspirated contaminants, if necessary.

Extracorporeal membrane oxygenation (ECMO): To oxygenate the blood and remove CO_2 when ARDS is severe enough that oxygen cannot be maintained even with high levels of PEEP.

Rewarming for hypothermia: Warm, moist oxygen 40°-43° C (104°-109.4° F) may be used to elevate core temperature. Peritoneal lavage also is used for rewarming. Fluid for lavage is warmed to 37° C (98.6° F). The goal is quick rewarming to achieve a normal core temperature. Intravenous fluids should also be warmed to prevent further exacerbation of the hypothermia.

Pharmacotherapy: Profound metabolic acidosis is treated with sodium bicarbonate, aggressive ventilation, and careful monitoring of arterial pH. If bronchospasm is present, aerosolized bronchodilators such as epinephrine or isoproterenol HCl may be used.

Note: Use of steroids and prophylactic antibiotics is controversial. Temperature elevation up to 38° C (100.4° F) during the first 24 hr can be a normal response to injury. Antibiotics may be prescribed if fever $\geq 38°$ C (100.4° F) persists for longer than 24 hr after the submersion.

Fluid and electrolyte management: Although uncommon, fluid and electrolyte abnormalities may occur. Usually no specific therapy is required for minor disturbances. Fluid volume may be replaced with crystalloid solutions (Ringer's lactate or normal saline).

Neurologic support: Depends on the severity of the neurologic impairment. Severe impairment may require intracranial pressure monitoring, steroids, osmotic diuretics (e.g., mannitol), mechanical ventilation, barbiturate coma, and deep hypothermia (core temperature <30° C). See "Traumatic Brain Injury," p. 98.

Management of event that precipitated the near drowning: Conditions such as substance abuse, seizure, myocardial infarction, or cervical spine fracture.

NURSING DIAGNOSES AND INTERVENTIONS

Impaired gas exchange related to alveolar-capillary membrane changes secondary to fluid accumulation in the lung or loss of surfactant

Desired outcomes: Within 12 hr of initiation of treatment, patient has adequate gas exchange as evidenced by the following ABG values: $PaO_2 \geq 60$ mm Hg and $PaCO_2 \leq 45$ mm Hg. Within 3 days of treatment, RR is ≤ 20 breaths/min with normal depth and pattern (eupnea); breath sounds are clear and bilaterally equal; and patient is oriented to time, place, and person (depending on degree of permanent neurologic impairment).

- Assess patient for increased respiratory effort: SOB, tachypnea (RR >20 breaths/min), change in the use of accessory muscles of respiration, nasal flaring, grunting, restlessness, and anxiety.
- Auscultate lung fields at frequent intervals. Note type of adventitious breath sounds (e.g., crackles, rhonchi, friction rubs); document findings. Consult physician if acute changes occur.
- Assess need for suctioning frequently. Document color, consistency, amount of sputum, frequency of suctioning needed to maintain a patent airway; and patient's response to the procedure.
- Monitor ABG values and/or oxygen saturation via pulse oximetry. Progressive hypoxia may require higher concentrations of oxygen or mechanical ventilation. Alert physician accordingly.
- Place patient in semi-Fowler's position to optimize lung expansion and decrease work of breathing.
- For PEEP therapy, be aware that alveoli collapse when PEEP is removed for suctioning. Oxygen levels achieved before suctioning will not return immediately after PEEP is reinstituted. A PEEP adapter on a manual resuscitator or an in-line suction device is recommended for patients receiving high levels of PEEP to help maintain PaO_2 when it is necessary to suction. (See "Mechanical Ventilation," p. 14, for details.)

- Provide rest periods between activities to decrease oxygen demands.
- Provide information and emotional support to decrease anxiety and reduce oxygen consumption.

Hypothermia related to prolonged exposure to cold water during submersion

Desired outcomes: Within 24 hr of initiating therapy, patient's core temperature increases to 35°-37° C (95°-98.6° F). BP, RR, and HR are within patient's normal limits.

- Use temperature probe or PA catheter to continuously measure patient's core temperature. The temperature of inspired gases may affect the accuracy of PA catheter measurements. Core temperature is also measured by bladder thermometry, rectal probe, or esophageal temperature probe (positioned in the lower third of the esophagus.)
- Monitor patient's response to rewarming. Assess temperature and humidity level of inspired oxygen. Monitor temperature of instilled peritoneal lavage fluid. Do not attempt surface or external warming until core temperature is within acceptable limits (i.e., 35°-37° C [95°-98.6° F]). Premature surface rewarming can lead to the return of cold blood to the heart and precipitate an "after-drop" in core temperature.
- After core temperature has reached acceptable limits, monitor patient's response to active rewarming of body surface. Rewarming can be achieved by warm baths, heating pads, or lights. Cover patient's head to prevent heat loss from this exposed area. Use of blankets alone is an inadequate method of rewarming surface areas except in cases of mild hypothermia.
- Be aware of the likelihood of decreased drug metabolism during patient's hypothermic period.

Risk for infection related to increased environmental exposure secondary to aspiration of water and contaminants present in water

Desired outcome: Patient is free of infection as evidenced by body temperature ≤37.5° C (99.5° F) after the first 24 hr; WBC count within normal limits for patient; clear sputum; and negative culture results.

- Monitor temperature q2h. Increases in temperature up to 38° C (100.4° F) are common during the first 24 hr. After 24 hr, an increased temperature may indicate infection.
- Monitor WBC count, being alert to increases from baseline values.
- Inspect sputum for changes in color, consistency, and amount.
- Use meticulous aseptic technique when suctioning patient's secretions.
- Collect sputum specimen for Gram's stain and culture and sensitivity as prescribed. These tests will identify the pathogen if infection is present.

NIC Acid Base Management; Acid Base Monitoring; Airway Management; Bedside Laboratory Testing; Laboratory Data Interpretation; Oxygen Therapy; Respiratory Monitoring; Temperature Regulation; Vital Signs Monitoring

ADDITIONAL NURSING DIAGNOSES

Also see "Posttrauma Response" in "Major Trauma," p. 97. See other nursing diagnoses and interventions in "Psychosocial Support," p. 68; and "Psychosocial Support for the Patient's Family and Significant Others," p. 78.

Cardiac Trauma

PATHOPHYSIOLOGY

Cardiac trauma may be caused by blunt or penetrating injuries to the heart. *Blunt cardiac trauma* may be caused by acceleration-deceleration injuries during a vehicular collision if the driver slams forward against the steering wheel. When this occurs, the heart muscle is injured by one or more of four mechanisms: compression of the heart between the sternum and vertebrae, bruising of heart tissue by bony structures, rupture or compression of coronary arteries by the blow, or cardiac rupture caused by intrathoracic or intraabdominal pressure. Other causes of blunt cardiac trauma are direct blows to the chest, falls from great heights, sporting and industrial injuries, and kicks by animals.

Blunt cardiac trauma was formerly classified as cardiac concussion or cardiac contusion. Neither condition had clear diagnostic criteria. Recent consensus among trauma surgeons is to describe the myocardial injury rather than use vague terms. Blunt cardiac trauma is considered significant when the patient has new findings, such as new dysrhythmias, abnormal cardiac wall motion, or injury to the heart.

The patient may exhibit signs and symptoms similar to individuals with myocardial infarction. The walls of the right ventricle are often injured since they are located behind the sternum. Blunt trauma may damage cardiac valves (aortic and mitral valves most often), the ventricular septum, or papillary muscle attachment. Rupture of the left ventricle generally leads to death in a few minutes. Rupture of the right ventricle can sometimes be successfully managed. Ventricular rupture may occur up to 2 wks following injury if a contused area of the heart fails to heal, weakens, and deteriorates to the point of rupture.

Penetrating cardiac trauma is caused by gunshot wounds, stab wounds, or foreign bodies entering the heart. The anteriorly located right ventricle is most vulnerable and commonly involved. Penetrating injuries are the most common cause of intrapericardial hemorrhage (see "Acute Cardiac Tamponade," p. 118).

Research Brief 2-1   Investigators at a level I trauma center found that over a 10-year span, of 70 patients with blunt cardiac trauma, only 12 required inotropes for management of cardiac pump problems, and only 3 patients died from causes directly attributable to the cardiac injury. Most frequently the myocardial contusion was of little importance clinically and did not affect the patient's outcome after injury

From Wijngaarden MH et al: Blunt cardiac injury: a 10-year institutional review, *Injury* 28(1):51-55, 1997.

ASSESSMENT

History and risk factors: Motor vehicle collision, assault, sporting injuries, car-pedestrian collision.

Clinical presentation

Blunt injury: Precordial chest pain (difficult to distinguish from angina), bradycardia, tachycardia or other dysrhythmia, hypotension, SOB, guarded breathing.

Penetrating injury: Tachycardia, SOB, weakness, diaphoresis, acute anxiety, cool and clammy skin, signs of shock.

Physical assessment

Blunt injury: Contusion marks on chest (may outline shape of steering wheel), flail chest (loss of continuity of bony thorax because of rib fracture) with resulting paradoxical movement of the chest wall with breathing, murmurs indicating valvular injury, atrial or ventricular gallops (if cardiac injury has decreased ventricular contractility). Upper body cyanosis with symptoms of cardiac tamponade may indicate cardiac rupture.

Penetrating injury: Protrusion of penetrating instrument (e.g., knife, ice pick), external puncture wound, signs of cardiac tamponade (see "Acute Cardiac Tamponade," p. 118).

ECG and hemodynamic measurements

Cardiac monitor: Sinus tachycardia, sinus bradycardia, premature ventricular contractions, ventricular tachycardia, ventricular fibrillation, asystole, and ST segment and T wave changes.

Arterial blood pressure: Decreased.

DIAGNOSTIC TESTS

Cardiac contusion is difficult to diagnose. The diagnostic methods lack sensitive and specific indicators of myocardial damage. The following diagnostic tests may demonstrate abnormal results with blunt cardiac trauma. None of the tests are universally accepted for confirmation of the diagnosis.

Chest x-ray: Findings may reveal damage to bony structures of the chest. Myocardial damage is not apparent on routine chest x-ray films.

Troponin: Cardiac markers, troponins I and t are used to diagnose cardiac injury. Cardiac troponins I (cTnI) and t (cTnt) are not present in adult skeletal muscles. Research indicates cTnI and cTnt, may be the most specific markers to indicate cardiac injury after blunt trauma if specimens are obtained 24 hr after injury.

Cardiac enzyme levels: Creatine kinase (CK) and the muscle-brain (MB) subfraction are unreliable in distinguishing cardiac trauma from other tissue injuries.

ECG: Cardiac injury may cause alterations in depolarization, repolarization, and muscle perfusion. The ECG may reveal: ST segment changes, T wave changes, prolongation of the QT interval, sinus tachycardia, heart block, and ventricular dysrhythmias. ECG may not be a reliable tool to determine myocardial contusion. ECG changes are detected in <40% of all contusions, possibly because the right ventricle is the most anterior chamber and thus most vulnerable. Routine 12-lead ECG does not view the right ventricle. Changes in 12-lead ECG reflect changes in the left ventricle rather than the right.

Multiple-gated acquisition (MUGA) scan: Used in the presence of a contusion to detect decreased ability of the heart to pump efficiently.

Echocardiography: Detects abnormal wall motion and valve function, intracavity thrombi, and pericardial effusion. Considered the gold standard for diagnosing blunt injury to the myocardium.

Transesophageal echocardiography (TEE): Useful in the hemodynamically compromised patient. Most helpful in differentiating severe right ventricular contusion from acute cardiac tamponade. High-frequency sound waves are emitted from a transducer fitted to the end of a standard gastroscope approximately 9 mm in diameter. When the gastroscope is introduced into the esophagus, the transducer produces clear posterior images of the heart.

Technetium pyrophosphate myocardial scan: Identifies localized area(s) of damaged myocardial cells by radioisotope uptake, which appear as "hot spot(s)" on the scan.

COLLABORATIVE MANAGEMENT

For blunt injuries

Treatment of dysrhythmias: Done using the Advanced Cardiac Life Support protocols of the American Heart Association. If rhythm disturbances do not appear in the first 5 days after trauma, they rarely occur later. (See Appendix 1 for resuscitation guidelines.)

Relief of acute pain: Usually with IV morphine sulfate in small increments unless hypotension occurs. Activity is restricted, and the patient is continuously observed.

Immediate corrective surgical repair: For ruptured valve, torn papillary muscle, or torn intraventricular septum accompanied by hemodynamic instability.

Treatment of shock: With fluid resuscitation, vasopressor drugs (i.e., norepinephrine, dopamine, vasopressin).

Treatment of myocardial failure: Oxygen, diuretics, positive inotropic agents, and monitoring with a pulmonary artery catheter for right- and left-sided heart pressures.

Research Brief 2-2   In a prospective study over 1 year, 60 patients with penetrating cardiac injuries were evaluated to determine the characteristics of survivors. More patients with stab wounds (68%) survived than did patients with gunshot wounds (14%). The presence of cardiac tamponade and the anatomic site of injury did not predict survival, but the mechanism of injury (stab vs gun shot wound) and the presence of sinus rhythm when the pericardium was penetrated were predictors of survival.

From Asensio JA et al: Penetrating cardiac injuries: a prospective study of variables predicting outcomes, *J Am Coll Surg* 186:24-34, 1998.

For penetrating injuries

Surgical intervention: Emergency thoracotomy for patients with probable cardiac tamponade unless already dead when found. Reasonably-sized foreign bodies can be seen by fluoroscopic examination and removed surgically.

Caution: Because of the potential for hemorrhage or pneumothorax, never remove a penetrating object until a surgeon is present.

Antimicrobial agents: To control infections secondary to contamination by the penetrating instrument.

NURSING DIAGNOSES AND INTERVENTIONS

Altered tissue perfusion: peripheral, cardiopulmonary, renal, and cerebral, related to interruption of arterial and venous flow secondary to decreased cardiac contractility

Desired outcome: Within 12 hr after injury, patient has adequate perfusion as evidenced by systolic BP ≥90 mm Hg (or within patient's normal range); HR ≤100 beats/min; RR 12-20 breaths/min with normal depth and pattern (eupnea); ease of respiration; clear lung fields; urine output ≥0.5 ml/kg/hr; brisk capillary refill (<2 sec); peripheral pulses >2+ on a 0-4+ scale; normal sinus rhythm; absence of neck vein distention with the HOB elevated to 30 degrees; and orientation to time, place, and person.

• Perform a complete cardiac assessment q4h, noting peripheral pulses, heart sounds, and capillary refill; assess heart rate and rhythm and BP hourly. For more assessment information, see

"Decreased Cardiac Output" in "Acute Cardiac Tamponade," p. 120; and "Impaired Gas Exchange" in "Pneumothorax," p. 200.

- Perform a complete pulmonary assessment q4h, noting respiratory rate, depth, and effort. Auscultate lung fields q4h and as needed to evaluate for pulmonary congestion.
- Consult physician for changes in mental status, systolic BP <90 mm Hg or a drop of >20 mm Hg from trend, delayed capillary refill, or absent or thready peripheral pulses.
- Administer fluids to maintain systolic BP at ≥90 mm Hg and urine output at ≥0.5 ml/kg/hr.
- Maintain continuous cardiac monitoring for the first 3-4 days after cardiac trauma.
- If dysrhythmias occur, administer antidysrhythmic agents or prepare for transvenous temporary pacemaker insertion.
- If hemodynamic instability occurs, place patient in supine position, if injuries allow, and prepare for initiation of pulmonary artery pressure (PAP) monitoring.

NIC   Cardiac Care: Acute; Circulatory Precautions; Emergency Care; Invasive Hemodynamic Monitoring; Dysrhythmia Management; Respiratory Monitoring; Shock Management; Vital Signs Monitoring; Oxygen Therapy; Fluid/Electrolyte Management

Pain   (acute precordial chest pain) related to biophysical injury secondary to myocardial damage and chest wall injury

Desired outcomes: Within 2 hr after initiation of analgesic therapy, patient's subjective evaluation of discomfort improves, as documented by a pain scale. Nonverbal indicators, such as grimacing or diaphoresis, are absent or reduced.

- Assess and document location, type, severity, and duration of discomfort. Devise a pain scale for the patient to rate discomfort from 0 (no pain) to 10. Administer IV morphine or other analgesic agent as prescribed, and record its effectiveness, using the pain scale. Pain may begin immediately after injury or after approximately 8 hr. Usually it is not affected by coronary vasodilators.
- Place patient in a position of comfort. Patients often prefer the HOB elevated at 30-45 degrees.
- If bony structures are damaged and pain limits coughing and deep breathing, assist patient with splinting during chest physiotherapy. Intercostal nerve blocks may be needed.
- Teach patient the signs of posttraumatic pericarditis (i.e., fever, diaphoresis, precordial chest pain) and to notify physician promptly if they occur.

NIC   Analgesic Administration; Pain Management; Positioning; Presence

ADDITIONAL NURSING DIAGNOSES

For other nursing diagnoses and interventions, see also "Major Trauma," p. 89; "Acute Cardiac Tamponade," p. 118; "Psychosocial Support," p. 68; and "Psychosocial Support of the Patient's Family and Significant Others," p. 78.

Acute Cardiac Tamponade

PATHOPHYSIOLOGY

Acute cardiac tamponade is a sudden accumulation of blood, fluid, clots, pus, and/or gas in the pericardial space, which compresses the heart and interferes with both ventricular filling (diastole) and ejection (systole). Acute and chronic tamponade may have the following causes:

1. Trauma: blunt or penetrating cardiac trauma
2. Iatrogenic: cardiac surgery, cardiac catheterization, pacemaker implant
3. Infection: viral, bacterial, or fungal
4. Carcinoma/neoplasm: most commonly breast and lung
5. Nontraumatic hemorrhage: aortic aneurysms or dissections, anticoagulation therapy
6. Left ventricular rupture following extensive myocardial infarction
7. Other: connective tissue disease or patient receiving radiation therapy

Hemodynamic compromise is the primary effect of sudden cardiac tamponade, resulting from inadequate CO and decreased tissue perfusion. The pericardial sac contains 20-50 ml of fluid to protect and provide a friction-free surface for the beating heart. The pericardial sac has limited stretching ability. A sudden addition of 50-100 ml of fluid can markedly increase intrapericardial pressure. Conversely, a slowly accumulating tamponade can result in 1.5 L of fluid collection without life-threatening cardiac compromise.

As intrapericardial pressure increases and exceeds CVP, the atria, ventricles, and coronary arteries are compressed. The compressed heart chambers are unable to expand, resulting in decreased end-diastolic volume, pressure, stroke volume and CO. Tissue perfusion is globally compromised as a result of the failure of the heart to fill and pump normal blood volume.

ASSESSMENT

Clinical presentation: *Shock:* tachycardia, decreased BP, pallor, confusion, restlessness, cold and clammy skin, dyspnea, oliguria, thready pulse. Unwillingness to lie supine is a cardinal sign of tamponade.

Classic signs: Beck's triad (distended neck veins, hypotension, muffled heart tones) occurs in 10%-33% of patients with acute cardiac tamponade. Distended neck veins may not be seen with acute traumatic tamponade (as compared with constrictive pericarditis) because of hypovolemia and increased blood to the right atrium during inspiration. Muffled heart tones may not be present if the patient is sitting upright, because gravity pulls the blood toward the bottom of the pericardial sac.

Presence of pulsus paradoxus when measuring blood pressure indicates possible tamponade. Stroke volume is reduced when intrathoracic pressure increases during inspiration. To assess for pulsus paradoxus:

1. Inflate BP cuff 20 mm above systolic BP while the patient breathes normally.
2. Begin to deflate cuff *slowly and evenly* until the first sound is heard. During deflation, it becomes evident the sounds are audible only during expiration. No sounds are heard during inspiration.
3. Continue deflating the cuff *slowly* until you hear sounds during both inspiration and expiration.
4. Pulsus paradoxus is measured as the difference between the first sound (even though only on expiration) and the sound when heard on both inspiration and expiration.

To assess for pulsus paradoxus with an intraarterial line: measure the distance between systole of the inspired breath and systole of the expired breath. A difference of >10 mm Hg may be used to assess for tamponade. Pulsus paradoxus may also be present when a patient is hypovolemic.

Physical assessment: See Table 2-7.

Note: In severe hypovolemic states, physical signs may be masked.

TABLE 2-7   Physical Signs of Acute Cardiac Tamponade

Physical sign	Explanation for findings
Muffled heart sounds	Accumulation of fluid surrounding the heart diminishes sounds of valve closure.
CVP elevated to >12 mm Hg	Mean right atrial pressure is elevated because diastolic filling is impeded by atrial compression.
Decreased BP	Compression by tamponade reduces ventricular filling, decreasing CO and BP.
Jugular venous distention	As atria and ventricles become compressed, there is less space for diastolic filling, causing impairment of venous return.
Pulsus paradoxus: a fall of ≥10 mm Hg in systolic BP during inspiration	Two possible explanations are: (1) during each inspiration, blood pools in pulmonary veins, reducing left ventricular filling and output; (2) with inspiration, intraventricular septum shifts toward left ventricle, causing more volume to be drawn to right side rather than to left side of heart.
Absence of Kussmaul sign: Kussmaul sign is a rise, rather than fall, in venous pressure during inspiration	On inspiration, blood is accelerated toward the right atrium because of septal shift toward left ventricle.

BP, Blood pressure; *CO,* cardiac output; *CVP,* central venous pressure.

ECG and hemodynamic measurements
Cardiac monitor: May show evidence of sinus tachycardia or electrical alternans (see "ECG," which follows).
Pulmonary artery pressure monitoring: *Early:* elevated right atrial pressure (if severe hypotension is not present).
Late: elevated left ventricular end-diastolic pressure.

DIAGNOSTIC TESTS

ECG: May reveal ST segment elevation, nonspecific ST and T wave changes (representing myocardial ischemia), and electrical alternans (alternation of the QRS axis from beat to beat) caused by a pendulum-like movement of the heart within the pericardial effusion.
Chest x-ray: If classic, reveals a widened mediastinum with a normal cardiac silhouette, clear lung fields, and dilation of the superior vena cava. Widened mediastinum may not be evident in early tamponade.
Echocardiography: May reveal an "echo-free area" located anterior to the right ventricle and posterior to the left ventricle. Right ventricular chamber size may be reduced. A right-to-left intraventricular septal shift is seen during inspiration.
TEE: See discussion with "Cardiac Trauma," p. 115.

COLLABORATIVE MANAGEMENT

Pericardiocentesis: Needle aspiration of the pericardium can be done using a subxiphoid or left parasternal approach to drain excess fluid from the pericardial space. The blood removed often will not clot, since the heart action can cause clotting factors within the pericardial sac to break down (defibrination). Pericardiocentesis alone may not suffice to manage acute pericardial tamponade. Surgical exploration with pericardial window is recommended because of the high incidence of recurrent bleeding if surgery is not performed. A drain may stay in place until fluid output decreases or ceases.
Surgical procedures: Subxiphoid pericardiostomy is a resection of the xiphoid process to drain the pericardial sac. It is performed using either local or general anesthesia. Other more extensive surgical procedures, including a pericardiectomy, can be used for cardiac decompression. An immediate thoracotomy can be done in the ICU or emergency department if the patient becomes suddenly bradycardic (HR <50 beats/min) or severely hypotensive (systolic BP <70 mm Hg), or has a cardiac arrest. Thoracotomy allows for pericardial sac evacuation, hemorrhage control, and internal cardiac massage if needed.
Fluid resuscitation: IV fluid infusion used to increase filling ventricular pressures during diastole. Should result in increased CO and BP. Blood products, colloids, or crystalloids may be used.
Inotropic agents: Medications used to increase myocardial contractility and CO, such as dopamine, dobutamine, norepinephrine, milrinone, isoproterenol, and amrinone. See Appendix 7.
Oxygen, intubation, mechanical ventilation: Oxygen is administered using the equipment that most effectively corrects each patient's hypoxia. Devices used range from nasal cannula to 100% nonrebreather masks to mechanical ventilators.

NURSING DIAGNOSES AND INTERVENTIONS

Decreased cardiac output (CO) related to decreased preload secondary to compression of ventricles by fluid in the pericardial sac
Desired outcome: Within 4-6 hr after fluid resuscitation or evacuation of tamponade, patient has adequate CO as evidenced by mean right atrial pressure (RAP) 4-6 mm Hg; mean PAWP 6-12 mm Hg; PAP 20-30/8-15 mm Hg; CO 4-7 L/min; CI >2.5 L/min; systolic BP ≥90 mm Hg (or within patient's normal range); HR 60-100 beats/min; normal sinus rhythm on ECG; and absence of new murmurs or gallops, distended neck veins, and pulsus paradoxus.
- Assess cardiovascular function by evaluating heart sounds and neck veins hourly. Consult physician for muffled heart sounds, new murmurs, new gallops, irregularities in rate and rhythm, and distended neck veins.
- Monitor all patients with blunt or penetrating trauma to the chest and abdomen for physical signs of acute cardiac tamponade (see Table 2-7), persistent hemodynamic instability, and shock symptoms more severe than expected for the blood loss.
- Evaluate patient for pulsus paradoxus: an abnormal decrease in arterial systolic BP during inspiration compared with that during expiration (Table 2-8).
- Measure and record hemodynamic parameters. Consult physician for sudden abnormalities or changes in trend. Early signs of tamponade include elevated RAP (CVP) with normal BP. Later signs include elevated PAP in the presence of hypotension.

T A B L E 2 - 8 **Measuring Paradoxic Pulse**

- After placing BP cuff on patient, inflate it above the known systolic BP. Instruct patient to breathe normally.
- While slowly deflating the cuff, auscultate BP.
- Listen for the first Korotkoff sound, which will occur during expiration with cardiac tamponade.
- Note the manometer reading when the first sound occurs, and continue to deflate the cuff slowly until Korotkoff sounds are audible throughout inspiration and expiration.
- Record the difference in millimeters of mercury between the first and second sounds. This is the pulsus paradoxus.

- Evaluate ECG for ST segment changes, T wave changes, rate, and rhythm. The optimal is sinus rhythm or sinus tachycardia. Maintain continuous cardiac monitoring.
- Administer blood products, colloids, or crystalloids as prescribed. For trauma patients, use large-bore IV lines in the periphery, if possible. Use pressure infusers and rapid-volume/warmer infusers for patients who require massive fluid resuscitation. Be prepared to administer pressor agents if fluid resuscitation does not support patient's BP.
- Have emergency equipment available for immediate pulmonary artery catheterization, central line insertion, pericardiocentesis, or thoracotomy.

NIC Cardiac Care; Cardiac Care: Acute; Emergency Care; Hemodynamic Regulation; Invasive Hemodynamic Monitoring; Fluid Monitoring; Fluid Management; Blood Product Administration; Medication Administration; Oxygen Therapy; Resuscitation; Shock Management: Cardiac; Vital Signs Monitoring; Dysrhythmia Management

Altered tissue perfusion: cardiopulmonary, peripheral, cerebral, and renal; related to interruption of arterial and venous flow secondary to compression of the myocardium by the collection of blood

Desired outcome: Within 4-6 hr after management with fluids or evacuation of tamponade, patient has adequate perfusion as evidenced by orientation to time, place, and person; systolic BP ≥90 mm Hg (or within patient's normal range); RR 12-20 breaths/min with normal depth and pattern (eupnea) and ease of respirations; SaO_2 >95%; peripheral pulses >2+ on a 0-4+ scale; equal and normoreactive pupils; warm and dry skin; brisk capillary refill (<2 sec); and urine output ≥0.5 ml/kg/hr.

- Assess tissue perfusion by evaluating the following at least hourly: LOC, BP, pulses, pupillary response, skin temperature, and capillary refill.
- Evaluate urine output hourly to ensure that it is at least 0.5 ml/kg/hr.
- Maintain tissue perfusion by delivering prescribed blood products, colloids, or crystalloids.
- If hypotension occurs, administer fluids and medication to maintain BP. Frequently assess peripheral IV lines for evidence of infiltration. If vasopressor agents infiltrate subcutaneous tissues, necrosis occurs. Follow appropriate management protocol for your institution.
- Have emergency oxygen, intubation and mechanical ventilation equipment available.
- Anticipate and prepare for emergent surgery and pericardiocentesis evacuation, if needed.

Note: Vasopressors (e.g., norepinephrine, dopamine) should be infused through a central line unless central venous access is not possible and/or the drugs are only needed for a few hours.

NIC Cardiac Care: Acute; Circulatory Care; Emergency Care; Invasive Hemodynamic Monitoring; Respiratory Monitoring; Shock Management; Vital Signs Monitoring; Cerebral Perfusion Promotion; Neurologic Monitoring; Medication Administration; Medication Management; Oxygen Therapy; Intravenous Therapy; Fluid/Electrolyte Management

ADDITIONAL NURSING DIAGNOSES

For other nursing diagnoses and interventions see also "Major Trauma," p. 89; "Cardiac Trauma," p. 115; "Hemodynamic Monitoring," p. 23; "Psychosocial Support," p. 68; and "Psychosocial Support for the Patient's Family and Significant Others," p. 78.

Renal and Lower Urinary Tract Trauma

PATHOPHYSIOLOGY

Injuries to the kidneys and lower urinary tract (LUT), including the ureters, urinary bladder, and urethra, occur in <1% of all trauma patients but have the potential for lifelong complications and death. These injuries are often overlooked in the initial trauma assessment because they frequently accompany life-threatening injuries that require aggressive and immediate management.

Blunt injuries caused by vehicular collisions, falls, sports-related injuries, and assaults are responsible for most renal and LUT trauma. Renal and LUT trauma can occur with penetrating injuries (stab and gunshot wounds). The pathophysiology for each type of renal and LUT trauma is discussed in Table 2-9.

Urethral injury may cause males long-term problems with sexual intercourse and voiding. Sexual dysfunction may be the result of damage to neural and vascular structures. Incontinence may result from damage to the sphincters or their innervation. In patients with complete urethral disruption, approximately 20% have voiding dysfunction and 25% have sexual dysfunction.

ASSESSMENT

Renal trauma
Clinical presentation: Abdominal or flank pain, back tenderness, colicky pain with passage of blood clots, hemorrhage (pallor, diaphoresis, hypotension, tachycardia, restlessness, confusion), gross hematuria.

> **Note:** Gross hematuria is present in only slightly more than half of patients with renal trauma and is considered an unreliable diagnostic sign.

Physical assessment: Hematoma over the flank of the eleventh or twelfth ribs; obvious wounds, contusions, or abrasions in the flank or abdomen; abdominal distention; Grey Turner's sign (bruising over the lower portion of the back and the flank caused by a retroperitoneal hemorrhage); pain at the costovertebral angle; flank or abdominal mass.

> **Note:** Physical signs may be masked because the kidneys are located beneath abdominal organs, back muscles, and bony structures.

Ureteral trauma
Clinical presentation: Microscopic or gross hematuria may be present. If the ureter is transected, normal urine from the unaffected kidney may still be voided. *Late signs* may include fever and flank or abdominal discomfort.
Physical assessment: Urine at the entrance or exit sites of penetrating wound, enlarging retroperitoneal mass.

Bladder trauma
Clinical presentation: Suprapubic tenderness, inability to void spontaneously, gross hematuria (present in approximately 95% of patients). *Late signs* may include fever and abdominal discomfort.
Physical assessment: Perineal or scrotal edema and hematoma, abnormal position of prostate, abdominal distention, palpable suprapubic mass, palpable and overdistended bladder.

Urethral trauma
Clinical presentation: Blood at the meatus, inability to void spontaneously, urethral bleeding, prostate tenderness, microscopic or gross hematuria, pain and tenderness of genitalia.
Physical assessment: Tracking of urine into tissues of the thighs or abdominal wall, bruised to discolored genitalia.

DIAGNOSTIC TESTS

Retrograde urethrogram: Used to diagnose urethral tears or rupture. A small urinary catheter is inserted and the balloon inflated in the distal anterior urethra. Contrast material is injected and a single x-ray film is taken to outline the inner size and shape of the urethra. In urethral rupture, extravasation of the contrast material occurs.

Cystogram: If no urethral tear is found on retrograde urethrogram, a catheter is inserted into the bladder. The bladder is filled with 300 ml of contrast material. After x-ray films are obtained to determine if intraperitoneal or extraperitoneal extravasation of contrast material occurs, the bladder is drained and repeat x-rays are taken to check for small posterior ruptures.

Caution: Check patient's history for allergy to iodine, iodine-containing foods, or contrast material. Hydration and sometimes diuretics are needed to facilitate excretion of contrast material after testing.

Excretory urogram/intravenous pyelogram (IVP): Contrast material is administered intravenously and is filtered by the kidneys before excretion through the urinary tract. X-ray films visualize the normal or injured structures of the kidneys, ureters, or bladder.

Renal ultrasound: Used to visualize the urinary tract. A transducer transmits high-frequency sound waves through the urinary tract. The resultant echoes are amplified and converted into electrical impulses displayed on an oscilloscope. The test is rarely used for early identification of injury because it is too imprecise.

Radionuclide imaging: Evaluates for injured LUT structures and alterations in renal blood flow. After IV injection of a radionuclide, a radioactivity-detecting device scans and records the radioactive uptake. The substance is excreted in 6-24 hr following the test.

Blood urea nitrogen values: Renal dysfunction causes insufficient excretion of urea, elevating nitrogenous wastes in the blood. In renal trauma, BUN level may increase because of body catabolism, dehydration, or from absorption of peritoneal extravasation of urine. When the BUN is elevated as a result of urine absorption, the serum creatinine levels remain normal. Normal BUN is 10-20 mg/dl.

Serum creatinine levels: Creatinine level is the most accurate measure of renal damage. Renal impairment is virtually the only cause of elevated serum creatinine. Creatinine production is fairly constant, since production is proportional to muscle mass. Creatinine is freely filtered at the glomerulus and minimally resorbed, so creatinine excretion is proportional to glomerular filtration rate. Normal value is 0.7-1.5 mg/dl.

Research Brief 2-3   Although ureteral injuries are rare, delay in diagnosis can lead to the loss of renal function. This study was performed to determine the effectiveness of preoperative testing after suspected ureteral injury. In 20 patients, a total of 10 diagnostic studies were performed, but only 2 were diagnostic for ureteral injury (1 IVP and 1 CT). The rest of the injuries were discovered during surgery by primary visualization. The authors concluded that direct visualization is the best and most accurate diagnostic modality in ureteral injury.

From Median D et al: *J Am Coll Surg* 186:641-644, 1998.

Note: If an intraperitoneal bladder rupture has occurred, hyperkalemia, hypernatremia, uremia, and acidosis may occur as a result of resorption of urine from the peritoneal cavity.

Clearance tests: Clearance is the volume of plasma that can be cleared of a specific substance during a specified period of time. Clearance tests evaluate the extent of injury by assessing renal filtration, resorption, secretion, and renal plasma flow. Creatinine, inulin (a plant starch), and urea may be tested.

Kidney-ureter-bladder (KUB) radiography: Evaluates position, size, structure, and defects of the urinary tract. May reveal foreign bodies, retroperitoneal hematoma, fracture of the lower ribs or pelvis, organ displacement, or fluid accumulation.

CT: Viewing the kidneys by a series of cross-sectional images interpreted by computer. May reveal hematomas, renal lacerations, renal infarcts, or extravasation of urine. Contrast-enhanced CT detects kidney laceration and arterial occlusion. CT is the method of choice to assess patients with severe renal trauma.

Renal angiography: Arterial injection of a contrast medium, permitting identification on x-ray film of renal vasculature and functional tissue. After renal trauma, angiography permits identification of renal pedicle injury, renal infarct, intrarenal hematoma, lacerations, and shattered kidney.

T A B L E   2 - 9   Pathophysiology for Renal and Lower Urinary Tract Trauma

Type of injury	Anatomic considerations	Pathophysiology and mechanism of injury	Result of injury
Renal trauma	Kidneys are well protected from injury posteriorly by muscles of the back, anteriorly by organs of the GI tract, and by a tough outer capsule and adipose tissue Kidneys are fixed in retroperitoneal space only by renal pedicle (vascular system in renal helium) and ureters Blunt renal injury is often caused by compression of kidney by the twelfth rib, which rotates inwardly and squeezes kidney into lumbar spine	Renal trauma can be divided into three classifications: **Minor trauma: Incidence 85%** Bruising of renal parenchyma; superficial lacerations of renal cortex without rupture of renal capsule **Major trauma: Incidence 10%-15%** Major lacerations through cortex and medulla; continuation of laceration through renal capsule **Critical trauma: Incidence <5%** Renal vascular trauma in which kidney is shattered and renal pedicle is injured; fragmentation (renal fracture)	**Minor trauma:** Hematuria and flank tenderness that will usually result in a full recovery with rest and observation **Major trauma:** Hematuria, flank pain, and possible hypotension that may require surgical intervention **Critical injury:** Severe blood loss and shock requiring immediate surgical intervention
Ureteral trauma	Injury to upper part of ureter is uncommon because of its location deep in retroperitoneum Ureteral lacerations are most common at ureteropelvic junction, where upper ureter joins renal pelvis	Ureteral injury is most commonly associated with iatrogenic injuries during gynecologic, colonic, and vascular surgery Blunt injury may occur when ureter becomes crushed against spinal column When ureteral injury is not associated with iatrogenic injury, it	Extravasation of urine or blood may lead to infection, abscess formation, hemorrhage, or shock; late complications include prolonged voiding time, ureteral strictures, and fistula formation

Bladder trauma	When bladder is distended, it extends above umbilicus and has less protection from trauma; the bladder ruptures at its point of least resistance (the dome), and blood and urine extravasate into the peritoneal cavity (intraperitoneal rupture) Extraperitoneal rupture occurs most often in conjunction with pelvic fractures; sharp bone fragments perforate bladder at its base, leading to extravasation of blood and urine into space surrounding bladder base	usually occurs in the setting of severe abdominal compression or significant penetrating abdominal injury Motor vehicle crashes are the most common cause of bladder rupture; bladder contusion often results from a direct blow or the cavitational effect of missiles (outward tissue acceleration away from the tract of the bullet); bladder rupture does not require extensive force, which may be a blunt blow to the lower abdomen	Bladder lacerations or rupture can lead to blood or urine extravasation outside of the peritoneal cavity (80%) and into the peritoneal cavity (20%); infection or hemorrhage can follow
Urethral trauma	Urethral injury is more common in males than females because the male urethra is 5 times longer; the male urethra is also rigidly fixed at the urogenital diaphragm (bulbous urethra), whereas the female urethra is short and mobile	Perineal trauma, straddle injuries, and pelvic fractures are often the causes of urethral injury; vehicular collisions with deceleration and shearing may also lead to injury of the posterior urethra	Urethral injury may lead to extravasation of blood and/or urine within penis; if disruption to Buck's fascia occurs, extravasation into upper thighs and peritoneum follows; hemorrhage or infection may also occur

Note: Assess patient for allergy to contrast medium. Hydrate patient during and after the procedure.

MRI: Used to identify the best surgical approach for more difficult injuries, such as traumatic posterior urethral injury. Identifies severity of injury and may help estimate time needed for recovery.

COLLABORATIVE MANAGEMENT

Pharmacotherapy
Antibiotics: Initiate for positive urine culture results, penetrating injuries, or peritonitis.
Analgesics: IV morphine sulfate is used to relieve pain and is easily reversed with naloxone if hypotension or respiratory depression are noted.
Management of complications
Hemorrhage shock: Volume resuscitation with crystalloids, colloids, or blood products as indicated.
Infections: Blood and urine cultures, antibiotics.
Renal dysfunction: Fluid restriction; dietary restrictions for renal impairment; peritoneal dialysis; continuous renal replacement therapy; or hemodialysis. See "Renal Replacement Therapies," p. 334, for more information.
Catheterization: If patient is unable to void. Catheter should be passed only as far as it will progress without undue force. If any resistance is met during catheterization, a urethrogram is indicated. If blood is present at the urethral meatus, the patient should not be catheterized until a urethrogram is obtained, since the blood may signal urethral injury. In the presence of urethral injury, an improperly placed catheter can cause subsequent incontinence, impotence, and urethral strictures. In renal trauma, diversion of urine may be required by nephrostomy tube, depending on location of injury or in cases of coexisting pancreatic and duodenal injury. A suprapubic catheter may be used to manage severe urethral lacerations and urethral disruption. Internal ureteral catheters (ureteral stents) may be indicated for ureteral trauma, particularly for gunshot wounds, to maintain ureteral alignment, ensure urinary drainage, and provide support during anastomosis.
Surgical correction: Indicated for transected ureter, partial ureteral tears of more than a third of the circumference of the ureter, bladder perforation with associated abdominal injuries or intraperitoneal rupture, and injuries accompanied by rapidly expanding, pulsating hematomas. See Table 2-10 for examples of procedures for the various types of renal and LUT injuries.

T A B L E 2 - 10 Surgical Procedures for Renal and Lower Urinary Tract Trauma	
Type of injury	**Surgical indications/surgical management**
Minor renal trauma	None needed. Rest and observation with careful follow-up to prevent progressive deformity and to evaluate BP.
Major renal trauma	Surgical intervention if hypotension and hemodynamic instability occur.
Critical renal trauma	Immediate surgical exploration; low rates of renal salvage.
Proximal ureteral injury	Primary ureterostomy with end-to-end anastomosis.
Distal ureteral injury	Ureteral stenting or percutaneous nephrostomy, depending on location and extent of injury.
Bladder injury	Use of suprapubic drainage versus indwelling urethral catheter drainage is controversial. Use of suprapubic catheter avoids complications of prolonged urethral catheterization, particularly in males who are prone to the development of urethral strictures.
Urethral injury	Suprapubic cystotomy and drainage for temporary urinary evacuation. Urethral splinting and surgical reconstruction usually are delayed for 3-6 mo to allow reduction in bruising and swelling, which could delay healing of urinary structures.

NURSING DIAGNOSES AND INTERVENTIONS

Altered urinary elimination related to mechanical trauma secondary to injury to the kidney and lower urinary tract structures

Desired outcome: Within 6 hr after immediate trauma management, patient has a urinary output of ≥0.5 ml/kg/hr with no evidence of bladder distention.

- Monitor urinary outflow. Encourage patient to void. If patient is unable to void, assess for full bladder. Urinary catheterization or suprapubic drainage may be needed. Report findings to the physician. Monitor for the following signs of kidney or LUT trauma:
  - ❑ Urge but inability to void spontaneously in spite of adequate volume replacement
  - ❑ Blood at the urethral meatus
  - ❑ Difficult or unsuccessful urinary catheterization
  - ❑ Anuria after urinary catheterization
  - ❑ Hematuria
- Do not catheterize patient if there is blood at the urethral meatus. Call physician for consultation if urethral injury is suspected.
- Monitor serum BUN and creatinine.
- Document I&O hourly. Consult physician if urine output is <0.5 ml/kg/hr.
- Assess whether clots may be occluding the drainage system. If indicated, obtain prescription for catheter irrigation or call physician to irrigate catheter. Sudden cessation of urine flow through the collection system (particularly if past output was >50 ml/hr) indicates possible catheter obstruction. If catheter irrigation does not resume urine drainage, consider changing the urinary catheter after discussion with physician.
- Ensure nephrostomy tubes are not occluded by patient's weight or external pressure. Irrigate the nephrostomy tube *only* if prescribed with ≤5 ml of fluid. The renal pelvis holds <10 ml of fluid.
- Assess entrance site of the nephrostomy tube for bleeding or leakage of urine. Catheter blockage or dislodging causes a sudden decrease in urine output. Inspect urine color and for blood clots. Hematuria is normal for 24-48 hr after nephrostomy tube insertion. Consult physician if gross bleeding (with or without clots) occurs.
- Hydrate to allow for clearing of contrast material from patient's system after diagnostic testing.

NIC Urinary Elimination Management; Urinary Catheterization; Fluid Management; Fluid Monitoring; Tube Care: Urinary

Risk for infection related to inadequate primary defenses and tissue destruction secondary to bacterial contamination of the urinary tract system occurring with penetrating trauma, rupture of the bladder into the perineum, or instrumentation

Desired outcome: Patient is free of infection as evidenced by normothermia; WBC count ≤11,000/mm^3; and negative results of urine and wound drainage testing for infective organisms.

- Use aseptic technique when caring for drainage systems. Keep catheters and collection container at a level lower than the bladder to prevent reflux; ensure that drainage tubing is not kinked.
- Record the color and odor of urine each shift. Culture urine specimen when infection is suspected.
- Monitor patient's WBC count daily and temperature q4h for elevations.
- Assess for signs of peritonitis: abdominal pain, abdominal distention with rigidity, nausea, vomiting, fever, malaise, and weakness.
- Assess catheter exit site each shift for the presence of erythema, swelling, or drainage.
- Assess thigh, groin, and lower portion of abdomen for indicators of urinary extravasation: swelling, pain, mass(es), erythema, and tracking of urine along fascial planes.
- Assess surgical incision for approximation of suture line and evidence of wound healing, noting presence of erythema, swelling, and drainage. Note color, odor, and consistency of drainage. Notify physician of purulent or foul-smelling drainage. Consider obtaining a culture.
- Assess skin at invasive sites for indicators of irritation: erythema, drainage, and swelling.
- Cleanse catheter insertion sites with antimicrobial solution. Manage catheter exit sites per protocol.

NIC Consider dressing changes q24h or as soon as noted they are wet. If skin is irritated from contact with urine, consider use of a pectin wafer skin barrier for extra protection.

Incision Site Care; Infection Protection; Wound Care; Infection Control; Surveillance; Tube Care: Urinary

Pain (acute tenderness in lower abdomen) related to physical injury associated with LUT structural injury, procedures for urinary diversion, or surgical incisions

Desired outcomes: Within 2 hr after giving analgesic agent, patient's subjective evaluation of discomfort improves, as documented by a pain scale. Nonverbal indicators of discomfort, such as grimacing, are absent.

- Assess patient for pain at least q4h. Devise a pain scale with patient, rating discomfort from 0 (no pain) to 10. Be alert to shallow breathing in the presence of abdominal pain, which can cause inadequate pulmonary excursion. Medicate promptly, and document patient's response to analgesic agent, using the pain scale. IV narcotics may be indicated if the injury is severe.
- Explain the cause of the pain to the patient.
- Assist patient into a position of comfort. Often knee flexion will relax lower abdominal muscles and help reduce discomfort.
- Implement nonpharmacologic measures for coping with pain: diversion, touch, and conversation. Also see discussion of pain, p. 51.

NIC   Analgesic Administration; Pain Management; Positioning; Presence

Pelvic Fractures

PATHOPHYSIOLOGY

The pelvis is composed of three bones: two innominate bones and the sacrum. The innominate bones are each composed of three bones (ilium, pubis, and ischium) that fuse after childhood. The two innominate bones are joined by the symphysis pubis, a fibrous cartilage joint that connects the two pubic bones anteriorly; they are attached posteriorly to a third bone, the sacrum, by a system of ligaments termed the *posterior osseous ligamentous* structures.

Motor vehicle collisions and auto-pedestrian trauma cause approximately two thirds of all pelvic fractures, which have mortality up to 50% in some studies. A large force is needed for a pelvic fracture to occur, because these bones are stabilized by a strong network of ligaments. Pelvic fractures have been classified by several systems, but perhaps the most helpful are the systems that classify fractures by their stability and the mechanism of injury (Table 2-11). Pelvic fractures are considered stable fractures when the posterior osseous ligamentous structures are intact. An unstable pelvic fracture occurs when the osseous ligamentous structures are disrupted posteriorly and portions of the pelvis can move in any direction.

Research Brief 2-4   After pelvic fractures, 255 women were interviewed to determine the effect of trauma on their genitourinary, sexual, and reproductive function. Urinary complaints occurred more frequently in women with residual pelvic fracture displacement of 5 mm or more compared with those without displacement, and more frequently in women with residual lateral and vertical displacement compared with those with medial displacement. Women with a fractured pelvis also reported more cesarean sections than controls, but there was no difference in the incidence of miscarriage or infertility. Pain during sex was most common in women with fractures displaced 5 mm or more.

From Copeland CE et al: *J Orthop Trauma* 11(2):73-81, 1997.

The most serious complications from a pelvic fracture are hemorrhage and exsanguination, which cause up to 60% of the deaths. The pelvis receives a rich supply of blood from a complex system of interconnected collateral arteries and the venous plexus of the iliac system, often called the *vascular sink*. The aorta and internal iliac artery are close to the pelvis. This vascular network can easily be damaged or disrupted by the same forces that injure the pelvis. Pelvic fragments can damage vascular structures. The retroperitoneal space can hold as much as 4 L of blood before spontaneous tamponade occurs. Acute blood loss is difficult to identify until systemic symptoms, such as those occurring with shock, appear. In addition, damage to the sciatic and sacral nerves may occur with sacral and sacroiliac disruption.

The most common cause of pelvic fractures in older adults is falls, as opposed to motor vehicle crashes in younger people. Older adults have more problems related to preexisting conditions. Cardiovascular disease often causes insufficient compensatory function to manage the stress of injury. Despite a less severe mechanism of injury, rates of sepsis and death are higher in older adults than in those trauma patients younger than 65 years with similar injuries.

ASSESSMENT

History and risk factors: Identify the cause of injury: motor vehicle or motorcycle crash, auto-pedestrian collision, fall, industrial accident, crush injury, or sports injury.
Clinical presentation: Suprapubic tenderness; pain over the iliac spines; signs and symptoms of hemorrhagic shock (tachycardia, delayed capillary refill, decreased urinary output, decreased extremity

TABLE 2-11 Classification of Pelvic Fractures

Classification of injury	Mechanism of injury	Description
Anteroposterior compression	External rotation is caused by a crushing force on the posterior superior iliac spines	"Open book injury"; the force causes the symphysis pubis to spring open. Rupture of anterior sacroiliac and sacrospinous ligaments occurs, but posterior ligaments are intact. Stable vertically but can rotate externally. May be associated with ruptured bladder (intraperitoneal) if injury occurs when bladder is full
Lateral compression	Internal rotation from a high-energy injury that causes direct pressure to crush anterior sacrum. Pressure on the greater trochanter causes the femoral head to displace the anterior pubic rami.	Most common type of injury. Often does not affect posterior ligamentous complex. Partially unstable fracture that is rotationally unstable but vertically stable. May have extensive soft tissue injury. May be associated with ruptured bladder (extraperitoneal).
Vertical shear (Malgaigne fracture)	Excessive force from trauma such as falls and crush injuries in a vertical plane leads to unstable disruption of the anterior and posterior ring.	Most severe injury with the highest mortality rates. Very unstable. Complete disruption of the posterior osseous ligamentous system. Often accompanied by injuries of the skin and subcutaneous tissues or injuries to the gastrointestinal, genitourinary, vascular, and neurologic systems.
Complex fracture	Excessive and powerful forces from many directions.	Pelvic ring disruptions resulting in bizarre fractures or dislocations in a combination of injury patterns. Usually very unstable.

temperature, pallor, hypotension); signs and symptoms of urinary injuries (as many as 15% of trauma victims with a pelvic fracture have associated renal and lower urinary tract injuries; see p. 122).

Note: Initial evaluation of a multiple trauma patient may reveal no obvious evidence of pelvic injury.

Note: Of patients with both pelvic fractures and urologic injuries, 50% have other abdominal injuries.

Accompanying abdominal injuries: in victims <65 years, upper and lower extremity fractures and head injuries; in victims >65 years, abdominal and chest trauma are more common.
Physical assessment: Groin, genitalia, and suprapubic swelling, ecchymosis, or lacerations; swelling, ecchymosis, or lacerations of medial thigh or lumbosacral area; increased diameter of the root of the thigh; pelvic instability (asymmetry or abnormal movement on downward pressure of

the iliac crests); crepitus; lower extremity shortening; abnormal lower extremity internal rotation; "frog-leg positioning" of the lower extremities; hematuria or urethral bleeding; vaginal bleeding; blood in the rectum; high-riding prostate; lower extremity paresis or hypoesthesia (in particular at the L5 and S1 levels); absence of plantar flexion and ankle jerk reflexes; unequal or weak peripheral pulses.

Note: Lacerations of the vagina, perineum, groin, or anus are assumed to be caused by compound open pelvic fractures until proven otherwise.

DIAGNOSTIC TESTS

Pelvic x-ray:
Anteroposterior view: Differentiates between a stable and unstable fracture; shows overall alignment, hip assessment, and location of fractures.
Inlet view: Determines rotational displacement, posterior displacement, and sacral fractures.
Outlet view: Demonstrates superior rotation, vertical migration, and sacral fractures.
CT: Determines the pattern of pelvic injury. This is the most reliable method for determining injury to the posterior portion of the pelvis and is particularly successful in identifying sacral and sacroiliac joint injury.
Angiography: Identifies bleeding, which often occurs at multiple points in the pelvic circulation. Two groups of patients need angiograms: those who undergo full laparotomy and are discovered to have an expanding pelvic retroperitoneal hematoma; and those with a pure pelvic injury who bleed internally. Commonly used for initial evaluation of patients with unstable pelvic fractures prior to surgery.
Hematocrit (Hct): Evaluates for ongoing bleeding. If Hct fails to stabilize, falls, or fails to rise with transfusion, ongoing bleeding is suspected. A falling Hct is a late sign of hemorrhage and occurs only after significant blood loss.
Excretory urography (intravenous pyelogram [IVP]), cystography, and urography: Used to determine associated injuries (see "Renal and Lower Urinary Tract Trauma," p. 125).

COLLABORATIVE MANAGEMENT

Pelvic stabilization
External immobilization: Defined as any device that is applied to immobilize the pelvis either externally or percutaneously through the skin into the bone. External fixation can be accomplished at the scene of injury to preserve function and prevent further orthopedic and neurovascular injury. When an unstable pelvis is identified, the pelvis should be stabilized. Stabilization can be achieved with a sheet wrapped around the pelvis and secured with towel clips. Emergency external fixation devices, consisting of one pin in each iliac wing connected by a bar, can be inserted to provide pelvic stability. If an emergency laparotomy is performed, more complex fixation devices may be applied. If abnormal shortening or rotation has occurred with the injury, the lower extremities should be supported and stabilized in the position in which they were found. A wooden backboard supported by pillows, towels, or blankets taped in place with cloth tape are used until a traction splint can be applied.

Note: Use of an external fixation device is not sufficient for maintaining reduction in the posterior pelvis or for stabilizing the pelvic posterior elements. As long as the patient is on bed rest or in traction, however, it can be used to manage the acute phase of the fracture.

Internal immobilization: Surgical open reduction and immobilization of unstable pelvic ring disruptions with surgically implanted plates, screws, or other devices. Permanent fixation requires closed reduction for final pelvic stabilization.
Surgical exploration: Done to identify blood vessels in need of ligation or repair for ongoing hemorrhage. Inflow of blood to the pelvic circulation can be limited by ligation of the internal iliac artery to control bleeding. Since many collateral vessels exist in the pelvic circulation, infarction rarely occurs with this procedure. Surgical exploration is not always recommended. When the peritoneal space is entered, the tamponade is released and bleeding can increase. The extensive vascular sink makes identification of bleeding vessels difficult. Some patients may undergo angiography and selective embolization of bleeding points with either an autologous blood clot or particulate gel foam instead of surgery.

Massive fluid resuscitation: Rapid fluid replacement with blood, colloids, or crystalloids. If >2 L of blood are required in the 8 hr after the initial resuscitation, additional measures to manage bleeding are indicated. Studies have revealed it may be appropriate to withhold aggressive fluid resuscitation until after operative repair. The increase in MAP will increase intravascular hydrostatic pressure and may increase bleeding from torn vessels.

Pharmacotherapy

Antibiotics: Initial use for prophylaxis against infection is controversial in patients with open fractures. Used later for positive cultures of wounds, blood, or urine.

Analgesics: IV morphine sulfate usually relieves pain and can be readily reversed with naloxone if hypotension or respiratory insufficiency are noted.

Vasopressors: For hypotension *only* after sufficient volume replacement has occurred (see Appendix 7).

Tetanus immunization: Booster is given if history is unknown or if a booster is needed (see Table 2-1).

NURSING DIAGNOSES AND INTERVENTIONS

Fluid volume deficit related to active blood loss secondary to injury to the pelvis and pelvic sink

Desired outcomes: Within 12 hr after injury, patient's fluid status is adequate as evidenced by regular HR ≤100 beats/min; bilaterally strong and equal peripheral pulses; warm and dry extremities; brisk (<2 sec) capillary refill; systolic BP ≥90 mm Hg (or within 10% of patient's normal range); and urine output ≥0.5 ml/kg/hr. If hemodynamic monitoring is present, PAWP is ≥6 mm Hg and CI is ≥2.5 L/min/m^2. Patient is awake, alert, and oriented to time, place, and person without restlessness or confusion.

- Perform a complete assessment of fluid balance hourly until patient is stable, noting all cardiac, hemodynamic, urinary, and CNS parameters. Consult physician for early signs of hemorrhage: decreased urinary output, delayed capillary refill, tachycardia, and changes in mental status.
- Prepare to move the patient to surgery rapidly for repair of pelvic vasculature if needed.
- Administer blood products, colloids, or crystalloids as prescribed through a large-bore peripheral IV or trauma catheter. Avoid using standard central lines or triple-lumen catheters for fluid resuscitation. Their length and narrow gauge increase resistance to flow and reduce the rate of fluid administration. Fluid resuscitation may occur only after surgical repair in some situations to reduce preoperative fluid loss from torn vessels.
- Use pressure infusers and rapid-warmer/infusers for patients who require massive fluid/blood resuscitation. Be prepared to administer vasopressor drugs, but only after fluid replacement is in progress. Vasopressors should not be used to maintain BP without fluid volume replacement.
- Keep the patient flat until fluid volume status is stabilized, unless contraindicated. Ensure that the patient has adequate airway and breathing while supine. Avoid Trendelenburg position, since it increases the risk of aspiration, may lower blood pressure or negatively alter circulation, and may impair breathing.

NIC Bleeding Reduction; Blood Products Administration; Shock Management: Volume; Fluid Management; Fluid/Electrolyte Management; Fluid Monitoring; Fluid Resuscitation; Electrolyte Monitoring; Hypothermia Treatment

Risk for infection related to inadequate primary defenses secondary to open pelvic fractures, percutaneous external fixation devices, or surgical procedure

Desired outcomes: Within 24 hr after injury, soft tissues begin to heal without purulent drainage or erythema; WBC count is ≤11,000/mm^3; cultures of blood and wounds are negative; pin insertion site is free of erythema, edema, or purulent drainage; and surgical wounds are well approximated and without erythema, edema, or purulent drainage.

- For initial wound care, remove any gross contamination from the wound and cover any exposed soft tissue and bone with wet sterile dressings. Avoid dressings soaked in povidone-iodine to minimize iodine absorption and local tissue irritation. Prevent reentry of a portion of dirty bone or soft tissue into a wound. See Appendix 8 for indications for use of sterile gloves, mask, and eye protection when managing large wounds.
- Perform pin care as prescribed (e.g., q4-6h). Pin care is controversial and may include removing dried exudate to allow the pin holes to drain freely. In contrast, some experts believe that exudate is a part of the normal healing process and provides a tight interface between the skin and pin, thereby limiting bacterial invasion into the wounds. Unless contraindicated, wrap a loose, open-gauze dressing around the insertion site of the pin.
- Monitor all wounds, incisions, and pin insertion sites on external fixation devices q4h for presence of warmth, erythema, drainage, edema, or purulence. Monitor patient for temperature ≥38.3° C (101° F) and increased WBC count.

NIC Incision Site Care; Infection Protection; Wound Care; Traction/Immobilization Care; Infection Control; Surveillance

Impaired physical mobility related to pelvic immobilization secondary to pelvic ring instability

Desired outcomes: Immediately after pelvic immobilization, patient maintains appropriate body alignment; external fixation devices and traction remain in place. At the time of hospital discharge, patient exhibits full ROM in uninjured extremities.

- Position patient in proper body alignment.
- Apply compression boots if appropriate to limit the effects of venous stasis. Remove boots at least every shift to provide skin care. Consider using compression boots on upper extremities if appropriate to aid in venous return.
- Provide active and passive ROM to uninjured extremities every shift as appropriate.
- Maintain traction by keeping it free-hanging. Do not remove weights even when repositioning.
- Use care when turning and positioning to maintain body alignment. If patient has an unstable fracture that has not yet been reduced, consult orthopedic surgeon before moving patient. Some patients can be turned from side to side until internal fixation is accomplished. Also consult physician regarding the appropriate HOB elevation, and put this information on the patient's individual plan of care.
- Do not turn patient by holding on to the external fixation.
- Provide pain relief appropriate to level of activity.

NIC Exercise Therapy: Joint Mobility; Positioning; Traction/Immobilization Care; Bed Rest Care; Body Mechanics Promotion; Pain Management; Pressure Management

Impaired skin integrity related to initial injury, physical immobility, and placement of external fixation or pneumatic antishock garment (PASG) secondary to pelvic injury

Desired outcomes: Within 12 hr of injury and throughout hospitalization, patient has timely wound healing. Patient does not develop pressure ulcers or experience tissue injury from the external fixation device.

- Cover the ends of all wires on the external fixation device with cork or gauze to protect the patient from injury.
- Apply padding to any traction slings.
- Use alternating air mattress or other specialty mattress.
- If patient can be positioned laterally, pad the external fixation device to prevent damage to the patient's skin. Provide padding over bony prominences and any body area that comes in contact with a rigid surface.
- Keep all skin areas clean and dry to minimize the risk of pressure ulcers.
- If cast is used, inspect cast for signs of drainage or odor from wounds under cast; pad rough cast edges.

Incision Site Care; Positioning; Pressure Management; Pressure Ulcer Prevention; Skin Surveillance;
NIC Traction/Immobilization Care; Wound Care; Cast Care: Maintenance

- See "Wound and Skin Care," p. 45, for more interventions.

Note: Also see "Pain," p. 51, for management of discomfort.

Compartment Syndrome (Ischemic Myositis)

PATHOPHYSIOLOGY

Compartment syndrome is defined as increased pressure within an anatomic compartment that compromises the circulation, viability, and function of tissues within the compartment. Failure to diagnose compartment syndrome is a frequent cause of litigation against the medical profession in North America. It is a surgical emergency that requires rapid intervention to prevent permanent cosmetic or functional deformity or loss of limb. Although compartment syndrome most commonly follows fractures, especially those of the tibia and fibula, it can occur from a variety of conditions (Table 2-12). Although compartment syndrome may be acute or chronic (exercise-related forms), this discussion focuses on acute forms.

The average interval between the initial injury to the compartment and the beginning symptoms of compartment syndrome is 2 hr. Compartmental tissue ischemia that lasts longer than 6 hr results in tissue necrosis and irreversible tissue changes. Neurologic injury begins within 30 min of inadequate blood supply and may become functionally irreversible after 4 to 6 hr.

TABLE 2-12   **Causes of Compartment Syndrome**

Localized compartmental trauma	Tissue reaction/ edema formation	Coagulation defects	Other
Fractures	Prolonged used of	Hemophilia	Compression during
Surgery	operative tourniquets	Anticoagulant	obtundation
Hematoma	Arterial or venous	therapy	(anesthesia, drug
Venomous bites	obstruction		overdose)
(snake, spider)	Limb reimplantation		Infiltrated IV therapy
Vascular injury	Burns (especially		Muscle hypertrophy
Postischemic swelling	when circumferential)		(e.g., skin splints)
Crush injuries	Excessive exercise		Constrictive dressings,
Electrical injuries	(e.g., march gangrene		inflatable splints or casts
	Nephritic syndrome		Closure of fascial defects
			Hypothermia
			or hyperthermia
			Clostridium
			perfringens infections
			Rocky Mountain
			spotted fever
			Use of pneumatic
			antishock garment
			(PASG)

Modified from Callahan J: *Orthop Nurs* 4(4):11-15, 1985.

Sustained hypotension and shock are associated with greater incidence of compartment syndrome. When systemic BP decreases, tissue ischemia may occur. It then takes less compartmental pressure to result in arteriolar spasm. Periods of hypotension may result in increased tissue injury at lower compartmental pressure. Persons in shock are more susceptible to compartment syndromes.

When compartmental tissue pressure increases, capillary blood flow is compromised. The increased pressure injures tissues. Histamine is released, producing vasodilation and increased capillary permeability. Fluids and proteins escape from the capillaries and contribute to higher tissue pressures. The higher tissue pressures eventually exceed both capillary and venous pressures, promoting further ischemia. Tissue ischemia results in the release of additional histamine, which further exacerbates the problem. As a result of impaired venous return, anaerobic metabolism creates more lactic acid, which stimulates vasodilation and decreases BP, and tissue pressure elevates further. As compartmental pressure continues to increase, arteriolar spasm occurs from vascular compression, further contributing to lower capillary hydrostatic pressure. Progressive ischemia leads to tissue necrosis, resulting in permanent tissue changes.

Late-onset compartment syndrome is seen in comatose or confused patients unable to communicate symptoms. Late-onset compartment syndrome is often more difficult to manage, sometimes worsening following treatment with fasciotomy. The late syndrome may occur in compartments already treated with fasciotomy. Healthy granulation tissue may cover necrotic muscle within partially opened compartments. With sufficient muscle tissue injury (e.g., after crush injuries), rhabdomyolysis can develop. The secondary myoglobinemia leads to acute tubular necrosis (ATN), which may progress to acute renal failure (ARF).

Abdominal compartment syndrome (ACS) may be associated with an exploration laparotomy. Recently identified as a complication of aggressive shock resuscitation in patients without abdominal trauma, the excessive pressure on the abdominal organs leads to multiple organ failure (MOF) and death. Even with decompression, the death rate from ACS has been reported as high as 55%.

ASSESSMENT

History and risk factors: Any patient with a peripheral injury listed in Table 2-11 is at risk for compartment syndrome. Patients admitted for acute renal failure after treatment for crush injuries or compartment syndrome should be suspected of having late-onset or continuing compartment syndrome. Patients with profound shock who receive aggressive fluid resuscitation are at risk for ACS.

Clinical presentation: compartment syndrome of the extremities

Early indicators: Unusually severe pain for an injury is a cardinal symptom. Passive motion of an involved muscle group significantly increases the pain. Palpation of the compartment reveals tension and slowed capillary refill. Tissue pressures vary with the method of measurement. Generally, normal tissue pressures vary from 0-10 mm Hg and sustained pressures >30 mm Hg result in tissue necrosis. Pressures >16 mm Hg may collapse thin-walled lower extremity veins, further contributing to the pathogenesis.

Late-onset syndrome indicators: Persistent peripheral edema or continued elevation of tissue pressures even after fasciotomy. If compartment syndrome is not treated, the necrosing muscles become fibrotic, contract, and can no longer function (e.g., Volkmann's ischemic contracture). Late decompression fasciotomy seldom restores lost myoneural function. Early recognition is the key to successful management and preservation of function.

Clinical presentation: abdominal compartment syndrome Manifests with progressive swelling of the abdomen associated with signs of multiple organ dysfunction syndrome. Decreased CI, increased SVR, decreased static lung compliance and increased bladder pressure may be noted.

Physical assessment

Muscle involvement: Inability to control pain with usual amounts of opiates in any patient at risk for compartment syndrome requires close monitoring. If use of opiates isn't enough to manage pain, the patient should be monitored for muscle involvement. Pain on passive extension or flexion of the digits is an early finding indicative of muscle tissue involvement.

Neurovascular involvement: Increasing extremity circumference, decrease in or loss of two-point discrimination, sluggish capillary refill, and tautness and tenderness over tissue compartments are early signs of neurovascular impairment. All neurovascular structures traversing the involved compartment may eventually show a deficit. *Late findings* include the *six P's: p*ain (increased with application of pressure over the compartment and passive movement of the digits), *p*allor, *p*olar (coolness), *p*ulselessness, *p*aresthesia, and *p*aralysis.

DIAGNOSTIC TESTS

Blood chemistries: Elevated creatine phosphokinase (CPK) is caused by the release of the enzyme by injured muscle tissue. Continued elevation in the course of treatment may indicate late-onset compartment syndrome. Extensive muscle necrosis may lead to myoglobinemia and myoglobinuria, and may lead to rhabdomyolysis. BUN and creatinine levels will be elevated if acute renal failure results from rhabdomyolysis.

Intracompartmental pressure monitoring: Compartment pressure and associated critical values may be monitored intermittently by inserting *needles* (pressure within 10-30 mm Hg of diastolic BP), which get obstructed by muscle tissue. *Continuous infusion catheters* (pressure >45 mm Hg) and *wick* or *slit catheters* (>30-35 mm Hg) monitor continuously via fluid-filled catheters and pressure monitors. In hypotensive patients at higher risk for compartment syndrome (see Table 2-11), the delta pressure should be calculated. Delta pressure equals MAP minus compartmental pressure. Delta pressures of ≤30 mm Hg for 6 hr or ≤40 for 8 hr require prompt consultation with the physician. Pressures warranting fasciotomy vary with clinical indicators, the patient's systemic condition, and measurement technique.

Bladder pressure: Reflects the intraabdominal pressure. Should be assessed when patients have undergone aggressive fluid resuscitation for shock and signs of early organ failure are present.

Arteriograms and venograms: Radiologic examination of blood vessels may be performed when embolus, thrombus, or other vascular injury is suspected.

Transcutaneous Doppler venous flow and/or duplex imaging: A noninvasive examination of blood vessels used to determine impaired venous flow.

MRI spectroscopy: Sometimes used to determine presence of muscle ischemia.

Pulse oximetry: Assesses perfusion of distal tissues. Readings should be compared with readings from a contralateral, uninvolved extremity.

Research Brief 2-5 Recent research by McQueen and Court-Brown suggests that a delta pressure of 30 mm Hg should be used as the definitive criterion in assessing the need for fasciotomy. The authors conclude that the absolute tissue pressures (e.g., the pressure within the compartment alone) is not sufficient to predict the need for fasciotomy.

From McQueen MM, Court-Brown CM: *J Bone Joint Surg Br* 78B(1)99-104, 1996.

COLLABORATIVE MANAGEMENT

Release of external pressure: Loosening or removing circumferential casts and padding or dressings; escharotomy for circumferential burns or frostbite.

Analgesia: Parenteral opiates often with sedative adjuncts (e.g., hydroxyzine HCl, promethazine HCl).

Ice and extremity elevation: Recommended with fractures to promote vasoconstriction when there is no evidence of impaired microcirculation (i.e., decreased capillary refill, pallor, pulselessness, or coolness of the extremity). However, once microcirculation has been impaired, use of ice and extremity elevation is *contraindicated* because further impairment of circulation may result.

Intravenous hypertonic mannitol: Used as a preventive measure to reduce compartmental pressure via systemic diuresis and to the help the kidneys excrete the large molecules of myoglobin if extensive tissue necrosis is present.

Fasciotomy of myofascial compartment: Treatment of choice for strongly suspected compartment syndrome to permit unrestricted swelling. In 7-10 days, primary surgical closure of the fasciotomy is performed. Skin grafting may be needed to ensure complete coverage of the exposed compartments. The affected compartment alone may be opened but more commonly, adjacent or all tissue compartments in the area are prophylactically incised. Persistent peripheral edema with elevated CPK, or the presence of ARF, may justify reexploration and wide excision of all necrotic muscle in involved and adjacent compartments. Complications of fasciotomy include wound infection, the potential for osteomyelitis, and large scars.

Surgeons may recommend other wound closure methods. Delayed wound closure may require several buttons, sutured on either side of the wound and held together with rubber bands, to provide tension that pulls wound edges together. Or, adhesive strips may be placed on either side of the wound to provide a base for more adhesive strips applied with tension across the wound, to help pull the wound edges together.

Compartment syndrome caused by vascular injury: The involved blood vessel is explored and treated. Papaverine, a vasodilating drug which relaxes smooth muscle, can be injected in a bolus of fluid to reestablish normal internal artery dynamics. Blood vessel lacerations can be repaired or severely damaged vessels can be resected.

NURSING DIAGNOSES AND INTERVENTIONS

Altered tissue perfusion (or risk for same): peripheral (compartment), related to interruption of capillary blood flow secondary to increased pressure within the anatomic compartment

Desired outcomes: Throughout hospitalization, patient has adequate perfusion to compartment tissues as evidenced by brisk (<2 sec) capillary refill; peripheral pulses >2+ on a 0-4+ scale; normal tissue pressures (0-10 mm Hg); and absence of edema, tautness, and the six P's for the involved compartment. Within 2 hr of admission, patient verbalizes understanding of reporting symptoms of impaired neurovascular status.

- Monitor neurovascular status of injured extremity at least q2h. Assess for increased pain on passive extension or flexion of the digits. Monitor for sluggish capillary refill, decrease in or loss of two-point discrimination, increasing limb edema, and tautness over individual compartments. Use pulse oximetry to help assess distal tissue perfusion, and report significant differences from oximetry readings taken from the uninvolved contralateral extremity. Assess for the six P's: *p*ain (especially on passive digital movement and with pressure over the compartment), *p*allor, *p*olar (coolness), *p*ulselessness, *p*aresthesia, and *p*aralysis.
- Report deficits in neurovascular status promptly. Loosen circumferential dressings as indicated. Apply ice only when appropriate.
- Teach patient the symptoms to be promptly reported: severe, unrelieved pain, paresthesias (diminished sensation, hyperesthesia, or anesthesia), paralysis, coolness, or pulselessness.
- Monitor tissue pressures continuously, with an intracompartmental pressure device if needed. Consult physician if pressures exceed normal or preestablished levels. Pressures >10 mm Hg may reflect significant elevation.
- Monitor closely for additional tissue injury if the patient becomes hypotensive.

NIC Cast care: Maintenance; Circulatory Precautions; Heat/Cold Application; Peripheral Sensation Management; Shock Management; Skin Surveillance; Teaching: Disease Process

Pain related to physical factors (tissue ischemia) secondary to compartment syndrome

Desired outcomes: Throughout the hospitalization, the patient's pain is controlled, as reflected by a pain scale. Nonverbal indicators of discomfort (e.g., grimacing) are reduced or absent. Within 2 hr of admission, patient verbalizes understanding of the need to report uncontrolled or increasing pain.

- Assess for pain: onset, duration, progression, and intensity. Devise a pain scale with patient, rating discomfort "0" for no pain to "10" for unbearable. Noncommunicative or low-level intellect patients may require a simpler or different pain scale.

- Determine if passive stretching of digits and pressure over limb compartments increase the pain. Both may indicate early compartment syndrome.
- Adjust the medication regimen to the patient's needs; document medication effectiveness. Promptly report uncontrolled pain.
- Prevent pressure being applied on involved compartment and neurovascular structures.
- Following a fasciotomy, pain that remains unrelieved may indicate that the fasciotomy is incomplete. Pain that increases several days after a fasciotomy may signal compartmental infection.
- Continue to monitor neurovascular function with each VS check to assess for recurring compartment syndrome or infection.

NIC Analgesic Administration; Anxiety Reduction; Coping Enhancement; Pain Management; Progressive Muscle Relaxation; Simple Guided Imagery

Risk for infection related to inadequate primary defenses secondary to necrotic tissue, wide-excision fasciotomy, and open wound

Desired outcomes: Throughout the hospitalization, patient is free of infection as evidenced by normothermia; WBC count ≤11,000/mm³; erythrocyte sedimentation rate (ESR) ≤20 mm/hr (women) or ≤15 mm/hr (men); and absence of wound erythema and other clinical indicators of infection. Within 24 hr of admission, patient verbalizes understanding of the need to report promptly any indicators of infection.

- Monitor patient for fever, increasing pain, and laboratory data indicative of infection (e.g., increased WBC count or ESR).
- Assess exposed wounds and dressings for erythema, increasing wound drainage, purulent wound drainage, increasing wound circumference, edema, and localized tenderness.
- Assess neurovascular deficits, which may signal infection or pressure in adjacent inflamed tissues.
- After primary closure or grafting of wound, assess for signs of infection beneath the closure.
- Assess for chronic infection and osteomyelitis: key complications of compartment syndrome.
- Instruct patient to report the following indicators of infection: fever, localized warmth, increasing pain, increasing wound drainage (especially if purulent), swelling, and redness.
- Consult with physician promptly regarding significant findings.

NIC Environmental Management; Infection Protection; Medication Management; Surveillance; Vital Signs Monitoring; Wound Care; Wound Care: Closed Drainage

Body image disturbance related to physical changes secondary to large, irregular fasciotomy wound and skin-grafted scar; loss of function in or change in appearance of an extremity; or amputation

Desired outcomes: Within the 24-hr period before discharge from ICU, patient acknowledges body changes and demonstrates movement toward incorporating changes into self-concept. Patient does not exhibit maladaptive response (e.g., severe depression) to wound or functional loss.

- Discuss compartment syndrome, therapeutic interventions, and long-term effects.
- Provide time for sharing the patient's feelings about his or her changed appearance and function. Encourage questions and discussion of these feelings with patient's significant others.
- Identify and emphasize patient's strengths. Help patient set realistic goals for recovery.
- Facilitate progression through the grieving process, as appropriate.
- Recognize when each patient is ready to view or discuss the injury. Adjustment time varies.
- Encourage self-care. Provide necessary adjunctive aids (e.g., built-up utensils, button hooks, orthotics) to facilitate independence in activities of daily living.
- Collaborate with physician regarding visit by an amputee who has successfully adapted and who can serve as patient's role model, as appropriate. For patients with functional loss or amputation, introduce use of orthotics and adjunctive devices to facilitate self-care.

NIC Active Listening; Amputation Care; Anxiety Reduction; Body Image Enhancement; Coping Enhancement; Emotional Support; Self-Care Assistance; Wound Care

Acute Spinal Cord Injury

PATHOPHYSIOLOGY

A spinal cord injury (SCI) results from concussion, contusion, laceration, transection, hemorrhage, or impairment of blood supply to the spinal cord, affecting 7800-10,000 people each year. The average age of victims is 33.4 years, of whom 75%-82% are males between ages 15-35. Two thirds of males sustain injury to the cervical spine. Approximately 85% of SCI patients who survive the initial 24 hours live at least 10 years. Pneumonia is the leading cause of death during the initial 15 years, followed by nonischemic heart disease and infections (decubitus ulcers, respiratory and urinary tracts). Unintentional injuries, suicides, and homicides result in more deaths than do infections. Motor vehicle crashes cause 44% of injuries, followed by acts of violence (24%), falls (22%), sports injuries (8%), and other causes (2%). The majority of the damage occurs at the time of injury. Subsequent ischemia results in further problems, including systemic hypertension and hypoxia.

SCI is classified in several ways according to *type and cause,* such as open (gunshot, stab wound) or closed (motor vehicle collision, fall, sports-related incident); *site* (which level of the spinal cord is involved); *mechanism,* such as flexion (e.g., occurring as a result of sudden deceleration in a head-on collision, backward fall down a flight of stairs, diving into a swimming pool) or extension (e.g., whiplash or fall involving hyperextension of the neck); *stability* (integrity of the supporting structures such as ligaments or bony facets); and whether the injury is *complete* or *incomplete* (complete meaning the absence of all voluntary motor, sensory, and vasomotor function below the level of injury, and incomplete meaning the presence of some percentage of voluntary motor or sensory function below the level of injury).

Fractures involving the vertebral bodies: These fractures may or may not cause SCI. Severe SCI can occur without damage to the vertebrae. With severe fractures, such as the "burst" fracture (fragmentation of a vertebral body with penetration of the spinal cord), paralysis almost always occurs. Penetration of the spinal cord with bony fragments may cause hemorrhage, infection, and leakage of CSF.

Spinal shock: A temporary loss of reflex function in all segments below the level of injury that occurs immediately after SCI, lasting several hours to weeks. Symptoms include the following: flaccid paralysis, loss of temperature control and vasomotor tone, loss of deep tendon reflexes, and bowel and bladder paralysis resulting in urinary retention and paralytic ileus. Spinal shock occurs following both complete and partial transection of the cord.

Neurogenic shock: Neurogenic shock occurs when sympathetic innervation to the vasculature is impaired, causing dilation of blood vessels and leading to hypotension and bradycardia. Patients who injure the cervical or upper thoracic cord may experience neurogenic shock and spinal shock. The loss of sympathetic innervation also causes venous pooling in the extremities and splanchnic vasculature. Venous return to the heart is decreased, resulting in decreased CO and poor tissue perfusion.

Autonomic dysreflexia (AD): A life-threatening condition affecting victims with lesions at or above T6, stemming from stimulation of the sympathetic nervous system by relatively minor events. The resultant uncompensated cardiovascular response may cause seizures, subarachnoid hemorrhage, fatal cerebrovascular accident, and myocardial infarction if not immediately recognized and treated. Once spinal shock resolves, AD may occur at any time from the acute phase to several years following the injury.

Causes: Most commonly, stimuli to the *bladder,* including from distention, infection, calculi, cystoscopy; or the *bowel,* such as from fecal impaction, rectal examination, suppository insertion; or the *skin,* such as from tight clothing or sheets, temperature extremes, sores, or areas of broken skin.

ASSESSMENT

Clinical presentation

Spinal shock: Flaccid paralysis of all skeletal muscles; absence of deep tendon reflexes (DTRs), cutaneous sensation, proprioception (position sense), visceral and somatic sensation, and penile reflex; urinary and fecal retention; anhidrosis (absence of sweating).

Neurogenic shock: Vasodilation, bradycardia, hypotension.

Note: Although spinal shock is seen in SCIs at *any* level, the loss of central control of peripheral vascular tone (neurogenic shock) occurs most dramatically in high cervical spine injuries, with interruption of the sympathetic nervous system. Profound bradycardia and hypotension are possible. With spinal cord injuries lower than the midthoracic area, the patient will experience a phase of neurogenic shock, with loss of sympathetic innervation to vasculature below the level of the lesion; however, the effects of that loss are not as dramatic.

Recovery phase of spinal shock: As spinal shock subsides, the patient may experience the following: (1) flexor spasms evoked by cutaneous stimulation, (2) reflex emptying of the bowel and bladder, (3) extensor or flexor rigidity, (4) hyperreflexic DTRs, and (5) reflex priapism or ejaculation in the male, evoked by cutaneous stimulation.

Autonomic dysreflexia: Pounding headache, paroxysmal hypertension (up to 300 mm Hg systolic), flushing of the skin with sweating above the level of the lesion, nasal congestion, blurred vision, nausea, bradycardia (30-40 beats/min), and chest pain. Below the level of the lesion, pilomotor erection (goose bumps), pallor, chills, and vasoconstriction will be present (Table 2-13).

TABLE 2-13   Levels of Cord Injury

Level of injury	Manifestation
C4 and above	Loss of muscle function, including respiratory function; fatal outcome unless ventilation is provided immediately
C4-C5	Same as above; phrenic nerve may be spared; assisted ventilation; quadriplegia/tetraplegia
C6-C8	Diaphragm and accessory muscles or respiration retained; movement of neck, shoulders, chest, and upper arms; quadriplegia
T1-T3	Neck, chest, shoulder, arm, hand, and respiratory function retained; difficulty maintaining a sitting position
T4-T10	More stability of trunk muscles; paraplegia
T11-L2	Use of upper extremities, neck, and shoulders; some function of upper thigh; reflex emptying of bowel; males may have difficulty achieving and maintaining an erection; decreased seminal emission
L3-S1	Reflex emptying of bowel/bladder; decreased/lack of ability to have an erection; decreased seminal emission; all muscle groups in upper body function; most muscles of lower extremities function
S2-S4	Flaccid bowel and bladder; lower extremity weakness; all muscle groups function; no ability to have a reflex erection

Cord syndromes

Anterior cord syndrome: This syndrome involves injury to the anterior portion of the spinal cord supplied by the anterior spinal artery and may be associated with acute traumatic herniation of an intervertebral disk. High-dose methylprednisolone is used in the acute phase, with surgical decompression as necessary. The prognosis varies with each patient and depends on the degree of structural damage and edema.
- *Clinical presentation:* Loss of varying degrees of motor function below the level of the injury. Clients may lose pain and temperature sensation below level of injury. Position, pressure, and vibration sensations remain intact.

Central cord syndrome: Generally seen in older adults with hyperextension injuries or interruption of blood supply to the cervical spinal cord. Associated with vertebral injury noted on radiograph. Motor and sensory deficits are less severe in the lower extremities than in the upper extremities because of the central arrangement of cervical fibers in the spinal cord. Incomplete injuries carry a relatively good prognosis. Steroids are used to decrease edema. Many patients can ambulate with an assistive device and may regain bowel and bladder function. There is a less favorable prognosis regarding regaining useful function in the hands.
- *Clinical presentation:* Motor and sensory deficits are usually severe in the upper extremities and profound in the hands and fingers. With sparing of sacral and some lumbar fibers there will be some motor and sensory function in the perineum, genitalia, and lower extremities. Bladder dysfunction varies with each patient.

Lateral cord (Brown-Séquard's) syndrome: Results from a horizontal hemisection of the spinal cord (e.g., from a gunshot or stab wound). Patients usually have bilateral motor and sensory impairment, with a relative difference in function from one side to the other. High-dose methylprednisolone is used for the acute phase, with treatment of fracture or dislocation as needed. Prognosis is usually good for recovery of upper and lower extremity function.
- *Clinical presentation:* Ipsilateral weakness and decrease in light touch, vibratory, and position senses, with contralateral hypalgesia. Usually there are bilateral motor and sensory deficits, but motor activity will be better on one side and sensory activity will be better on the other.

DIAGNOSTIC TESTS

Spinal x-ray: AP and lateral films are obtained to detect fractures or dislocations of vertebral bodies, narrowing of the spinal canal, and hematomas. Additional views (odontoid (open-mouth, bilateral oblique, or flexion-extension) or tomograms may be necessary to view some levels of the spinal cord, particularly in obese and heavily muscled patients. CT and MRI scans are also used, along with myelographic exam.

Caution: This stage in the evaluation of the patient with a possible SCI is extremely danger-ous, because any sudden or incorrect movement of the injured area could cause further trauma to the spinal cord.

COLLABORATIVE MANAGEMENT

Immobilization of the injured site: Additional injury to the spinal cord from inadequate stabiliza-tion after injury is suffered by 10%-25% of SCI patients. Decompression and surgical fixation may be needed.

Cervical spine injury: Cervical traction to immobilize and reduce the fracture or dislocation is most often achieved through the use of a halo system. Traction may also be achieved by means of Vinke, Gardner-Wells, or Crutchfield tongs, which are inserted through the outer table of the skull. These tongs are attached to ropes and pulleys with weights to achieve bony reduction and proper alignment. The patient may be placed on a special frame or bed (e.g., RotoRest kinetic treatment table). The use of the halo device and a plaster or fiberglass jacket for skeletal fixation of the head and neck allows for earlier mobilization and rehabilitation.

Surgical intervention during the immediate postinjury phase is controversial. Surgery may be per-formed if (1) the neurologic deficit is progressing, (2) there are compound fractures, (3) the injury involves a penetrating wound of the spine, (4) there are bone fragments in the spinal canal, or (5) there is acute anterior spinal cord trauma. Surgeries may include decompression laminectomy, closed or open reduction of the fracture, or spinal fusion for stabilization.

Thoracic and lumbar spine injuries: May require surgical stabilization with laminectomy with or without fusion and insertion of Harrington or Cotrel-Dubousset (CD) rods. If the injury is stable, it may be treated with closed reduction. Some patients with lumbar spine injury may be immobilized with a halo device with femoral distraction. This device may be connected to traction with weights for reduction and stabilization before surgery.

Respiratory management: The need for assisted ventilation is based on level of injury, ABG val-ues, and the results of pulmonary function tests, pulmonary fluoroscopy, and physical assessment data. The need for mechanical ventilation is likely with injuries at C4 and above, patients older than 40, smokers, and with associated chest trauma and immersion injuries. Initially, the patient may require intubation, and later, tracheotomy. Persons with high cervical injury who survive the initial injury but have paralysis of the muscles of respiration may require permanent tracheostomy and mechanical ventilation.

Aggressive pulmonary care: To prevent, detect, and treat atelectasis, pulmonary infection, and res-piratory failure, inasmuch as pulmonary problems are a major source of morbidity and mortality in the patient with SCI. Chest physiotherapy, noninvasive positive pressure ventilation (NPPV) using bilevel continuous positive airway pressure (BiPAP) may provide support, but intubation with mechanical ventilation is sometimes required.

Fluid management: In patients with neurogenic shock, blood volume is normal but the vascular space is enlarged, causing peripheral pooling, decreased venous return, and decreased CO. Careful fluid repletion, usually with crystalloids, is indicated. Pressor therapy is initiated for patients unre-sponsive to fluid volume replacement (see discussion under "Pharmacotherapy," which follows). For fluid management in patients with multisystem trauma, see "Major Trauma," p. 89.

Gastric tube placement: To decompress the stomach, prevent aspiration of gastric contents, and decrease the risk of paralytic ileus (often seen within 72 hr of injury in patients with lesions higher than T6).

Urinary catheterization: Insertion of an indwelling or intermittent catheter to decompress an atonic bladder in the immediate postinjury phase (spinal shock). With the return of the reflex arc after spinal shock subsides, a reflex neurogenic bladder that fills and empties automatically will develop in patients with lesions above T12. Patients with lesions at or below T12 generally will have an atonic, areflexic neurogenic bladder that overfills, distending the bladder and causing overflow incontinence. Intermittent catheterization may be necessary.

Pharmacotherapy: Because neuromembranes are 40% fat (compared with 5%-10% fat for other body cell membranes), administration of methylprednisolone within 8 hr of injury inhibits lipid peroxidation, which in turn protects the neuromembrane from further destruction. In addition, it improves blood flow to the injury site, facilitating tissue repair. A loading dose (30 mg/kg) is administered by IV bolus over a 15-min period. After a 45-min wait, 5.4 mg/kg/hr is then admin-istered in a continuous IV infusion over a 23-hr period and then stopped. If the infusion is inter-rupted for any reason, it must be recalibrated so that the entire dose can be completed within the original 23 hr.

Other useful agents currently under investigation include ganglioside (GM1) and 4-aminopyridine. GM1 may prevent secondary damage and help to recover damaged nerve cells. Nerve function may be improved by 4-aminopyridine, possibly by remyelation of demyelinated axons.

Ulcer prevention

Antacids (e.g., Maalox): To prevent gastric ulceration, which may occur after SCI because of hyperacidity of gastric secretions and increased production of gastric acid. The risk of ulceration with hemorrhage is further increased if steroids are used. Maintain gastric pH >5.0 by using Maalox 30 ml q3h.

Histamine H$_2$-receptor antagonists (e.g., cimetidine, ranitidine): To suppress secretion of gastric acid and to prevent or treat ulcers in the patient with increased production of gastric acid and an increased susceptibility to gastric ulceration and perforation.

Bowel retraining

Stool softeners (e.g., docusate sodium): Prevent fecal impaction and distention of the bowel, which could stimulate an episode of AD.

Hyperosmolar laxatives (e.g., glycerin suppository): To facilitate movement of the bowels on a regular basis and prevent fecal impaction.

Irritant or stimulant laxatives (e.g., bisacodyl): To stimulate bowel movements as part of a bowel training program.

Relief of pain and anxiety

Analgesics (e.g., acetaminophen or acetaminophen with codeine): To decrease pain associated with the injury or surgery.

Sedatives: To decrease anxiety caused by the injury, hospitalization, or fear of the prognosis.

Blood pressure regulation

Antihypertensives (e.g., hydralazine hydrochloride, methyldopa, nitroprusside sodium): To treat the severe hypertension that occurs in AD.

Note: Orthostatic hypotension may be a permanent problem, especially in patients with cervical and high thoracic injuries. Caregivers should move the patient slowly into the upright position to avoid a sudden drop in BP, prompting cerebral hypoxia and loss of consciousness. Abdominal binders and Ace bandages or thigh-high antiembolic stockings also may help prevent orthostatic hypotension.

Vasopressors (e.g., norepinephrine): To treat the hypotension during the immediate postinjury stage caused by loss of vasomotor control below the level of injury, with resultant vasodilation and a relative hypovolemia (see Appendix 7).

Respiratory support

Bronchodilators (e.g., theophylline): To dilate bronchioles and facilitate removal of secretions. Early use of theophylline is recommended in patients with a history of COPD or smoking, and who show evidence of difficulty moving secretions. Some research indicates that theophylline may increase diaphragmatic contractility and reduce respiratory fatigue.

Mucolytic agents (e.g., guaifenesin, acetylcysteine): To reduce tenacity and viscosity of purulent and nonpurulent secretions.

Control of infection, inflammation, and coagulation

Anticoagulants (heparin or low-molecular-weight heparins such as enoxaparin [Lovenox]): To prevent thrombophlebitis, deep vein thrombosis, and pulmonary emboli.

Note: Patients with SCI are at high risk for development of vascular complications because they are immobilized, have lost vasoconstrictive capabilities below the level of injury, and cannot constrict the muscles in the lower extremities to facilitate venous flow. Patients who are not candidates for anticoagulation therapy may have an inferior vena cava umbrella or Greenfield filter inserted to trap emboli traveling from the lower extremities to the lungs.

Antibiotics: To prevent or treat respiratory infection or UTI.

NURSING DIAGNOSES AND INTERVENTIONS

Impaired gas exchange related to altered oxygen supply associated with hypoventilation secondary to paresis or paralysis of the muscles of respiration (diaphragm, intercostals) occurring with high cervical spine injury or ascending cord edema

Desired outcomes: Within 24 hr of this diagnosis and throughout remaining hospitalization, patient has adequate gas exchange as evidenced by orientation to time, place, and person; Pao_2 ≥80 mm Hg; and $Paco_2$ ≤45 mm Hg. RR is 12-20 breaths/min with normal depth and pattern (eupnea), HR is 60-100 beats/min, BP is stable and within patient's normal range, and vital capacity (depth or volume of inspiration) is ≥1 L. Motor and sensory losses remain at the same spinal cord level as the initial findings.

Note: Patients with cervical injuries usually arrive in the ICU already intubated. However, with some high thoracic or low cervical lesions, patients who ventilate independently in the emergency department may arrive in the ICU without assisted ventilation. Such a patient is at risk for an increasingly higher level of cord damage because of hemorrhage and edema, which can result in a higher level of dysfunction and a change in respiratory status that requires assisted ventilation.

- Assess for signs of respiratory dysfunction: shallow, slow, or rapid respirations; poor cough; vital capacity <1 L; changes in sensorium; anxiety; restlessness; tachycardia; pallor
- Monitor ABG studies; report abnormalities. Be particularly alert to Pao_2 <60 mm Hg, $Paco_2$ >50 mm Hg, and decreasing pH, inasmuch as these findings indicate the need for assisted ventilation possibly caused by atelectasis, pneumonia, or respiratory fatigue.
- Monitor vital capacity at least q8h. If it is <1 L, Pao_2/PAo_2 ratio is ≤0.75, or copious secretions are present, intubation is recommended.
- Monitor chest x-ray films, and consult physician for abnormalities.
- Monitor patient for evidence of ascending cord edema: increasing difficulty with swallowing secretions or coughing, presence of respiratory stridor with retraction of accessory muscles of respiration, bradycardia, fluctuating BP, and increased motor and sensory loss at a higher level than the initial findings.
- Before attempting oral intubation with neck flexion, ensure that cervical x-ray studies have confirmed the absence of cervical involvement. Use either nasal intubation or orotracheal intubation with manual cervical spine immobilization if cervical spine injury is not ruled out.
- If patient has cranial tongs or traction with a halo apparatus in place, monitor patient's respiratory status q1-2h for the first 24-48 hr and then q4h if patient's condition is stable. Be alert to absent or adventitious breath sounds, and inspect chest movement to ensure that the plaster or fiberglass vest is not restricting diaphragmatic movement.
- If intubation via ET tube or tracheostomy becomes necessary, explain the procedure to patient and significant others.

NIC Airway Management; Oxygen Therapy; Respiratory Monitoring; Mechanical Ventilation
Ineffective airway clearance (or risk for same) related to decreased or absent cough reflex secondary to cervical or high thoracic spine injury
Desired outcome: Within 24-48 hr of this diagnosis, patient has a clear airway as evidenced by absence of adventitious breath sounds.
- Monitor patient's respiratory status, and be alert to the following indicators of ineffective airway clearance: adventitious breath sounds (i.e., crackles, rhonchi), decreased or absent breath sounds (bronchial, bronchovesicular, vesicular), increased HR (>100 beats/min) and BP (>10 mm Hg over patient's normal), decreased tidal volume (<75%-85% of predicted value) or vital capacity (<1 L), shallow or rapid respirations (>20 breaths/min), pallor, cyanosis, increased restlessness, and anxiety.
- Monitor and report abnormal ABG values and chest x-ray results.

Note: Be alert for bradycardia associated with tracheal suctioning. Some authorities suggest giving atropine before suctioning.

- Suction secretions as needed, according to auscultation findings. Always hyperoxygenate before suctioning.
- If indicated by the assessment findings, prepare patient for intubation or tracheostomy with mechanical ventilation. See "Mechanical Ventilation," p. 14, for more information.
- If patient does not require intubation with mechanical ventilation, implement the following measures to improve airway clearance:
  ❏ Place patient in semi-Fowler's position unless it is contraindicated (e.g., patient is in cervical tongs with traction).
  ❏ Turn patient from side to side at least q2h to help mobilize secretions.

❑ Keep room humidified to help loosen secretions.

❑ Unless contraindicated, keep patient hydrated with at least 2-3 L fluid/day.

❑ If patient has respiratory muscle control, teach coughing and deep-breathing exercises, which should be performed at least q2h.

❑ If patient's cough is ineffective, implement the following method, known as *quad coughing:* Place palm of hand under patient's diaphragm, and push up on the abdominal muscles as patient exhales.

Note: Be aware that using the *quad cough* maneuver in patients with intracaval filters to prevent pulmonary emboli has been reported to have significant complications, including bowel perforation and filter migration and deformation.

NIC Airway Management; Cough Enhancement; Respiratory Monitoring

Autonomic dysreflexia (AD) (or risk for same) related to abnormal response of the autonomic nervous system to a stimulus

Desired outcomes: Patient has no symptoms of AD as evidenced by dry skin above the level of injury; BP within patient's normal range; HR ≥60 beats/min; and absence of headache and other clinical indicators of AD. ECG demonstrates normal sinus rhythm.

• Assess for the classic triad of AD: throbbing headache, cutaneous vasodilation, and sweating above the level of injury. In addition, extremely elevated BP (e.g., ≥250-300/150 mm Hg), nasal stuffiness, flushed skin (above the level of the injury), blurred vision, nausea, bradycardia, and chest pain can occur. Be alert to the following signs of AD that occur below the level of injury: pilomotor erection, pallor, chills, and vasoconstriction.

• Assess for cardiac dysrhythmias, via cardiac monitor during initial postinjury stage (2 wks).

• Be aware of and implement measures to prevent factors that may precipitate AD: *bladder stimuli* (i.e., distention, calculi, infection, cystoscopy); *bowel stimuli* (i.e., fecal impaction, rectal examination, suppository insertion); and *skin stimuli* (i.e., pressure from tight clothing or sheets, temperature extremes, sores, areas of broken skin).

• If indicators of AD are present, implement the following measures:

  ❑ Elevate HOB, or place patient in a sitting position. This will decrease BP by promoting cerebral venous return.

  ❑ Monitor BP and HR q3-5min until patient stabilizes.

  ❑ Determine and remove offending stimulus. If the patient's bladder is distended, catheterize cautiously, using sufficient lubricant containing a local anesthetic. If patient has an indwelling urinary catheter, check for obstruction, such as granulation in catheter or kinking of tubing; as indicated, irrigate catheter, using no more than 30 ml normal saline. If UTI is suspected, obtain a urine specimen for culture and sensitivity once the crisis stage has passed. Check for fecal impaction; perform the rectal examination gently, using an ointment containing a local anesthetic (e.g., Nupercainal). Check for sensory stimuli, and loosen clothing, bed covers, or other constricting fabric as indicated.

• Consult physician for severe or prolonged hypertension or other symptoms that do not abate. Severe or prolonged elevations of BP may result in life-threatening consequences: seizures, subarachnoid or intracerebral hemorrhage, fatal cerebrovascular accident.

• As prescribed, administer antihypertensive agent and monitor its effectiveness.

• Remain calm and supportive of patient and significant others during these episodes.

• Upon resolution of the immediate crisis, answer patient's and significant others' questions regarding cause of the AD. Provide patient and family teaching regarding signs and symptoms and methods of treatment of AD. This is particularly critical for the patient with SCI who has sustained injury above T6, because these patients are at risk for AD for life.

NIC Dysreflexia Management

Decreased cardiac output (CO) related to relative hypovolemia secondary to enlarged vascular space occurring with neurogenic shock

Desired outcome: Within 24 hr of this diagnosis, patient has adequate CO as evidenced by orientation to time, place, and person; systolic BP ≥90 mm Hg (or within patient's normal range); HR 60-100 beats/min; RAP 4-6 mm Hg; PAP 20-30/8-15 mm Hg; PAWP 6-12 mm Hg; SVR 900-1200 dynes/sec/cm^{-5}; normal amplitude of peripheral pulses (>2+ on a 0-4+ scale); urinary output ≥0.5 ml/kg/hr; and normal sinus rhythm on ECG.

• Monitor patient for indicators of decreased CO: drop in systolic BP <20 mm Hg, systolic BP >90 mm Hg, or a continuous drop of 5-10 mm Hg with each assessment; HR >100 beats/min, irregular HR, lightheadedness, fainting, confusion, dizziness, flushed skin; diminished amplitude of peripheral pulses; change in BP, HR, mental status, and color associated with a change in position. Monitor I&O; urine output <0.5 ml/kg/hr for 2 consecutive hours should be reported. Assess hemodynamic measurements. In the presence of neurogenic shock, anticipate decreased RAP, PAP, PAWP, and SVR. (See Table 1-13)

- Continuously assess cardiac rate and rhythm; report changes in rate and rhythm.
- Prevent episodes of decreased CO caused by orthostatic hypotension:
  - ❑ Change patient's position slowly.
  - ❑ Perform ROM exercises q2h to prevent venous pooling.
  - ❑ Apply elastic antiembolic hose as prescribed to promote venous return.
  - ❑ Avoid placing pillows under patient's knees, "gatching" the bed, or allowing patient to cross the legs or sit with legs in a dependent position.
  - ❑ Collaborate with physical therapy personnel in progressing patient from a supine to upright position, using a tilt table.
- As prescribed, administer fluids to control *mild* hypotension.
- Administer and monitor for therapeutic effects of vasopressors (see Appendix 7).
- Ensure adequate volume repletion before or concurrent with pressor therapy.

NIC Cardiac Care; Hemodynamic Regulation; Fluid Management

Risk for injury related to risk of development of gastric ulcer (Cushing's) or gastritis secondary to increased gastric acid production

Desired outcome: Result of patient's gastric pH test is >5, and patient has no symptoms of gastric ulcer as evidenced by gastric aspirate and stool culture that are negative for blood; BP within patient's normal range; HR ≤100 beats/min; and absence of midepigastric or referred shoulder pain.

> **Note:** Patients sustaining major trauma are at high risk for development of gastritis/gastric ulcers caused by increased production of gastric acid. Although ulceration can occur at any time in the patient with SCI, it is most likely to occur within 3 wks of the injury.

- Assess for indicators of GI ulceration or hemorrhage: midepigastric pain (dull, gnawing, burning ache) if patient has sensation; and hematemesis, melena, constipation, anemia, pallor, decreased BP, increased HR, and complaints of shoulder pain.
- Test gastric aspirate and stools for blood q8h. Promptly consult physician if blood is present.
- Monitor CBC for signs of anemia: decreases in Hct, Hgb, and RBCs. Normal values are as follows: Hct 40%-54% (male) or 37%-47% (female); Hgb 14-18 g/dl (male) or 12-16 g/dl (female); and RBCs 45-60 million/mm^3 (male) or 40-55 million/mm^3 (female).
- As prescribed, implement measures to treat or prevent ulceration and hemorrhage:
  - ❑ Monitor gastric pH q2h; administer antacids q2-4h or as prescribed to maintain gastric pH >5.
  - ❑ Administer histamine H$_2$-receptor antagonists to suppress secretion of gastric acids, decrease irritating effects of gastric secretions, and facilitate healing.
  - ❑ Insert gastric tube and attach to low, intermittent suction to remove gastric contents.
  - ❑ Prepare patient for surgery as indicated.
- For the patient with GI ulceration and hemorrhage, bowel perforation is an added risk. Be alert to the following indicators: pallor, shock state, abdominal distention, vomiting of material that resembles coffee grounds, absent bowel sounds, elevated WBC count (>11,000/mm^3), and presence of air on abdominal x-ray view. In some cases the only indicators are tachycardia and shoulder pain. Bowel perforation is an emergency situation, requiring immediate surgical intervention.

NIC Surveillance; Medication Administration; Bleeding Precautions; Risk Identification

Altered tissue perfusion (or risk for same): peripheral and cardiopulmonary, related to interruption of blood flow associated with thrombophlebitis, deep vein thrombosis (DVT), and pulmonary emboli (PE) secondary to venous stasis, vascular intimal injury, and hypercoagulability occurring as a result of decreased vasomotor tone and immobility

Desired outcome: Patient is free of symptoms of thrombophlebitis, DVT, and PE within 48 hr of initiation of therapy as evidenced by absence of heat, swelling, discomfort, and erythema in the calves and thighs; HR ≤100 beats/min; RR ≤20 breaths/min with normal pattern and depth (eupnea); BP within patient's normal range; Pao$_2$ ≥80 mm Hg; and absence of chest or shoulder pain.

- The high-risk interval for this diagnosis is the 6-12-wk period after injury. Assess for indicators of thrombophlebitis and DVT: unusual heat and erythema of calf or thigh, increased circumference of calf or thigh, tenderness or pain in extremity (depending on patient's level of injury and whether injury is complete or incomplete), pain in the calf area with dorsiflexion (positive reaction for Homan's sign).

- Assess for indicators of pulmonary emboli: sudden chest or shoulder pain, tachycardia, dyspnea, tachypnea, hypotension, pallor, cyanosis, cough with hemoptysis, restlessness, increasing anxiety, and low Pao$_2$.
- Implement measures to prevent development of thrombophlebitis, DVT, and PE:
  - ❏ Change patient's position at least q2h to prevent venous pooling.
  - ❏ Perform ROM exercises on all extremities q1-2h to promote venous return and prevent stasis.
  - ❏ Avoid use of knee gatch or pillows under the knees, which can compromise circulation.
  - ❏ If patient is out of bed and in a chair, do not allow patient to cross legs at the knee or sit with legs dependent for longer than 0.5-1 hr. For the patient experiencing some return of spinal reflexes below the lesion with spasticity of lower extremities, instruct patient to alert nurse should legs become crossed.
  - ❏ Apply sequential compression devices or antiembolic hose as prescribed.
  - ❏ Maintain adequate hydration of at least 2-3 L/day, unless contraindicated, to prevent dehydration and concomitant increase in blood viscosity, which can promote thrombus formation.
  - ❏ Administer prophylactic low-dose, low molecular–weight heparin as prescribed.
- If the patient exhibits signs of thrombophlebitis or DVT:
  - ❏ Consult physician.
  - ❏ Maintain bed rest unless otherwise directed.
  - ❏ Maintain rest of affected extremity, keeping extremity in a neutral or elevated position. Administer anticoagulants and antiplatelet aggregating agents as prescribed.

> **Note:**   Patients with SCI who are not candidates for anticoagulation therapy may require surgical intervention (insertion of intracaval filter) to prevent pulmonary emboli as a result of thrombophlebitis or DVT.
> Apply warm, moist heat as prescribed. Use of heat is controversial, however, because of concern that heat causes vasodilation, which may mobilize a thrombus.

- If patient exhibits evidence of PE, perform the following, in addition to the aforementioned interventions for thrombophlebitis and DVT:
  - ❏ Elevate HOB if not contraindicated.
  - ❏ Administer oxygen.
  - ❏ As prescribed, administer vasopressors (for hypotension) and analgesics (for pain).
  - ❏ Prepare patient for diagnostic procedure (i.e., perfusion lung scan) or surgical intervention (e.g., insertion of intracaval filter).
  - ❏ Remain calm, and provide support and reassurance to patient and significant others.
- See "Pulmonary Emboli," p. 192, for more information.

NIC Circulatory Care: Arterial Insufficiency; Circulatory Care: Venous Insufficiency; Peripheral Sensation Management; Cardiac Care: Acute; Respiratory Monitoring; Shock Management: Cardiac

Risk for impaired skin integrity related to prolonged immobility secondary to immobilization device or paralysis

Desired outcome: Patient's skin remains intact during hospital course.

- Perform a complete skin assessment at least q8h. Pay close attention to skin that is particularly susceptible to breakdown (i.e., skin over bony prominences and around halo vest edges). Be alert to erythema, warmth, open or macerated tissue, and foul odors (indicative of infection with tissue necrosis).
- Turn and reposition patient and massage susceptible skin at least q2h. Post a turning schedule, and include patient in the planning and initiating of this schedule.

> **Caution:**   Do not turn patient without a written prescription until the injured area of the spinal cord has been stabilized. If turning is allowed before immobilization with tongs, halo, or surgery, use logrolling technique only, using at least three people to turn patient: *one to support the head and neck and keep them in alignment during the procedure, and two to turn the patient.*

- Keep skin clean and dry.
- Pad halo jacket edges (e.g., with sheepskin) to minimize irritation and friction.
- Provide pressure-relief mattress most appropriate for patient's injury.
- For more information related to the maintenance of skin and tissue integrity, see "Wound and Skin Care," p. 45.

NIC Pressure Management; Pressure Ulcer Prevention; Skin Surveillance

Altered nutrition: less than body requirements, related to decreased oral intake secondary to anorexia, difficulty eating in prone position, fear of choking and aspiration, and inability to feed self because of paralysis of upper extremities; decreased GI motility secondary to autonomic nervous system dysfunction

Desired outcome: Within 24-72 hr of this diagnosis, patient has adequate nutrition as evidenced by balanced nitrogen state per nitrogen balance studies; serum albumin 3.5-5.5 g/dl; thyroxine-binding prealbumin 20-30 mg/dl; and retinol-binding protein 4-5 mg/dl.
- Perform a complete baseline assessment of nutritional status. See "Nutritional Support," p. 1.
- Assess patient's readiness for oral intake: presence of bowel sounds, passing of flatus, or bowel movement.

Note: Next to fecal impaction, paralytic ileus is the second most common GI disorder of patients with SCI. It usually occurs within 72 hr of the injury and is associated with gastric distention. (See "Constipation," p. 147.)

- When the patient begins an oral diet, progress slowly from liquids to solids as tolerated.
- Monitor and record percentage of each meal eaten by patient.
- Implement measures to maintain or improve patient's intake.
  - ❑ Obtain dietary consultation to provide patient with his or her favorite foods, as well as those that are highly nutritious.
  - ❑ Make mealtime pleasant: provide oral hygiene before and after meals, and decrease external stimuli (which also will help patient concentrate on chewing and swallowing and thus minimize the risk of aspiration).
  - ❑ Provide small, frequent feedings, inasmuch as they may be more readily digested; less likely to cause abdominal distention, which may compromise respiratory movement; and less fatiguing.
  - ❑ If patient is on a Stryker wedge frame or Foster frame, feed in a prone position to minimize the risk of aspiration. If patient is in a halo device or has been stabilized, feed in high Fowler's position.
  - ❑ Feed patient slowly, providing small, bite-size pieces, which facilitate digestion and help prevent choking.
  - ❑ Provide straws for liquids; teach patient to sip slowly.
- Once patient's condition has been stabilized, consult with occupational therapy personnel for selection of assistive devices that will enable patient to feed him- or herself.

NIC Fluid/Electrolyte Management; Nutrition Management; Swallowing Therapy; Self-Care Assistance: Feeding

Urinary retention related to inhibition of the spinal reflex arc secondary to spinal shock after SCI

Desired outcome: Within 24 hr of this diagnosis, patient has urinary output ≥0.5 ml/kg/hr with output comparable to intake.

Caution: Urinary retention with stretching of the bladder muscle may trigger AD. Therefore it is critical to assess for retention and to treat it promptly.

- Assess for indicators of urinary retention: suprapubic distention and intake greater than output.
- Catheterize patient as prescribed. Patients usually have an indwelling catheter for the first 48-96 hr after injury. Then, intermittent catheterization is used to try to retrain the bladder.
- Ensure continuous patency of the drainage system to prevent reflux of urine into the bladder or blockage of flow, which could lead to urinary retention or UTI, which may cause AD.
- Maintain a fluid intake of at least 2.5-3 L/day to prevent early stone formation caused by mobilization of calcium.
- Tape the catheter over the pubis to prevent traction on the catheter, which can lead to ulcer formation in the urethra and erosion of the urethral meatus.
- If an episode of AD is triggered by a distended bladder, obstructed catheter, kinked tubing, or UTI, implement the following:
  - ❑ Have someone notify physician.
  - ❑ If patient is not already catheterized, catheterize patient, using an anesthetic jelly.
  - ❑ If the catheter is obstructed, gently instill <30 ml normal saline to try to open the catheter.
  - ❑ If the catheter remains obstructed, remove it and insert another, using anesthetic lubricant.
  - ❑ If a UTI is the suspected triggering factor, obtain a specimen for culture and sensitivity testing.
  - ❑ For other treatment interventions, see "Dysreflexia," p. 142.

NIC Urinary Catheterization; Urinary Retention Care

Reflex incontinence related to uninhibited activity of the spinal reflex arc secondary to recovery phase from spinal shock in patients with cord lesions above T12

Desired outcome: Patient does not experience urinary incontinence.

- As prescribed, catheterize patient on a regularly scheduled basis (e.g., q3-4h).
- If episodes of urinary incontinence occur, catheterize more frequently. If >400 ml of urine is obtained, catheterize more often and reduce fluid intake.
- Measure the amount of residual urine, and attempt to increase the length of time between catheterizations as indicated by decreased amounts (e.g., <50-100 ml urine).

Note: Recent studies recommend continuing 3- to 4-hr intermittent catheterizations to prevent >300-400 ml of urine from accumulating in the bladder. Amounts of urine >400 ml are associated with a significant increase in the rate of infection.

- Monitor and record I&O. Encourage a consistent intake of fluids, evenly distributed throughout the day, to prevent overdistention, which can increase the risk for AD.
- Decrease fluid intake before bedtime to prevent nighttime incontinence.
- Discourage intake of caffeine-containing beverages and foods (e.g., colas, chocolate, coffee, and tea) because they have a diuretic effect and may stimulate increased urine production, bladder spasms, and reflex incontinence.
- Teach patient and significant others the procedure for intermittent catheterization. Alert them to the indicators of UTI (restlessness, incontinence, malaise, anorexia, fever, and cloudy or foul-smelling urine) and the importance of adequate fluid intake, regular urine cultures, good hand-washing technique, and cleansing of the urinary catheter before catheterization. (The patient with a lesion above T12 whose bladder indicates a neurogenic reflex eventually may be able to empty the bladder automatically and may not require catheterization.)

Caution: UTI is one of the leading causes of morbidity and mortality in the patient with SCI. This patient may not be aware of the presence of UTI until he or she is severely ill as a result of pyelonephritis (calculi, infection, septicemia).

Urinary retention (with overflow incontinence) related to loss of reflex activity for micturition and bladder flaccidity secondary to cord lesion at or below T12

Desired outcome: Patient has urinary output without incontinence.

- Insert an indwelling urinary catheter or catheterize patient intermittently on a regularly scheduled basis (e.g., q3-4h).
- If intermittent catheterization is used and episodes of urinary incontinence occur, catheterize more frequently. If >400 ml of urine is obtained, catheterize more often and reduce fluids.
- Measure the amount of residual urine, and attempt to increase the length of time between catheterizations, as indicated by decreased amounts (i.e., <50-100 ml urine).
- Monitor and record I&O. Distribute fluids evenly throughout the day to prevent overdistention, which can cause incontinence and increase the risk for AD.
- Decrease fluid intake before bedtime to prevent nighttime incontinence.
- Discourage intake of caffeine-containing beverages and foods (e.g., colas, chocolate, coffee, and tea) because they have a diuretic effect and may stimulate increased urine production.
- Teach bladder-emptying techniques such as straining or Credé's method.

Note: Even with these techniques, patients may experience dribbling of urine, which will necessitate catheterization or incontinence undergarments.

- Teach patient and significant others the procedure for intermittent catheterization. Alert them to the indicators of UTI (restlessness, incontinence, malaise, anorexia, fever, and cloudy or foul-smelling urine) and the importance of adequate fluid intake, regular urine cultures, good hand-washing technique, and cleansing of the urinary catheter before catheterization.

Caution: UTI is one of the leading causes of morbidity and mortality in the patient with SCI. This patient may not be aware of the presence of UTI until he or she is severely ill as a result of pyelonephritis (calculi, infection, septicemia).

Ineffective thermoregulation related to inability of the body to adapt to environmental temperature changes secondary to poikilothermic reaction occurring with SCI
Desired outcome: Within 2-4 hr of this diagnosis, patient becomes normothermic.

> **Note:** With SCI the patient may become poikilothermic, meaning that the patient adapts his or her own body temperature to that of the environment and cannot control core body temperature by means of vasodilation to lose heat, or vasoconstriction to conserve heat.

- Monitor patient's temperature at least q4h, and assess patient for signs of ineffective thermoregulation: complaints of being too warm, excessive diaphoresis, warmth of skin above level of injury, complaints of being too cold, pilomotor erection (goose bumps), or cool skin above the level of injury.
- Implement measures to attain normothermia:
  ❏ Regulate room temperature.
  ❏ Provide extra blankets to prevent chills.
  ❏ Protect patient from drafts.
  ❏ Provide warm food and drink if patient is chilled; provide cool drinks if patient is warm.
  ❏ Use fans or air conditioners to prevent overheating.
  ❏ Remove excess bedding to facilitate heat loss.
  ❏ Provide a tepid bath or cooling blanket to facilitate cooling.

NIC Temperature Regulation; Environmental Management

Risk for injury related to potential of paralytic ileus with concomitant risk of AD secondary to SCI
Desired outcomes: Patient remains free of symptoms of paralytic ileus, as evidenced by auscultation of normal bowel sounds, and free of symptoms of AD, as evidenced by BP within patient's normal range; vision normal for patient; dry skin above the level of injury; HR ≥60 beats/min; and absence of headache, nasal congestion, flushed skin above the level of injury, and nausea; as well as absence of the following findings below the level of injury: pilomotor erection (goose bumps), pallor, chills.

> **Note:** Paralytic ileus occurs most often in patients with SCI at T6 and above and usually within the first 72 hr after injury.

- Assess for indicators of paralytic ileus: decreased or absent bowel sounds, abdominal distention, anorexia, vomiting, and altered respirations as a result of pressure on the diaphragm. Report significant findings promptly.
- Observe closely for signs of AD, which can be triggered by distention of the abdomen (for assessment and treatment of AD, see interventions with "Dysreflexia," p. 142).
- If indicators of paralytic ileus appear, implement the following, as prescribed:
  ❏ Restrict oral or enteral intake.
  ❏ Insert gastric tube to decompress the stomach; attach to suction.
  ❏ Insert a rectal tube if prescribed.

> **Caution:** Stimulation of the rectum by a rectal tube may precipitate an episode of AD; therefore application of anesthetic ointment before insertion is recommended.

- If patient has a rectal tube in place, he or she may not have sensation in the rectal area. Therefore special care is necessary to prevent damage to the rectal mucosa and anal sphincter. Remove the tube as soon as possible.

NIC Surveillance: Safety; Dysreflexia Management; Tube Care

Constipation or fecal impaction related to neuromuscular impairment secondary to spinal shock
Desired outcome: Within 24-48 hr of this diagnosis and subsequently q2-3 days (or within patient's preinjury pattern), patient has bowel elimination of soft and formed stools.
- Monitor patient for indicators of constipation (nausea, abdominal distention, and malaise) and fecal impaction (nausea, vomiting, increasing abdominal distention, palpable colonic mass, or presence of hard fecal mass on digital examination).
- Until bowel sounds are present and paralytic ileus has resolved, maintain patient on nothing by mouth (NPO) status, with gastric suction.
- Perform a gentle digital examination for fecal impaction and check for rectal reflexes.
- Before the return of rectal reflexes, manual removal of feces may be needed. If a fecal impaction is present in an atonic bowel, administration of a small-volume enema may be necessary.

> **Caution:** Be aware that overdistention of the bowel or stimulation of the anal sphincter caused by impaction, rectal examination, or enema may precipitate AD. Use generous amounts of anesthetic lubricant when performing a rectal examination or administering an enema.

Constipation related to lack of voluntary control of the anal sphincter and lack of sensation of a fecal mass after return of reflex arc associated with neuromuscular impairment
Desired outcome: Within 24-48 hr of this diagnosis and subsequently q2-3 days (or within patient's preinjury pattern), patient has bowel elimination of soft and formed stools.
- Obtain history of patient's preinjury bowel elimination pattern.
- Assist patient with selection of menu items that are high in fiber.
- Unless contraindicated, maintain a minimum fluid intake of 2-3 L/day.
- Administer stool softeners (e.g., docusate sodium) daily.
- If possible, avoid enemas for long-term bowel management, because the patient with SCI cannot retain the enema solution. However, if impaction occurs, a gentle, small-volume cleansing enema may be necessary, followed by manual removal of fecal material.
- Assess patient's readiness for bowel retraining program, including neurologic status and current bowel patterns, noting frequency, amount, and consistency. Bowel retraining is initiated when the patient is neurologically stable and can resume a sitting position.
- Provide a bedside commode to facilitate better bowel evacuation, if allowed.
  - ❑ Provide ample time for elimination. The gastrocolic reflex occurs 30 minutes after eating.
  - ❑ Ensure patient's privacy.
  - ❑ Stimulate the rectal sphincter with digital stimulation or insert suppository (i.e., bisacodyl) to initiate reflex peristalsis with reflex evacuation.

> **Caution:** See precautions with "Autonomic Dysreflexia," p. 142.

- If patient has upper extremity function, teach him or her how to perform digital rectal stimulation, insert suppository, and massage abdomen to facilitate bowel movement.

NIC Constipation/Impaction Management

Risk for infection related to inadequate primary defenses (broken skin) secondary to presence of invasive immobilization devices
Desired outcome: Patient is free of infection at insertion site for tongs or halo device as evidenced by normothermia; negative culture results; and absence of erythema, swelling, warmth, purulent drainage, or tenderness at insertion site.
- Assess insertion sites q8h for indicators of infection: erythema, swelling, warmth, purulent drainage, and increased or new tenderness. Note pin migration. If the pin appears to be loose, consult physician and instruct patient to remain still until the pin can be secured.
- Perform pin care as prescribed. One possibility is to cleanse the site with povidone-iodine or half-strength normal saline and hydrogen peroxide, leaving any superficial crust intact, followed by application of an antibiotic ointment. An alternative regimen involves cleansing with povidone-iodine or hydrogen peroxide and no antibiotic ointment. Sterile dressings may be applied around the pins, or the area may be left open to air per orders or policy. Use sterile applicators, and follow aseptic technique during all pin care procedures.

NIC Infection Control; Infection Protection; Skin Surveillance

Sensory/perceptual alterations: visual, related to presence of immobilization device; use of therapeutic bed
Desired outcome: After intervention(s), patient expresses satisfaction with visual capabilities.
- Assess for factors that limit the patient's visual capabilities: presence of tongs, cervical traction, halo device; and use of Stryker wedge frame, Foster frame, or RotoRest kinetic treatment table.
- Provide for increased visualization of patient's surroundings:
  - ❑ Obtain prism glasses for patient who must remain supine or cannot turn his or her head because of halo traction device. If prism glasses are unavailable, provide a hand mirror for patient with upper extremity function.
  - ❑ Position mirrors to increase the amount of area that can be visualized from patient's position.
  - ❑ Approach patient and converse within patient's visual field.
  - ❑ Keep clocks, calendars, and other personal objects within patient's visual field.

NIC Environmental Management; Positioning

Sexual dysfunction or altered sexuality patterns related to trauma associated with SCI

Desired outcome: Patient verbalizes sexual concerns before discharge from ICU.

- Assess patient's level of sexual function or loss from a neurologic and psychologic perspective. The general rule for men is that the higher the lesion, the greater the chance of maintaining the ability to have an erection, but with less chance for ejaculation. For women, ovulation may stop for several months because of stress after the injury. Ovulation usually returns, however, and the woman can become pregnant and have a normal pregnancy. Both men and women with high lesions may experience feelings of excitement similar to a preinjury orgasm.
- Evaluate your own feelings about sexuality. Arrange for a knowledgeable staff member to speak with patient about his or her concerns.
- Check level of patient's knowledge, and elicit questions about his or her sexual function after the SCI.
- It is normal for men to experience a reflex erection upon resolution of the spinal shock, particularly for individuals with lesions in the cervical and thoracic areas. Reassure patient that this is normal and therefore nothing to be embarrassed about.
- Expect acting-out behavior related to the patient's sexuality. This is a normal response to the patient's concern regarding his or her sexual prognosis.
- Provide accurate information regarding expected sexual function in an open, interested manner, based on your assessment of the patient's readiness for information.
- Facilitate communication between the patient and his or her partner.
- Refer patient and his or her partner to a sex therapist or other knowledgeable rehabilitation professional upon resolution of the critical stages of SCI.
- Also provide patient with the following addresses and phone numbers:
    National Spinal Cord Injury Association, 1-800-962-9629; e-mail/URL: www.spinalcord.org
    Spinal Cord Injury Network International; 1-800-548-CORD (2673), 1-707-577-8796; fax:1-707-577-0605; URL: www.sonic.net/?spinal/; e-mail: spinal@sonic.net

NIC Sexual Counseling; Anxiety Reduction; Body Image

ADDITIONAL NURSING DIAGNOSES

Also see nursing diagnoses and interventions as appropriate under "Nutritional Support," p. 1; "Mechanical Ventilation," p. 14; "Prolonged Immobility," p. 61; "Psychosocial Support," p. 68; and "Psychosocial Support for the Patient's Family and Significant Others," p. 78.

Abdominal Trauma

PATHOPHYSIOLOGY

The abdomen consists of three distinct but overlapping areas: the peritoneal cavity (contains diaphragm, liver, spleen, stomach, some small bowel, and transverse colon), the retroperitoneum (contains aorta, vena cava, pancreas, kidneys, adrenal glands, ureters, some of the duodenum, small bowel, and colon), and the pelvis (contains rectum, bladder, iliac vessels, and in women, the genitalia). The upper region of the peritoneal cavity is covered by the bony thorax.

The degree of abdominal injury is related to the type of force applied to the organs suspended inside the peritoneum. Forces may be blunt or penetrating. Organs are either solid (pancreas, kidneys, adrenal glands, liver, and spleen) or hollow (stomach, small bowel, and colon). Penetrating forces injure the organ(s) in the direct path of the instrument or missile, while shock waves from high-velocity weapons (e.g., high-powered rifles) may also injure adjacent organs. Stab wounds are generally easier to manage than gunshots, but may be fatal if a major blood vessel (aorta) or highly vascular organ (liver) is penetrated. Blunt trauma is more likely to damage solid organs, but hollow organs are at risk for rupture if suddenly and severely compressed.

Management of hemorrhagic shock is the initial priority for the trauma nurse. Metabolic failure, acidosis, hypothermia, coagulopathy, and abdominal compartment hypertension (abdominal compartment syndrome) may also occur and must be subsequently managed. Blood loss results in an initial compensatory tachycardia with vasoconstriction. A normal BP usually is maintained in early hemorrhagic shock. When blood loss is severe, the BP deteriorates to a MAP <70 mm Hg as shock progresses. SVR remains high. Right (CVP) and left (PCWP) ventricular filling pressures should reflect volume status, but may appear falsely elevated due to tachycardia. Volume status, as reflected by blood pressure, may appear adequate as hypovolemia ensues, due to the powerful vasoconstrictor response. Blood pressure should be interpreted with caution.

Base deficit and serum lactate level should be closely monitored. Lactic acid is a by-product of anaerobic metabolism, which signifies poor perfusion and is an indicator of hemorrhagic shock. When base is in deficit, acid is in excess. Bases are "proton acceptors." For every 1 mEq/L decrease in base, there is a 10 mEq/L increase in acid. If acid level increases, pH decreases. If pH falls below 7.15, medications such as catecholamines (e.g., norepinephrine, dopamine) may not be effective in the extremely acidic environment. Aggressive efforts should be made to augment perfusion and ventilation, in addition to administering bicarbonate for pH correction.

Other pathophysiologic changes associated with abdominal trauma include: (1) massive fluid shifts related to tissue damage, blood loss, and shock; (2) systemic inflammation and metabolic changes associated with stress and catecholamine release; (3) coagulation problems associated with massive hemorrhage and multiple transfusions; (4) inflammation, infection, and abscess formation caused by release of GI secretions and bacteria into the peritoneum; and (5) nutritional and electrolyte alterations that develop as a consequence of disruption of GI tract integrity.

The following overview summarizes common injuries:

Diaphragm: The diaphragm is commonly injured at the left posterior portion after blunt trauma. The tear is best visualized by chest x-ray, which reveals an elevation of the left hemidiaphragm and a bubble of air in the chest.

Spleen: The organ most frequently injured after blunt trauma and the most common cause of major abdominal injury. Massive hemorrhage from splenic injury is common. Damage to the spleen may occur with the most trivial of injuries, so index of suspicion should be high. Splenic injury is often associated with hepatic or pancreatic injury. Splenectomy is the treatment of choice for major spleen injuries. Minor splenic injuries may be managed with direct suture techniques.

Liver: The organ most frequently involved in penetrating trauma (80%) because of its large size and location, the liver is less often affected by blunt injury (20%). Control of bleeding and bile drainage are the priorities with hepatic injury. Mortality from liver injuries is about 10%. In most patients, bleeding from a liver injury can be controlled with conventional techniques. Hemorrhage is controlled by perihepatic packing. About 5% of injuries require packing for bleeds. Major arterial bleeding from the liver parenchyma will require further attention. Biliary tree injuries may require surgical repair and should be suspected with liver injury. The patient may be asymptomatic or have mild to moderate abdominal discomfort with biliary tree injury.

Lower portion of esophagus and stomach: Occasionally the lower portion of the esophagus is involved in penetrating trauma. The stomach is usually not injured with blunt trauma since it is flexible and readily displaced, but may be injured by direct penetration. Injury to either the esophagus or stomach results in the escape of irritating gastric fluids (gastric perforation) and the release of free air below the level of the diaphragm. Esophageal injuries often are associated with thoracic injuries. Once hemorrhage has been controlled, attention is turned to prevention of further contamination by controlling spillage of gut contents.

Pancreas and duodenum: Traumatic pancreatic or duodenal injury is uncommon, but associated with high morbidity and mortality. These injuries are difficult to detect and may be associated with massive injury to nearby organs, prompting spillage of irritating fluids, activated enzymes, and bile, which augments the inflammatory response. Pancreatic injury rarely requires or allows definitive surgery in the damage control setting. Clinical indicators of injury to these retroperitoneal organs may not be obvious for several hours.

Small bowel and mesentery: The three most common injuries associated with penetrating abdominal trauma are to small bowel, liver, and colon. With blunt trauma, injury to the liver, spleen, and kidney are more common. Undetected mesenteric damage may cause compromised blood flow, with eventual bowel infarction. Perforations or contusions result in release of bacteria and intestinal contents into the abdominal cavity, causing serious infection.

Colon: Injury is most frequently caused by penetrating forces, although lap belts, direct blows, and other blunt forces cause a small percentage of colonic injuries. Because of the high bacterial content, infection is even more a concern than it is with small bowel injury. Most patients with significant colon injuries require a temporary colostomy.

Pelvis: See "Renal and Lower Urinary Tract Trauma," p. 122.

Major vessels: Injuries to the abdominal aorta and inferior vena cava most often are caused by penetrating trauma, but also occur with deceleration injury. Hepatic vein injuries frequently are associated with juxtahepatic vena caval injury and result in rapid hemorrhage. Blood loss after major vascular injury is massive. Survival depends on rapid transport to a trauma center and immediate surgical intervention.

Retroperitoneal vessels: Tears in retroperitoneal vessels associated with pelvic fractures or damage to retroperitoneal organs (pancreas, duodenum, and kidney) can cause bleeding into the retroperitoneum. Although the retroperitoneal space can accommodate up to 4 L of blood, detection of retroperitoneal hematomas is difficult and sophisticated diagnostic techniques may be required.

The initial focus should be stabilization and supporting hemodynamics, but the highest priority is to diagnose and repair causes of hemorrhage. Timely provision of needed surgery, preferably in a trauma center, is the critical factor impacting survival. Prolonged hypovolemia and shock result in organ ischemia and ultimately failure (see "Major Trauma," p. 89; "Acute Respiratory Distress Syndrome," p. 189; "Cardiogenic Shock," p. 290; "Acute Renal Failure," p. 315; "Hepatic Failure," p. 427; and "Disseminated Intravascular Coagulation," p. 489).

INITIAL ASSESSMENT

Physical examination of the trauma patient: The *ABCD*and*Es* (*A*—airway with cervical spine protection; *B*—breathing: oxygenation and ventilation; *C*—circulation with hemorrhage control; *D*—disability: brief neurologic examination (usually Glasgow Coma Scale [see Appendix 3]); *E*—exposure/environment) of the trauma patient are evaluated as soon as the patient arrives. Immediate overview assessment is performed to ensure the basic stability. (See "Major Trauma," p. 89.)

History: Details regarding circumstances of the accident and mechanism of injury are invaluable in detecting the presence of specific injuries. Other information, including the time of the patient's last meal, previous abdominal surgeries, and use of safety restraints (if appropriate) should be noted. Hollow viscous injury is often missed but should always be suspected with a visible contusion on the abdomen. Medical information including current medications, allergies (particularly to contrast material and antibiotics), and last tetanus-toxoid immunization, should be obtained. The history is sometimes difficult to obtain because of alcohol or drug intoxication, head injury, breathing difficulties, or impaired cerebral perfusion. Family members and emergency personnel may be valuable sources of information.

Clinical presentation: Mild tenderness to severe abdominal pain may be present, with the pain either localized to the site of injury or diffuse. Blood or fluid collection within the peritoneum causes irritation that results in involuntary guarding, rigidity, and rebound tenderness. Fluid or air under the diaphragm may cause referred shoulder pain. Kehr sign (left shoulder pain caused by splenic bleeding) also may be noted, especially when the patient is recumbent. Nausea and vomiting may occur, and the conscious patient who has sustained blood loss often complains of thirst—an early sign of hemorrhagic shock. Symptoms of abdominal injury may be minimal or absent in the patient who is intoxicated or has sustained head or spinal cord injury.

Note: The absence of signs and symptoms does not exclude the presence of major abdominal injury. Blood in the peritoneum does not produce peritoneal signs. Outward signs of injury are absent in as many as 36% of patients with abdominal trauma.

Because metabolic failure may be evolving, actual physical assessment will be limited initially to rapid scanning for penetrating wounds (entrance and exit) and significant hematoma or ecchymotic lesions. Careful evaluation of the patient including log roll, counting the bullet wounds, and exploration of the body creases and perineum is essential. Abdominal assessment is highly subjective, and serial evaluations by the same examiner are strongly recommended to detect subtle changes. Abdominal assessment after blunt injury is often unreliable. Diagnosis of intraabdominal or intraperitoneal hemorrhage may be assumptive and is supported by visualization techniques.

Physical assessment: In the traditional perspective of the "Golden Hour of Trauma," rapid assessment of hemorrhage includes aggressive volume resuscitation. The American College of Surgeons (ACS) guidelines for assumptive blood loss are seen in the following list.

Vital signs and hemodynamic measurements:
- Pulse >100, decreased pulse pressure, oliguria: blood loss 750-1500 ml
- Pulse >120, hypotension, oliguria, confusion: blood loss 1500-2000 ml
- Pulse > 140, severe oliguria, lethargy: blood loss >2000 (data from the ACS Definition of Trauma Response [1997])

Persistent tachycardia should always be considered a clue to tissue hypoxia. As the neuroendocrine response ensues, persistent tachycardia should warn all observers that there is response to tissue signals of inadequate resuscitation.

Although the presence of hypotension is a sign of impending doom, absence of hypotension does not always accurately reflect an absence of hemorrhage. After an injury, a profound neuroendocrine response ensues to activate the beta receptors (sinus node and ventricular contractile tissue), the α-receptors (smooth muscle in the arteries), and the renal tubules (promoting preservation of fluid), resulting in significant tachycardia, profound vasoconstriction and progressive oliguria. These responses may mask the severity of hemorrhage. Patients on α- or β-antagonists or those with acute spinal cord injuries (above C5) will not manifest these responses and therefore will have few compensatory mechanisms.

Pulse pressure may be effectively used to determine the amount of volume in the arteries (SBP-DBP normal >40 mm Hg). Pulse pressure generally correlates with the volume ejected by the left ventricle, and therefore gives one a valuable tool for indication of volume in the vascular bed. Presence of pulsus paradoxus (see Table 2-8) may be visualized with either the invasive arterial pressure trace or the plethysmograph of the pulse oximeter and is an invaluable tool in evaluating arterial volume.

DELAYED ASSESSMENT

Inspection: Abrasions and ecchymoses may indicate underlying injury. Ecchymosis over the left upper quadrant (LUQ) suggests splenic rupture, and erythema and ecchymosis across the lower portion of the abdomen suggest intestinal injury caused by lap belts. Grey Turner's sign, a bluish discoloration of the flank, may indicate retroperitoneal bleeding from the pancreas, duodenum, vena cava, aorta, or kidneys. Cullen's sign, a bluish discoloration around the umbilicus, may be present with intraperitoneal bleeding from the liver or spleen. Ecchymosis may take hours to days to develop, depending on the rate of blood loss. The absence of ecchymosis does not exclude major abdominal trauma and massive internal bleeding. In the event of gunshot wounds, entrance and exit (if present) wounds should be identified.

Auscultation: It is important to auscultate before palpation and percussion, because these maneuvers can stimulate the bowel and confound assessment findings. Bowel sounds are likely to be decreased or absent with abdominal organ injury or intraperitoneal bleeding. The presence of bowel sounds, however, does not exclude significant abdominal injury. Immediately after injury, bowel sounds may be present, even with major organ injury. Bowel sounds should be auscultated in each quadrant q1-2h in patients with suspected abdominal injury. Absence of bowel sounds is expected immediately after surgery. Failure to auscultate bowel sounds within 24-48 hr after surgery suggests ileus, possibly caused by continued bleeding, peritonitis, or bowel infarction.

Palpation: Tenderness to light palpation suggests pain from superficial or abdominal wall lesions, such as that occurring with seatbelt contusions. Deep palpation may reveal a mass in the area of hematoma. Internal injury with bleeding or release of GI contents into the peritoneum results in peritoneal irritation and certain assessment findings. Table 2-14 describes signs and symptoms that suggest peritoneal irritation. Subcutaneous emphysema of the abdominal wall is usually caused by thoracic injury but also may be produced by bowel rupture. Measurements of abdominal girth may be helpful in identifying increases in girth attributable to gas, blood, or fluid. Visual evaluation of abdominal distention is a late and unreliable sign of bleeding.

Percussion: Unusually large areas of dullness may be percussed over ruptured blood-filled organs. For example, a fixed area of dullness in the LUQ suggests a ruptured spleen. An absence (or decrease in the size) of liver dullness may be caused by free air below the diaphragm, a consequence of hollow viscous perforation, or, in unusual cases, displacement of the liver through a ruptured diaphragm. The presence of tympany suggests gas; dullness suggests that the enlargement is caused by blood or fluid.

Caution: Massive intestinal edema is common following laparotomy and prolonged shock. Inflammatory response, neuroendocrine stimulation, aggressive crystalloid resuscitation, bowel handling, intraabdominal packing, and retroperitoneal hematomas may cause a delay in abdominal closure. If the abdomen is closed, the intraabdominal volume may compress arteries, capillaries, the bladder, and the ureters. This compartment hypertension (abdominal compartment syndrome) may cause a significant hypotension, oliguria and base deficit that will be difficult to combat.

TABLE 2-14   Signs and Symptoms That Suggest Peritoneal Irritation

- Generalized abdominal pain and tenderness
- Involuntary guarding of the abdomen
- Abdominal wall rigidity
- Rebound tenderness
- Abdominal pain with movement or coughing
- Decreased or absent bowel sounds

ASSESSMENT FINDINGS WITH ABDOMINAL COMPARTMENT SYNDROME

Cardiovascular: The swollen abdomen will compress the inferior vena cava and limit the venous return to the heart. Along with this compression syndrome, the shift of the diaphragmatic floor upward further compresses the cardiac structures. Filling pressures will reflect a loss of compliance of the heart, with a corresponding elevation of right (CVP) and left (PCWP) ventricular pressures. False elevation limits the use of these values to guide volume resuscitation.

Respiratory: Both peak and plateau airway pressures increase as the diaphragm shifts upward into the thoracic cage. The patient will exhibit refractory hypoxemia, and as the functional lung surface decreases, volume ventilation may cause significant barotrauma.

Renal: The renal vein, renal parenchyma, ureters, and bladder are compressed. Glomerular filtration decreases, prompting signs of acute renal failure.

Cerebral: As abdominal and thoracic pressures rise, cerebral venous outflow will be decreased. As venous engorgement occurs, intracranial pressure will rise and limit arterial blood flow.

DIAGNOSTIC TESTS

Hct level: Serial levels reflect the amount of blood lost. If measured immediately after the injury, the Hct level may be normal, but serial levels will reveal dramatic decreases during resuscitation and as extravascular fluid mobilizes during the recovery phase. Major blood loss is common with intraabdominal injury.

WBC count: Leukocytosis is expected immediately after injury. Splenic injuries in particular result in the rapid development of a moderate to high WBC count. A later increase in WBCs or a shift to the left reflects an increase in the number of neutrophils, which signals an inflammatory response and possible intraabdominal infection. In the patient with abdominal trauma, ruptured abdominal viscera must be considered as a potential source of infection.

Platelet count: Mild thrombocytosis occurs immediately after traumatic injury. Spontaneous bleeding and a very low platelet count ($<20,000$-$30,000/mm^3$) signal the need for platelet transfusion.

Glucose levels: Initially elevated because of catecholamine release and insulin resistance associated with major trauma. Glucose metabolism is abnormal after major hepatic resection, and patients with significant hepatic injury should be monitored at frequent intervals to prevent severe hypoglycemic episodes.

Electrolytes: Sodium, potassium, and chloride levels may drop because of gastric suctioning or vomiting.

BUN: Elevations are associated with shock, dehydration, GI bleeding, infection, and impaired kidney function.

Amylase levels: Elevated serum levels are associated with pancreatic or upper small bowel injury, but values may be normal even with severe injury to these organs. Delayed elevation suggests traumatic pancreatitis.

Liver enzymes: Elevations of aspartate aminotransferase (AST), alanine aminotransferase (ALT), and alkaline phosphatase (ALP) reflect hepatic dysfunction as a result of liver ischemia during prolonged hypotensive episodes or as a result of direct traumatic damage. Fluctuations in these enzyme levels during the postoperative period can be used to detect evidence of liver necrosis.

Bilirubin: Elevated direct (conjugated) indicates the liver's inability to excrete bilirubin. Elevated indirect (unconjugated) indicates rapid destruction of RBCs or possible retroperitoneal hematoma.

X-ray: Flat and upright chest x-ray films exclude chest injuries (frequently associated with abdominal trauma) and establish a baseline, inasmuch as surgery is likely. In addition, chest, abdominal, and pelvic x-ray studies may reveal fractures, missiles, free intraperitoneal air, hematoma, or hemorrhage.

Occult blood: Gastric contents and stool should be tested for blood in the initial and recovery periods because GI bleeding can occur as a result of both direct injury and later complications, including gastric erosion.

Focused assessment with sonography (FAST): In light of the difficulty in initial assessment of the injury, FAST can be a useful tool for rapid evaluation of intraperitoneal hemorrhage or pericardial tamponade. FAST is directed solely at identifying the presence of free intraperitoneal or pericardial fluid.

FAST examines four areas for free fluid:
• Perihepatic and hepatic-renal space
• Perisplenic
• Pelvis
• Pericardium

With traumatic injury, free fluid is usually due to hemorrhage. The average time for an experienced operator to perform a FAST is 2-3 minutes. FAST may be performed by any credentialed and qualified physician or sonographer. It is done for trauma patients who give a history of abdominal trauma, are hypotensive, or are unable to provide adequate history. Ultrasound should not interfere with ongoing patient assessment. Ultrasound is poor at identifying and grading solid organ injury, bowel injury, and retroperitoneal trauma.

If the initial FAST is negative, but the patient is hemodynamically unstable, a judgment will have to be made based on mechanism of injury, clinical signs, injury pattern, and physiologic response. A diagnostic peritoneal lavage may be necessary to exclude intraperitoneal injury. If the FAST is positive or indeterminate and the patient is hemodynamically stable, a CT scan of the abdomen and pelvis is indicated.

Hollow-organ injury may be missed on ultrasound examination if there has not been leakage of enough gut contents to detect free fluid. Retroperitoneal injuries are also difficult or impossible to detect with ultrasonography. An unstable patient with a positive FAST is transported immediately to the operating room for damage control surgery

Diagnostic peritoneal lavage (DPL): Insertion of a peritoneal dialysis catheter into the peritoneum to check for intra-abdominal bleeding. DPL is indicated for confirmed or suspected blunt abdominal trauma for any *unstable* patient with equivocal assessment findings and a negative FAST. DPL is unnecessary for patients with obvious intraabdominal bleeding or other indications for immediate laparotomy (see "Surgical Considerations," p. 155.

If gross blood is recovered when the catheter is inserted, immediate laparotomy is indicated. If blood is not recovered, 1 L of normal saline or Ringer's lactate is infused rapidly through the catheter and then drained into a sterile bedside drainage device. If possible, the patient is moved from side to side after fluid instillation to distribute the lavage fluid evenly. If the drained lavage is grossly bloody, intraperitoneal bleeding is confirmed. Other indicators of positive lavage results are >100,000 RBC/:l; >500 WBC/:l; amylase >175 U/dl; presence of bile or bacteria; or obvious intestinal contents in the drainage.

> **Note:** An indwelling urinary catheter is inserted before DPL to prevent inadvertent puncture of a full bladder. The stomach is decompressed with a gastric tube to check for bleeding and avoid pressure on a full stomach and prevent vomiting and aspiration.

CT: Can detect intraperitoneal and retroperitoneal bleeding and free air (associated with rupture of hollow viscera). It is most useful in assessing injury to solid abdominal organs.

Angiography: Performed selectively to evaluate injury to spleen, liver, pancreas, duodenum, and retroperitoneal vessels when other diagnostic findings are equivocal.

> **Caution:** Because of the large amount of contrast material used during this procedure, monitor urine output closely for several hours for a decrease and ensure adequate hydration.

Diagnosis of abdominal compartment syndrome: Abdominal compartment syndrome should be suspected in any patient who has undergone abdominal surgery, received aggressive crystalloid resuscitation or vasopressors, or suffered significant periods of hypoxia. The common presenting signs include the following: increasing peak pressures, hypotension, base deficit, and decreasing urine output. The diagnosis can be confirmed by the measurement of intrabladder pressure as a reflection of bladder compression in a fluid-filled compartment. Typically, the bladder can distend to hold up to 4-5 L of urine. When the abdomen is engorged, the compression on the bladder limits filling, and when fluid is introduced, a higher-than-normal pressure may be evaluated. The simplest method is to introduce 50 ccs of fluid into the infusion port of the Foley catheter when clamped. The system is connected to a pressure transducer, which is zero-referenced at the symphysis pubis. Normal intraabdominal pressure is zero or subatmospheric. A pressure of >25 cm H_2O with clinical symptoms is suggestive of ACS, and a pressure >35 is diagnostic.

COLLABORATIVE MANAGEMENT

Managing the abdominal injury trial

Hypothermia: Trauma patients are often profoundly hypothermic on arrival in the emergency department as a result of inadequate protection, intravenous fluid administration, ongoing blood loss, and environmental exposure. Hemorrhagic shock leads to decreased cellular perfusion and oxygenation and impoverished heat production. Hypothermia interferes with coagulation and platelet aggregation, and therefore exacerbates hemorrhage. The patient should be actively warmed with blankets, air-warming devices, or possibly continuous arteriovenous warming techniques. A simple method is to cover all extremities and the abdomen with plastic (e.g., blue side of underpads or trash bags) to trap all heat produced.

Acidosis: Hemorrhagic shock reduces perfusion, resulting in hypoxemia, anaerobic metabolism and lactic acidosis. The compensatory vasoconstrictive response shunts blood to the heart, lungs, and brain from the skin, muscles, and abdominal organs. Base deficit or lactate levels should be used to guide fluid resuscitation, ventilation, and blood pressure support.

Hypoxia: Abdominal injury may result in poor ventilatory efforts caused by pain or compression of thoracic structures. High-flow supplemental oxygen is indicated initially and then titrated according to ABG values. Mechanical ventilation may be necessary.

Hypervolemia and anemia: Because massive blood loss is associated with most abdominal injuries, immediate volume resuscitation is critical. Initially, Ringer's lactate or a similar balanced salt solution is given. Colloid solutions may be helpful in the postoperative period if there are low filling pressures and evidence of decreased plasma oncotic pressure. Typed and cross-matched fresh blood is the optimal fluid for replacement of large blood losses. However, since fresh whole blood is rarely available, a combination of packed cells and fresh frozen plasma often is used. Overaggressive use of colloids and PRBC may increase third spacing and SIRS. See "Major Trauma," p. 89, for more information.

Gastric distention: Gastric intubation permits gastric decompression, aids in removal of gastric contents, prevents accumulation of gas or air in the GI tract, and enhances respiratory excursion by allowing the diaphragm to fully descend. Aspirated contents can be checked for blood to aid in the diagnosis of lower esophageal, gastric, or duodenal injury or bleeding. The tube usually remains in place until bowel function returns.

Coagulopathy: Hypothermia, acidosis, and massive blood transfusion all lead to coagulopathy. The top priority is to stop the bleeding. Coagulopathy is treated by the administration of fresh frozen plasma, cryoprecipitate, and platelets and correcting the hypothermia and acidosis. If bleeding persists, consider vasopressin infusion (promotes platelet aggregation) and calcium chloride.

Surgical considerations for penetrating abdominal injuries: Removing penetrating objects can result in additional injury; thus attempts at removal should be made only under controlled situations with a surgeon and operating room immediately available. The issue of mandatory surgical exploration versus observation and selective surgery, especially with stab wounds, remains controversial. There is a trend toward observation of patients without obvious injury or peritoneal signs. Indications for laparotomy include one or more of the following: (1) penetrating injury suspected of invading the peritoneum; (2) positive peritoneal signs (e.g., tenderness, rebound tenderness, involuntary guarding); (3) shock; (4) GI hemorrhage; (5) free air in the peritoneal cavity as seen on x-ray film; (6) evisceration; (7) massive hematuria; and (8) positive findings on diagnostic peritoneal lavage.

Note: The patient should be evaluated for peritoneal signs at least hourly by the same examiner. Consult surgeon immediately if the patient shows peritoneal signs, evidence of shock, gastric or rectal bleeding, or gross hematuria.

Surgical considerations for blunt, nonpenetrating abdominal injuries: Physical examination usually is reliable in determining the necessity for surgery in alert, cooperative, unintoxicated patients. Additional diagnostic tests such as abdominal ultrasound, DPL, or CT are necessary to evaluate the need for surgery in the patient who is intoxicated or unconscious or who has sustained head or spinal cord trauma. Immediate laparotomy for blunt abdominal trauma is indicated under the following circumstances: (1) clear signs of peritoneal irritation (see Table 2-14); (2) free air in the peritoneum; (3) hypotension caused by suspected abdominal injury, or persistent and unexplained hypotension; (4) positive DPL findings; (5) GI aspirate or rectal smear positive for blood; (6) other positive findings in diagnostic tests such as CT or arteriogram; (7) abdominal gunshot wound; and/or (8) abdominal stab wound with evisceration, hypotension, or peritonitis. Carefully evaluated, stable patients with blunt abdominal trauma may be admitted to a critical care unit for observation. These patients should be evaluated in the same manner as that described in the previous section, "Surgical Considerations for Penetrating Abdominal Injuries." It is important to note that damage to retroperitoneal organs such as the pancreas and duodenum may not cause significant signs and symptoms for 6-12 hr or longer. Relatively slow bleeding from abdominal viscera may not be clinically apparent for 12 hr or longer after the initial injury. In addition, the nurse should be aware that complications such as bowel obstruction caused by adhesions or narrowing of the bowel wall from localized ischemia, inflammation, or hematoma may develop days or weeks after the traumatic event. The need for vigilant observation in the care of these patients cannot be overemphasized.

Need for immediate surgery vs. triad of failure
Once in the operating room, it may become apparent that the patient cannot survive a long procedure, or that the *"triad of failure"* (acidosis, hypothermia, and coagulopathy) may cause death. At this point the surgeon may do limited repair and packing, choosing to "fight another day." The patient is transferred to the ICU, where the triad may be corrected. Survival from abdominal trauma and surgery requires an integrated team effort. The focus is to limit the effects of hemorrhage, acidosis, and coagulopathy and to promote perfusion of all organs.

Closure of abdominal incision
During closure after surgery, if the bowel (intestines) can be visualized with an abdominal horizontal view, the abdomen fascia should not be closed
    There are multiple methods discussed in the literature to supplement closure.
1. Silo bag closure: A 3-L sterile plastic irrigation bag is emptied and cut to lie flat. The edges are trimmed and sutured to the skin.
2. Vacuum pack: A 3-L sterile plastic irrigation bag is emptied and cut to lie flat, then placed into the abdomen, and the edges placed under the sheath. Two suction drains are placed on top of the bag and a large adherent steridrape is then placed over the whole abdomen. The catheters are placed to suction, providing continuous drainage.
3. Vacuum-Assisted Closure (V.A.C.™KCl): A sterile sponge dressing with an adherent dressing and a continuous negative pressure. Promotes closure, blood flow, and collagen formation.
If the abdomen has been closed, it may become necessary to open it again either in the ICU or the operating room.
    Sudden release of the abdominal pressure may lead further injuries such as ischemia-reperfusion, acute vasodilatation, and cardiac dysfunction and arrest. The nurse should hydrate the patient with at least 2 L of volume and may consider a cellular protection cocktail, such as mannitol 12.5% and 2 ampules of bicarbonate. IV fluids and vasopressors should be immediately available in case severe hypotension occurs.
Nutrition: Patients with abdominal trauma have complex nutritional needs because of the hypermetabolic state associated with major trauma and traumatic or surgical disruption of normal GI function. Often infection and sepsis contribute to a negative nitrogen state and increased metabolic needs. Prompt initiation of parenteral or postpyloric feedings, as appropriate, in patients unable to accept conventional enteric feedings and the administration of supplemental calories, proteins, vitamins, and minerals are essential for healing. For additional information, see "Nutritional Support," p. 1.

Pharmacotherapy
Antibiotics: Abdominal trauma is associated with a high incidence of intraabdominal abscess, sepsis, and wound infection, particularly with injury to the terminal ileum and colon. Persons with penetrating or blunt trauma and suspected intestinal injury are started on parenteral antibiotic therapy immediately. Broad-spectrum antibiotics are continued postoperatively and stopped after approximately 72 hr unless there is evidence of infection.
Analgesics: Because opiates alter the sensorium, making evaluation of the patient's condition difficult, they seldom are used in the early stages of trauma. Analgesics are used in the immediate postoperative period to relieve pain and promote ventilatory excursion.

NURSING DIAGNOSES AND INTERVENTIONS

Fluid volume deficit related to active loss secondary to physical injury
Desired outcome: Within 12 hr of this diagnosis, patient becomes normovolemic as evidenced by MAP ≥70 mm Hg; HR 60-100 beats/min; normal sinus rhythm on ECG; CVP 2-6 mm Hg; PAWP 6-12 mm Hg; CI ≥2.5 L/min/m^2; SVR 900-1200 dynes/sec/cm^{-5}; urinary output ≥0.5 ml/kg/hr; warm extremities; brisk capillary refill (<2 sec); and distal pulses >2+ on a 0-4+ scale. Although hemodynamic parameters are helpful to determine adequacy of resuscitation, serum lactate and base deficit are essential to evaluate cellular perfusion.
• Monitor BP q15min, or more frequently in the presence of obvious bleeding or unstable VS. Be alert to changes in MAP of >10 mm Hg. Even a small but sudden decrease in BP signals the need to consult the physician, especially with the trauma patient in whom the extent of injury is unknown.
• Monitor HR, ECG, and cardiovascular status q15min until volume is restored and VS are stable. Check ECG to note HR elevations and myocardial ischemic changes (i.e., ventricular dysrhythmias, ST segment changes), which can occur because of dilutional anemia in susceptible individuals.

- In the patient with evidence of volume depletion or active blood loss, administer pressurized fluids rapidly through several large-caliber (16-gauge or larger) catheters. Use short, large-bore IV tubing (trauma tubing) to maximize flow rate. Avoid use of stopcocks, because they slow the infusion rate. Fluids should be warmed to prevent hypothermia.

Caution: Evaluate patency of IV catheters continuously during rapid-volume resuscitation.

- Measure central pressures and thermodilution CO q1-2h or more frequently if blood loss is ongoing. Calculate SVR and PVR q4-8h or more often in unstable patients. Be alert to low or decreasing CVP and PAWP. An elevated HR, along with decreased PAWP, decreased CO/CI, and increased SVR, suggests hypovolemia (see Table 4-24 for hemodynamic profile of hypovolemic shock). Anticipate slightly elevated HR and CO caused by hyperdynamic cardiovascular state in some patients who have undergone volume resuscitation, particularly during the preoperative phase. Also anticipate mild to moderate pulmonary hypertension, especially in patients with concurrent thoracic injury, such as pulmonary contusion, smoke inhalation, or early ARDS. ARDS is a concern in patients who have sustained major abdominal injury, inasmuch as there are many potential sources of infection and sepsis that make the development of ARDS more likely (see "Acute Respiratory Distress Syndrome," p. 189).
- Measure urinary output q1-2h. Be alert to output <0.5 ml/kg/hr for 2 consecutive hours. Low urine output usually reflects inadequate intravascular volume in the patient with abdominal trauma.
- Monitor for physical indicators of arterial hypovolemia, which may include cool extremities, capillary refill >2 sec, absent or decreased amplitude of distal pulses, elevated serum lactate, and base deficit (see Table 4-22).
- Estimate ongoing blood loss. Measure all bloody drainage from tubes or catheters, noting drainage color (e.g., coffee grounds, burgundy, bright red [Table 2-15]). Note the frequency of dressing changes as a result of saturation with blood to estimate amount of blood loss by way of the wound site.

NIC Electrolyte Management; Fluid Management; Fluid Monitoring; Hypovolemia Management
Pain related to physical injury secondary to external trauma or surgery
Desired outcomes: Within 2 hr of this diagnosis, patient's subjective evaluation of discomfort improves, as documented by use of a pain scale. Nonverbal indicators of discomfort, such as grimacing, are absent.
- Evaluate patient using a pain scale for presence of preoperative and postoperative pain. Preoperative pain is anticipated and is a vital diagnostic aid. The nature of postoperative pain also

---

TABLE 2-15 Characteristics of Gastrointestinal Drainage

Source	Composition and usual character
Mouth and oropharynx	Saliva; thin, clear, watery; pH 7
Stomach	Hydrochloric acid, gastrin, pepsin, mucus; thin, brown to green, acidic
Pancreas	Enzymes and bicarbonate; thin, water, yellowish brown; alkaline
Biliary tract	Bile, including bile salts and electrolytes; bright yellow to brownish green
Duodenum	Digestive enzymes, mucus, products of digestion; thin, bright yellow to light brown, may be green, alkaline
Jejunum	Enzymes, mucus, products of digestion; brown, watery with particles
Ileum	Enzymes, mucus, digestive products, greater amounts of bacteria; brown, liquid, feculent
Colon	Digestive products, mucus, large amounts of bacteria; brown to dark brown, semiformed to firm stool
Postoperative (GI surgery)	Initially, drainage expected to contain small amounts of fresh blood appearing bright to dark; later, drainage mixed with old blood appearing dark brown (coffee-ground); and then approaches normal composition
Infection present	Drainage cloudy, may be thicker than usual; strong or unusual odor, drain site often erythematous and warm

can be important. Incisional and some visceral pain can be anticipated, but intense or prolonged pain, especially when accompanied by other peritoneal signs, can signal bleeding, bowel infarction, infection, or other complications.

- Recognize that opiate analgesics can decrease GI motility, causing nausea, vomiting, and delay of bowel activity. These factors are especially significant if the patient has had a recent laparotomy.
- See this diagnosis in "Major Trauma," p. 89, and in Pain, p. 51, for additional pain interventions.

NIC Pain Management; Bowel Management

Risk for infection related to inadequate primary defenses secondary to physical trauma or surgery; inadequate secondary defenses caused by decreased hemoglobin or inadequate immune response; tissue destruction and environmental exposure (especially to intestinal contents); multiple invasive procedures

Desired outcome: Patient is free of infection as evidenced by core or rectal temperature <37.7° C (100° F); HR ≤100 beats/min; CI ≤4 L/min/m^2; SVR ≥900 dynes/sec/cm^{-5}; orientation to time, place, and person; and absence of unusual redness, warmth, or drainage at surgical incisions and drain sites.

- Note color, character, and odor of all drainage. Report the presence of foul-smelling or abnormal drainage. See Table 2-15 for a description of the *usual* character of GI drainage.
- As prescribed, administer pneumococcal vaccine to patients with total splenectomy to minimize the risk of postsplenectomy sepsis.
- If evisceration occurs initially or develops later, do not reinsert tissue or organs. Place a saline-soaked gauze over the evisceration, and cover with a sterile towel until the evisceration can be evaluated by the surgeon.
- For more interventions, see this diagnosis in "Major Trauma," p. 89.

NIC Infection Control; Infection Protection

Altered tissue perfusion: gastrointestinal, related to interruption of arterial or venous blood flow or hypovolemia secondary to physical injury

Desired outcome: By the time of hospital discharge, patient has adequate GI tract tissue perfusion as evidenced by normoactive bowel sounds; soft, nondistended abdomen; and return of bowel elimination.

- Auscultate for bowel sounds hourly during the acute phase of abdominal trauma and q4-8h during the recovery phase. Report prolonged or sudden absence of bowel sounds during the postoperative period, because these signs may signal bowel ischemia or mesenteric infarction.
- Evaluate patient for peritoneal signs (see Table 2-14), which may occur initially as a result of injury or may not develop until days or weeks later, if complications caused by slow bleeding or other mechanisms occur.
- Ensure adequate intravascular volume (see "Fluid Volume Deficit," p. 156).
- Evaluate laboratory data for evidence of bleeding (e.g., serial Hct) or organ ischemia (e.g., AST, ALT, lactic dehydrogenase [LDH]). Desired values are as follows: Hct >28%-30%, AST 5-40 IU/L, ALT 5-35 IU/L, and LDH 90-200 U/L.
- Document amount and character of GI secretions, drainage, and excretions. Note changes that suggest bleeding (presence of frank or occult blood), infection (e.g., increased or purulent drainage), or obstruction (e.g., failure to eliminate flatus or stool within 3-4 days after surgery).
- Stress the importance of seeking medical attention if indicators of infection or bowel obstruction occur (e.g., fever, severe or unusual abdominal pain, nausea and vomiting, unusual drainage from wounds or incisions, change in bowel habits).

NIC Circulatory Care

Impaired tissue integrity related to mechanical factors (including physical injury); increased metabolic needs secondary to trauma/stress response; altered circulation secondary to hemorrhage or direct vascular injury; exposure to irritants (gastric secretions)

Desired outcome: Patient has adequate tissue integrity by the time of hospital discharge as evidenced by wound healing within an acceptable time frame (according to extent of injury) and absence of skin breakdown caused by GI drainage.

- Protect the skin surrounding tubes, drains, or fistulas, keeping the areas clean and free from drainage. Gastric and intestinal secretions and drainage are highly irritating and can lead to skin excoriation. If necessary, apply ointments, skin barriers, or drainage pouches to protect the surrounding skin. If available, consult ostomy nurse for complex or involved cases.
- For other interventions, see this diagnosis in "Major Trauma," p. 89.

NIC Wound Care; Skin Surveillance; Tube Care

Altered nutrition: less than body requirements, related to decreased intake secondary to disruption of GI tract integrity (traumatic or surgical); increased need secondary to hypermetabolic posttrauma state

Desired outcome: Within 5 days of this diagnosis, patient has adequate nutrition as evidenced by maintenance of baseline body weight and state of nitrogen balance on nitrogen studies.
- Collaborate with physician, dietitian, and pharmacist to estimate patient's metabolic needs on the basis of type of injury, activity level, and nutritional status before injury.
- Consider patient's specific injuries when planning nutrition. For example, expect patients with hepatic or pancreatic injury to have difficulty with blood sugar regulation. Patients with trauma to the upper GI tract may be fed enterally, but feeding tube must be placed distal to the injury. Disruption of the GI tract may require a feeding gastrostomy or jejunostomy. Patients with major hepatic trauma may have difficulty with protein tolerance.
- Ensure patency of gastric or intestinal tubes to maintain decompression and encourage healing and return of bowel function. Avoid occlusion of the vent side of sump suction tubes, because this may result in vacuum occlusion of the tube. Use caution when irrigating gastric or other tubes that have been placed in or near recently sutured organs.
- For additional information, see this diagnosis in "Major Trauma," p. 89.

NIC Electrolyte Management; Feeding; Nutrition Management; Nutrition Therapy; Tube Feeding

Body image disturbance related to creation of stoma (often without the patient's prior knowledge); mutilating physical injury

Desired outcomes: By the time of hospital discharge, patient acknowledges body changes, views and touches affected body part, and demonstrates movement toward incorporating changes into self-concept.
- Evaluate the patient's reaction to the stoma or missing/mutilated body part by observing and noting evidence of body image disturbance (see Table 1-40).
- Anticipate feelings of shock and disbelief initially. Be aware that trauma patients usually do not receive the emotional preparation for ostomy, amputation, and other disfiguring surgery that the patient undergoing elective surgery receives.
- Anticipate and acknowledge normalcy of feelings of rejection and isolation (and uncleanliness in the case of fecal diversion).
- Offer patient opportunity to view stoma/altered body part. Use mirrors if necessary.
- Encourage patient and significant others to verbalize feelings regarding altered/missing body part.
- Offer patient the opportunity to participate in care of ostomy, wound, or incision.
- Confer with surgeon regarding advisability of a visit by an ostomate or a patient with similar alteration in body part.
- Be aware that most colostomies are temporary in persons with colonic trauma. This fact can be reassuring to the patient, but it is important to verify the type of colostomy with the surgeon before explaining this to the patient.

NIC Body Image Enhancement; Ostomy Care

ADDITIONAL NURSING DIAGNOSES

Also see "Major Trauma" for "Hypothermia," p. 96, and "Posttrauma response," p. 97. For additional information, see other diagnoses under "Major Trauma," as well as nursing diagnoses and interventions in the following sections, as appropriate: "Hemodynamic Monitoring," p. 23; "Prolonged Immobility," p. 61; "Psychosocial Support," p. 68; "Psychosocial Support for the Patient's Family and Significant Others," p. 78; "Peritonitis," p. 454; "Enterocutaneous Fistulas," p. 465; "Septic Shock," p. 501; and "Arterial Blood Gas Monitoring," p. 568.

Burns

INTRODUCTION AND PATHOPHYSIOLOGY

Major burn injuries involve damage to the skin, but other organ systems are often affected. The cause of injury may be thermal (flame/flash), electrical, chemical, contact with hot liquids, semi-liquids or objects, or radiation. The risk of injury and precise cause are often related to the victim's age, occupation, and recreational activities. Estimates for burn injuries in the United States range from 1.4 to 2 million injuries annually, and of those, approximately 70,000 require hospitalization. The burning agent, intensity and duration of exposure, location and depth of burn, percentage of body exposure, age of the patient, and preinjury health are factors in determining injury severity and ultimately, outcome.

Burn injuries are categorized based on depth and extent (size of injury). The longer and more intense the exposure to the burning agent, the greater the depth of injury. A burn injury is medically described as either a partial-thickness or full-thickness injury, relative to the layer(s) of skin and tissues involved. Partial-thickness injuries are further differentiated into superficial and deep partial-thickness burns. *Superficial injury,* commonly referred to as "first-degree" burn (e.g., sunburn), damages only the epidermis. These burns typically heal within 3-5 days and without permanent scarring. *Partial-thickness injury,* called a "second-degree" burn, involves varying levels of the dermis, which contain structures essential to skin function (e.g., sweat and sebaceous glands, hair follicles, sensory and motor nerves, capillary network). These burns heal within 14-21 days or longer, depending on the depth. *Full-thickness injury,* a "third-degree" burn, exposes the poorly vascularized fat layer, which contains adipose tissue, roots of sweat glands, and hair follicles; this injury destroys all epidermal elements. These wounds may heal by granulation and migration of healthy epithelium from the wound margins (small wounds only); if wounds require more than 2-3 wks to heal, surgical excision and skin grafting may be required to improve functional and cosmetic outcomes. Some clinicians may also subdivide full-thickness injuries and include a description of "fourth-degree" burns. These injuries are the deepest and require excision, possibly amputation of extremities, and skin grafting to heal. Refer to Table 2-16 for detailed burn wound classification and descriptions.

Care for the patient with a major burn injury is based on the patient's stage of recovery from the pathophysiologic changes resulting from the burn. The resuscitative period lasts from the time of injury until capillary membrane integrity is restored, typically 48-72 hr after the burn occurs. The second stage, or acute phase, may last for days to months. It begins with resolution of the fluid shifts and continues until all wounds are closed or, until open wound areas are <10% of the total body surface area (TBSA). The last stage, or rehabilitative stage, can continue for many years and is seldom a focus for critical care nurses. Early rehabilitative efforts such as patient positioning, exercise, and patient and family teaching begin in the critical care unit.

ASSESSMENT

The American Burn Association (ABA) has developed an injury severity classification system that categorizes burn injuries as minor, moderate, and major (Table 2-17). The ABA advocates that patients with major burns be treated in a burn center or a facility with expertise in burn care. Moderate burns usually require hospitalization, although not necessarily in a burn center, and minor burns are often treated on an outpatient basis.

History and risk factors: Several factors affect survival after a major burn injury. The patient's age is a determining factor with those at the extremes of age (<2 years and >65 years of age) being at highest risk of death. Patients who sustain a thermal injury in a confined area may have a concomitant smoke inhalation injury. Preexisting cardiac or lung disease (e.g., COPD) or history of smoking increase susceptibility to respiratory distress. Patients with diabetes, or preexisting cardiac, vascular, renal, or respiratory conditions may not tolerate aggressive fluid resuscitation therapy and may experience complications. Conditions such as immunosuppression, diabetes mellitus, collagen vascular disease, invasive procedures, history of cardiopulmonary or vascular disease, and delayed antimicrobial therapy contribute to the likelihood of infection, sepsis, and prolonged healing. Those patients with a history of drug and/or alcohol abuse have an increased mortality risk and often have longer hospital stays.

General clinical presentation: The primary patient survey should include the basic *ABCDEs,* with the addition of *F: A*—airway, *B*—breathing, *C*—circulation, *D*—disability or neurologic deficit, and *E*—exposure and evaluation. The secondary survey includes a detailed head-to-toe assessment, exploration of the circumstances of the injury, and the patient's medical history. Injury severity is assessed according to percentage of body surface area burned, burn depth and location, potential for inhalation injury, and patient's age and past medical history.

The extent of the burn wound is reported as a percent of the TBSA injured. In adults, this measure can be estimated by using the *rule of nines* (Figure 2-1). In children, this rule is altered slightly, reflecting the difference in body surface area between adults and children. The rule of nines technique is often used in emergency departments when a quick assessment is necessary. For very small and/or irregularly shaped burns, it helps to remember that the surface area of the patient's palm (palm plus fingers) equals 1% of the TBSA. A more accurate assessment tool is the Lund-Browder chart (Figure 2-2), which is more detailed and accounts for changes in body parts according to age. This chart may be used for both children and adults and is frequently used in the acute care setting.

Electrical burn injuries often reveal only superficial injury on initial inspection, but extensive damage may occur to deep and underlying tissues, nerves, blood vessels, and muscles along the conduction path and at the electrical current contact site. Careful assessment is needed to determine the full extent of these injuries.

Respiratory system: Check for airway obstruction as a result of swelling caused by heat, smoke, or chemical injury to nasopharyngeal mucosa or by constriction around the neck or chest caused by eschar (burned, devitalized tissue) formation. Assess for singed nasal hairs, perioral burns, change in

TABLE 2 - 16 Burn Wound Description and Characteristics

	Cause of injury	Depth	Characteristics	Treatment and recovery
First-degree burn	Prolonged ultraviolet light exposure (sun); brief exposure to hot liquids	Limited damage to epithelium; skin remains intact	Erythematous, hypersensitive, no blister formation	Complete healing within 3-5 days without scarring
Superficial partial-thickness (second degree)	Brief exposure to flash, flame, or hot liquids	Epidermis destroyed; minimal damage to superficial layers of dermis; epidermal appendages intact	Moist and weepy, pink or red, blisters, blanching, hypersensitive	Complete healing within 21 days with minimal to no scarring
Deep partial-thickness (second degree)	Intense radiant energy; scalding liquids, semi-liquids (e.g., tar), or solids; flame	Epidermis destroyed; underlying dermis damaged; some epidermal appendages remain intact	Pale; decreased moisture; blanching absent or prolonged; intact sensation to deep pressure but not to pinprick	Prolonged healing (often longer than 21 days); may require skin graft to achieve complete healing with better functional outcome
Full-thickness (third degree)	Prolonged contact with flame, scalding liquids; steam; hot objects; chemicals; electrical current	Epidermis, dermis, and epidermal appendages destroyed; injury through dermis	Dry, leather-like; pale, mottled brown, or red; thrombosed vessels visible; insensate	Requires skin grafting

Modified from Carrougher GJ, editor: *Burn care and therapy*, St Louis, 1998, Mosby.

| **T A B L E 2 - 17** American Burn Association Injury Classification Scheme | |
Severity classification	Criteria
Major	>25% TBSA burn in adults <40 years >20% TBSA burn in adults >40 years and children <10 years *or*>10% TBSA full-thickness burn in all age groups *or* Injuries involving the face, eyes, ears, hands, feet, or perineum that may result in functional or cosmetic disability; high-voltage electrical injury; all injuries with concomitant inhalation injury or major trauma
Moderate	15%-25% TBSA burn in adults <40 years 10%-20% TBSA burn in adults >40 years and children <10 years *and* <10% TBSA full-thickness burn without cosmetic or functional risk
Minor	<15% TBSA burn in adults < 40 years <10% TBSA burn in adults > 40 years and children <10 years *and* <2% TBSA full-thickness burn without cosmetic or functional risk

Modified from Carrougher GJ, editor: *Burn care and therapy,* St Louis, 1998, Mosby.

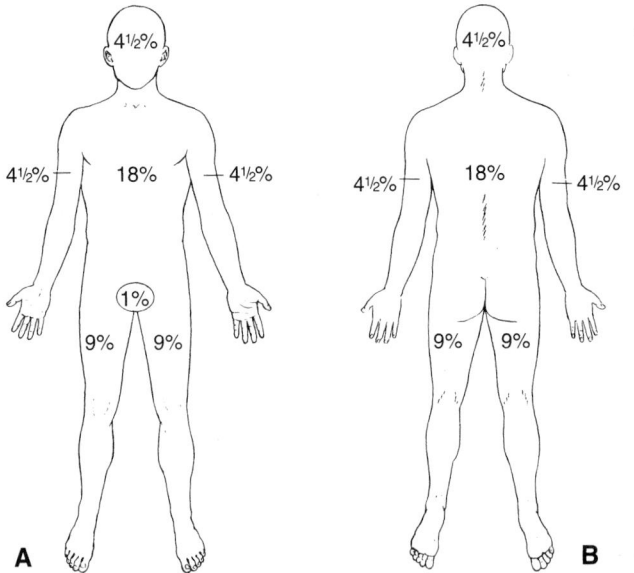

Figure 2-1: Estimation of adult burn injury: rule of mines, **A,** Anterior view. **B,** Posterior view. From Thompson M et al: *Mosby's clinical nursing,* ed 4, St Louis, 1997, Mosby.

voice, or coughing, especially if productive for soot. The lower respiratory tract can be damaged by contact with products of combustion and inhalation of vaporized caustic substances, such as sulfur, nitrogen, aldehydes, and hydrochloric acid. Damage may not appear immediately. Epithelial sloughing with bronchitis and respiratory distress may occur 6-72 hr after the burn occurs. Carbon monoxide (CO), a by-product of combustion, displaces oxygen from hemoglobin, resulting in hypoxia. Refer to Table 2-18 for signs and symptoms of CO poisoning.
Clinical indicators: Crackles, rhonchi, stridor, severe hoarseness, hacking cough, labored breathing, dyspnea, tachypnea, and possible altered LOC caused by hypoxia. Headache, decreased visual acuity, tinnitus, vertigo, and convulsions may be signs of CO poisoning.

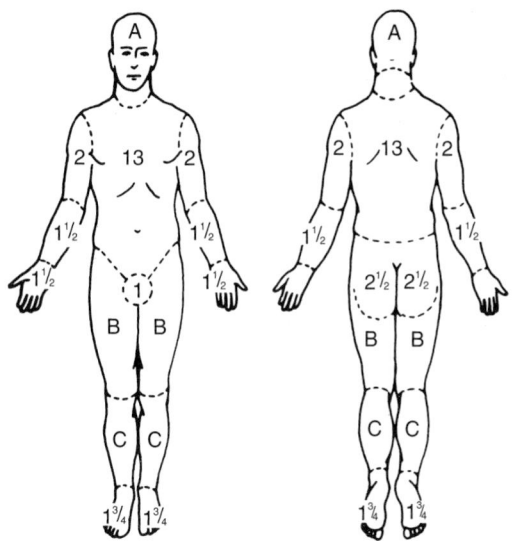

Relative percentages of areas affected by growth
(age in years)

	0	1	5	10	15	Adult
A: Half of head	$9\frac{1}{2}$	$8\frac{1}{2}$	$6\frac{1}{2}$	$5\frac{1}{2}$	$4\frac{1}{2}$	$3\frac{1}{2}$
B: Half of thigh	$2\frac{3}{4}$	$3\frac{1}{4}$	4	$4\frac{1}{4}$	$4\frac{1}{2}$	$4\frac{3}{4}$
C: Half of leg	$2\frac{1}{2}$	$2\frac{1}{2}$	$2\frac{3}{4}$	3	$3\frac{1}{4}$	$3\frac{1}{2}$

Second degree_____and
Third degree_____=
Total percent burned___

Figure 2-2: Estimation of burn injury: Lund and Browder chart. Areas represent percentages of body surface area that vary according to age. The accompanying table indicates the relative percentages of these areas in various stages of life.
From Sabeston DC, Jr, editor: *Textbook of surgery: the biographical basis of modern surgical practice,* ed. 11, Philadelphia, 1977, Saunders.

> **Note:** Physical and radiographic evidence of respiratory compromise may be absent initially, despite pulmonary injury. Progression to airway obstruction and acute respiratory distress can occur rapidly, especially in the presence of smoke inhalation.

Cardiovascular system: Circulatory compromise results from the fluid shifts that occur following a significant burn injury. Increased capillary permeability caused by the inflammatory response results in a shift of intravascular fluid into the interstitial spaces during the resuscitative phase. This causes a decrease in circulating volume and increased blood viscosity. Other systemic responses include increases in catecholamines, cortisol, renin-angiotensin, ADH, and aldosterone production as the body struggles to retain sodium and water to replenish intravascular fluid. Rapid fluid shifts can result in hemoconcentration and thrombus formation.

Clinical indicators: Signs of shock, such as thirst, pallor, dry mucous membranes, decreased LOC, and cool skin temperature; tachycardia, hypotension, and decreased filling pressures (CVP, PAP, PAWP); decreased or absent peripheral pulses and delayed capillary refill; impaired peripheral perfusion with possible obstruction caused by vascular compression with circumferential full-thickness burns or thrombus formation; cardiac dysrhythmias caused by direct cardiac damage (electrical burns) and electrolyte imbalance (e.g., hyperkalemia caused by cellular hemolysis); and peripheral edema as a result of fluid shifts and hypoproteinemia.

TABLE 2 - 18   Carbon Monoxide Poisoning

Carboxyhemoglobin saturation (%)	Signs and symptoms
<10	Impaired vision
11-20	Headache, facial flushing
21-30	Nausea, trouble with dexterity
31-40	Nausea, vomiting, dizziness, syncope
41-50	Tachypnea, tachycardia, loss of consciousness
>50	Coma, death

Gastrointestinal system: Initially, blood flow is shunted away from the GI tract and peristalsis is slowed or stopped completely, causing a gastric ileus (usually resolves within 72 hr after burn injury). Prior to the initiation of early enteral feedings, life-threatening stomach and intestinal ulcerations (Curling's ulcers) and hemorrhage (associated with a gastric pH of ≤5) often occurred. With enteral feedings, the incidence of Curling's ulcer is rare.
Clinical indicators: Diminished or absent bowel sounds; presence of nausea and vomiting; abdominal distention caused by accumulated flatus.
Renal system: Hemoconcentration and reduced circulatory volumes result in decreased renal blood flow and low urinary output. A high myoglobin or hemoglobin load may be reflected by dark, concentrated urine. Continued poor renal perfusion can result in acute tubular necrosis and renal failure with buildup of metabolic waste products and electrolyte imbalances (see "Acute Renal Failure," p. 315).
Clinical indicators: Urine output <30 ml/hr in adults and ≤0.5 ml/kg/hr in children; dark, amber-colored urine.
Integumentary system: Loss of skin integrity results in fluid loss through evaporation, hypothermia, and increased risk of infection. Circumferential full-thickness burns can cause constriction of underlying tissue, blood vessels, and muscles (see "Compartment Syndrome," p. 132) with circulatory compromise to underlying muscles and distal extremities. Scar formation can result in contractures that limit ROM.
Clinical indicators: See Table 2-16 for a complete description of partial-thickness and full-thickness burn wound injuries.
Invasive wound infection: Ongoing evaluation for wound sepsis is imperative as sepsis is a serious complication. Typically, the larger the wound, the greater the risk for wound infection.
Clinical indicators: Early clinical signs of wound infection include fever, redness, cellulitis, increased wound pain, change in exudates or wound appearance, and loss of previously healed skin grafts. Invasive wound infection is indicated by rapid eschar separation (invasive fungal infections); focal, dark red, brown, or black discolorations in the eschar; rapid conversion of an area of partial- to full-thickness injury; and hemorrhagic fat necrosis.
Signs of systemic inflammatory response syndrome (SIRS)/septic shock: Tachycardia, tachypnea, decreased BP with low SVR, labile core body temperature, changes in LOC (confusion, disorientation, agitation), hyperglycemia, gastric distention, and gastric ileus. (See "Systemic Inflammatory Response Syndrome," p. 501.)

DIAGNOSTIC TESTS

Arterial blood gases: Early ABGs may be normal. Later studies may reflect hypoxemia secondary to respiratory failure, with progressive metabolic acidosis in patients with impending shock or systemic inflammatory response syndrome.
Carboxyhemoglobin level: Elevated if carbon monoxide (CO) is present in the blood following inhalation of smoke and the by-products of combustion. Cigarette smokers may also have an elevated carboxyhemoglobin level.
Pulse oximetry: For continuous monitoring of oxygenation. Probe placed on uninjured area. Not reliable in patients who are profoundly hypovolemic or in shock.
Serial chest x-rays: Usually normal on admission; 24-48 hr after injury may show atelectasis or increased lung water, reflecting fluid shifts, ARDS, or pulmonary edema in susceptible individuals.
Laryngoscopy and bronchoscopy: Not routine, but may help determine presence of extramucosal carbonaceous material and the state of the mucosa (e.g., edema, denudation, erythema, blistering) in patients with inhalation injury.

Culture and sensitivity studies: To evaluate sputum, blood, urine, and wound tissue for evidence of infection. Burn wound infection is defined as $>10^5$ microorganisms/g of burn wound tissue with active invasion of adjacent, viable, unburned skin. Typical gram-negative organisms include *Pseudomonas aeruginosa, Klebsiella, Serratia, Escherichia coli,* and *Enterobacter cloacae.* Less frequently, gram-positive organisms *(Staphylococcus* and *Streptococcus)* and fungal pathogens *(Candida* and *Aspergillus)* may be present.

> **Note:** If a burn wound culture is positive for a group A *Streptococcus* sp., an epidemiologic investigation may be needed. The facility's infection control department should assist, especially if more than one patient is involved.

Urine collections: Culture and sensitivities (C&S) performed for early detection of UTI. Urinalysis and 24-hr urine collection for total nitrogen, urea nitrogen, creatinine, and amino acid nitrogen values may indicate return of capillary integrity (3-5 days after burn occurs) and mobilization of third-spaced fluids (fluid extravasating from the intravascular to the extravascular space), the degree of catabolism present, and the onset or resolution of acute renal failure. Myoglobinuria may be present as a result of muscle injury.

Hematology: Hct increased due to hemoconcentration. Hgb decreased secondary to hemolysis or multiple laboratory blood samples drawn. WBCs may be elevated due to systemic inflammatory response or sepsis. Burn patients will typically be leukopenic initially as WBCs migrate to areas of injured tissue.

Electrolytes: Sodium is decreased secondary to large fluid shifts into interstitial spaces. Potassium may be elevated as a result of cell lysis, fluid shifts, or renal insufficiency. BUN is elevated because of hypovolemic state, increased protein catabolism, or possible acute renal failure. Persistent elevation of BUN and creatinine signals inadequate fluid intake or acute renal failure. Total protein and albumin are decreased secondary to leakage of plasma proteins into interstitial spaces. Creatine kinase (CK) is sometimes used as index of muscle damage, but a burn injury that damages even a small quantity of muscle tissue will result in markedly elevated CK levels in the first 24 hr.

ECG: Tachycardia secondary to hypovolemia or pain. Myocardial damage secondary to electrical burn injury may be evident. Dysrhythmias related to electrolyte imbalance may occur.

COLLABORATIVE MANAGEMENT

Humidified oxygen therapy: Treats hypoxemia and prevents drying and sloughing of the mucosal lining of the tracheobronchial tree. If patient is awake, oxygen administration by mask may be sufficient; intubation may be required if the patient is stuporous. Any patient with suspected carbon monoxide poisoning/inhalation injury should receive humidified 100% oxygen by mask immediately until the carboxy hemoglobin level falls below 10%.

Intubation and mechanical ventilation: Indicated for respiratory distress or to maintain airway patency. Because laryngeal edema typically resolves in 3-5 days after burn occurrence, tracheostomy is avoided for upper airway distress unless there is acute obstruction.

Bronchodilators and mucolytic agents: Aid in the removal of secretions.

Escharotomy: Procedures to relieve constriction caused by circumferential, full-thickness burns. Relieves respiratory distress secondary to circumferential, full-thickness burns of the trunk. Lessens pressure in extremities from underlying edema to restore adequate perfusion. May be performed at the bedside or in the emergency room by trained personnel. Indicated when patients have cyanosis and cold temperature of distal unburned skin, prolonged capillary filling, decreased sensation and movement, or weak or absent peripheral pulses (mimics compartment syndrome), and for burns of thorax, when respiratory motion may be restricted. See "Compartment Syndrome," p. 132 for more information.

Fluid resuscitation: Fluid replacement protocols are based on body weight and percentage of body surface area burned. Various formulas are used to estimate fluid requirements for burn patients during the resuscitative phase of injury (Table 2-19). Colloids generally are avoided during the first 24 hr after injury because increased capillary permeability causes leakage of protein into the interstitial tissues. In general, lactated Ringer's solution are used in the first 24 hr, with small amounts of colloid fluids added during the second 24 hr after injury. The Consensus formula recommends administration of 2-4 ml fluid/kg body weight/percent TBSA burned. The first half of the calculated volume is infused over the first 8 hr, when fluid shifts are greatest. Infants and young children should receive fluid with 5% dextrose at a maintenance rate in addition to the lactated Ringer's resuscitation fluid.

T A B L E 2 - 19   **Adult Burn Resuscitation Formulas**

Formula name	Recommended solutions	Formula for estimating fluid needs
Initial 24 hr after injury		
Evans*	0.9% Normal saline plus colloid solution	1 ml/kg/% TBSA burn 1 ml/kg/% TBSA burn
Brooke*	Lactated Ringer's solution plus colloid solution	1.5 ml/kg/% TBSA burn 0.5 ml/kg/% TBSA burn
Hypertonic saline (Monafo)	Na⁺ 250 mEq/L	Volume to maintain urine output at 30 ml/hr
Modified Brooke*	Lactated Ringer's solution	2 ml/kg/% TBSA burn
Parkland*	Lactated Ringer's solution	4 ml/kg/% TBSA burn
Consensus	Lactated Ringer's solution	Adults: 2-4 ml/kg/% TBSA burn Children: 3-4 ml/kg/% TBSA burn
Second 24 hr after injury		
Modified Brooke	Colloid solution (diluted to physiologic concentration) plus 5% dextrose in water	0.3-0.5 ml/kg/% TBSA burn (0.3 ml/kg/% TBSA burn for injuries of 30% to 50%; up to 0.5 ml/kg/% TBSA burn for injuries >50% TBSA Volume to maintain desired urine output
Parkland	25% Albumin plus 5% dextrose in water	20% to 60% of calculated plasma volume Volume to maintain desired urine output

From Gordon MD, Winfree JH: Fluid resuscitation after a major burn. In Carrougher GJ: *Burn care and therapy,* St Louis, 1998, Mosby.
*The total estimated volume is calculated with one-half administered over the initial 8 hours after injury and the remaining half over the subsequent 16 hours.
TBSA, Total body surface area.

Note: Calculate fluid infusion time from the time of injury, not the time of hospital admission. Fluid formulas should be modified, based on individual patient responses and needs. Patients with electrical injuries, inhalation injury, and ethanol intoxication and those with concomitant trauma (e.g., crushing injuries) may have greater fluid needs than suggested by their cutaneous burn injury alone (see Table 2-19).

Indwelling urinary catheter: Essential for accurate measurement of urine output and evaluation of renal status in patients with a major burn injury.
Gastric suction: Allows aspiration of gastric contents, which may be necessary during the resuscitative phase because of the potential for gastric ileus in patients with a ≥30% TBSA burn and in patients with intubated airway.
Tetanus-toxoid prophylaxis: Given intramuscularly to prevent tetanus.
IV morphine sulfate: Common agent for pain management. Administered in small, frequent intravenous doses, as needed for comfort and before painful procedure.

Note: During the resuscitative phase of care, all medications, except tetanus-toxoid, are administered intravenously to avoid sequestration of medication, which then would "flood" the vascular system with the return of capillary integrity and the diuresis of third-spaced fluids.

Gastric acid suppression therapy: Maintain gastric pH >5.0 and prevent development of Curling's ulcer. Early initiation of enteral tube feedings also helps to prevent Curling's ulcer.
Nutritional support: High metabolic activity and increased protein catabolism related to burn injury result in dramatic increases in energy requirements and nutritional needs. Energy requirements are estimated using one of several formulas based on body size and extent of burn with adjustment for age. Additional injury or poor nutritional status before the burn may increase nutri-

tional needs. The appropriate mix of protein, fat, and carbohydrates is controversial, but a positive nitrogen state has been achieved with patients who are administered high-protein, moderate-carbohydrate diets. To facilitate weaning of patients from the ventilator, it has been suggested that the use of higher-fat, lower-carbohydrate diets may be beneficial since excess carbohydrate increases CO_2 production. Oral, enteral, or parenteral methods of delivery are used, based on patient tolerance. Enteral tube feedings may decrease GI acidity and ulcer formation. Either gastric or postpyloric jejunal feedings may be used. Elemental jejunal feedings may be tolerated when conventional feedings are not. Bowel sounds are unnecessary when elemental feedings are used. Total parenteral nutrition (TPN) may be initiated for the patient with gastric ileus or inability to tolerate an adequate amount of enteral feedings.

Multivitamin and mineral supplements: Many vitamins and minerals affect immune function, protein synthesis, and wound healing. Vitamins A and C and zinc are especially important for promoting wound healing.

IV antibiotics: As indicated according to culture and sensitivity findings and clinical indicators suggestive of infection.

Wound care: Wound cleansing is accomplished with dilute antimicrobial skin cleansers (e.g., chlorhexidine) and water. Burns are débrided using manual, enzymatic, or surgical techniques. Topical antimicrobial agents such as silver sulfadiazine (Silvadene), mafenide acetate (Sulfamylon), and silver nitrate control bacterial proliferation and promote tissue granulation. Burn wounds may be covered and ultimately closed with various temporary and permanent coverings as in the following list. Care of the patient with these coverings depends on the type of wound closure technique used.

Wound coverage and closure techniques:
- Cutaneous autograft—includes split-thickness skin (STSG) and cultured epithelial autograft (CEA) (permanent)
- Cutaneous allograft—fresh or preserved donated cadaver skin (temporary)
- Cutaneous xenograft— harvested porcine epidermis (pigskin) (temporary)
- Biosynthetic coverings—artificial skin (e.g., Integra) (permanent)
- Synthetic coverings—various dressings often used to cover partial-thickness burns and/or donor sites (temporary)

NURSING DIAGNOSES AND INTERVENTIONS

Impaired gas exchange (or risk for same) related to smoke inhalation with tracheobronchial swelling and carbonaceous debris; competition of carbon monoxide (CO) with O_2 for hemoglobin; hypoventilation associated with constricting circumferential burns to the thorax

Desired outcome: Within 1 hr of treatment/intervention, patient exhibits adequate gas exchange as evidenced by $PaO_2 \geq 80$ mm Hg; oxygen saturation $\geq 95\%$; CO_2 35-45 mm Hg, RR 12-20 breaths/min with a normal pattern and depth (eupnea); absence of adventitious breath sounds and other signs of respiratory dysfunction; and orientation to time, place, and person.

- Assess and document respiratory status hourly, noting rate and depth, breath sounds, and LOC. Be alert to a declining respiratory status as evidenced by indicators of upper airway distress (e.g., severe hoarseness, stridor, dyspnea) and lower airway distress (e.g., crackles, rhonchi, hacking cough, labored or rapid breathing). Consult physician promptly for all significant findings. Prepare for intubation and mechanical ventilation and thoracic escharotomies, if needed.
- Administer humidified oxygen therapy, mechanical ventilation, or bronchodilator treatment as prescribed.
- Monitor for hypoxemia with serial ABG values, noting decreasing PaO_2 or oxygen saturation, or increased $PaCO_2$. Declining vital capacity, tidal volume, and/or inspiratory force indicate respiratory insufficiency.
- Place patient in high Fowler's position to enhance respiratory excursion.
- Teach patient the necessity of coughing and deep-breathing exercises q2h, including incentive spirometry.

NIC Airway Management; Respiratory Monitoring; Oxygen Therapy; Bedside Laboratory Testing; Cough Enhancement: Laboratory Data Interpretation

Ineffective airway clearance (or risk for same) related to increased pulmonary secretions and inflammation and swelling of nasopharyngeal mucous membranes secondary to smoke irritation and impaired cough; constricting neck and thorax burns and decreased expansion of alveoli secondary to circumferential thorax burns

Desired outcome: Patient has a clear airway within 10-30 min of treatment/intervention as evidenced by auscultation of normal breath sounds over the lung fields; a state of eupnea; and orientation to time, place, and person.

- Assess and document respiratory status hourly, noting breath sounds, rate and depth of respirations, and LOC. Be alert to a declining respiratory status as evidenced by crackles, rhonchi, stridor, labored breathing, dyspnea, tachypnea, restlessness, and decreasing LOC. Consult physician promptly for all significant findings.

- Assess and document character and amount of secretions after each coughing and deep-breathing exercise.
- Reposition patient from side to side q1-2h to help mobilize secretions; specialized rotation bed may be used.
- As prescribed, administer percussion and postural drainage to facilitate airway clearance (this is contraindicated with fresh skin grafts over thorax). Perform oropharyngeal or ET suctioning as indicated by the presence of adventitious breath sounds and the patient's inability to clear the airway effectively by coughing.

NIC Airway Management; Airway Suctioning; Artificial Airway Management; Aspiration Precautions; Cough Enhancement; Mechanical Ventilation

Fluid volume deficit related to active loss through the burn wound and leakage of fluid, plasma proteins, and other cellular elements into the interstitial space

Desired outcome: Within 24-72 hr of this diagnosis, patient becomes normovolemic as evidenced by BP 110-130/70-80 mm Hg (or within patient's normal preinjury baseline); peripheral pulses >2+ on a 0-4+ scale; urine output ≥0.5 ml/kg/hr (children) or >30 ml/hr (adult); and urine specific gravity 1.010-1.030.

- Monitor patient for evidence of fluid volume deficit, including tachycardia, decreased BP, decreased amplitude of peripheral pulses, urine output <0.5 ml/kg/hr or <30 ml/hr (adult), thirst, and dry mucous membranes.
- Monitor I&O; administer fluid therapy using formula or as prescribed. Adjust infusion to maintain urine output at a minimum of 30 ml/hr. Avoid colloids during first 24 hr of burn injury.
- Monitor weight daily; report significant gains or losses. Recognize that weight loss also may be caused by catabolism and an increased metabolic rate as the body attempts to heal itself.
- Monitor urine specific gravity. An elevated value occurs with hypovolemia and reflects the need for additional volume.
- Monitor serial Hct, and Hgb, values. During the first 24 hr postburn, neither the Hct or Hgb levels are reliable guides to fluid recuscitation. As the circulating volume is restored, hemoconcentration is no longer present and Hct returns to within normal limits (WNL). Be aware that Hgb values may decrease secondary to hemolysis within the first 1-2 hr after burn injury. Consult physician for significant anemia or electrolyte imbalance.
- Monitor patient for evidence of fluid volume excess secondary to rapid fluid resuscitation, especially in patients with preexisting respiratory or cardiac disease. Be alert to crackles, SOB, tachypnea, and excessive urine output. Central hemodynamic monitoring is recommended for patients who have preexisting heart or lung disease.
- In presence of myoglobinuria, confer with physician regarding the need to increase the rate of fluid administration and for the use of mannitol to promote osmotic diuresis and prevent renal tubular sludging. Other diuretics are avoided because they further deplete an already compromised intravascular volume.
- With the onset of spontaneous diuresis, decrease infusion rates as prescribed. Continue to reduce rates gradually according to intake/output ratio and clinical status.

NIC Fluid/Electrolyte Management; Fluid Monitoring; Hypovolemia Management; Shock Prevention; Venous Access Devices Maintenance

Pain related to burn injury

Desired outcomes: Within 1 hr of treatment/intervention, patient's subjective evaluation of discomfort improves as documented by a pain scale. Nonverbal indicators of discomfort are absent or diminished.

- Assess patient's level of discomfort at frequent intervals. Using a pain scale, ask patient to rate discomfort from 0 (no pain) to 10 (worse pain imaginable). Patients with partial-thickness burns may experience severe pain because of damage and exposure of sensory nerve endings. Pain tolerance often decreases with prolonged hospitalization, multiple painful procedures, and sleep deprivation.
- Monitor patient for clinical indicators of pain: increased BP, tachypnea, shivering, rigid muscle tone, or guarded position.
- Administer opioid analgesia and anxiolytics as prescribed. Time dosage for optimal effectiveness before painful procedures.
- Provide a full explanation of procedures.
- Employ nonpharmacologic interventions as indicated: relaxation breathing, guided imagery, distraction, music.
- Ensure that patient receives periods of uninterrupted sleep (optimally 90 min at a time) by grouping care procedures when possible.
- See "Pain," p. 51, for additional information about pain management.

NIC Analgesic Administration; Anxiety Reduction; Environmental Management: Comfort; Pain Management

Impaired tissue integrity/altered tissue perfusion: peripheral, related to thermal injury; circumferential burns; edema; hypovolemia
Desired outcomes: Patient's wound exhibits evidence of healing. Tissue healing occurs without hypertrophic scarring (late outcome).

Note: Healing time varies with the extent and depth of injury. Tissue perfusion in burned extremities is adequate when peripheral pulses are >2+ on a scale of 0-4+, capillary refill is brisk (<2 sec), and skin is warm to the touch.

- Assess and document time and circumstances, extent and depth of burn wound. (See Table 2-16.)
- Monitor tissue perfusion hourly in burned extremities. Note capillary refill, temperature, and peripheral pulses. Report signs of impaired tissue perfusion to the physician immediately, including coolness of the extremity, weak or absent peripheral pulses, pain or paresthesias, and delayed capillary refill.
- Cleanse and débride wound as prescribed. Control ambient temperature carefully to prevent hypothermia.
- Apply topical antimicrobial treatments as prescribed, using aseptic technique.
- Elevate burned or recently grafted extremities at or above heart level to promote venous return and to prevent excessive dependent edema formation.
- Help prevent graft loss by expressing fluid from between graft and recipient bed as prescribed by using a rolling motion with sterile applicators. Always roll the applicator toward the nearest graft juncture.
- Monitor type and amount of drainage from wounds. Promptly report the presence of bright red bleeding, which would inhibit graft take, and purulent exudate, which indicates infection.
- Maintain immobility of grafted site for 3-5 days or as prescribed. This is achieved with a combination of positioning, splinting, or light pressure and sedation. In some instances, restraints, stents, bulky dressings, or occlusive dressings may be required to maintain immobilization and promote hemostasis of graft.
- Apply elastic wraps as prescribed to legs that have grafts to promote venous return.
- Use bed cradle to prevent bedding from coming in contact with burned or grafted area.
- Provide donor site care as prescribed, and be alert to signs of donor site infection (see "Risk for infection," p. 171.)
- Apply compression dressing to graft and incision sites. Teach patient about need for extended compression to prevent hypertrophic scarring.

NIC Infection Protection; Positioning; Wound Care

Altered tissue perfusion: gastrointestinal, related to hypovolemia and interruption in blood flow associated with splanchnic vasoconstriction secondary to fluid shifts and catecholamine release
Desired outcome: Patient has adequate GI tissue perfusion as evidenced by auscultation of bowel sounds/min within 48-72 hr after burn injury; bowel elimination and appetite within patient's normal pattern; and absence of nausea and vomiting.

Note: Be aware that prolonged impaired perfusion to GI organs increases the likelihood of such complications as impaired gastric motility, adynamic ileus, gastritis, and Curling's ulcer.

- Assess bowel function q2-4h. Be alert to abdominal distention and decreasing or absent bowel sounds, which occur with adynamic ileus.
- During period of absent bowel sounds, maintain gastric tube to intermittent low suction as prescribed. Check at intervals to ensure patency and position of the tube. Before removing tube, clamp for several hours to be certain patient has sufficient GI motility. Abdominal distention, nausea, vomiting, or return of a large volume of gastric contents when tube is reconnected indicates insufficient motility to tolerate tube removal.
- Maintain NPO status until return of bowel sounds. Provide mouth care for comfort and hygiene.
- Administer histamine H$_2$-receptor antagonists, antacids, and other agents prescribed to reduce formation of gastric acids. If prescribed, start enteral feedings to protect the patient's gastric mucosa from irritation.
- Test gastric aspirate for occult blood q8h. Promptly report presence of blood to physician.

NIC Gastrointestinal Intubation; Hemodynamic Regulation; Nutritional Management; Tube Care: Gastrointestinal

Altered nutrition: less than body requirements of protein, vitamins, and calories, related to hypermetabolic state secondary to burn wound healing

Desired outcome: Patient has adequate nutrition as evidenced by stable weight; balanced nitrogen state per nitrogen studies; serum albumin ≥3.5 g/dl; thyroxine-binding prealbumin 20-30 mg/dl; retinol-binding protein 4-5 mg/dl; and evidence of burn wound healing and graft take within an acceptable time frame.

- Record all intake for daily calorie counts. Measure weight initially and then daily. Evaluate on the basis of patient's weight before the burn. Minimize error by weighing patient without dressings or splints, if possible.
- Monitor serum albumin, thyroxine-binding prealbumin, retinol-binding protein, and urine nitrogen measurements. Long periods of catabolism cause serum values to decrease. Be alert to measures of protein deficiencies, weight loss, and poor wound healing, all of which are signals that nutritional needs are not being met.
- Provide high-protein, high-calorie diet as prescribed. When patient can take foods orally, promote supplemental feedings/snacks between meals.
- Patients with burns >10% BSA, preinjury illness, or associated injuries have greatly increased calorie requirements and are likely to require nutritional supplements. Patients with ileus that persists for more than 4 days or those unable to meet caloric needs enterally may require TPN.
- Assess individual food preferences, and encourage those high in protein and carbohydrates. As appropriate, encourage family members to provide desired foods.
- For additional information, see "Nutritional Support," p. 1.

NIC Nutrition Management; Nutrition Therapy; Nutritional Monitoring; Weight Gain Assistance

Sensory/perceptual alterations: tactile and visual, related to altered reception secondary to medications, sleep pattern disturbance, pain, swollen eyelids, and full-thickness burn wounds.

Desired outcomes: Within 24-48 hr of this diagnosis, patient verbalizes orientation to time, place, and person and describes rationale for necessary treatments.

- Assess patient's orientation to time, place, and person.
- Answer patient's questions simply and succinctly, providing information regarding immediate surroundings, procedures, and treatments. During the emergent phase of the burn injury, anticipate the necessity of having to repeat information at frequent intervals.
- For patient with full-thickness injury, explain why tactile sensation is decreased or absent.
- If patient's eyelids are swollen shut because of facial edema, reassure patient that he or she is not blind and that swelling will resolve within 3-5 days.
- Touch patient often on unburned skin to provide nonpainful tactile stimulation.
- For additional information, see this nursing diagnosis in "Psychosocial Support," p. 68.

NIC Peripheral Sensation Management; Surveillance: Safety; Communication Enhancement: Visual Deficit; Environmental Management

Body image disturbance related to biophysical changes secondary to burn injury

Desired outcomes: Patient begins to acknowledge body changes and demonstrates movement toward incorporating changes into self-concept. Patient does not exhibit maladaptive responses such as severe depression.

- Assess patient's perceptions and feelings about the burn injury and changes in lifestyle and relationships, especially those with significant others.
- Involve significant others in as much care as possible to maintain bond with patient.
- Respect patient's need to express anger over body changes.
- Provide information concerning eventual appearance of grafts and donor sites.
- Provide names and telephone numbers of local and national support groups for burn survivors: The American Burn Association, National Headquarters Office, website: www.ameriburn.org; phone: (800) 548-2876; The Phoenix Society for Burn Survivors, Inc., National Headquarters Office, website: www.phoenix-society.org, phone: (800) 888-2876.

NIC Anxiety Reduction; Body Image Enhancement; Coping Enhancement; Grief Work Facilitation; Self-Esteem Enhancement; Support System Enhancement; Wound Care

Risk for disuse syndrome related to immobilization from pain, splints, or scar formation

Desired outcome: Patient displays complete ROM without verbal or nonverbal indicators of discomfort.

- Provide ROM exercises q4h while awake. When possible, combine when medicated with analgesics for other procedures and during activities of daily living (ADLs).
- Apply splints as prescribed to maintain body parts in functional positions and to prevent contracture formation.
- For patient with graft, institute ROM exercises and ambulation on prescribed postgrafting day (often 3-7 days postgrafting). Premedicate with analgesic to aid in mobility and reduce discomfort.

NIC Exercise Therapy: Ambulation; Exercise Therapy: Joint Mobility; Exercise Promotion; Nutrition Management; Positioning; Surveillance

Risk for infection related to inadequate primary and secondary defenses secondary to traumatized tissue, bacterial proliferation in burn wounds, presence of invasive intravenous lines or urinary catheter, and immunocompromised status

Desired outcome: Patient is free of infection as evidenced by normothermia; WBC count ≤11,000/mm^3; negative culture results; and absence of purulent matter and other clinical indicators of burn wound infection.

- Except for eyebrows, shave all hair within wound to prevent wound contamination.
- Monitor temperature q2h. Report temperatures >38.8° C (102° F).
- Assess burn wound daily for signs of infection. Report to the physician: fever, elevated WBC count, rapid eschar separation, increased amount of wound exudate, purulent material. Also report signs of wound deterioration: loss of previously healed wounds, disappearance of a well-defined burn margin with edema formation and hemorrhagic discoloration.
- Assess appearance of grafted site, including adherence to recipient bed, appearance, and color. Be alert to erythema, hyperthermia, increasing tenderness, purulent drainage, and swelling around the grafted site.
- Observe for clinical indicators of sepsis: tachypnea, hypothermia, hyperthermia, ileus, subtle disorientation, unexplained metabolic acidosis, and glucose intolerance (see "Systemic Inflammatory Response Syndrome," p. 501). If sepsis is suspected, obtain wound, blood, sputum, and urine culture specimens as prescribed.
- Administer antipyretic and antimicrobial agents as prescribed. Ensure aseptic technique when administering care to burned areas and performing invasive techniques. Rotate intravenous access sites at regular intervals.
- Practice standard precautions to reduce the risk of transmission of microorganisms. Consult the hospital's infection control professional to assist with placement of patients with contagious infections, if private rooms are not available.
- For patients with skin grafts, monitor donor site for evidence of infection, including purulent drainage, poorly defined borders, and foul odor.

NIC Environmental Management; Infection Control; Infection Protection; Surveillance; Wound Care; Shock Management

Knowledge deficit: self-care during the acute care and rehabilitative stages

Desired outcome: Within the 24-hr period before discharge from the burn unit, patient and significant others verbalize knowledge about prescribed medications and demonstrate and verbalize knowledge about techniques that facilitate continued wound healing and limb mobility.

- Review the splinting and exercise program for contracture prevention, as directed by physical therapist. Teach patient and significant others to monitor for pain or pressure caused by improperly applied splint and to assess splinted extremity for coolness, pallor, cyanosis, decreased pulses, and impaired function.
- Discuss skin care, emphasizing the following:
  - ❏ Explain that a lubricating cream without alcohol should be applied several times a day and after bathing to healed skin to promote soft and pliant skin and assist with control of pruritus.
  - ❏ Teach patient to avoid exposure to sun, because healed skin is highly sensitive to ultraviolet rays for up to 1 year following injury and that pigmentation changes may occur.
  - ❏ Explain to a darker-skinned patient that permanent pigmentation changes may occur.
- Review wound care. Provide simplified dressing change procedure; explain indicators of infection and importance of notifying physician should they appear. Have patient or caregiver demonstrate wound care before hospital discharge.
- Teach patient the importance of wearing pressure garments as prescribed to prevent hypertrophic scarring (raised, erythematous, and hardened scar tissue).
- Review nutrition needs: explain the importance of maintaining an adequate intake of protein and calories for optimal wound healing.
- Provide a list of medications, including drug name, purpose, dosage, schedule, precautions, and potential side effects.
- Discuss home care, including resources to provide support for adjustment to life outside the hospital environment.
- Provide addresses and telephone numbers of local support groups for burn patients.
- Stress the importance of follow-up care; confirm date and time of first appointment if it has been established.

NIC Learning Facilitation; Learning Readiness Enhancement; Teaching: Individual

ADDITIONAL NURSING DIAGNOSES

For other nursing diagnoses and interventions, see the following, as appropriate: "Nutritional Support," p. 1; "Mechanical Ventilation," p. 14; "Wound and Skin Care," p. 45; "Pain," p. 51; "Prolonged Immobility," p. 61; "Psychosocial Support," p. 68; "Psychosocial Support for the Patient's Family and Significant Others," p. 78; and Appendix 8.

Bibliography

Adams JE: Utility of cardiac troponins in patients with suspected cardiac trauma or after cardiac surgery, *Clin Lab Med* 17(4):613-623, 1997.

Alost T, Waldrop RD: Profile of geriatric pelvic fractures presenting to the Emergency Department, *Am J Emerg Med* 15(6):576-578, 1997.

American College of Surgeons: *Advanced trauma life support for doctors—first impression,* Chicago, 1997, ACS.

American College of Surgeons: *Resources for optimal care of the injured patient: 1999,* Chicago, 1998, ACS.

Ball JB, Morrison WL: Cardiac tamponade, *Postgrad Med J* 73:141-145, 1997.

Balough, Z et al.: Secondary abdominal compartment syndrome is an elusive early complication of traumatic shock resuscitation, *Am J Surg* 184:538-544, 2002.

Banning AP, Pillai R: Non-penetrating cardiac and aortic trauma, *Heart* 78:226-229, 1997.

Beachly M, Farrar J; Abdominal trauma: putting the pieces together, *Am J Nurs* 93(11):26-34, 1993.

Better OS, Rubinstein I: Management of shock and acute renal failure in casualties suffering from crush syndrome, *Ren Fail* 19(5):647-653, 1997.

Brain Trauma Foundation: Guidelines for cerebral perfusion pressure, *J Neurotrauma* 13(11):693-698, 1996.

Brain Trauma Foundation: Intracranial pressure threshold, *J Neurotrauma* 13(11):681-684, 1996.

Brain Trauma Foundation: Nutritional support of brain-injured patients, *J Neurotrauma* 13(11):721-730, 1996.

Brain Trauma Foundation: Resuscitation of blood pressure and oxygenation, *J Neurotrauma* 13(11):661-666, 1996.

Brain Trauma Foundation: The role of antiseizure prophylaxis following head injury, *J Neurotrauma* 13(11):731-734, 1996.

Brain Trauma Foundation: The role of glucocorticoids in the treatment of severe head injury, *J Neurotrauma* 13(11):715-718, 1996.

Brain Trauma Foundation: The use of barbiturates in the control of intracranial hypertension, *J Neurotrauma* 13(11):711-714, 1996.

Brain Trauma Foundation: The use of hyperventilation in the acute management of severe traumatic brain injury, *J Neurotrauma* 13(11):699-704, 1996.

Brain Trauma Foundation: The use of mannitol in severe head injury, *J Neurotrauma* 13(11):705-710, 1996.

Canobbio M: *Pericarditis, handbook of patient teaching,* ed 3, St Louis, 2003, Mosby.

Carrougher GJ: Burn wound assessment and topical treatment. In Carrougher GJ, editor: *Burn Care & Therapy,* St Louis, 1998, Mosby.

Carrougher GJ et al: Comparison of patient satisfaction and self-reports of pain in adult burn-injured patients, *J Burn Care Rehabil* 24(1):1-8, 2003.

Coates TJ et al: Prehospital resuscitative thoracotomy for cardiac arrest after penetrating trauma: rationale and case series, *J Trauma* 50(4):670-673, 2001.

Crosby L, Parsons C: Cerebrovascular response of closed head-injured patients to a standardized endotracheal tube suctioning and manual hyperventilation procedure, *J Neurosci Nurs* 24(1):40-49, 1992.

Darovic GO: *Hemodynamic monitoring: invasive and non-invasive clinical application,* ed 3, Philadelphia, 2002, Saunders.

Davis A: Mechanisms of traumatic brain injury: biomechanical, structural, and cellular considerations. *Crit Care Nurs Q* 23(3):1-13, 2000.

Davis A, Briones T: Intracranial disorders. In Kinney M et al: *AACN Clinical Reference,* St Louis, 1998, Mosby.

Davis A, Briones T: Neurological clinical physiology. In Kinney M et al: *AACN Clinical Reference,* St Louis, 1998, Mosby.

Davis A, Hinkle J: Constructing cerebral dynamic profiles, Unpublished data, 2000.

DeBoer S: Neurologic outcomes after near drowning, *Crit Care Nurse* 17(4):19-25, 1997.

Dillard TA, Grathwohl KW: Near drowning and diving accidents. In Baum GL et al, editors: *Textbook of pulmonary diseases,* ed 6, Philadelphia, 1998, Lippincott-Raven.

Dochterman JM, Bulechek GM: *Nursing interventions classification (NIC),* ed 4, St Louis, 2004, Mosby.

Eastridge BJ et al: The importance of fracture pattern in guiding therapeutic decision-making in patients with hemorrhagic pelvic ring disruptions, *J Trauma* 53(3):446-451, 2002.

Evans-Murray A: Adult respiratory distress syndrome after near drowning, *Crit Care Nurs* 17(2): 41-44, 1997.

Fratianne RB, Brandt CP: Improved survival of adults with extensive burns, *J Burn Care Rehabil* 18:347-351, 1997.

Gennarelli T: The pathobiology of brain injury, *Neuroscientist* 3:73-80, 1997.

Goff CD, Collin GR: Management of renal trauma at a rural, level I trauma center, *Am Surg* 64(3):226-230, 1998.

Goldman SM et al: Blunt urethral trauma: a unified, anatomical mechanical classification, *J Urol* 157:85-89, 1997.

Gordon M, Goodwin CW: Initial assessment, management, and stabilization, *Nurs Clin North Am* 32(2):237-249, 1997.

Gottschlich MM et al: An evaluation of the safety of early vs delayed enteral support and effects on clinical, nutritional, and endocrine outcomes after severe burns, *J Burn Care Rehabil* 23(6):401-415, 2002.

Greenfield, LJ: *Surgery,* ed 3, Philadelphia, 2001, Lippincott Williams & Wilkins.

Heath FR, Blum F, Rockwell S: Physical examination as a screening test for pelvic fractures in blunt trauma patients, *W V Med J* 93(5):267-269, 1997.

Hinkle J, Davis A: Positioning effects on intracranial and cerebral perfusion pressures: an integrated review. (Unpublished data, 2000.)

Howard CA: Chest trauma. In Keen JH, Swearingen PL, editors: *Mosby's critical care nursing consultant,* St Louis, 1997, Mosby.

Howard CA: Flail chest. In Keen JH, Swearingen PL, editors: *Mosby's critical care nursing consultant,* St Louis, 1997, Mosby.

Iowa Outcomes Project. Johnson M, Maas M, editors: *Nursing outcomes classification (NOC),* ed 4, St Louis, 2004, Mosby.

Ibsen LM, Koch T: Submersion and asphyxial injury, *Crit Care Med* 30(11):S402-S408, 2002.

Jacobs BB, Hoyt KS: Brain and craniofacial trauma. In Emergency Nurses Association: *Trauma nurse core course: provider manual,* ed 5, 2000, Emergency Nurses Association.

Jacobs BB, Hoyt KS: Abdominal trauma. In Emergency Nurses Association: *Trauma nurse core course: provider manual,* ed 5, 2000, Emergency Nurses Association.

Jordan BS, Harrington DT: Management of the burn wound, *Nurs Clin North Am* 32(2):251-271, 1997.

Kerr M, Lovasik D: Evaluating cerebral oxygenation using jugular venous oximetry in head injuries, *AACN Clin Issues Nurs* 6:11-20, 1995.

Kaiser L, DiPierro F: Thoracic trauma. In Fishman AP: *Fishman's pulmonary diseases and disorders,* New York, 1998, McGraw-Hill.

Kirby RR, Taylor RW, Civetta JM: Primary triage of the trauma patient. In Kirby RR, Taylor RW, Civetta JM: *Handbook of critical care,* ed 2, Philadelphia, 1997, Lippincott-Raven.

Kotkin L, Koch MO: Impotence and incontinence after immediate realignment of posterior urethral trauma: result of injury or management? *J Urol* 155:1600-1603, 1996.

Lynn-McHale D, Carlson K: *AACN Procedure manual for critical care,* ed 4, Philadelphia, 2001, Saunders.

MacLeod M, Powell JN: Evaluation of pelvic fractures: clinical and radiologic, *Orthop Clin North Am* 28(3):331-344, 1997.

Mattox KL, Feliciano DV, Moore EE: *Trauma,* ed 4, New York, 2002, McGraw-Hill.

Mbubaegbu CE, Stallard MC: A method of fasciotomy wound closure, *Injury* 27(9):613-615, 1996.

McCance KL, Huether SE: *Pathophysiology: the biologic basis for disease in adults and children,* ed 3, St Louis, 1998, Mosby.

McQueen MM, Court-Brown CM: Compartment monitoring in tibial fractures, *J Bone Joint Surg Br* 78B(1):99-104, 1996.

McQuillan KA et al: *Trauma nursing: from resuscitation through rehabilitation,* ed 3, Philadelphia, 2002, Saunders.

Montgomery KD et al: Thromboembolic complications in patients with pelvic trauma, *Clin Orthop* 329:68-87, Aug 1996.

Naranja RL Jr et al: Treatment considerations in patients with compartment syndrome and inherited bleeding disorder, *Orthopedics* 20(8):706-709, 1997.

Patterson DR, Sharar S: Treating pain from severe burn injuries, *Adv Med Psychother* 9:55-71, 1997.

Porter JM, Ivatury RR: Unwillingness to lie supine? A sign of pericardial tamponade, *Am Surg* 63:365-366, April 1997.

Price S, Wilson L: *Pathophysiology and clinical concepts of disease processes*, ed 6, St Louis, 2003, Mosby.

Ragnarson K: Restorative treatment of persons with spinal cord injury: current trends. *J Rehab Res Dev* 35 (4):11-14, 1998.

Rogers FB, Leavitt BJ: Upper torso cyanosis: a marker for blunt cardiac rupture, *Am J Emerg Med* 15:275-276, 1997.

Sachdeva RC: Near drowning, *Crit Care Clin* 15(2):281-295, 1999.

Saffle JR: Predicting outcomes of burns, *N Engl J Med* 338(6):387-389, 1998.

Salim A et al: Clinically significant blunt cardiac trauma: role of serum troponin levels combined with electrocardiographic findings, *J Trauma* 50(2):237-243, 2001.

Seidl E: Promising pharmacologic agents in the management of acute spinal cord injury, *Crit Care Nurs Q* 22(2):44-50, 1999.

Shaw CJ, Spencer JD: Late management of compartment syndromes, *Injury* 26(9):633-635, 1995.

Solar-Solar J, Sagrista-Sauleda J, Permanyer-Miralda G: Management of pericardial effusion, *Heart* 86:235-240, 2001.

Spodick DH: Pathophysiology of cardiac tamponade, *Chest* 113:1372-1378, 1998.

St. John RE: Near drowning. In Alspach JG, editor: *American Association of Critical Care Nurses core curriculum for critical care nurses,* ed 5, Philadelphia, 1998, Saunders.

Stoffer G et al: Diagnosis and management of chronic pericardial effusions, *Am J Med Sci* 322: 79-97, 2001.

Swaanenburg JC et al: Troponin I, troponin T, CKMB-activity and CKMB-mass as markers for the detection of myocardial contusion in patients who experienced blunt trauma, *Clin Chim Acta* 272:171-181, 1998.

Taffet R: Management of pelvic fractures with concomitant urologic injuries, *Orthop Clin North Am* 28(3):389-396, 1997.

Tremblay LC, Feliciano DV, Rozycki GS: Secondary extremity compartment syndrome, *J Trauma* 53(5):833-837, 2002.

Thalmann M et al: Resuscitation in near drowning with extracorporeal membrane oxygenation, *Ann Thorac Surg* 72:607-608, 2001.

Turner JG et al: The effect of the therapeutic touch on pain and anxiety in burn patients, *J Adv Nurs* 28(1):10-20, 1998.

Ward RS: Physical rehabilitation. In Carrougher GJ, editor: *Burn care and therapy*, St Louis, 1998, Mosby.

Warden GD: Fluid resuscitation and early management. In Herndon DN, editor: *Total burn care*, Philadelphia, 1996, WB Saunders.

Warden GD: Burn shock resuscitation, *World J Surg* 16:16-23, 1992.

Weber JM: Epidemiology of infections and strategies for control. In Carrougher GJ, editor: *Burn care and therapy*, St Louis, 1998, Mosby.

Wessel LC, Cunningham BL: Patient with compartment syndrome of the lower extremity, *J Vasc Nurs* 21:24-29, 2003.

Williams A, Coyne S: Effects of neck position on intracranial pressure, *Am J Crit Care* 2(1):68-71, 1993.

Winfree J, Barillo DJ: Nonthermal injuries, *Nurs Clin North Am* 32(2):275-287, 1997.

Available Websites

American Association of Critical Care Medicine: www.aacn.org
American College of Surgeons: www.acs.org
American Nurses Association: www.ana.org
Center for Disease Control: www.cdc.org
Emergency Nurses Association: www.ena.org
International Trauma Anesthesia and Critical Care Society: www.itaccs.com
Johns Hopkins Center for Injury Research & Policy: www.jhsph.edu
National Study on Cost and Outcomes of Trauma Care: www.nscot.org
Society of Critical Care Medicine: www.sccm.org

CHAPTER 3

Respiratory Dysfunctions

Status Asthmaticus: Refractory Severe Asthma

PATHOPHYSIOLOGY

Asthma is a problem affecting over 13 million people in the United States. A severely asthmatic person is unable to complete expiration due to increased airway resistance and limited expiratory time resulting from tachypnea. Asthmatics eventually develop air trapping, increased functional residual capacity, and decreased forced vital capacity. Status asthmaticus (SA) is a severe, life-threatening condition resulting from bronchial smooth muscle contraction (bronchospasm), bronchial inflammation leading to airway edema, and mucous plugging. The diameter of the patient's bronchial network is markedly reduced. When an episode of bronchospasm (critical airway narrowing) is not reversed after 24 hr of maximal doses of traditional inhaled beta-(β-)adrenergic agonist, theophylline, inhaled ipratroprium, and steroid therapy, the patient is diagnosed with SA. Common triggers for asthma exacerbations include air pollutants, smoke, allergens (airborne or ingested), physical irritants (e.g., cold air, exercise), and respiratory tract infections. Anxiety or "panic" attacks and use of β-adrenergic blocking agents and nonsteroidal antiinflammatory agents may predispose patients to development or exacerbation of severe asthma.

Two clinical patterns for development of status asthmaticus are recognized. An "attack" can happen suddenly (over several hours), or it may take several days to reach a critical airway obstruction. The more common gradual presentation manifests increasing symptoms of sputum production, coughing, wheezing, and dyspnea. As air trapping increases, lung hyperinflation prompts increased work of breathing. Rapid exhalations increase insensible water loss through exhaled water vapor and diaphoresis. Oral intake may be decreased, contributing to hypovolemia. Without adequate oral intake to promote hydration, mucous becomes thick and begins to plug the airways. Terminal bronchioles can become occluded completely from mucosal edema and tenacious secretions. Ventilation-perfusion mismatch or shunting occurs as poorly ventilated alveoli continue to be perfused, which leads to hypoxemia. Tachycardia is an early compensatory mechanism to increase oxygen delivery to the body cells, but increases myocardial oxygen demand. Oxygen requirements and work of breathing increase, leading to respiratory failure and respiratory arrest if not managed promptly and appropriately.

ASSESSMENT

Clinical presentation: Coughing, wheezing, diaphoresis, orthopnea, dyspnea, chest tightness, labored breathing with use of accessory muscles, increased sputum production, increased respiration rate (RR) (>40 breaths/min), fatigue, insomnia, anorexia, restlessness, and confusion. Absence of wheezing in a severely asthmatic patient may signal minimal air movement and impending respiratory arrest.
Physical assessment: Agitation, inability to recline or talk, chest retractions, nasal flaring, and decreased tactile fremitus are present. Hyperresonance over lung areas in which there is air trapping

and dullness over areas of atelectasis can be percussed. Wheezing may be inspiratory or expiratory and correlates with the amount of airway obstruction if the patient is able to move adequate air. If moving air, coarse rhonchi may be auscultated. In addition, the patient may have hypotension and pulsus paradoxus >15 mm Hg, Cyanosis of the lips and nail beds is a late sign of respiratory compromise.

Research Brief 3-1   The investigators assessed the impact of an evidence-based multidisciplinary asthma pathway on patient outcomes and expenses. Data were collected over a 6-month period and included demographics about the patients, as well as health-related information such as peak expiratory flow rates, pulse oximetry measurements, and length of stay (LOS). Nineteen patients were placed into the study group and were placed on the pathway. Twenty-three patients were not treated according to the pathway, and 38 patients were in the historical control group. The results showed that, although there was not a significant reduction in LOS, use of the pathways was associated with a significant increase in conversion from nebulizer treatments to metered-dose inhaler use, resulting in a substantial cost savings.

From Bailey R et al: Impact of clinical pathways and practice guidelines on management of acute exacerbations of bronchial asthma, *Chest* 113(1):28-33, 1998.

Note: Patients with severe wheezing who have not been diagnosed with asthma should be evaluated for other causes of upper airway obstruction and "cardiac asthma." Patients with left ventricular failure may wheeze if interstitial fluid increases to the point where bronchioles are compressed or if the pulmonary interstitial edema is severe enough to cause bronchospasm. Asymmetric breath sounds or chest pain may signal that the patient has a pneumothorax.

DIAGNOSTIC TESTS

Arterial blood gas (ABG) analysis: Evaluates status of oxygenation and acid-base balance. Initially PaO_2 is normal and then decreases as the ventilation-perfusion mismatch becomes more severe. Rising PCO_2 is an ominous sign in a patient with severe asthma, since it signals severe hypoventilation which can lead to respiratory arrest. A normal PCO_2 in a distressed asthma patient receiving aggressive treatment may indicate respiratory fatigue, prompting a progressively ineffective breathing pattern, which can also lead to respiratory arrest.

Pulse oximetry (SpO2): Noninvasive technology that measures the oxygen saturation of arterial blood intermittently or continuously using a probe placed on the patient's finger or ear. Normal reading is >90%. Correlation of SpO_2 with SaO_2 (arterial saturation) is within 2% when SaO_2 is >50%. Temperature, pH, $PaCO_2$, anemia, and hemodynamic status may reduce the accuracy of pulse oximetry measurements. Presence of other forms of Hgb in the blood (carboxyhemoglobin, a byproduct of smoking and CO, or methemoglobin, formed by the use of drugs such as lidocaine and nitroglycerin) can produce falsely high readings. When using pulse oximetry, it is helpful to obtain ABG values to compare the oxygen saturation and evaluate the PaO_2, $PaCO_2$, and pH.

Pulmonary function testing: Forced expiratory volume (FEV) is decreased during acute episodes because severely narrowed airways prevent forceful exhalation of inspired volume (Table 3-1). The hallmark sign of asthma is a decreased FEV_1 (forced expiratory volume in the first second)/FVC (forced vital capacity.) Peak expiratory flow rate (PEFR) <100-125 L/min in a normal-sized adult indicates severe obstruction to air flow. If PEFR does not improve with initial aggressive inhaled bronchodilator treatments, morbidity increases.

Chest x-ray: Useful in ruling out other causes of respiratory failure (e.g., foreign body aspiration, pulmonary edema, pulmonary embolism, pneumonia). The x-ray usually shows lung hyperinflation caused by air trapping and a flat diaphragm related to increased intrathoracic volume.

Sputum: Gross examination may show increased viscosity or actual mucous plugs. Culture and sensitivity may show microorganisms if infection is the precipitating event.

Complete blood cell count (CBC): Differential will show increased eosinophils in patients not receiving corticosteroids, which is indicative of inflammatory response. White blood cells (WBCs) may be increased by asthma in the absence of infection. The hematocrit (Hct) may be increased because of hypovolemia and hemoconcentration.

Serum theophylline level: Important baseline indicator for patients who take theophylline regularly. Acceptable therapeutic range is 10-20 mcg/ml. Since the therapeutic level is close to the toxic level, the patient should be monitored for side effects (e.g., nausea, nervousness, dysrhythmias). If additional theophylline is given, serial levels should be measured within the first 12-24 hr of treatment

TABLE 3-1   Pulmonary Function Tests in Status Asthmaticus

Test	Description	Normal values	Parameters in SA
FVC	Total amount of gas exhaled as forcefully and rapidly as possible after maximal inspiration	≥80% of predicted normal	Normal or slightly decreased because of air trapping
FEV_1	Volume of gas exhaled over first second of FVC	≥75% of predicted normal	Decreased because of obstruction; may return to normal after inhalation of aerosolized bronchodilator
FEF	Average rate of flow during middle half of FEV; an accurate estimate of airway resistance	≥80% of predicted normal	Decreased because of small airways obstruction; may return to normal after inhalation of aerosolized bronchodilator

FEF, Forced expiratory flow; *FEV_1,* forced expiratory volume in 1 sec; *FVC,* forced vital capacity; *SA,* status asthmaticus.

and daily thereafter. There is little evidence to support clinical benefit for adding theophylline to inhaled β-adrenergic blocking agents and steroids for patients with acute, severe asthma who were not already using theophylline regularly.

Electrocardiogram (ECG): Presence of sinus tachycardia is an important baseline indicator, because the use of some bronchodilators (e.g., metaproterenol) may produce cardiac stimulant effects and dysrhythmias.

COLLABORATIVE MANAGEMENT

The potential for respiratory failure in SA is high. Management is directed toward decreasing bronchospasm and increasing ventilation. Other interventions are directed toward treatment of complications.

Oxygen therapy: Patients with SA have profound hypoxia and can tolerate high doses of oxygen (FiO_2) unless they retain CO_2 and breathe by hypoxic drive. Oxygen dosage must be limited in non-intubated, mechanically ventilated patients who breathe by hypoxic drive to avoid hypoventilation and respiratory arrest. Humidified oxygen therapy is begun immediately to correct hypoxemia and thin secretions. PaO_2 is kept slightly above normal unless the patient retains CO_2, to compensate for the increased oxygen demands imposed by the increased work of breathing. The degree of hypoxemia and patient response determine the method of oxygen delivery. A high-flow device (e.g., 100% nonrebreather mask) delivers more precise and higher FiO_2. Comfort must be considered, especially if the patient will not wear a mask because of feelings of suffocation.

Heliox therapy: A blended mixture of helium and oxygen, available in mixtures of 60:40, 70:30, and 80:20, which is delivered either through a tight-fitting face mask or through a mechanical ventilator circuit. Use results in decreased inspiratory and expiratory airway resistance, may increase removal of CO_2, and may improve oxygenation.

Intubation and mechanical ventilation: Strongly considered when the patient has significant confusion, somnolence, agitation, or central cyanosis, or if patient experiences intolerable respiratory distress. When these clinical signs are evident, the patient is going into respiratory failure. Mechanical ventilation ensures adequate alveolar ventilation, and the endotracheal (ET) tube provides a pathway for clearing airway secretions by means of suctioning. Initial ventilator settings may include a tidal volume of 8-10 ml/kg and a rate of 12-15 breaths/min. Controlled mandatory ventilation may be required, along with heavy sedation, analgesia, and possibly, neuromuscular blockade.

Pharmacotherapy: Vigorous therapy is initiated to improve bronchospasm. Treatment is continued until wheezing is eliminated and pulmonary function tests return to baseline.

Bronchodilators: Dilate smooth muscles of the airways (Table 3-2).

Corticosteroids: Given intravenously during the acute phase of SA to decrease the inflammatory response. Dosage varies according to severity of episode and whether patient currently is taking steroids. The patient may be converted to inhaled corticosteroids once the acute phase has been

T A B L E 3 - 2   Medications Used For Status Asthmaticus/Refractory Asthma

Drug type	Medication and dosage	Action	Side effects
β_2 Selective-adrenergic therapy	*Albuterol* 2.5-5 mg (0.5-1.0 ml of 0.5% solution in 5 ml normal saline solution) by nebulizer every 20 min for three doses, followed by 2.5-10 mg every 1-4 hr as needed for symptoms.	Immediate adrenergic effects; activates β_2 adrenergic receptors; relaxes smooth muscle to relieve bronchospasm	Slightly increased heart rate, possible anxiety, nervousness, tremors, palpitations
Non-selective β-agonist therapy	*Epinephrine* 0.3-0.5 ml of a 1:1000 dilution SC; may be repeated every 15 min for patients at risk of respiratory arrest *Terbutaline* 0.25 mg SC; may repeat in 15-30 min; max 5 mg in 4 hr	Stimulates both α- and β-adrenergic receptors; relaxes bronchial smooth muscle; *epinephrine* may cause peripheral vasoconstriction; *terbutaline* is the drug of choice in pregnant women	Increased HR (>120 beats/min), nervousness, tremor, palpitations, nausea, vomiting, headache Paradoxical bronchospasm
Corticosteroids	*Methylprednisolone* 120-180 mg/day in three or four divided doses for 48 hours; tapered as clinically tolerated	Antiinflammatory effects help to decrease both swelling and reactivity of airways	Mood swings, insomnia, agitation; GI upset: nausea, heartburn; if tapered improperly, pt. may experience adrenal insufficiency
Anticholinergics	*Ipratroprium (Atrovent):* 0.5 mg by nebulizer every 30 min for three doses; then every 2-4 hr as needed for symptoms; generally used in conjunction with β-agonist therapy	Blocks action of acetylcholine at parasympathetic sites of bronchial smooth muscle to cause inhibition of nasal secretions and bronchodilation	Dry mouth, dizziness, transient increased bronchospasm; may cause narrow angle glaucoma if eyes are contaminated in susceptible patients. Use of mouthpiece nebulizer is safer than face mask.

Note: Recommendations originate from the NIH expert panel on the diagnosis and management of asthma. *IV Theophylline and magnesium are not recommended for general use* in a hospitalized patient with acute asthma. All patients receiving theophylline prior to hospitalization should have a theophylline level determined before a loading dose is given. *BP,* Blood pressure; *GI,* gastrointestinal; *HR,* heart rate; *IV,* intravenous; *SC,* subcutaneous.

resolved. Acute adrenal insufficiency can develop in patients who take steroids routinely at home, if these drugs are not given to the patient during hospitalization.

Anticholinergics: Recent studies support use of ipratroprium (Atrovent) in combination with inhaled β-adrenergic agonists for severe, acute asthma. The National Institutes of Health (NIH) expert panel recommends nebulized ipratroprium 0.5 mg every 30 min for 3 doses, then every 2-4 hr as needed to relieve bronchospasm.

Sedatives and analgesics: Used in more limited doses in patients who are neither intubated nor mechanically ventilated, unless the person is extremely agitated and unable to cooperate with therapy. These agents depress the central nervous system (CNS) response to hypoxia and hypercapnia. Once mechanical ventilation is in place, the dosage is titrated until the patient is comfortable and/or hypoxemia or hypercapnia begins to resolve.

Buffers: Sodium bicarbonate may be given to correct severe acidosis not corrected by intubation and mechanical ventilation. The physiologic response to bronchodilators improves with correction of metabolic acidosis.

Antibiotics: Given if a respiratory infection is suspected, as evidenced by fever, purulent sputum, or leukocytosis.

Fluid replacement: To liquefy secretions and replace insensible losses. Generally, crystalloid fluids (e.g., D_5W, D_5NS) are used.

Chest physiotherapy: Generally contraindicated in acute phases of SA because of acute respiratory decompensation and hyperreactive airways. Once the crisis is over, the patient may benefit from percussion and postural drainage q2-4h to help mobilize secretions.

NURSING DIAGNOSES AND INTERVENTIONS

Impaired gas exchange related to altered oxygen supply secondary to decreased alveolar ventilation present with narrowed airways

Desired outcomes: Within 2-4 hr of initiation of treatment, patient has adequate gas exchange as evidenced by Pao_2 >60 mm Hg; $Paco_2$ 35-45 mm Hg; and pH 7.35-7.45 (or ABG values within 10% of patient's baseline), with mechanical ventilation, if necessary. Within 24-48 hr of initiation of treatment, patient is weaning or weaned from mechanical ventilation, and RR is 12-20 breaths/min with normal baseline depth and pattern.

- Monitor for hypoxia (e.g., restlessness, agitation) and hypercapnea (e.g., confusion, somnolence). Cyanosis of the lips (central) and nail beds (peripheral) are late indicators of hypoxia.
- Auscultate breath sounds at frequent intervals. Monitor for decreased or adventitious sounds (e.g., wheezes, rhonchi). Absent breath sounds in a distressed asthma patient may indicate impending respiratory failure and arrest.
- Position patient for comfort and to promote optimal gas exchange. High Fowler's position, with the patient leaning forward and elbows propped on the over-the-bed table to promote maximal chest excursion, may reduce use of accessory muscles and diaphoresis due to work of breathing.
- Deliver oxygen as prescribed; monitor Fio_2 to ensure that oxygen is within prescribed concentrations. If patient does not retain carbon dioxide, 100% nonrebreather mask may be used to provide maximal oxygen support. If the patient retains CO_2 and is unrelieved by positioning, lower-dose oxygen, bronchodilators, and steroids, intubation and mechanical ventilation may be necessary sooner than in patients who are able to receive higher doses of oxygen by mask.
- Monitor ABG and pulse oximetry values. Be alert to decreasing Pao_2 and increasing $Paco_2$ or decreasing O_2 saturation levels, indicative of impending respiratory failure.
- Monitor patients with respiratory failure who are intubated and mechanically ventilated for auto-PEEP, wherein the next breath is delivered prior to complete emptying of the first breath. Each subsequent breath failing to completely empty increases lung volume and predisposes the patient to barotrauma, pneumothorax, and/or increased intrathoracic pressure (auto-PEEP), which may decrease cardiac output (CO). Low CO (resulting from decreased venous return) can lead to hypotension. Auto-PEEP should be suspected in an intubated asthmatic patient who is hypotensive following intubation and initiation of mechanical ventilation, when there is no other obvious cause (e.g., tension pneumothorax). If auto-PEEP is suspected, consult with the respiratory therapist and the physician to modify ventilator settings.

Ineffective airway clearance related to presence of increased tracheobronchial secretions; decreased ability to expectorate secondary to fatigue

Desired outcome: Within 24-48 hr of initiating treatment, patient's airway has reduced secretions as evidenced by return to baseline RR (12-20 breaths/min) and absence of excessive coughing.

- At frequent intervals, assess patient's ability to clear tracheobronchial secretions. Set up suction equipment at the bedside.
- Encourage oral fluid intake or administer IV fluids within patient's prescribed limits to help decrease viscosity of the secretions.
- If patient is not coughing uncontrollably or going into respiratory failure, encourage patient to cough to clear secretions.
- After crisis phase of SA has been resolved, ensure that patient receives chest physiotherapy as prescribed; document patient's response to treatment. If appropriate, teach significant others to perform chest physiotherapy.
- Ensure that oxygen is humidified to aid in liquefying tracheobronchial secretions.

Activity intolerance related to imbalance between oxygen supply and demand secondary to decreased alveolar oxygen supply and greater metabolic oxygen demands caused by increased work of breathing

Desired outcome: Within 24-48 hr of resolution of severe, refractory asthma, patient reports an increased energy level with decreased fatigue and associated symptoms.

- Teach patient progressive muscle relaxation technique (see "Health-Seeking Behavior," p. 259). Teach significant others how to coach patient in using relaxation techniques.
- Teach patient and family how to decrease metabolic demands for oxygen by limiting or pacing patient's activities and procedures.
- If patient is restless (increases oxygen demand), ascertain and alleviate the cause of the restlessness (e.g., if restlessness is related to anxiety, help reduce anxiety by providing reassurance, enabling family members to stay with patient, and offering distractions such as soft music or television). Be aware that restlessness may be an early sign of hypoxemia.
- Explain all procedures and offer support to minimize fear and anxiety, which can increase oxygen demands.
- Encourage patient to breathe slowly and deeply. Teach pursed-lip breathing technique to assist patient with controlling his or her respirations as appropriate:
  - ❑ Inhale through the nose.
  - ❑ Form lips in an O shape as if whistling.
  - ❑ Exhale slowly through pursed lips.
  - ❑ Record patient's response to breathing technique. Educate significant others in coaching.
- Teach patient proper coughing technique for effective management of secretions.
  - ❑ Instruct patient to take several deep breaths. Instruct significant others in coaching this technique.
  - ❑ After the last inhalation, teach patient to perform a succession of coughs (usually three to four) on the same exhalation until most of the air has been expelled.
  - ❑ Explain that patient may need to repeat this technique several times before the cough becomes productive.
- Schedule rest times after meals to avoid competition for oxygen supply during digestion.
- Monitor Spo_2 by pulse oximetry during activity to evaluate limits of activity, set future activity goals, and recommend optimal positions for oxygenation.
- Assess temperature q2-4h. Consult physician for increases, and provide treatment as prescribed to decrease temperature and thus oxygen demands.

Refer to the Nursing Interventions Classification (NIC) for the following: Acid-Base Management; Acid-Base Monitoring; Airway Management; Anxiety Reduction; Bedside Laboratory Testing; Cough Enhancement; Emotional Support; Energy Management; Fluid Management; Fluid Monitoring; Laboratory Data Interpretation; Oxygen Therapy; Positioning; Respiratory Monitoring; Vital Signs Monitoring

ADDITIONAL NURSING DIAGNOSES

Also see "Risk for infection" (nosocomial pneumonia) in "Acute Pneumonia," p. 185, and "Acute Respiratory Failure," p. 201, for information about support of breathing. For other nursing diagnoses ▮NIC and interventions, see "Psychosocial Support," p. 68, and "Psychosocial Support for the Patient's Family and Significant Others," p. 78.

Research Brief 3-2   The investigators studied 181 ICU patients to determine if the practice of oral decontamination proved to be cost effective to prevent ventilator-associated pneumonia (VAP). Patients who received oral decontamination had a mean total cost of $16,119, whereas those patients without the strategy had mean total cost of $18,268. This study provides strong evidence that oral decontamination is cost effective.

From van Nieuwenhoven CA et al: Oral decontamination is cost saving in the prevention of ventilator-associated pneumonia in intensive care units, *Crit Care Med* 32(1):1260130, 2004.

Acute Pneumonia

PATHOPHYSIOLOGY

Pneumonia is the sixth leading cause of death in the United States and the leading cause of death due to infectious disease. Pneumonia is an acute infection that causes inflammation of the parenchyma (alveolar spaces and interstitial tissue) of the lung. As a result of the inflammation, the involved lung tissue becomes swollen and the air spaces fill with liquid. Pneumonias can be classified into two groups: community-acquired (CAP) and hospital-associated/nosocomial (HAP). (See Table 3-3 for a detailed discussion by pneumonia type.)

TABLE 3-3 Assessment Guidelines by Pneumonia Type

Type/pathogen	Risk groups	Onset	Defining characteristics	Complication/comments
Community acquired				
Pneumococcal (*Pneumococcus pneumoniae, Streptococcus pneumoniae*)	Persons >40 yr, especially males. Risk increases with alcoholism and debilitating diseases (e.g., COPD, heart failure, multiple myeloma, sickle cell disease). Viral upper respiratory tract infections often precede this pneumonia.	Abrupt	Single shaking chill, fever, pleuritic chest pain, severe cough, SOB, rust-colored sputum, and diaphoresis. Many patients also have herpes labialis, abdominal pain and distention, and paralytic ileus.	Pleural effusions, empyema, impaired liver function, bacteremia, and meningitis. Incidence of pneumococcal pneumonia peaks in winter and early spring. Mortality rate increases if more than one lobe is involved.
Mycoplasma (*Mycoplasma pneumoniae*)	School-age children to young adult (5-30 yr). Intrafamilial spread is common.	Gradual	Cough, sore throat, fever, headache, chills, malaise, anorexia, nausea, vomiting, diarrhea. In children, arthralgia involving the large joints is common.	Rare. Persistent cough and sinusitis are possible. Pulse-temperature dissociation is common.
Legionnaires (*Legionella pneumophila*)	Middle-age, elderly (males at increased risk) populations; smokers; individuals with malignancy, immunosuppression, or chronic renal failure; exposure to contaminated construction site. Hgb not elevated.	Abrupt	Malaise, headache within 24 hr, fever with normal HR, shaking chills, progressive dyspnea, cough that may become productive; GI symptoms, including anorexia, vomiting, diarrhea; arthralgia, myalgia.	Respiratory failure, hypotension, shock, acute renal failure.
Viral influenza A	Elderly persons with chronic diseases (e.g., COPD, diabetes mellitus, heart failure); pregnancy	1 wk after onset of influenza symptoms	Severe dyspnea, cyanosis, scant sputum occasionally with blood, fever, persistent and dry cough.	Rapid course leading frequently to acute respiratory failure; secondary bacterial pneumonia.

Continued

T A B L E 3 - 3   Assessment Guidelines by Pneumonia Type—cont'd

Type/pathogen	Risk groups	Onset	Defining characteristics	Complication/comments
Community acquired—cont'd				
Haemophilus influenzae	Adults (especially ≥50 yr of age) with chronic diseases (e.g., diabetes mellitus, COPD, chronic alcohol ingestion)	2-6 wk after URI	Fever, chills, dyspnea, cough, nausea, vomiting, pain.	Fever may be minimal or absent; HR and RR may be normal.
Nosocomial				
Klebsiella (*Klebsiella pneumoniae*) (also may be acquired in the community). Enterobacter, Serratia	Males >40 yr of age, chronic disease (e.g., diabetes mellitus, COPD, chronic alcohol ingestion, heart disease); those previously treated with antibiotics or ET intubation	Abrupt	Chills, fever, productive cough (copious), purulent, green or "currant jelly" sputum). Severe pleuritic chest pain, dyspnea, cyanosis, jaundice, vomiting, and diarrhea.	Lung abscess and empyema, necrotizing pneumonitis with cavitation, acute respiratory failure. High mortality rate (up to 50%). Aspiration of oropharyngeal flora believed responsible for many nosocomial and community-acquired cases.
Pseudomonas (also may be acquired in the community)	Patients neutropenic from chemotherapy or immunosuppressed secondary to cortisone therapy or other illnesses.	Gradual	Fever, chills, confusion, delirium, bradycardia, purulent sputum (green, foul smelling).	Rarely occurs in previously healthy adults; high mortality rate.
Proteus	Older adults with debilitating underlying diseases	Abrupt	High fever, chills, pleuritic chest pain.	Rare. Localizes to areas that already are damaged. Occurs as a mixed infection; has four pathogenic species with differing antibiotic susceptibilities.

Organism	Patients	Onset	Clinical Features	Comments
Staphylococcus aureus, methicillin-resistant *S. aureus* (MRSA)	Patients with debilitating diseases (e.g., diabetes mellitus, renal failure, liver disease, COPD); prior viral influenza infection; IV drug abusers.	Abrupt with community acquired; insidious with hospital associated	Cough, chills, high fever, pleuritic pain, progressive dyspnea, cyanosis, bloody sputum.	Pulmonary abscesses, empyema, pleural effusions; slow response to antibiotics.
Aspiration of gastric contents	Patients with impaired gag/cough reflexes; general anesthesia; presence of NG/ET tube.	Gradual: latent period between aspiration and onset of symptoms	Fever, wheezes, crackles (rales), rhonchi, dyspnea, cyanosis.	Physiologic response depends on pH of material aspirated; ≥2.5, little necrosis occurs; <2.5, atelectasis, pulmonary edema, hemorrhage, and necrosis can occur.
Immunocompromised patient				
Pneumocystis (*Pneumocystis carinii*)	Patients with AIDS or organ transplants	Insidious	Several weeks of fever, nonproductive cough, night sweats, dyspnea; hypoxemia with few auscultatory signs.	Bronchoscopy with transbronchial biopsy usually required for diagnosis.
Aspergillosis (*Aspergillus*)	Patients with AIDS, COPD, and transplants (especially autologous bone marrow transplant); also those receiving cytotoxic agents or steroids	Abrupt with immunosuppression; insidious with COPD	High fever; fungal ball within lung cyst or cavity; nonproductive cough; pleuritic chest pain	Cavitation frequently occurs; hematogenous spread common in immunocompromised patients.

AIDS, Acquired immunodeficiency syndrome; *COPD*, chronic obstructive pulmonary disease; *ET*, endotracheal; *GI*, gastrointestinal; *HR*, heart rate; *IV*, intravenous; *NG*, nasogastric; *RR*, respiratory rate; *SOB*, shortness of breath; *URI*, upper respiratory infection.

Community-acquired (CAP): Can vary from a mild to a severe illness. Less than 20% of CAP patients require hospitalization. Patients are seen in intensive care areas in two general circumstances: when an underlying medical condition is present such as chronic obstructive pulmonary disease (COPD), cardiac disease, diabetes mellitus, liver, renal or cerebrovascular disease, malignancy, or an immunocompromised state; or when the pneumonia leads to septic shock and respiratory failure. Patients with underlying, chronic illnesses are more likely to experience sepsis.

Hospital-associated/nosocomial (HAP): Is the hospital acquired infection most likely to lead to the death of patients? The Centers for Disease Control and Prevention defines nosocomial pneumonia as a condition occurring at least 72 hr after hospital admission, reflecting an infiltrate on chest x-ray studies, lung crackles on auscultation, or dullness with chest percussion. Either purulent sputum, a pathogenic organism in the sputum or blood, a virus from the lower respiratory tract, or serologic/pathologic evidence must be present to confirm HAP. Nosocomial pneumonias result from an impairment of host defenses caused by coexisting illnesses, especially chronic illnesses such as COPD, diabetes mellitus, chronic organ failure (e.g., heart, liver, renal), or malignancy, or by therapeutic interventions (e.g., use of antibiotics, corticosteroids, sedatives, agents to neutralize gastric pH, artificial airway in the trachea). HAP is caused by increased bacterial exposure, such as from the use of respiratory therapy equipment (e.g., mechanical ventilation where bacteria can be inhaled from aerosols), or is acquired from the caregiver's hands. Gastric overgrowth with gram-negative organisms occurs when pH-altering agents are used. Pneumonias often occur after aspiration of oropharyngeal flora in an individual whose resistance is altered or whose coughing mechanisms are impaired. A patient who acquires pneumonia while on mechanical ventilation may be classified as having **ventilator associated pneumonia (VAP)**, a subgroup of HAP. **Aspiration pneumonia** that occurs when gastric contents are aspirated can lead to acute respiratory distress syndrome (ARDS). Critically ill patients are at high risk for HAP.

Immunocompromised patient: Immunosuppression and neutropenia are predisposing factors in the development of nosocomial and community-acquired pneumonias, from both common and unusual pathogens. Severely immunocompromised patients are affected not only by bacteria but also by fungi *(Candida, Aspergillus)*, viruses *(Cytomegalovirus)*, and protozoa *(Pneumocystis carinii)*. Most commonly, *P. carinii* is seen in patients with HIV disease or in those who have received organ transplants.

ASSESSMENT

Findings are influenced by patient's age, extent of the disease process, underlying medical condition, and pathogen involved.

Risk factors: In addition to the risk factors listed in Table 3-3, any factor that alters the integrity of the lower airways, thereby inhibiting ciliary activity, increases the likelihood of pneumonia. These factors include hypoventilation, hyperoxia (increased Fio_2), hypoxia, airway irritants such as smoke, and the presence of an artificial airway.

Clinical presentation: Cough (productive and nonproductive), sputum (rust colored, purulent, bloody, or mucoid), fever, pleuritic chest pain (more common in community-acquired bacterial pneumonias), dyspnea, chills, headache, and myalgia. The older adult may be confused or disoriented and run low-grade fevers, but initially may have few other signs and symptoms.

Physical assessment: Presence of nasal flaring and expiratory grunt, use of accessory muscles of respiration, restricted chest expansion caused by pleuritic pain, dullness to percussion, tachypnea (RR >20 breaths/min), tachycardia (heart rate [HR] >100 beats/min), decreased or bronchial breath sounds, high-pitched and inspiratory crackles (increased by or heard only after coughing), and low-pitched inspiratory crackles caused by airway secretions.

DIAGNOSTIC TESTS

ABG analysis: Hypoxemia (Pao_2 <80 mm Hg) and hypocapnea ($Paco_2$ <35 mm Hg), with a resultant respiratory alkalosis (pH >7.45), will be seen in the absence of an underlying pulmonary disease. In severe cases the $Paco_2$ can be >45 mm Hg because CO_2 elimination may be affected by underlying diseases of ventilation. If pneumonia results in respiratory acidosis, the patient may require ET intubation and mechanical ventilation for respiratory failure.

Pulse oximetry (Spo_2): O_2 saturation is reduced from the patient's baseline.

CBC: Increased WBC count (>11,000/mm^3) is seen in the presence of bacterial pneumonias. Normal or low WBC count will be seen with viral or mycoplasma pneumonias.

Sputum for Gram's stain and/or culture and sensitivity tests: Expectorated sputum specimens may not originate from the lower airways and are therefore unreliable. A sputum culture should be obtained from the lower respiratory tract before initiation of antimicrobial therapy. The most reliable specimens are obtained via bronchoalveolar lavage (BAL) during bronchoscopy, a protected telescoping catheter (miniBAL), or open-lung biopsy (used only in extreme cases).

Blood culture and sensitivity: Secondary bacteremia is a frequent finding, and blood cultures help to identify the causative organism. Patients with bacteremia are at higher risk for developing respiratory failure.

Diagnostic fiberoptic bronchoscopy: Two diagnostic techniques (protected specimen brush [PSB] and BAL) make it possible to obtain specimens during simple bronchoscopy without contaminating the aspirate.

Serologic studies: Acute and convalescent titers are drawn to diagnose viral pneumonia. Rises in antibody titers are a positive sign for viral infection.

Acid-fast stain: To rule out mycobacterial infection (e.g., tuberculosis).

Chest x-ray: To identify anatomic involvement, extent of disease, presence of consolidation, pleural effusions, or cavitation:

- *Lobar:* Entire lobe involved
- *Segmental (lobular):* Only parts of a lobe involved
- *Bronchopneumonia:* Affects alveoli contiguous to the involved bronchi

Thoracentesis: Removal of pleural effusion fluid from the pleural space using a needle to drain the chest cavity. Pleural effusion fluid may be cultured following thoracentesis to identify the causative organism.

COLLABORATIVE MANAGEMENT

Oxygen therapy: Administered when patient is seen to have hypoxemia. Special care must be taken not to abolish the hypoxic drive needed for effective breathing if patient has COPD and is known to retain CO_2. For patients with chronic CO_2 retention, oxygen is delivered in low concentrations while oxygen saturation (SpO_2) is closely monitored. The physician should be consulted for parameters of "acceptable" oxygen saturation values in any patient with CO_2 retention.

Intubation and mechanical ventilation: Intubation may be necessary if a patient experiences progressive respiratory distress despite treatments. Mechanical ventilation is required if patient is unable to maintain adequate ABG values (PaO_2 >60 mm Hg) with supplemental oxygen. High concentrations of oxygen and positive end-expiratory pressure (PEEP) may be necessary in severe cases of pneumonia that lead to acute respiratory failure. See "Acute Respiratory failure, p. 201.

Pharmacotherapy

Antibiotics: Prescribed empirically on the basis of presenting signs and symptoms, clinical findings, and chest x-ray results until sputum or blood culture results are available. *Pneumococcus* is the most common pathogen associated with CAP, whereas enteric gram-negative bacteria are the most common pathogens identified with HAP. *Pseudomonas aeruginosa* and methicillin-resistant *Staphylococcus aureus* are the most common organisms seen in patients on long-term mechanical ventilation. Antimicrobial therapy in critically ill patients usually is parenteral and guided by sensitivity of the causative organism. Many of the organisms responsible for nosocomial pneumonias are resistant to multiple antibiotics. Proper identification of the organism, determination of antibiotic sensitivity, and attainment of therapeutic drug levels are critical for effective therapy.

Antitussives: Used to control coughing. Occasionally narcotics such as codeine are required to control coughing unrelieved by other agents.

Antipyretics and analgesics: To reduce temperature and provide relief for pleuritic pain. Patients with pneumonia may have significant pleuritic pain that requires administration of opioid analgesics for relief. When opiates (e.g., codeine, morphine sulfate, meperidine) are given, varying degrees of respiratory depression occur, but these agents are often effective in controlling severe coughing. Careful and frequent monitoring of the patient's RR and depth, as well as oxygen saturation via pulse oximetry, is necessary.

Nutritional therapy: Malnutrition is a causative factor in development of infections. In severely ill patients, enteral nutrition may provide the best protection against development of sepsis, owing to probable prevention of bacterial translocation from the gut. A nutritional therapy consultation is warranted for all patients who have developed an infection and those at high risk of infection.

Hydration: Intravenous (IV) fluids may be necessary to replace fluids lost from insensible sources (e.g., tachypnea, diaphoresis with fever).

Isolation: Some patients with pneumonia may require isolation and transmission-based precautions. See Appendix 8.

Percussion and postural drainage: Indicated if deep breathing, coughing, and moving about in bed or ambulation are ineffective in raising and expectorating sputum. Consult with respiratory therapy as indicated.

NURSING DIAGNOSES AND INTERVENTIONS

Risk for infection (nosocomial pneumonia) related to inadequate primary defenses (e.g., decreased ciliary action); invasive procedures (e.g., intubation); chronic disease

Desired outcome: Patient is free of infection as evidenced by normothermia and negative cultures; WBC count within normal limits for patient; and sputum clear to white in color.

- Perform good hand-washing procedure before and after any patient contact (even though gloves were worn). Use special care with patient with tracheostomy or intubation. Inform visitors of effective precautions or pertinent isolation procedures.
- Identify the presurgical candidate who is at increased risk for nosocomial pneumonia: age >70 yr; obesity; diabetes mellitus; COPD; history of smoking; abnormal pulmonary function tests (especially decreased forced expiratory flow rate); tracheostomy; prolonged intubation; abdominal or thoracic surgery.
  - ❑ Before surgery, provide patient and significant others with verbal and written instructions and demonstrations of turning, coughing, and deep-breathing exercises to perform after surgery to prevent respiratory tract infection.
  - ❑ Postoperatively, at frequent intervals encourage lung expansion: deep breathing; coughing if secretions are present; turning in bed; and walking (may not be possible in critical care). In addition, use of incentive spirometry promotes periodic, voluntary lung expansion to prevent atelectasis. Educate significant others to encourage these activities.
  - ❑ If pain interferes with lung expansion, control it by administering prn analgesics 0.5 hr before deep-breathing exercises, and provide splint support of wound areas with hands or pillows placed firmly across site of incision.
  - ❑ For patients who cannot remove secretions effectively by coughing, perform procedures that stimulate coughing such as chest physiotherapy, which includes breathing exercises, postural drainage, and percussion.
- Recognize the following ways in which nebulizer reservoirs can contaminate patient: introduction of nonsterile fluids or air; manipulation of nebulizer cup; or backflow of condensation into reservoir or into patient when delivery tubing is manipulated.
- Use only sterile fluids, and dispense them aseptically.
  - ❑ Change breathing circuits according to Centers for Disease Control and Prevention (CDC) guidelines.
  - ❑ Fill fluid reservoirs immediately before use.
  - ❑ Discard any fluid that has condensed in tubing; do not allow it to drain back into reservoir or into patient.
- Recognize risk factors for patients with tracheostomy or ET tubes: presence of underlying lung disease or other serious illness; colonization of oropharynx or trachea by aerobic gram-negative bacteria; greater access of bacteria to lower respiratory tract; and cross-contamination as a result of manipulation of these tubes.
  - ❑ Use "no-touch" technique, or use sterile gloves on both hands until tracheostomy wound has healed or formed granulation tissue around the tube.
- Suction on an "as needed" rather than a routine basis, inasmuch as frequent suctioning increases the risk of trauma and cross-contamination. Consider use of an in-line suction device to reduce the risk of infection or contamination.
- Always wear gloves on both hands when suctioning to protect against transmission of the herpes simplex virus (HSV) from the patient's oral secretions; transmission of HSV into openings in the skin (e.g., a hangnail) can cause herpetic whitlow. The use of eye protection is recommended if the patient has a tracheostomy.

Risk for aspiration related to individuals who have a depressed LOC or dysphagia or who have a gastric tube in place

Desired outcome:
- Identify patients who are at high risk for aspiration:
- For patients with depressed level of consciousness (LOC) who are unable to eat normally, consult physician regarding need for a method of feeding in which risk of aspiration is minimal such as postpyloric feeding (e.g., small-bore, weighted feeding tube that imports total parenteral nutrition [TPN] to the duodenum; or percutaneous endoscopic gastrostomy (PEG tube).
- For patients with a gastric tube in place provide continuous, rather than bolus, feedings. Elevate head of bed (HOB) to at least 30 degrees during feedings and for 1 hr after any feeding or medication.

Risk for fluid volume deficit related to increased insensible loss secondary to hyperventilation, fever, and use of supplemental oxygen; reduced fluid intake

Desired outcome: Patient is normovolemic as evidenced by no clinical evidence of hypovolemia (e.g., furrowed tongue); stable weight; blood pressure (BP) within patient's normal range; central venous pressure (CVP) 2-6 mm Hg; pulmonary artery pressure (PAP) 20-30/8-15 mm Hg; cardiac output (CO) 4-7 L/min; mean arterial pressure (MAP) 70-105 mm Hg; HR 60-100 beats/min; and systemic vascular resistance (SVR) 900-1200 dynes/sec/cm^{-5}.

- Monitor I&O hourly. Initially, intake should exceed output during volume replacement therapy. Consult physician for urine output <0.5 ml/kg/hr for 2 consecutive hours.
- Monitor VS and hemodynamic pressures for signs of continued hypovolemia. Be alert to decreased values in BP, CVP, PAP, CO, and MAP, as well as increased HR and SVR.
- Weigh patient daily, at the same time of day (preferably before breakfast), on a balanced scale, with the patient wearing the same type of clothing.
- Administer fluids by mouth (PO) and IV as prescribed. Document patient's response to replacement therapy.
- Monitor for signs and symptoms of fluid overload or too-rapid fluid administration: crackles (rales); shortness of breath (SOB); tachypnea; tachycardia; increased CVP; increased PAPs; jugular vein distention; and edema.

NIC Aspiration Precautions; Chest Physiotherapy; Cough Enhancement; Environmental Management; Fluid/Electrolyte Management; Fluid Monitoring; Hypovolemia Management; Infection Control; Intravenous Therapy; Mechanical Ventilation; Nutrition Management; Positioning; Surveillance; Respiratory Monitoring, Vital Signs Monitoring

ADDITIONAL NURSING DIAGNOSES

Also see "Impaired Gas Exchange" in "Near Drowning," p. 114. See "Status Asthmaticus" for "Ineffective Airway Clearance," p. 179, and "Activity Intolerance," p. 179. As appropriate, see nursing diagnoses and interventions in "Nutritional Support," p. 1; "Acute Respiratory Failure," p. 201; "Mechanical Ventilation," p. 14; "Prolonged Immobility," p. 61; "Psychosocial Support," p. 68; and "Psychosocial Support for the Patient's Family and Significant Others," p. 78.

Pulmonary Hypertension

PATHOPHYSIOLOGY

Pulmonary hypertension is defined as a mean pulmonary artery pressure (MPAP) >20 mm Hg. Primary pulmonary hypertension (also known as *idiopathic* or *unexplained pulmonary hypertension*) is less common than secondary pulmonary hypertension, which can occur as a result of many pulmonary, cardiac, vascular, and other disorders. See Table 3-4 for a discussion of etiologic factors. The treatment of secondary pulmonary hypertension is directed at treating the underlying cause.

Rising PAP increases pulmonary vascular resistance (PVR), which in turn causes two responses in the vasculature: standby vessels open to increase the surface area available for perfusion; and the capillaries distend to accommodate the increased blood flow. Although these responses reduce PVR initially, the system eventually fails if the increased pressure becomes chronic as a result of vasoconstriction that occurs in response to chronic alveolar hypoxia. Though most of the vascular system responds to hypoxia by dilating in an effort to increase blood flow to vital organs, the pulmonary vasculature responds to alveolar hypoxia by vasoconstriction, a beneficial mechanism that shunts blood away from underventilated areas in the lungs to better ventilated areas, thereby improving oxygenation. This regional mechanism is not strong enough to correct the ventilation/perfusion imbalance, however. Generally, Pao_2 decreases to ≤60 mm Hg before vasoconstriction occurs; the lower the Pao_2, the more severe the vasoconstriction.

The rise in PAP and the resulting increase in PVR from acute hypoxia are completely reversible once the hypoxia has been resolved. However, in the presence of chronic hypoxia the pulmonary vasculature undergoes permanent changes (i.e., hypertrophy, hyperplasia), causing thickening of the vessel and narrowing of the lumen. In addition, polycythemia develops as a compensatory mechanism to increase oxygen transport; this condition increases blood viscosity, which in turn increases PVR.

The functions of the heart and lungs are interdependent. Increased PVR stimulates the right ventricle to increase the pumping force to maintain adequate CO. The right ventricle dilates and hypertrophies under the constant strain and workload. Eventually, the right side of the heart weakens and is unable to accommodate venous blood returning to the heart. As a result, pressure in the systemic venous circulation increases, causing cor pulmonale, or right-sided heart failure. See "Right Ventricular Heart Failure/Pulmonary Edema," p. 220, for further discussion of right-sided heart failure.

TABLE 3-4 Etiologic Factors in the Development of Pulmonary Hypertension	
Cause	**Clinical examples**
Congenital heart disease with left-to-right shunt	Ventricular septal defect, atrial septal defect, patient ductus arteriosus
Congenital heart disease with diminished pulmonary blood flow	Tetralogy of Fallot, transposition of the great vessels
Obstruction to pulmonary venous outflow (congenital and acquired)	Mitral valve disease, left ventricular failure, stenosis of large pulmonary veins, portal hypertension
Pulmonary embolism	Thrombotic embolism, fat embolism
Chronic alveolar hypoxia	High-altitude hypoxia, COPD, obstructive sleep apnea, obesity (hypoventilation syndrome), neuromuscular disease processes
Diffuse pulmonary fibrosis	Lupus erythematosus, systemic sclerosis, sarcoidosis, idiopathic interstitial fibrosis

COPD, Chronic obstructive pulmonary disease.

ASSESSMENT

Because the low-resistance pulmonary vascular bed is clinically silent until late in the disease process, onset is insidious.

Clinical presentation

Early indicators: Hyperventilation, vague chest discomfort.

Late indicators: Tachypnea, dyspnea, orthopnea, chest congestion.

Physical assessment: Cyanosis of the lips and nail beds, edema of the hands and feet, increasing abdominal girth, anasarca (generalized, massive edema), distended jugular veins, right ventricular heave (visible left parasternal systolic lift), accentuated pulmonary component of the second heart sound, right ventricular diastolic gallop, pulmonary ejection click, distant breath sounds, basilar crackles.

Hemodynamic measurements: Mean pulmonary artery pressure (MPAP) will be >20 mm Hg. Normally, PAP ranges from 8-15 mm Hg during diastole to 20-30 mm Hg during systole.

DIAGNOSTIC TESTS

ABG values: Will vary but are important to the differential diagnosis of the cause of pulmonary hypertension. Generally Pao_2 will be <60 mm Hg, whereas $Paco_2$ will be within normal limits (35-45 mm Hg) unless COPD is the cause of the pulmonary hypertension, in which case $Paco_2$ is usually elevated.

Chest x-ray: Will confirm anatomic abnormalities associated with chronic right ventricular failure (right ventricular dilation or hypertrophy), enlarged pulmonary artery secondary to increased pressure, and diminished diaphragmatic excursion.

ECG: May show right ventricular hypertrophy, right-axis deviation, right bundle-branch block, and enlarged P waves.

Echocardiography: Reveals elevated pulmonary pressures; may reveal enlarged right atrium and right ventricle, diminished wall motion, and pulmonic valve malfunction (midsystolic closure or delayed opening).

Pulmonary function tests: Also important for the differential diagnosis of the underlying pathologic condition; will vary according to cause. For normal values, see Table 3-1.

Pulmonary angiography and perfusion scans: To rule out an embolic event as the underlying cause.

Hemodynamic monitoring: Pressures in the pulmonary vasculature are measured by way of the flow-directed pulmonary artery (e.g., Swan-Ganz) catheter. Data will differentiate or quantify the contribution of the left or right ventricular failure and measure the response to pharmacotherapy.

Red blood cell (RBC)/Hct values: May be increased above normal.

COLLABORATIVE MANAGEMENT

The goal of medical management is to diagnose and treat the underlying disorder or process causing the pulmonary hypertension. Treatment is directed primarily toward increasing myocardial contractility or reducing right ventricular afterload caused by the high pulmonary vascular resistance.

Oxygen therapy: To eliminate hypoxia, a cause of pulmonary vascular vasoconstriction, and the resulting right ventricular afterload.

Nitric oxide therapy: Nitric oxide gas is administered through either a face mask, a tracheostomy, or an ET tube to promote pulmonary vasodilation. The vasodilation reduces blood pressure in the pulmonary circulation. Available in a limited number of centers. Use is increasing across the United States.

Pharmacotherapy

Diuretics: Reduce circulating volume via loss of sodium and water, which may decrease PAP and right ventricular workload. In turn, this reduces leftward septal bulging seen with right ventricular overload.

Digitalis: Generally used only with biventricular failure. The inotropic effects of digitalis can increase CO and pulmonary resistance, which are deleterious in the presence of right ventricular failure.

Bronchodilators (e.g., aminophylline, isoproterenol, terbutaline): Act as afterload reducers by decreasing pulmonary vascular resistance and increasing right ventricular ejection fraction. By improving gas exchange, bronchodilators may decrease hypoxic vasoconstriction of the pulmonary vascular bed.

Vasodilators (e.g., nitrates, hydralazine, calcium channel blockers, prostaglandins): Reverse pulmonary vasoconstriction, to reduce right ventricular afterload and enhance pulmonary blood flow. The prostaglandin epoprostenol (Flolan) is given as a continuous IV infusion both in hospital and on an outpatient basis.

NURSING DIAGNOSES AND INTERVENTIONS

Note: See "Activity Intolerance," in "Status Asthmaticus," p. 179. Refer to "Heart Failure/ Pulmonary Edema," p. 223, for nursing diagnoses and interventions related to the care of patients with heart failure. See "Impaired Gas Exchange" in "Near Drowning," p. 114. As appropriate, see nursing diagnoses and interventions in "Prolonged Immobility," p. 61; "Psychosocial Support," p. 68; and "Psychosocial Support for the Patient's Family and Significant Others," p. 78.

NIC Activity Therapy; Airway Management; Acid-Base Monitoring; Anxiety Reduction; Cardiac Care: Acute; Coping Enhancement; Invasive Hemodynamic Monitoring; Medication Administration: Intravenous; Medication Administration: Inhalation; Medication Administration: Oral; Self Care Assistance; Sleep Enhancement; Support Group

Acute Lung Injury and Acute Respiratory Distress Syndrome

PATHOPHYSIOLOGY

Acute lung injury (ALI) is a continuum of lung damage that includes ARDS. ARDS is often fatal, with a mortality rate of >60%, sometimes approaching 90%. Although ARDS often is a result of ALI due to trauma or infection, it is more likely related to an indirect insult to the lung. ARDS is also known as noncardiogenic pulmonary edema. Both ARDS and ALI include acute respiratory failure with bilateral effusions, refractory hypoxemia, and retention of CO_2. Pao_2/Fio_2 is <300 mm Hg with ALI, and <200 mm Hg with ARDS. The alveolar-capillary membrane sustains an injury, and hyaline membrane formation occurs and eventually results in pulmonary fibrosis. All of the etiologic factors that lead to the development of ARDS (see "History and Risk Factors," p. 190) cause an increase in the permeability of the alveolar-capillary membrane, either by altering hydrostatic or osmotic pressure or by injuring the alveolar epithelium or capillary endothelium. This enables the passing of larger molecules (e.g., albumin, globulin) across the membrane ("leaky membrane" or capillary leak), leading to an accumulation of protein-rich fluid in the interstitial and intraalveolar spaces and reducing gas exchange at this critical level. As the capillary permeability continues to increase, the interstitium, the alveoli, and the terminal airways become filled with fluid, blood, and protein. Surfactant activity is reduced, and gas exchange worsens. The alveoli tend to collapse and resist reexpansion in the absence of surfactant. These areas become a mass of interstitial and alveolar edema, hemorrhage, and focal atelectasis. Ventilation-perfusion mismatching, with resultant hypoxia, occurs as areas of the lung are perfused but not ventilated. Arterial oxygen tension (Pao_2) begins to fall, shunt fraction increases (the amount of blood returning to the arterial system without passing through ventilated regions of the lung), and physiologic dead space increases.

ASSESSMENT

History and risk factors: Trauma, hemorrhagic shock, sepsis, inhalation of toxic substances, severe pneumonitis, aspiration of gastric contents, near drowning, air or fat embolus, acute pancreatitis, postperfusion cardiopulmonary bypass, oxygen toxicity, drug overdose, neurologic injury, immunosuppression, massive blood transfusion, and multiple liters of intravascular volume replacement.

Clinical presentation: Will vary, depending on the pathophysiology contributing to the ARDS. The goals are to diagnose ALI early to reduce additional insults to the lungs leading to ARDS.

Indicators of ALI: Initially, dyspnea, restlessness, hyperventilation, cough, increased work of breathing, chest clear on auscultation. Symptoms can worsen and lead to respiratory failure.

Indicators of ARDS: Respiratory failure including cyanosis, pallor, grunting respirations, adventitious breath sounds, rapid and shallow breathing, intercostal-suprasternal retractions, tachypnea, tachycardia, diaphoresis, mental obtundation.

DIAGNOSTIC TESTS

ABG analysis: Essential to the diagnosis of ARDS. Severe refractory hypoxemia is a key indicator (decreasing PaO_2 that is unresponsive to increasing FiO_2). PaO_2/FiO_2 <200 mm Hg. In early ALI, the pH may be above normal (>7.45) because the patient hyperventilates and exhales greater-than-normal levels of CO_2. As respiratory failure ensues, the pH falls below 7.35 (respiratory acidosis), which may be further complicated by metabolic acidosis resulting from the anaerobic metabolism induced by global hypoxia.

Pulse oximetry: Used for continuous monitoring of oxygenation (see discussion, p. 176).

Mixed venous oxygen saturation (Svo2): Svo_2 is a more sensitive indicator of oxygen available for tissue oxygenation. Normal values range from 60%-80%. A value <50% is associated with impaired tissue oxygenation.

Serial chest x-rays: May be normal in the early stages. As ARDS progresses, the lung shows bilateral diffuse infiltrates. In later stages, few air spaces may be left in the lung—a condition that gives the lung a completely white (opaque) appearance on the x-ray study.

Pulmonary function tests: Static and dynamic lung compliance will be decreased. Lung volumes also will be decreased, particularly functional residual capacity (FRC).

Hemodynamic monitoring: Measurements of pulmonary artery wedge pressure (PAWP) are important to the differential diagnosis. PAWP is normal in ARDS (noncardiogenic pulmonary edema), but high (>12 mm Hg) in cardiogenic pulmonary edema.

Tracheal-protein/plasma-protein ratio: A relatively new diagnostic tool used to differentiate between cardiogenic and noncardiogenic pulmonary edema (ARDS). It compares total protein in tracheal aspirate with total protein in plasma. Ratio in cardiogenic pulmonary edema is <0.5, whereas the ratio in ARDS generally is >0.7.

Lactic acid (lactate) level: Lactic acid is a byproduct of anaerobic metabolism and will accumulate in the serum in the presence of hypoxemia. The presence of arterial lactate contributes to acidosis.

A-a gradient/A-a $Do_2/P(A-a)o_2$: Alveolar-arterial oxygen tension difference. Normally it increases approximately 4 mm Hg with each decade of life. Will be increased above the baseline in ARDS and reflects the intrapulmonary shunting that occurs secondary to alveolar flooding.

QS/QT: Ratio of shunt to cardiac output. Measures intrapulmonary shunting. Normal physiologic shunt is 3%-4%; may increase to 15%-20% with ARDS. The routine measurements of ABG, CXR, OP/F ratio and the patient's clinical presentation are much more routinely used than invasive hemodynamic monitoring.

COLLABORATIVE MANAGEMENT

The goals for management: first, maintenance of adequate arterial oxygenation and ventilation; second, treatment of the underlying pathophysiologic condition that caused the ARDS; third, therapy is initiated aimed at treating the lung injury.

Oxygen therapy: Goal is to provide acceptable PaO_2 levels (>60 mm Hg) with FiO_2 <0.50, but FiO_2 up to 1.00 may be necessary.

Mechanical ventilation: Mechanical ventilation is indicated for patients with ARDS. Decreased lung compliance significantly increases work of breathing, Increased physiologic dead space causes a compensatory increase in ventilatory requirements. The goal of mechanical ventilation is to preserve arterial oxygen saturation while preventing complications of increased airway pressures and/or high concentration of oxygen. Many clinicians have successfully employed strategies to treat ARDS by reducing the delivered tidal volume (4-8 ml/kg) and increasing the set RR (12-40) to maintain adequate minute ventilation and reduce peak inspiratory pressures. Ventilator modes such as pressure control (PCV) or inverse ratio pressure control ventilation (IRPCV) can also be used. See "Mechanical Ventilation," p. 14.

Positive end-expiratory pressure: Used in conjunction with mechanical ventilation, PEEP or other means of maintaining positive airway pressure to allow better arterial oxygenation (PaO_2) with administration of lower levels of inspired oxygen tension (FiO_2). It also increases FRC by recruiting or maintaining open alveoli that are otherwise collapsed. High pressures (5-24 cm H_2O) are mechanically maintained at the end of the expiratory cycle, allowing alveoli to remain open and thus participate in gas exchange. For a more complete discussion of PEEP, see "Mechanical Ventilation," p. 15.

Patient positioning: continuous lateral rotation therapy: Lung edema is proposed to be in the dependent areas of the lung. Repositioning the patient at least q2h is indicated in patients with hypoxemia. Continuous lateral motion therapy beds can be used to continuously turn the patient. Motion therapy assists in the redistribution of interstitial edema and may improve oxygenation.

Patient positioning: prone: Prone positioning of the patient improves the oxygenation of many patients with ARDS. There are various methods to turn the patient prone: pillows, foam wedges, or the Vollman prone positioner.

Corticosteroids: Although use of steroids is controversial and their efficacy is not well established, short-term, stress-dose corticosteroids may be useful in stabilizing the alveolar-capillary membrane to prevent further deterioration.

Fluid therapy: Primary goal is to maintain a minimal PAWP to provide adequate CO. Usually, the patient's fluid volume is kept slightly depleted to minimize leakage of excess fluids into the interstitium through damaged capillary membrane. The use of crystalloid versus colloid fluids has been and remains controversial. Both types of fluid have been shown to leak across the alveolar-capillary membrane. Generally, colloids are reserved for those patients with hypoalbuminemia, and crystalloids are used for all other patients.

Anxiety reduction: Most patients require anxiety reduction with medication such as morphine sulfate or anxiolytics. Those patients who are not able to be adequately oxygenated and ventilated with mechanical ventilation may be given anxiety-reducing agents such as midolazam or lorazepam. Patients who are unable to be ventilated and are unstable may have to be heavily sedated with agents such as propofol (Diprivan) or, in extreme cases, paralyzed with a neuroblocking agent such as vecuronium bromide (Norcuron). A sedation scale and protocol should be used to standardize this practice.

The caregiver must recognize that, although the paralyzed patient may appear comatose, he or she may be alert and extremely anxious because of the total lack of muscle control. These patients must receive appropriate sedation (e.g., lorazepam [Ativan]) and analgesia (e.g., morphine), and they will require expert psychosocial nursing interventions. See "Sedating and Paralytic Agents," p. 32. The routine use of analgesics first, followed by anxiety-relieving medications, should be encouraged.

Nutritional support: Energy outlay with respiratory failure is high, in part because of the increased work of breathing. If the patient is unable to consume adequate calories with enteral feedings, TPN is added. It is important to do an occasional evaluation of the patient's caloric and metabolic needs to make certain that the patient is being adequately nourished, but not overfed. All efforts should be made to feed enterally so the gut is used. Newer elemental feedings require no digestion and can be used in the stomach or jejunum.

Research Brief 3-3   This multicenter, randomized, crossover trial studied the effects of alveolar recruitment maneuvers in ALI/ARDS patients receiving lung protective mechanical ventilation using both smaller tidal volumes and higher levels of PEEP than traditionally used. Patients receiving recruitment maneuvers (RMs) experienced greater decreases in systolic BP and SpO_2 during the first 10 minutes. RMs were terminated in three instances. RMs did not cause greater and sustained improvements in SpO_2 and FiO_2/PEEP. Most patients in this study had ALI/ARDS from pneumonia or aspiration. There may be greater potential for lung recruitment in sepsis or trauma-induced ALI/ARDS.

The ARDS Clinical Trials Network, National Heart, Lung and Blood Institute; National Institures of Health: Effects of recruitment maneuvers in patients with acute lung injury and acute respiratory distress syndrome ventilated with high positive end-expiratory pressure, *Crit Care Med* 31(11):2592-2597, 2003.

NURSING DIAGNOSES AND INTERVENTIONS

Impaired gas exchange related to alveolar-capillary membrane changes secondary to increased permeability with alveolar injury and collapse

Desired outcomes: On initiation of therapy, and the titration of ventilatory support, the patient has adequate gas exchange as evidenced by the following ABG values: PaO_2 >60 mm Hg; $PaCO_2$ <45 mm Hg; pH 7.35-7.45. Within 4-6 days of initiation of therapy, patient's RR is 12-20 breaths/min with a normal pattern and depth (eupnea) and there are no adventitious breath sounds.

- Assess and document character of respiratory effort: rate, depth, rhythm, and use of accessory muscles of respiration.
- Assess patient for signs and symptoms of respiratory distress: restlessness, anxiety, confusion, tachypnea (RR >20 breaths/min).
- Assess breath sounds with each vital signs (VS) check. Adventitious sounds, which usually are present in the later stages of ARDS, are not as likely to occur during the early stage.
- Monitor serial ABG values, and consult physician for significant changes. Explain need for frequent analysis to patient and significant others.
- Compare ABG saturation with pulse oximetry saturation for accuracy. Consult physician for pulse oximetry values <90%.
- Administer oxygen and monitor Fio_2 as prescribed.
- Monitor and record pulmonary function tests as prescribed, especially tidal volume and minute ventilation. Expect decreased tidal volume and increased minute ventilation with respiratory distress.
- Position patient for comfort and to promote adequate gas exchange. Usually, semi-Fowler's to high Fowler's position is therapeutic.
- Keep oral airway and self-inflating manual ventilating bag at the bedside for emergency use. Keep emergency intubation equipment at the bedside for use should patient's condition deteriorate.

Risk for injury related to dislodging of life-sustaining equipment during positioning or repositioning

Desired outcome: Patient is able to be turned, placed prone, or repositioned without dislodging life-sustaining equipment or devices. When PaO_2 and SpO_2 return to an acceptable level, or the chest x-ray shows improvement, the bed may be discontinued.

- Secure the ET tube/other devices to prevent accidental movement or dislodging.
- Provide the appropriate length ventilator tubing to facilitate positioning of the patient without risk of pulling on the ET tube.
- Facilitate tolerance of rotational therapy by managing anxiety and promoting sleep with medications.
- Assess oxygenation once patient is prone. Typical responders will demonstrate at least 10 mm Hg increase in PaO_2 within 10 min of being placed prone.
- Collaborate with the respiratory care practitioner to decrease the delivered oxygen as the patient's oxygenation status improves.

NIC Acid-Base Management; Airway Management; Bedside Laboratory Testing; Laboratory Data Interpretation; Mechanical Ventilation; Oxygen Therapy; Positioning; Respiratory Monitoring; Ventilation Assistance; Vital Signs Monitoring

ADDITIONAL NURSING DIAGNOSES

Also see "Activity Intolerance" in "Status Asthmaticus," p. 179. As indicated, see nursing diagnoses and interventions in "Nutritional Support," p. 1; "Mechanical Ventilation," p. 14; and "Prolonged Immobility," p. 61.

Pulmonary Embolus (PE)

PATHOPHYSIOLOGY

Pulmonary perfusion disorders are the result of any obstruction of blood flow in the pulmonary vasculature. The two most common abnormalities of pulmonary perfusion are thrombotic emboli and fat emboli. Emboli related to venous air and rarer sources (amniotic fluid, sepsis/infection, and tumors) are also discussed.

Thrombotic embolus (TE): The most common pulmonary perfusion abnormality, thrombotic emboli (TEs), are caused by a dislodged blood clot from the systemic circulation, typically the deep veins of the legs, the iliofemoral system, or pelvis. Many patients with TEs do not experience symptoms of deep vein thrombosis (DVT). Thrombus formation can result from blood stasis, alterations in clotting factors, and injury to vessel walls. The formed thrombus becomes dislodged and travels to the pulmonary circulation, where it obstructs one or both branches of the pulmonary artery or a smaller, distal vessel. Total obstruction leading to pulmonary infarction is rare. Early diagnosis and appropriate treatment reduce mortality to less than 10%. Although most thrombotic emboli resolve completely, leaving no residual deficits, some patients may be left with chronic pulmonary hypertension.

Fat emboli: The most common nonthrombotic cause of pulmonary emboli (PEs), fat emboli generally result from the release of free fatty acids prompting toxic vasculitis followed by thrombosis and obstruction of small pulmonary arteries by fat. The syndrome occurs within 12-24 hr after skeletal trauma or major orthopedic surgery.

Venous air emboli: Almost always an iatrogenic complication caused by a large volume of air that is introduced into the venous circulation and travels to the pulmonary circulation. Smaller amounts of air may be completely unproductive of symptoms, since air can be rapidly resorbed. Surgical procedures, insertion of pulmonary artery catheters, central venous catheters, hemodialysis, endoscopy, and use of automatic injectors such as those used for contrast media can prompt symptomatic air emboli. A larger bolus of air into the right ventricle may completely obstruct pulmonary blood flow, leading to cardiac arrest. In severe cases, venous air embolus has a mortality >50%. Rapid diagnosis and treatment are essential.

Other pulmonary emboli: *Amniotic fluid embolism* occurs in less than one in 8000 women, but results in death during delivery in many of the affected mothers. *Septic pulmonary emboli* are infected clots dislodged from either peripheral or abdominal vein septic thrombophlebitis or right heart endocarditis. Prognosis is dependent on the overall patient condition and severity of the sepsis. *Tumor embolism* occurs with many types or carcinoma and sarcoma, but cause significant respiratory symptoms in less than 3% of affected patients.

ASSESSMENT
Thrombotic emboli
History and risk factors
Prolonged immobilization: Especially significant when coexisting with surgical or nonsurgical trauma, carcinoma, or cardiopulmonary disease. Risk increases as length of immobilization increases.
Cardiac disorders: Atrial fibrillation, congestive heart failure, myocardial infarction, rheumatic heart disease, or any low CO state.
Surgical intervention: Risk increases in postoperative period, especially for patients with pelvic, thoracic, and abdominal surgery and for those with extensive burns or musculoskeletal injuries of the hip or knee.
Pregnancy: Especially during the postpartum period.
Trauma: Especially fractures of the lower extremities, hip fracture in the older adult, burns, and acute head and spinal cord injuries. The degree of risk is related to the severity, site, and extent of trauma.
Carcinoma: Particularly neoplasms involving the breast, lung, pancreas, and genitourinary (GU) and gastrointestinal (GI) tracts.
Obesity: Patients with a ≥20% increase in ideal body weight have an increased incidence of TEs.

Varicose veins or prior thromboembolic disease
Age: Risk of thromboembolism is greatest between 55 and 65 yr of age.

Note: Low-dose heparin prophylaxis (e.g., 5000 units subcutaneously q8-12h) frequently is initiated in high-risk groups (except for neurosurgical patients). Low–molecular weight (LMW) heparins (e.g., dalteparin [Fragmin] and enoxaparin [Lovenox]) may be used for DVT prophylaxis in certain high-risk surgical patients, such as those who have abdominal and orthopedic surgery.

Clinical presentation: Often nonspecific but may involve sudden onset of dyspnea, tachypnea, restlessness, and anxiety. The patient also may have a nonproductive cough, palpitations, nausea, and syncope. With a large embolism, oppressive substernal chest discomfort will be present. Fever, pleuritic chest pain, and hemoptysis are present with pulmonary infarction. Saddle embolus is the largest, most dangerous PE. The embolus lodges at the bifurcation of the right and left pulmonary arteries, occludes blood flow into both lungs and can result in cardiopulmonary arrest within minutes.

Physical assessment: RR >20 breaths/min, HR >100 beats/min, crackles, decreased chest wall excursion secondary to splinting, S_3 and S_4 gallop rhythms, diaphoresis, edema, and cyanosis. Temperature may be elevated if pulmonary infarction has occurred, and transient pleural friction rub may be present. With saddle embolus, patient experiences acute respiratory failure, which may progress to cardiopulmonary arrest.

Fat emboli
History and risk factors
Multiple long bone fractures: Especially fractures of the femur and pelvis (see p. 128).
Trauma to adipose tissue or liver
Burns: See p. 159.
Osteomyelitis
Hemolytic crisis: See p. 473.

Clinical presentation: Typically, patient is without symptoms for a period lasting 12-24 hr after embolization; this period ends with sudden cardiopulmonary and neurologic deterioration: dyspnea, restlessness, confusion, delirium, and coma. Petechial rash may appear over the body, especially the upper body. This is secondary to thrombocytopenia, which may be related to platelet aggregation by circulating fats.

Physical assessment: RR >20 breaths/min; HR >100 beats/min; increased BP; elevated temperature; petechiae, especially of the upper torso and axillae; inspiratory crowing; and expiratory wheezes.

Venous air emboli
History and risk factors
Recent surgical procedure
Pulmonary artery/central venous catheter insertion
Misuse of closed-wound suction unit
Cardiopulmonary bypass
Hemodialysis
Endoscopy

Clinical presentation: Depends on severity of the bolus. Agitation, confusion, cough, dyspnea, and chest pain.

Physical assessment: RR >20 breaths/min, HR >100 beats/min, wheezing, hypotension, mill wheel heart murmur.

DIAGNOSTIC TESTS

Thrombotic emboli

ABG values: Initially, hypoxemia (Pao_2 <80 mm Hg), hypocapnia ($Paco_2$ <35 mm Hg), and respiratory alkalosis (pH >7.45). A normal Pao_2 does not rule out the presence of TE. Pulse oximetry is used for continuous monitoring of oxygen saturation (see p. 176). If embolus is large, patient may experience acute respiratory failure, with Po_2 <60 mm Hg, Pco_2 >45 mm Hg, and pH <7.35.

Alveolar-arterial oxygen pressure difference: $P(A-a)o_2$ usually will be >10 mm Hg, depending on the severity of the perfusion disorder and the degree of ventilation-perfusion mismatch.

Chest x-ray: Initially the chest x-ray shows normal findings, or an elevated hemidiaphragm will be present. After 24 hr the x-ray may reveal small infiltrates secondary to atelectasis from decrease in surfactant. If pulmonary infarction is present, infiltrates and pleural effusions may be seen within 12-36 hr.

ECG: If TEs are extensive, signs of acute pulmonary hypertension may be present: right-shift QRS axes, tall and peaked P waves, ST segment changes, and T wave inversion in leads V_1-V_4.

Pulmonary ventilation-perfusion scan: A key diagnostic test used to detect the presence of abnormalities of ventilation or perfusion in the pulmonary system. The patient inhales radioactive-tagged gases, and radioactive particles are injected peripherally. If there is a mismatch of ventilation and perfusion (e.g., normal ventilation with decreased perfusion), vascular obstruction is likely. Results may not be definitive.

Pulmonary angiography: This is the definitive study for TEs. It is an invasive procedure involving catheterization of the right ventricle and injection of dye into the pulmonary artery (PA) to visualize pulmonary vessels. An abrupt vessel "cut off" may be seen at the site of embolization. Usually, filling defects are seen.

Hemodynamic studies: If TEs lead to increased pulmonary vascular resistance, PA pressure will be elevated. PA pressures increase significantly (>20 mm Hg) if 30%-50% of the pulmonary arterial tree is affected. If massive TEs are present and PA pressure increases to >40 mm Hg, right ventricular failure can develop, leading to a decrease in CO and hypotension.

Fat emboli

ABG values: Hypoxemia (Pao_2 <80 mm Hg) and hypercapnia ($Paco_2$ >45 mm Hg) will be present with a respiratory acidosis (pH <7.35).

Chest x-ray: A pattern similar to ARDS is seen: diffuse, extensive, bilateral interstitial and alveolar infiltrates.

CBC count: May reveal decreased hemoglobin (Hgb) and Hct secondary to hemorrhage into the lung, in addition to thrombocytopenia.

Venous air emboli

ABG values: Hypoxemia (Pao_2 <80 mm Hg), hypercapnia ($Paco_2$ >45 mm Hg), and respiratory acidosis (pH <7.35) generally are present in severe cases.

Chest x-ray: Reveals changes consistent with pulmonary edema or air-fluid levels in the main pulmonary artery system.

Pulmonary artery pressure: Systolic, diastolic, and mean pressure are acutely elevated, but slight elevation of PAWP remains within normal limits (WNL).

Evolving diagnostic tests for pulmonary emboli: Spiral computerized tomography, magnetic resonance angiography, echocardiography, and whole blood D-dimer levels are being evaluated for effectiveness in diagnosis of pulmonary emboli.

COLLABORATIVE MANAGEMENT

Thrombotic emboli

Oxygen therapy: Delivered at an appropriate concentration to maintain a Pao_2 of >60 mm Hg.

IV heparin (unfractionated) therapy: Treatment of choice. It is started immediately in patients without bleeding or clotting disorders and in whom TE is strongly suspected.

Initial dose: 80 units/kg IV bolus.

Maintenance dose: Following initial dose, a continuous IV infusion of approximately 18 units/kg/h is usually indicated, regulated by serial activated partial thromboplastin time (aPTT) values to determine level of anticoagulation. Heparin requirements are the largest in the initial 72 hr of therapy. Maintenance continues for 7-14 days, during which time the patient is placed on bed rest to ensure the thrombus is firmly attached to the vessel wall before ambulation. Platelets should be monitored, as patients sometimes experience heparin-induced thrombocytopenia (HIT), or low platelets.

Low–molecular weight heparin (dalteparin, enoxaparin): An alternative to unfractionated heparin with longer half-life, greater bioavailability, and more predictable anticoagulant activity when given subcutaneously in fixed doses.

Goals of therapy: To inhibit thrombus growth, promote resolution of the formed thrombus, and prevent further embolus formation. These goals are achieved by keeping aPTT at 1½-2½ times the normal. In addition, platelet counts should be obtained q3days, because thrombocytopenia and paradoxic arterial thrombosis can occur as a result of heparin therapy. (See "Heparin-Induced Thrombocytopenia," p. 482.)

Protamine sulfate: Heparin antidote, which should be readily available during heparin therapy. Fatal hemorrhage occurs in 1%-2% of patients undergoing heparin therapy. Risk of bleeding is greatest in women >60 yr of age.

Oral anticoagulants (warfarin sodium): Started within 72 hr of initiation of heparin therapy. Both agents are given simultaneously for 4-6 days to allow time for warfarin to inhibit vitamin K-dependent clotting factors before heparin is discontinued. Daily warfarin dose is adjusted according to International Normalized Ratio (INR), and correct dosage is individualized per patient based on frequent INR determinations. An INR of 2.0-3.0 is desirable.

Prothrombin time (PT): Monitored daily, with a goal of 1¼-1½ times normal. Once the patient's condition has stabilized and the heparin is discontinued, weekly monitoring of INR is acceptable. After hospital discharge the PT should be monitored q2wk for as long as the patient continues to take warfarin.

Maintenance: Usually 10 mg/day, continued for 3-6 months and based on the continued presence of risk factors. Certain tumors (e.g., Trousseau's syndrome) necessitate lifetime therapy.

> **Note:** Subcutaneous heparin therapy is an effective alternative to warfarin, with less risk of bleeding. The dose of heparin must be adjusted while the patient is hospitalized to ensure a PTT of 1½ times normal.

Vitamin K: Reverses the effects of warfarin in 24-36 hr. Fresh-frozen plasma may be required in cases of serious bleeding.

> **Caution:** Warfarin crosses the placental barrier and can cause spontaneous abortion and birth defects.

Thrombolytic therapy: These drugs lyse clots via conversion of plasminogen to plasma and may be given within 72 hr of TE to speed the process of clot lysis. Used immediately when severe cardiopulmonary compromise or arrest has occurred. Heparin therapy is used following thrombolytic infusion. As many as 33% of patients who receive thrombolytic therapy have hemorrhagic complications. The drug should be discontinued, and fresh-frozen plasma infusion may be initiated for severe bleeding complications.

Research Brief 3-4   The investigators attempted to determine the risk factors and frequency of intracranial hemorrhage in patients receiving thrombolysis for documented pulmonary embolism. There were 312 cases reviewed for incidence of intracranial hemorrhage, as well as background information that might support or not support the use of such therapy. It was found that intracranial hemorrhage with thrombolytic therapy occurred infrequently but that risk factors such as diastolic hypertension or previous history of intracranial disease must be screened for in this population.

From Kanter DS et al: Thromboembolytic therapy for pulmonary embolism: frequency of intracranial hemorrhage and associated risk factors, *Chest* 111(5):1241-1245, 1997.

Streptokinase: Loading dose of 250,000 IU in normal saline or D_5W given IV over a 30-min period. Maintenance dose is 100,000 IU/hr given IV for 24-72 hr.

Tissue plasminogen activator: Given 50 mg/h for 2 hr. Followed by heparin therapy.

Thrombin time: Monitors therapy for both drugs. The test is repeated q4h during therapy to ensure adequate response, which should be 2-5 times normal. An aPTT can be used instead of thrombin time and should be 2-5 times the control. Once thrombolytic therapy is stopped, thrombin time or aPTT should be checked frequently until values fall below twice the normal. When the values are below twice the normal, heparin is started.

Contraindications: Active internal bleeding, stroke, or intracranial bleeding within 2 months of TE. Other contraindications include trauma or surgery within 15 days of TE, diastolic hypertension >100 mm Hg, recent cardiopulmonary resuscitation, pregnancy, and <10 days postpartum.

Surgical interventions: Inferior vena caval interruption (IVC filter insertion) in severe or recurrent cases of pulmonary embolism. Inferior vena caval interruption most often involves the transvenous insertion of an umbrella filter (e.g., Greenfield filter) that prevents the passage of major emboli from deep venous thrombi in the lower extremities. Pulmonary embolectomy may be indicated in select cases of massive pulmonary embolism.

Fat emboli

Oxygen: Concentration of oxygen is based on clinical presentation, ABG results, and the patient's prior respiratory status. Intubation and mechanical ventilation may be required.

Steroids: Cortisone, 100 mg, or methylprednisolone, 30 mg/kg, is used to decrease local injury to pulmonary tissue and pulmonary edema.

Diuretics: Pulmonary edema develops in approximately 30% of patients with fat emboli, necessitating use of diuretics.

Venous air emboli

Emphasis is on prevention. Ensure that central venous catheter is inserted with the patient in Trendelenburg position. Use Luer-Lok connectors on all IV tubing to prevent a disconnection. Should venous air embolus occur despite precautions, the following measures are anticipated.

Oxygen therapy: 100% Fio_2 is initiated immediately.

Trendelenburg position with a left decubitus tilt: To minimize further movement of air bolus through the heart and into the pulmonary vasculature and beyond.

Aspiration of air: If a central venous catheter is in place near the right atrium, an attempt is made to aspirate the air.

NURSING DIAGNOSES AND INTERVENTIONS

Impaired gas exchange related to altered blood flow secondary to presence of pulmonary emboli

Desired outcomes: Within 12 hr of initiation of therapy, patient has adequate gas exchange as evidenced by the following ABG values: Pao_2 >60 mm Hg; $Paco_2$ 35-45 mm Hg; and pH 7.35-7.45. Within 2-4 days of initiating therapy, patient's RR is 12-20 breaths/min with normal depth and pattern (eupnea).

- Monitor serial ABG values, assessing for the desired response to treatment: increased Pao_2 (>60 mm Hg) and correction of respiratory alkalosis ($Paco_2$ 35-45 mm Hg and pH 7.35-7.45). Report lack of response to treatment or worsening ABG values. Monitor oxygen saturation via continuous pulse oximetry.
- Monitor patient for signs and symptoms of increasing respiratory distress, and consult physician for significant findings: RR increased from baseline, increasing dyspnea, anxiety, cyanosis.
- Ensure delivery of prescribed concentrations of oxygen.
- Position patient for comfort and optimal gas exchange. Ensure that the area of the lung affected by the emboli is not dependent when patient is in the lateral decubitus position. Position patient with

the unaffected side down, and elevate HOB 30 degrees. This will ensure a better ventilation-perfusion match, thereby improving Pao$_2$.

- Avoid positioning patient with knees bent (i.e., "gatching" the bed), because this impedes venous return from the legs and can increase the risk of TE.
- Ensure that patient performs deep-breathing exercises 3-5 times q2h.
- Decrease metabolic demands for oxygen by limiting or pacing patient's activities and procedures.
- Explain all procedures, and offer support to minimize fear and anxiety, which can increase oxygen demands.
- Schedule rest times after meals to avoid competition for oxygen supply during digestion.

Altered protection related to risk of clotting anomalies secondary to anticoagulation or thrombolytic therapy

Desired outcome: Patient is free of bleeding signs; or if bleeding occurs, it is not prolonged.

- Monitor serial coagulation or thrombin times. Report values outside the desired therapeutic ranges. Optimal range for aPTT is 1½-2½ times control value. A therapeutic INR is 2.0-3.0. Optimal range for thrombin time is 2-5 times normal.
- Ensure easy access to antidotes for prescribed treatment:
  ❏ *Protamine sulfate:* 1 mg counteracts 100 units of heparin. Usually, the initial dose is 50 mg.
  ❏ *Vitamin K:* 20 mg given subcutaneously.
  ❏ *Epsilon-aminocaproic acid* (e.g., Amicar): Reverses the fibrinolytic condition related to thrombolytic therapy.

Note: Although use of epsilon-aminocaproic acid as an antidote has not been approved, it has been used in some emergency situations.

- Inspect the following sites for evidence of bleeding: any entry site of an invasive procedure, oral mucous membranes, wounds, and nares; inspect the torso and extremities for evidence of petechiae or ecchymoses. Also check stool, urine, sputum, and vomitus for occult blood. Be alert to complaints of back pain or other site-specific pain (e.g., headache), which may signal occult bleeding.
- Apply pressure over puncture sites until bleeding stops—usually 5-10 min for venous site and 10-20 min for arterial site. Apply pressure dressing over arterial puncture sites to stop oozing of blood.
- To prevent hematoma formation, avoid giving intramuscular (IM) injections.
- Monitor Hgb and Hct. Consult physician for significant findings, including decreases in values or failure to see appropriate increases after transfusion.
- To avoid negative interactions with anticoagulants or thrombolytic therapy, establish compatibility of all drugs before administering them:
  ❏ *Heparin:* Digitalis, tetracyclines, nicotine, and antihistamines decrease the effect of heparin therapy. Establish compatibility before infusing other IV drugs through heparin IV line.
  ❏ *Warfarin sodium:* Numerous drugs result in a decrease or an increase in response to treatment with warfarin. Consult with pharmacist to obtain specific information about patient's medication profile.
  ❏ *Thrombolytic therapy:* Do not infuse other medications through the same IV line.
- Because aspirin and nonsteroidal antiinflammatory drugs (e.g., ibuprofen) are platelet-aggregation inhibitors and can prolong episodes of bleeding, avoid use of *any* drug that contains these agents.
- Discuss with patient and significant others the importance of reporting promptly the presence of bleeding from any source.
- Teach patient the necessity of using sponge-tipped applicators (instead of toothbrush) and mouthwash for oral care to minimize the risk of gum bleeding during hospitalization when anticoagulant therapy is most intensive. Instruct patient to shave with an electric razor.
- If patient is restless and combative, provide a safe environment: pad the side rails; obtain prescription to restrain patient as necessary to prevent falls; and use extreme care when moving patient to avoid bumping extremities into side rails.

Knowledge deficit: oral anticoagulant therapy: potential side effects and complications; foods and medications to avoid during therapy

Desired outcome: Within 24 hr of initiation of oral anticoagulant therapy, patient and/or significant others verbalize knowledge of patient's prescribed anticoagulant drug, the potential side effects, and foods and medications to avoid during oral anticoagulant therapy.

- Determine patient's knowledge of oral anticoagulant therapy. As appropriate, discuss the drug name, purpose, dosage, schedule, potential side effects, and complications of therapy.
- Inform patient of the potential side effects and complications of anticoagulant therapy: easy bruising; prolonged bleeding from cuts; spontaneous nose bleeds; black and tarry stools; blood in urine and sputum.

- Teach the rationale and application procedure for antiembolism stockings. Explain that patient should put them on in the morning before getting out of bed.
- Stress the importance of preventing impairment of venous return from the lower extremities by avoiding prolonged sitting, crossing the legs, and wearing constrictive clothing.
- Teach patient about foods high in vitamin K (e.g., fish, bananas, dark-green vegetables, tomatoes, cauliflower), which can interfere with anticoagulation.
- Caution patient that a soft-bristle toothbrush, rather than a hard-bristle one, and an electric razor, rather than a safety razor, should be used during anticoagulant therapy while at home.
- Instruct patient to consult with physician before taking any new over-the-counter (OTC) or prescribed drugs. The following are among many drugs that enhance the response to warfarin: aspirin, ibuprofen, cimetidine, and trimethoprim. Drugs that decrease the response include antacids, diuretics, oral contraceptives, and barbiturates, among others.

█NIC Acid-Base Management; Acid-Base Monitoring; Bedside Laboratory Testing; Bleeding Precautions; Health Education; Oxygen Therapy; Respiratory Monitoring; Surveillance; Teaching: Individual; Teaching: Prescribed Medication; Respiratory Monitoring, Vital Signs Monitoring

ADDITIONAL NURSING DIAGNOSIS
See "Activity Intolerance" in "Status Asthmaticus," p. 179.

Pneumothorax

PATHOPHYSIOLOGY
Pneumothorax is an accumulation of air between the parietal and visceral pleura with secondary lung collapse. There are three types of pneumothorax.

Spontaneous: A type of closed pneumothorax in which the chest wall remains intact with no leak to the atmosphere. It results from the rupture of a bleb or bulla on the visceral pleural surface, usually near the apex. In a *primary* spontaneous pneumothorax, the cause of the rupture is unknown, although it may result from a weakness related to a respiratory infection. The affected individual is usually a young male (20-40 yr of age), previously healthy, and a smoker. Generally onset of symptoms occurs at rest rather than with vigorous exercise or coughing. The potential for recurrence is great, with the second pneumothorax occurring an average of 2-3 yr after the first. A primary spontaneous pneumothorax is rarely life-threatening. A *secondary* spontaneous pneumothorax results as a complication of an underlying lung disease (COPD, cystic fibrosis, tuberculosis, malignant neoplasm). The symptoms are more severe than with the primary spontaneous pneumothorax, and this disorder may be life-threatening because of the underlying lung disease. In addition, recurrence rates are high in this population.

Traumatic: Can be open or closed. An *open* pneumothorax occurs when air enters the pleural space from the atmosphere through an opening in the chest wall, such as with a penetrating injury or an invasive medical procedure (e.g., lung biopsy, thoracentesis, placement of a central line into a subclavian vein). A *closed* pneumothorax occurs when the visceral pleura is penetrated but the chest wall remains intact, with no atmospheric leak. This usually occurs with blunt trauma that results in a fracture and dislocation of the ribs. It also may occur from the use of high level PEEP therapy or after cardiopulmonary resuscitation (CPR). For more information about blunt chest injuries, see "Chest Trauma," p. 110.

Tension: Occurs when air enters the pleural space through a pleural tear during inspiration. Air continues to accumulate but cannot escape during expiration because of intrapleural pressure, which is greater than alveolar pressure. This leads to a one-way or flap-valve effect. As the pressure increases, it is transmitted to the mediastinum. This results in a mediastinal shift toward the unaffected side, which further impairs ventilatory efforts. The increase in pressure also compresses the vena cava, which impedes venous return, leading to a decrease in CO and, ultimately, to circulatory collapse if it is not diagnosed and treated quickly. Tension pneumothorax is a life-threatening medical emergency. Although it can occur with a spontaneous pneumothorax, it most often is associated with trauma or infection, or it can occur during mechanical ventilation in patients who require positive-pressure ventilation.

ASSESSMENT
The clinical presentation will vary in degree, depending on the type and size of pneumothorax.

Spontaneous or traumatic: Sudden onset of sharp, stabbing chest pain on the affected side, which may radiate to the shoulder; moderate to severe dyspnea; anxiety.

Inspection: Decreased chest wall movement on affected side.

Palpation: Tracheal shift toward unaffected side; subcutaneous emphysema (crepitus); tactile and vocal fremitus decreased or absent on affected side.
Percussion: Hyperresonance on affected side.
Auscultation: Absent or decreased breath sounds on affected side; increased RR. Moderate tachycardia (HR >140 beats/min) may be present.
Tension: Severe dyspnea; chest pain on affected side; cool, clammy, mottled skin; anxiety and restlessness.
Inspection: Decreased chest wall movement on affected side; expansion of affected side throughout respiratory cycle; jugular vein distention.
Palpation: Tracheal shift toward unaffected side; subcutaneous emphysema in neck and chest.
Percussion: Hyperresonance on affected side.
Auscultation: Absent or decreased breath sounds on affected side; distant heart sounds; increased RR (>20 breaths/min); decreased BP; increased HR (may be >140 beats/min).

Caution: Tension pneumothorax is life-threatening. Immediate medical intervention is critical.

DIAGNOSTIC TESTS

Chest x-ray: Will show size of the pneumothorax and any tracheal shift. The affected side will show air in the pleural space, expansion of the chest wall, lowering of the diaphragm, and partial to total collapse of the lung. A small pneumothorax (<20%) may not be detectable on physical examination.
ABG analysis: Hypoxemia (PaO_2 <80 mm Hg) will be evident immediately after a moderate to large pneumothorax that occupies ≥15% of the hemithorax. As the pneumothorax resolves, arterial oxygen saturation returns to normal. Hypoxemia may be accompanied by respiratory acidosis (pH <7.35) and hypercapnia ($PaCO_2$ >45 mm Hg).
ECG: May reveal decrease in QRS amplitude, precordial T wave inversion, rightward shift of frontal QRS axis, and small precordial R voltage.

COLLABORATIVE MANAGEMENT

Oxygen therapy: Administered when ABG values demonstrate the presence of hypoxemia, which usually occurs with a large pneumothorax.
Analgesic: Provides relief of pain of pneumothorax or its treatment.
Thoracentesis: Performed immediately in tension pneumothorax to remove air from the chest cavity. A large-bore needle is inserted into the second intercostal space, midclavicular line, which correlates to the superior portion of the anterior axillary lobe. A sudden rushing out of air confirms the diagnosis of tension pneumothorax. To decrease the risk of further pleural laceration as the chest reexpands, a stylet introducer needle with a plastic sheath may be used. The needle is removed after penetration, and the plastic catheter sheath is left in place to allow decompression of the chest cavity. After air aspiration, chest tubes are inserted.
Chest tube placement: A chest tube may be inserted in a patient who has a pneumothorax, depending on the severity of collapse. Chest tube placement may follow a needle decompression. Chest tubes cause inflammation, ultimately scarring the pleura to help prevent recurrent spontaneous pneumothoraces. Patients with recurrent pneumothoraces require chest tubes rather than needle decompression because their visceral pleura does not seal promptly. Chest tubes (26-30 Fr) are inserted in the second or third lateral intercostal space, midclavicular line. During insertion, the patient should be in an upright position so that the lung falls away from the chest wall. A small (1-2 cm) incision is made, and the chest tube is placed, sutured in place, and connected to an underwater-seal drainage system. Usually simple underwater-seal drainage is all that is necessary for 6-24 hr. Suction may be used, depending on the size of the pneumothorax, the patient's condition, and the amount of drainage. A one-way flutter valve may be used with the chest tube instead of the underwater-seal drainage system. The flutter valve allows air to escape but prevents its reentry. The flutter valve (e.g., Heimlich valve) is placed on the end of the chest tube. Suction can be applied with the flutter valve in place. After chest tube insertion and removal of air from the pleural space, the lung begins to reexpand. A chest tube may cause pleuritic pain, slight temperature elevation, and pleuritic friction rub. The nurse should administer analgesics and monitor the patient's response to the procedure.
Thoracotomy: Often indicated because of the risk of continuous recurrence if patient has had two or more spontaneous pneumothoraces on one side or if resolution of the pneumothorax does not occur within 7 days. Thoracotomy may involve mechanical abrasion of the pleural surfaces with a dry, sterile

sponge or chemical abrasion via an agent such as tetracycline solution or talc, both of which result in pleural adhesions to prevent recurrence. A partial pleurectomy may be performed instead of mechanical or chemical abrasion.

NURSING DIAGNOSES AND INTERVENTIONS

Impaired gas exchange related to decreased alveolar blood flow and decreased oxygen supply secondary to increased pleural pressure

Desired outcome: Within 2-6 hr of initiation of treatment, patient exhibits adequate gas exchange as evidenced by Pao_2 ≥60 mm Hg and $Paco_2$ ≤45 mm Hg (or values within 10% of patient's baseline values, which depend on underlying pathophysiology); RR <20 breaths/min with normal depth and pattern (eupnea); and orientation to time, place, and person.

- Monitor serial ABG results to detect continued presence of hypercapnea or hypoxemia. Monitor O_2 saturation via pulse oximetry as indicated. Consult physician for new or persistent hypoxemia or hypercapnea.
- Observe for indicators of hypoxia, including increased restlessness, anxiety, and changes in mental status.
- Assess patient for increasing respiratory distress: increased RR; diminished or absent movement of chest wall on affected side; complaints of increased dyspnea; cyanosis.
- Position patient to allow for full expansion of unaffected lung. Semi-Fowler's position usually provides comfort and allows adequate expansion of chest wall. The patient also can be turned unaffected side-down with the HOB elevated to ensure a better ventilation-perfusion match.
- Change patient's position q2h to promote drainage and lung reexpansion and to facilitate alveolar perfusion.
- Encourage patient to take deep breaths, providing necessary analgesia to decrease discomfort during deep-breathing exercises. Deep breathing will promote full lung expansion and may decrease the risk of atelectasis.
- Ensure delivery of prescribed concentrations of oxygen.
- Assess and maintain closed chest-drainage system:
  - ❏ Tape all connections, and secure chest tube to thorax with tape.
  - ❏ Avoid all kinks in the tubing, and ensure that the bed and equipment are not compressing any component of the system.
  - ❏ Maintain fluid in underwater-seal chamber, and suction chamber at appropriate levels.
  - ❏ Be aware that the suction apparatus does not regulate the amount of suction applied to the closed drainage system. The amount of suction is determined by the water level in the suction control chamber. Minimal bubbling is optimal. Excessive bubbling causes rapid evaporative loss.

Note: Suction aids in the reexpansion of the lung, but removing suction for short periods, such as for transporting, will not be detrimental or disrupt the closed drainage system.

  - ❏ Be aware that fluctuations in the long tube of the underwater-seal chamber indicate a patent chest tube. Fluctuations stop when either the lung has reexpanded or there is a kink or obstruction in the chest tube.
  - ❏ Bubbling in the underwater-seal chamber occurs on expiration and is a sign that air is leaving the pleural space.
  - ❏ Continuous bubbling on both inspiration and expiration in the underwater-seal chamber is a signal that air is leaking into the drainage system. Locate and seal the system's air leak, if possible.
- Keep necessary emergency supplies at the bedside: (1) petroleum gauze pad to apply over insertion site if the chest tube becomes dislodged; and (2) sterile water in which to submerge the chest tube if it becomes disconnected from the underwater-seal system. *Never* clamp a chest tube without a specific directive from the physician: clamping may lead to tension pneumothorax because the air can no longer escape.

Caution: Follow your institutional policy regarding chest tube stripping. Be aware that this mechanism for maintaining chest tube patency is controversial and has been associated with high negative pressures in the pleural space, which can damage fragile lung tissue. Chest tube stripping may be indicated when bloody drainage or clots are visible in the tubing. Squeezing alternately hand-over-hand along the drainage tube may generate sufficient pressure to move fluid along the tube.

Pain related to biophysical injury as a result of chest tube placement and pleural irritation

Desired outcomes: Within 1-2 hr of initiating analgesic therapy, patient's subjective evaluation of discomfort improves as documented by a pain scale. Nonverbal indicators of discomfort, such as grimacing and splinting on inspiration, are absent.

- Give patient and significant others appropriate information regarding chest tube placement and maintenance.
- At frequent intervals, assess patient's degree of discomfort, using patient's verbal and nonverbal cues. Devise a pain scale with patient, rating discomfort on a scale of 0 (no pain) to 10 (worst pain). Medicate with analgesics as prescribed, evaluating and documenting the effectiveness of the medication on the basis of the pain scale.
- Position patient on unaffected side to minimize discomfort from chest tube insertion site. Administer medication 30 min before initiating movement.
- Teach patient to splint affected side during coughing, moving, or repositioning. Move patient as a unit to enhance stability and comfort.
- Schedule activities to provide for periods of rest, because fatigue may lower patient's pain threshold.
- Stabilize chest tube to reduce pull or drag on latex connector tubing. Tape chest tube securely to thorax, and loop latex tubing on bed beside patient.
- Teach patient to maintain active ROM on the involved side to prevent development of a stiff shoulder from the immobility.

NIC Acid-Base Management; Acid-Base Monitoring; Analgesic Administration; Environmental Management: Comfort; Exercise Promotion; Laboratory Data Interpretation; Medication Administration; Medication Management; Oxygen Therapy; Pain Management; Positioning; Respiratory Monitoring; Vital Signs Monitoring

ADDITIONAL NURSING DIAGNOSES

Also see "Activity Intolerance" in "Status Asthmaticus," p. 179. See appropriate nursing diagnoses and interventions in "Psychosocial Support," p. 68; and "Psychosocial Support for the Patient's Family and Significant Others," p. 78.

Acute Respiratory Failure

PATHOPHYSIOLOGY

Acute respiratory failure is defined as the inability of the respiratory system to meet the ventilation, oxygenation, or metabolic needs of the patient. *Type I (hypoxemic)* is oxygenation failure, whereas *type II (hypercapneic)* is ventilation failure. Some patients may manifest respiratory failure of types I and II simultaneously. Clinically, type I failure exists when Pao_2 is <50 mm Hg with the patient at rest and breathing room air. $Paco_2$ >50 mm Hg or pH <7.35 is significant for acute respiratory acidemia, more reflective of type II. Although a variety of diseases can lead to respiratory failure, three basic mechanisms are involved in creating right to left intrapulmonary shunting, which leads to poor tissue level oxygenation:

Alveolar hypoventilation (type II respiratory failure): Occurs as a result of reduction in alveolar minute ventilation. Because initial indicators of hypercapnea (CO_2 retention) such as lethargy and somnolence are subtle changes, the condition may go unnoticed until hypoxia is severe and cyanosis is present. Patients with brain injuries or neuromuscular diseases can have hypercapneic respiratory failure without lung disease present.

Ventilation-perfusion mismatch (type I respiratory failure): Considered the most common cause of hypoxia. Normal alveolar ventilation occurs at a rate of 4 L/min, with normal pulmonary vascular blood flow occurring at a rate of 5 L/min. The normal ventilation/perfusion ratio is 0.8:1. Any disease process that interferes with either side of the equation upsets the physiologic balance and can lead to respiratory failure as a result of reduction in arterial oxygen levels.

Diffusion disturbances (type I respiratory failure): Processes that physically impair gas exchange across the alveolar-capillary membrane. Diffusion is impaired because of the increase in anatomic distance the gas must travel from the alveoli to the capillaries and from the capillaries to the alveoli.

Right to left shunting (intrapulmonary shunt): Occurs when the aforementioned processes go untreated. Large amounts of blood pass from the right side of the heart to the left and out into the general circulation without adequate ventilation; therefore blood is poorly oxygenated. This process occurs when alveoli are atelectatic or fluid-filled, inasmuch as these conditions interfere with gas exchange.

Note: See Table 3-5 for a description of some of the disease processes that can lead to acute respiratory failure.

T A B L E 3 - 5   Disease Processes Leading to the Development of Respiratory Failure

Impaired alveolar ventilation
- COPD (emphysema, bronchitis, asthma, cystic fibrosis)
- Restrictive pulmonary disease (interstitial fibrosis, pleural effusion, pneumothorax, kyphoscoliosis, obesity, diaphragmatic paralysis)
- Neuromuscular defects (Guillain-Barré syndrome, myasthenia gravis, multiple sclerosis, muscular dystrophy, polio, brain/spinal injury)
- Depression of respiratory control centers (drug-induced cerebral infarction, inappropriate use of high-dose oxygen therapy, drug/toxic agents)
- Chest trauma (rib fractures)

Ventilation or perfusion disturbances
- Pulmonary emboli
- Atelectasis
- Pneumonia
- Emphysema
- Chronic bronchitis
- Bronchiolitis
- ARDS

Diffusion disturbances
- Pulmonary/interstitial fibrosis
- Pulmonary edema
- ARDS
- Anatomic loss of functioning lung tissue (pneumonectomy)

ARDS, Acute respiratory distress syndrome; *COPD,* chronic obstructive pulmonary disease.

ASSESSMENT

Clinical presentation: Indicators of acute respiratory failure vary according to the underlying disease process and severity of the failure. Acute respiratory failure is one of the most common causes of impaired LOC. Respiratory failure is often associated with heart failure, pneumonia, or stroke. Sometimes the onset of acute respiratory failure is so insidious it is missed. Staff members do not want to disturb patients who appear to be sleeping, when in reality, a patient may be somnolent due to hypercapnea (CO_2 retention) from ventilatory failure.

Early indicators: Dyspnea, restlessness, anxiety, headache, fatigue, cool and dry skin, increased BP, tachycardia, and cardiac dysrhythmias.
Intermediate indicators: Confusion, lethargy, tachypnea, hypotension caused by vasodilation, cardiac dysrhythmias.
Late indicators: Cyanosis, diaphoresis, coma, respiratory arrest.

DIAGNOSTIC TESTS

ABG analysis: Assesses adequacy of oxygenation and effectiveness of ventilation. Typical results are Pao_2 <60 mm Hg, $Paco_2$ >45 mm Hg, and pH <7.35, which are consistent with severe respiratory acidosis. Pulse oximetry is used for continuous monitoring of oxygen saturation (see p. 176).

Mixed venous oxygen saturation (Svo_2): Mixed venous blood gases are drawn intermittently or measured continuously from the distal tip of the pulmonary artery catheter. A blood sample taken from this site ensures complete mixing of the blood returned from all parts of the body. Changes in Svo_2 provide an early indication of perfusion failure or increased tissue demands for oxygen. Svo_2 is a more sensitive indicator of oxygen available for tissue oxygenation than Spo_2. Normal values are 60%-80%. A value <50% is associated with impaired tissue oxygenation.

Chest x-ray: Ascertains presence of underlying pathophysiology or disease process that may be contributing to the failure.

COLLABORATIVE MANAGEMENT

Correction of hypoxemia: First treatment priority. Pao_2 levels <30 mm Hg for longer than 5 min may cause permanent brain damage or death. High-concentration oxygen therapy, in conjunction with pharmacotherapy (e.g., bronchodilators, steroids, antibiotics), often improve ABG levels sufficiently to remove the patient from danger. Patients with COPD who retain CO_2 (chronic hypercapnia) are unable to receive high concentrations of oxygen unless on positive pressure ventilation (bilevel continuous positive airway pressure [BiPAP].

Correction of hypercapnia leading to respiratory acidosis: May be corrected using noninvasive positive pressure ventilation (NPPV), such as BiPAP, or mechanical ventilation following ET intubation. Adequate cellular and metabolic functioning is hindered when pH level remains outside the normal range of 7.35-7.45. When the pH is <7.20, IV sodium bicarbonate may be used conservatively and usually only when the patient is mechanically ventilated. A pH >7.45 may be managed by placing a rebreathing mask on the patient or increasing dead space on mechanical ventilator circuitry.

Intubation and mechanical ventilation: The purposes of intubation and mechanical ventilation are to restore alveolar ventilation, restore pH level within normal limits, and decrease work of breathing. Early intubation can prevent further airway collapse and tissue injury. In most cases the patient will require intubation and mechanical ventilation to support adequate respiratory function and stabilize ABG levels. Noninvasive (NPPV) or invasive mechanical support is used until the underlying cause of the failure can be corrected and the patient can resume ventilatory efforts independently. Mechanical ventilation is discussed in greater depth in Chapter 1.

Research Brief 3-5 The investigators studied 14 patients with acute respiratory failure on the first day of mechanical ventilation in the volume-controlled mode. Increasing respiratory rate did not improve CO_2 clearance, produced hyperinflation, and impaired right ventricular ejection. Increasing respiratory rate is proposed to improve CO_2 clearance in this population. Efficacy may be limited by dead space ventilation coupled with induced hemodynamic instability related to alveolar hyperinflation.

Viellard-Baron A et al: Increasing respiratory rate to improve CO_2 clearance during mechanical ventilation is not a panacea in acute respiratory failure, *Crit Care Med* 30(7):1407-1412, 2002.

NURSING DIAGNOSES AND INTERVENTIONS

See sections relating to patient's underlying pathologic condition. Refer to Mechanical Ventilation, p. 14 for further information.

Bibliography

Acute Respiratory Distress Syndrome Network: Ventilation with lower tidal volumes as compared with traditional tidal volumes for acute lung injury and the acute respiratory distress syndrome, *N Engl J Med* 42:1301-1308, 2000.

American Heart Association: Primary or unexplained pulmonary hypertension, www.american-heart.org, retrieved March 1, 2003.

American Lung Association: Fact sheet: primary pulmonary hypertension, retrieved 2001 from www.lungusa.org.

Balas MC: Prone positioning of patients with acute respiratory distress syndrome: applying research to practice, *Crit Care Nurs* 20(1):24-35, 2000.

Barst RJ: Medical therapy of pulmonary hypertension: an overview of treatment and goals, *Clin Chest Med* 22(3):509-515, 2001.

Buckley JD, Popovich Jr J: Pulmonary embolism. In Parrillo JE, Dellinger RP: *Critical care medicine*, ed 2, St Louis, 2002, Mosby.

Dellinger RP: Life-threatening asthma. In Parrillo JE, Dellinger RP: *Critical care medicine*, ed 2, St Louis, 2002, Mosby.

Frakes MA: Measuring end tidal carbon dioxide: clinical applications and usefulness, *Crit Care Nurs* 21(5):23-35, 2001.

Galie N et al: Effects of beraprost sodium, an oral prostacyclin analogue, in patients with pulmonary arterial hypertension: a randomized, double-blind, placebo-controlled trial, *J Am Coll Cardiol* 39(9):1496-1502, 2002.

Gerbeaux P et al: Use of heliox in patients with severe exacerbation of chronic obstructive pulmonary disease, *Crit Care Med* 29(12):2322-2324, 2001.

Goss CH et al: Incidence of acute lung injury in the United States, *Crit Care Med* 31(6):1607-1611, 2003.

Grap MJ: Ventilator-associated pneumonia: clinical significance and implications for nursing, *Heart Lung* 26(6):419-429, 1997.

Gurka DP, Balk RA: Acute respiratory failure, including acute lung injury and ARDS. In Parrillo JE, Dellinger RP: *Critical care medicine*, ed 2, St Louis, 2002, Mosby.

Harris JR, Miller TH: Preventing nosocomial pneumonia: evidence based practice, *Crit Care Nurs* 20(1):51-68, 2000.

Henneman E et al: Effect of a collaborative weaning plan on patient outcome in the critical care setting, *Crit Care Med* 29:297-303, 2001.

Hynes-Gay P, MacDonald R: Using high frequency oscillatory ventilation to treat adults with acute respiratory distress syndrome, *Crit Care Nurs* 21(5):38-47, 2001.

Kirby RR, Taylor RW, Civetta JM: *Handbook of critical care,* ed 2, Philadelphia, 1997, Lippincott-Raven.

Lode hr et al: Nosocomial pneumonia in the critical care unit, *Crit Care Clin* 14(1):119-133, 1998.

Luce JM. Acute lung injury and the acute respiratory distress syndrome *Crit Care Med* 26:369-376, 1998.

Mandell, LA et al: Update of practice guidelines for the management of community acquired pneumonia in immunocompetent adults, *Clin Infect Dis* 37:1405-1427, 2003.

McCloskey JC, Bulechek GM: *Nursing interventions classification (NIC),* ed 3, St Louis, 2000, Mosby.

Meade MO et al: Agreement between alternative classifications of acute respiratory distress syndrome, *Am J Resp Crit Care Med* 163:490-493, 2001.

Misasi R, Keyes J: Matching and mismatching ventilation and perfusion in the lung, *Crit Care Nurs* 16(3):23-40, 1996.

Moss M, Mannino DM: Race and gender differences in acute respiratory distress syndrome deaths in the United State: an analysis of multiple-cause mortality data (1979-1996), *Crit Care Med* 30:1679-1685, 2002.

Misasi R, Keyes J: Matching and mismatching ventilation and perfusion in the lung, *Crit Care Nurs* 16(3):23-40, 1996.

Nauser TD, Stites SW: Diagnosis and treatment of pulmonary hypertension, *Am Fam Physician* 63:1789-1800, 2001.

Niederman MS: Pneumonia: considerations for the critically ill patient. In Parrillo JE, Dellinger RP: *Critical care medicine,* ed 2, St Louis, 2002, Mosby.

Pierce LNB: Traditional and non-traditional modes of mechanical ventilation, *Crit Care Nurs* 22(4):56-59, 2002.

Rich S, Kaufmann E, Levy PS: The effect of high doses of calcium-channel blockers on survival in primary pulmonary hypertension, *N Engl J Med* 327(2):76-81, 1992.

Siela D: Using chest radiography in the intensive care unit, *Crit Care Nurs* 22(4):18-29, 2002.

Silverboard H, Martin GS, Moss IM: Evaluating ARDS: a fresh look at a difficult diagnosis, *J Resp Dis* 24(8):340-348, August, 2003.

St. John RE: The pulmonary system. In Alspach JG, editor: *American Association of Critical Care Nurses core curriculum for critical care nursing,* ed 5, Philadelphia, 1998, Saunders.

Thelan LA et al: *Critical care nursing: diagnosis and management,* ed 3, St Louis, 1998, Mosby.

Nauser TD, Stites SW: Diagnosis and treatment of pulmonary hypertension, *Am Fam Physician* 63(9):1789-1802, 2001.

U.S. Department of Health and Human Services, National Institutes of Health, National Heart, Lung and Blood Institute: Practical Guide for the diagnosis and management of asthma, NIH Publication No 97-4053, October 1997.

Villar J, Perez-Mendez L, Kacmarek RM: Current definitions of acute lung injury and the acute respiratory distress syndrome do not reflect their true severity and outcome, *Intensive Care Med* 25:930-935, 1999.

Ware LB, Matthay MA: The acute respiratory distress syndrome, *N Engl J Med* 342:1334-1339, 2000.

CHAPTER 4

Cardiovascular Dysfunctions

Acute Coronary Syndromes: Chest Pain—Angina Pectoris and Myocardial Infarction

PATHOPHYSIOLOGY

Acute or unstable coronary syndromes include chest discomfort caused by either myocardial ischemia or pain associated with myocardial infarction. *Angina pectoris* is chest discomfort or pain associated with myocardial ischemia, caused by insufficient coronary blood flow to meet myocardial oxygen demands (e.g., during exercise). If the pain has a predictable pattern, it is considered stable. Those with ischemic pain that occurs at rest or with normal activity have *unstable angina.* Angina may occur when the coronary blood flow is reduced as a result of vessel lumen narrowing by plaque or when perfusion pressure is low, as in sudden hypotension. Angina may also be due to increased myocardial workload as in aortic stenosis, when oxygen demands are greatly elevated. The heart's workload is significantly increased by pumping against the tremendous resistance to ejection created by the narrowed aortic valve. Dysrhythmias may also cause chest discomfort caused either by increased workload (e.g., with tachycardias) or coronary perfusion deficit (e.g., with bradycardias).

Acute myocardial infarction (AMI) is necrosis of myocardial tissue resulting from relative or absolute lack of blood supply to the myocardium. Most AMIs are caused by atherosclerosis, which results in plaque formation within the coronary arteries. Plaque deposition results in endothelial changes, which over time cause narrowing of the lumen of the coronary artery. If an unstable plaque ruptures, the immune system responds with localized inflammation, platelets aggregate at the site of the injured plaque, and a thrombus forms; and if the lesion is large enough to fill the vessel lumen, this process results in total occlusion of blood flow. Occlusion can also be caused by coronary artery spasm. The site and size of myocardial infarction is determined by the location of the arterial occlusion. Research has revealed that the presence of specific inflammatory substrates may be an effective tool to help diagnose progressive coronary vascular disease.

American Heart Association (AHA) and American College of Cardiology (ACC) standards recommend treatment protocols for three types of acute coronary syndromes: unstable angina, myocardial infarction (MI) with ST segment elevation (STEMI) and MI without ST segment elevation (NSTEMI or nonSTEMI). Patients with STEMI and NSTEMI evolve to an electrocardiogram (ECG) with or without Q waves. The type of clot present in the coronary artery determines the appropriate treatment. Platelet-rich clots often result in unstable angina or NSTEMI, whereas fibrin-rich clots result in STEMI.

The cause of acute chest pain may not be related to myocardial ischemia. Differential diagnosis of cardiac pain versus other origins is critical and can challenge the most experienced clinician. Extracardiac causes of chest pain include pulmonary embolus, pneumonia, bronchitis, pneumothorax, aortic arch or high thoracic aortic aneurysm, esophagitis, hiatal hernia, cholecystitis, cholelithiasis, gastroesophageal reflux disease (GERD), costochondritis, musculoskeletal strain, anemia, hypoglycemia, fractured ribs or sternum, hyperthyroidism, hypothyroidism, obstipation, and bowel obstruction. Cardiac causes of chest pain not directly related to ischemia include valvular disease, cardiac trauma, cardiac tamponade, pericarditis, and endocarditis.

The diagnostic process should initially focus on ruling out MI. It is the most common cause of severe, unrelieved chest pain and requires immediate reperfusion therapy to minimize loss of myocardium. Left unchecked, patients with large areas of necrosis can progress to cardiogenic shock quickly. The patient's history and physical examination provide the initial framework for treatment decisions, coupled with the initial diagnostic ECG and assessment of serum enzyme levels and, more recently, of the presence of inflammatory substrates to evaluate for acute or impending MI. If MI does not appear likely from these findings, differential diagnosis of chest pain should then focus on identification of other life-threatening events such as dissecting thoracic or aortic arch aneurysms, large pulmonary embolism, or cardiac tamponade.

ASSESSMENT

History and risk factors: Familial history of coronary artery disease (CAD), age >70 yr, male sex (risk for females increases after menopause), cigarette smoking, hypercholesterolemia, hyperlipidemia, hypertension, diabetes, obesity, increased stress, sedentary lifestyle.

Clinical presentation

Angina pectoris

Chest pain caused by myocardial ischemia, which may result from exertion or emotional upset; usually subsides with rest; lasts for about 1-4 min but generally not longer than 30 min; should subside gradually when precipitating factor is removed; should be relieved by nitroglycerin, usually within 45-90 sec. Can be an abrupt or gradual onset of substernal discomfort described as deep, visceral, squeezing, choking, burning, heavy, tight, or aching. Many patients will deny the presence of chest "pain" but will admit to severe chest "discomfort" or "pressure." Pain may radiate to the jaw, neck, arms, or hands. Certain patients have pain in the teeth and may be referred from an emergent dental visit. Diabetic patients, particularly those taking beta (β)-adrenergic blocking agents, can experience myocardial ischemia leading to myocardial infarction entirely without pain. Diabetic neuropathy coupled with the β-adrenergic blocking drugs masks symptoms of MI.

Forms of angina

Stable: Has not increased in frequency or severity over a period of several months. Does not occur at rest.

Unstable: A broad category that includes several types. Usually the quality of pain has changed or increased in frequency, duration, or severity; can occur at rest.

- Wellen's syndrome: unstable angina, usually associated with left anterior descending (LAD) coronary artery lesions.
- Rest angina: chest discomfort which occurs without an increase in activity.
- New-onset angina: chest discomfort which has not occurred previously.
- Preinfarction or crescendo: unstable angina with the potential for progression to infarction. Patients with preinfarction angina may exhibit a rise in troponin level if microemboli from an enlarging clot in a coronary vessel clot break off and lodge in the coronary microvasculature. Microembolization markedly increases the possibility of MI. Mild ST segment elevation is noted in many of these patients.

Prinzmetal (variant): May occur at rest, long after exercise, and during sleep; usually caused by coronary vasospasm.

Myocardial infarction

Chest pain with ST segment elevation, or without ST segment elevation and lasting for >30 minutes and/or is unrelieved by nitroglycerin, is indicative of myocardial infarction. These patients may or may not form Q waves on their ECG. Presence of new bundle branch block (especially left bundle branch block) also indicates MI. Diabetics may have a "silent MI," free of symptoms. Approximately 25% of AMIs are silent. Many characteristics of ischemic pain apply to infarct pain. Other associated signs and symptoms include nausea, vomiting, dyspnea, orthopnea, anxiety, apprehension, diaphoresis, unexplained weakness and fatigue, cyanosis, and denial. Sometimes the presentation can be vague, manifesting with symptoms of gastrointestinal (GI) upset such as heartburn, no chest discomfort, with only arm or shoulder pain, or jaw/dental pain. The elderly with acute MI are more frequently first seen with symptoms of fatigue, shortness of breath (SOB), nausea/vomiting, syncope, weakness, falls, congestive heart failure, and pain in areas other than the chest. Women's symptoms are often more vague than men.

Older patients have a higher risk of stroke—both with and without thrombolytic therapy. Thrombolytic-eligible women have been offered reperfusion strategies significantly less frequently than men, as women are more difficult to diagnose, are older than men with acute MI, and may have more comorbidities. The AHA and the ACC developed the first set of evidenced-based guidelines for management of women with heart disease in 2004.

Physical assessment: Blood pressure (BP) may be elevated related to the sympathetic response to the patient's pain experience. BP may also decrease when pain is caused by ischemia or infarction, because the loss of myocardial perfusion results in decreased myocardial contractile strength and decreased cardiac output. Heart rate (HR) may increase in response to hypoxia and enhanced sympathetic tone, or the patient may have other dysrhythmias such as sinus bradycardia, atrioventricular (AV) blocks, or ventricular ectopy. S_4 heart sound may be audible during ischemic and infarction episodes. Infarcting patients may have an elevated temperature because of inflammation and may develop abnormal heart sounds including split S_1 and S_2, as well as S_3 if left-sided heart failure ensues. Other chest sounds may include a pericardial friction rub, crackles in lung fields, and new murmurs. The elderly may manifest sensorimotor and cognitive deficits if stroke is also present.

DIAGNOSTIC TESTS
Electrocardiogram (ECG)

Angina pectoris: myocardial ischemia
Characteristic changes may establish diagnosis of ischemic heart disease, although the absence of abnormality does not rule out this disease. In the absence of pain and with the patient at rest, the 12/15/18-lead ECG may be normal; therefore this test must be obtained during an episode of chest pain. ST segment and T wave changes, which occur during spontaneous chest pain and disappear with relief of the pain, are significant. The most characteristic change is depression of the ST segment with or without T wave inversion. In variant or Prinzmetal angina, the ST segments may be elevated during the chest pain episode. If chest pain persists for more than 30 min, serial ECGs should be repeated approximately every 30 min for 2 hr to determine if the patient is having an MI. With Wellen's syndrome, characteristic changes include inverted symmetric T waves with little or no ST elevation.

Acute myocardial infarction
The first ECG is done immediately and is used as part of the process to differentiate AMI from angina pectoris or other causes of chest pain, and to help determine suitability for antiplatelet medications (often given to patients with unstable angina and NSTEMI) versus thrombolytic therapy or other reperfusion strategy (e.g., coronary angioplasty) for MI. Reperfusion strategies should be implemented immediately for STEMI patients. The standard 12-lead ECG is designed for evaluation of the anterior, inferior, and lateral walls of the left ventricle (LV). Infarcts that extend to the right ventricle (RV) and/or the posterior wall of the LV cannot be clearly detected by the 12-lead. Indications for performing additional ECG evaluation with 15 or 18 leads include: ST segment elevation suggestive of an inferior wall MI (II, III, AVF); isolated ST segment elevation in V_1 or ST segment elevation in V_1 is greater than in V_2; borderline ST segment elevation in V_5 and V_6 or in V_1 through V_3; and ST segment depression or suspicious isoelectric ST segments in V_1 through V_3. ECGs are then done in a series (initially, and then every 30 min for the first 2 hr). Characteristic changes in certain lead groups identify the area and evolution of infarct. After the initial evaluation phase, ECGs may be done every 8-24 hr. Changes include:

Q waves: May or may not be present with patients having an MI. Are indicative of MI or are "pathologic" if they meet one of two criteria: wide (>.04 sec) and/or deep (>25% of the total voltage of the QRS). Q waves have been used as one of the diagnostic criteria for acute MI to determine if a reperfusion strategy is appropriate for the patient. Patients who initially are without Q waves may develop them later, or the tissue necrosis may extend itself if a reperfusion strategy is withheld. In the past, non-Q wave MIs often were left untreated, because it was thought the risk of thrombolysis outweighed the benefits.

ST segment changes and new bundle branch block: Should be elevated in the leads "over" or facing the infarcted area. Reciprocal changes (ST segment depressions) will be found in leads 180 degrees from the area of infarction. Not all patients experience ST segment elevation with MI. New bundle branch block, especially left bundle branch block, coupled with other findings, may also indicate MI is present.

> **Note:** Fewer than 42% of patients with acute MI have diagnostic ST segment elevation on their emergency department admission 12-lead ECG. Also, bundle branch blocks can distort the 12-lead ECG, making recognition of ST segment elevation difficult to impossible. Mild ST segment elevation is seen in some patients before MI, related to microemboli breaking off the ruptured plaque where the clot is evolving in the damaged coronary vessel.
>
> For posterior wall MI, ECG diagnosis is made only by notation of the reciprocal changes apparent in the anterior leads. Diagnosis of this type MI is difficult with solely a 12-lead ECG. For right ventricular MI, only changes in the V_1 lead suggest a problem in this area. Use of 15- or 18-lead ECGs that provide a more direct view of the posterior and right ventricular walls of the heart is recommended for more accurate diagnosis of both posterior wall and right ventricular MI.

T wave changes: May occur hours to weeks after infarction. Within the initial hour of infarction, tall, peaked, "hyperacute" upright T waves may be seen in leads over the infarct. Within several hours to days, the T wave becomes inverted. Gradually over time, the ST segment becomes isoelectric and the T wave may remain inverted. T wave changes may last for weeks and return to normal or remain inverted for the rest of the patient's life. T wave changes reflective of posterior and right ventricular MI are not clearly seen in the 12-lead ECG. Use of 15- or 18-lead ECG should provide clearer information about these areas (Table 4-1).

Serial cardiac enzyme levels (biochemical cardiac markers): Serum cardiac enzymes should be measured on all patients who experience chest pain of any etiology at the onset of pain and at least q8h × 3 to assess for signs of MI. See Table 4-2 for biochemical marker information.

TABLE 4-1   12-18 Lead ECG Location of Myocardial Infarction

MI Location	Leads reflecting MI	Reciprocal leads	Affected artery(ies)
Intraventricular septum	V1, V2	Not seen	Left coronary, LAD septal branch
Anterior LV	V3, V4	II, III, AVF	Left coronary, LAD diagonal branch
Lateral LV	V5, V6	V1-V3	Left coronary circumflex branch
Posterior LV	V7-V9 *	V1-V4	Right coronary or circumflex branch
Right ventricle (RV)	V1R-V6R *	Not seen	Right coronary with proximal branches
Inferior LV	II, III, AVF	I, AVL	Right coronary posterior descending branch

*Leads must be added to normal 12-lead ECG.
LAD, Left anterior descending artery; *LV,* left ventricle.

TABLE 4-2   Myocardial Infarction Biochemical Marker Information

Cardiac enzyme	Elevation begins	Elevation peaks	Normalizes
Myoglobin	1-3 hr	6-7 hr	24 hr
CK-MB Isoform	2-6 hr	18 hr	Unknown
CK-MB	3-12 hr	24 hr	48-72 hr
Troponin I	3-12 hr	24 hr	5-10 days
Troponin T	3-12 hr	12 hrs-2 days	5-14 days

Generally a creatine kinase-myocardial band (CK-MB) isoenzyme level that is >10% of the total CK is indicative of myocardial muscle damage. The ratio of the MB2 (cardiac) to MB1 (all muscle) types of CK-MB is also diagnostic for MI if the ratio becomes >2.5. Normal levels may vary from one institution or laboratory instrument to another. If MI is strongly suspected and CK total and MB are within normal limits (WNL), testing for troponin will provide the best diagnostic information.

C-reactive protein (highly sensitive or hs-CRP) studies: If elevated (normal range 0.03-1.1 mg/dl), indicate coronary artery plaques are inflammatory, placing the patient at higher probability of an imminent acute coronary event.

B-type ("brain") natriuretic peptide (BNP): A cardiac neurohormone secreted in response to ventricular volume expansion and pressure overload. Levels may be obtained in patients with MI to assess for presence/degree of ventricular dysfunction. If elevated, ventricular dysfunction is present.

Homocysteine: A toxic, highly reactive amino acid synthesized during protein catabolism. Patients lacking folate and vitamins B_6 and B_{12} have been shown to have elevated levels (>15mmol/L in critically ill patients), which can lead to accelerated arterial plaque formation.

Chest x-ray: May reveal cardiac enlargement or new infiltrates indicative of heart failure in MI patients. Cardiomegaly indicates myocardial ischemia and decreased myocardial contractility in patients with ischemic heart disease. May also provide information regarding other anomalies that cause chest pain such as pneumonia, pneumothorax, thoracic fractures, and aortic aneurysm.

Echocardiography (ECHO): Ultrasound technique used on the chest wall above the heart to detect abnormalities of left ventricular wall motion, measure ejection fraction, evaluate valve function, and estimate left ventricular end-diastolic pressure (LVEDP). Normal ejection fraction is >60%. Wall motion abnormalities or reduced ejection fraction may indicate an MI and will help define any risk of heart failure.

Transesophageal echocardiography (TEE): Ultrasound technique done via a high-frequency transducer attached to an endoscope inserted into the esophagus as the patient swallows. Provides clearer ultrasonic images of the heart.

Complete blood cell count (CBC): May provide useful information regarding possible anemia or infection/inflammation. Can assist in differential diagnosis of chest discomfort.

Serum electrolytes: May provide information regarding potential for development of dysrhythmias or the cause of dysrhythmias occurring with chest discomfort.

Coagulation studies: Obtained as part of screening for thrombolytic therapy in acute MI patients, wherein a question exists about potential for bleeding. More extensive coagulation studies may provide information about hematologic problems associated with an increased risk of thrombosis formation.

Multiple-gated acquisition (MUGA) scanning: Intravenous (IV) injection of the isotope *technetium pertechnetate* to evaluate left ventricular function and detect aneurysms, wall motion abnormalities, and intracardiac shunting. In the stress MUGA test, the same test is performed at rest and after exercise.

Stress test: Patient exercises while being monitored by electrocardiography. Its purpose is to elicit chest pain and document any associated ECG changes. Positive stress test results elicit at least 1-mm horizontal depression or downsloping ST segment in one or more leads that lasts 0.08 sec. In addition, frequent premature ventricular complexes (PVCs) or runs of ventricular tachycardia are suggestive of ischemia. Not indicated if acute MI is suspected.

Thallium treadmill stress test: Normal myocardial tissue will accumulate thallium, whereas infarcted or ischemic areas will have decreased uptake, appearing as "cold spots" on the scan. To identify areas of decreased uptake, the patient exercises after an injection of thallium. A scan is obtained both immediately after exercise and 4 hr later to determine if areas with decreased uptake fill in after 4 hr. Ischemic areas that fill in are considered to have viable tissue and reversible damage, whereas areas that remain as "cold spots" are diagnosed as infarcted. For MI patients, generally used after the acute phase of MI.

Thallium stress test with medications: Used when exercise is not possible because of physical disabilities or exercise intolerance. Either dypyridamole (Persantine), dobutamine, or adenosine has been used to "stress" the patient. Not generally used for patients at high risk for infarction or those who are experiencing acute MI, because the test can prompt MI.

Technetium 99m pyrophosphate radionuclide imaging: May help to localize area of infarction and demonstrate necrotic tissue. IV pyrophosphate will bind with calcium, which is found in high concentrations within the cells of necrotic tissue, and appears as a darkened area or "hot spot" on the scan up to 10 days after MI.

Technetium 99m sestamibi radionuclide imaging: Enhances nuclear imaging to allow clearer views of myocardial tissue perfusion, ventricular function, and gated pool ejection fractions.

Magnetic resonance imaging (MRI) and computed tomography (CT) scan: Used to assess ventricular size, morphology, function, and status of cardiac valves and coronary circulation. Magnetic resonance imaging (MRI) generally provides more detail than does computed tomography (CT).

Coronary angiocardiography or cardiac catheterization (cardiac cath): To determine presence and extent of CAD or valvular disease as the cause of the chest pain or myocardial infarction. Reliably determines the status of coronary perfusion to the left and right sides of the heart. A radiopaque catheter is inserted through a peripheral vessel and advanced to the heart, where measurements are done of ejection fraction, degree of stenosis of vessels and valves, status of pressures in the major vessels and chambers (atria and ventricles), and wall motion. Characteristics of lesions can be described for prescription of most appropriate treatment. Cardiac cath also allows for direct injection of thrombolytics (e.g., streptokinase, tissue plasminogen activator [t-PA]) into the coronary system during acute MI.

Positron emission tomography (PET): Use of isotopes to assess metabolic activity of areas of infarction to determine if viable, but jeopardized, myocardial tissue is present. Viable tissue has metabolic activity as seen by increased uptake of the glucose tracer and decreased uptake of the blood flow tracer, which is ammonia.

Indium 111 antimyosin imaging: Technique in which antibodies (antimyosin) are labeled with radioactive indium 111 and injected to permit visualization of damaged areas. The antibody is taken up by damaged myocardial cells as white blood cells rush to the area as part of the inflammatory process.

Serum lipid tests

Cholesterol analysis: A total cholesterol test measures the circulating levels of free cholesterol and cholesterol esters. Concentrations vary with age. Many physicians prefer patients to have a total cholesterol level of <200 mg/dl, but if fractionation is used, other risk factors are considered prior to recommending patients lower their cholesterol level if >200 mg/dl.

Lipoprotein-cholesterol fractionation: Measures the major lipids in the serum, including very low–density lipoproteins (VLDLs), low-density lipoproteins (LDLs), and high-density lipoproteins (HDLs). There is lower incidence of CAD when patients have higher levels of HDL. Normal HDL levels range 40-77 mg/dl; normal LDL levels range 62-130 mg/dl. High LDL levels increase the risk of CAD. Various fractionation systems are available, wherein the significant cardiac risk factors are analyzed before prescribing appropriate treatments. Acceptable lab values vary for patients, depending on their other risk factors.

Triglyceride analysis: Analyzes the storage form of lipids, which constitute 95% of fatty tissue. Although not diagnostic of CAD, enables early identification of individuals who may have increased risk of CAD. Triglyceride values are age-related, but a generally accepted range is 40-150 mg/dl in individuals aged 50-59 yr.

Serum magnesium level: Often drops in AMI. Low levels are associated with dysrhythmias.

COLLABORATIVE MANAGEMENT

Relief of acute pain: Drugs are administered and titrated to reduce or eliminate chest pain. Morphine, oxygen, nitrates and aspirin (MONA) are considered primary treatment modalities.

Oxygen: Usually 2-4 L/min by nasal cannula, or mode and rate as directed by arterial blood gas (ABG) values. Used to promote both myocardial and generalized increases in oxygenation. As oxygen (O_2) delivery to the heart is enhanced, pain can be relieved. If the patient deteriorates, other methods of O_2 delivery may be implemented (e.g., nonrebreather mask with reservoir and mechanical ventilation for those who deteriorate markedly).

Note: Patients with chest discomfort that is unrelieved by O_2 and nitrates are in all probability having an acute MI and should be evaluated immediately for a reperfusion strategy.

Oral, sublingual, and other forms of nitrates/nitroglycerin (NTG): Can be used for short-term therapy or longer-lasting prophylactic effects. These non-IV medications are used for management of myocardial ischemia or angina pectoris rather than for MI.

IV nitrates/NTG: For unstable angina or evolving MI, it is titrated until relief is obtained, generally up to 200 mcg/min as long as the patient maintains a systolic BP of at least 80 mm Hg.

IV or oral immediate release morphine sulfate: Given in small increments (e.g., 2 mg) until relief is obtained. This medication is usually not necessary unless an MI is occurring. Low BP may contraindicate administration.

Antithrombin therapy: Heparin (unfractionated) or low–molecular weight heparin (fractionated) infusion is sometimes implemented to prevent clot extension and/or formation, particularly if significant ST depression (>1 mm) is noted or troponins are slightly positive. Dosage should be weight-based and follow a titration protocol based on ongoing studies of PTT/aPTT (partial thromboplastin time/activated partial thromboplastin time). If patients experience a drop in platelets with heparins, a direct thrombin inhibitor (i.e., Argatroban) may be used.

Antiplatelet therapy: Infusion of glycoprotein IIB/IIIA inhibitors (e.g., abciximab, eptifibatide, tirofiban) is implemented more regularly since receiving support of the AHA and ACC year 2000 advanced cardiac life support (ACLS) standards of emergency cardiac care. In patients with marked ST segment depression (>1 mm) or progressively unstable angina, antiplatelet therapy may halt the vessel occlusion process by interrupting platelet aggregation. Clots are unable to form without the "white clot scaffolding" provided by platelet aggregation. Aspirin is an antiplatelet drug.

Calcium channel blockers (e.g., nifedipine, diltiazem): No longer recommended for management of patients with acute coronary syndromes unless coronary artery spasms are strongly suspected.

Reduction of cardiac workload to decrease oxygen demand

β-Adrenergic blocking agents (e.g., metoprolol, carvedilol, propranolol): To decrease HR, BP, and myocardial contractility. Strongly recommended as part of primary pharmacologic therapy for acute MI patients.

Angiotensin-converting enzyme (ACE) inhibitors (e.g., enalapril, ramipril, quinapril): To decrease BP and thus reduce the resistance to ventricular ejection. Used for patients with myocardial ischemia and after MI if patients need long-term BP control. Effective in prevention of heart failure.

AT1 receptor antagonists (candesartan, eposartan, irbesartan, olmesartan, losartan, telmisartan: Have similar effects to ACEIs but have not proved to reduce mortality. AT1 receptor blocking agents are used in patients who are ACEI intolerant.

Fenoldopam: Used to help prevent contrast-induced nephropathy in azothemc patients undergoing cardiac catheterization. Recent studies indicate Mucomyst may be more effective.

Prevention, recognition, and treatment of dysrhythmias: ACLS algorithms (see Appendix 1) or agency protocol used.

Caution: Caution should be exercised in use of antidysrhythmic agents in acute MI patients, especially with management of reperfusion dysrhythmias.

Instability of the conduction system with acute MI is sometimes aggravated by use of antidysrhythmic agents. Electrical therapies such as synchronized cardioversion, defibrillation, external/transthoracic pacing, or transvenous pacing may provide a safer management strategy for these patients.

Limit activities: Restrictions based on patient's activity tolerance. Bed rest with bedside commode privileges generally is recommended for patients with acute MI for up to 12 hr after symptom onset. Longer periods of bed rest can promote development of orthostatic intolerance, which is preventable by elevation of the head of the bed, dangling the lower extremities, and other low-exertion activities. Patients should be instructed to avoid the Valsalva maneuver when toileting, because it may predispose them to ventricular dysrhythmias.

Management of unstable angina and non-ST segment elevation myocardial infarction (NSTEMI)

Prevention of initial or further coronary thrombus formation: May include administration of an anticoagulant/antithrombin (i.e., heparin or low–molecular weight heparin infusion) and antiplatelet drugs (e.g., aspirin, ticlopidine, GPIIb/IIIa inhibitors such as abciximab, eptifibatide, tirofiban) to prevent thrombus formation. In patients evolving towards MI, these agents are thought to abate complete closure of the coronary arteries or to prevent more extensive clot formation. Cardiac cath is often done to assess the size and location of coronary lesions.

Management of unstable acute MI with ST segment elevation (STEMI)

Hemodynamic monitoring: Used in a patient with a complicated MI resulting in ventricular failure with threat of cardiogenic shock. Pulmonary artery (PA) and capillary pressures are measured, along with cardiac output (CO) and systemic vascular resistance (SVR). Unstable patients may manifest increased pulmonary artery pressure (PAP), increased pulmonary artery wedge pressure (PAWP), decreased CO, and increased SVR.

Percutaneous transluminal coronary angioplasty (PTCA): The original percutaneous coronary intervention (PCI) performed for improving blood flow through stenotic coronary arteries. A balloon-tipped catheter is inserted into the coronary arterial lesion, and the balloon is inflated to compress the plaque material against the vessel wall, thereby opening the narrowed lumen. PTCA is performed on individuals with acute MI, postinfarction angina, postbypass angina, and chronic stable angina. The ideal candidate has single-vessel disease with a discrete, proximal, noncalcified lesion. As technology has improved, patients with more complex conditions have become routine candidates for the procedure if performed by an experienced invasive cardiologist.

During the procedure the patient is sedated lightly and is given a local anesthetic at the insertion site—usually the femoral artery. ECG electrodes are placed on the chest. A PA catheter is passed through the vena cava and right atrium into the heart for pressure measurements. A pacing wire may be inserted as well. An introducer sheath is inserted into the femoral artery, a guidewire is passed into the aorta and coronary artery, and the balloon catheter is passed over the guidewire to the stenotic site. The patient may be asked to take deep breaths and cough to facilitate passage of the catheter. Heparin is given to prevent clot formation. The balloon is inflated repeatedly for 60-90 sec at a pressure of 4-15 atmosphere (atm). Subsequently, radiopaque dye is injected to determine whether the stenosis has been reduced to less than 50% of the vessel diameter, which is the goal of the procedure. The introducer sheath is left in the femoral artery for up to 12 hr after PTCA for heparin infusion or in the event of the need for repeat angiography.

Complications after PTCA include acute coronary artery occlusion, coronary artery dissection, reocclusion in acute MI patients, AMI, coronary artery spasm, bleeding, circulatory insufficiency, renal hypersensitivity to contrast material, hypokalemia, vasovagal reaction, dysrhythmias, and hypotension. Restenosis can occur 6 wk-6 mo after PTCA, although the patient may not experience angina.

Coronary artery atherectomy: A PCI which removes atherosclerotic plaque from coronary arteries using a special catheter equipped with a cutting device that shaves the lesion. Fragments from the technique are collected into the "nose cone" of the device (directional atherectomy); pulverized and dispersed into the circulation (rotational or "rotoblade" atherectomy); or aspirated (transluminal extraction catheterization [TEC]). May be used for patients with myocardial ischemia and during or after an acute MI.

Intracoronary stent procedure: A PCI wherein endovascular stents (metal-mesh tubes) are used to keep arteries open. A variety of designs, materials, and deployment procedures are available. Newer "drug eluting" stents are coated with drugs to help prevent restenosis of the affected artery. Balloon-expanded stents are most commonly used in the United States and are inserted during PTCA. May be used for stenosed coronary arteries or to reopen stenotic coronary artery bypass graft (CABG) replacement vessels (grafts).

Laser coronary angioplasty: A PCI that enables debulking of distal coronary lesions in tortuous arteries to allow for reperfusion. The laser is a part of the coronary artery catheter (similar to the device used in PTCA) and ablates only the tissue it contacts.

Additional interventions for management of acute myocardial infarction

Thrombolytic therapy (lysis of coronary arterial clot): Used for reperfusion of the occluded coronary vessel(s) that causes AMI. Drugs include tenecteplase (TNK-tpa), alteplase (r-TPA, Activase); reteplase (Retavase); streptokinase; urokinase; and anisoylated plasminogen streptokinase activator complex (APSAC, Eminase). Thrombolytic therapy is an AHA and ACC class I intervention for patients with ST segment elevation in two or more contiguous leads, bundle branch block (obscuring ST segment analysis), and history suggestive of acute MI, who present within 12 hr of symptom onset and are <75 yr of age. Patients must be carefully screened for risk of bleeding before administration of these IV medications. Time from the entry of the patient into the emergency department of the hospital to treatment with thrombolytics should be no longer than 1 hr and, ideally, within 30 min of arrival. Thrombolytics are also used for direct injection into the coronary arteries as part of coronary angiography during cardiac catheterization and angioplasty.

Surgical revascularization: Surgical revascularization procedures are seldom used as the primary management strategy for acute MI. Several approaches are available for myocardial revascularization, including CABG via median sternotomy or minimally invasive technique. Patients with multivessel or diffuse CAD are the most appropriate candidates for these procedures. Surgical indications include (1) stable angina with 50% stenosis of the left main coronary artery, (2) stable angina with three-vessel CAD, (3) unstable angina with three-vessel disease or severe two-vessel disease, (4) recent MI, (5) ischemic heart failure with cardiogenic shock, and (6) signs of ischemia or impending MI after angiography procedure. Robotics have been used recently to assist the surgeon with the procedure.

Cardiac surgery should be readily available for patients who experience complications undergoing any diagnostic or treatment procedures in the cardiac cath laboratory.

NURSING DIAGNOSES AND INTERVENTIONS

Pain (chest) related to biophysiologic injury secondary to decreased oxygen supply to the myocardium

Desired outcomes: Within 30 minutes of intervention, patient's subjective evaluation of discomfort improves, as documented by a pain scale. Nonverbal indicators, such as grimacing, are absent. Vital signs (VS) return to baseline. ECG changes present during event resolve.

- Assess and document the character of the patient's chest pain, including location, duration, quality, intensity, precipitating and alleviating factors, presence or absence of radiation, and associated symptoms. Devise a pain scale with patient, rating discomfort from 0 (no pain) to 10 or any system that assists in objectively reporting pain level.
- Measure BP and HR with each episode of chest pain. BP and HR may increase because of sympathetic stimulation as a result of pain. If the chest pain is caused by ischemia, the heart muscle may not be functioning normally and cardiac output may decrease, resulting in a low BP. In addition, dysrhythmias such as bradycardia and ventricular ectopy may be noted with ischemia. If BP is low, it may not be advisable to administer nitrates and morphine, which can further reduce BP, adding to myocardial ischemia.
- Obtain a 12/15/18-lead ECG during patient's episode of chest pain. During angina, ischemia usually is demonstrated on the ECG by ST segment depression and T wave inversion.
- Administer nitrates as prescribed, titrating IV NTG so that chest pain is relieved yet SBP remains >90 mm Hg. NTG drip is usually 100 mg NTG in 250 ml D_5W. Begin with 3 ml/min, which is 20 mcg/min. Titrate by increments of 3 ml q5min (or 20 mcg/min q5min) up to a maximum dosage determined by agency protocol or physician.
- After each titration of IV NTG, evaluate patient's BP and the effects of therapy in relieving patient's chest pain. If slight hypotension occurs (80-90 mm Hg systolic), reduce the flow rate to one-half or less of the infusing dose. If severe hypotension (<80 mm Hg systolic) occurs, stop the infusion and contact the physician for further directions. In either situation the physician may prescribe a low-dose positive inotropic agent (e.g., dopamine, dobutamine) to enhance cardiac contractility. For additional information, see "Inotropic and Vasoactive Agents," Appendix 7.
- Monitor for side effects of NTG, including headache, hypotension, syncope, facial flushing, and nausea. If side effects occur, place patient in a supine position and consult physician for further interventions.
- As prescribed, administer β-blockers and possibly calcium channel blockers, which relieve chest pain by (1) diminishing coronary artery spasm, causing coronary and peripheral vasodilation and (2) decreasing myocardial contractility and oxygen demand. Monitor for side effects, including bradycardia and hypotension. Be alert to indicators of heart failure, including fatigue, SOB, weight gain, and edema, and to indicators of heart block, such as syncope and dizziness.
- Administer heparin, GPIIb/IIIa inhibitors (e.g., abciximab, tirofiban, eptifibatide), and ASA as prescribed. Heparin infusion usually should be administered using a weight-based protocol, which is titrated according to PTT results. These patients are predisposed to bleeding and may need to be placed on bleeding precautions.
- Administer oxygen per nasal cannula at 2-4 L/min, as prescribed.
- Position patient according to his or her comfort level.
- Provide care calmly and efficiently; reassure patient during chest pain episodes.
- Maintain a quiet environment, and group patient care activities to allow for periods of uninterrupted rest. Consider healing touch therapy, relaxation exercises, or music therapy.
- Ensure that activity restrictions and bed rest are maintained; teach patient about activity limitation and its rationale: to minimize oxygen requirements and thus decrease chest pain. Reassure patient that activities are allowed based on individual response. Often, patients may be afraid to engage in activities for fear of further deterioration.
- Instruct patient to report any further episodes of chest pain.
- For more information about pain, see Pain, p. 51.

NIC Pain Management; Analgesic Administration; Cardiac Care: Acute; Hemodynamic Regulation; Oxygen Therapy

Decreased cardiac output (or risk for same) related to negative inotropic changes secondary to vessel occlusion, infarction, coronary artery spasm, and cardiac tamponade; electrical factors secondary to dysrhythmias

Desired outcomes: Within 24 hr of this diagnosis, patient exhibits adequate cardiac output, as evidenced by BP within normal limits for patient; HR 60-100 beats/min; normal sinus rhythm on ECG; peripheral pulses >2+ on a 0-4+ scale; warm and dry skin; hourly urine output ≥0.5 ml/kg; measured CO 4-7 L/min; right atrial pressure (RAP) 4-6 mm Hg; PAP 20-30/8-15 mm Hg; PAWP 6-12 mm Hg; and patient awake, alert, oriented, and free from anginal pain.

- Monitor BP, RAP/CVP, and PAP continuously; monitor PAWP and CO hourly. Be alert to the following indicators of decreased cardiac output: decreased BP, increased HR, increased PAP, increased PAWP, decreased measured CO, and decreased RAP.
- Monitor ECG continuously for evidence of dysrhythmias and ST and T wave changes. Observe for bradycardia during sheath removal. Run a 12/15/18-lead ECG daily.
- Monitor urinary output hourly for the first 4 hr, and thereafter according to agency protocol. Consult physician for hourly output <0.5 ml/kg/hr for 2 consecutive hr.
- Measure CK-MB and troponin levels immediately after PTCA and then q8h for 24 hr; report elevations. Optimally, CK-MB will be 0%-5% of total CK and troponins will no longer be elevated. Some physicians may choose to monitor BNP (B-type natriuretic peptide) levels to assess if ventricular dysfunction is present and/or increasing.
- Monitor patient for hypotension caused by antianginal and coronary vasodilator medications. As a result of vessel occlusion, consult physician and treat hypotension immediately, as prescribed. Usually, fluids are given and the patient is placed in supine position. If the patient has left ventricular heart failure and pulmonary congestion, the supine position may prompt respiratory distress.
- When patient first sits up, ensure that it is done in stages to minimize the likelihood of postural hypotension. Monitor VS at frequent intervals during this stage.
- Monitor patient continuously for bleeding at sheath insertion site. Monitor hematocrit (Hct) level for decrease from baseline values.
- Monitor patient for evidence of cardiac tamponade: hypotension, tachycardia, pulsus paradoxus, jugular venous distention, elevation and plateau pressuring of PAWP and RAP, and possibly an enlarged heart silhouette on chest x-ray study.
- When heparin and antiplatelet drugs are discontinued, monitor patient closely for indicators of coronary occlusion: ST segment elevation on ECG, angina, hypotension, tachycardia, dysrhythmias, and diaphoresis.
- Monitor peripheral pulses (radial and pedal) and color and temperature of extremities q4h for first 4 hr.
- Monitor patient's mental alertness on an ongoing basis.

Additional interventions for decreased cardiac output for myocardial infarction

- Assess for and document the following as evidence of myocardial dysfunction with decreasing cardiac output: presence of jugular venous distention, dependent edema (e.g., sacral), hepatomegaly, fatigue, weakness, decreased activity level, and SOB with activity. In addition, assess and document the following:
  - ❏ *Mental status:* Be alert to restlessness, decreased responsiveness.
  - ❏ *Lung sounds:* Monitor for crackles, rhonchi.
  - ❏ *Heart sounds:* Note presence of gallop, murmur, increased HR.
  - ❏ *Urinary output:* Be alert to output <0.5 ml/kg/hr.
  - ❏ *Skin:* Monitor for pallor, mottling, cyanosis, coolness, diaphoresis.
  - ❏ *Vital signs:* Note BP <90 mm Hg systolic, HR >100 beats/min, respiratory rate (RR) >20 breaths/min, and temperature >38.5° C (101.3° F). The temperature of patients with MI may spike as a result of the body's reaction to necrotic tissue.
- Keep accurate intake and output (I&O) records, and weigh patient daily. Be alert to fluid volume excess. A 1-kg acute weight gain can signal retention of 1 L of fluid.
- Help minimize cardiac workload by administering prescribed β-blockers, positioning patient in Fowler's or semi-Fowler's position, and encouraging bed rest.
- Have patient perform active range-of-motion (ROM) exercises, along with level I activities (Table 4-3) to help prevent deleterious effects of bed rest on oxygen supplies.
- If a PA catheter is present, record hemodynamic readings q1-2h and prn. Be alert to PAWP >18 mm Hg, CO <4 L/min, and cardiac index (CI) <2.5 L/min/m^2.
- Administer and titrate prescribed medications: nitrates and afterload-reducing agents, such as nitroprusside, and preload-reducing agents, such as nitroglycerin, to maintain SVR within 900-1200 dynes/sec/cm^{-5} and PAWP ≤18 mm Hg; diuretics, such as furosemide and metolazone, to keep PAWP ≤18 mm Hg and urine output ≥0.5 ml/kg/hr; and inotropic agents, such as milrinone, dobutamine, and dopamine, to keep SBP >90 mm Hg.
- Monitor patient continuously in modified chest lead (MCL) V_1 to detect ventricular ectopy versus aberrancy. Monitor on V_2 if supraventricular dysrhythmias are present or if it is imperative to identify axis deviations. Keep alarms on at all times (e.g., 50-100).
- Assess apical HR hourly. Monitor for irregularities in rhythm.
- Document rhythm strip every shift and prn if dysrhythmias occur. Measure PR segment, QRS complex, and QT interval with each strip. Note and report any deviations from the patient's baseline.

T A B L E   4 - 3   Activity Level Progression for Hospitalized Patients*

Level		Activity
I	Bed rest	Flexion and extension of extremities qid, 15 times each extremity; deep breathing qid, 15 breaths; position change from side to side q2h
II	OOB to chair	As tolerated, tid for 20-30 min
III	Ambulate in room	As tolerated, tid for 20-30 min
IV	Ambulate in hall	Initially, 50-200 ft bid; progressing to 50-200 ft qid

Signs of activity intolerance: Decrease in BP <20 mm Hg; increase in HR to >120 beats/min (or >20 beats/min above resting HR in patients receiving β-blocker therapy).
BP, Blood pressure; *HR,* heart rate; *OOB,* out of bed.

Normal intervals are PR 0.10-0.20 sec and QRS 0.10 sec. The QT interval is rate-related, and the upper limits of normal usually correspond to approximately one-half the RR interval.
- Monitor serum potassium for levels >5 mEq/L or <3.5 mEq/L. Hypokalemia or hyperkalemia can cause dysrhythmias. Replace potassium as prescribed.

NIC Cardiac Care; Cardiac Care: Acute; Shock Prevention; Hemodynamic Regulation; Dysrhythmia Management

Activity intolerance related to imbalance between oxygen supply and demand secondary to decreased cardiac output associated with CAD
Desired outcome: Within the 12- to 24-hr period before discharge from critical care unit (CCU), patient exhibits cardiac tolerance to increasing levels of activity as evidenced by RR <24 breaths/min; normal sinus rhythm on ECG; BP within 20 mm Hg of patient's normal range; HR <120 beats/min (or within 20 beats/min of resting HR for patients on β-blocker therapy); and absence of chest pain.
- Assist patient with identifying activities that precipitate chest pain, and teach patient to use NTG prophylactically before the activity.
- Assist patient as needed in progressive activity program, beginning with level I and progressing to level IV, as tolerated (Table 4-3).
- Assess patient's response to activity progression. Be alert to presence of chest pain, SOB, excessive fatigue, and dysrhythmias. Monitor for a decrease in BP >20 mm Hg and an increase in HR to >120 beats/min (>20 beats/min above resting HR in patients receiving β-blocker therapy).
- Teach patient about measures that prevent complications of decreased mobility, such as active ROM exercises. (For additional details, see p. 61).

NIC Activity Therapy; Energy Management

Knowledge deficit: disease process and its lifestyle implications
Desired outcome: Within the 24-hr period before discharge from the step-down unit, patient verbalizes understanding of his or her disease, as well as the necessary lifestyle changes that may modify risk factors.
- Teach patient about ischemia and its resultant chest pain, referred to as *angina pectoris.*
- Discuss the pathophysiologic process underlying patient's angina, using drawings or heart models as indicated.
- Assist patient in identifying his or her own risk factors (e.g., cigarette smoking, high-stress lifestyle, high-fat diet).
- Teach patient about risk factor modification:
  - ❑ *Diet low in cholesterol and saturated fat:* Provide sample diet plan for meals that are low in cholesterol and saturated fat. Teach patient about foods that are high in cholesterol and those that are low in cholesterol and saturated fat (see Tables 4-4 and 4-5). Stress the importance of reading food labels.
  - ❑ *Smoking cessation:* Teach patient that smoking causes the coronary arteries to constrict, thus decreasing blood flow to the heart.
  - ❑ *Blood pressure control*: If patient was found to have hypertension associated with MI, the patient should be taught the importance of taking appropriate medications to control BP and to follow recommended dietary guidelines to minimize sodium intake. Sodium promotes water retention, which can increase the BP. Higher systemic BP increases the workload of heart, demanding more myocardial oxygen to be consumed. (See Table 4.6 for low-sodium dietary guidelines.)

❑ *Stress management:* Discuss the role that stress plays in angina. Explain that stress increases sympathetic tone, which can cause the BP and HR to increase, resulting in increased oxygen demand. By employing relaxation techniques such as imagery, meditation, or biofeedback, one can decrease the effects of stress on the heart. For a sample relaxation technique, see p. 259.
- Teach patient about the medications prescribed, including name, purpose, dosage, action, schedule, precautions, and potential side effects.
- Teach patient the actions that should be taken if chest pain is unrelieved or increases in intensity. If chest pain occurs:
  1. Stop and rest.
  2. Take one NTG; wait 5 min. If pain is not relieved, take a second NTG; wait 5 min. If pain is not relieved, take a third NTG.
  3. Lie down if headache occurs. (NTG lowers BP, causing headache and dizziness upon standing.)
  4. If the pain is not relieved after three NTGs are taken over a 15-min period, dial 911 or local emergency number.
- Review activity limitations and prescribed progressions (see Table 4-3; see also Table 4-7) and provide the following information:
  1. Depending on how you feel, you may only be able to stay at one level or you may progress to 2 miles quickly.
  2. Remember to warm up and cool down with stretches for 5-7 min and to walk 3-5 times each week.
  3. In addition:
  ❑ Avoid sudden energetic activities.
  ❑ Plan for regular rest periods in the afternoon.
  ❑ Let your body guide you regarding whether to increase or decrease activity.
  ❑ Inform your physician of any changes in activity tolerance, such as the development of new symptoms with the same activity.
  ❑ Avoid exercising outdoors in very cold, hot, or humid weather. Extreme weather places an additional stress on the heart. If you do exercise in extremes of weather, decrease the pace and monitor your response carefully.
- Pulse monitoring: Teach patient how to take pulse, including target heart rates and limits.
- Sexual activity guidelines: Because sexual activity is a physical activity, certain guidelines can help the patient and his or her partner enjoy a satisfying sexual relationship while minimizing the workload of the heart:
  ❑ Rest is beneficial before engaging in intercourse.
  ❑ Find a position that is comfortable for you and your partner. Assuming a different position that is uncomfortable to both may increase the workload of the heart.
  ❑ Medications such as NTG may be taken prophylactically by the patient before intercourse to prevent chest pain.
  ❑ Postpone intercourse for 1-1½ hr after eating a heavy meal.
  ❑ Report the following symptoms to your physician if they are experienced after sexual relations: SOB, increased HR that persists for more than 15 min, unrelieved chest pain.

▌NIC Teaching: Disease Process; Teaching: Prescribed Activity/Exercise; Teaching: Prescribed Medication; Teaching: Sexuality

For patients undergoing percutaneous transluminal coronary angioplasty
Knowledge deficit: angioplasty procedure and postprocedure care
Desired outcome: Within the 24-hr period before the procedure, patient describes the rationale for the procedure, how it is performed, and postprocedure care. Patient relates discharge instructions within the 24-hr period before discharge from the CCU.
- Assess patient's understanding of CAD and the purpose of angioplasty. Evaluate patient's style of coping and degree of information desired.
- As appropriate for coping style, discuss the following with patient and significant others:
  ❑ Location of patient's CAD, using heart drawing.
  ❑ Use of local anesthesia and sedation during procedure.
  ❑ Insertion site of catheter: groin or arm.
  ❑ Sensations that may occur: mild chest discomfort; a feeling of heat as the dye is injected.
  ❑ Use of fluoroscopy during procedure. Ask about prior sensitivity to contrast material.
  ❑ Ongoing observations done after procedure: BP, HR, ECG, leg or arm pulses, blood tests.
  ❑ Lying flat in bed for 6-12 hr after procedure unless a vascular closure device was used. Patients are able to get out of bed sooner when a closure strategy is used.
  ❑ How to ask for nursing assistance with eating, drinking, and toileting after procedure.
  ❑ Drinking lots of fluid after procedure to flush dye from system.

❑ Discharge instructions: importance of taking antiplatelet drugs to prevent restenosis, avoidance of strenuous activity during first few weeks at home, follow-up visit with cardiologist 1 wk after hospital discharge, signs and symptoms to report to physician (e.g., GI upset, repeat of angina, fainting).

• If patient and significant others express anxiety regarding the procedure, try to arrange for them to meet with another patient who has had a successful angioplasty.

NIC Teaching: Procedure/Treatment; Anxiety Reduction; Support Group

Altered tissue perfusion (or risk for same): peripheral: involved limb, related to interruption of arterial blood flow secondary to presence of angioplasty sheath; risk of clot formation in vessel after sheath removal

Desired outcome: On admission to CCU and continuously thereafter, patient has adequate tissue perfusion in the involved limb as evidenced by warm skin; peripheral pulses >2+ on a 0-4+ scale; normal skin color; ability to move the toes; and complete sensation.

• Monitor circulation to affected limb q30min for 2 hr and then q2h thereafter. Assess pulses, temperature, color, sensation, and mobility of toes. Be alert to weak or thready pulses, coolness and pallor of the extremity, and patient complaints of numbness and tingling. Consult physician immediately if any of these signs or symptoms are present.
• Inspect sheath site for signs of external or subcutaneous bleeding.
• Keep sandbag at insertion site until discontinued by physician.
• Maintain immobilization of limb for at least 6 hr or until discontinued by physician. *Requirements may differ per institutional protocols.*
• Keep head of bed (HOB) no higher than 15 degrees to prevent kinking of sheath.
• Monitor sheath patency by evaluating for continuous IV infusion into the involved vessel.
• Instruct patient to notify staff immediately if numbness, tingling, or pain occurs at the affected extremity.

NIC Peripheral Sensation Management; Surveillance

Knowledge deficit: myocardial infarction and its implications for lifestyle changes

Desired outcome: Within the 24-hr period before discharge from CCU, patient and significant others verbalize an understanding of heart attack and the necessary lifestyle changes that must be made.

• Discuss the following with patient and significant others, providing both oral instructions and written materials:
   ❑ Anatomy and functions of the heart muscle.
   ❑ Coronary arteries and the atherosclerotic process.
   ❑ Definition of "heart attack."
   ❑ Healing process of the heart and the role of collateral circulation.
• Assist patient with identifying his or her own risk factors.
• Assist patient with devising a plan for risk factor modification (e.g., diet, smoking cessation, stress-reduction techniques).
• Provide guidelines for a diet low in cholesterol and saturated fat (Tables 4-4 and 4-5) and high in vitamins B_6, B_{12} and folate; refer patient to nutritionist. Patient may consider supplemental multivitamins containing 0.4 mg of folic acid, 2 mg of B_6 (pyridoxine) and 6 mcg of B_{12} (cyanocobalamin).
• Discuss post-MI activity progression (e.g., a progressive walking program). See Tables 4-3 and 4-7.
• Discuss guidelines for resuming post-MI sexual activity. Explain that sexual activity requires the same amount of oxygen as that needed to walk briskly up two flights of stairs; consequently, patients usually are instructed to wait 2 wk after hospital discharge before resuming sexual activity.
• Teach patient about medications that will be taken after hospital discharge, including name, purpose, dosage, schedule, precautions, and potential side effects.

NIC Teaching: Prescribed Diet; Anxiety Reduction; Support Group; Teaching: Disease Process; Teaching: Prescribed Activity/Exercise; Teaching: Prescribed Medication; Teaching: Sexuality

For patients undergoing coronary artery bypass grafting (CABG) for myocardial revascularization

Risk for fluid volume deficit related to loss of fluid through normal and abnormal routes secondary to postoperative diuresis and excessive bleeding

Note: Diuresis is common in the early postoperative period because of the hormonal changes that accompany surgery.

Desired outcome: Patient is normovolemic as evidenced by intake equal to output plus insensible losses; RAP ≥4 mm Hg; PAWP ≥6 mm Hg; and urinary output between 30 and 120 ml/hr.

TABLE 4-4 Low-Cholesterol Dietary Guidelines

Foods to avoid	Foods allowed
Egg yolks (no more than 3/wk)	Egg whites; cholesterol-free egg substitutes
Foods made with many egg yolks (e.g., sponge cakes)	Lean, well trimmed meats; minimize servings of beef, lamb, and pork
Fatty cuts of meat, fat on meats	Fish (except shellfish), chicken, and turkey (without the skin)
Skin on chicken and turkey	
Luncheon meats or cold cuts	Dried peas and beans as meat substitutes
Sausage, frankfurters	Nonfat (skin) or low-fat (2%) milk
Shellfish (e.g., lobster, shrimp, crab)	Low-fat cheese
Whole milk, cream, whole milk cheese	Ice milk, sherbet, low-fat yogurt
Ice cream	Mono-saturated oils for cooking and food preparation: canola, safflower, olive
Commercially prepared foods with hydrogenated shortening, which is saturated fat	Margarines that list one of the above oils as their first ingredients
Coconut and palm oils and products made with them (e.g., cream substitutes)	Foods prepared "from scratch" with the above suggested oils
Butter, lard, hydrogenated shortening	Meats (in acceptable quantity) and vegetables prepared by broiling, steaming, or baking (never frying)
Meats and vegetables prepared by frying	
Seasonings containing large amounts of sugar and saturated fats	Spices, herbs, lemon juice, wine, flavored wine vinegars
Sauces and gravies	
Salad dressings containing cream, cheese, or mayonnaise	

TABLE 4-5 Guidelines for a Diet Low in Saturated Fat

Foods to avoid	Foods to choose
Red meat especially when highly "marbled"; salami, sausages, bacon	Lean cuts of meat, fresh fish, poultry from which skin was removed before cooking; meats that have been grilled
Whole milk, whipping cream	
Tropical oils (coconut, palm oils; cocoa butter)	Low-fat or skim milk
	Monosaturated cooking oils, such as olive or canola oil
Candy	Fresh fruit, vegetables
Sweet rolls, donuts	Whole grain breads, cereals
Ice cream	Nonfat yogurt, sherbet
Salad dressings	Vinegar, lemon juice
Peanut butter, peanuts, hot dogs, potato chips	Unbuttered popcorn
Butter	Margarine (safflower oil listed as the first ingredient)

- Measure I&O hourly. Consult physician for imbalance in I&O ratio (i.e., urinary output ≥120 ml/hr and chest tube drainage ≥100 ml/hr). Replace excessive chest tube drainage with packed red blood cells (RBCs) as prescribed.
- Monitor RAP and PAP mean hourly. Correlate PAP mean to PAWP. Consult physician for PAP/PAWP <6 mm Hg and RAP <4 mm Hg.
- As prescribed, administer IV fluids in the early postoperative period to equal the amount of diuresis.
- Monitor clotting studies (i.e., prothrombin time [PT], PTT, activated clotting time [ACT], platelet count) immediately after surgery and then q12h for 24 hr. Be alert to prolongation of PT, PTT, ACT;

decreased platelet count; and low fibrinogen value. Optimal values are the following: PT 11-15 sec; PTT 30-40 sec (activated); ACT ≤120 sec; platelet count 150,000-400,000/mm^3; and fibrinogen 200-400 mg/dl.
- Replace clotting factors as prescribed with platelets, fresh-frozen plasma, or cryoprecipitate; administer protamine or aminocaproic acid as prescribed.
- Assess chest x-ray films immediately after surgery and daily for signs of bleeding into the pericardial sac and mediastinum, as evidenced by an increase in the cardiac silhouette.

NIC Fluid Management; Fluid Monitoring; Blood Products Administration; Shock Management: Volume; Hypovolemia Management

Hypothermia related to prolonged cooling of body during surgery

Desired outcomes: Patient's body temperature is returned to normal at a rate not greater than 1° C/hr as evidenced by warm extremities and absence of shivering. Within 8 hr of treatment, oxygen saturation is ≥95%; CO is 4-7 L/min; SVR is ≥900 dynes/sec/cm^{-5}; HR is 60-100 beats/min; and BP is within patient's normal range.

Note: The danger of postoperative hypothermia in heart surgery is that the patient will warm too quickly and shiver, causing hypertension or hypotension, increased or decreased SVR, metabolic acidosis, and hypoxia. Each of these problems can increase cardiac workload and may potentiate ischemia, dysrhythmias, or hemorrhage in the early postoperative period.

- On a continuous basis, measure core temperature via rectal, tympanic, or thermodilution catheter. If temperature is <36° C (96.8° F), initiate warming measures such as warm blankets, thermal garment, heating lamps, heating blankets, or warm inspired gases.
- Continue to monitor patient during rewarming phase, maintaining rewarming rate at 1° C/hr.
- Monitor skin temperature, particularly that of the extremities, q30min-1h during rewarming. Once extremities are warm, patient should be close to normothermia and warming measures should be discontinued.
- Monitor BP, pulse, CO, and SVR continuously during rewarming for sudden changes related to rewarming. SVR may fall along with BP as the peripheral vascular bed dilates. This can precipitate sudden hypotension.
- If shivering caused by hypothermia develops, treat immediately with warming measures and drug therapy as prescribed. Drugs used to treat shivering may include meperidine (Demerol), diazepam or other benzodiazepines, or, in extreme instances, an intubated, mechanically ventilated patient may receive a neuromuscular blocking agent (e.g., vecuronium). During shivering episodes, monitor VS for changes and assess oxygen saturation continuously with oximeter.

NIC Hypothermia Treatment; Temperature Regulation; Vital Signs Monitoring

Impaired gas exchange (or risk for same) related to altered oxygen supply, alveolar-capillary membrane changes, and altered oxygen-carrying capacity of the blood secondary to central nervous system (CNS) depression from anesthesia, atelectasis, and decreased hemoglobin

Desired outcomes: Within 12-24 hr of treatment, patient has adequate gas exchange as evidenced by Pao$_2$ ≥80 mm Hg; Paco$_2$ 35-45 mm Hg; pH 7.35-7.45; presence of normal breath sounds; and absence of adventitious breath sounds. RR is 12-20 breaths/min with normal pattern and depth (eupnea).
- During intubation/mechanical ventilation period, provide supportive measures to ensure optimal aeration: perform suctioning when need for it is determined by auscultatory findings, turn patient q2h, and maintain HOB at an elevation of 45 degrees, if tolerated.
- Assess breath sounds, RR, and amount and character of mucus production hourly during the first 12 hr after surgery. Be alert to crackles and rhonchi, labored breathing, and subjective complaints of breathing difficulties. Copious, tenacious secretions place the patient at risk for airway obstruction caused by mucus plugging.
- Monitor Spo$_2$ continuously. Report sustained levels <90% to the physician.
- Assess ABG values upon admission and prn during periods of respiratory distress. Consult physician for significant findings, including a decreasing Pao$_2$, increased Paco$_2$, and the presence of acidosis or alkalosis.
- As prescribed, perform ventilator weaning and extubation as early as possible. Use nonopiate analgesics (e.g., ketorolac [Toradol]), and closely monitor the effects of incremental doses of opiate analgesics and sedatives to avoid excessive sedation during the weaning process.

❑ Explain weaning procedure to patient. Stay with patient during first 15 min after each ventilatory change, and reassure patient about his or her ability to breathe independently. Instruct
patient to take slow, deep breaths.

❑ Monitor patient's RR, tidal volume, expiratory pressure, BP, HR, and ECG during weaning.
Consult physician for changes, inasmuch as they may be indicative of weaning intolerance.

❑ Assess for indicators that suggest hypoxemia during weaning: agitation, irritability, tachycardia,
and diaphoresis.

• After extubation, turn patient q2h. Have patient deep breathe and cough q2h, and use incentive
spirometry hourly. As prescribed, perform chest physiotherapy qid.

• Have patient dangle lower extremities over the side of bed and sit in chair as tolerated.

• Instruct patient to sit upright as much as possible and to perform deep-breathing exercises.

NIC Airway Management; Acid-Base Monitoring; Acid-Base Management; Oxygen Therapy;
Respiratory Monitoring

ADDITIONAL NURSING DIAGNOSES

Also see nursing diagnoses and interventions as appropriate in "Nutritional Support," p. 1;
"Mechanical Ventilation," p. 14; "Hemodynamic Monitoring," p. 23; "Prolonged Immobility," p. 61;
"Psychosocial Support," p. 68; "Psychosocial Support for the Patient's Family and Significant
Others," p. 78; "Acute Cardiac Tamponade," p. 118; "Heart Failure/Pulmonary Edema," p. 220;
"Dysrhythmias and Conduction Disturbances," p. 231; "Acute Pericarditis," p. 275; and "Cardiogenic
Shock," p. 290.

Heart Failure/Pulmonary Edema

PATHOPHYSIOLOGY

Heart failure is the leading cause of death in the United States. One in five patients dies within a year
of diagnosis. The annual medical cost is over $30 billion. Heart failure is a complex clinical syn-
drome characterized by an impaired ability of the heart to fill with or to eject blood. It is a degenerative process manifested by progressive changes in the cardiac geometry. The affected chamber wall
dilates, hypertrophies, and becomes more spherical—a process known as remodeling. The remodeling process itself increases the wall stress, causing further remodeling. Therefore, reduction of
remodeling is an important goal of therapy.

Effective pumping of the heart depends on the cardiac cycle: preload (end-diastolic volume in the
ventricles), which stretches the myocardial fibers; afterload (resistance to ejection); and contractility
of the myocardium. Myocardial contractility depends heavily on the delivery of oxygen and nutrients
to the heart. Patients with cardiomyopathy, valvular disease, hypertension, or CAD may have oxygen
deprivation to a portion of the myocardium (local) or across the entire ventricle (global), resulting in
alterations in both ventricular wall motion and contractility. Deprived areas can become hypokinetic
(weakly contractile), akinetic (noncontractile), or dyskinetic (moving opposite from the normal tissues). Compromised patients may also have dysrhythmias that disturb the cardiac cycle, resulting
from damage to the conduction pathways. Less frequently, the heart cannot compensate for greatly
increased metabolic demands caused by disease states such as with thyroid storm. These metaboli-
cally deranged patients manifest symptoms of heart failure as a result of oxygen delivery that is insufficient to compensate for an elevated metabolic rate.

One ventricle typically fails before the other, so pump failure is discussed as either the left-sided
or right-sided ventricular or both ventricles (biventricular).

Left-sided heart failure: Patients may have left-sided heart failure resulting from problems with
either ventricular systole or diastole. CAD is the cause of left-sided heart failure in about two thirds
of patients with left ventricular systolic dysfunction (LVSD). With inadequate contraction of the heart
during systole, blood cannot move forward effectively through the arterial system to deliver oxygen
and nutrients to the rest of the body systems. Problems with diastole are related to failure of the ventricle to effectively "relax" during diastole, resulting in inadequate filling. Either cause of heart failure can result in pulmonary vascular congestion and edema.

Right-sided heart failure: Failure of the right side of the heart results from increased resistance to
right ventricular ejection, most often due to left-sided heart failure, pulmonary hypertension, or lung
disease. Right ventricular MI, cardiomyopathy, or trauma often result in ineffective, abnormal right
ventricular wall motion, resulting in reduced ejection into the pulmonary circulation with subsequent
congestion in the venous system (inferior and superior vena cava and branching vessels). Perfusion

to the left ventricle is also compromised because blood does not flow at the normal rate from the right ventricle through the pulmonary vasculature into the left side of the heart.

Biventricular failure: Patients who experience both left and right ventricular MI (a combination often seen with inferior wall MI) experience hemodynamics that are extremely complex to manage. The impaired right ventricle needs volume infusion to promote better expansion, or "more stretch," of the ventricle, whereas the left ventricle may be unable to accommodate a normal or pre-MI volume and requires volume reduction. Deviation of the intraventricular septum associated with right-sided heart failure caused by distention of the ventricle can significantly reduce the size of the left ventricle. Ultimately, failure in either side of the heart will affect both sides, because the ventricles are interdependent.

ASSESSMENT

History and risk factors: History of CAD and MI, familial history of CAD, age >65 yr, male sex (risk for females increases after menopause), cigarette smoking, alcohol use, hypercholesterolemia, hypertension, diabetes, obesity, increased stress, and sedentary lifestyle. Other important data include understanding of and compliance with low-sodium diet, fluid restriction or medications, and a decreased exercise tolerance.

Left-sided heart failure (pulmonary edema/congestion)
Clinical presentation: Anxiety, air hunger, tachypnea, nocturnal dyspnea, dyspnea on exertion (DOE), orthopnea, moist cough with frothy sputum, tachycardia, diaphoresis, cyanosis or pallor, insomnia, palpitations, weakness, fatigue, anorexia, and changes in mentation.
Physical assessment: Decreased BP, orthostasis (drop in BP with sitting or standing), tachycardia, dysrhythmias, tachypnea, crackles or bibasilar (or dependent) rales, S_3 or summation gallop.
Monitoring parameters: Decreased CO/CI, Spo_2 and Svo_2; elevated PAP, PAWP, SVR; dysrhythmias.

Right-sided heart failure (cor pulmonale/systemic congestion)
Clinical presentation: Fluid retention, peripheral edema, weight gain, decreased urinary output, abdominal tenderness, nausea, vomiting, constipation, and anorexia. Because the edema of heart failure is dependent, patients on bed rest may have edema of the feet, ankles, legs, hands, and/or sacrum.
Physical assessment: Hepatomegaly, splenomegaly, dependent pitting edema, jugular venous distention, positive hepatojugular reflex, and ascites.
Monitoring parameters: Dysrhythmias, elevated RAP and CVP, precipitous drop in Svo_2 with minimal activity, and possibly decreased CO/CI, caused by failure of right ventricle to pump adequate blood through the pulmonary vasculature to maintain adequate left ventricular filling volumes for normal cardiac output.

Biventricular failure (systemic and pulmonary congestion)
Clinical presentation: All signs of both right- and left-sided heart failure, as stated, along with possible signs of cardiogenic shock in acutely ill patients: peripheral cyanosis, fatigue, decreased tissue perfusion, decrease in metabolism, and low urinary output.
Physical assessment: Hypotension, tachycardia, tachypnea, pulmonary edema, dependent pitting edema, hepatosplenomegaly, distended neck veins, pallor, and cyanosis.
Monitoring parameters: Elevated PAP, PAWP, SVR, pulmonary vascular resistance (PVR), RAP, and CVP, decreased CO/CI, dysrhythmias, and decreasing Spo_2 and Svo_2, despite increasing administered oxygen.

DIAGNOSTIC TESTS

Chest x-ray: May reveal pulmonary edema, increased interstitial density, infiltrates, engorged pulmonary vasculature, and cardiomegaly.
ECG: May reveal atrial and/or ventricular hypertrophy, dysrhythmias such as atrial fibrillation, which may precipitate heart failure by decreasing cardiac output, and dysrhythmias associated with electrolyte imbalance.
Serum electrolyte levels: May reveal hyponatremia (dilutional); hypokalemia, which can result from use of diuretics; or hyperkalemia, if glomerular filtration is decreased. Hyperkalemia can also be a side effect of angiotensin-converting enzyme inhibitors (ACEIs) and potassium-sparing diuretics.
Blood urea nitrogen (BUN) and creatinine levels: Rising BUN and creatinine indicate undesirable renal response to diuretic therapy.
B-type natriuretic peptide: B-type natriuretic peptide (BNP), a hormone secreted by the ventricles, can be useful in distinguishing dyspnea due to heart failure from dyspnea due to pulmonary

causes and in monitoring response to therapy. Levels >100 pg/ml support the diagnosis of heart failure. However, though the BNP level decreases with effective therapy, it may remain chronically >100, even when the patient is no longer symptomatic.

Hepatic enzymes and serum bilirubin levels: Serum glutamate oxaloacetate transaminase/aspartate aminotransferase (SGOT/AST), serum glutamate pyruvate transaminase/alanine aminotransferase (SGPT/ALT), and serum bilirubin levels may be elevated because of hepatic venous congestion.

CBC: May reveal decreased hemoglobin (Hgb) and Hct levels in the presence of anemia or dilution.

ABG values: May reveal hypoxemia caused by the decreased oxygen available from fluid-filled alveoli.

Digitalis levels: Chronic heart failure predisposes the patient to digitalis toxicity because of the low cardiac output state, which also causes decreased renal excretion of the drug.

Echocardiogram: May reveal a reduced ejection fraction, ventricular wall motion disorders, valvular dysfunction, cardiac chamber enlargement, pulmonary hypertension, or other cardiac dysfunction.

COLLABORATIVE MANAGEMENT

Treatment of underlying cause and precipitating factors: Initial therapy focuses is focused on stabilizing the hemodynamic and respiratory status and searching for reversible causes of heart failure. The goals of long-term therapy focus on improvement of the quality of the patient's life and management of the compensatory mechanisms causing the patient's symptoms. ACEI and β-blockers have been shown to improve mortality and morbidity and are now the standard of care.

Diseases/conditions causing left-sided heart failure: Atherosclerotic heart disease, AMI, dysrhythmias, cardiomyopathy, increased circulating volume, systemic hypertension, aortic stenosis, aortic regurgitation, mitral regurgitation, coarctation of the aorta, atrial septal defect, ventricular septal defect, cardiac tamponade, and constrictive pericarditis.

Diseases/conditions causing right-sided heart failure: Left-sided heart failure, pulmonary hypertension, atherosclerotic heart disease, AMI, dysrhythmias, pulmonary embolism, fluid overload or excess sodium intake, chronic obstructive pulmonary disease (COPD), mitral stenosis, pulmonary stenosis, and myocardial contusion.

Diseases/conditions causing biventricular failure: Any combination of the diseases that cause either right- or left-sided heart failure.

Oxygen therapy: Supplemental oxygen as required to optimize the patient's oxygen saturation, as determined by pulse oximetry.

Pulse oximetry: Device placed on the patient's finger or ear to determine efficacy of ventilation through measurement of oxygen saturation.

Pharmacotherapy

Diuretics: To reduce blood volume and decrease preload.

Morphine: To induce vasodilation and decrease venous return, preload, sympathetic tone, anxiety, myocardial oxygen consumption, and pain.

Inotropic agents: Digitalis to slow heart rate, giving the ventricles more time to fill, and to strengthen contractions; dopamine or dobutamine to support BP and enhance contractility (see Appendix 7). Dopamine and dobutamine may cause tachycardia, reducing ventricular filling time.

Vasodilators: Nitrates (oral, topical, or IV) to dilate venous or capacitance vessels, thereby reducing preload and cardiac and pulmonary congestion. Nesiritide, nitroprusside, and hydralazine will dilate the resistant vessels and reduce afterload, thus increasing forward flow (see Appendix 7).

Inodilators (amrinone and milrinone): Phosphodiesterase-inhibiting drugs increase contractility of the heart and lower systemic vascular resistance by vasodilation. This allows the failing heart to pump against less pressure (reduced afterload), resulting in increased cardiac output.

Cardiac neurohormones: Infusion of BNP (Nesiritide) induces diuresis, natriuresis and vasodilation to assist in management of heart failure. Chronic heart failure patients sometimes require fewer hospital admissions for congestive heart failure (CHF) when periodic infusions are employed.

ACEIs (benazepril, captopril, enalapril, fosinopril, lisinopril, moexipril, perindopril, quinapril, ramipril, trandolapril): ACEIs affect the renin-angiotensin system by inhibiting the conversion of circulating angiotensin I into angiotensin II. They reduce remodeling, and both preload and afterload, to decrease the work of the ventricles while resulting in increased cardiac output and systemic perfusion/oxygenation.

AT$_1$ receptor antagonist (candesartan, eposartan, irbesartan, olmesartan, losartan, telmisartan): Have effects similar to ACEIs, but have not proved to reduce mortality. AT$_1$ receptor blocking agents are used in patients who are ACEI intolerant.

β-Adrenergic blocking agents (acebutolol, atenolol, betaxolol, carteolol, carvedilol, esmolol, labetalol, metoprolol, nadolol, oxprenolol, propanolol, penbutolol, sotalol, pindolol, timolol):

Block the effects of circulating catecholamines released during heart failure. Catecholamines cause peripheral vasoconstriction, increased resistance to ventricular ejection, increased HR, and increased myocardial oxygen consumption, and may precipitate myocardial ischemia and ventricular dys-rhythmias. β-Blockers also reduce contractility, resulting in decreased myocardial oxygen consumption and demand. The combination of ACEI, diuretics, and β-blockers given at the same time may cause hypotension. Spacing the drug administration times usually relieves this effect.

Treatment of acute pulmonary edema: Immediate interventions include:

- Monitoring for signs and symptoms of respiratory failure.
- Titrating supplemental oxygen to maintain adequate oxygenation.
- Elevating HOB as needed to promote oxygenation.
- Possible endotracheal (ET) intubation with mechanical ventilation.
- Diuretic therapy: in severely ill patients, furosemide and bumetanide may be used as continuous IV infusions to assist with constant fluid removal. Patients with renal impairment/failure may require infusions of appropriate diuretics or ultrafiltration if other efforts to remove fluid fail.
- Pharmacologic therapy, including continuous IV infusions of inotropic agents, vasodilators, β-blockers, and IV morphine. If cardiogenic shock ensues, vasopressors and intraaortic balloon pumping may also be necessary. If the person has evidence of renal insufficiency or failure, ACEI dosage may be reduced or the drug discontinued.

Low-calorie diet (if weight control is necessary) and low-sodium diet: Extra salt and water are held in the circulatory system, causing increased strain on the heart. Limiting sodium (Table 4-6) will reduce the amount of fluid retained by the body. In addition, fluids may be limited to 1500-2000 ml/day.

NURSING DIAGNOSES AND INTERVENTIONS

Fluid volume excess related to compromised regulatory mechanism secondary to decreased cardiac output

T A B L E 4 - 6 Low-Sodium Dietary Guidelines

Foods high in sodium*	Foods low in sodium
Beans and frankfurters	Bread
Bouillon cubes	Cereal (dry or hot); read labels
Canned or packaged soups	Fresh fish, chicken, turkey, veal, beef, and lamb
Canned, smoked, or salted meats; salted fish	(if limiting fats, avoid the latter two)
Dill pickles	Fresh fruits and vegetables
Fried chicken dinners and other fast foods	Fresh or dried herbs
Monosodium glutamate (e.g., Accent)	Gelatin desserts
Olives	Oil, salt-free margarine
Packaged snack foods	Peanut butter
Pancake or waffle mix	Tabasco sauce
Processed cheese	Low-salt tuna packed in water
Seasoned salts (e.g., celery, onion, garlic)	
Sauerkraut	
Soy sauce	
Vegetables in brine or cans	
Additional suggestions	
Do not add table salt to foods.	
Season with fresh or dried herbs.	
Avoid salts or powders that contain salt.	
Do not buy convenience foods; remember that fresh is best.	
Read all labels for salt, sodium, or sodium chloride content.	

*Many of these foods now are available in low-salt or salt-free versions.

Desired outcome: Within 24 hr of treatment, patient becomes normovolemic as evidenced by absence of adventitious lung sounds; decreased peripheral edema; increased urine output; weight loss; PAWP ≤18 mm Hg (reasonable outcome for these patients); SVR ≤1200 dynes/sec/cm^{-5}; and CO ≥4 L/min.

- Auscultate lung fields for presence of crackles and rhonchi or other adventitious sounds.
- Monitor I&O closely. Report positive fluid state or decrease in urine output to <0.5 mg/kg/hr.
- Weigh patient daily; report increases in weight. An acute gain in weight of 1 kg can signal a 1-L gain in fluid.
- Note changes from baseline assessment to detect worsening of heart failure, such as increased pedal edema, increased jugular venous distention, development of S_3 heart sound or new murmur, and dysrhythmias.
- Monitor hemodynamic status q1-2h and prn. Note response to drug therapy as well as indicators of the need for more aggressive therapy, including increasing PAWP and SVR and decreasing CO.
- Administer diuretics, positive inotropes, inodilators, β-blockers, and vasodilators as prescribed. (See Appendix 7 for more information about inotropic and vasoactive drugs.)
- Watch for signs and symptoms of renal insufficiency.
- Limit oral fluids as prescribed, and offer patient ice chips or frozen juice pops to decrease thirst and relieve discomfort of dry mouth.

▌NIC Fluid/Electrolyte Management; Invasive Hemodynamic Monitoring; Medication Management; Nutrition Counseling; Surveillance; Teaching: Disease Process; Hemodialysis Therapy

Cardiac output decreased, related to disease process that has resulted in decreased ability of the heart to provide adequate pumping to maintain effective oxygenation and nutrition of body systems.

Desired outcomes: Within 24 hr of initiating treatment, the patient has attained a CI of at least 2.0; PAP is reduced to within 10% of patient's normal baseline; BP has stabilized to within 10% of baseline; and HR is controlled to within 10% of normal baseline.

- Monitor cardiac rhythm and rate continuously.
- Monitor CO, CI, pulmonary and systemic vascular pressures, and other hemodynamic values at least hourly, as appropriate. Implement continuous CO and Svo$_2$ monitoring if available.
- Monitor neurologic status to assess for adequate cerebral perfusion.
- Monitor renal function (BUN and creatinine) daily, as appropriate.
- Monitor liver studies (SGOT/AST, SGPT/ALT, and/or bilirubin), as appropriate.
- Monitor the other determinants of oxygen delivery, including level of Hgb and oxygen saturation.
- Refrain from taking rectal temperatures, to prevent bradycardias.
- Control tachycardia as soon as possible with β-blockers or other appropriate measure as determined by the physician and ACLS guidelines.
- Obtain 12/15/18-lead ECG to assess new dysrhythmias or profound instability.
- Intraaortic balloon pumping may be necessary; prepare needed equipment for insertion of the balloon catheter and implementation of pumping.
- If patient has atrial fibrillation, ensure that patient has been receiving appropriate anticoagulants or antiplatelet agents to prevent thrombus formation.

▌NIC Cardiac Care: Acute; Circulatory Care: Mechanical Assist Device; Hemodynamic Regulation; Shock Management: Cardiac; Neurologic Monitoring; Medication Management; Dysrhythmia Management

Impaired gas exchange related to alveolar-capillary membrane changes secondary to fluid collection in the alveoli and interstitial spaces

Desired outcome: Within 24 hr of initiation of treatment, patient has improved gas exchange as evidenced by Pao$_2$ ≥80 mm Hg; RR 12-20 breaths/min with normal pattern and depth (eupnea); and absence of adventitious breath sounds.

- Monitor respiratory rate, rhythm, and character q1-2h. Be alert to RR >20 breaths/min, irregular rhythm, use of accessory muscles of respiration, or cough.
- Auscultate breath sounds, noting presence of crackles, wheezes, and other adventitious sounds.
- Provide supplemental oxygen as prescribed and titrate to Spo$_2$.
- Monitor Spo$_2$ for decreases to <90%-92%.
- Assess ABG findings; note changes in response to oxygen supplementation or treatment of altered hemodynamics.
- Suction patient's secretions as needed.
- Establish a protocol for deep breathing, coughing, and turning q2h.
- Place patient in semi-Fowler's or high Fowler's position to maximize chest excursion.
- If mechanical ventilation is necessary, monitor ventilator settings, ET tube function, and respiratory status.

NIC Airway Management; Anxiety Reduction; Cardiac Care: Acute; Medication Management; Oxygen Therapy; Respiratory Monitoring

Activity intolerance related to imbalance between oxygen supply and demand secondary to decreased functioning of the myocardium.

Desired outcome: Within the 12- to 24-hr period before discharge from CCU, patient exhibits cardiac tolerance to increasing levels of activity as evidenced by RR <24 breaths/min; normal sinus rhythm on ECG; HR ≤120 beats/min (or within 20 beats/min of resting HR); BP within 20 mm Hg of patient's normal range; and absence of chest pain.

- Maintain prescribed activity level, and teach patient the rationale for activity limitation.
- Organize nursing care so that periods of activity are interspersed with extended periods of uninterrupted rest.
- To help prevent complications of immobility, assist patient with active/passive ROM exercises, as appropriate. Encourage patient to do as much as possible within prescribed activity allowances.
- Note patient's physiologic response to activity, including BP, HR, RR, and heart rhythm. Signs of activity intolerance include chest pain, increasing SOB, excessive fatigue, increased dysrhythmias, palpitations, HR response >120 beats/min, SBP >20 mm Hg from baseline or >160 mm Hg, and ST segment changes. If activity intolerance is noted, instruct patient to stop the activity and rest.
- Administer medications as prescribed, and note their effect on patient's activity tolerance.
- As needed to help prevent muscle loss and wasting, refer patient to physical therapy department.

NIC Activity Therapy; Energy Management; Teaching: Prescribed Activity/Exercise; Dysrhythmia Management; Pain Management; Medication Management

Knowledge deficit: disease process with heart failure; need to stop smoking, if applicable; activity requirements and limitations; need for daily weight log; symptoms to report; prescribed diet and fluid restriction and medications.

Desired outcome: Within the 24-hr period before discharge from CCU, patient and significant others verbalize understanding of patient's disease, as well as the prescribed diet and medication regimens.

- Teach patient the physiologic process of heart failure, discussing in terms appropriate to the patient how fluid volume increases because of poor heart function.
- Teach the patient about the adverse effects of smoking and how smoking cessation may benefit him or her.
- Teach patient about the importance of a low-sodium diet to help reduce volume overload. Provide patient with a list of foods that are high and low in sodium. Teach patient how to read and evaluate food labels.
- Teach patient the signs and symptoms of fluid volume excess that necessitate medical attention: irregular or slow pulse, increased SOB, orthopnea, decreased exercise tolerance, and steady weight gain (≥1 kg/day for 2 successive days).
- Advise patient about the need to keep a journal of daily weight. Explain that an increase of ≥1 kg/day on 2 successive days of normal eating necessitates notification of physician.
- If patient is taking digitalis, teach the technique for measuring pulse rate. Provide parameters for withholding digitalis (usually for pulse rate <60/min) and notifying the physician.
- Instruct patient regarding the prescribed activity progression after hospital discharge, signs of activity intolerance that signal the need for rest, and use of prophylactic NTG to reduce congestion of the heart and lungs. General activity guidelines are as follows:
  ❑ Get up and get dressed every morning.
  ❑ Space your meals and activities to allow time for rest and relaxation.
  ❑ Perform activities at a comfortable, moderate pace. If you get tired during any activity, stop to rest for 15 min before resuming.
  ❑ Avoid activities that require straining or lifting.
  ❑ Plan at least two periods a day of walking, following the guidelines in Table 4-7.
  ❑ Warning signals to stop your activity and rest: chest pain, SOB, dizziness or faintness, unusual weakness.

NIC Cardiac Care: Rehabilitation; Exercise Promotion; Smoking Cessation Assistance; Teaching: Prescribed Activity/Exercise; Emotional Support; Progressive Muscle Relaxation; Weight Management; Mutual Goal Setting; Teaching: Prescribed Diet; Teaching: Prescribed Medication

ADDITIONAL NURSING DIAGNOSES

Also see nursing diagnoses and interventions in "Hemodynamic Monitoring," p. 23; "Prolonged Immobility," p. 61; "Psychosocial Support," p. 68; and "Psychosocial Support for the Patient's Family and Significant Others," p. 78.

T A B L E 4 - 7   Activity Progression After Hospital Discharge

Week	Distance walked	Time
1-2	¼ mi	Leisurely; twice daily
2-3	½ mi	15 min
3-4	1 mi	30 min
4-5	1½ mi	30 min
5-6	2 mi	40 min

Cardiomyopathy

PATHOPHYSIOLOGY

Cardiomyopathy (CM) is a disease process affecting the myocardial structure and function. CM may occur as a primary (idiopathic) or secondary problem (Table 4-8). Classifications of cardiomyopathy are based on disease-induced structural changes of the heart. All classifications may lead to heart failure.

Functional classification

Dilated cardiomyopathy (DCM) (previously referred to as congestive): DCM is characterized by marked, progressive dilation of the ventricles, resulting in decreased myocardial contractility and reduced systolic ejection fraction (<40%). Heart failure occurs secondary to decreased systolic ejection fraction. DCM is the most frequently diagnosed cardiomyopathy. Ventricular hypertrophy is minimal or absent. In the United States, *ischemic cardiomyopathy* associated with a history of AMI or >70% luminal narrowing of a major coronary artery is the most common cause of DCM.

Hypertrophic cardiomyopathy (HCM): Characterized by hypertrophy of the ventricular muscle, leading to left ventricular diastolic dysfunction. Hypertrophy affects the ventricular septum and the ventricular free wall. Though the hypertrophy results in a decreased left ventricular volume, ejection fraction may increase. *Obstructive* HCM occurs when the enlarged heart muscle obstructs the ventricular outflow channel. *Nonobstructive* HCM is more common. Although cardiac function may remain normal initially, deterioration and poor ventricular compliance known as *idiopathic hypertrophic subaortic stenosis* (IHSS) may occur.

Restrictive cardiomyopathy (RCM): Manifests as ventricular walls become rigid from fibrosis, resulting in inadequate left ventricular filling with atrial dilatation. LV diastolic dysfunction occurs, often associated with very high end-diastolic pressures. Systolic function remains normal. Treatment is difficult, and prognosis is poor. It is important to discern the difference between RCM and constrictive pericarditis, since both clinical pictures are similar while management is markedly different.

Arrhythmogenic right ventricular cardiomyopathy (ARVC): A recently recognized cardiomyopathy characterized by replacement of normal myocardial cells with fibrous and fatty tissue. Primarily

T A B L E 4 - 8   Secondary Causes of Cardiomyopathy

Dilated	Hypertrophic	Restrictive
Ischemic insult	Inherited: autosomal-dominant	Amyloidosis
Infection: viral and bacterial	trait	Cardiac transplant
Chronic alcohol consumption		Endocardial fibroelastosis
Childbirth/postpartum period		Sarcoidosis
Drug therapy (daunorubicin,		Radiation exposure
doxorubicin)		
Kawasaki syndrome		
Autoimmune response		
Genetic defect		

affects the right ventricle (RV), causing ventricular dysrhythmias and ultimately RV failure. AVRC is rare and etiology is unknown, but linked to an autosomal dominant gene. Sudden death in young adults is often the initial presenting symptom.

ASSESSMENT

Clinical presentation: Will vary based on classification, extent, and severity of CM.
Physical assessment: Decreased BP, increased HR, and dysrhythmias. Mild to severe cardiomegaly may be present, causing a displaced and diffuse point of maximal impulse (PMI). Ascites, hepatomegaly and peripheral hypoperfusion may be present. Perfusion deficit is seen as diminished pulses, cool skin, and mottling or cyanosis. (Table 4-9).
Monitoring parameters: See Table 4-10.

DIAGNOSTIC TESTS

Cardiac catheterization: Does not confirm cardiomyopathy but can be used to rule out other disorders, such as ischemic heart disease. Findings in DCM may include decreased CO, abnormal ventricular wall motion, and decreased ejection fraction; increased filling pressure; and valvular regurgitation.
Endomyocardial biopsy: Used to determine the classification and/or cause of CM through histologic studies, to identify the pathologic agent, and in some cases, to identify genetic disorders. May be performed during cardiac catheterization.
Chest x-ray: For *DCM:* may detect cardiomegaly with enlarged left ventricle, pulmonary venous congestion, and characteristic lines of interstitial edema; for *HCM:* normal cardiac silhouette, may show pulmonary venous hypertension; for *RCM:* may show mild cardiac enlargement.
ECG: Dysrhythmias such as supraventricular tachycardias, atrial fibrillation, and ventricular dysrhythmia occur with DMC, HMC, and RMC. Other changes may include left ventricular hypertrophy, left bundle-branch block, left anterior hemiblock, left axis deviation, AV conduction delays, nonspecific ST segment changes, and Q waves that resemble those that occur with MI.
Echocardiography: Assesses for left ventricular impairment and dilation of the cardiac chambers. Ventricular wall and septal contractility can be evaluated, as well as valvular motion. Two-dimensional echo can detect thrombus formation, estimate ejection fraction, and detect the location and degree of hypertrophy.
Radionuclide studies: For *DCM:* may show diffuse left ventricular hypokinesis, left ventricular ejection fraction <40%, and elevated end-diastolic and systolic volumes; for *HCM:* reveal vigorous systolic function, hypertrophy, and a small LV volume; for *RCM:* reveal normal systolic function and a small to normal LV.

COLLABORATIVE MANAGEMENT

Pharmacotherapy: To maintain or reestablish hemodynamic stability.
ACE inhibitor/Angiotensin II receptor blocker: For *DCM:* to block the compensatory response of the renin-angiotensin system to heart failure, decreasing preload and afterload.
Diuretics: For *DCM:* to reduce preload and pulmonary congestion; for *HCM:* may be contraindicated or given cautiously in obstructed *HCM.*
Inotropic therapy: For *DCM:* to enhance contractility (see Appendix 7).

Note: Digitalis is contraindicated in the treatment of obstructive *HCM,* as it may be ineffective or worsen the condition.

Vasodilators: Decrease preload and afterload, resulting in improved cardiac output.
β-Blockers: For *DCM:* to block the compensatory response of the adrenergic system to heart failure. Though the exact mechanism is not known, left ventricular ejection fraction is improved, symptoms are reduced, and survival rate is increased. For *HCM:* to decrease outflow obstruction during exercise and reduce sympathetic cardiac stimulation.
Antidysrhythmic agents: To control atrial and ventricular dysrhythmias (see Table 4-12) common to DCM and HCM.
Calcium channel blockers: For *DCM:* to produce vasodilation and decrease cardiac workload; for *HCM:* to improve diastolic filling and increase exercise capacity.
Spironolactone: A potassium-sparing diuretic; blocks the action of aldosterone, which has been shown to contribute to the development of fibrosis in the remodeling and development of left ventricular hypertrophy (LVH). Potassium level must be closely monitored to avoid hyperkalemia.

TABLE 4 - 9　Signs and Symptoms of Cardiomyopathy

	Dilated	Hypertrophic	Restrictive
Source of initial Clinical presentation	*Systolic dysfunction* S & S caused by biventricular failure: exertional dyspnea, fatigue, weakness, orthopnea, PND, ascites, peripheral edema. May have changes in mentation; i.e., confusion, restlessness	*Diastolic dysfunction* Wide spectrum of S & S, depending on extent and severity of dysfunction; most common: dyspnea (caused by increasing LV diastolic pressure) and angina (caused by hypertrophy and relative ischemia); also: decreased exercise tolerance, fatigue, syncope, exertional dyspnea, orthopnea, palpitations	*Diastolic dysfunction* Exercise intolerance, exertional dyspnea, fatigue, nocturnal dyspnea, plus other signs of pulmonary edema and heart failure
Physical assessment	PMI displaced down and to left, heave palpated; S_3 and S_4 gallops, systolic murmur of AV valves; basilar rales; hepatomegaly; extremities cool, mottled, cyanotic; peripheral pulses weak with pulsus alternans; BP normal or low; sinus tachycardia, atrial fibrillation, ventricular dysrhythmias	Harsh systolic murmur: S_4 gallop: basilar rales; supraventricular dysrhythmias, especially atrial fibrillation; ventricular dysrhythmias are common and sudden death can be the first symptom	Jugular venous distention; PMI typically in normal position and of normal character; S_3 gallop; peripheral edema; ascites; hepatomegaly, atrial fibrillation is very common

AV, Atrioventricular; *PMI,* point of maximal impulse; PND, paroxysmal nocturnal dyspnea; *S & S,* signs and symptoms.

TABLE 4-10 **Hemodynamic Presentation With Cardiomyopathy**

Pressure	Effect	Normal values
Right atrial pressure	Increased	4-6 mm Hg
Pulmonary artery pressure	Increased	20-30/8-15 mm Hg
Pulmonary wedge pressure	Increased	6-12 mm Hg
Cardiac output	Decreased	4-7 L/min
Cardiac index	Decreased	2.5-4 L/min/m^2
Pulmonary vascular resistance	Unchanged or increased	60-100 dynes/sec/cm^{-5}
Systemic vascular resistance	Increased	900-1200 dynes/sec/cm^{-5}

Anticoagulants: To prevent thrombus formation related to decreased ventricular contraction and emptying, as well as atrial fibrillation.

Potassium supplements: To replace potassium lost in the urine as a result of diuresis. Maintenance of serum levels in the high normal range (4.3-5 mEq/L) is optimal.

Hemodynamic monitoring: To guide and evaluate therapeutic interventions.

Activity level: Initially reduced to decrease oxygen demand, but then increased gradually to prevent complications of immobility.

Dual chamber pacemakers: To improve CO and treat cardiac dysrhythmias.

Implantable cardioverter-defibrillator (ICD): To treat life-threatening ventricular dysrhythmias (see Intervention for Ventricular Fibrillation, p. 257).

Intraaortic balloon pump: In the presence of a failing myocardium, may be used to decrease afterload and increase coronary artery perfusion (see Intraaortic Balloon Pump, p. 293).

Ventricular assist devices: Used in the presence of a failing myocardium to increase cardiac output (see Ventricular Assist Device, p. 294).

Alcohol ablation: During cardiac catheterization, ethanol is injected into the septal branches of the LAD coronary artery. Reduces myocardial mass through a limited, therapeutic septal infarction, which reduces outflow obstruction in HCM.

Surgical interventions

Ventricular septal myotomy-myectomy: For removal of the hypertrophied ventricular septum in obstructive HCM.

Heart transplantation: For advanced CM that is refractory to medical therapy to manage progression and symptoms of heart failure. Each institution has criteria that must be met before transplantation is considered as alternative treatment (see Cardiac Transplantation, p. 299).

NURSING DIAGNOSES AND INTERVENTIONS

> **Note:** Care must be based on the type of cardiomyopathy, its associated pathology, and the patient's clinical manifestations. Because DCM is the most commonly occurring cardiomyopathy, the primary aspects of care related to DCM are outlined.

Decreased cardiac output related to negative inotropic changes in the heart secondary to myocardial cellular destruction and dilation

Desired outcomes: Within the 24-hr period before discharge from CCU, patient has adequate cardiac output as evidenced by SBP ≥90 mm Hg; CO 4-7 L/min; CI 2.5-4 L/min/m^2; RR 12-20 breaths/min; HR ≤100 beats/min; urinary output ≥0.5 ml/kg/hr; warm and dry skin; peripheral pulses >2+ on a 0-4+ scale; and orientation to time, place, and person. PAWP is ≤18 mm Hg, and RAP is 4-6 mm Hg.

- Assess for and document the following factors as evidence of decreasing CO: the degree of exertional dyspnea, jugular venous distention, dependent edema, and hepatomegaly. In addition, assess and document the following:
  - ❑ *Mental status:* Be alert to restlessness, decreased responsiveness.
  - ❑ *Lung sounds:* Auscultate for crackles, rhonchi, wheezes.
  - ❑ *Heart sounds:* Note presence of S$_3$ gallop, murmur.
  - ❑ *Urinary output:* Be alert to output <0.5 ml/kg/hr.
  - ❑ *Skin:* Monitor for pallor, mottling, cyanosis, coolness, diaphoresis.

- ❏ *Vital signs:* Note BP <90 mm Hg systolic, HR >100 beats/min, RR >20 breaths/min, and elevated temperature. Increasing HR and BP may reflect compensatory mechanisms in response to sodium and water retention.
- If a PA catheter is present, record hemodynamic readings q1-2h and prn. Be alert to PAWP >18 mm Hg and RAP >6 mm Hg. Although normal PAWP is 6-12 mm Hg, these patients may need increased filling pressures for adequate preload, with wedge pressure at 15-18 mm Hg.
- Measure CO/CI q2-4h and prn. Optimally, CO should be 4-7 L/min and CI should be 2.5-4 L/min/m^2; for some patients the best CO/CI will be below expected normal values.
- Keep accurate I&O records and weigh patient daily, noting trends. Individuals with cardiomyopathy may be on strict fluid restriction (e.g., 1000 ml/day).
- Assess peripheral pulses and rate on a scale of 0-4+.
- Monitor cardiac rhythm continuously for dysrhythmias that may further decrease CO, such as sinus or atrial tachycardias, atrial fibrillation, or ventricular ectopy.
- Assist patient with activities of daily living (ADL) when necessary to minimize patient's cardiac workload.
- Administer medications as prescribed. Observe for the following desired effects:
  - ❏ *Vasodilators:* Decreased BP, decreased SVR, increased CO/CI.
  - ❏ *Diuretics:* Decreased PAWP.
  - ❏ *ACE inhibitors:* Decreased SVR, RAP, PAWP.
  - ❏ *Inotropes:* Increased CO/CI, increased BP.
  - ❏ *β-Blockers:* Increased CO/CI, decreased PAWP. NOTE: These effects are not immediate and may take days to weeks for positive effects to be noted.
- Be alert to the following undesirable effects:
  - ❏ *Vasodilators:* Postural hypotension, dizziness, headache, nausea, vomiting.
  - ❏ *Diuretics:* Weakness, postural hypotension, hypokalemia (see Hypokalemia, p. 549).
  - ❏ *ACE inhibitors:* Headache, dizziness, postural hypotension.
  - ❏ *Inotropes:* Dysrhythmias, headache, angina.
  - ❏ *β-Blockers:* Initial or increased dosing may cause bradycardia and vasodilation and worsen symptoms of heart failure, such as increased dyspnea and edema. The vasodilator and heart failure side effects are typically transient and can be managed by adjusting diuretic and vasodilator medications until the patient is stabilized on the β-blocker. Bradycardia side effects are not transient and will not resolve with time. Not all patients with cardiomyopathy can tolerate β-blockers.

NIC Cardiac Care; Dysrhythmia Management; Electrolyte Management: Hypokalemia; Fluid Monitoring; Fluid Management; Hemodynamic Regulation; Medication Administration; Medication Management; Shock Management: Cardiac

Activity intolerance related to imbalance between oxygen supply and demand secondary to decreased myocardial contractility

Desired outcome: Within the 12- to 24-hr period before discharge from CCU, patient exhibits cardiac tolerance to increasing levels of activity as evidenced by RR <24 breaths/min; normal sinus rhythm on ECG; BP within 20 mm Hg of patient's normal range; HR within 20 beats/min of patient's resting HR; and patient report of decreased fatigue level and absence of chest pain.

- Monitor patient's physiologic response to activity, reporting any symptoms of chest pain, new or increasing SOB, increases in HR >20 beats/min above resting HR, and increase or decrease in SBP >20 mm Hg.
- Monitor cardiac rhythm for the occurrence of dysrhythmias during activity.
- Observe for and report any signs of decreased cardiac output, e.g., changes in mentation.
- Plan nursing care so that patient is assured of extended periods of rest (at least 90 min).
- To prevent complications of immobility, perform or teach patient and significant others active, passive, and assistive range-of-motion (ROM) exercises. For a discussion of an in-bed exercise program, see Table 4-3 and interventions in "Prolonged Immobility," p. 61. Consult physician to ensure that exercises are within patient's prescribed limitations.

NIC Energy Management; Cardiac Care: Rehabilitative

ADDITIONAL NURSING DIAGNOSES

Also see nursing diagnoses and interventions in "Hemodynamic Monitoring," p. 23; "Heart Failure/Pulmonary Edema," p. 220; "Prolonged Immobility," p. 61; "Patients With Implantable Cardioverter-Defibrillator," p. 257; "Psychosocial Support," p. 68; "Psychosocial Support for the Patient's Family and Significant Others," p. 78; and "Ventricular Assist Device," p. 294.

Dysrhythmias and Conduction Disturbances

PATHOPHYSIOLOGY

Cardiac dysrhythmias reflect abnormal function of the heart's electrical system. Cardiac electrophysiology involves studying the electrical impulses and their conduction across the atria and throughout the ventricles to provide power and coordination for the cardiac cycle. Electrical dysfunction can markedly change the cardiac output and cause prompt deterioration in the patient's VS (Figure 4-1).

Dysrhythmias may originate in any part of the electrical system, from the pacing cells (SA node, AV junction) to any portion of the conduction system (atria, His-Purkinje system, bundle branches, and ventricles). Myocardial ischemia, electrolyte or other chemical imbalance, and an abnormally configured electrical system are factors likely to stimulate dysrhythmias. The normal flow of impulses depends on properly nourished, well-oxygenated electrical tissues with an anatomically correct pacing and conduction system. The cardiac cycle depends on a balance of basic regulatory substances: electrolytes such as sodium, potassium, calcium, glucose; and appropriate amounts of catecholamines. Imbalance of these regulators can cause a disturbance in pacing (automaticity), conduction, or myocardial contractility (Figure 4-2).

Disturbances in automaticity: May involve an increase or decrease in the pacing function (automaticity) in the sinus node, such as sinus tachycardia (HR >100 beats/min) or sinus bradycardia (HR <60 beats/min). Premature beats or possibly an escape or compensatory heart rhythm may arise from the atria, junction, or ventricles. Escape rhythms occur when the sinus node ceases to function or arrests. Abnormal rhythms, such as atrial or ventricular tachycardia, also may occur, especially if there is an excess of catecholamines. Without excessive catecholamines, escape rhythms generated from the AV junction or the ventricles are usually bradycardic (HR <60 beats/min).

Disturbances in conduction: Conduction may be too rapid, as in conditions that prompt excessive catecholamines (e.g., severe/critical illness, certain endocrine diseases, profound emotional stress) or in the presence of an accessory pathway (e.g., Wolff-Parkinson-White syndrome). Accessory pathways are extra conduction fibers that provide a direct connection between the atria and the ventricles, circumventing the AV node. Rhythms generated from these anatomically incorrect conduction systems are called *AV reciprocating tachycardias* and may have rates >250 beats/min. Impulse conduction

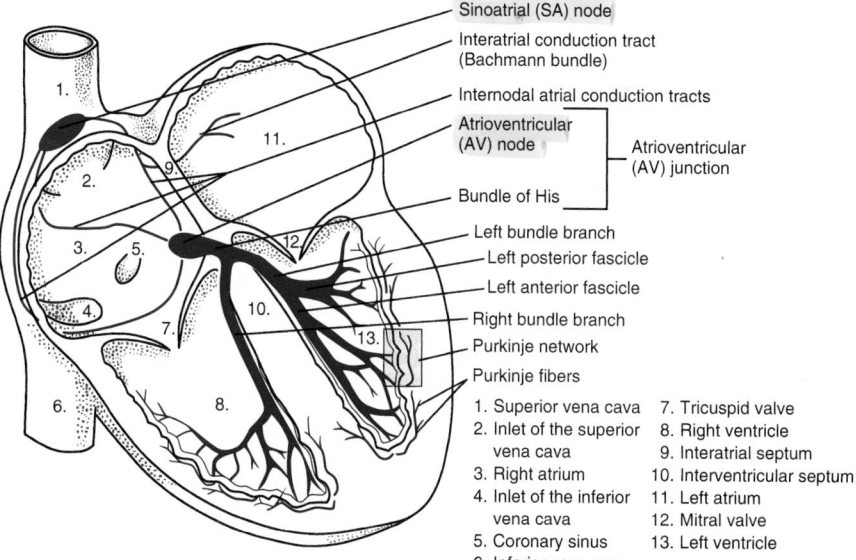

Figure 4-1: Electrical conduction system.
From Huszar *RJ: Basic dysrhythmias: interpretation and management,* ed 3, St Louis, 2002, Mosby.

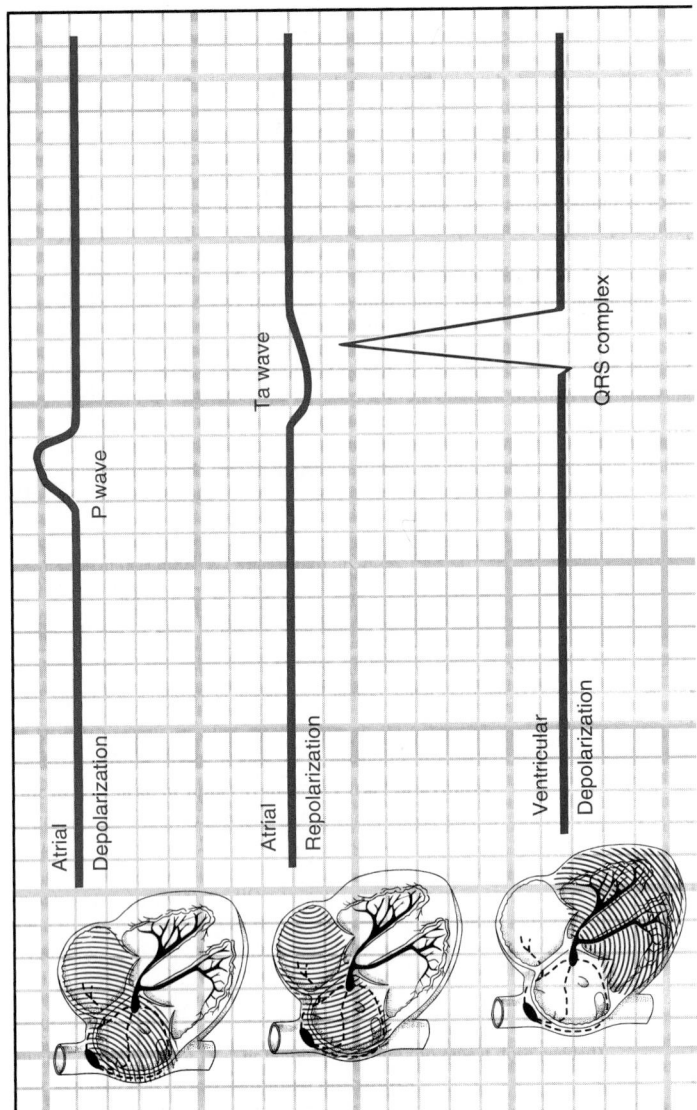

Figure 4-2:   Electrical basis on the ECG.
From Huszar RJ: *Basic dysrhythmias: interpretation and management,* ed 3, St Louis, 2002, Mosby.

may be delayed or too slow (e.g., first- and second-degree AV block). Reentry is a situation in which a misdirected electrical impulse reexcites a conduction pathway through which it has already passed. Once started, this impulse may circulate through the same area repeatedly, prompting an AV reentrant tachycardia. The trapped impulse becomes the pacemaker in this circumstance. Impulses may also be totally blocked from continuing down the pathway by abnormal electrical tissues (e.g., third-degree or complete heart block) (Figure 4-3)

Combinations of disturbed automaticity and conduction: Observed when several dysrhythmias are noted (e.g., first-degree AV block [disturbance in conductivity]; premature atrial complexes [PACs] [disturbance in automaticity]).

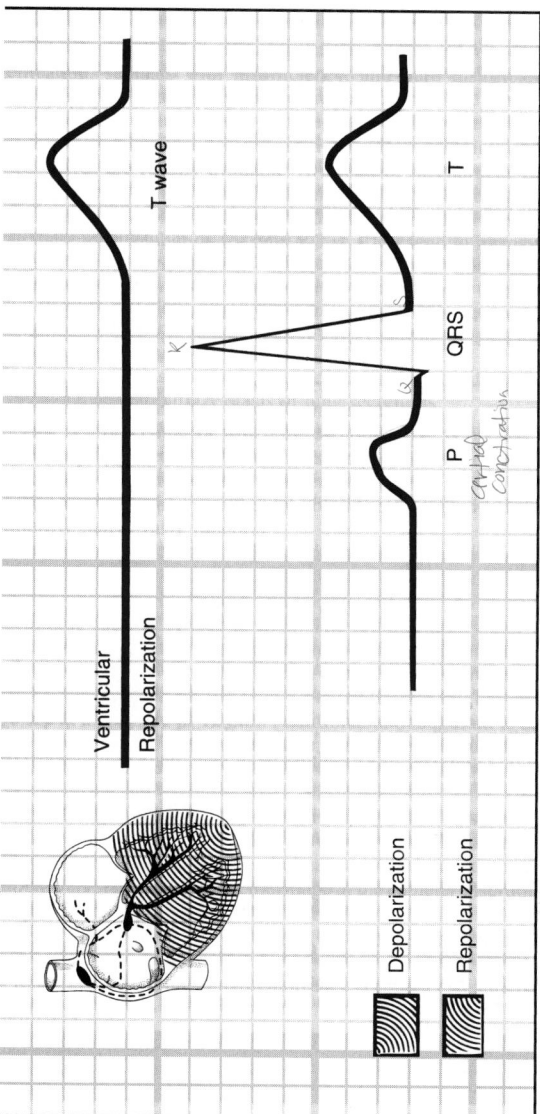

Figure 4-2: cont'd

ASSESSMENT

History and risk factors: Coronary atherosclerotic heart disease (CASHD), acute MI, recent MI, current use of antidysrhythmic or bronchodilating drugs, electrolyte disturbances (especially potassium, glucose, or magnesium), endocrine disease (thyroid, adrenal, or pancreas), low BP/shock, increased intracranial pressure, valvular heart disease, cardiomyopathy, unstable angina, acid-base imbalance, hypoxemia, pulmonary disease, respiratory failure, anemia, drug overdose.

Clinical presentation: Varies from absence of symptoms to complete cardiopulmonary arrest. Most commonly: activity intolerance, weakness, hypotension, dizziness, SOB, dyspnea, palpitations, chest discomfort or pressure, sensation of "racing heart" or "skipped beats." More serious symptoms include: altered mental status, anxiety, respiratory insufficiency, syncope, and seizures, which may

1. Prolonged PR interval (>0.20 sec)
(first-degree AV block)

Delay of
conduction of the
electrical impulse
through the:

AV node or
bundle of His

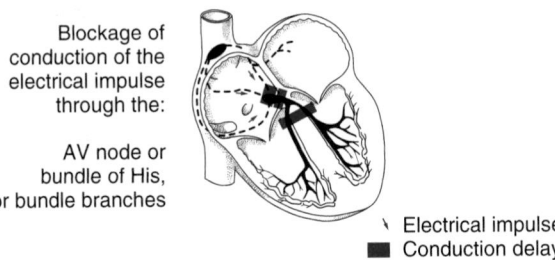

\ Electrical impulse
▨ Conduction delay

2. Absence of a QRS after a P wave
(second- and third-degree AV block)

Blockage of
conduction of the
electrical impulse
through the:

AV node or
bundle of His,
or bundle branches

\ Electrical impulse
■ Conduction delay

3. Short PR interval (<0.12 sec)

a. Ectopic
pacemaker in
the atria or
AV junction

OR

b. Conduction of the
electrical impulse
through abnormal
AV conduction
pathways

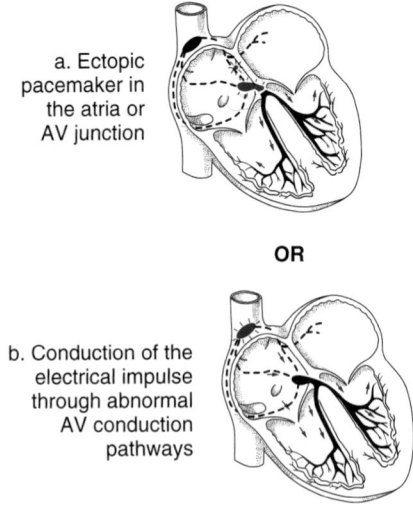

\ Electrical impulse

Figure 4-3:   Anomalous AV conduction.
From Huszar RJ: *Basic dysrhythmias: interpretation and management,* ed 3, St Louis, 2002, Mosby.

lead to heart failure and cardiopulmonary arrest. Pulseless ventricular tachycardia, ventricular fibrillation, asystole, and electromechanical dissociation result in immediate cardiac arrest.

Physical assessment: Symptomatic dysrhythmias most often result in a very rapid, slow, or irregular pulse, changed pulse quality, hypotension, pallor, possibly a variable heart rate (fast, then slow), and tachypnea. If the cardiac output is markedly decreased, shocklike symptoms ensue including cold, clammy skin, dusky or cyanotic appearance, decreased urine output, and feeling of impending doom or imminent death. If heart failure is present, heart sounds may include S_3 and S_4; basilar crackles or rales are audible with lung auscultation; jugular veins are distended; and peripheral edema and a wet cough with frothy sputum may be present.

ECG and hemodynamic measurements: Hemodynamic measurements will vary, depending on the effect of the dysrhythmia on the cardiac output. If patient has heart failure, CO is decreased and PAP is elevated. Tachycardias usually increase CO initially, unless the rate is too fast to allow adequate ventricular filling, in which case CO decreases and may lead to heart failure. ECG findings seen with various dysrhythmias include abnormalities in rate such as sinus bradycardia or sinus tachycardia; irregular rhythm such as atrial fibrillation; extra beats such as PACs and premature junctional complexes (PJCs); wide and bizarre-looking beats such as premature ventricular complexes (PVCs) and ventricular tachycardia (VT); a fibrillating baseline such as ventricular fibrillation (VF); and a straight line as with asystole (Figure 4-4). Figures 4-5 through 4-25 give an overview of common rhythms, dysrhythmias, and conduction disturbances and their treatment. Occasionally, patients have an electrical rhythm without corresponding mechanical pumping. This condition is known as *pulseless electrical activity (PEA)* or *electrical-mechanical dissociation (EMD)*. Initially, the rhythm may appear nearly normal but rapidly deteriorates as the conduction pathway becomes hypoxic.

DIAGNOSTIC TESTS

12-lead ECG: Accepted standard method used to detect and analyze dysrhythmias, including those associated with myocardial ischemia, injury, and infarction. Leads are attached to the patient's limbs and on the chest over the left ventricle (Figure 4-26).

15/18-lead ECG: Expanded method used to detect and analyze dysrhythmias, in which leads are added to the 12-lead ECG on the right side of the chest and/or left posterior subscapular area to better detect problems with the perfusion to the right ventricle and posterior wall of the left ventricle.

Serum electrolyte levels: Identify key chemical imbalances that may precipitate dysrhythmias. Both elevations and deficits of electrolytes can create an electrically unstable environment.

Therapeutic drug levels: Toxic levels of many cardiac, pulmonary, neurologic, and antidysrhythmic medications may prompt development of new, possibly more dangerous dysrhythmias. All antidysrhythmic agents are proarrhythmic in toxic amounts or when certain electrolyte imbalances are present, especially the class I agents (e.g., quinidine, mexiletine, disopyramide).

Stress testing: Continuous ECG monitoring of the patient while a stressor (e.g., exercise on the treadmill, Persantine, dobutamine or adenosine injection) is induced. The test continues until the patient reaches the target heart rate or becomes symptomatic (e.g., chest pain, severe fatigue, dysrhythmias). Results determine the ability of the heart to compensate for various amounts of stress.

Electrophysiologic studies (EPS): Invasive test in which two or three catheters are placed into the heart at suspected proarrhythmic sites, to give a pacing stimulus at those sites with various voltages of electricity to induce dysrhythmias. Various medications and electrical therapies are then implemented to terminate the induced dysrhythmias. Results help to determine the type of device and medications the patient may need to maintain cardiac electrical stability.

Toxicology screening: Toxic levels of "recreational" or "street" drugs (e.g., "crack," cocaine, amphetamines, barbiturates) or mood-altering drugs (e.g., tricyclic antidepressants, sedative/hypnotics) can induce lethal dysrhythmias.

Ambulatory monitoring (e.g., 24-hr Holter monitor or cardiac event recorder): Continuous cardiac monitor worn for 24 hr by the patient so that ECG changes that occur during normal daily activities (including sleeping) can be determined. The patient keeps a timed log of all activities/ events/symptoms, which is later compared with the ECG recording to analyze the relationship of dysrhythmias to symptoms and activities.

Atrial electrogram (AEG): Specialized and somewhat invasive ECG used to diagnose atrial dysrhythmias, wherein a needle is inserted into the patient's chest over the right atrium; through a single wire, the atrial activity can be more thoroughly analyzed.

ABG values: May reflect hypoxemia or pH abnormality that can interfere with electrolyte balance, both of which can cause dysrhythmias. Hypoxemia can also result from dysrhythmias that significantly decrease cardiac output.

Text continued on page 254

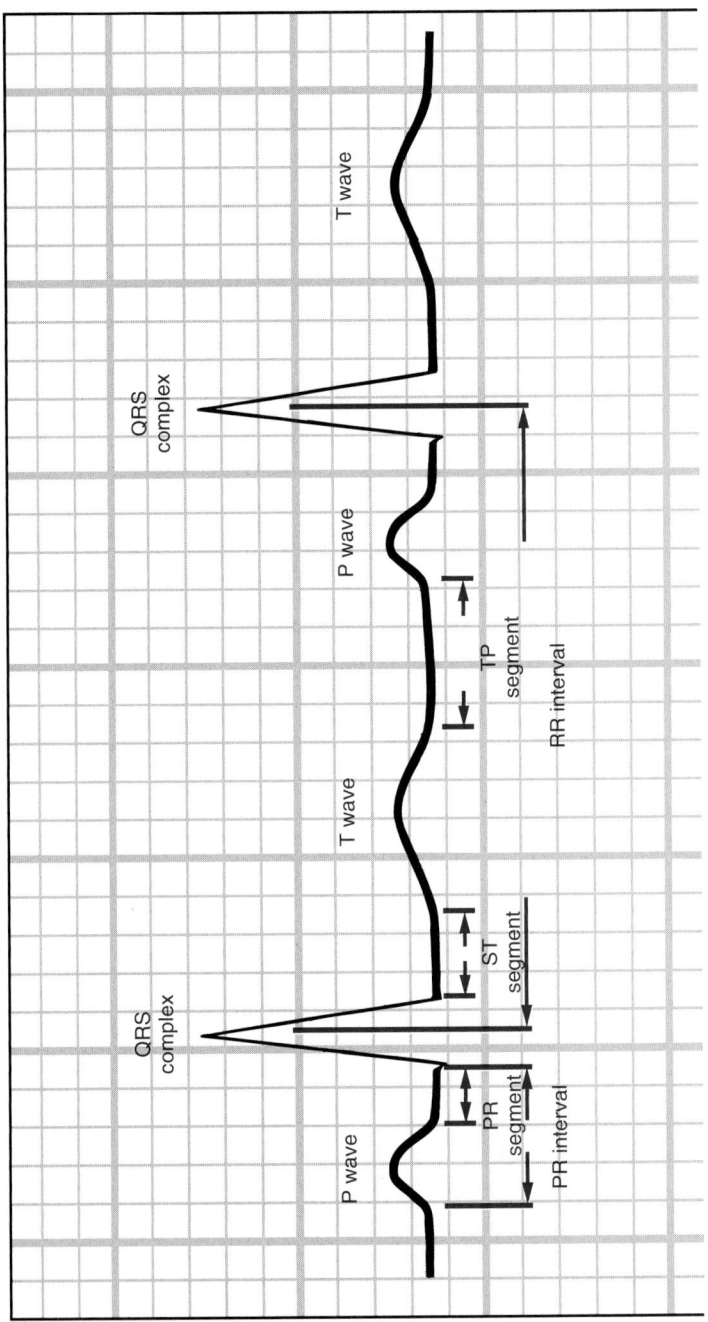

Figure 4-4:   Components of the ECG.
From Huszar RJ: *Basic dysrhythmias: interpretation and management,* ed 3, St Louis, 2002, Mosby.

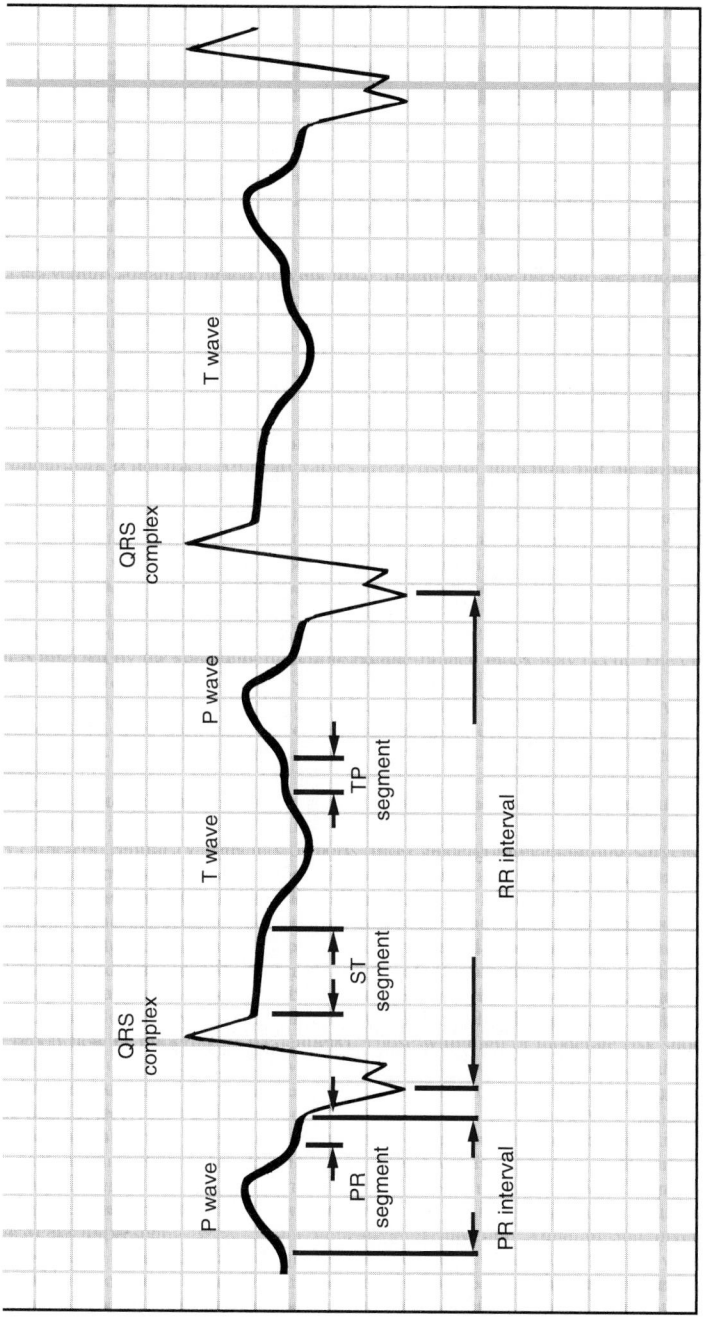

Figure 4-4: cont'd

Normal Sinus Rhythm

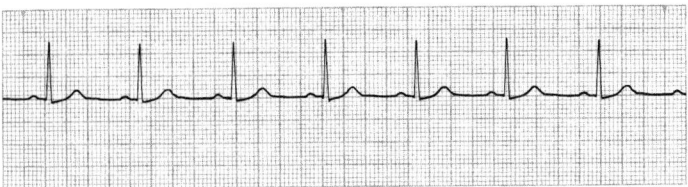

- Rhythm: regular
- Atrial rate: 60-100 beats/min
- Ventricular rate: 60-100 beats/min
- P waves: before each QRS
- QRS: normal and of normal width
- PR interval: normal
- P: QRS: 1:1

Significance: Usual, normal rhythm and conduction.
Intervention: None.

Figure 4-5: Normal sinus rhythm.
From Huszar RJ: *Basic dysrhythmias: interpretation and management,* ed 3, St Louis, 2002, Mosby.

Sinus Tachycardia

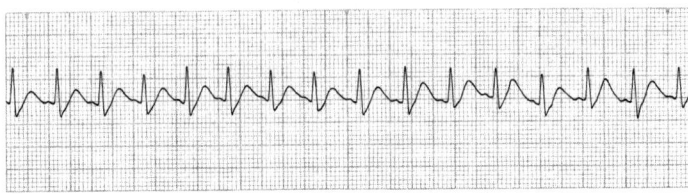

- Rhythm: regular
- Atrial rate: >100 beats/min; usually <160 beats/min
- Ventricular rate: >100 beats/min; usually <160 beats/min
- P waves: before each QRS
- QRS: normal duration
- PR interval: normal
- P: QRS: 1:1

Significance: Increased rate usually caused by sympathetic stimulation.
Causes may include pain, fever, anxiety, hypovolemia, heart
failure, caffeine intake, use of theophylline or sympathomimetic agents.
Intervention: Treat cause.

Figure 4-6: Sinus tachycardia.
From Huszar RJ: *Basic dysrhythmias: interpretation and management,* ed 3, St Louis, 2002, Mosby.

Sinus Bradycardia

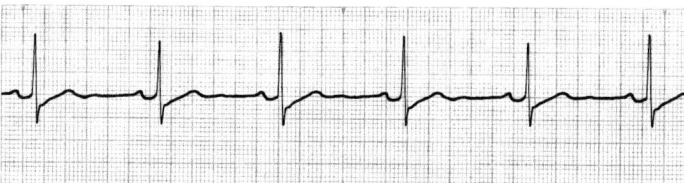

- Rhythm: regular
- Atrial rate: <60 beats/min
- Ventricular rate: <60 beats/min
- P waves: before each QRS
- QRS: normal duration
- PR interval: normal
- P: QRS: 1:1

Significance: Slow rate usually caused by increased parasympathetic stimulation. Causes may include vagal stimulation, β-adrenergic blocking agents and other drugs, AMI, increased intracranial pressure (IICP). This rhythm may be "normal" in some people.

Intervention: No treatment necessary unless patient's BP drops and/or LOC is altered or PVCs occur. Initial treatment is atropine and oxygen. See "Bradycardia Algorithm" in Appendix 1.

Figure 4-7: Sinus bradycardia.
From Huszar RJ: *Basic dysrhythmias: interpretation and management,* ed 3, St Louis, 2002, Mosby.

Sinus Dysrhythmia

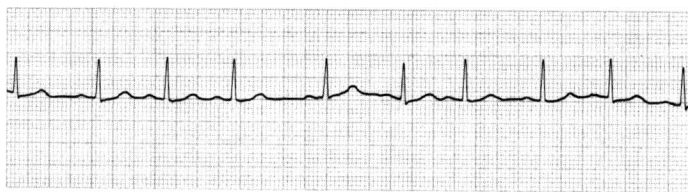

- Rhythm: regular
- Atrial rate: 60-100 beats/min
- Ventricular rate: 60-100 beats/min
- P waves: before each QRS
- QRS: normal duration
- PR interval: normal
- P: QRS: 1:1

Significance: This rhythm usually increases in rate with respiration and decreases with expiration. It can be a normal finding in children. As an abnormal finding, it may be caused by drugs, IICP, or heart disease.

Intervention: Observation; usually no treatment necessary.

Figure 4-8: Sinus dysrhythmia.
From Huszar RJ: *Basic dysrhythmias: interpretation and management,* ed 3, St Louis, 2002, Mosby.

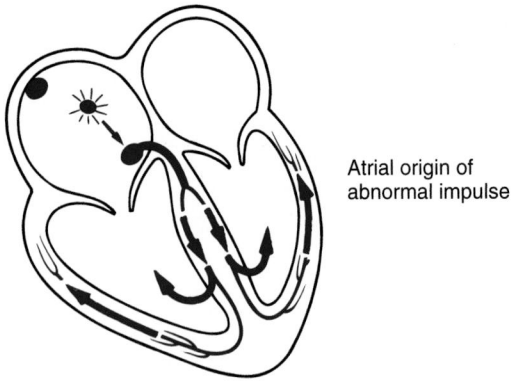

Atrial origin of
abnormal impulse

Premature Atrial Complexes (PACs)

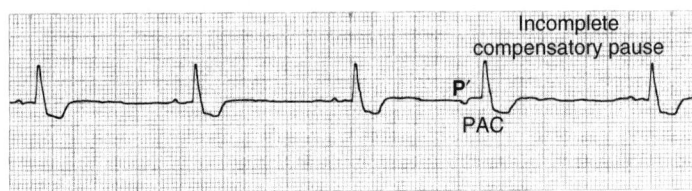

- Rhythm: irregular
- Atrial rate: depends on underlying rhythm
- Ventricular rate: depends on underlying rhythm
- P waves: early beat P looks different from sinus P
- QRS: normal duration
- PR interval: variable in premature complexes
- P: QRS: 1:1

Significance: PACs come from an ectopic atrial focus. Causes often are the same as sinus tachycardia. May progress to atrial fibrillation or atrial tachycardia.

Intervention: Observation. Limit caffeine, alcohol, and smoking. If symptoms occur (decreased BP, dizziness), treatment may include β-blockers, verapamil, or diltiazem.

Figure 4-9:   Premature atrial complexes (PACs).
Top illustration modified from Sheehy SB, Lenehan GP: *Manual of emergency care,* ed 5, St Louis, 1999, Mosby. Bottom illustration from Huszar RJ: *Basic dysrhythmias: interpretation and management,* ed 3, St Louis, 2002, Mosby.

Atrial Tachycardia

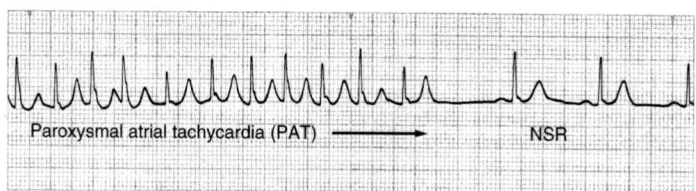

- Rhythm: mostly regular
- Atrial rate: 160-240 beats/min
- Ventricular rate: depends on AV conduction ratio
- P waves: may be difficult to identify because of fast rate
- QRS: normal; may be wide if aberrant conduction is present

Significance: Can precipitate chest pain and ischemia. Patients often experience dizziness, diaphoresis, and nausea. Many patients diagnosed with wide-complex atrial tachycardia (SVT) are found to have ventricular tachycardia when electrophysiology studies are done.

Intervention: Vagal maneuvers, verapamil, adenosine. Other agents include digoxin, β-blockers, and procainamide. See "Narrow QRS Tachycardia Algorithm" in Appendix 1. If the patient has an accessory pathway with AV reciprocating tachycardia, catheter ablation may be necessary to correct the problem.

Figure 4-10:   Atrial tachycardia.
From Huszar RJ: *Basic dysrhythmias: interpretation and management,* ed 3, St Louis, 2002, Mosby.

Wandering Atrial Pacemaker

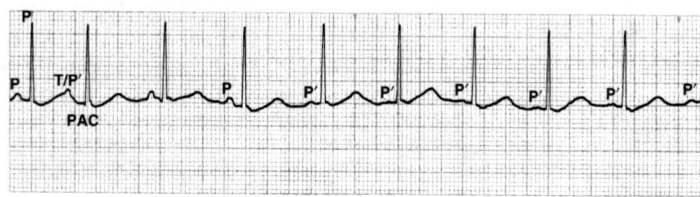

- Rhythm: irregular
- Atrial rate: usually 60-100 beats/min
- Ventricular rate: usually 60-100 beats/min
- P waves: before each QRS
- QRS: normal duration
- PR interval: usually normal; some variation
- P: QRS: 1:1

Significance: An ectopic atrial focus. Causes may include drugs, COPD, inflammatory disorders.

Intervention: Observation. If cause can be determined, treat cause. If patient is receiving digoxin, check serum level.

Figure 4-11:   Wandering atrial pacemaker.
From Huszar RJ: *Basic dysrhythmias: interpretation and management,* ed 3, St Louis, 2002, Mosby.

Atrial Flutter (Type I)

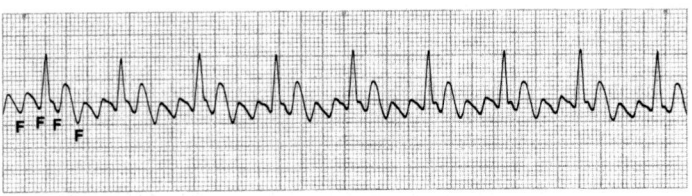

- Rhythm: regular if block is regular; may be irregular
- Atrial rate: 240-340 beats/min (type I); 340-430 beats/min (type II)
- Ventricular rate: depends on AV conduction
- P waves: saw-toothed; F waves
- QRS: normal
- PR interval: not measurable
- P: QRS: P > QRS

Significance: An atrial ectopic focus. AV conduction ratios can be variable, usually at least 2:1. The ineffective contraction can cause thrombus formation in the atria, which may subsequently embolize to the lungs, brain, and possibly other distal vessels.

Intervention: IV diltiazem, verapamil, or β-blockers. For type I, rapid atrial pacing or cardioversion if unstable. Other agents may include IV ibutilide or amiodarone. PO flecainide, amiodarone, propafenone, or sotalol may also be used. Patients with an atrial rate of >240 may need to be anticoagulated to prevent atrial thrombus formation. See "Atrial Fibrillation/Atrial Flutter Algorithm" in Appendix 1.

Figure 4-12:   Atrial flutter (type I).
From Huszar RJ: *Basic dysrhythmias: interpretation and management,* ed 3, St Louis, 2002, Mosby.

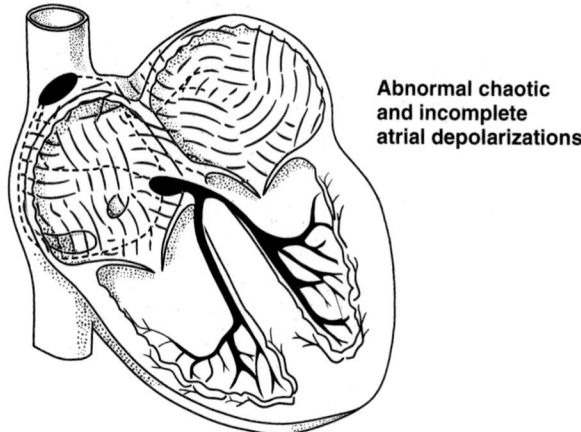

Abnormal chaotic and incomplete atrial depolarizations

Atrial Fibrillation

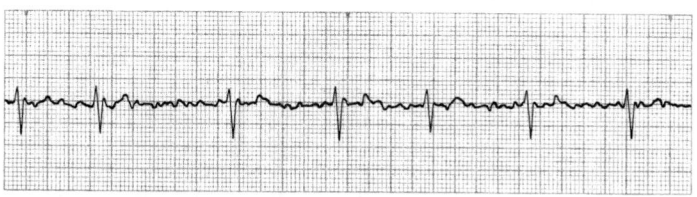

- Rhythm: irregularly irregular
- Atrial rate: >350 beats/min
- Ventricular rate: variable
- P waves: coarse or fine fibrillatory waves
- QRS: normal
- PR interval: not measurable
- P: QRS: P > QRS

Significance: Chaotic atrial firing and ineffective atrial contraction. Cardiac output usually drops because of loss of atrial "kick." Ineffective atrial contraction makes clot formation a danger.

Intervention: Patients in chronic AF with controlled ventricular response may not require intervention. For new-onset AF with a rapid ventricular response, use the same protocol as recommended for atrial flutter. See "Atrial Fibrillation/Atrial Flutter Algorithm" in Appendix 1. Patients should be anticoagulated to prevent atrial thrombus formation, unless contraindication because of other medical problems.

Figure 4-13: Atrial fibrillation (AF).
From Huszar RJ: *Basic dysrhythmias: interpretation and management,* ed 3, St Louis, 2002, Mosby.

AV Junctional Rhythm or Junctional Escape Rhythm

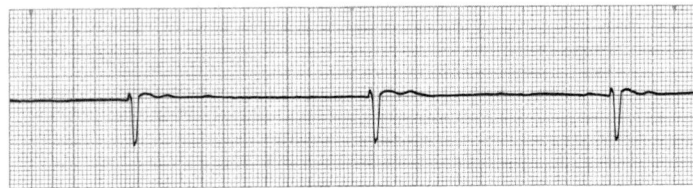

- Rhythm: regular
- Atrial rate: cannot determine
- Ventricular rate: 40-60 beats/min
- P waves: inverted before or after QRS or not present
- QRS: normal
- PR interval: <0.2 sec if P precedes QRS
- P: QRS: P ≤ QRS

Significance: AV node assumes primary pacing function from atria.
Intervention: Usually no specific therapy indicated. If patient becomes symptomatic because of a slow rate, see "Symptomatic Bradycardia Algorithm" in Appendix 1.

Figure 4-14:   AV junctional rhythm or junctional escape rhythm.
From Huszar RJ: *Basic dysrhythmias: interpretation and management,* ed 3, St Louis, 2002, Mosby.

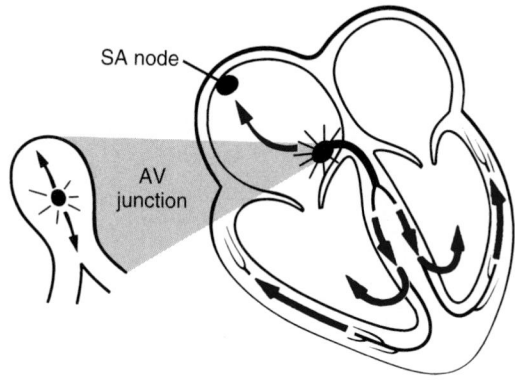

Premature Junctional Complexes

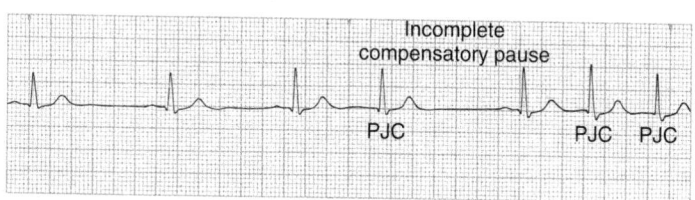

- Rhythm: irregular
- Atrial rate: cannot determine
- Ventricular rate: depends on underlying rhythm
- P waves: before, during, and after QRS
- QRS: normal
- PR interval: <0.2 sec if present
- P: QRS: P ≤ QRS

Significance: Less common than PACs; may precede blocks.

Intervention: Observation. Usually no treatment is necessary. If indicated, therapy is similar to that for PACs.

Figure 4-15: Premature junctional complexes.
Top illustration modified from Sheehy SB, Lenehan GP: *Manual of emergency care,* ed 5, St. Louis, 1999, Mosby. Bottom illustration from Huszar RJ: *Basic dysrhythmias: interpretation and management,* ed 3, St Louis, 2002, Mosby.

Junctional Tachycardia

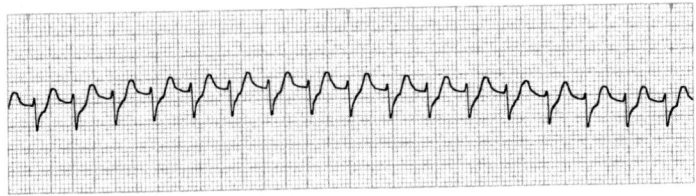

- Rhythm: regular
- Atrial rate: cannot determine
- Ventricular rate: 100-250 beats/min
- P waves: inverted before or after QRS
- QRS: normal
- PR interval: cannot determine
- P: QRS: P < QRS

Significance: This rhythm is essentially the same as junctional rhythm (JR),
except that an increase in sympathetic stimulation
results in increased HR. Causes may include heart disease,
electrolyte disturbances, COPD, or hypoxia.
Intervention: See "Wide QRS Tachycardia of Unknown Origin Algorithm" in Appendix 1.

Figure 4-16:   Junctional tachycardia (JT).
From Huszar RJ: *Basic dysrhythmias: interpretation and management,* ed 3, St Louis, 2002, Mosby.

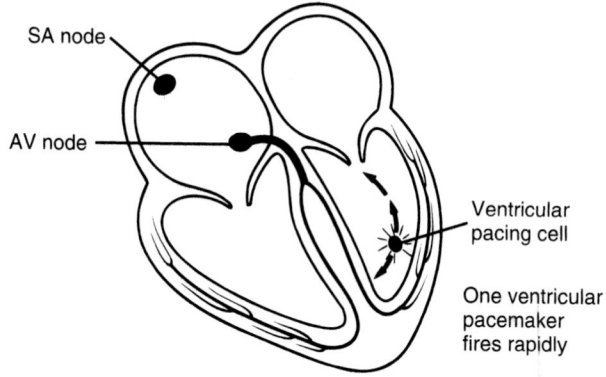

Ventricular Tachycardia

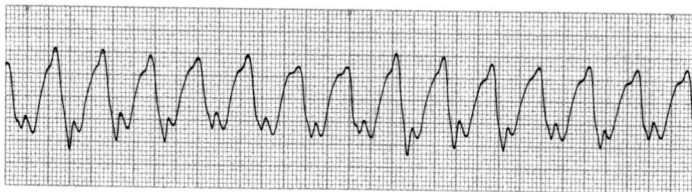

- Rhythm: slightly irregular
- Atrial rate: cannot determine
- Ventricular rate: 150-250 beats/min
- P waves: not visible
- QRS: wide (>0.12 sec)
- PR interval: cannot determine
- P: QRS: absent

Significance: Cardiac output falls significantly, cannot be tolerated for long, and will deteriorate into VF and asystole. May be monomorphic (same form repeated) or polymorphic (more than one type present).

Intervention: If pulseless, patient requires immediate defibrillation. Recent studies indicate patients who survive sudden cardiac death and those with sustained VT should be considered for an implantable cardioverter-defibrillator (ICD). See "Polymorphic Ventricular Tachycardia Algorithm" and "Ventricular Fibrillation (VF)/Pulseless Ventricular Tachycardia (VT)/Algorithm" in Appendix 1.

Figure 4-17: Ventricular tachycardia.
Top illustration modified from Sheehy SB, Lenehan GP: *Manual of emergency care,* ed 5, St. Louis, 1999, Mosby. Bottom illustration from Huszar RJ: *Basic dysrhythmias: interpretation and management,* ed 3, St Louis, 2002, Mosby.

Premature Ventricular Complexes (PVCs)

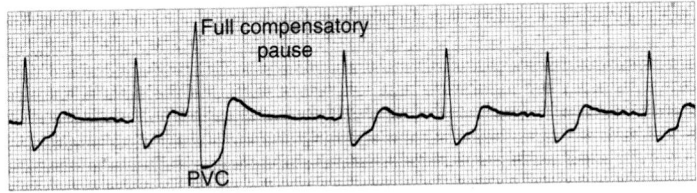

- Rhythm: irregular
- Atrial rate: not determined with PVCs
- Ventricular rate: depends on underlying rhythm
- P waves: not seen
- QRS: wide (>0.12 sec); bizarre
- PR interval: not determined
- P: QRS: P < QRS

Significance: PVCs signal an irritable focus in the ventricle. Causes may include AMI, hypoxia, hypovolemia, electrolyte imbalance. PVCs may be monomorphic (same form repeated) or polymorphic (more than one type present) and may occur in patterns. They may precipitate lethal dysrhythmias.

Intervention: PVCs are common in AMI, and there is controversy regarding treatment. Antidysrhythmic agents may not be used for asymptomatic patients. Treatment should include correction of electrolyte abnormality, specifically hypokalemia and hypomagnesemia.

Figure 4-18:   Premature ventricular complexes (PVCs).
From Huszar RJ: *Basic dysrhythmias: interpretation and management,* ed 3, St Louis, 2002, Mosby.

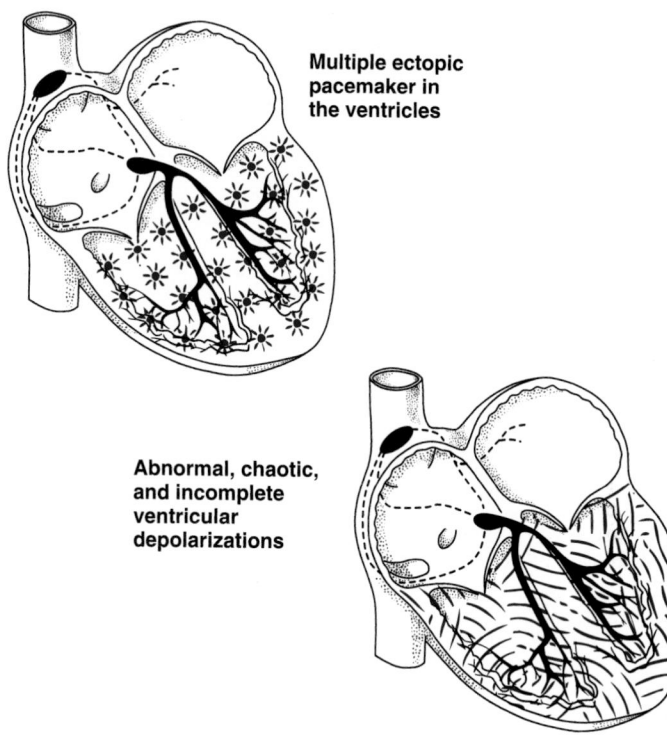

Multiple ectopic pacemaker in the ventricles

Abnormal, chaotic, and incomplete ventricular depolarizations

Ventricular Fibrillation

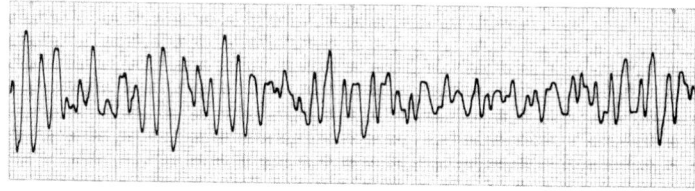

- Rhythm: irregular
- Atrial rate: cannot determine
- Ventricular rate: rapid
- P waves: not seen
- QRS: absent; fibrillatory waves
- PR interval: none
- P: QRS: none

Significance: Most common cause of sudden cardiac death. VF produces no cardiac output.

Intervention: Current research indicates Amiodarone is useful in conversion of unstable VT to sinus rhythm. Patients who survive sudden cardiac death (VF) should be considered for an implantable cardioverter-defibrillator (ICD). See Pulseless Ventricular Tachycardia (VT) / Ventricular Fibrillation (VF) Algorithm" in Appendix1.

Figure 4-19: Ventricular fibrillation.
From Huszar RJ: *Basic dysrhythmias: interpretation and management,* ed 3, St Louis, 2002, Mosby.

Idioventricular Rhythm

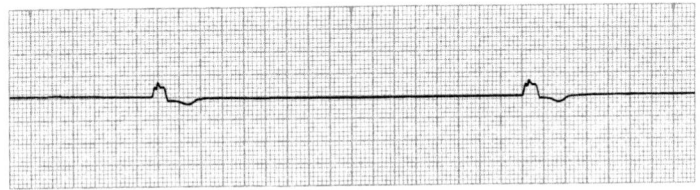

- Rhythm: regular or irregular
- Atrial rate: none
- Ventricular rate: <40 beats/min
- P waves: none
- QRS: wide (>0.12 sec); bizarre
- PR interval: none
- P: QRS: none

Significance: Usually lethal. Pulse may be present but usually is not.
Intervention: See "Pulseless Electrical Activity (PEA) Algorithm" in Appendix 1.

Figure 4-20:   Idioventricular rhythm.
From Huszar RJ: *Basic dysrhythmias: interpretation and management,* ed 3, St Louis, 2002, Mosby.

Asystole

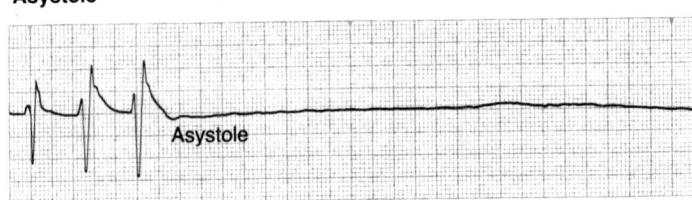

- No electrical activity
- May see a rare, wide, bizarre QRS

Significance: Mortality >95%. Always confirm asystole in 2 leads.
Intervention: See "Asystole Algorithm" in Appendix 1.

Figure 4-21:   Asystole.
From Huszar RJ: *Basic dysrhythmias: interpretation and management,* ed 3, St Louis, 2002, Mosby.

First-Degree AV Block

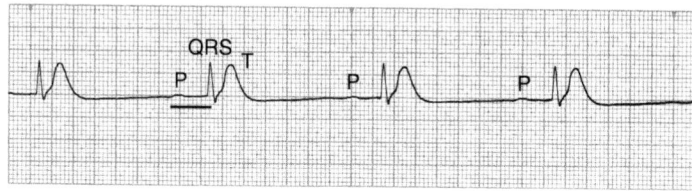

- Rhythm: regular
- Atrial rate: 60-100 beats/min
- Ventricular rate: 60-100 beats/min
- P waves: present; precede each QRS
- QRS: normal
- PR interval: prolonged (>0.2 sec)
- P: QRS: 1:1

Significance: Impulse conduction is delayed through the AV node. Causes are varied and may include heart disease, ischemia, digitalis toxicity, other drug effect, and myocarditis.

Intervention: Observation; usually no treatment needed. If hypotensive,see Symptomatic Bradycardia Algorithm in Appendix 1.

Figure 4-22:   First-degree AV block.
From Huszar RJ: *Basic dysrhythmias: interpretation and management,* ed 3, St Louis, 2002, Mosby.

Second-Degree AV Block Type I (Wenckebach)

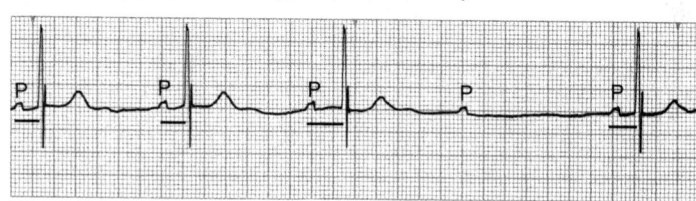

- Rhythm: irregular
- Atrial rate: exceeds ventricular rate
- Ventricular rate: less than sinus rate
- P waves: one P wave precedes each QRS except during nonconducted P waves, which occur regularly
- QRS: normal
- PR interval: lengthens progressively with each cycle until one is nonconducted

Significance: Usually a transient block that does not progress to complete heart block.

Intervention: Observation; treatment usually not necessary. If hypotensive, see Symptomatic Bradycardia Algorithm in Appendix 1.

Figure 4-23:   Second-degree AV block (type I) (Wenckebach).
From Huszar RJ: *Basic dysrhythmias: interpretation and management,* ed 3, St Louis, 2002, Mosby.

Second-Degree AV Block Type II

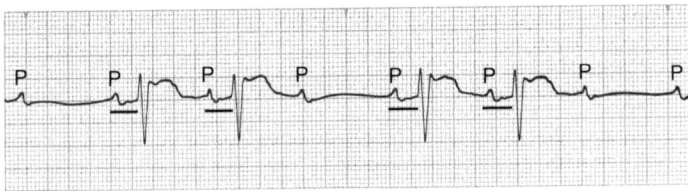

- Rhythm: irregular
- Atrial rate: exceeds ventricular rate
- Ventricular rate: depends on degree of block
- P waves: 2 or more for each QRS
- QRS: normal duration
- PR interval: normal or prolonged on the conducted complex
- P: QRS: P > QRS

Significance: This block may occur with anterior wall AMI and may progress rapidly to complete heart block.

Intervention: Observation if patient is asymptomatic. If symptoms occur, see "Symptomatic Bradycardia Algorithm" in Appendix 1.

Figure 4-24:   Second-degree AV block (type II).
From Huszar RJ: *Basic dysrhythmias: interpretation and management,* ed 3, St Louis, 2002, Mosby.

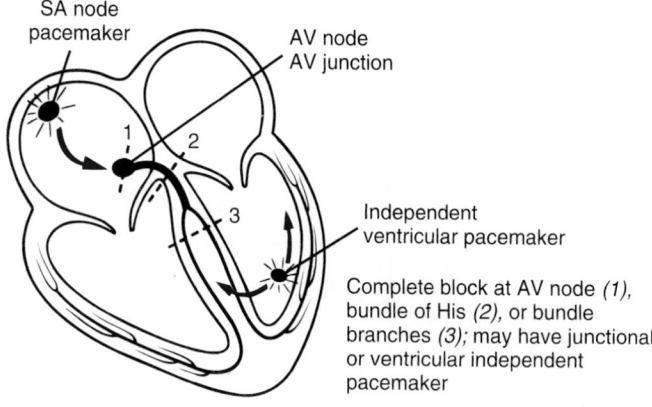

SA node
pacemaker

AV node
AV junction

Independent
ventricular pacemaker

Complete block at AV node *(1),*
bundle of His *(2),* or bundle
branches *(3);* may have junctional
or ventricular independent
pacemaker

Complete Heart Block

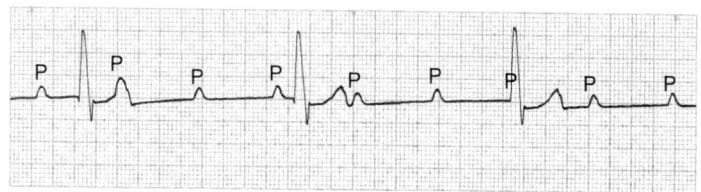

- Rhythm: usually regular
- Atrial rate: exceeds ventricular rate
- Ventricular rate: <60 beats/min
- P waves: occur at regular intervals
- QRS: <0.12 sec if pacemaker is in the AV node; >0.12 sec if ventricular
  pacemaker
- PR interval: no relationship between P and QRS
- P: QRS: no relationship

Significance: No conduction of SA node impulses. The atria and ventricles
beat independently of each other. The slow rate can cause
myocardial ischemia.

Intervention: Pacemaker insertion necessary. See "Symptomatic
Bradycardia Algorithm" in Appendix 1.

Figure 4-25: Complete (third-degree) AV block.
Top illustration modified from Sheehy SB, Lenehan GP: *Manual of emergency care,* ed 5, St. Louis,
1999, Mosby. Bottom illustration from Huszar RJ: *Basic dysrhythmias: interpretation and management,* ed 3, St Louis, 2002, Mosby.

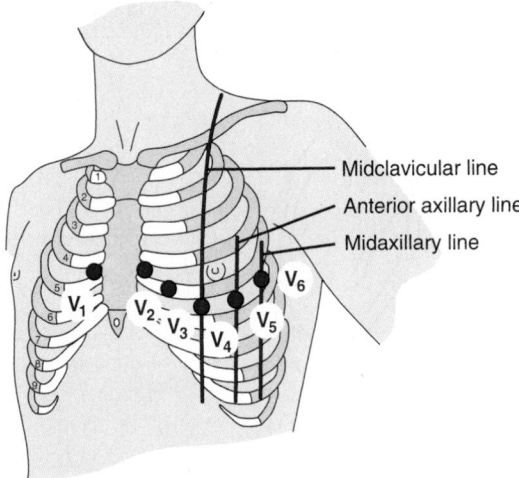

Midclavicular line

Anterior axillary line

Midaxillary line

Figure 4-26:   Placement of precordial electrodes.
From Huszar RJ: *Basic dysrhythmias: interpretation and management,* ed 3, St Louis, 2002, Mosby.

COLLABORATIVE MANAGEMENT

Antidysrhythmic drugs: Pharmacologic management of dysrhythmias is based on providing and/or balancing electrolytes, catecholamines, and other regulators of the cardiac cycle. Provision of these substances is the basis of the antidysrhythmic drug classification system, which has evolved from the original Vaughan Williams classification system. Toxic levels of any antidysrhythmic medication can prompt development of different and sometimes lethal dysrhythmias. All antidysrhythmic agents have the potential for proarrhythmic effects (Table 4-11).

Defibrillation and cardioversion: Delivery of electrical shocks to the heart through the chest wall via use of an external defibrillator. Shocks may be synchronized with the patient's R waves (QRS complexes) or may be given as random/unsynchronized countershocks. Used to convert sympto- matic, rapid atrial or ventricular rhythms to sinus rhythm. The operator must set the desired amount of electricity, apply the defibrillator paddles with conductive gel or gel pads to protect the patient from electrical burns, apply at least 80 lb of pressure to the paddles, and discharge the device. Defibrillators may use monophasic or the newer biphasic technology. Biphasic defibrillation gener- ally requires lower energy settings than recommended for monophasic defibrillation. Newer defibril- lators include a "hands free" feature. These devices use a special cable and defibrillator pads instead of the conventional paddles. The operator is not required to apply the paddles with pressure if "hands free" is available.

Automatic external defibrillation (AED): Defibrillation technique designed for families of patients and others (including health care providers untrained in ECG interpretation), in which the device is programmed to interpret the patient's dysrhythmia and deliver an unsynchronized countershock if deemed necessary. The operator must be able to assess for pulselessness and apnea, along with apply- ing "hands free" defibrillator pads in the proper position at the right sternal border and anterior axil- lary line, fifth intercostal space. Devices may be semiautomatic or fully automatic.

Cardiac pacing (internal): Temporarily inserted or permanently placed, battery-powered device that provides an artificial pacing or electrical pacing stimulus for the heart. Used in situations where the heart is unable to either generate an appropriate number of pacing impulses or conduct the impulses, or both. Most often used for management of symptomatic bradycardias including second- and third-degree heart block, and may be used for patients with ventricular asynchrony. Specialized devices may also be used to correct rapid atrial and ventricular rhythms via antitachy- cardia pacing (ATP). Third-generation implantable cardioverter defibrillators (ICDs) may also be programmed for cardiac pacing. Temporary pacing can be done via transvenous catheter insertion with positioning of leads into the endocardium or via surgically inserting epicardial wires with leads during open heart surgery. Pacemakers are named or coded based on the functions they are able to perform. (See Table 4-12, p. 256, for various pacing options.) If cardiac output is disturbed

TABLE 4-11　Antidysrhythmic Drugs

Class I (sodium channel blockers)

Block the rapid, inward sodium current. Local anesthetics and other drugs that decrease automaticity of ventricular conduction, delay ventricular repolarization, decrease conduction velocity, increase conduction via AV node, and suppress ventricular automaticity. Class IA decreases depolarization moderately and prolongs repolarization. Class IB decreases depolarization and shortens repolarization. Class IC significantly decreases depolarization with minimal effect on repolarization.

Class IA	Class IB	Class IC
Disopyramide (PO)	Lidocaine (IV, IM)	Encainide (PO)
Procainamide (PO, IV, IM)	Mexiletine (PO)	Flecainide (PO)
Quinidine (PO, IV)	Phenytoin (PO)	Propafenone (PO)
	Tocainide (PO)	
	Moricizine (PO)	

Class II (β-adrenergic blockers)

Block stimulation of β_1- and β_2-receptors by catecholamines. Slow sinus node automaticity, slow conduction via AV node, control ventricular response to supraventricular tachycardias, and shorten the action potential of Purkinje fibers.

Acebutolol (PO)	Metoprolol (PO,IV)
Atenolol (PO)	Nadolol (PO, IV)
Betaxolol (PO)	Oxyprenolol (PO)*
Bisoprolol (PO)	Penbutolol (PO)
Carteolol (PO)	Pindolol (PO)
Carvedilol (PO)	Propranolol (PO, IV)
Esmolol (IV)	Timolol (PO, IV)
Labetalol (PO, IV)	

Class III (potassium channel/IK1 blockers)

Block the outward current of potassium. Increase the action potential and refractory period of Purkinje fibers, increase ventricular fibrillation threshold, restore injured myocardial cell electrophysiology toward normal, and suppress reentrant dysrhythmias.

Amiodarone (PO, IV)	Dofetilide (PO)
Azimilide (PO)	Ibutelide (IV)
Bretylium (IV, IM)	Sotalol (PO, IV)

Class IV (calcium channel blockers)

Depress automaticity in the SA and AV nodes, block the slow calcium current in the AV junctional tissue, reduce conduction via the AV node, and are useful in treating tachydysrhythmias due to AV junctional reentry.

Diltiazem (PO, IV)
Verapamil (PO, IV)

Unclassified

Depress activity of the AV node.
Adenosine (IV)

AV, Atrioventricular; β, beta; *PO,* by mouth; *IV,* intravenous; *IM,* intramuscular; *SA,* sinoatrial.
*Available in Great Britain.

---

by ventricular asynchrony, biventricular pacing may be used. Biatrial pacing has been used to help control atrial fibrillation.

Transthoracic cardiac pacing (external): Cardiac pacing done by a device that delivers electrical stimulation to the heart via two conductive pads positioned over the anterior and posterior walls of the heart. One pad is near the left sternal border and the other near the left paraspinal line beneath the scapula. The device includes an ECG monitor so that efficacy of pacing can be assessed. Resistance of all muscles and bones of the chest wall must be overcome for impulses to reach the heart. The technique is usually quite uncomfortable for the patient, and sedation may be required. Certain defibrillators include capability for transthoracic cardiac pacing.

TABLE 4-12 NBG Pacemaker Codes

The pacemaker code is written in a five-letter format as in the table below, using no more letters than necessary. For example, the DDDR pacemaker is a dual-chamber paced, dual-chamber sensed, dual response, rate modulated device. At least one pacemaker mode, the DVIC mode variation, does not conform to the NBG identification code and may sometimes be written DVI(C).

In the 1970s and 1980s, before the NBG codes came into being, the Inter-Society Commission for Heart Disease (IHCD) established standardized codes for pacemakers. Information on these older pacemaker codes can be found at NASPE.

Chambers paced (1)	Chambers sensed (2)	Modes of response (3)	Programmable functions (4)	Antitachycardia functions (5)
V = Ventricle	V = Ventricle	T = Triggered	R = Rate Modulated	O = None
A = Atrium	A = Atrium	I = Inhibited	C = Communicating	P = Paced
D = Dual (A & V)	D = Dual (A & V)	D = Dual Triggered/Inhibited	M = Multiprogrammable	S = Shocks
O = None	O = None	O = None	P = Simple Programmable	D = Dual (P & S)
—	—	—	O = None	—

NASPE, North American Society of Pacing and Electrophysiology, and BPEG, British Pacing and Electrophysiology Group, and generic. www.MeDiCaLeSe.org/pacemakers.html.

Implantable cardioverter-defibrillator (ICD): A battery-powered pulse generator (electrical device) implanted into the pectoral area, with lead systems positioned inside the heart and superior vena cava, which can recognize and terminate potentially lethal dysrhythmias. Newer, third-generation devices do not require thoracotomy for insertion and may also provide antitachycardia pacing (ATP), low-energy cardioversion, antibradycardia pacing, and ability to score performance data. Algorithms for treatment of recognized dysrhythmias are programmed into the device. Maximal energy output is 30-40 joules, which can defibrillate malignant or lethal rhythms such as pulseless ventricular tachycardia and ventricular fibrillation. Magnets may be used for emergency deactivation/activation or suppression of all or part of programmed therapies in newer devices.

Risks and complications of thoracotomy (T) versus nonthoracotomy (NT) approaches are outlined in Table 4-13.

Catheter ablation: A procedure in which a catheter is placed in the heart via cardiac catheterization and an electrical heat stimulus is applied to the area in which the dysrhythmia originates. The heat stimulus causes controlled, localized necrosis of the area.

Transesophageal echocardiography (TEE): Ultrasound technique to monitor atrial and ventricular wall motion through a sound-sensitive lead that the patient swallows. Can also detect clots that are present in the heart as a result of stasis of blood secondary to dysrhythmias (e.g., atrial fibrillation).

Anticoagulation: Use of warfarin (Coumadin) and/or platelet inhibitors (e.g., ticlodipine, clopidogrel) may be recommended for patients at higher risk for development of blood clots within the heart secondary to dysrhythmias that decrease either atrial or ventricular wall motion.

Dietary guidelines: Patients with recurrent dysrhythmias are usually placed on a diet that restricts or reduces caffeine and is low in fat and cholesterol (see Tables 4-5 and 4-6).

Surgical procedures

Left ventricular aneurysmectomy and infarctectomy: Excision of possible focal spots of ventricular dysrhythmias.

T A B L E 4 - 13   Implications for Patient Care and Costs: Implantable Cardioverter Defibrillators (ICD)

NOTE: Magnetic fields are measured in units (gauss) or 1000th of a gauss, milligauss (MG). 10 gauss will affect an ICD or some programmable pacemakers. Common household electrical appliances (interferences) are less than 50 MG. Electrical fields are measured in volts per meter. 750 volts is approximately 30 joules.

Complication	*Thoracotomy (T)*	*Non-thoracotomy (NT)*	*Patient care implications*
Pneumothorax or hemothorax	Higher risk	Lower risk	ICU monitoring required for **T**. ICU unnecessary for **NT**. Length of hospital stay decreases with **NT**.
Pocket hematoma, seroma, wound adhesions	Higher risk	Lower risk	Wound care and home care less complex for **NT**.
Wound infection	Higher risk	Lower risk	If wound infection, **T** more likely to require IV antibiotics, which will increase costs and length of hospital stay.
Blood loss/ bleeding	Higher risk	Lower risk	**T** may need type and screen for blood products. **NT** does not.
Pneumonia	Higher risk	Lower risk	**T** may have decreased activity tolerance and requires pulmonary toilet.
Pain	Higher risk	Lower risk	**NT** requires less analgesia to manage pain.

Myocardial revascularization: Performed alone or in conjunction with electrophysiologic mapping, with excision or cryoablation of the dysrhythmia focus. Newer surgical techniques are less invasive than the more standard median sternotomy approach.

Encircling ventriculotomy: Excises the diseased portion of the ventricle without compromising myocardial blood supply.

Stellate ganglionectomy and block: Alters the electrical stability of the myocardium and predisposition to ventricular dysrhythmias.

NURSING DIAGNOSES AND INTERVENTIONS

Decreased cardiac output related to altered rate, rhythm, or conduction or negative inotropic changes secondary to cardiac disease

Desired outcomes: Within 15 min of development of serious dysrhythmias, patient has adequate cardiac output as evidenced by BP ≥90/60 mm Hg; HR 60-100 beats/min; and normal sinus rhythm on ECG. PAP is 20-30/8-15 mm Hg; PAWP is ≤18 mm Hg (a reasonable outcome for these patients); RAP is ≤7 mm Hg; and CO is 4-7 L/min.

- Monitor patient's heart rhythm continuously; note BP and symptoms if dysrhythmias occur or increase in occurrence.
- If a PA catheter is present, note PAP, PAWP, and RAP; monitor for a reduced CO in response to dysrhythmias.
- Document dysrhythmias with rhythm strip. Use a 12/15/18-lead ECG as necessary to identify the dysrhythmia.
- Monitor patient's laboratory data, particularly K^+, Mg^{++}, glucose, and digoxin levels.
- Administer antidysrhythmic agents as prescribed; note patient's response to therapy.
- Provide oxygen as prescribed. Oxygen may be beneficial if dysrhythmias are related to ischemia.
- Maintain a quiet environment, and administer pain medications promptly. Both stress and pain can increase sympathetic tone and cause dysrhythmias.
- If life-threatening dysrhythmias occur, initiate immediate unit protocols or standing orders for treatment, as well as cardiopulmonary resuscitation (CPR) and ACLS algorithms (see Appendix 1) as necessary.
- When dysrhythmias occur, stay with patient; provide support and reassurance while performing assessments and administering treatment.
- Administer inotropic agents (see Appendix 7) as prescribed to support patient's BP and CO.

NIC Cardiac Care; Hemodynamic Regulation; Medication Management; Oxygen Therapy; Respiratory Monitoring; Vital Signs Monitoring

Risk for activity intolerance related to imbalance between oxygen supply and demand secondary to dysrhythmias that reduce cardiac output

Desired outcomes: During activity, patient rates exertion <3 on a scale of 0-10 and exhibits tolerance of the dysrhythmia by a RR <20 breaths/min; SBP within 20 mm Hg of baseline; HR within 20 beats/min of resting HR; and absence of chest discomfort and/or new dysrhythmias.

- Monitor patient's response to activity. Instruct patient to report chest discomfort and SOB. Note new dysrhythmias associated with activity or other stressors.
- Administer medications as prescribed.
- Observe and report signs of acute decreased cardiac output, including oliguria, decreasing BP, altered mentation, and dizziness.
- Monitor BP and other VS frequently, and as soon as possible report to the physician changes such as irregular HR, HR >120 beats/min, or decreasing BP.
- Assess integrity of peripheral perfusion by monitoring peripheral pulses, distal extremity skin color, and urinary output. Report changes such as decreased pulse amplitude, pallor or cyanosis, and decreased urine output.

NIC Activity Therapy; Cardiac Care; Energy Management; Surveillance

Knowledge deficit: mechanism by which dysrhythmias occur; lifestyle implications

Desired outcome: Within the 24-hr period before discharge from CCU, patient and significant others verbalize knowledge about causes of dysrhythmias and the implications for modification of patient's lifestyle.

- Discuss causal mechanisms for dysrhythmias, including resulting symptoms. Use a heart model or diagrams as necessary.
- Teach the signs and symptoms of dysrhythmias that necessitate medical attention: unrelieved and prolonged palpitations, chest pain, SOB, rapid pulse (>150 beats/min), dizziness, and syncope. Teach patient and significant others how to check pulse rate for a full minute.
- Teach patient and significant others about medications that will be taken after hospital discharge, including drug name, purpose, dosage, schedule, precautions, and potential side effects. Stress that

patient will be maintained on long-term antidysrhythmic therapy and that it could be life-threatening to stop or skip these medications without physician approval, because doing so may decrease blood levels required for dysrhythmia suppression.

- Advise patient and significant others about the availability of support groups and counseling; provide appropriate community referrals. Patients who survive sudden cardiac arrest may experience nightmares or other sleep disturbances at home. Explain that anxiety and fear, along with periodic feelings of denial, depression, anger, and confusion, are normal following this experience.
- Stress the importance of leading a normal and productive life, even though patient may fear break-through of life-threatening dysrhythmias. If patient is going on vacation, advise him or her to take along sufficient medication and to investigate health care facilities in the vacation area.
- Advise patient and significant others to take CPR classes; provide addresses of community programs.
- Teach the importance of follow-up care; confirm date and time of next appointment, if known. Explain that outpatient Holter monitoring is performed periodically.
- Explain that individuals with recurrent dysrhythmias should follow a general low-fat and low-cholesterol diet (see Tables 4-5 and 4-6) and reduce intake of products containing caffeine, including coffee, tea, chocolate, and colas.
- As indicated, teach patient relaxation techniques, which will reduce stress and enable patient to decrease sympathetic tone (see next nursing diagnosis section).

NIC Surveillance; Teaching: Individual; Teaching: Prescribed Medication; Vital Signs Monitoring

Health-seeking behavior: relaxation technique effective for stress reduction and facilitation of ability to take deep breaths slowly to relax. See Appendix 9 for a sample relaxation technique.

Desired outcome: Within the 24-hr period after instruction, patient verbalizes and demonstrates the following relaxation technique.

- Explain that to decrease sympathetic tone, some patients with dysrhythmias may benefit from practicing a relaxation response. Many different techniques can be used, including use of breathing alone or in conjunction with muscle group contraction and relaxation. Other techniques incorporate use of imagery.

NIC Anxiety Reduction; Calming Technique; Meditation; Music Therapy; Simple Guided Imagery; Simple Relaxation Therapy; Teaching: Prescribed Activity/Exercise

For patients with an implantable cardioverter-defibrillator and permanent pacemaker

Knowledge deficit: ICD or pacemaker insertion procedure and follow-up care

Desired outcomes: Within the 24-hr period before the procedure, patient and significant others describe rationale for the procedure and method of insertion. Within the 24-hr period before discharge from CCU, patient and significant others describe postinsertion care and need for continued physician and nurse follow-up.

- Assess patient's understanding of his or her medical condition (dysrhythmias) and the amount of detailed information desired.
- Discuss the following with the patient and significant others:
  - ❏ Type of dysrhythmia patient has, using rhythm strip and heart model or drawings/illustrations/charts to promote understanding.
  - ❏ Possible need for temporary transvenous pacemaker insertion before ICD or permanent pacemaker procedure.
  - ❏ Use of appropriate anesthesia throughout procedure.
  - ❏ Testing of the ability of the device to control lethal dysrhythmias, which will occur in the operating room/catheterization lab after implantation and before the incision is closed.
  - ❏ Reassurance that should the mechanism fail to control the dysrhythmia, the device can be adjusted or reprogrammed to do so.
  - ❏ Continuous observation of patient in a cardiac care unit for ≈24 hr, with ongoing monitoring of BP, HR, and RR.
  - ❏ Importance of deep breathing, coughing (as necessary), and incentive spirometry exercises as appropriate. Explain that patient is at increased risk for respiratory tract and incisional infection if thoracic surgery was done, which tends to cause patient to avoid deep breathing and coughing to guard against pain. Have patient return demonstrations of breathing exercises. Reassure patient that analgesics can be administered before pulmonary toilet exercises, if needed.
  - ❏ Discharge instructions: Follow-up visit within 10-14 days, need for obtaining an automatic external defibrillator (AED)/"home defibrillator," and importance of CPR/defibrillator classes for significant others.
- Describe the procedure should ICD device deliver a "shock." If the patient is aware of the shocks,

the physician should be notified as soon as possible that the device is firing. With newer devices, patients may be unaware of shocks but may become symptomatic (e.g., become intolerant of activity, dizzy, have chest discomfort) with prolonged or serious dysrhythmias. Teach patient to record the number of "shocks" experienced.
- Explain use of the AED/ "home defibrillator," which is available commercially from several companies. It is designed to allow the nonmedical person or care providers untrained in dysrhythmia interpretation to effect defibrillation, and its purpose is to convert lethal dysrhythmias should the ICD fail.
- Explain that "shocks" during sinus rhythm may indicate a lead fracture in the ICD system. Usually this is detected while the patient is being monitored (e.g., by ECG in physician's office, hospital monitor, or Holter monitor).

NIC Learning Facilitation; Learning Readiness Enhancement; Risk Identification; Teaching: Disease Process; Teaching: Prescribed Medication; Teaching: Psychomotor Skill

Risk for infection related to invasive procedure into thorax

Desired outcome: Patient is free of infection as evidenced by normothermia; WBC count ≤11,000/mm^3; negative culture results; and absence of the clinical indicators of infection at the incision site and of the respiratory tract.
- Encourage and assist with deep breathing, coughing (if needed), and incentive spirometry exercises q2h, and encourage early ambulation to the chair. As indicated, assist patient with splinting the incision site with hands or pillow to promote pain control. Administer prescribed analgesics 20 min before scheduled breathing exercises. For more information, see this nursing diagnosis in "Acute Pneumonia," p. 180.
- Assess incision site q2h for warmth, erythema, swelling, and drainage. The presence of a seroma, which has the same symptoms as incision site infection, is confirmed by decubitus chest x-ray studies or CT.
- Monitor patient's temperature q2-4h, being alert to elevation >38.6° C (101.5° F).
- Monitor CBC for elevation of WBCs.
- Consult physician for significant findings.
- Teach patient and significant others the signs and symptoms of infection, both of the incision site and respiratory tract: cough, sputum production, fever, dyspnea, chills, headache, myalgia. Explain that the older adult with an infection may be confused and disoriented and may run low-grade fevers even though other indicators are present.

NIC Infection Control; Infection Protection; Cough Enhancement; Exercise Promotion; Surveillance; Medication Prescribing; Home Maintenance Assistance

For patients with a pacemaker (temporary or permanent) or patients with third-generation ICDs with cardiac pacing

Decreased cardiac output related to malfunction of cardiac pacemaker

Desired outcome: Within the 24-hr period preceding hospital discharge or throughout the duration of temporary cardiac pacing, patient has adequate cardiac output as evidenced by SBP >90 mm Hg; RR 12-20 breaths/min; HR <100 beats/min; urinary output >0.5 ml/kg/hr; warm and dry skin; and ECG indicative of effective capture, sensing, response to sensing, and function of antitachycardia pacing (if operational).
- Recognize and document paced rhythms. Events to document include the following: (1) recognition of pacing spike preceding P wave and/or QRS complex as appropriate for settings; (2) sensing of patient's inherent pacing; (3) response of pacemaker when triggering and/or inhibiting pacing; (4) response of HR to activity if pacemaker is programmed "rate responsive"; and (5) initiation of antitachycardia pacing or electric shock (with ICD) for dysrhythmias.
- Promptly detect problems with pacemaker functions. Include assessment of potential electromagnetic interference (EMI) (Table 4-14). Ensure that temporary pacemaker battery is still functional or changed as needed, and that cable connectors for temporary pacemakers are appropriately connected to the pulse generator (pacemaker box). For problems with functions of permanent pacemakers and ICDs, the physician should be notified immediately.
- Provide electrical safety measures for temporary cardiac pacing to include proper grounding and protection of exposed catheter tips and/or heart wires. Caregiver must wear rubber/nonconductive gloves when handling pacing lead wires/catheter so that microshocks are avoided. Microshocks can induce lethal dysrhythmias.
- Observe for complications of temporary pacing, which include dysrhythmias, lead displacement or fracture, lead perforation of the heart that could lead to cardiac tamponade, pericarditis, infection, and bleeding.

NIC Cardiac Care; Dysrhythmia Management; Vital Signs Management; Surveillance; Environmental Management: Safety

T A B L E 4 - 14   Electromagnetic Interference and the Third-Generation ICD and Some Programmable Pacemakers

Unsafe hospital procedures/equipment	Unsafe home equipment: use caution	Safe home equipment
MRI (magnetic resonance imaging)	Large magnets: junkyards, construction sites, other areas that may have large magnets	Microwave ovens
Nerve stimulator	Hand-held wands at airport security	Refrigerator magnets
Electrocautery	Bingo wands	Electric blankets
Diathermy	Certain slot machines	Tanning bed
Lithotripsy	Large stereo speakers (unsafe to carry)	Riding lawnmower
	Cellular telephones	Jacuzzi
	High-tension wires	CB radio
	Industrial transformers	HAM radio (except for antennas)
	Robotic jacks	Table saw
	Arc welders	Gas welder
	Power generators in dams	Electric drill
	Industrial motors	Weed Eater™
	Large boat motors	Small boat motors

ICD, Implantable cardioverter defribillator.

For patients with an implantable cardioverter-defibrillator
Altered sexuality patterns (or risk for same) related to fear of inducing dysrhythmias during sexual activity
Desired outcome: Within the 24-hr period before discharge from CCU, patient and significant other verbalize understanding of interventions during and alternatives for sexual intercourse.
• Ask patient to describe any symptoms of dysrhythmias during presurgical sexual experiences.
• Explain the following interventions or alternatives that can be made if patient continues to experience dysrhythmias during sexual intercourse:
  ❏ Patient may need to take a less active role.
  ❏ Patient may find that taking a prescribed vasodilator before engaging in sexual intercourse will prevent dysrhythmias.
  ❏ Suggest that during periods when dysrhythmias are a problem, less stressful forms of sexual activity, such as caressing and hugging, are positive alternatives.
• As appropriate, advise patient that stressful situations, such as extramarital relations or unfamiliar environment, may contribute to symptoms during sexual activity.
• Explain that the device may "shock" at any time. If the patient's partner is in contact with the patient's body at that time, the shock may be experienced as a tingling sensation by the partner.
NIC Sexual Counseling; Teaching: Sexuality; Anxiety Reduction; Coping Enhancement; Support Group

ADDITIONAL NURSING DIAGNOSES
The patient with ICD is at risk for pneumothorax. As indicated, also see "Pneumothorax," p. 198, for information related to this disorder. Also see nursing diagnoses and interventions in "Hemodynamic Monitoring," p. 23; "Psychosocial Support," p. 68; and "Psychosocial Support for the Patient's Family and Significant Others," p. 78.

Valvular Heart Disease

PATHOPHYSIOLOGY
Valvular heart disease manifests as either stenosis (i.e., narrowed valve opening) or incompetency/insufficiency (i.e., incomplete closure of valve leaflets). Stenosis impairs forward

blood flow. Increased resistance to ventricular ejection is created by the smaller valve opening. An incompetent valve allows backward flow of blood during systole (i.e., regurgitation), and this reduces the amount of forward flow of blood. One or more valves may be diseased. When a valve is compromised, symptoms of heart failure may develop.

Stenosis of a valve is caused by sclerosing, thickening, and calcification of the valve leaflets. A stenotic valve obstructs blood flow from the affected atrium or ventricle, which leads to hypertrophy of the chamber. Increased muscle mass is needed to pump through the narrowed valve. A lower percentage of volume in the ventricle is ejected, so that an increased amount of blood is retained with each contraction. A stenotic aortic or pulmonic valve results in increased intramyocardial wall tension. Persistent increase in wall tension leads to ventricular hypertrophy, as more muscle is needed for the increased work. The heart must remodel its structure to compensate for the work of pumping blood through the highly resistant valve opening. If stenosis is unrelieved, the enlarged ventricle eventually fails. When either ventricle fails, blood "backs up" into the atrium, leading to either pulmonary congestion from left ventricular failure or peripheral edema from right ventricular failure. Ventricular hypertrophy and high intramyocardial wall tension diminish blood flow to the endocardium. Patients may have angina and ventricular dysrhythmias. Both mitral and tricuspid stenosis can be severely debilitating, causing the easy fatigability and limited activity typical of heart failure.

An incompetent or regurgitant valve may be caused by rheumatic heart disease, dilation of the valve ring, or damage to the nearby valve structures. Regurgitation results in increased volume into the affected chamber (Figure 4-27). Mitral and tricuspid regurgitation can occur with the remodeling and enlargement of the ventricles.

The aortic valve has three cusps. People can be born with a bicuspid aortic valve, rendering them at higher risk for the development of either stenosis or regurgitation. Acute or sudden failure of a valve is more problematic, as the patient does not have time to develop compensatory mechanisms. If the person with valvular disease is asymptomatic, able to maintain adequate activity level, and has not developed ventricular dysfunction, medical management may be possible. Eventually valvular replacement or repair may be needed.

Valvular disorders have been reported from the use of the diet drug combinations of fenfluramine, dexfenfluramine, and phentermine. From one to four of the heart valves have been found to be diseased in persons who took these drugs. Aortic regurgitation was the most frequently noted finding and should be explored in patients presenting with this drug history.

ASSESSMENT

See Table 4-17, p. 270.

Many persons with long-standing valvular disease leading to atrial enlargement develop atrial fibrillation and should be monitored. Note irregularly irregular heart sounds with auscultation and/or heart movements with palpation. Aortic valve stenosis often manifests with syncope during activity. Chest pain occurs with aortic valve dysfunction totally independent of CAD, often due to low diastolic pressure and insufficient coronary perfusion pressure. Aortic regurgitation is indicated by three findings: Corrigan's pulse, DeMusset's sign, and Quincke's sign. Corrigan's pulse is a palpated pulse with rapid and forceful distention of the artery followed by quick collapse. DeMusset's sign is forward and backward bobbing of the head. Quincke's sign is visible pulsation seen with slight compression of nail-beds. The presence of pulmonic or tricuspid valve disease may be manifested by hepatic tenderness and enlargement from venous congestion due to right ventricular failure. Tricuspid regurgitation is associated with abnormal venous pulsations and elevated jugular pressure. Cardiac cachexia may be seen in persons with long-standing valvular dysfunction.

DIAGNOSTIC TESTS

Cardiac catheterization: A ventriculogram may assist in visualization of blood flow. Measurement of chamber pressures assists in determining the type of disorder present and the degree of severity. Gradients across valves can indicate severity of stenosis. Abnormal or giant V wave on the pulmonary artery occlusive pressure (PAOP) waveform (right-sided heart catheterization) is seen with mitral regurgitation. Visualizing the coronary arteries also provides information about concomitant CAD, which may require revascularization at the time of surgical valve repair or replacement.

Echocardiography: To determine ventricular function, chamber size, and valve function.
- *Doppler flow studies:* Continuous wave or pulsed wave frequencies used to determine blood flow.
- *Color flow mapping studies:* Uses colors (red and blue) to enhance the image of blood flowing through the heart.
- *TEE:* Uses an endoscope to produce an image unimpeded by the chest wall. The esophagus is close to the heart, so images are clearer or less distorted.

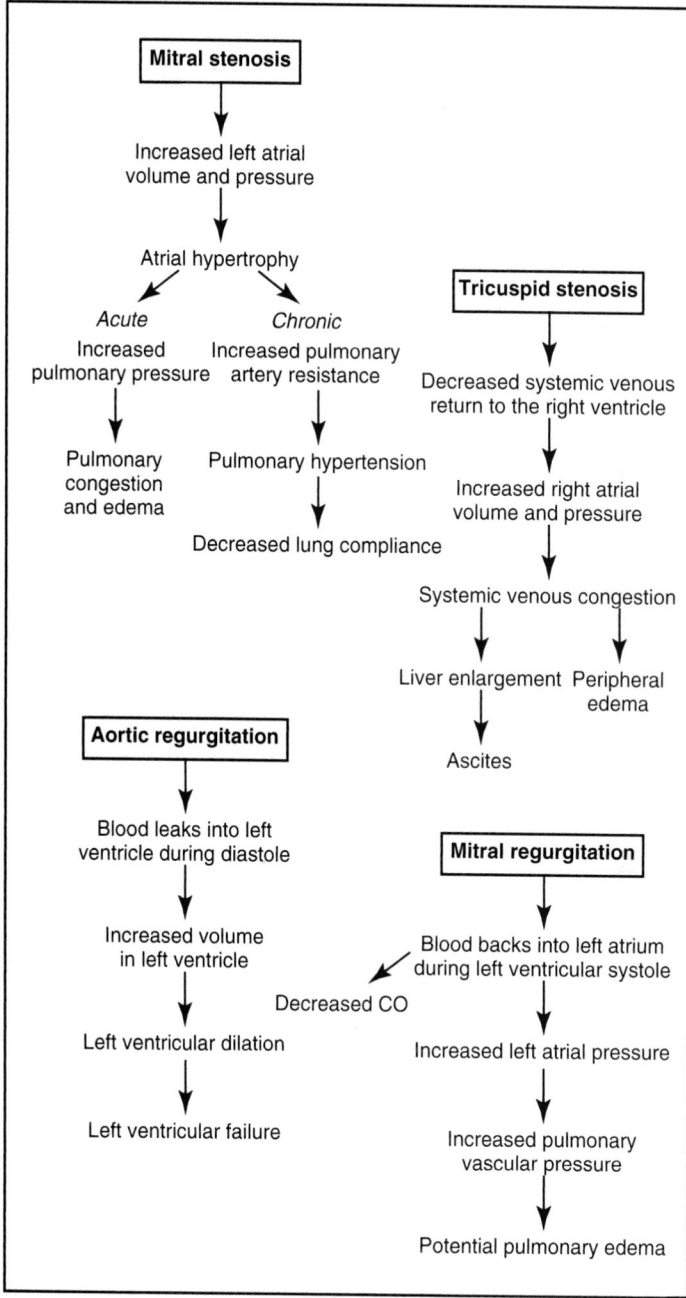

Figure 4-27: Disease progression with valvular disorders. (*CO*, Cardiac output.)

Laboratory test: B-type natriuretic peptide (BNP) elevation may be an early marker of heart failure resulting from the valvular stenosis or regurgitation.
ECG: See Table 4-18, p. 272.

MEDICAL INTERVENTIONS

Prophylaxis for infective endocarditis is mandatory medical therapy for all persons with valvular stenosis, regurgitation, or replacement (Table 4-15). Generally aortic stenosis is treated surgically. It is important to recognize that until the procedure is performed, vasodilators are contraindicated. They can further reduce peripheral vascular resistance and because the cardiac output is fixed, the fall in BP can lead to syncope or death. Nitrates may be avoided for treatment of chest pain. ACE inhibitors and β-blockers are poorly tolerated in these patients.

Asymptomatic patients with mild, chronic aortic regurgitation should undergo annual follow-up, including echocardiography at 2-3 yr intervals. Symptomatic patients with abnormal left ventricular function on echocardiography are surgical candidates.

Mild mitral stenosis may be managed medically. If present, atrial fibrillation must be rate-controlled and the patient should be anticoagulated to reduce the risk of stroke. β-Adrenergic blockers, calcium channel blockers, or digitalis may be used for rate control. Sodium restriction and diuretics may be added when pulmonary congestion is present.

In acute mitral regurgitation, vasodilators are used to reduce aortic pressure and impedance; this results in less regurgitation with improved forward flow of blood during systole. In chronic mitral regurgitation, vasodilators may not be used since afterload is not elevated.

Research Brief 4-1 Twenty-four persons with aortic stenosis and left ventricular dysfunction (mean ejection fraction of 0.25) underwent dobutamine stress echocardiograms. The subjects with non-severe aortic stenosis did well on the test; those with severe aortic stenosis did poorly. Authors suggest that this diagnostic test be used to decide who should undergo valve replacement.

Schwammenthal E et all: Dobutamine echocardiography in patients with aortic stenosis and left ventricular dysfunction: predicting outcome as a function of management strategy, *Chest* 119:1766-1777, 2001.

T A B L E 4 - 15   Antibiotic Prophylaxis With Infective Endocarditis

Regimen for dental, oral, or upper respiratory tract procedures

Standard regimen for those at risk who can take oral medications

Amoxicillin	2 g PO 1 hr before procedure*

If allergic to amoxicillin/penicillin

Clindamycin	600 mg PO 1 hr before procedure*
Cefazolin	1 g IM or IV 30 min before procedure

Alternate regimen for those unable to take oral medications

Ampicillin	2 g IV or IM 30 min before procedure

If allergic to amoxicillin/penicillin

Clindamycin	600 mg IV 30 min before procedure* or
Vancomycin	1 g IV 1 hr before procedure (no repeat dose needed)

Regimen for genitourinary/gastrointestinal procedures

Standard regimen

Ampicillin	2 g IM or IV† *and*
Gentamicin	1.5 mg/kg (not >80 mg) IV 30 min before before procedure† *and*
Amoxicillin	1.5 g orally q6h after initial dose of other medications

If allergic to ampicillin/amoxicillin/penicillin

Vancomycin	1 g IV over 1 hr before procedure† *and*
Gentamicin	1.5 mg/kg (not >80 mg) 1 hr before procedure‡

Alternative low-risk patient regimen

Amoxicillin	1 g PO before procedure*

Modified from Dajani AN et al: Prevention of bacterial endocarditis: recommendations by the American Heart Association, *JAMA* 264:2919-2922, 1990; *Circulation* 96:358-364, 1997.
*Give half of original dose q6h after initial dose.
†Optional to give same dose IV or IM q8h after initial dose.
‡May repeat once, 8 hr after initial dose.
P.O, By mouth; *IV,* intravenous; *IM,* intramuscular.

SURGICAL INTERVENTIONS

Valve replacement: Procedure with a mortality rate of about 6%, performed in patients with moderate to severe calcification, stenosis with insufficiency, and pure insufficiency. Three types of replacement valves are available: homografts and heterografts, which are tissue grafts, and artificial valves. *Homografts* are specially treated human cadaver valves. They are seldom used because of a lack of availability. A *heterograft* is a specially prepared valve from an animal, usually a pig or a cow. These commonly used valves are readily available. *Artificial or mechanical valves* are made from stainless steel, carbon, plastic and other durable materials. Natural tissue grafts are advantageous because there is less of a tendency for clots to form and adhere to them. Patients do not require anticoagulant therapy, but these valves function for only 5-8 yr. Clots tend to form on artificial valves, so these patients receive lifetime anticoagulant therapy for valves that function for 10-15 yr. Postoperative care of the patient who has had valve surgery is similar to that of the patient who has undergone CABG (see p. 217). Patients undergoing valve surgery are at increased risk for thrombosis and embolism (particularly with mechanical mitral valves and in patients with atrial fibrillation) and for valvular endocarditis.

Postoperative considerations specific to these patients are discussed later in this section under "Nursing Diagnoses and Interventions after Valve Replacement."

Commissurotomy: This is a procedure in which the stenotic valve is opened by a dilating instrument. When performed early in the course of the disease, chances of success are good, although the procedure may result in valve regurgitation and recurrent stenosis.

Surgical valvuloplasty: Valvular repair may be possible in select patients. In addition, insertion of a valvular ring can improve native valve function.

Percutaneous balloon valvuloplasty: For dilation of stenotic heart valves. Candidates for this procedure (1) are at high risk for surgery, (2) refuse surgery, (3) are older adults (often >80 yr of age), or (4) are informed of treatment choices and choose this procedure over others. The procedure parallels the technique for PTCA (see p. 211). The femoral artery and vein are cannulated, and the patient receives anticoagulation therapy. For aortic valve dilation, a catheter is passed into the femoral artery to measure supravalvular and left ventricular pressures before valvuloplasty. A balloon valvuloplasty catheter is then passed over a guidewire into the left ventricle. It is inflated three times for 12-30 sec at a pressure of 12 atm. Additional anticoagulant is administered, and the valve gradient is remeasured. To reach the mitral valve, the balloon valvuloplasty catheter is passed via the femoral vein and through the atrial septum to the mitral valve opening. The inflation procedure is the same.

With both aortic and mitral dilation, initial clinical improvement has been demonstrated in the valve gradient and in blood flow across the valve. However, benefits may not even last 6 months. Complications that have been observed include embolization to the brain, disruption of the valve ring, acute valve regurgitation, valvular restenosis, hemorrhage at the catheter insertion site, guidewire perforation of the left ventricle, and dysrhythmias.

NURSING DIAGNOSES AND INTERVENTIONS AFTER VALVE REPLACEMENT

Altered protection related to risk of bleeding/hemorrhage secondary to anticoagulation

---

Note: Patients undergoing aortic valve replacement are at a higher risk for postoperative hemorrhage than those undergoing CABG.

Desired outcome: Throughout hospitalization, patient is free of symptoms of bleeding or hemorrhage as evidenced by RAP ≥4 mm Hg; PAWP ≥6 mm Hg; BP within patient's normal range; CO ≥4 L/min; CI ≥2.5 L/min/m²; urine output ≥0.5 ml/kg/hr; urine specific gravity 1.010-1.030; and chest tube drainage ≤100 ml/hr.

- Measure chest tube drainage hourly. Report chest tube drainage >100 ml/hr. Maintain patency of chest tubes at all times.
- Monitor clotting studies. Be alert to and report prolonged PT, PTT, and ACT and decreased platelet count. Optimal values are as follows: PT 11-15 sec; PTT 30-40 sec (activated); and ACT ≤120 sec. For patient with prolonged PT, PTT, or ACT, administer IV protamine sulfate as prescribed if heparin was the anticoagulant used. After discharge from the hospital, the international normalized ratio (INR) should be maintained at 2.5.
- Assess VS hourly, and monitor patient for physical indicators of hemorrhage or hypovolemia: RAP <4 mm Hg; PAWP <6 mm Hg; decreased BP; decreased measured CO/CI; urine output <0.5 ml/kg/hr; increased urine specific gravity; and excessive chest tube drainage (>100 ml/hr). Be alert to a decreased Hct. Optimal values are: Hct ≥37% (female) and ≥40% (male).

- Assess postoperative chest x-ray for a widened mediastinum, which may indicate hemorrhage and possible cardiac tamponade.
- As prescribed, administer platelets, fresh-frozen plasma, or cryoprecipitate to replace clotting factors and blood volume.
- Administer packed RBCs as prescribed to replace blood volume, or use chest tube drainage for autotransfusion.
- To correct hyperfibrinolytic state (increased fibrin degradation products), aminocaproic acid is sometimes given slowly per IV bolus as prescribed (Table 4-16).

NIC Bleeding Reduction; Autotransfusion; Hemorrhage Control

Decreased cardiac output (or risk for same) related to negative inotropic changes secondary to intraoperative subendocardial ischemia and administration of myocardial depressant drugs

> **Note:** After cardiac surgery some myocardial depression is always present, usually lasting 48-72 hr. Patients with long-standing aortic stenosis or ventricular failure caused by mitral valve disease are at an even greater risk for postoperative low cardiac output.

Desired outcomes: Within 48-72 hr of this diagnosis, patient has adequate cardiac output as evidenced by normal sinus rhythm on ECG; measured CO of 4-7 L/min; CI $\geq$2.5 L/min/m^2; BP within patient's normal range; PAP 20-30/8-15 mm Hg; PAWP 6-12 mm Hg (or range specified by physician); Svo$_2$ 60%-80%; SVR 900-1200 dynes/sec/cm^{-5}; peripheral pulses >2+ on a 0-4+ scale; warm and dry skin; and hourly urine output $\geq$0.5 ml/kg/hr. Patient is awake, alert, and oriented.

- Monitor BP, PAP, RAP, Svo$_2$, HR, and heart rhythm continuously. Monitor PAWP, SVR, and CO hourly. Be alert to and report the following: elevated PAWP; decreased CO; decreased Svo$_2$; or elevated SVR.
- Monitor urinary output, noting output that is <0.5 ml/kg/hr for 2 consecutive hr.
- Monitor peripheral pulses and color and temperature of extremities q2h.
- Provide oxygen therapy as prescribed.
- Maintain an adequate preload (i.e., PAWP >6 mm Hg; RAP >4-6 mm Hg) via administration of IV fluids.

> **Note:** With aortic stenosis and severe left ventricular hypertrophy, a high filling pressure (i.e., PAWP >18 mm Hg) may be necessary to ensure an adequate cardiac output.

- Maintain a normal or reduced afterload (SVR <1200 dynes/sec/cm^{-5}) by administering prescribed IV vasodilating drugs such as nitroprusside and NTG.
- Maintain normal sinus rhythm by administering antidysrhythmic agents as prescribed. Atrial fibrillation is common in aortic and mitral valve disease and may result in a 20%-50% decrease in CO. If a junctional rhythm or bradycardia occurs, a pacemaker may be necessary.
- Administer inotropic agents as prescribed to maintain CI $\geq$2.5 L/min/m^2 and SBP >90 mm Hg. Commonly used agents include dobutamine, dopamine, milrinone, and amrinone. Monitor for side effects, including tachydysrhythmias, ventricular ectopy, headache, and angina.

NIC Cardiac Care; Hemodynamic Regulation

TABLE 4-16   Nursing Implications for Administration of Epsilon-Aminocaproic Acid (EACA)

- Be aware that rapid administration may induce hypotension, bradycardia, or cardiac dysrhythmias.
- Monitor for and report the following side effects: nausea, cramps, diarrhea, dizziness, tinnitus, headache, skin rash, malaise, nasal stuffiness, postural hypotension.
- Be alert to clotting or thrombosis, which can be precipitated by this medication. Assess for indicators of thrombophlebitis: calf erythema, warmth, tenderness, or increase in size or positive reaction for Homan's sign. Provide pneumatic compression stockings as prescribed.
- Assess for indicators of pulmonary emboli: chest pain, dyspnea, fever, tachycardia, cyanosis, falling BP, restlessness, agitation.
- Monitor and report blood levels of EACA via use of chromatography, which is available in some institutions.
- Consult physician promptly for significant findings.

Altered tissue perfusion (or risk for same): cerebral, related to impaired blood flow to the brain secondary to embolization resulting from cardiac surgery

> **Note:** An air embolus, particulate emboli from calcified valves, and thrombotic emboli from prosthetic valves may lodge in the brain, leading to varying degrees of stroke.

Desired outcome: Throughout hospitalization, patient has adequate or baseline brain perfusion as evidenced by orientation to time, place, and person; equal and normoreactive pupils; and ability to move all extremities, communicate, and respond to requests (or comparable to patient's preoperative baseline).
- Monitor patient immediately after surgery and hourly for signs of neurologic impairment: diminished LOC, pupillary response, ability to move all extremities, and response to verbal stimuli.
- Assess patient's orientation and ability to communicate, answer yes-no questions, point to objects, write responses and requests, identify family members, and state his or her location. Inform other health care personnel about patient's LOC and communication deficits.
- Assess patient's PT, PTT, and INR as heparin is tapered off and Coumadin therapy is instituted. Heparin and Coumadin may be initiated simultaneously to reduce the time needed to stabilize the lab values.
- If CNS impairment is noted, report findings to the physician and administer medications for brain resuscitation as prescribed.
- In the presence of CNS impairment, implement the following measures:
  ❏ Assist patient with turning and moving as needed. Teach patient to use unaffected extremities to assist with moving.
  ❏ Perform ROM to all extremities QID. Have patient assist as much as possible.
  ❏ Progress patient's activity level, as tolerated, with the assistance of a physical therapist.
- Assess patient's ability to swallow food and fluids. If patient's voice is hoarse or patient coughs when swallowing, consult physician. Patient may require nothing-by-mouth (NPO) status and an enteric tube until the swallowing reflex has improved.

NIC Surveillance; Cerebral Perfusion Promotion

Knowledge deficit: risk of infective endocarditis after valve surgery and preventive strategies

> **Note:** All patients with valve surgery are at risk for infective endocarditis (IE) as a result of bacteria entering the bloodstream and traveling to the heart, leading to destruction of a new tissue valve or obstruction of a new artificial valve.

Desired outcome: Within the 24-hr period before discharge from CCU, patient verbalizes knowledge about the risk of IE after valve surgery and the precautions that must be taken to prevent it.
- Teach patient about IE (see "Acute Infective Endocarditis," p. 269), describing what it is, how it develops, and how it may affect the repaired valve.
- Teach patient to caution dentists and other health care providers so antibiotics can be prescribed to prevent development of endocarditis after valve surgery. Antibiotics must be taken before any dental work or examination by instrument, including teeth cleaning, fillings, extractions, cystoscopy, endoscopy, or sigmoidoscopy.
- Instruct patient to cleanse all wounds and apply antibiotic ointments to help prevent infection.

NIC Teaching: Prescribed Medication; Surveillance

Knowledge deficit: risk of bleeding or clotting caused by excessive or insufficient anticoagulation therapy

> **Note:** Finding and maintaining the dose of Coumadin to maintain target INR is difficult. Foods, medications, vitamins, and food supplements can enhance or inhibit the efficacy.

Desired outcome: Within the 24-hr period before discharge from the hospital, patient or significant others verbalize knowledge about the risk of Coumadin therapy after valve surgery and the precautions that must be taken to prevent embolism or hemorrhage.
- Teach patient how to institute bleeding precautions after discharge. Shave with an electric razor. Take care when handling sharp objects. Prevent injury through an annual safety home check. Use soft-bristle toothbrush.
- Teach patient to call physician if bleeding or bruising noted.

- Teach patient and significant others to report all changes in medication to health care provider who is managing Coumadin or other anticoagulant therapy.
- Teach patient and significant others to avoid altering the intake of foods that may be high in vitamin K. Excessive intake of vitamin K can block Coumadin and lower the INR.

■ NIC   Teaching: Prescribed Medication; Teaching: Prescribed Diet; Surveillance

For patients undergoing percutaneous balloon valvuloplasty (PBV)

Knowledge deficit: procedure for percutaneous balloon valvuloplasty (PBV) and postprocedural assessment

Desired outcome: Within the 24-hr period before PBV, patient verbalizes rationale for the procedure, the technique, and postprocedural care.

- Assess patient's understanding of aortic stenosis and the purpose of valvuloplasty. Evaluate patient's style of coping and the degree of information desired.
- As appropriate for patient's coping style, discuss with patient and significant others the valvuloplasty procedure, including the following:
  - ❏ Location of diseased valve, using heart drawing.
  - ❏ Use of local anesthesia and sedation during procedure.
  - ❏ Insertion site of catheter: femoral artery and vein.
  - ❏ Use of fluoroscopy during procedure. Evaluate patient for a history of sensitivity to contrast material.
  - ❏ Postprocedural observations made by nurse: BP, HR, ECG, pulses, and catheter insertion site.
  - ❏ Importance of lying flat for 6-12 hr after the procedure to minimize the risk of bleeding.

■ NIC   Teaching: Procedure/Treatment

Decreased cardiac output (or risk for same) related to altered preload and negative inotropic changes associated with valve regurgitation or hemorrhage secondary to PBV; altered rate, rhythm, or conduction associated with dysrhythmias secondary to PBV.

Desired outcomes: Throughout the postoperative course, patient has adequate cardiac output as evidenced by normal sinus rhythm; CO 4-7 L/min; CI $\geq$2.5 L/min/m^2; HR 60-100 beats/min; RAP 4-6 mm Hg; PAWP 6-12 mm Hg; PAP 20-30/8-15 mm Hg; BP within patient's normal range; urinary output $\geq$0.5 ml/kg/hr; peripheral pulses >2+ on a 0-4+ scale; orientation to time, place, and person; and absence of new murmurs, pulsus paradoxus, or jugular vein distention.

- Monitor ECG continuously after procedure. Document any changes. Consult physician for dysrhythmias, and treat according to hospital protocol.
- Monitor CO/CI, HR, RAP, PAWP, and PAP hourly or as prescribed. Report a fall in CO/CI, a change in HR, and an increase or decrease in RAP, PAWP, or PAP.
- Monitor Hct and electrolyte values. Observe for a decrease in Hct or any change in electrolyte levels (particularly potassium) that could precipitate dysrhythmias. Optimal values are: Hct >37% (female) or >40% (male); and serum potassium 3.5-5 mEq/L.
- Assess heart sounds immediately after procedure and q4h. Report the development of a new murmur.
- Monitor patient for evidence of cardiac tamponade: hypotension, tachycardia, pulsus paradoxus, jugular vein distention, elevation and plateau pressuring of PAWP and RAP, and possibly an enlarged heart silhouette on chest x-ray study. For more information, see "Acute Cardiac Tamponade," p. 118.

■ NIC   Cardiac Care; Hemodynamic Regulation

Altered protection related to risk of hemorrhage or hematoma formation secondary to heparinization with PBV

Desired outcomes: Throughout the postoperative course, patient has minimal or absent bleeding or hematoma formation at the catheter insertion site. PTT is within therapeutic anticoagulation range (per physician or agency protocol).

- Monitor catheter insertion site for evidence of bleeding. Report hematoma formation, and outline the bleeding on the dressing for subsequent comparison.
- Keep patient's catheterized leg straight for the prescribed amount of time.
- Monitor heparin drip as prescribed. Usually heparin drip is maintained until 1-2 hr before the sheaths are removed.
- Monitor PTT for therapeutic range, which is usually 1½ times that of normal.
- When IV or invasive lines (arterial or venous sheaths) are removed, apply firm pressure either manually or with a mechanical clamp for 30 min.

■ NIC   Surveillance; Bleeding Reduction: Wound

ADDITIONAL NURSING DIAGNOSES

Also see "Knowledge Deficit" in "Pulmonary Emboli," p. 197. Also see "Altered Tissue Perfusion (or risk for same)" in "For Patients Undergoing Percutaneous Transluminal Coronary Angioplasty" under "Acute Coronary Syndromes," p. 217. See all nursing diagnoses in the discussion of "Coronary Artery Bypass Graft" in "Acute Coronary Syndromes," p. 217. Also see nursing diagnoses and interventions in "Hemodynamic Monitoring," p. 23; "Prolonged Immobility," p. 61; "Psychosocial Support," p. 68; and "Psychosocial Support for the Patient's Family and Significant Others," p. 78.

Acute Infective Endocarditis

PATHOPHYSIOLOGY

Infective endocarditis (IE) is infection of the endocardium (the innermost layer of the heart), often involving the natural or prosthetic valve; it is caused by bacteria, viruses, fungi, or rickettsiae. Four mechanisms are known to contribute to the development of IE. The first is a congenital or acquired defect of the heart valve or the septum (i.e., septal defect, stenotic or insufficient valve), often accompanied by a jet-Venturi stream of blood flowing from a high- to a low-pressure area through a narrow opening. The low-pressure area beyond the narrowed jet-flow site provides an ideal site for colonization by any infecting organism. The second mechanism is the formation of a sterile thrombus at the low-pressure site, which gives rise to vegetation. Third, a bacteremia occurs as a result of colonization in the vegetation. Fourth, a high level of agglutinating antibodies promotes growth of the vegetation, which usually develops on the low-pressure side of the valve leaflet within 1-2 cm of the tip of the leaflet.

Portals of entry for the infecting organism include the mouth and GI tract, upper airway, skin, and external genitourinary (GU) tract. All heart valves are at risk for infection, but the aortic and mitral valves are more commonly affected than the right-sided pulmonic and tricuspid valves. IV drug abuse increases the possibility of tricuspid IE. Once the infection process begins, valvular dysfunction, manifested by insufficiency with regurgitant blood flow, can occur, ultimately resulting in a decrease in cardiac output. The vegetation may enlarge and obstruct the valve orifice, further reducing cardiac output. The vegetation may break apart and embolize to vital organs. In severe cases, the affected valve may necrose, develop an aneurysm, and rupture or the infection may extend through the myocardium and epicardium to cause a pericarditis (see "Acute Pericarditis," p. 275). If the conduction system is affected by the spreading infection, bundle-branch block may occur. The chordae tendonae can become infected and rupture resulting in severe acute mitral or tricuspid regurgitation. Complications of IE occur suddenly, with a dramatic change in the clinical picture. Mortality rates between 20% and 50% have been reported. Recurrence of the infection occurs at a rate of 10%-20%.

ASSESSMENT

History and risk factors: Patients at higher risk for bacteremia leading to IE include those with valvular disease undergoing invasive procedures and insertion of devices including temporary pacemakers, PA catheters, central IV catheters or ports; those undergoing endoscopy, surgery, or dental work, and immunosuppressed patients (e.g., with organ transplants, carcinoma, burns, or diabetes mellitus). Users of illicit IV drugs are at risk of IE involving the tricuspid valve.

The American Heart Association recommends prophylactic antibiotics for patients with valvular disease, before and after selected invasive procedures and dental work to prevent or reduce the risk of IE. The current guidelines identify high risk individuals (bioprosthetic valve replacement, valvular repair, complex congenital repairs, and previous IE); moderate risk (other congenital defects, valvular dysfunction, hypertrophic cardiomyopathy, and mitral valve prolapse with evidence of regurgitant blood flow or thickened valve leaflets). Those with high or moderate risk should receive prophylaxis. Those at low risk (cardiac revascularization, pacemaker insertion, atrial septal defect repair, mitral valve prolapse with normal leaflets and no regurgitation) no longer require antibiotic prophylaxis. See Table 4-15.

Clinical presentation (acute infective stage): Fever, diaphoresis, fatigue, anorexia, joint pain, weight loss, and abdominal pain. The severity of symptoms varies depending on the infective organism. (For example, *Staphylococcus aureus* infection is more severe than that with *Streptococcus viridans*.) Acute presentation is defined onset within 1 week of infection, while subacute infections may take up to 4 weeks to present.

Physical assessment: A new or changed murmur may be heard as a result of the valvular dysfunction. (See Table 4-17 for a description of the types of murmurs heard, depending on the valve and the type of dysfunction present.) If heart failure is present, fine crackles may be auscultated at the lung bases and an S_3 or S_4 heart sound may be audible. The skin is often pale. If right-sided heart failure is present, skin and sclera may be jaundiced and edematous, with neck vein distention, a positive hepatojugular reflex, and ascites. Late assessment findings include anemia, petechiae, and clubbing

T A B L E 4 - 17   Assessment Findings With Valvular Heart Disease

Valve dysfunction	Murmur	Pathology	Hemodynamic changes
Aortic stenosis	Systolic, blowing murmur at second ICS, RSB; may radiate to the neck	Reduced flow across aortic valve with ↑ LV volume and pressure, with ↓ CO; LV hypertrophy eventually occurs	↑ LV pressure; ↑PAEDP; ↓ CO and aortic pressure with a narrow pulse pressure reflecting the decreased stroke volume
Aortic insufficiency	Diastolic blowing murmur at second ICS, RSB, beginning immediately with S₂	Regurgitant blood flow from aorta to LV during diastole	↑ LV pressure and PAEDP; ↓ CO; ↑ systolic BP and widened pulse pressure
Mitral stenosis	Loud, long, diastolic rumbling murmur at fifth ICS, MCL; may radiate to axilla; S₁ is loud and there is an opening snap with S₂	Reduced flow across mitral valve with left atrial and pulmonary congestion	↑ Mean PAP; ↓ CO
Mitral insufficiency	Systolic murmur at fifth ICS, MCL	Regurgitant blood flow from LV to left atrium, resulting in pulmonary congestion	Giant V waves in the PA occlusive tracing; ↑ systolic PAP; ↓ CO; mean PAP may be normal
Pulmonic stenosis	Systolic blowing murmur at second ICS, LSB; may radiate to neck	Reduced flow across pulmonic valve with ↑ RV volume and pressure, with diminished LV return, resulting in ↓ CO	↑ RV systolic pressure, mean RAP, PAEDP, and mean PAP
Pulmonic insufficiency	Diastolic murmur at second ICS, LSB that starts later and is lower pitched than aortic murmur	Regurgitant blood flow from pulmonary artery to RV during diastolic, resulting in RV overload	↑ Systolic RV pressure with wide pulse pressure; LVEDP and CO often normal but may ↓ if disorder is severe
Tricuspid stenosis	Diastolic murmur at fourth ICS	Reduced flow across tricuspid valve with ↑ right atrial and venous congestion	CVP ↑ with accentuated A wave on the RA waveform
Tricuspid insufficiency	Pansystolic murmur at fourth ICS, LSB that increases in intensity with inspiration	Regurgitant blood flow from RV to RA; right atrial and venous congestion occurs	↑ CVP with prominent V wave on the RA tracing; normal or low PAP, LVEDP, and CO

BP, Blood pressure; *CO,* cardiac output; *CVP,* central venous pressure; *ICS,* intercostal space; *LSB,* left sternal border; *LV,* left ventricle/ventricular; *LVEDP,* left ventricular end-diastolic pressure; *MCL,* midclavicular line; *PA,* pulmonary artery; *PAEDP,* pulmonary artery end-diastolic pressure; *PAP,* pulmonary artery pressure; *RA,* right atrium; *RAP,* right atrial pressure; *RSB,* right sternal border; *RV,* right ventricle/ventricular.

of the fingers. Splenomegaly occurs by 10 days due to the activation of the reticuloendothelial system. If marked, a splenic infarct may have occurred.

CLASSIC FINDINGS

Splinter hemorrhages: Small red streaks on the distal third of the fingernails or toenails.
Janeway lesions: Painless, small, hemorrhagic lesions found on the fingers, toes, nose, or earlobes, probably occurring as the result of immune complex deposition with inflammation.
Osler nodes: Painful, red, subcutaneous nodules found on the pads of the fingers or on the feet, probably occurring as a result of emboli producing small areas of gangrene or vasculitis.
Roth spots: Retinal hemorrhages with pale centers seen on fundoscopic examination.

> **Note:** If emboli of the vegetations occur in other areas, signs and symptoms of stroke or peripheral, myocardial, renal, or mesenteric insufficiency or infarct will be seen.

Hemodynamic measurements: Invasive monitoring devices are used cautiously with these patients, as they may cause further valvular dysfunction, embolization, and infection. PA catheters are used to assess hemodynamic function if necessary. Elevations of pulmonary artery and central venous pressures, with reduced cardiac output, are expected in most patients with IE.

DIAGNOSTIC TESTS

Blood cultures: Provide definitive diagnosis of the infecting organism. Antibiotics are prescribed based on organism sensitivity. The most common bacteria found in native (the patient's) valve IE are: *Streptococcus viridans* (60%), *Staphylococcus aureus* (25%), and the HACEK group (*Haemophilus, Actinobacillus, Cardiobacterium, Eikenella,* and *Kingella* species). Manipulations of the GI or genitourinary (GU) tract may result in IE from *Enterococcus faecalis.* Early prosthetic valve infections are caused by *Staphylococcus epidermidis* (33%), gram-negative bacteria (19%) and *Staphylococcus aureus* (17%). *Candida* is the most common fungal source of IE, accounting for 8% of prosthetic valve endocarditis and 1% of native valve endocarditis.

For low suspicion of IE, 3-6 sets of aerobic and anaerobic blood cultures should be drawn from different venipuncture sites over 24 hr. If suspicion is high, cultures should be drawn within 1-2 hr and empiric antibiotic treatment begun. Unfortunately, cultures can be negative when IE is present as a result of slow-growing organisms, prior antibiotic use, failure to obtain adequate number of specimens, or the organism's failure to grow in standard culture media.

Echocardiography: Reveals valvular involvement and vegetation size and defines severity of valvular dysfunction. M-mode, two-dimensional, Doppler, and transesophageal echocardiograms (TEE) are used. TEE is the preferred test, as it more accurately detects vegetation, especially with prosthetic valves. Obtained within 2 hr of acute presentation, the test is 90% specific and sensitive. Preexisting IE may be indistinguishable from new vegetations.

ECG: Frequently performed to determine if conduction system defects are present. Heart block may manifest if the AV node or bundle of His is affected by the infection. Atrial and/or ventricular enlargement may be seen from the prolonged effects of valve disease. Chambers may be enlarged or muscle walls thickened (Table 4-18). Atrial dysrhythmias including PACs, paroxysmal atrial tachycardia (PAT), and atrial fibrillation (AF) are frequently seen as chambers enlarge from volume overload. Also see Figures 4-5 through 4-25.

Hematology studies: Increased WBCs and eosinophils, with reduced RBCs.

Cardiac enzyme levels: Elevated if MI occurs from embolization of vegetations into the coronary arteries.

ABG values: Determine effectiveness of oxygenation, indicative of cardiac and pulmonary status.

Additional studies: Renal, mesenteric, and peripheral arteriograms or CT may be done to assess for embolization to other organs. Rheumatoid factor and erythrocyte sedimentation (ESR) are elevated. IE gamma globulins may be present. BNP will be elevated if heart failure is present.

COLLABORATIVE MANAGEMENT

Antibiotic treatment: Patients usually require 4-6 wk of IV antibiotics. The first 2 wk may be initiated during hospitalization and the remaining therapy done on outpatient status. The vegetation must be sterilized, abscesses treated, and spread of infection prevented. Initial antibiotic selection is empirical followed by therapy based on the results of the blood/tissue culture and sensitivity studies.

Fluid and sodium restriction: Used for optimal fluid balance with reduced heart function or heart failure. Specific restrictions must be individualized and based on severity of symptoms.

Bed rest: May be used initially, with activity as tolerated for the remainder of treatment.

TABLE 4-18   ECG Changes Frequently Found With Ventricular and Atrial Hypertrophy

Chamber	ECG Change
Left ventricular enlargement	"R" voltage increases in V_{4-6}; "S" voltage increases (deeper inflection) in V_{1-2}; the sum of "S" in V_1 or V_2 and "R" in V_5 or V_6 will be >35 mm, or "R" in any V lead will be >25 mm
Left atrial enlargement	"P mitrale" in leads II, III, aV_F, and V_1; P wave is m-shaped with a duration >0.1 sec
Right ventricular enlargement	"R" voltage increases in V_1 or V_2; "S" voltage increases in V_5, V_6; sum of "R" in V_1 or V_2 and "S" in V_5 or V_6 will be ≥35 mm
Right atrial enlargement	"P pulmonale" in leads II, III, aV_F, and V_1; P wave is >2.5 mm voltage and <0.1 sec duration

Diet: High in protein and calories to prevent cardiac cachexia and support the immune system.

Pharmacotherapy

Diuretics: May be used to decrease symptoms of heart failure by reducing intravascular volume.

Positive inotropic agents (e.g., digoxin, dobutamine, milrinone, amrinone): Used to increase contractility and cardiac output. For more information, see Appendix 7.

Vasodilators: nitroprusside, nitroglycerin: Reduce cardiac work and improve coronary arterial perfusion. Both preload and afterload (end-diastolic ventricular volume and pressure) may be reduced to help relieve symptoms of heart failure. Aggressive vasodilation is not well tolerated by all patients.

Sedation: May be necessary to allay anxiety and to reduce myocardial oxygen consumption.

Oxygen therapy with pulse oximetry (SpO$_2$): Oxygen (FiO$_2$) to maintain PaO$_2$>60 mm Hg, and pulse oximetry to monitor oxygen saturation continuously or intermittently to keep SpO$_2$ >95%.

Treatment of other signs and symptoms: If heart failure is present, see "Heart Failure," p. 220. See "Cardiogenic Shock," p. 290, for management of heart failure that has deteriorated into shock.

Prophylaxis regimen: Provides prophylactic antibiotics for those individuals at risk who undergo invasive procedures. See Table 4-16.

Surgical valve replacement: Required when heart failure worsens or if the infection fails to respond to antibiotics. See "Valvular Heart Disease," p. 261. An abscess or infected tissue may be surgically removed if there is no response to long-term antibiotics. If the patient is hemodynamically stable, surgery may not be needed. A surgeon is usually consulted in case of a heart failure emergency.

Research Brief 4-2   Body piercing is increasing in popularity among teenagers and young adults. This report provides a review of the literature on infective endocarditis resulting from tongue, nipple, and nasal piercing. In addition, a case study is provided. This report cautions health care providers to look to this increasingly popular fashion statement as a potential source for the development of infective endocarditis. Also, high and moderate IE risk individuals should be instructed to avoid undergoing these procedures.

Akhond H, Rahimi AR: *Haemophilus aphrophilus* endocarditis after tongue piercing, *Emerg Infect Dis*, vol 8, no 8, 2002. ©2002 Centers for Disease Control and Prevention (CDC).

NURSING DIAGNOSES AND INTERVENTIONS

Decreased cardiac output related to altered preload, afterload, or contractility secondary to valvular dysfunction

Desired outcomes: Within 72 hr after initiation of therapy, patient has adequate hemodynamic function with normal sinus rhythm or controlled atrial fibrillation as evidenced by the following: HR ≤100 beats/min; BP ≥90/60 mm Hg; stable weight; intake equal to output plus insensible losses; RR ≤20 breaths/min with normal depth and pattern (eupnea); and absence of S_3 or S_4 heart sounds, crackles, distended neck veins, and other clinical signs of heart failure. Optimally, the following normal parameters will be achieved: CO 4-7 L/min; CVP 2-6 mm Hg; PAP 20-30/8-15 mm Hg; RAP 4-6 mm Hg; and MAP 60-105 mm Hg.

- Assess heart sounds q2-4h. A change in the characteristics of a heart murmur may signal progression of valvular dysfunction, which can occur with insufficiency, stenosis, dislodgment of vegetation, or unseating of a prosthetic valve.
- Assess heart sounds. A new S_3 or S_4 sound may signal heart failure.
- Monitor heart rhythm continuously. Report dysrhythmias which may indicate the spread of infection to the conduction system or atrial volume overload.
- Monitor for signs of left-sided heart failure: crackles, S_3 or S_4 sounds, dyspnea, tachypnea, digital clubbing, decreased BP, increased pulse pressure, increased serum BNP levels, increased LVEDP, and decreased CO.
- Monitor for signs of right-sided heart failure: increased CVP, distended neck veins, positive hepatojugular reflex, edema, jaundice, increased serum BNP levels, and ascites.
- Monitor I&O hourly, and measure weight daily. Use the same scale and amount of clothing, and weigh patient at the same time of day for accuracy. Consult physician if patient's weight increases by more than 1 kg (2.2 lb) per day.
- If patient's PAP or RAP is high, decrease preload by limiting fluid and sodium intake and administer diuretics and venous dilators (e.g., NTG) as prescribed.
- If patient's MAP is high, decrease afterload with prescribed arterial dilators (e.g., nitroprusside).
- For low preload or afterload, consult with physician. Vasopressors may be prescribed.

Note: See "Cardiogenic Shock," p. 293, for a discussion of preload and afterload medications.

- If afterload is low, coronary artery perfusion may be reduced. Prevent further reductions by avoiding administration of morphine sulfate or rapid warming of hypothermic patients. Increase contractility with inotropic drugs, as prescribed.
- Provide activities as tolerated. Intolerance indicates ineffective oxygenation.
- Help patient reduce stress and myocardial oxygen consumption by teaching stress-reduction techniques such as imagery, meditation, or progressive muscle relaxation. For description of a relaxation technique, see "Health-Seeking Behavior," p. 259.
- Provide sedation as needed.
- Prevent orthostatic hypotension by changing patient's position slowly.

NIC Energy Management; Cardiac Care

Impaired gas exchange related to alveolar-capillary membrane changes with decreased diffusion of oxygen secondary to pulmonary congestion

Desired outcome: Within 24 hr of initiation of oxygen therapy and during the weaning process, patient has adequate gas exchange as evidenced by RR ≤20 breaths/min with normal pattern and depth (eupnea); Svo_2 60%-80%; Pao_2 ≥80 mm Hg; Sao_2 ≥95%; and natural skin color.

- Assess rate, effort, and depth of respirations. RR increases in response to inadequate oxygenation. Tachypnea may indicate pulmonary congestion.
- Assess color of skin and mucous membranes. Pallor signals impaired oxygenation.
- Auscultate lungs q2h. Report crackles, rhonchi, and wheezing.
- If hemodynamic monitoring with oximetry is used, assess Svo_2. It may fall because increased metabolic demands have increased oxygen uptake, or because the patient has increased extraction as a result of reduced perfusion/oxygen delivery. Svo_2 values may fall before the patient is symptomatic; they correlate with CO.
- Monitor ABG values for evidence of hypoxemia (Pao_2 <80 mm Hg), respiratory acidosis ($Paco_2$ >45 mm Hg, pH <7.35), or respiratory alkalosis ($Paco_2$ <35 mm Hg, pH >7.45) from tachypnea. Either may indicate impending respiratory failure.
- Deliver oxygen as prescribed. Observe respiratory rate of COPD patients if O_2 is increased to avoid hypoventilation and/or respiratory arrest.
- Assess arterial oxygen saturation with pulse oximetry. Normal oxygen saturation is 95%-99%. Levels of 90%-95% necessitate frequent assessment. Levels <90% require aggressive interventions to increase oxygen saturation. Consider increasing Fio_2, decreasing preload, and taking measures to improve ventilation.
- Place patient in high Fowler's position to facilitate gas exchange as tolerated.
- Have patient cough, deep breathe, and use incentive spirometry to prevent atelectasis.

NIC Invasive Hemodynamic Monitoring; Oxygen Therapy; Respiratory Monitoring

Risk for infection related to presence of invasive catheters and lines; inadequate secondary defenses secondary to prolonged antibiotic use

Desired outcomes: Patient is free of secondary infection as evidenced by clear urine with normal odor; wound healing within acceptable time frame; and absence of erythema, warmth, and purulent drainage at insertion sites for IV lines. On resolution of acute stage of IE, patient remains normothermic with WBC count ≤11,000/mm³; negative culture results; and HR ≤100 beats/min. SVR is ≥900 dynes/sec/cm⁻⁵; CO is ≤7 L/min; and Svo₂ is 60%-80%. No yeast overgrowth infections are present. Patient and significant others verbalize rationale for antibiotic therapy and identify where and how to obtain guidelines.

- Use strict aseptic technique to care for all invasive monitoring device insertion sites and IV lines. Rotate central lines per hospital protocol. Discuss feasibility of a tunneled catheter or peripherally inserted central catheter (PICC) line with physician.
- Change tubing, containers, and peripheral insertion sites per agency protocol. Inspect all catheter insertion sites daily for redness, drainage, or other evidence of infection. Rotate site immediately if infection is suspected.
- Provide mouth care at least q4h to minimize fungal and other infections. Women may require antifungal medications to manage vaginal yeast infections.
- Provide perineal care with soap and water for patients with indwelling urinary catheters. Inspect urine for evidence of infection, such as casts, cloudiness, or foul odor. Be alert to patient complaints of burning with urination after catheter is removed.
- Monitor temperature, WBC count, and HR. Increases may be signs of infection.
- Calculate SVR with CO measurements. Symptoms of septic shock include increased CO, decreased SVR, and increased Svo₂ during the early stages.
- Teach patient and significant others the importance of reporting signs and symptoms of recurring infections (e.g., fever, malaise, flushing, anorexia) or heart failure (e.g., dyspnea, tachypnea, tachycardia, weight gain, peripheral edema).
- Stress the importance of prophylactic antibiotics before invasive procedures such as dental examinations or surgery. The AHA publishes general guidelines for prophylactic antibiotic treatment for preventing IE (see Table 4-15).

NIC Fever Treatment; Surveillance; Infection Control

Altered tissue perfusion (or risk for same) renal, gastrointestinal, peripheral, cardiopulmonary, and cerebral, related to interrupted arterial blood flow secondary to emboli caused by vegetations

Desired outcome: Patient has adequate perfusion as evidenced by urine output ≥0.5 ml/kg/hr; 5-34 bowel sounds/min; peripheral pulses >2+ on a 0-4+ scale; warm and dry skin; BP ≥90/60 mm Hg; RR 12-20 breaths/min with normal pattern and depth (eupnea); normal sinus rhythm on ECG; and orientation to time, place, and person.

> **Note:** Unlike peripheral venous emboli, these emboli are caused by the vegetations; therefore prevention is difficult. Interventions are aimed at early detection of embolization and supportive therapies.

- Monitor I&O at frequent intervals. Be alert to urinary output <0.5 ml/kg/hr for 2 consecutive hr. Report oliguria, as it may signal impending acute renal failure.
- Monitor bowel sounds q2h. Report hypoactive or absent bowel sounds. Patients are at risk for decreased mesenteric perfusion and mesenteric or bowel infarction.
- Assess peripheral pulses, color, and temperature of extremities. Weak pulses (≤2+ on a 0-4+ scale) with pale, cool limbs/hands/feet may denote peripheral embolization.
- Monitor patient for confusion and changes in sensorimotor capabilities or cognition, which may signal cerebral emboli.
- Assess for chest pain, decreased BP, SOB, ischemic or injury pattern on 12-lead ECG, or elevated cardiac enzyme levels indicative of MI caused by vegetation emboli that have migrated to the coronary arteries (see "Acute Coronary Syndromes," p. 206).
- Assess for and report appearance of splinter hemorrhages, Osler's nodes, Janeway's lesions, and Roth's spots (see "Assessment," p. 271).

NIC Circulatory Care; Cardiac Care: Acute

ADDITIONAL NURSING DIAGNOSES

As appropriate, also see nursing diagnoses and interventions in "Nutritional Support," p. 1; "Hemodynamic Monitoring," p. 23; "Prolonged Immobility," p. 61; "Psychosocial Support," p. 68; "Psychosocial Support for the Patient's Family and Significant Others," p. 78; "Heart Failure," p. 220; and "Cardiogenic Shock," p. 290.

Acute Pericarditis

PATHOPHYSIOLOGY

Pericarditis is the general term for an inflammatory process involving the pericardium and the epicardial surface of the heart. Inflammation can occur as the result of an MI, an infection, chronic renal failure, or an immunologic, chemical, or mechanical event (Table 4-19). Often early pericarditis manifests as a dry irritation, whereas late pericarditis (after 6 wk) involves pericardial effusions that can lead to cardiac tamponade if severe. Pericarditis is most often seen in the intensive care unit (ICU) as a secondary finding. Astute assessment and recognition are essential for appropriate treatment, as symptoms can be masked by the primary condition. Patients sometimes come to be seen at the ICU with cardiac decompensation caused by the effusions.

The initial pathophysiologic findings of pericarditis include infiltration of polymorphonuclear leukocytes, increased vascularity, and fibrin deposition. Inflammation may spread from the pericardium to the epicardium or pleura. The visceral pericardium may develop exudates or adhesions. Large effusions can lead to cardiac tamponade (see p. 118). The excess fluid compresses the heart within the pericardial sac, which impairs filling of the chambers and ventricular ejection.

ASSESSMENT

Clinical presentation: The chief complaint is chest pain, but location and quality can vary. Usually the pain is aggravated by a supine position, coughing, deep inspiration, and swallowing. Dyspnea develops because of shallow breathing to prevent pain.

Early indicators: Fatigue, pallor, fever, and anorexia.

Late indicators (evident after development of effusions): Increased dyspnea, crackles, and neck vein distention. Heart sounds can be distant, and the pulmonic component of the second heart sound will be accentuated. Joint pain may be present when inflammation is generalized.

Physical assessment: Auscultation of heart sounds may reveal an intermittent friction rub with one, two, or three components: atrial systole, ventricular systole, and rapid ventricular filling. The rub is heard best with the diaphragm of the stethoscope positioned at the left lower sternal border. The rub is often positional so auscultation should be done with the patient in several positions (i.e., supine, sitting and leaning forward, lying on the left lateral side).

> **Note:** A friction rub may not be heard, even in the presence of pericarditis.

Pulsus paradoxus: BP should be checked for a paradox pressure >10 mm Hg. Normally the systolic pressure is slightly higher during the expiration and lower during inspiration. When effusions are present, this difference in systolic pressure across the respiratory cycle will be >10 mm Hg. For procedure, see "Acute Cardiac Tamponade," p. 119.

ECG findings: During acute episodes, atrial dysrhythmias such as PAT, PACs, atrial flutter, or atrial fibrillation may occur. Late dysrhythmias include ventricular ectopy or bundle-branch blocks if the inflammatory process involves the ventricles. Pericardial effusion may decrease the voltage of the QRS complex on the ECG. Diffuse ST segment elevation can be documented as described in Table 4-20.

TABLE 4-19   Conditions Associated With the Development of Pericarditis

Autoimmune cardiac injury	Neoplasms
Dressler syndrome (post-MI)	Radiation injury
Postpericardiotomy syndrome	Rheumatologic disease
Drug-induced	Rheumatic fever
Procainamide, hydralazine	Rheumatoid arthritis
Idiopathic	Systemic lupus erythematosus
Infection	Trauma
Myocardial infarction	Uremia

MI, Myocardial infarction.

TABLE 4-20   ECG Changes With Pericarditis

Stage	Time of change	Pattern
1	Onset of pain	ST segments have a concave elevation in all leads except a V_L and V_1; T waves are upright
2	1-7 days	Return of ST segments to baseline with T wave flattening
3	1-2 wk	Inversion of T waves without R or Q changes
4	Weeks to months	Normalization of T waves

Hemodynamic measurements: PA catheter reveals elevated CVP, PAP, and PAWP. As effusions increase, CO will decrease. If adhesions are present, the filling of the chambers may be restricted, resulting in reduced end-diastolic volumes and pressures. If cardiac tamponade is developing, the pressures in all heart chambers eventually equalize and the patient has a cardiac arrest.

DIAGNOSTIC TESTS

ECG: Will show ST segment or T wave changes, which often are confused with ischemic changes. In pericarditis they are more diffuse and follow a four-stage pattern (see Table 4-20).

Echocardiography: Will show absence of echoes in the areas of effusion. This test, which is essential for quantifying and evaluating the trend of effusions, will appear normal if the pericarditis is present without effusions. TEE may be helpful in identifying some areas of effusion.

Computed tomography (CT): Will differentiate restrictive pericarditis from constrictive cardiomyopathy by means of the appearance of thickened pericardium on the cross-sectional views of the thorax, which occurs with pericarditis.

Cardiac enzyme levels: May reveal elevation of the CK and MB bands if the epicardium is inflamed.

Cardiac technetium pyrophosphate scan: May show a diffuse regional uptake ("hot spot") in an area of epicardial inflammation.

Hematologic studies: Antistreptolysin O (ASO) titer is elevated when the cause of the pericarditis is an immunologic disorder. If the pericarditis is the result of an infection, blood cultures will identify the infecting organism. Other markers of inflammation can be seen (elevated WBC, C-reactive protein [CRP], or ESR) unless the pericarditis is secondary to uremia.

COLLABORATIVE MANAGEMENT

Bed rest: Until pain and fever have disappeared. Activity is increased as tolerated.

Pharmacotherapy

Nonsteroidal antiinflammatory drugs (NSAIDs): Preferred for reducing inflammation, particularly if the patient has had an MI or cardiac surgery, since these drugs do not delay healing as do corticosteroids. NSAIDs have fewer side effects than do steroids. Examples include aspirin, indomethacin, and ibuprofen. NSAIDs can increase fluid retention and may cause renal insufficiency and worsen heart failure.

Prednisone: Given at 60-80 mg daily for 5-7 days if there is no response to NSAIDs. Must be tapered gradually to avoid adrenal insufficiency.

Immunosuppressive medications: In resistant and chronic pericarditis, immunosuppressive medications or colchicine may be effective in reducing the inflammatory response.

> **Note:** In the presence of effusions, anticoagulants are contraindicated because of the high risk of cardiac tamponade, which can result from bleeding into the pericardium.

Subxiphoid pericardiocentesis: Performed if effusions persist and cardiac status decompensates. A needle (used in a tamponade emergency) or catheter is used to remove the fluid compressing the heart. Echocardiography is used to guide the catheter tip and assess the amount of effusion remaining. The pericardial catheter may be removed after the fluid has been withdrawn or may be left in place for several days to allow for gradual removal of fluid. Usually ≥100 ml is withdrawn q4-6h. The catheter is flushed with saline q4-6h after withdrawal of the effusion to prevent clotting. Strict aseptic technique is essential for preventing infection.

Pericardiectomy: To prevent cardiac compression or relieve the restriction. It may be necessary in chronic pericarditis for patients with recurrent effusions or adhesions. This procedure is often required in severe and recurrent pericarditis associated with uremia.

Research Brief 4-3   As part of the civilian preparation for possible terrorist attack before the Iraq military encounter of 2003, the small pox vaccination was administered to 31,297 civilian health care and public health workers in 54 jurisdictions. Because the Vaccine Adverse Event Reporting System (VAERS) now tracks all adverse effects of a vaccine, the Centers for Disease Control and Prevention (CDC) was able to promptly identify seven cases of pericarditis that occurred subsequent to vaccination. Although this is a small number, it bears watching in those with a cardiac history. Caution should be taken as to who is administered the vaccine. Further tracking of this information will be available through the CDC and found at their website: www.cdc.gov.

Update on adverse events following civilian smallpox vaccination—United States, *MMWR*, posted 4-21-03.

NURSING DIAGNOSES AND INTERVENTIONS

Ineffective breathing pattern related to guarding as a result of chest pain
Desired outcome: Within 48 hr of this diagnosis, patient demonstrates RR 12-20 breaths/min with normal depth and pattern (eupnea) and reports that chest pain is controlled.
- Assess the character and intensity of the chest pain. Provide prescribed pain medication as needed.
- Teach patient to avoid aggravating factors such as a supine position. Encourage patient to alter his or her position to minimize the chest pain. The following positions may be helpful: side-lying, high Fowler's, or sitting and leaning forward.
- Assess lung sounds q4h. If breath sounds are decreased, encourage patient to perform incentive spirometry exercises q2-4h along with coughing and deep-breathing exercises.
- To facilitate coughing and deep breathing, teach the patient to support the chest by splinting with pillows, or by holding the arms around the chest.

NIC Positioning; Pain Management

Activity intolerance related to bed rest, weakness, and fatigue secondary to impaired cardiac function, ineffective breathing pattern, or deconditioning
Desired outcome: Within 72 hr of this diagnosis, patient exhibits cardiac tolerance to increasing levels of exercise as evidenced by peak HR ≤20 beats/min over patient's resting HR; peak SBP ≤20 mm Hg over patient's resting SBP; Svo_2 ≥60%; RR <24 breaths/min; normal sinus rhythm on ECG; warm and dry skin; and absence of crackles, murmurs, and chest pain during or immediately after activity.

Note: Steroid myopathy may develop in patients who receive high doses or long-term treatment with steroids. Muscle weakness occurs in the large proximal muscles. Patients experience difficulty in lifting objects and moving from a sitting position to a standing position. Steroids also increase the risk of developing osteoporosis and bone fracture.

- Assess the patient for evidence of muscle weakness; assist with activities as needed.
- Modify the activity plan for the patient with post-MI pericarditis who is receiving steroids. A lower activity level may help prevent thinning of the ventricular wall and reduce the risk of an aneurysm or rupture of the ventricle.
- Teach patient to resume activities as tolerated, resting between activities.
- For other interventions, see this nursing diagnosis in "Prolonged Immobility," p. 61.

NIC Energy Management; Cardiac Care: Rehabilitative; Teaching: Prescribed Activity/Exercise

ADDITIONAL NURSING DIAGNOSES

Also see "Decreased Cardiac Output" in "Acute Cardiac Tamponade," p. 120. See "Renal Transplantation" for "Knowledge Deficit: Immunosuppressive Medications and Their Side Effects," p. 332, "Impaired Skin Integrity," p. 334, and "Risk for Infection," p. 333. For other nursing diagnoses and interventions, see "Prolonged Immobility," p. 61.

Hypertensive Emergencies

PATHOPHYSIOLOGY

Hypertension is sustained elevation of the resting arterial pressure. In 2003 the AHA estimated that more than 50 million Americans have hypertension defined as elevation of BP above 140/90 mm Hg. Because fatal stroke or other cardiac event can occur as a result of hypertension, the impact of this disease on mortality is greater than that of any other health problem. Recent studies have demonstrated that even high normal BP increases the risk of stroke. Table 4-21 describes the blood pressure classifications and the recommendations for follow-up.

Most often, hypertension occurs as a primary disorder of unknown etiology. Secondary hypertension is the result of other disorders that alter the mechanisms that control BP. Many factors contribute to the development of secondary hypertension: (1) increase in secretion of catecholamines; (2) increase in secretion of renin by the kidneys; (3) increase in serum sodium and blood volume; (4) increase in plasma and extracellular fluid volume; (5) reduction in kidney perfusion pressure; (6) impairment of control mechanisms in the kidney; and (7) alteration in adrenal cortical hormone secretion. Table 4-22 lists the causes of secondary hypertension.

Hypertensive crisis is seen in about 1% of the population with hypertension. When it occurs, immediate vascular necrosis is a threat that can occur if the diastolic pressure exceeds 120 mm Hg, although necrosis also has been seen with mean arterial pressures (MAPs) ≥150 mm Hg.

The rapidity of the rise in pressure may be more destructive than the actual BP level recorded. If left untreated, hypertensive crisis is fatal in 75% of affected persons within 1 yr. With current treatment techniques, 1-yr mortality is 30% and 5-yr mortality is 50%. Hypertensive crisis can lead to hypertensive encephalopathy as cerebral blood vessels dilate because of their inability to effect autoregulation. Blood flow is increased, and the excessive pressure drives fluid into the perivascular tissue, resulting in cerebral edema. The extreme pressure can cause arteriolar damage, as demonstrated by fibrinoid necrosis of the intima and media of the vessel wall. Although any organ is vulnerable, the eyes and the kidneys are most likely to suffer damage, leading to blindness and renal failure.

Patients with hypertension who are admitted to the ICU may have a rebound elevation of the BP if their usual antihypertensive regimen is interrupted. In addition, a loss of BP control can occur because of the nature of the primary disorder, trauma, or the stress of the ICU. Complications of hypertension include nephrosclerosis, aortic dissection, CAD, heart failure, stroke, and peripheral vascular disease.

Pheochromocytoma is a chromaffin-cell tumor of the adrenal medulla that causes secretion of high levels of catecholamines (epinephrine and norepinephrine). The surge of catecholamines causes episodic elevations of BP, increased metabolism, and hyperglycemia. These surges can occur as often

TABLE 4-21   Classification of Blood Pressure for Adults Age 18 and Older*

Category	Systolic pressure (mm Hg)		Diastolic pressure (mm Hg)	Follow-up
Normal [†]	<120	and	<80	
Prehypertension [‡]	130-139	or	80-89	Begin lifestyle modification
Hypertension [§]				
Stage I	140-159	or	90-99	Begin pharmcologic therapy along with lifestyle change
Stage II	>160	or	>100	Evaluate or refer to source of care within 1 mo

Modified from National Institutes of Health: the Seventh Report of the Joint National Committee on Prevention, Detection, Evaluation, and Treatment of High Blood Pressure (JNCVII), NIH Pub. No. 03-5231, May 2003.

*Not taking hypertensive drugs and not actually ill.

[†] Optimal blood pressure with respect to cardiovascular risk is below 120/80 mm Hg. However, unusually low readings should be evaluated for clinical significance.

[‡] Begin instructions on life-style modification, including:

Lose weight if overweight.

Limit alcohol intake <1 oz ethanol/day (24 oz beer, 8 oz wine, or 2 oz whiskey).

Reduce sodium intake to <100 mmol/day (2.3 g sodium or 6 g sodium chloride).

Maintain adequate dietary potassium, calcium, and magnesium intake.

Stop smoking.

Reduce dietary saturated fat and cholesterol intake for general cardiovascular health.

[§] Based on the average of two or more readings taken at each of two or more visits.

[¶] In the presence of diabetes and kidney disease, treat to a goal at 130/80.

TABLE 4 - 22 Causes of Secondary Hypertension

Renal disease	Endocrine disorders	Congenital disorders	Pregnancy-induced disorders	Drug-induced disorders	Other
Acute glomerulonephritis	Cushing's syndrome	Adrenal hyperplasia	Pregnancy-induced hypertension (PIH)	Cyclosporine	Sleep apnea
Chronic pyelonephritis	Pheochromocytoma	Coarctation of the aorta	Preeclampsia	Oral contraceptives	
Hydronephrosis	Primary aldosteronism		Eclampsia	Steroids	
Renal tumors	Thyroid/parathyroid disease				
Renovascular hypertension					

as 25 times a day or as infrequently as every 2 months. Although pheochromocytoma accounts for only 0.5% of all new cases of hypertension, it is found in a much larger proportion of individuals who experience hypertensive crisis. The tumor is most often benign (90% of cases).

ASSESSMENT

History and risk factors: Psychologic stress, diet high in sodium, and cigarette smoking increase the risk of developing high BP. Hypertension is a familial disease; genetic and environmental factors contribute to its etiology. Hypertension is a risk factor for angina and MI. See "Acute Coronary Syndromes," p. 206.

Clinical presentation

Early indicators: Although most patients are free of symptoms, vague discomfort, fatigue, dizziness, and headache can occur.

Late indicators (nearly always present during a hypertensive crisis): Throbbing suboccipital headache, irritability, confusion, somnolence, stupor, visual loss, focal deficits, and coma. The patient also may have signs of heart failure, including dyspnea on exertion, orthopnea, and paroxysmal nocturnal dyspnea. If CAD is present, angina may occur as a result of increased myocardial oxygen consumption caused by the high vascular resistance, which is evidenced by high BP. Chest pain may also indicate a dissecting aortic aneurysm. Renal symptoms include hematuria, nocturia, and azotemia. Nausea and vomiting also may occur.

Physical assessment: An accurate cuff pressure must be obtained after 5 min of rest, with two or more measurements taken at least 2 min apart. Average these readings unless there is a 5 mm Hg or greater difference. Greater differences warrant additional readings. A well-calibrated manometer with a properly fitting cuff or an automatic BP recorder should be selected for use. The bladder of the cuff must encircle 80% of the arm and cover two thirds of the length of the upper portion of the arm. Note when the patient last smoked or used any nicotine product, how much caffeine was consumed during the previous 4 hr, and whether adrenergic stimulants (e.g., over-the-counter [OTC] decongestants or bronchodilators) have been used within the past 24 hr, as they elevate BP.

Cardiac assessment: Evaluates for left ventricular hypertrophy, which results from the need of the heart to pump against the high SVR or afterload. A left ventricular heave may be palpated with the palm of the hand at the mitral area (fifth intercostal space [ICS] at the midclavicular line [MCL]). A fourth heart sound or S_4 gallop may be auscultated in the same site with the stethoscope bell. If cardiac failure is present or the left ventricle is enlarged, the apical impulse will be felt nearer to the anterior axillary line (AAL) instead of the MCL. In addition, crackles may be auscultated in the presence of cardiac failure. Pulsus alternans, an alteration in pulse pressure with a regular rhythm, may be palpated at any of the major pulse points. All peripheral pulses should be palpated bilaterally. With coarctation of the aorta, the femoral pulses will be bilaterally weak with a slow up-stroke, whereas the radial and brachial pulses will be normal or bounding.

Eye assessment: A funduscopic exam is performed to determine whether hemorrhage, fluffy cotton exudates, or arterial-venous nicking of the vessels has occurred. When these changes occur, visual perception is decreased. Nurses should assess the patient's gross visual acuity by the ability to read and recognize objects and people.

Neurologic assessment: May reveal evidence of a residual neurologic deficit from a cerebral infarct or ischemic event, as manifested by a positive Babinski reflex (up-going toe), hemiparesis, hemiplegia, ataxia, confusion, or cognitive alterations.

Pheochromocytoma assessment: Paroxysmal elevations of BP associated with palpitations, tachycardia, headache, diaphoresis, pallor, warmth or flushing, tremor, excitation, fright, nervousness, feelings of impending doom, tachypnea, abdominal pain, nausea, and vomiting. Episodes also are associated with hyperglycemia and hypermetabolism. Postural hypotension and paradoxic response to antihypertensive medications may occur.

DIAGNOSTIC TESTS

The definitive test for hypertension is BP measurement. Once hypertension has been documented, many tests may be performed to determine the amount of end-organ damage or to diagnose the condition responsible for the development of secondary hypertension.

ECG: Left ventricular hypertrophy (LVH) is demonstrated by an increase in voltage in the LV precordial lead (V_{5-6}). In addition, a strain pattern of ST segment depression and T wave inversion reflects repolarization abnormalities caused by the endocardial fibrosis that accompanies hypertrophy. General voltage criteria for LVH are (1) "R" in V_5 or V_6 plus "S" in V_1 >35 mm or (2) voltage of "R" in any precordial lead >25 mm.

Echocardiography: LVH with or without dilation will be demonstrated on echocardiogram by an increase in the wall thickness with or without increased chamber size.

Chest x-ray: If dilation of the left ventricle is present, the cardiac silhouette will be enlarged. If failure is present, there will be evidence of pulmonary congestion and pleural effusions. Notching of the aorta and a distended aortic root are indicative of coarctation of the aorta. If widening of the aorta is seen, dissection is suspected (see p. 288).

Urinalysis/urine culture: Urinalysis results will be normal until hypertension causes renal impairment. Specific gravity may be low (<1.010), and proteinuria may be present. Glomerulonephritis is suspected if the urine contains granular or red cell casts or if the patient has hematuria. Pyelonephritis is suspected if there is bacterial growth in the urine. Elevations of the 24-hr urine vanillylmandelic acid (VMA) and urinary catecholamines (10-50 times normal) are indicative of pheochromocytoma. The VMA level is elevated only during episodes of hypertension. If the patient has Cushing's disease, the urine cortisol or adrenocorticotropic hormone (ACTH) level will be elevated.

Blood studies: If renal parenchymal disease is present, the patient may have serum creatinine >1.3 mg/dl and BUN >20 mg/dl. The RBC count may fall because of hematuria caused by acute tubular necrosis (ATN).

Radiographic studies to detect pheochromocytoma: Angiography may identify an adrenal medullary tumor. An intravenous pyelogram (IVP) with nephrotomography or CT may identify the adrenal tumor.

COLLABORATIVE MANAGEMENT

Treatment of hypertensive crisis: Immediate and rapid reduction in BP. Lower MAP no more than 25% within 2 hr. Try to reach 160/100 within 2-6 hr.

Nitroprusside: A rapid arterial and venous dilator. Usual initial dose is 10-25 mcg/min, with increases of 5-10 mcg q5min. Maintenance dosage for nitroprusside ranges from 0.25-10 mcg/kg/minute until oral medications are effective. This drug is short acting, and BP will rise almost immediately if the drip is stopped. Direct arterial pressure monitoring is essential for titration of this drug, with constant vigilance to prevent hypotension. When oral antihypertensives begin to affect the BP, weaning is done carefully to prevent hypotensive episodes. Nitroprusside is metabolized to thiocyanate, a toxin, which can cause fatigue, nausea, tinnitus, blurred vision, and delirium. Serum thiocyanate levels should be drawn after 48 hr of use and regularly thereafter. Levels <10 mg/dl are considered safe.

Fenoldopam: This new alternative to nitroprusside has a similar antihypertensive profile. Fenoldopam is a selective dopamine-1 receptor agonist with a half-life of 9.8 min. It has few side effects other than hypotension and does not require thiocyanate monitoring. Initial dose is 0.1 mcg/kg/min and it can be increased by 0.05 mcg/kg/min. The patient must still be kept in the ICU and undergo arterial monitoring with this drug.

Labetalol hydrochloride: A fast-acting alpha-(α-) and β-blocker, which also can be used to treat the patient in hypertensive crisis. Given slowly by IV push, beginning with a 20- to 80-mg dose, repeated q10min; or a continuous infusion of 2 mg/min can be administered. The usual cumulative dose is 50-200 mg. Keep the patient supine during the injection and until stable. Check BP q5min × 6 and then q30min × 4. Monitor for bronchospasm, heart block, or orthostatic hypotension.

Esmolol: A fast-acting β-blocker with an onset of action of 1-2 min and a duration of 10-20 min. Initial dose is 250-500 mcg/kg/min for 1 min; then 50-100 mcg/kg/min for 4 min. May repeat the sequence. Observe for hypotension, nausea, and vomiting and with asthmatics, for bronchospasm.

Nicardipine: A potent calcium channel blocker given 5-15 mg/hr. Onset is 5-10 min, duration is 1-4 hr. May cause tachycardia, headache, and flushing. It has been noted to aggravate angina.

Enalaprilat: An ACE inhibitor. Usual dose is 1.25-5 mg by IV bolus, administered over a 5-min period. Dose may be repeated q6h. Patients on diuretics should receive a lower standard dose. Peak effect from the first IV dose should be at 4 hr, but for subsequent doses, the peak effect occurs 1 hr after administration. Enalaprilat should be used with caution in patients with renal failure or those with bilateral renal artery stenosis (because of high renin states). Avoid in acute MI.

Hydralazine: A potent vasodilator administered as a 10- to 20-mg IV bolus or a 10- to 40-mg intramuscular (IM) injection. The onset is 10-30 min, with a duration of 2-6 hr. Adverse effects include tachycardia, headache, vomiting, and aggravation of angina.

Nitroglycerin: A coronary and peripheral vasodilator supplied in a 50-mg vial, which is added to a 250-ml glass bottle of D_5W. The IV infusion may be concentrated to prevent fluid overload if higher doses are needed to control BP. Nitroglycerin (NTG) is administered via an infusion pump starting at 5 mcg/min. Onset is rapid, so BP must be monitored closely during titration of the drug. Increase by 5-10 mcg q3-5 min. Headache is common and controlled with analgesics.

Phentolamine: An α-adrenergic blocking agent that drug reduces afterload. Has minimal effect in reducing BP except for secondary hypertension caused by pheochromocytoma. A dose of 5-15 mg is administered via IV push. Onset is 1-2 min. Used with caution in patients with CAD.

Nifedipine:

> **Caution:**   In the past, Nifedipine had been given sublingually by piercing the capsule to provide rapid treatment for hypertension. Effects were variable and dangerous. Serious side effects such as stroke were reported. Not recommended for management of hypertensive emergency.

Oral antihypertensive medications: Added as soon as the patient responds to oral medications, including captopril, clonidine, and labetalol. As the patient is adjusted to a routine antihypertensive regimen, hydrochlorothiaze, ACE inhibitors, calcium channel blockers, β-blockers, α-blockers, or angiotensin receptor blockers may be used in various combinations. For persons with severe hypertension, 3-5 medications are often needed to achieve normal BP.

> **Note:**   The latest guideline for the treatment of hypertension, *The Seventh Report of the Joint National Committee on Prevention, Detection, Evaluation, and Treatment of High Blood Pressure* (JNC 7), was published in 2004. The report is available at the National Heart, Lung, and Blood Institute website (www.nhlbi.nih.gov/guidelines/hypertension/index.htm).

Lifestyle alterations: Behavioral changes are the cornerstones of medical treatment for early and established hypertension. Normal body weight should be maintained. Alcohol consumption should be <1 oz ethanol a day. Daily intake of sodium for the average adult should be modified to 2-3 g for the person with hypertension. Smoking cessation is imperative (1) to halt the injury to the intima of the coronary and peripheral vessels and (2) to reduce the workload of the heart. A regular aerobic program has been proved beneficial in maintaining better control of BP. This should consist of 30 min of exercise 3-5 times per wk at a target heart rate of 60%-80% maximum. Maintenance of adequate potassium, calcium, and magnesium intake is important.

Pharmacotherapy: Maintenance pharmacotherapy for hypertension is now approached by evaluating on an individual basis the best treatment option based on the patient's other disease states or demographic factors. This approach has been accepted and promoted by the Joint National Committee VI (JNC VII) and the AHA. After an adequate trial of the first drug, a second drug from a different category may be tried. Figure 4-28 identifies the algorithm, and Table 4-23 lists the medications, the usual dosage, the schedule, and potential side effects of the antihypertensive agents commonly used.

Surgical treatment: Although there is no surgical intervention for primary hypertension, several forms of secondary hypertension respond well to the surgical correction of the primary problem. A coarctation of the aorta can be repaired by removing the narrowed area of the vessel and inserting a Teflon aortic graft. Renal artery stenosis may be corrected by grafting or by renal artery angioplasty. For patients with pheochromocytoma, surgical removal of the tumor(s) will return the patient to a normotensive state.

> **Research Brief 4-4**   The investigators evaluated the records of 171 surgical ICU patients with sinus tachycardia treated with diltiazem who had contraindications for beta-blockers or in whom beta-blockers were ineffective. Diltiazem effectively achieved short-term heart rate control in 56% without significant adverse effects in nearly all patients studied.
>
> Gabrielli A et al: Diltiazem to treat sinus tachycardia in critically ill patients: a four-year experience, *Crit Care Med* 29(10): 1874-1879, 2001.

NURSING DIAGNOSES AND INTERVENTIONS

Altered tissue perfusion: cardiopulmonary, cerebral, and renal, related to interruption of arterial flow secondary to vasoconstriction that occurs with interruption of the normal BP control mechanism; interruption of venous flow secondary to vasodilation or tissue edema that occurs with loss of autoregulation

Desired outcomes: Tissue perfusion is established within 24 hr as evidenced by systemic arterial BP 110-160/70-110 mm Hg (or within patient's normal range); MAP 70-105 mm Hg; equal and normoreactive pupils; strength and tone of the extremities bilaterally equal and normal for patient;

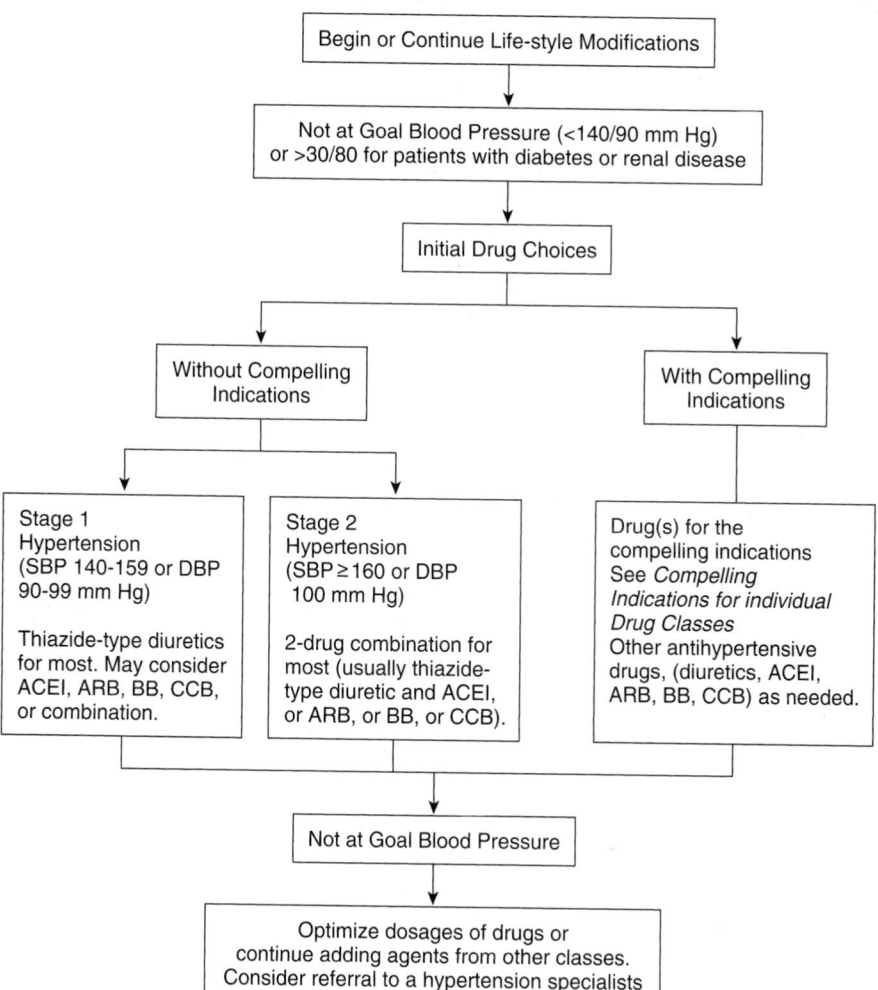

Begin or Continue Life-style Modifications

↓

Not at Goal Blood Pressure (<140/90 mm Hg)
or >30/80 for patients with diabetes or renal disease

↓

Initial Drug Choices

Without Compelling Indications

Stage 1
Hypertension
(SBP 140-159 or DBP
90-99 mm Hg)

Thiazide-type diuretics
for most. May consider
ACEI, ARB, BB, CCB,
or combination.

Stage 2
Hypertension
(SBP ≥160 or DBP
100 mm Hg)

2-drug combination for
most (usually thiazide-
type diuretic and ACEI,
or ARB, or BB, or CCB).

With Compelling Indications

Drug(s) for the
compelling indications
See *Compelling
Indications for individual
Drug Classes*
Other antihypertensive
drugs, (diuretics, ACEI,
ARB, BB, CCB) as needed.

↓

Not at Goal Blood Pressure

↓

Optimize dosages of drugs or
continue adding agents from other classes.
Consider referral to a hypertension specialists

ACE, Angiotensin-converting enzyme; *ISA*, intrinsic sympathomimetic activity,
* Unless contraindicated.
† Based on randomized controlled trials.

Key: ACEI, angiotensin converting enzyme inhibitor, ALDO ANT, aldosterone antagonist, ARB,
    angiotensin receptor blocker, BB, beta blocker, CCB, calcium channel blocker,
    THIAZ, thiazide diuretics.

Compelling Indications for Individual Drug Classes	Initial Therapy Options
• Heart failure	THIAZ, BB, ACEI, ARB, ALDO ANT
• Post myocardial infarction	BB, ACEI, ALDO ANT
• High CVD risk	THIAZ, BB, ACEI, CCB
• Diabetes	THIAZ, BB, ACEI, ARB, CCB
• Chronic kidney disease	ACEI, ARB
• Recurrent stroke prevention	THIAZ, ACEI

Figure 4-28:   Algorithm for the treatment of hypertension.
Modified from the Joint National Committee: The Seventh Report of the Joint National Committee
on Prevention, Detection, Evaluation, and Treatment of High Blood Pressure (JNC VII), NIH Pub.
No. 03-5231, May, 2003.

orientation to time, place, and person; urinary output ≥0.5 ml/kg/hr; and stable weight. Within 48 hr, SBP is <140 mm Hg and diastolic BP is <90 mm Hg, with MAP 70-105 mm Hg.
- Monitor BP and MAP q1-5min during titration of the medications. As patient's condition stabilizes, perform these assessments q15min-1h. Be alert to sudden drops or elevations in BP. As the oral medications begin to affect BP, gradually wean IV nitroprusside and other potent vasodilators to prevent hypotensive episodes. Continuous monitoring is recommended.
  ❏ Correlate cuff pressure with pressure from arterial cannulation.
  ❏ Determine ideal range for BP control and maximal nitroprusside dose with physician. Usually the following guidelines are used: SBP <140-160 mm Hg; MAP <110 mm Hg; diastolic BP <90 mm Hg.
  ❏ If hypotension develops, decrease or stop nitroprusside infusion until the pressure rises.
- Assess patient for neurologic deficit by performing hourly neurostatus checks. Be alert to sensori-motor deficit if MAP is >140 mm Hg. As patient's condition stabilizes and BP becomes controlled, perform neurostatus checks at least q4h.
- Monitor patient for changes in funduscopic examination. Consult physician if hemorrhages or fluffy cotton exudates are present.
- Assess patient for evidence of decreasing renal perfusion by monitoring I&O and weighing patient daily. Consult physician if urinary output is <0.5 ml/kg/hr for 2 consecutive hr or if weight gain ≥1 kg (2.2 lb). Be alert to azotemia (increasing BUN), decreasing creatinine clearance, and increasing serum creatinine. Optimal laboratory values are: BUN ≤20 mg/dl; creatinine clearance ≥9.5 ml/min; and serum creatinine ≤1.5 mg/dl.

NIC Hemodynamic Regulation; Medication Administration; Cardiac Care; Circulatory Care

Pain related to headache secondary to cerebral edema occurring with high perfusion pressures
Desired outcomes: Patient's subjective evaluation of pain improves within 12-24 hr, as documented by a pain scale. Nonverbal indicators, such as grimacing, are absent or diminished.
- Monitor patient for headache pain at frequent intervals. Devise a pain scale with patient, rating discomfort from 0 (no pain) to 10 (severe pain).
- Provide pain medications as prescribed. A variety of analgesics may be used, ranging from acetaminophen with codeine to morphine, depending on the severity of the symptoms. Assess effectiveness of the pain medication, using the pain scale to determine degree of relief obtained.
- Teach patient relaxation techniques to use in conjunction with the medications. Guided imagery, meditation, progressive muscle relaxation, and music therapy often are effective. See "Health-Seeking Behavior," p. 259.
- Maintain a quiet, low-lit environment that is free of extensive distraction and stimulation. Limit visitations as indicated.

NIC Analgesic Administration; Pain Management; Environmental Management: Comfort; Progressive Muscle Relaxation

Sensory/perceptual alterations related to decreased visual acuity secondary to retinal damage occurring with high perfusion pressures; pain secondary to cerebral edema
Desired outcome: Within 24-48 hr of this diagnosis, patient reads print, recognizes objects or people, and demonstrates coordination of movement.
- Assess patient for signs of decreased visual acuity by monitoring patient's ability to read and recognize objects or people. Evaluate patient's coordination of movement to determine depth perception. Perform a funduscopic examination q8h for evidence of findings discussed on p. 280. Consult physician for significant findings.
- If patient has decreased visual acuity, assist with feeding and other ADL and keep patient's personal effects within his or her visual field.
- Reassure patient and significant others that visual problems usually resolve when the BP is lowered sufficiently.

NIC Surveillance: Safety

ADDITIONAL NURSING DIAGNOSES

For other nursing diagnoses and interventions, see the following as appropriate: "Hemodynamic Monitoring," p. 23; "Psychosocial Support," p. 68; and "Psychosocial Support for the Patient's Family and Significant Others," p. 78.

T A B L E 4 - 23 Medications Used in the Treatment of Hypertension

Drug type	Medication	Dosage/schedule	Side effects
Diuretics			
Thiazides/related compounds	Chlorothiazide	12.5-50 mg; daily	Hypokalemia and hyperuricemia in the first two categories; hypercholesterolemia, hypoglycemia, impotence, *** and indigestion in all categories of diuretics
	Chlorthalidone	12.5-100 mg; daily	
	Cyclothiazide	1-2 mg; daily	
	Hydrochlorothiazide	12.5-50 mg; daily	
	Hydorflumethiazide	12.5-50 mg; daily	
	Methylchlorthiazide	2.5-5 mg; daily	
	Metolazone	2.5-5 mg; daily	
	Polythiazide	2-4 mg; daily	
Loop diuretics	Bumetanide	0.25-2.5 mg; q12h	
	Ethacrynic acid	25-200 mg; q12h	
	Furosemide	20-200 mg; q6-24h	
	Torsemide	2.5-10 mg; q12-24h	
Potassium-sparing agents	Amiloride	5-10 mg; q12-24h	Hyperkalemia, gynecomastia, menstrual abnormalities
	Eplerenone	25-100 mg; daily	
	Spironalactone	25-200 mg; q8-24h	
	Triamterene	100-300 mg; q12-24h	
Adrenergic-inhibiting agents			
β-Blockers	Atenolol*	25-100 mg; daily	Fatigue, drowsiness, depression, fluid retention, heart failure, impotence, hypoglycemia, flushing, bronchospasm (diminished with cardioselective β1-blockers)
	Betaxolol*	5-20 mg; daily	
	Bisoprolol*	2-20 mg; daily	
	Metoprolol*	25-100 mg; q12-24h	
	Nadolol	20-120 mg; daily	
	Propranolol	40-160 mg; q12h	
	Timolol	20-40 mg; q12h	
with ISA	Acebutolol*	200-800 mg; bid	
	Carteolol	2.5-10 mg; daily	
	Penbutolol	10-40 mg; daily	
	Pindolol	10-40 mg; bid	

Continued

ACE, Angiotensin-converting enzyme; *BP,* blood pressure; *ISA,* intrinsic sypathomimetic activity; *IV,* Intravenous; *PO,* by mouth. Drug abbreviations: *ACEI,* Angiotensin-converting enzyme inhibitor; *ARB,* angiotensin receptor blocker; *CCB,* calcium channel blocker. Some drug combinations available in multiple fixed doses. Each drug dose is reported in milligrams.
*Cardioselective.

T A B L E 4 - 23 Medications Used in the Treatment of Hypertension—cont'd

Drug type	Medication	Dosage/schedule	Side effects
Adrenergic-inhibiting agents—cont'd			
α- and β-Blocker	Labetalol	200-800 mg; bid	May cause severe postural hypertension; dose adjustments should be made based on standing BP
	Carvedilol	12.5-50 mg; bid	
α-Receptor blocker	Doxazosin	1-16 mg; daily	Hypoglycemia, diarrhea, hypertension, flashing, first-dose syncope, blurred vision
	Phentolamine	50 mg; bid	
	Prazosin HCl	1-7 mg; tid	
	Terazosin	1-20 mg; daily	
ACE inhibitors	Benazepril	10-40 mg; bid	To prevent severe hypotension, reduce dose of diuretic; may cause hyperkalemia in person with renal failure; may cause acute renal failure in bilateral renal artery stenosis; also may cause profound postural hypotension; dose adjustments should be made based on standing BP.
	Captopril	25-50 mg; bid	
	Enalapril	2.5-40 mg; bid	
	Fosinopril	10-40 mg; daily	
	Lisinopril	10-40 mg; daily	
	Moaxipril	7.5 mg; daily	
	Perindopsil	4-8 mg; qd, bid	
	Quinapril HCl	10-40 mg; daily	
	Ramipril	25 mg; daily	
	Trandolapril	1-4 mg; daily	
Angiotensin receptor blockers (ARB) (Angiotensin II antagonists)	Candesartan (Atacand)	8-32 mg; daily	Hepatoxicity, hyperkalemia, agranulocytosis, leukopenia, neutropenia. Less risk of angioedema and cough than with ACE inhibitors.
	Eprosartan (Tavetan)	400-800 mg; daily; may divide doses	
	Irbesartan (Avapro)	150-300 mg; daily	
	Losartan (Cozaar)	25-100 mg; daily; may divide doses	
	Olmesartan (Benicar)	20-40 mg; daily	
	Telmisartan (Micardis)	20-80 mg; daily	
	Valsartan (Diovan)	80-320 mg; daily	
Calcium channel blockers	Dilitazem	30-90 mg; qid	Constipation, peripheral edema
	Verapamil	80-120 mg; qd-tid	

Dihydropyridines			Dihydropyridines are more potent peripheral vasodilators and may cause more flushing, peripheral edema, tachycardia, dizziness, and headache.
	Amlodipine	2.5-10 mg; daily	
	Felodipine	5-50 mg; daily	
	Isradipine	2.5-10 mg bid	
	Nicardipine	60-120 mg; bid	
	Nifedipine LA	30-60 mg; tid	
	Nisoldipine	10-40 mg; daily	

Combination type	Trade name	Fixed dose combinations
ACEIs and CCBs	Lotrel	Amlodipine/benazepril hydrochloride (2.5/10, 5/10, 5/20, 10/20)
	Lexxel	Enalapril maleatre/felodipine (5/5)
	Tarla	Tradolapril/verapamil (2/180, 1/240, 2/240, 4/240)
ARBs and diuretics	Atacand HCT	Candesartan cilexeti/hydrochlorothiazide (16/12.5,32/12.5)
	Teveten/HCT	Eprosartan mesylate/hydrochlorothiazide (600/12.5, 600/25)
	Avalide	Irbesartan/hydrochlorothiazide (150/12.5, 300/12.5)
	Hyzaar	Losartan potassium/hydrochlorothiazide (50/125, 100/25)
	Micardis/HCT	Telmisartan/hydrochlorothiazide (40/12.5, 80/12.5)
	Diovan/HCT	Telmisartan/hydrochlorothiazide (40/12.5, 80/12.5)
β-Blockers and diuretics	Tenorectic	Atenolol/chlorthalidone (50/25, 100/25)
	Ziac	Bisoprolol fumarate/hydrochlorothiazide (2.5/6.25, 5/6.25, 10/6.25)
	Inderide	Propranolol LA/hydrochlorothiazide (40/25, 80/25)
	Lopressor HCT	Metoprolol tartrate/hydrochlorothiazide (50/25, 100/25)
	Corzide	Nadolol/bandrofluthlazide (40/5, 80/5)
	Timolide	Timolol maleate/hydrochlorothiazide (10/25)
Centrally acting drug and diuretic	Aldoril	Methyldopa/hydrochlorothiazide (250/15, 250/25, 500/30, 500/50)
	Diupres	Reserpine/chlorothiazide (0.125/250, 0.25/500)
	Hydropres	Reserpine/hydrochlorothiazide (0.125/25, 0.125/50)
Diuretic and diuretic	Moduretic	Amiloride HCl/hydrochlorothiazide (5/50)
	Aldactone	Spironolactone/hydrochlorothiazide (25/25, 50/50)
	Dyazide, Maxzide	Triamterene/hydrochlorothiazide (37.5/25, 50/25, 75/50)

Aortic Aneurysm/Dissection

PATHOPHYSIOLOGY

An aneurysm is any abnormal dilation of an artery. Complications related to the aorta can be life threatening, owing to the potential for disruption of blood flow to a large portion of the body, including vital organs such as the brain, the heart, the kidneys, and the GI tract. A true aneurysm involves all three layers of the arterial wall (intima, media, adventitia). The two forms of true aneurysm are fusiform (a concentric, spindle-shaped deformity) and saccular (an eccentric, balloon-shaped deformity). A false aneurysm is a pulsatile hematoma caused by disruption of the intimal layer or the intimal and medial layers only.

Most often, aneurysms develop at the site of an atherosclerotic lesion, which initially involves only the intimal layer of the aorta. As the lesion becomes more complicated, there is hemorrhage into the media, which weakens and allows the arterial wall to dilate. With advancing age, the elastin in the aorta is decreased, which further weakens the vessel wall. Acute hypertension may decrease flow into the media, leading to ischemia, which weakens this layer yet further. The abdominal, thoracic, or ascending arch of the aorta may be affected. The rate at which the aneurysm increases is not predictable; however, the likelihood of rupture or dissection increases dramatically when the size exceeds 6 cm.

Rupture of an abdominal aneurysm may lead to extravasation of blood either anteriorly into the peritoneal cavity or posteriorly into the retroperitoneal space. Anterior bleeds often occur rapidly and are associated with a high mortality because of rapid circulatory collapse. Posterior bleeds may lead to tamponade on the spinal cord, with neurologic deficits. Either form of rupture can lead to mesenteric ischemia. Surgical repair is the only treatment for rupture.

An *aortic dissection* is a longitudinal tear in the intimal layer of the aortic wall caused by the degeneration of the medial layer with hemorrhage. An intimal tear develops at the proximal end of the medial degeneration and dissection. The column of blood drives the dissection distally with the force of systole, and the diastolic recoil within the aorta forces the dissection in the proximal direction. Precipitating factors include medial necrosis from other disorders, trauma, or hypertension (see "Hypertensive Emergencies," p. 280). The three types of aortic dissections first described by DeBakey are differentiated by the site of the intimal tear and the direction of dissection. In type I, which accounts for 60%-80% of all cases, the tear begins in the ascending aorta and the dissection extends beyond the aortic arch. Type II is the rarest form, with the intimal tear and entire dissection confined to the ascending aorta. Type III occurs in 20%-30% of all cases and involves a tear in the descending aorta, with distal dissection only. The Stanford Classification of Aortic Dissections combines DeBakey types I and II into a new group called class A, and type III becomes Stanford class B.

Aortic dissection is sudden and life threatening. The disruption of the vessel may continue along any arterial branch of the aorta, compromising organs such as the heart, the brain, and the kidneys if the coronary, subclavian, innominate, and renal arteries are involved. Approximately 2000 episodes occur annually, with a mortality approaching 100% if the dissection is left untreated.

ASSESSMENT

History and risk factors: Hypertension and related risk factors, connective tissue disorders, coarctation of the aorta, blunt chest trauma, medial necrosis of the aorta, pregnancy, family history of aortic aneurysm.

Clinical presentation: The major symptom is a sudden onset of severe, tearing chest or abdominal pain that is unrelieved by position or respiratory change. The pain may radiate to the back if the dissection is moving distally or to the neck if the dissection is moving proximally. With rupture of an abdominal aneurysm, pain will occur along the flank or lumbar back. Vasovagal responses such as diaphoresis, apprehension, nausea, vomiting, and faintness may occur. Signs of acute left ventricular failure may be seen if the dissection involves the coronary arteries or the aortic valve. Neurologic deficits such as confusion, sensorimotor changes, and lethargy may be the result of a dissection along the branches of the ascending aorta. Urine output will fall if the dissection extends to the renal arteries.

Physical assessment: Pulse deficits or BP differences between extremities are classic findings. A drop in BP or pulse at a site helps identify the location of the dissection, inasmuch as both will be decreased beyond the area of dissection. Usually the skin is pale and cool and capillary refill is sluggish as a result of poor tissue perfusion. If bleeding extends to the pericardium, cardiac tamponade can occur (see p. 118).

DIAGNOSTIC TESTS

Chest/abdominal x-ray: Will demonstrate widening of the aortic arch or descending aorta. Film taken with patient in upright position is necessary to demonstrate widening of the mediastinum.

Echocardiography of the aortic arch or descending aorta or TEE: Will locate the site of dissection, inasmuch as the hemorrhage within the vessel will be an area of absent echoes and the total diameter of the vessel will be enlarged.

Aortography or digital subtraction angiography: Will locate actual site of the tear and dissection by use of contrast material. This is the only way to identify tears into the coronary arteries.

CT: Often as useful as an aortogram in locating the dissection; its advantage over an aortogram is that it is noninvasive. Spiral and ultrafast CT are more accurate and allow complete imaging of the thoracic aorta with a single injection of contrast material.

COLLABORATIVE MANAGEMENT

Antihypertensive therapy: Initiated as soon as possible to prevent further aortic dissection. Usually nitroprusside or labetolol is started, as described in "Hypertensive Crisis," p. 281. A MAP of 70-80 mm Hg is desired. After control of the pressure is achieved, oral antihypertensive therapy is begun, along with gradual weaning from the IV infusion.

Propranolol therapy: To reduce velocity of the left ventricular ejection, HR, and BP. Usually it is administered intravenously in increments of 1 mg at 5-min intervals until the HR is reduced to 60-80 beats/min. The maximal initial dosage should not exceed 0.15 mg/kg body weight. Additional doses of 2-6 mg are then administered q4-6h until the condition can be managed with oral medications.

Complete bed rest: To prevent further dissection. This may continue for days to weeks until the dissection has stabilized. A gradual resumption of activity is recommended.

Pain relief: Usually achieved with IV morphine sulfate, 2-10 mg.

Sedation: To prevent sympathetic stimulation, which can increase BP. Lorazepam or midazolam used for sedation.

Long-term medical management: Aimed at maintaining SBP <130 mm Hg to prevent redissection. It is important to instruct patients to stop smoking to prevent the increases in BP that can result from nicotine. Most often patients with type B dissections are candidates for medical therapy.

Surgical treatment: Recommended for proximal dissection, distal dissection when vital organ compromise occurs, impending rupture, or when pain and BP are refractory to medications. The surgery involves removal of the dissected vessel sections and replacement of the vessel sections with Teflon grafts.

NURSING DIAGNOSES AND INTERVENTIONS

Altered tissue perfusion: peripheral, cardiopulmonary, renal, and cerebral, related to interruption of arterial blood flow secondary to narrowed aortic lumen

Desired outcome: Within 48 hr of this diagnosis, patient has adequate tissue perfusion as evidenced by distal pulses bilaterally equal and >2+ on a 0-4+ scale; brisk capillary refill (<2 sec); warm skin; bilaterally equal sensations in the extremities; bilaterally equal SBP; BP within patient's normal range; HR ≤100 beats/min; normal sinus rhythm on ECG; urine output ≥0.5 ml/kg/hr; equal and normoreactive pupils; and orientation to time, place, and person.

- Perform bilateral assessment of BP and distal pulses (particularly radial, femoral, and dorsalis pedis) hourly during initial phase of dissection and then q4h as the patient's condition stabilizes. Note changes in strength or symmetry of distal pulses. Correlate cuff pressures with arterial monitor recordings. Be alert to any change in color, capillary refill, and temperature of each extremity. Report significant findings.
- If the difference in SBP between the extremities exceeds 10 mm Hg, consult physician immediately.
- Monitor for paresthesias of the extremities—a sign of decreased peripheral perfusion.
- Assess for signs of pericardial tamponade: distended neck veins; muffled heart sounds; decreased SBP (<90 mm Hg or >20 mm Hg drop in systolic trend); and pulsus paradoxus.
- Assess cardiovascular status by monitoring heart rate and rhythm, ECG, and cardiac enzyme levels. A dissection along the coronary arteries will result in an MI.
- Monitor urine output hourly. Consult physician if urine output is <0.5 ml/kg/hr for 2 consecutive hr.
- Assess neurologic status hourly. Report restlessness and changes in LOC, pupil size, or reaction to light.
- Use relaxation techniques such as guided imagery or meditation to reduce BP. Avoid techniques that involve exercise, such as progressive muscle relaxation.

NIC Hemodynamic Regulation; Cardiac Care: Acute; Circulatory Care; Surveillance

Pain related to biophysical injury secondary to necrosis at the aortic media and distal tissue hypoperfusion

Desired outcomes: Within 24-48 hr of this diagnosis, patient's subjective evaluation of pain improves, as documented by a pain scale. Nonverbal indicators, such as grimacing, are decreased or absent.

- Monitor patient at frequent intervals for the presence of discomfort. Devise a pain scale with patient, rating discomfort from 0 (no pain) to 10 (severe pain). Medicate with analgesics as prescribed, and rate relief obtained, using the pain scale.
- Teach patient relaxation techniques to use in conjunction with analgesics. Examples include guided imagery and meditation. Avoid progressive muscle relaxation, which may increase cardiac and aortic workload. For guidelines, see "Health-Seeking Behavior," p. 259.
- During episodes of pain, assess for a change in peripheral pulses or altered hemodynamics (i.e., BP, PAP, PAWP, CO, SVR), because such changes often are associated with an increase in aortic dissection.
- Control BP during episodes of pain by titrating nitroprusside to maintain specified parameters.
- Immediately consult physician for any increase in the severity of pain, because it may indicate the need for emergency surgery.

NIC Pain Management; Anxiety Reduction; Simple Relaxation Therapy

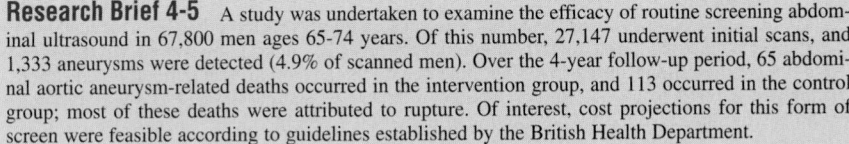

Research Brief 4-5   A study was undertaken to examine the efficacy of routine screening abdominal ultrasound in 67,800 men ages 65-74 years. Of this number, 27,147 underwent initial scans, and 1,333 aneurysms were detected (4.9% of scanned men). Over the 4-year follow-up period, 65 abdominal aortic aneurysm-related deaths occurred in the intervention group, and 113 occurred in the control group; most of these deaths were attributed to rupture. Of interest, cost projections for this form of screen were feasible according to guidelines established by the British Health Department.

Ahston HA et al: for the Multicentre Aneurysm Screening Study Group: The Multicentre Aneurysm Screening Study (MASS) into the effect of abdominal aortic aneurysm screening on mortality in men: a randomized controlled trial, *Lancet* 360:1531-1539, 2002.

ADDITIONAL NURSING DIAGNOSES

For other nursing diagnoses and interventions, also see the following as appropriate: "Hemodynamic Monitoring," p. 23; "Prolonged Immobility," p. 61; "Psychosocial Support," p. 68; "Psychosocial Support for the Patient's Family and Significant Others," p. 78; and "Chest Trauma," p. 110.

Cardiogenic Shock

PATHOPHYSIOLOGY

Cardiogenic shock results from significantly impaired cardiac function that leads to profound reduction in peripheral blood flow and oxygenation. Cardiogenic shock occurs in 15%-20% of all patients experiencing MI, with a mortality rate of more than 80%. When at least 40% of the myocardium becomes necrotic or severely ischemic, the heart no longer has enough healthy tissue to pump adequate blood through the systemic circulation. With cardiac output markedly reduced, BP decreases and all tissues suffer from inadequate perfusion. Decreased diastolic BP reduces coronary flow, which further impairs the ability of the heart to pump. Other causes of cardiogenic shock include a "stunned heart" following cardiac surgery, massive pulmonary embolism, severe valvular dysfunction, end-stage cardiomyopathy, congestive heart failure, and cardiac tamponade.

Heart failure prompts development of early shock. Decreased BP prompts an increased sympathetic discharge by the baroreceptors in the carotid sinus and aortic arch. Epinephrine and norepinephrine are released to help increase cardiac output and BP. HR and force of contraction of the uninjured myocardium increase. Vasoconstriction increases BP. Blood is diverted from the skin, the abdominal organs, and the skeletal muscles to the vital organs: brain, heart, and lungs. As heart failure worsens, the shock state intensifies, and the patient's condition deteriorates. Perfusion is reduced to all organs and body tissues. Lactate and pyruvic acid accumulate as anaerobic metabolism occurs in the cells deprived of oxygen. Metabolic acidosis results from accumulated tissue acids and early acute renal failure. In the late stage of shock, compensatory mechanisms become ineffective and multiple organ failure occurs.

At the cellular level, massive endothelial dysfunction ensues. Injury begins with hypoxia and lack of intracellular glucose. Without these substances, adenosine triphosphate (ATP), the energy source for all cellular functions, cannot be produced. The mitochondria and endoplasmic reticulum are rendered dysfunctional. The final phase of cellular damage is marked by swelling, rupture of the cell membrane, and complete cellular degradation. Cellular changes are similar in all body organs and types of tissue.

ASSESSMENT

Clinical presentation: The assessment section in "Acute Coronary Syndromes" (see p. 206) describes early cardiogenic shock. As shock progresses, cerebral perfusion is compromised and the patient's LOC deteriorates. Agitation, restlessness, lethargy, confusion, or unresponsiveness may be noted. Urine output falls to <0.5 ml/kg/hr as renal perfusion is reduced. The kidneys initially compensate by triggering the renin-angiotensin-aldosterone system to help increase BP by vasoconstriction and fluid retention.

Physical assessment: HR increases; pulses are weak and possibly irregular. Pulsus alternans may be palpated. SBP is <90 mm Hg or at least 30 mm Hg below the patient's normal resting level. Skin is cold, clammy, and mottled because of reduced peripheral perfusion. Cardiac auscultation may reveal S_3 or S_4 sounds, reflecting an overdistended, noncompliant ventricle. Crackles are auscultated over the lung fields as heart failure worsens, resulting in pulmonary congestion and tachypnea. Peripheral pulse amplitude is decreased. Capillary refill is prolonged to greater than 3 sec. A murmur of mitral regurgitation may be auscultated.

Hemodynamic measurements: Cuff blood pressures are unreliable in shock states. Direct or invasive arterial pressure monitoring should be considered. Pulmonary artery pressure monitoring should be used to guide therapy. Arterial systolic and mean arterial pressures are decreased. Pulse pressure is narrowed or decreased. Because contractility is greatly reduced, the stroke volume, ejection fraction, and CO are decreased. CVP, RAP, PAP, and PAWP all are elevated, demonstrating increased preload secondary to pulmonary congestion. SVR is increased because of the initial compensatory vasoconstriction. Coronary perfusion pressure (diastolic BP minus PAWP) will be less than the normal 60 mm Hg.

An oximetric (Svo_2) catheter may be used to provide continuous measurement of mixed venous oxygen saturation in the pulmonary artery. Svo_2 indicates how well oxygen supply meets tissue demand for energy production. If the tissue demand is increased (as in exercise) or oxygen supply is decreased (perfusion is reduced), Svo_2 falls below the normal range of 60%-80%. Tissues begin to extract more oxygen from the "less available" RBCs or hemoglobin; fewer RBCs reach the cellular level when blood flow is reduced. Svo_2 has a positive correlation with CO. Continuous Svo_2 monitoring provides an indirect but continuous assessment of cardiac output and perfusion. See Table 4-24 for details about Svo_2.

DIAGNOSTIC TESTS

The diagnosis of cardiogenic shock is made by both physical assessment and analysis of the hemodynamic profile. If the primary problem is MI, cardiac enzymes are elevated and the ECG changes to reflect location of the heart damage (see discussion, p. 208). Other diagnostic tests are used to assess the effect of hypoperfusion on other organs.

ABG values: Hypoxemia (Pao_2 <80 mm Hg) and metabolic acidosis (pH <7.35; $Paco_2$ usually <35 mm Hg) are seen because of impaired oxygen diffusion in the alveoli and tissue lactic acidosis from anaerobic metabolism. Aerobic metabolism ceases when perfusion becomes inadequate.

Serum chemistry values: Moderate hyperglycemia may result from epinephrine-induced glycogenolysis and/or glucocorticoid-induced hyperglycemia during the stress response. Insulin release is reduced as the pancreas is hypoperfused. Serum lactate levels may be elevated as a result of anaerobic metabolism. Electrolyte studies may reveal hypernatremia reflective of a water deficit or early renal insufficiency. Hyperkalemia may be seen with acute renal failure secondary to lack of perfusion during hypotension, which causes tissue destruction and end-organ dysfunction.

Urinalysis: Urine sodium, osmolality, and creatinine levels are reflective of the patient's renal status.

Coagulation profile: Coagulation studies become progressively abnormal as the shock state deteriorates as a result of capillary and/or endothelial dysfunction.

ECG: Although not specific for cardiogenic shock, dysrhythmias may occur as a result of infarction or injury to areas of the conduction system and/or myocardium or as a result of electrolyte imbalance.

COLLABORATIVE MANAGEMENT

Oxygen therapy: To maximize tissue oxygenation, because perfusion is impaired. If dyspnea, hypoxemia, acidosis, or pulmonary congestion worsens, intubation and mechanical ventilation will be necessary. Morphine sulfate 2 mg administered by IV push may assist in reducing pulmonary congestion, thereby relieving dyspnea and increasing Pao_2.

Correction of acidosis: Sodium bicarbonate delivered by IV push and guided by serial ABG checks to assess effectiveness of treatment.

TABLE 4-24   Hemodynamic Profile of Shock

Values	RAP (mm Hg)	RVP (mm Hg)	PAP (mm Hg)	PAWP (mm Hg)	SVR (dynes/sec/cm^{-5})	Svo$_2$(%)	CO (L/min)	CI (L/min/m^2)
Normal	4-6	25/0-5	20-30/8-15	6-12	900-1200	60-80	4-7	2.5-4
Shock values								
Cardiogenic	6-10	40-50/6-15	50/25-30	25-40	>1200	≤50	<4	≤1.5
Hypovolemic	0-2	15-20/0-2	15-20/2-8	2-6	>1200	65	<4	2.5
Neurogenic	0-2	20-25/0-2	20-25/0-8	0-6	≤1000	60-80	≥4-7	2.5
Septic								
Early	0-2	20-25/0-2	20-25/0-8	0-6	≤900	≥60	>7	≥4
Late	0-4	25/0-4	25/4-10	>12	>1200	≤60	<4	<2.5

CO, Cardiac output; *CI*, cardiac index; *PAP*, pulmonary artery pressure; *PAWP*, pulmonary artery wedge pressure; *RAP*, right atrial pressure; *RVP*, right ventricular pressure; *SVR*, systemic vascular resistance; *Svo$_2$* mixed venous oxygen saturation.

Correction of electrolyte imbalance: Replacement of potassium, sodium, chloride, magnesium, or calcium as indicated by serum chemistry findings.

Diuretics/vasodilators: To decrease preload (or venous blood return) and improve stroke volume and cardiac output. Diuretics such as furosemide 40-200 mg by IV push or ethacrynic acid 25-100 mg by IV push may be given. Bumetanide (Bumex) is another frequently used diuretic similar in action to furosemide. One mg of bumetanide is equal to 40 mg of furosemide. Morphine sulfate also reduces preload. Oral or topical nitrates or IV nitroglycerin and IV nitroprusside (Nipride) may be used to decrease filling pressures by means of venous dilation.

Note: It may be necessary to increase preload if the patient is hypovolemic. In this situation, fluids are increased cautiously, the patient's hemodynamics are monitored carefully, and diuretics are avoided.

Positive inotropic agents and inodilators: To improve contractility of the uninjured myocardium and to increase cardiac output. Dopamine infusions at 2-20 mcg/kg/min are titrated to accomplish the desired effect. Higher doses increase HR and SVR, which increase the myocardial workload. Dobutamine infusions of 2-20 mcg/kg/min increase contractility and decrease preload with less of an increase in HR, but renal perfusion may decrease at the higher dosage range. Infusion of milrinone 0.375 to 0.75 mcg/kg/min provides similar inotropic effects.

Vasopressors: To increase BP to a mean pressure level (usually ≥70 mm Hg) that will perf' tissues. This is accomplished by stimulating the α-adrenergic receptors in the blood vessel causes vasoconstriction. Vasopressors that may be used include dopamine, norepinephrine, rine, phenylephrine, and methoxamine (see Appendix 7).

Intraaortic balloon pump (IABP) or balloon counterpulsation therapy: A counterpulsation device that assists the failing heart by decreasing afterload and increasing coronary artery perfusion. It may be used before and after cardiac surgery and in cases of cardiogenic shock, heart failure, unstable angina, refractory ventricular dysrhythmias, cardiomyopathy, and post-PTCA complications, as well as in patients awaiting heart transplantation. IABP is a temporary measure that supports the heart and circulation for up to 30 days. It is used as an adjunct to medical therapy.

Balloon insertion can be performed emergently at the bedside or under controlled conditions during fluoroscopic examination. A local anesthetic agent is injected over the femoral artery, the introducer sheath is inserted, and the balloon is passed through the sheath into the thoracic aorta. The catheter is placed so that the balloon is below the left subclavian artery and above the renal artery. If the balloon migrates in either direction, arterial flow can be obstructed. The balloon is then unwrapped and connected to the pump console. Pumping is timed according to the ECG or arterial pressure waveform. Balloon inflation occurs with diastole, and deflation occurs with systole.

The patient derives benefits from both phases of balloon pumping. The first phase, balloon inflation, is termed *diastolic augmentation*. During this phase, both antegrade and retrograde blood flow is increased within the aorta. Coronary artery blood flow increases during diastole, resulting in increased oxygen supply to the myocardium. Blood flow to the kidneys also increases, improving urinary output. The second phase is *systolic unloading* or balloon deflation. Aortic pressure decreases rapidly. Afterload, the resistance to left ventricular ejection, and ventricular wall tension are reduced. With reduced afterload, the ventricle empties more completely, stroke volume rises, and myocardial oxygen use diminishes. Balloon counterpulsation therapy increases BP, CO, and systemic perfusion. Urinary flow increases, mental status improves, extremities become warmer to touch, peripheral pulses are stronger, chest discomfort is relieved, and ECG changes that denote ischemia may be lessened.

Complications of IABP therapy include aortic dissection, thrombus formation, impaired circulation to the involved leg, sepsis, obstruction to the left subclavian artery blood flow, obstruction to the renal and mesenteric arteries, and paraplegia (caused by spinal artery thrombosis). In addition, problems such as pneumonia and dermal ulcers can occur as a result of prolonged immobility.

Note: Pulmonary artery balloon counterpulsation (intrapulmonary artery balloon pump) is available for support of the right ventricle after cardiac surgery. The catheter usually is inserted during surgery and involves creation of an artificial diverticulum on the pulmonary artery. During systole, the balloon is deflated and right ventricle stroke volume is directed into the diverticulum, which reduces afterload. During diastole, the balloon inflates and the cardiac output is propelled into the pulmonary vessels.

Ventricular assist device: A mechanical ventricular assist device (VAD) is used to support the patient with massive left ventricular and/or right ventricular dysfunction. The VAD provides a conduit that diverts blood from the ventricle to an artificial pump. The VAD can maintain circulation and decreased myocardial workload to promote ventricular recovery. Candidates for this device include individuals with acute ventricular dysfunction; shock after cardiotomy, angioplasty, or myocardial infarction; cardiac arrest; or massive pulmonary embolism.

In general, the right ventricle recovers within 5 days and the left ventricle recovers within 10 days. This device is used as a temporary measure to promote rest and healing of the damaged myocardium. Left ventricular assistance is provided through either percutaneous cannulation of the femoral artery or direct cannulation of the atrium and ascending aorta, whereas a right VAD is used in the right atrium and the main pulmonary artery. In individuals with right and left ventricular failure, biventricular assistance is available. As the patient's overall condition improves, the goal is to gradually wean the patient from the device by decreasing the flow rate. Some devices are implanted for prolonged periods and used as a bridge to transplant procedures. Studies of permanent assist devices for severe heart failure are in progress.

Complications of the assist device include coagulopathy, bleeding, embolization, infection, sepsis, right ventricular failure (with left-sided heart assist only), and renal failure. These patients are severely ill and need constant monitoring by means of a myriad of highly complex, technical equipment and meticulous administration of medications. Highly specialized nursing care is imperative.

Emergency cardiac catheterization: To determine patient's suitability for emergency PTCA, CABG, or arthrectomy.

Emergency coronary artery bypass grafting (CABG) or surgical reperfusion: Surgical procedure which adds blood vessels to improve myocardial perfusion. This procedure may not be as beneficial if a large area of necrosis is present. Other problems, such as ventricular aneurysm due to MI, may be corrected in addition to reperfusion. See p. 212.

Emergency percutaneous transluminal coronary angioplasty (PTCA): A specially designed balloon catheter is used to mechanically alter plaque within the coronary artery. Often used with coronary artery stents or rotoblade atherectomy. See p. 253.

Thrombolytic therapy: Intravenous "clot buster" drugs used to lyse or "break up" the fibrin portion of blood clots in the coronary vessels. These drugs reperfuse the injured myocardium. See p. 304).

Heart transplantation: To replace the failing heart with a suitably matched donor organ. The recipient is screened carefully to ensure that all other organs are still functional. Refer to "Cardiac Transplantation," p. 299.

NURSING DIAGNOSES AND INTERVENTIONS

Decreased cardiac output related to increased afterload, increased preload, or decreased contractility secondary to loss of ≥40% of myocardial functional mass

Desired outcome: Before weaning from assist device or pharmacologic agents is attempted, the patient's hemodynamic function is as near the acceptable limits as possible as evidenced by CO ≥4 L/min; BP ≥90/60 mm Hg; SVR ≤1200 dynes/sec/cm^{-5}; and PAWP ≤12 mm Hg.

- Monitor arterial BP, PAP, S$\bar{v}$o$_2$, and heart rate and rhythm continuously. Titrate vasoactive drugs to achieve a CO between 4-7 L/min; arterial BP ≥90/60; and PAWP ≤12 mm Hg.
- Assess CO and SVR q1-4h and after every change in pharmacologic therapy. Consult physician if SVR increases (>1200 dynes/sec/cm^{-5}). A vasodilating drug such as nitroprusside or similar medication may be needed to decrease excessive afterload.
- Auscultate lung sounds q1-2h, and monitor urinary output. Report changes, including an increase in crackles and decreased urine output. An adjustment in IV fluid therapy or additional diuretics may be necessary.
- Keep HOB elevated less than 30 degrees to prevent further decreases in BP.
- Treat ventricular dysrhythmias with prescribed antidysrhythmic medications.
- Be prepared for temporary cardiac pacing for bradycardia. Second or third degree heart block may occur. Transcutaneous or transvenous pacing may be used.
- If preload (CVP or RAP) is low, administer prescribed IV fluids according to fluid challenge protocol (see Table 4-25 for sample protocol) and note response.
- If medical management is ineffective, prepare patient for insertion of IABP (see p. 293) or left VAD above.

NIC Cardiac Care: Acute; Circulatory Care: Mechanical Assist Device; Hemodynamic Regulation; Shock Management: Cardiac

Altered tissue perfusion: cardiopulmonary, cerebral, peripheral, and renal, related to interrupted arterial blood flow to vital organs secondary to inadequate arterial pressure

T A B L E 4 - 25 **Fluid Challenge Guidelines in Cardiogenic Shock**

Assessment	PAWP (mm Hg)	Fluids
CO low, and PAWP low or normal	<6	200 ml infused over 10 min
	6-12	100 ml infused over 10 min
	≥12	50 ml infused over 10 min
PAWP increases during infusion	>6	Return to KVO rate
	≤3	Continue infusion
Assess PAWP after 10 min	If >3 or <6	Repeat challenge

CO, Cardiac output; *KVO,* keep vein open; *PAWP,* pulmonary artery wedge pressure.

Desired outcome: Within 96 hr of this diagnosis, patient has adequate tissue perfusion as evidenced by orientation to time, place, and person; equal and normoreactive pupils; normal reflexes; urine output ≥0.5 ml/kg/hr; warm and dry skin; peripheral pulses >2+ on a 0-4+ scale; brisk capillary refill (<2 sec); and BP >90/60 mm Hg or within patient's normal range.
- Check neurologic status q1-2h to assess cerebral perfusion. Be alert to changes in LOC, orientation, perception, motor activity, reflexes, and pupillary response to light. Consult physician for any changes.
- Monitor I&O hourly to assess renal perfusion; report urine output <0.5 ml/kg/hr for 2 consecutive hr. Assess extremities q1-2h, noting changes in skin color, temperature, capillary refill, BP, and distal pulses.
- Titrate vasoactive drugs to maintain SBP >90 mm Hg.

NIC Circulatory Care: Peripheral, Cerebral, Cardiac, Gastrointestinal

Impaired gas exchange related to alveolar-capillary membrane changes secondary to pulmonary congestion; altered oxygen-carrying capacity of the blood secondary to acidosis occurring with anaerobic metabolism

Desired outcome: Before weaning from supplemental oxygen or ventilatory assistance is attempted, the patient has adequate gas exchange as evidenced by Pao_2 ≥80 mm Hg; RR 12-20 breaths/min with normal depth and pattern (eupnea); oxygen saturation ≥95%; and Svo_2 60%-80%.
- At least hourly, assess rate, depth, and effort of patient's respirations. Note tachypnea or labored breaths. Inspect skin and mucous membranes for pallor or cyanosis (a late sign of hypoxia). Consult physician promptly for significant findings.
- Auscultate lung fields q1-2h. Be alert to crackles, rhonchi, or wheezes.
- Monitor ABG values for hypoxemia (Pao_2 <80 mm Hg) or metabolic acidosis (pH <7.35 and HCO_3^- <24 mEq/L).
- Deliver oxygen as prescribed.
- Monitor transcutaneous oxygen saturation with a pulse oximeter. Consult physician if oxygen saturation falls <90%.
- Monitor and manage Svo_2 by supporting cardiac output. When cardiac output drops, perfusion decreases and oxygen extraction increases, resulting in a lower Svo_2.
- If patient's condition deteriorates, prepare for intubation and mechanical ventilation.

NIC Acid-Base Management; Airway Management; Oxygen Therapy; Mechanical Ventilation

For patients undergoing intraaortic balloon pump procedure

Decreased cardiac output (or risk for same) related to negative inotropic changes and rate, rhythm, and conduction alterations secondary to ischemia or injury

Desired outcomes: Within 24 hr of this diagnosis, patient's cardiac output is effectively supported as evidenced by adequate BP to support peripheral perfusion; improved ECG rhythm; HR 60-100 beats/min; peripheral pulses audible with Doppler or palpable; hourly urinary output ≥0.5 ml/kg/hr or renal support strategy in place; measured CO 4-7 L/min; CI ≥2 L/min/m²; PAWP ≤15 mm Hg; SVR ≤1200 dynes/sec/cm⁻⁵; Svo_2 60%-80%; and patient awake, alert, oriented, and free from chest discomfort.
- Monitor BP, PAP, RAP, Svo_2, and HR and rhythm on a continuous basis. Monitor PAWP, SVR, and CO/CI hourly. Report the following to the physician: increased PAWP; decreased CO; new ST segment elevation or depression; deterioration in heart rhythm; decreased Svo_2; or elevated SVR.
- Monitor hourly urinary output. Report output that is <0.5 ml/kg/hr for 2 consecutive hr. Monitor BUN and creatinine values daily. Report increased BUN (>20 mg/dl) and serum creatinine (>1.5 mg/dl), indicative of acute renal failure.

- Monitor bilateral peripheral pulses and color and temperature of extremities q2h.
- Provide oxygen therapy or maintain ventilator settings as prescribed.
- Regulate IV inotropic agents such as dobutamine, dopamine, and milrinone to maintain CI ≥2.5-4 L/min/m^2. Monitor for side effects, including tachyarrhythmias, ventricular ectopy, headache, and angina. (See Appendix 7 for more information.)
- Regulate afterload-reducing agents such as nitroprusside and nitroglycerin to maintain SVR <1200 dynes/sec/cm^{-5}. Monitor for drug side effects, including hypotension, headache, dizziness, nausea, vomiting, and cutaneous flushing.
- Administer diuretic agents as prescribed for elevated PAWP (>12 mm Hg). Monitor for signs and symptoms of hypokalemia (e.g., weakness, dysrhythmias), a potential side effect of diuretics.
- Provide a quiet environment conducive to stress reduction.
- Administer prescribed pain medications to keep patient comfortable. Stress increases workload of the heart.
- Monitor Hgb and Hct values daily. Loss of blood reduces oxygen delivery to the cells, prompting tachycardia and tachypnea to help correct cellular oxygen deficit.

NIC Circulatory Care: Mechanical Assist Device; Surveillance

Altered tissue perfusion (or risk for same): peripheral: involved leg, related to interrupted arterial blood flow secondary to arterial wall dissection by sheath; thrombus formation

Desired outcome: Throughout hospitalization, patient has adequate perfusion in the involved leg as evidenced by Doppler or palpable peripheral pulses; normal color and sensation; warmth; full motor function; and absence of bleeding, abdominal pain, and tingling in the involved leg.

- Monitor circulation in affected leg q30min × 4 and q2h thereafter if assessment is within normal limits. Assess pulses, temperature, color, sensation, and mobility of the toes in the involved leg. Consult physician immediately for significant changes.
- Instruct patient to notify staff member if pain, numbness, or tingling occurs in the involved leg.
- Provide protection to heel of involved foot, using sheepskin, occlusive opaque dressing, or heel protector. Place lamb's wool between the toes to minimize their pressure against each other.
- To enhance perfusion in the involved leg, have patient perform passive foot exercises qid, without bending leg at the hip: foot flexion/extension, foot circles, and quadriceps setting. A pneumatic compression device may be beneficial.
- Administer IV medications (e.g., heparin) as prescribed to prevent clots from forming on the balloon. Monitor patient for signs of bleeding, including decreased Hct (optimal values are ≥37% [female] or ≥40% [male]), abdominal pain, hematuria, oral bleeding, or blood-tinged mucus.
- Monitor PTT if heparin is used (optimal value is 30-40 sec [activated]). Therapeutic anticoagulation is usually 1½ times that of normal. Maintain adequate hydration (2-3 L/day) to minimize risk of clot formation.
- Keep HOB at 30 degrees or less to prevent upward migration of the balloon catheter, which may occlude subclavian artery.
- Assess for the following signs of balloon migration: decreased left radial pulse, sudden decrease in urine output (<0.5 ml/kg/hr), flank pain, and dizziness.
- When the balloon is no longer needed, maintain regular balloon inflation timing to prevent clot formation until balloon can be removed.

NIC Positioning; Circulatory Care: Peripheral

Impaired tissue integrity (or risk for same) related to external factors (pressure and immobilization); internal factors (altered circulation, possible insulin resistance, and decreased nutritional intake)

Desired outcome: Throughout hospitalization, patient's tissue remains intact.

- Position patient on low-pressure protective bed to enhance blood flow to dependent areas and allow air circulation across the skin, promoting evaporation of moisture.
- Reposition patient q2h, especially when spontaneous movement is diminished. When turning patient, keep involved leg extended and log-roll patient onto side.
- Provide meticulous care to keep skin clean and dry. Inspect pressure areas (e.g., coccyx, ischial tuberosity, calcaneus, malleolus) at least tid.
- Ensure that patient's diet is high in protein and calories, with blood glucose 80-110 mg/dl to promote an anabolic or "building" state. If patient's oral intake is inadequate, consider nutritional support (i.e., enteral or parenteral nutrition.)
- Teach patient how to move in bed while minimizing flexion of involved hip.
- See pp. 45 and 61, for more information.

NIC Bedrest Care; Positioning; Self-Care Assistance

Ineffective breathing pattern related to fatigue and decreased energy secondary to heart failure; decreased lung expansion secondary to medically imposed position (HOB no higher than 30 degrees)

Desired outcome: Within 4 hr of this diagnosis, patient has an effective breathing pattern as evidenced by Pao_2 ≥80 mm Hg; Spo_2 >90%; absence of adventitious breath sounds; and RR 12-20 breaths/min with normal pattern and depth (eupnea).

- Monitor breath sounds q2h. Assess anterior and posterior lung fields for adventitious (e.g., crackles, rhonchi) or absent sounds.
- Monitor oxygen saturation by pulse oximetry. Be alert to levels <90%.
- Monitor respiratory rate, rhythm, and breathing pattern hourly.
- Assess for atelectasis (e.g., dyspnea, elevated temperature, weakness, absent or decreased breath sounds) and respiratory infection (e.g., elevated temperature, SOB, increased sputum production or coughing, altered color of sputum).
- Monitor temperature q4h and WBC count daily for signs of infection. Be alert to low-grade fever of ≤37.8° C (≤100° F) and increased WBC count.
- Provide supplemental oxygen and chest physiotherapy as prescribed.
- Encourage patient to perform deep-breathing exercises or incentive spirometry with coughing q1-2h while awake to reduce the possibility of atelectasis.
- If coughing is ineffective in raising secretions, consider suctioning if indicated.
- Reposition patient at least q2h to minimize stasis of lung secretions.
- Monitor patient's fluid volume status to ensure adequate hydration to keep secretions thin and mobile. Fluid intake goal may be 2-3 L/day.
- Elevate HOB 30 degrees at tolerated, to promote effective breathing pattern.
- If patient has respiratory insufficiency despite other measures, prepare for endotracheal intubation and mechanical ventilation.

NIC Airway Management; Oxygen Therapy; Respiratory Monitoring; Mechanical Ventilation

Altered protection related to risk of bleeding/hemorrhage secondary to coagulopathy or IV anticoagulants needed to maintain therapeutic equipment, such as ventricular assist devices

Desired outcome: Throughout hospitalization, patient's bleeding is controlled as evidenced by secretions and excretions negative for blood; chest tube drainage within acceptable amounts (<100 ml/hr); and absence of abdominal pain or ecchymoses. Hct is ≥37% (female) or ≥40% (male); PTT is in the range of therapeutic anticoagulation established by physician or protocol; ACT is ≤120 sec; and platelet count is 150,000-400,000/mm^3.

- Monitor PTT, ACT, and platelet level daily. Report and manage levels not within therapeutic range. Anticoagulation and decreased platelet level increase the risk of bleeding and hemorrhage.
- Monitor Hct and Hgb daily. Decreased levels may signal the presence of bleeding.
- Test GI drainage and stool daily for blood.
- Protect patient from injury. Pad side rails, if necessary, and turn patient carefully. Use sponge-tipped applicators for oral care.
- Test gastric pH q4h. Administer gastric acid-neutralizing drugs, such as antacids or histamine H_2-receptor antagonists as prescribed to maintain gastric pH >5.

NIC Bleeding Precautions

Patients with ventricular assist devices

Risk for disuse syndrome related to imposed restrictions against movement secondary to presence of assist device or debilitated state

Desired outcome: Patient maintains baseline ROM without evidence of muscle atrophy or contracture formation.

- Be aware that patient can be turned gently from side to side when the heart assist device is in place. Do this q2h, observing assist device cannulas closely to ensure that tension is not placed on them during patient repositioning.
- Provide passive ROM to extremities qid.
- See "Prolonged Immobility," p. 61, for more information.

NIC Energy Management

Decreased cardiac output (or risk for same) related to altered preload and negative inotropic changes secondary to reduced right ventricular contraction occurring with left-sided heart assist device

---

Note: This is a complication of the left-sided heart assist device, particularly when the outflow cannula is located in the left ventricle. When the left ventricle is decompressed, septal wall motion is diminished, thereby reducing right ventricular contraction. Patients who have pulmonary hypertension or impaired right ventricular function caused by AMI or cardiopulmonary bypass are especially prone to developing this problem.

Desired outcome: Within 24 hr of this diagnosis, patient's cardiac output is adequate as evidenced by measured CO 4-7 L/min; RAP 4-6 mm Hg; PVR 60-100 dynes/sec/cm^{-5}; and LAP ≥10 mm Hg.
- Monitor patient for a decrease in CO with associated increases in RAP and PVR, which are diagnostic of the complication just described.
- Ensure that patient attains prescribed IV fluid intake to maintain a minimal LAP of 10 mm Hg. An adequate preload is necessary to prevent a vacuum effect from the device, which would aggravate this problem.

NIC Circulatory Care: Mechanical Assist Device; Hemodynamic Regulation

Risk for infection related to inadequate primary defenses secondary to presence of multiple invasive lines, movement restrictions, and stasis of body fluids

Desired outcome: Patient is free of infection as evidenced by normothermia; WBC count ≤11,000/mm^3; negative culture results; and absence of erythema, swelling, warmth, tenderness, and purulent drainage at incision or cannulation sites.
- On a daily basis, monitor temperature, WBC count, and all incisions and cannulation sites for evidence of infection. Be alert to low-grade fever of approximately 37.8° C (100° F); WBC count >11,000/mm^3; and incision that is erythematous, warm, swollen, and tender to the touch or that has purulent discharge.
- Culture any suspicious drainage or secretions; report positive findings.
- Change IV tubing q72h (or per agency protocol), using aseptic technique.
- Change all dressings over catheter insertion sites per agency protocol, using aseptic technique. Apply antimicrobial ointment (e.g., povidone-iodine).
- Administer prophylactic IV antibiotics as prescribed.
- Provide nutritional support to ensure that nitrogen balance is attained.
- Monitor breath sounds q2h. Assess for the presence of crackles, rhonchi, or signs of consolidation. Following extubation, perform coughing and deep-breathing exercises.
- If patient is incapable of raising secretions independently, suction as often as a need for it is determined by auscultation. Inspect the mucus, noting color and consistency. Be alert to secretions that are yellow or green or thickened.
- Provide gentle chest physiotherapy as prescribed. Percussion and vibration can be performed over the posterior and lateral lung lobes during every positioning change, or at least qid.

NIC Infection Protection

Altered nutrition: less than body requirements, related to decreased intake secondary to oral intubation; increased need secondary to debilitated state and impaired tissue perfusion with concomitant nitrogen malabsorption

Desired outcome: Within the 24- to 48-hr period before discharge from ICU, patient has adequate nutrition as evidenced by a balanced nitrogen state; stable weight; urine nitrogen 10-20 g/24 hr; thyroxine-binding prealbumin 20-30 mg/dl; and retinol-binding protein 4-5 mg/dl.
- Provide nutrition via tube feedings, or total parenteral nutrition, to ensure minimum of 1-5 g protein/kg/day and a calorie intake of 100 kcal/kg/day, along with other essential elements. Ask dietitian to monitor daily calorie and protein intake.
- Weigh patient daily for trend. Report continuing decreases in weight.
- Monitor 24-hr urinary nitrogen q3days for increase in excretion.
- Monitor I&O hourly. Report positive or negative fluid state of 300 ml/hr.
- Assess patient for signs of cardiac cachexia: muscle atrophy, weakness, anorexia, and weight loss.
- For more information, see "Nutritional Support," p. 1.

NIC Nutritional Monitoring; Nutrition Therapy

Research Brief 4-6 Cardiogenic shock is the most frequent reason of death for patients with acute myocardial infarction. The Should We Emergently Revascularize Occluded Coronaries for Cardiogenic Shock (SHOCK) trial was conducted to see if acute revascularization or initial medical stabilization resulted in better outcomes in this vulnerable group of patients. To study this, 302 patients with predominant left ventricular failure following an acute myocardial infarction were randomly assigned to a strategy of emergency revascularization within 6 hours or to medical stabilization and perhaps later surgical intervention. The primary end point of the study was 30-day all-cause mortality, and results found no statistical significant difference. However, at the 6- and 12-month follow up there was a significant survival benefit with early revascularization (50% vs. 37%, p = 0.027, and 47% vs. 34%, p = 0.025, respectively). Those who demonstrated the greatest benefit were less than 75 years of age. Based on the results of the SHOCK trial, the American College of Cardiology/America Heart Association guidelines for myocardial infarction have been revised to recommend emergency revascularization for patients younger than 75 years with cardiogenic shock.

Menon V, Fincke R: Cardiogenic shock: a summary of the randomized SHOCK trial, *Congest Heart Failure* 9(1): 35-39, 2003.

ADDITIONAL NURSING DIAGNOSES

Also see the following, as appropriate: "Mechanical Ventilation," p. 14; "Hemodynamic Monitoring," p. 23; "Prolonged Immobility," p. 61; "Psychosocial Support," p. 68; and "Psychosocial Support for the Patient's Family and Significant Others," p. 78.

Cardiac Transplantation

PATHOPHYSIOLOGY

Cardiac transplantation is the treatment of choice for patients with end-stage heart failure. The discovery of cyclosporine in 1980 improved patient outcomes, and success rates prompted a growing number of transplant centers. In the United States, 25,000 patients are candidates for cardiac transplantation. Approximately 4000 persons are actively awaiting a donor heart on the United Network of Organ Sharing (UNOS) list. Since an average of only 2200 hearts are donated annually, 20%-40% of the actual transplant candidates expire before receiving an organ. Of the cardiac transplant recipients, 80% survive more than 1 yr and 50% live more than 5 years.

The three types of transplant procedures are orthotopic, heterotopic, and xenotransplantation.
- *Orthotopic/homotopic/allotransplantation:* recipient's heart, except for the posterior atria, is replaced with a donor heart. This most commonly done procedure is the focus of this chapter.
- *Heterotopic:* donor heart is "piggy backed" to the right of the recipient's heart. An anastomosis allows for both hearts to function.
- *Xenotransplantation:* donor heart is from a different species.

Functional classifications for the etiologies of heart failure or cardiomyopathy are numerous but can be categorized as follows:
- *Idiopathic dilated:* gross dilation of the heart as a result of damaged myofibrils causing cellular hypertrophy and fibrosis. The precise etiology is unclear, but related factors include alcohol abuse, pregnancy, viral infection, ischemia, immunologic disorders, muscular dystrophy, myocarditis, and a positive family history (35%).
- *Hypertrophic/obstructive:* abnormal muscle fiber organization. There is thickening and hypertrophy of the interventricular septum with ventricular wall rigidity. The stiff ventricular wall results in poor ventricular filling (diastole) and sometimes obstruction of the outflow tract (systole). Etiology: unknown but probably genetically transmitted. 50% of patients have a familial link.
- *Restrictive/constrictive:* endocardial scarring of ventricle. Impairment of diastolic function. Least common. Etiology: amyloid, hemochromatosis, glycogen deposition, environment, genetic background (not familial), modifier genes of the reninangiotensin, adrenergic, and endothelin system.

Although the primary indication for cardiac transplantation is cardiomyopathy, additional indications include valvular disease and congenital heart defects.

With the imbalance between supply and demand, patients must meet selection criteria before they can be considered for transplantation (Table 4-26). Those same criteria considered relative are risk factors for an increase in mortality at 1 yr (Box 4-1).

Once the patient is selected as a candidate for cardiac transplantation, he or she is placed on a waiting list and given a status code. The status code is assigned to all transplant candidates and identifies the level of urgency for transplantation (Table 4-27).

LEFT VENTRICULAR ASSIST DEVICE (LVAD)

Implantation, as a "bridge to transplant," is increasingly common for patients awaiting transplantation. The "bridge" provides more time to await a donor, and patients are healthier, more physically fit, and have increased quality of life. Destination therapy (long-term or permanent use) is in the final stages of research.

T A B L E 4 - 26   Selection Criteria for Transplantation Consideration

Inclusion criteria	Exclusion criteria
End-stage heart failure	*Relative*
Refractory and intolerable symptoms;	Active substance abuse
New York Heart Association	Active infection associated with ventricular assist
classes III-IV	Psychologic-social issues related to support or finances
Failure of maximal medical treatment	Age <65-70 yr
(e.g., digoxin, diuretics, vasodilators,	History of cancer in remission
ACE inhibitors, β-blockers)	*Absolute*
1-year survival expectancy <50% and	Complicated IDDM with end-organ damage
poor short-term prognosis or poor	Poor compliance
functional capacity	Severe obesity
Age >60-70	Pulmonary hypertension: PVR >6 Wood units
Left ventricular ejection fraction 20%-35%	Comorbid diseases
Chronic, unstable angina	Active infection (until resolved)
Peak O_2 consumption 14 ml/kg/min	Irreversible liver and kidney dysfunction
Onset of atrial fibrillation	Active peptic ulcer disease
Decreasing cardiac output	Coexisting cancer
Cachexia	Symptomatic peripheral and cerebral vascular disease
Refractory ventricular dysrhythmias	Severe osteoporosis
Otherwise good health	Amyloidosis

IDDM, Insulin-dependent diabetes mellitus; *PVR,* pulmonary vascular resistance.

BOX 4-1   RISK FACTORS THAT INCREASE 1-YEAR MORTALITY RATES

Mechanical circulatory support (IABP, VAD)
Advanced age >55
Female recipient
Increase in troponin I levels
LVEF <40%
Increase in serum creatinine
Ischemic cardiomyopathy
Previous sternotomy
Liver failure
Preoperative physical wasting
Repeat transplant
Sensitization
Donor age
Donor inotropic support

IABP, Intraaortic balloon pump; *LVEF,* left ventrivular ejection fractions; *VAD,* ventricular assist device.

DONOR PROCUREMENT

During surgery, the donor heart is exposed and then inspected to assess viability. The heart is cooled with a high-potassium cardioplegic agent, excised, and protected in plastic bags containing ice-cold normal saline. It is then transferred via an ice chest to the waiting recipient.

POSTOPERATIVE CLINICAL PRESENTATION

Physical assessment: Varies depending on time of postoperative assessment.
Neurologic: Initially somnolent related to anesthesia. As cerebral perfusion improves, alertness increases and neurologic status improves relative to baseline.
Cardiovascular: HR maintained at 110 beats/min, usually atrially paced at 110/min; SBP maintained at >100 mm Hg; MAP >65; CI should be >2.5, and CI will improve as heart is warmed and

TABLE 4-27 Allocation of Thoracic Organs*

Status IA

A patient is admitted to the transplant center and has at least one of the following:

A Mechanical circulatory support for acute hemodynamic decompensation that includes at least one of the following:
- Left or right ventricular assist device implanted <30 days
- Total artificial heart
- Intraaortic balloon pump
- Extracorporeal membrane oxygenator

B Mechanical circulatory support for >30 days with significant device-related complications such as thromboembolism, device infection, mechanical failure, or life-threatening ventricular arrhythmias

C Mechanical ventilation

D Continuous infusion of a single high-dose inotrope or multiple inotropes with hemodynamic monitoring

E Patient does not meet the above criteria but has a life expectancy without a heart transplant of <7 days

Status 1B

A patient listed as status 1B has at least one of the following devices or therapies in place:

A Left and/or right ventricular assist device implanted for >30 days

B Continuous infusion of inotropes

Status 2

A patient who does not meet the criteria for status 1A or 1B is listed as a status 2.

Status 7

A patient listed as status 7 is considered temporarily unsuitable to receive a thoracic organ transplant.

From United Network for Organ Sharing (UNOS) for allocation of Thoracic Organs.
*For complete detailed criteria, see actual policy at www.UNOS.org.

perfused. Skin warm, dry, and intact; color appropriate for race; mucous membranes pink. All pulses palpable. S_1, S_2 without murmur. If rejecting, CI will be <2.2; BP will be decreased; and atrial (most common) or other dysrhythmias may be present. Generalized edema expected until postoperative diuresis. Initially, patient may be placed on isoproterenol (Isuprel) to increase HR and decrease PVR.

Respiratory: Clear throughout unless in rejection; then rales and rhonchi are possible. Chest tubes set to 20-cm suction for first 24 hr or until output <100 ml/8 hr. Ventilator initially, with extubation expected 4-6 hr postoperative. RR 12-20/min and unlabored.

Gastrointestinal: Initially bowel sounds (BS) inactive because of anesthesia, with gradual resumption of normal BS. May have some nausea and vomiting related to anesthetic agent and medications.

Genitourinary: Urine output initially decreased and then increased after warming as diuresis ensues.

Musculoskeletal: Weak but may experience more energy because of increase in cardiac output from new heart. HOB should be flat until patient is extubated because of potential air trapped in the circulatory system when the donor heart was attached.

Pain: Incisional pain is expected.

Vital signs/hemodynamics: BP initially decreased and then normal; HR maintained at ≥110. Temperature initially decreased and then normal with rewarming. CVP and PAWP initially increased or decreased and then normal. CO initially may be decreased and then normal. ECG shows normal sinus tachycardia with possible native P wave along with donor P wave.

Diagnostic studies

Laboratory studies: immediate postoperative period

- CBC: watch for increase in WBC count indicative of infection. (Imuran and mycophenolate mofetile can cause leukopenia.)
- Hgb, Hct, and platelets: may be decreased as a result of postoperative bleeding.
- Chemistry panel: assess electrolyte balance. Carefully monitor potassium (prevent dysrhythmias) and glucose (promote tissue healing).
- BUN/creatinine: assess renal function, especially with cyclosporine use.
- ABGs: initially, then pulse oximetry and end-tidal CO_2 for weaning purposes from ventilator.

- 12-Lead ECG: watch for atrial dysrhythmias and ventricular hypertrophy. May see the native P wave along with the donor P wave.

Daily laboratory studies
- Chemistry panels: electrolytes, liver, and renal function. Steroids bind with albumin; may need less steroids if albumin low.
- PT and PTT: assessment of coagulation status.
- Chest x-ray: assessment of cardiac enlargement and pulmonary complications.
- Electrolytes plus BUN/creatinine or BUN/creatinine alone every afternoon to adjust pm dose of cyclosporine, if on that immunosuppressive drug.
- Urine and sputum culture and sensitivity 1-3 times a week to monitor for infection.
- Cytomegalovirus (CMV) and toxoplasmosis cultures.
- Cyclosporine level daily, if applicable.

COLLABORATIVE MANAGEMENT

Infection control: Infection control is paramount because of immunosuppression therapy.
- Betadine scrub for 5 min to initially enter room; then good hand washing thereafter.
- Keep door closed, and limit visitors; no employees or visitors with active infection; avoid taking care of other patients with infections.
- Use leukocyte filter for blood administration or use leukocyte-reduced blood.
- Remove lines and tubes as soon as possible.
- Sterile dressing changes for lines and wounds q24h and prn.
- Clean large equipment brought into room with hospital disinfectant.
- Monitor temperature: >99.2° F may be sign of infection.

Rejection: The major complication of organ transplantation is rejection. When the recipient's body detects the new heart as a foreign object (antigen), the immune response is triggered. This inflammatory response causes infiltrates with fibrosis and scar formation in the heart muscle. Untreated rejection results in complete destruction of the heart (see p. 000 for more details). Signs of rejection include fever (>99.5° F); atrial dysrhythmias; decreased cardiac output/heart failure with syncope; peripheral edema; S_3, S_4 sounds; decreased urine output; jugular vein distention (JVD); hypotension; and rales. Patient symptoms might include malaise, weakness, anorexia, nausea, vomiting, SOB, and decreased activity tolerance.

Myocardial biopsy: Tiny pieces of muscle tissue are removed from the endocardium for pathologic examination to assess for tissue rejection. Performed in a cardiac cath lab/biopsy lab. Prophylactic antibiotics may be given. The cannulation site is generally the right internal jugular or sometimes the femoral vein. Biopsies are graded according to one of several grading systems. (See Organ Rejection, p. 520). Biopsies are generally performed at 7 and 14 days after surgery and at specified intervals thereafter.

Oxygenation: Extubate as soon as tolerated; prolonged mechanical ventilation is to be avoided. Supplemental oxygen is administered as needed. Encourage frequent coughing and deep breathing.

Fluid management: Monitor I&O q1-2h. Evaluate urine output to assess volume status and kidney function. Fluid retention is common because of steroids and cyclosporine therapy, which may cause renal failure. Restrict fluids to 2000-3000 ml/day. Weigh patient daily.

Other:
- Initially NPO with nasogastric tube (NGT) set to low intermittent suction. Clear liquids are provided after extubation if bowel sounds present. Advance to a low-fat, 4-gm sodium diet as tolerated.
- Activity: turn patient from side to side q2h if stable. On first postoperative day or after extubation patient can sit up in chair. Advance activity as tolerated.
- Chest tubes set to 20-cm suction. Assess for bleeding. Discontinue when drainage is <100 ml in an 8-hr period.
- Use atrial/ventricular pacing prn to keep heart rate >110/min. Commonly used to improve cardiac output and to avoid bradycardia as a result of an anoxic heart during transport. In addition, mild tachycardia reduces filling time, keeps the heart from excessive stretching, prevents right-sided failure, and decreases tension on suture lines.

Pharmacotherapy
Postoperative immunosuppression

Steroids: Solu-Medrol and prednisone: antiinflammatory agents used to suppress both T- and B-lymphocyte function, to reduce or prevent edema, to promote normal capillary permeability, and to prevent vasodilation. Can be used for maintenance to prevent rejection or as part of an acute rejection protocol. Side effects are numerous, including mood changes, sodium retention, blurred vision, fragile skin, bleeding, glucose intolerance, increase in appetite and subsequent weight gain, osteoporosis, and "moon face" appearance from an accumulation of fatty tissue on cheeks and upper back.
- ❏ Solu-Medrol—dosage: 125 mg IV q12h for 3 doses.
- ❏ Prednisone—30-35 mg by mouth (PO) q12h. Taper to as low a dose as tolerated.

Mycophenolate mofetile (Cellcept): Currently a first-line immunosuppressant that inhibits immunologically mediated inflammatory responses. An inhibitor of purine synthesis that inhibits lymphocyte proliferation. Dosed at 1.5 g every 12 hr IV/PO. Preferred administration is on an empty stomach, if given PO. Side effects include diarrhea, vomiting, headache, tremor, insomnia, dizziness, leukopenia, and anemia.

Research Brief 4-7 Salyer, Flatlery, Joyner, and Elswick (2003) studied 93 cardiac transplant recipients with greater than 1-yr survival regarding quality of life after transplantation. Although their perception of health was good and they experienced a moderately satisfactory life, patients were uncertain of how well they could manage their lives and cited barriers such as physical disability, fatigue, lack of money, bad weather, and a lack of support that interfered in their ability to practice health-promoting behavior. Patients were most satisfied with family life, psychosocial and spiritual aspect, and least satisfied with their health and functioning. Predictors of a better quality of life included less education, longer time since transplantation, ischemic etiology of heart failure, fewer barriers, higher perceived health competence, and a health promoting lifestyle.

Sayler J et al: Lifestyle and quality of life in long-term cardiac transplant recipients, *J Heart Lung Transplant* 22(3):309-321, 2003.

Tacrolimus: Prograf FK 506: Immunosuppressant similar to but more potent than cyclosporine. Replaces cyclosporine if there are multiple rejections while on cyclosporine. Inhibits T-lymphocyte activation. Dosage depends on trough blood levels, organ function, and rejection status. Cleared through the liver and depends on liver function. Dosage 0.15 mg/kg/day IV given in two divided doses 12 hr apart, followed by a PO dose of 0.3 mg/kg/day after GI function has returned. Should be given on an empty stomach without other medications. Side effects are dose-related and diminish when dose is decreased. They include hyperkalemia, nephrotoxicity, glucose intolerance, hypertension, nausea, diarrhea, infections, and lymphoproliferative disorders. Consult pharmacist before administering.

Cyclosporine: Immunosuppressant. Dosage adjusted according to daily blood levels and body weight. Dosage: 0.5 mg/kg/day is adjusted to maintain blood levels between 300 and 500 ng/ml. Side effects include kidney and renal dysfunction, excessive hair growth, hypertension, diarrhea, swelling and tenderness in gums, hand tremors, and increased risk of infections and tumors.

Azathioprine (Imuran): Immunosuppressant. WBC counts monitored, and dosage adjusted accordingly. Taken daily at bedtime. Maintenance dosage is 2 mg/kg/day, maximum of 150-175 mg/day. Side effects include decreased WBC count, bone marrow suppression, toxic hepatitis, hair loss, mouth sores, and muscle wasting. Decrease or hold if WBC is <5.

OKT3: Orthoclone OKT 3 is substituted for cyclosporine if patient is in perioperative hepatorenal dysfunction. Strong immunosuppressant is used in acute rejection. 5-mg dose is given IV for 10 days. CD3 levels are measured daily to maintain adequate levels of OKT3. Side effects, usually seen after the first 1-3 days, include alterations in temperature control, bronchial smooth muscle tone, and GI tract. Fever, chills, nausea, vomiting, diarrhea, and pulmonary edema can result. During the first 1-3 days of OKT3 therapy, steroids are given at much higher doses. When receiving OKT3, patients are premedicated with acetaminophen, H_2-receptor antagonist, and hydrocortisone (before) and diphenhydramine (after).

Others

Antibiotics: Kefzol or similar antibiotic is given until chest tubes are removed. Ganciclovir: prophylaxis and treatment for CMV. Given IV postoperatively and changed to PO when tolerated. CMV remains the major cause of morbidity and mortality with cardiac transplantation patients.

Mycostatin: 5 ml swish-and-swallow or Mycelex troche tid beginning after extubation, for potential secondary *Candida* infections related to immunosuppression.

H_2-blocker: For gastric secretion suppression.

Inotropic medications: Nitroglycerin to decrease preload; nitroprusside (Nipride) to decrease afterload; dobutamine to increase contractility/cardiac output; epinephrine to increase HR and contractility; norepinephrine (Levophed) to increase BP; milrinone (Primacor) to increase contractility/cardiac output and decrease afterload; dopamine for renal perfusion in smaller doses (controversial), and increase HR and BP at higher doses; and isoproterenol (Isuprel) to increase HR and decrease pulmonary vascular resistance. Theophylline may also be used for increasing HR and decreasing PVR.

Pain: Fentanyl is commonly used because it is short acting and does not cause histamine-mediated hypotension as morphine does.

Pretransplant and posttransplant sensitization: Poor outcomes, such as CAD, and an increased incidence of rejection have been associated with pretransplant sensitization. Positive panel-reactive antibody (PRA) levels detect circulating human leukocyte antigens (HLA) and reflect level of sensitization. Pregnancy, blood transfusion, or previous transplants can trigger sensitization. Elevated PRA levels increase the difficulty of finding an HLA-compatible donor heart. HLA-compatible hearts will enhance graft survival and reduce infection and malignancies related to aggressive immunosuppression. Plasmapheresis may decrease sensitization and reduce PRA levels.

NURSING DIAGNOSES AND INTERVENTIONS

Risk for injury: (rejection) related to inadequate immunosuppressant drug levels
Desired outcomes: No signs of rejection (clinical or with biopsy); patient and staff are compliant with immunosuppression therapy.
- Assess patient's knowledge of drug therapy.
- Monitor blood levels as appropriate for drug.
- Instruct patient to take medication at designated time(s) each day. Never withhold immunosuppressant without consulting with physician.
- Monitor for signs of rejection: atrial fibrillation or other dysrhythmias; hypotension; increase in temperature; decrease in CO; or malaise.
- Reinforce necessity of regularly scheduled appointments with transplant coordinator. Encourage patient to bring a significant other to the visit.

Risk for infection (lungs and heart most common) related to immunosuppression
Desired outcomes: Infections will be absent or minimized; if signs and symptoms occur, the patient will report within 1-4 hr.
- Patient is to wear mask when outside immediate living area, in public areas, or near construction.
- Notify physician/transplant coordinator immediately if temperature >99.5° F; WBC increasing; patient complaints of malaise; or any obvious infection.
- Avoid placement of indwelling catheters; if necessary, remove as soon as possible.

NIC Infection Control; Infection Protection

Decreased cardiac output related to rejection; inadequate donor pump/long ischemic time
Desired outcomes: The patient will have an adequate cardiac output as evidenced by a SBP >90-100; MAP 65-85; CI >2.2 L/min; RR 12-20 breaths/min; and HR >100 beats/min; regular sinus rhythm without ectopy; urinary output >0.5 ml/kg/hr; intake equals output; and ejection fraction >60%.
- Consult physician for the following:
  - ❏ Signs and symptoms of infection: temperature >99.5° F; increased WBC count; or changes in drainage from incisions.
  - ❏ Signs and symptoms of rejection: atrial or ventricular dysrhythmias; temperature >99.5° F; decreased BP; decreased CO/CI; malaise; anorexia; nausea and vomiting, activity intolerance, or SOB.
  - ❏ Increase in chest tube output to >400 ml/hr or sudden cessation of chest tube output.
  - ❏ Svo_2 <60%; SBP <90; CI <2.2.
  - ❏ Any other abnormal lab results.

NIC Hemodynamic Regulation

Caring for Patients Undergoing Coronary Artery Thrombolysis

PATHOPHYSIOLOGY

Acute thrombus formation with coronary artery occlusion is the most common cause of AMI. Early reperfusion of an ischemic myocardium can prevent or reduce myocardial injury. Therefore the ability to dissolve (lyse) fresh coronary thromboses early in the course of infarction is essential to salvage myocardial tissue and preserve ventricular function. The goal of thrombolysis is to reduce infarct size, improve left ventricular function, and minimize morbidity and mortality. Thrombolytic therapy is a safe and effective way to establish reperfusion for patients with AMI secondary to complete or partial coronary arterial thrombotic occlusion.

Thrombolytic agents act to dissolve or lyse existing clots. A clot, or thrombus, is formed when deposits of fibrin collect within the artery and form an insoluble matrix. The fibrin clot eventually is broken down by the naturally occurring enzyme, *plasmin*. Thrombolytic agents work to accelerate this natural process by converting plasminogen to plasmin, which rapidly dissolves the fibrin clot. However, plasmin also breaks down circulating clotting proteins, thus producing excessive fibrin/fibrinogen degradation products (FDPs). The presence of large amounts of FDPs results in significant systemic anticoagulation and can trigger bleeding complications.

First-generation thrombolytics (streptokinase, anistreplase) are nonfibrin selective and activate both fibrin-bound and nonfibrin bound plasminogen. They are also antigenic. Second-generation thrombolytics are fibrin-selective or "clot-specific" and preferentially activate fibrin-bound plasminogen. They are also approved for use in management of acute ischemic stroke and massive pulmonary embolism.

Indications that lysis has taken place include decreased chest pain; rapid resolution of ST segment depression; and a new onset of dysrhythmias. As many as 80% of patients are reported to have had reperfusion dysrhythmias, primarily accelerated idioventricular rhythm and PVCs. Bradycardia and heart block also are seen.

After clot lysis occurs, thrombin is released into the circulation. The thrombin induces platelet clumping and increases the potential for reocclusion. Use of thrombolytic agents results in excessive circulating thrombin and increases the risk of coronary artery reocclusion. Heparin, antiplatelet agents, and glycoprotein IIb/IIIa inhibitors are used as adjuncts to thrombolytic therapy to inhibit the action of free thrombin and prevent reocclusion.

ASSESSMENT

History and risk factors: Presence of cardiac risk factors (see "Acute Coronary Syndrome," p. 206). Assess patient for absolute and relative contraindications for thrombolytic therapy (Table 4-28). Assess for recent (within 6 months) streptococcal infection when use of streptokinase or anistreplase is anticipated. Assess for aspirin allergy, since antiplatelet therapy with aspirin is usually initiated.

Subjective findings: Candidates for thrombolytic therapy include patients with clear symptoms of AMI: usually, sudden onset of chest pain/pressure that is unrelieved by sublingual nitrates and lasts >30 min but <6-12 hr. The pain may radiate to the neck, jaw, and arms. Intermittent, severe chest pain over hours or days can indicate subtotal occlusion secondary to coronary thrombosis, and these patients also may be considered for thrombolytic therapy. Diaphoresis, nausea, vomiting, anxiety, and other symptoms consistent with the diagnosis of AMI may be present.

T A B L E 4 - 28   Contraindications and Warnings for Thrombolytic Therapy

Contraindications
   Known hypersensitivity to thrombolytic agents
   Active internal bleeding
   History of stroke
   Recent intracranial or intraspinal surgery or trauma
   Known bleeding diathesis
   Severe, uncontrolled hypertension

Warnings (risks may be increased and should be weighed against anticipated benefits)
   Recent major surgery (e.g., coronary artery bypass graft, obstetric delivery, organ biopsy)
   Previous puncture of noncompressible vessels
   Cerebrovascular disease
   Recent gastrointestinal or genitourinary bleeding
   Recent trauma
   Hypertension (systolic BP ≥180 mm Hg and/or diastolic BP ≥110 mm Hg)
   High likelihood of left-sided heart thrombus (e.g., mitral stenosis with atrial fibrillation)
   Acute pericarditis
   Subacute bacterial endocarditis
   Hemostatic defects including those secondary to severe hepatic or renal disease
   Severe hepatic or renal dysfunction
   Pregnancy
   Diabetic hemorrhagic retinopathy or other hemorrhagic ophthalmic conditions
   Septic thrombophlebitis or occluded AV cannula at a seriously infected site
   Advanced age
   Currently receiving anticoagulants (e.g., warfarin sodium)
   Any other condition in which bleeding constitutes a significant hazard or would be particularly
      difficult to manage because of its location

AV, Arteriovenous.

Selection of candidates for thrombolytic therapy relies heavily on clinical history, ECG, and physical examination. The presentation of aortic dissection and acute pericarditis is similar to that of AMI, and these diagnoses must be excluded before proceeding with thrombolytic therapy.

Objective findings: The patient may experience tachycardia, bradycardia, irregular pulse, hypotension, and other findings consistent with AMI (see p. 207). Assess patient for absolute and relative contraindications for thrombolytic therapy (see Table 4-28). Assess for and note all venipuncture attempts and superficial injuries that could become active bleeding sites after thrombolysis. Perform a careful baseline neurologic assessment for comparison of subsequent examinations, which are indicated to detect neurologic changes associated with acute stroke.

DIAGNOSTIC TESTS

ECG: 12/15/18-lead ECG is performed to determine presence, location, and extent of myocardial injury. Localized ST segment elevation of 1 mm in 2 contiguous leads, significant Q waves, and T wave inversion are findings associated with AMI. Because left bundle branch block (LBBB) obscures ECG evidence of AMI, patients with presumed new LBBB are also candidates for thrombolytic therapy. ST segment elevation that decreases after administration of sublingual NTG suggests coronary artery spasm (Prinzmetal angina), and thrombolytic therapy is not indicated.

Laboratory studies: Serum enzymes, including cardiac enzymes, troponins, myoglobin and isoenzymes, electrolytes, CBC, and clotting studies are evaluated before initiating thrombolytic therapy. A heparin-lock device is used for specimen collection. Do not delay therapy for confirmation of laboratory values.

COLLABORATIVE MANAGEMENT

Thrombolytics: Prompt identification of candidates for thrombolytic therapy and rapid initiation of therapy increase the effectiveness of all thrombolytic agents. Because time is crucial, initiation of thrombolytic therapy may occur in the prehospitalization setting or in the emergency department of a smaller hospital before transfer to a definitive care center. In these settings the thrombolytic agents are administered peripherally. Ideally, thrombolytic therapy is initiated within 30 min of the patient's arrival at the hospital's emergency department. Patients with AMI must be identified expediently and treated rapidly. Table 4-29 compares thrombolytic agents that are in general use and gives dosing regimens.

First-generation thrombolytics:
- *Streptokinase:* An enzyme derived from group C β-hemolytic streptococci. Because it is an antigen, patients who have had previous exposure to streptococcal organisms may have antibodies against streptokinase. Therefore steroids or antihistamines are administered before streptokinase therapy to prevent a hypersensitivity reaction.
- *Anistreplase:* A plasminogen activator that induces clot lysis with fewer systemic lytic effects than does streptokinase. Allergic and anaphylactic reactions are possible.

Second-generation thrombolytics:
- Second-generation thrombolytics are fibrin-specific, decrease systemic activation of plasminogen and the resulting degradation of circulating fibrinogen as compared to a first-generation thrombolytics, and are nonantigenic.
- *Alteplase:* A recombinant tissue plasminogen activator (rt-PA) with the same amino acid sequence as endogenous tissue plasminogen activator (t-PA). Has a shorter half-life than do the other agents, less than 5 min. Several dosage regimens are approved for coronary thrombolysis.
- *Reteplase:* A recombinant deletion mutein of t-PA. Catalyzes cleavage of endogenous plasminogen to generate plasmin. Is not clot-specific, so fibrinogen levels fall to lower than those seen with rt-PA (alteplase), with a return to baseline value within 48 hr after infusion. The half-life is 13-16 min, and the drug is cleared by the liver and kidneys. Dosage: given as two boluses 30 minutes apart, each over 2 min.
- *Tenecteplase:* A modified form of human tissue plasminogen activator (tPA) that binds to fibrin and converts plasminogen to plasmin. In the presence of fibrin, conversion of plasminogen to plasmin is increased relative to its conversion in the absence of fibrin. This fibrin-specificity decreases systemic activation of plasminogen and the resulting degradation of circulating fibrinogen as compared to a molecule lacking this property. Following administration of tenecteplase there are decreases in circulating fibrinogen and plasminogen. Tenecteplase is given as a single 5-sec bolus and is dosed by weight.

Adjunctive therapy: Standard therapy for AMI is initiated including oxygen administration, continuous ECG monitoring, nitrates, IV analgesia, β-blockade, and other therapies as indicated. Heparin and antiplatelet agents are given concurrently with thrombolytic therapy to prevent reocclusion.

Coronary angiography: May be performed to assess for patency or reocclusion or in preparation for an attempt to open occluded vessels with angioplasty and stent when thrombolytic therapy fails.

T A B L E 4 - 29 **Thrombolytic dosage regimens**

Name of agent: generic and brand	Streptokinase (Streptase)	Anistreplase (APSAC, Eminase)	Reteplase (Retavase)	Alteplase (Activase)	Alteplase (Activase)	Tenecteplase (TNKase)
Regimen	Original	Original	Double bolus	Accelerated	Original	Single bolus
Total time of regimen	30-60 min	2-5 min	30 min	90 min	180 min	5 seconds
Initial IV bolus		30 units over 2-5 min	10 units over 2 min	15 mg	6-10 mg	Weight Dose <60 kg 30 mg ≥60 to <70 kg 35 mg ≥70 to <80 kg 40 mg ≥80 kg 50 mg
Second IV bolus at time: 30 min			10 units over 2 min			
Infusion from time 0 to ≥30 min	1.5 million units IV over 30-50 min			0.75 mg/kg max dose 50 mg		
Infusion from time 0 to 60 min					50-54 mg; 1hr total 60 mg	
Infusion from 30 to 90 min				0.50 mg/kg max dose 35 mg		
Infusion from 60 to 120 min					20 mg	
Infusion from 120 to 180 min					20 mg	
Total dose	1.5 million units	30 units	20 units	Varies by weight, max dose 100 mg	100 mg	50 mg

Because of the systemic lytic effects of all thrombolytics, it is best to wait 24-48 hr after initial thrombolytic therapy. See "Coronary Angiography," p. 210.

NURSING DIAGNOSES AND INTERVENTIONS

Pain related to myocardial ischemia; injury; infarction
Desired outcome: Patient's subjective perception of pain decreases within 30 min of onset, as documented by a pain scale.
- Assess location, character, intensity, and duration, using a pain scale. Assess associated symptoms including SOB, restlessness, diaphoresis, and grimacing.
- Run an ECG rhythm strip and consider obtaining a 12/15/18-lead ECG, per hospital protocol, for episodes of chest discomfort or arm, shoulder, back, or jaw pain.
- Record VS during each episode of pain associated with myocardial ischemia.
- Administer prescribed analgesics (e.g., morphine sulfate) as necessary or per protocol, and document, compare, and report results of analgesia.
- Administer oxygen as prescribed, with humidity to reduce the drying effects on oral and nasal mucosa.
- Position the patient in semi-Fowler's position to reduce cardiac workload, unless the patient is intolerant of having HOB elevated because of hypotension.
- Provide reassurance during episodes of discomfort; stay with the patient to assess for acute changes in assessment or VS.

▌NIC Analgesic Administration; Anxiety Reduction; Calming Technique; Cardiac Care: Acute; Cardiac Precautions; Oxygen Therapy

Knowledge deficit: the atherosclerotic process and the rationale, procedure, and expected outcomes of thrombolytic therapy
Desired outcome: Before initiation of the thrombolytic therapy, patient verbalizes basic knowledge about the atherosclerotic process and thrombolytic therapy.
- Assess patient's knowledge about the atherosclerotic process and the rationale, procedure, and expected outcome of thrombolytic therapy. Explain the goal of therapy: to reduce injury to the heart muscle.
- Explain the need for monitoring and close observation after the procedure.
- Ask patient to report any signs or symptoms of bleeding.
- Provide emotional support during the procedure, keeping the patient informed about the events that are taking place.
- After the procedure, discuss potential long-term outcomes and the possibility of reocclusion, including interventions the patient can take to prevent it: take prescribed antiplatelet medications; exercise; comply with dietary modifications; and manage or eliminate risk factors such as smoking, hyperlipidemia, hypertension, stress, and obesity.
- Before discharge, instruct patient to report any signs and symptoms of MI that occur after hospitalization: unrelenting chest heaviness or pressure; pain that radiates to the arm, neck, or jaw; accompanying nausea and diaphoresis; and lightheadedness or dizziness.

▌NIC Teaching: Individual; Teaching: Disease Process

Altered protection related to risk of bleeding/hemorrhage secondary to nonspecific thrombolytic effects of therapy
Desired outcome: Symptoms of bleeding complications are absent as evidenced by BP within patient's normal range; HR ≤100 beats/min; blood-free secretions and excretions; natural skin color; baseline or normal LOC; and absence of back and abdominal pain, hematoma, headache, dizziness, and vomiting.
- When patient is admitted, obtain a thorough history, assessing for the following:
  - ❏ Risk factors for intracranial hemorrhage: uncontrolled hypertension; cerebrovascular pathology; CNS surgery within previous 6 months.
  - ❏ Bleeding risks: recent or active GI bleeding; recent trauma; recent surgery; bleeding diathesis; advanced liver or kidney disease.
  - ❏ Risk of systemic embolization: suspected left-sided heart thrombus.
  - ❏ History of streptococcal infection or previous streptokinase therapy.
- Monitor clotting studies per agency protocol. Regulate heparin drip to maintain PTT at 1½-2 times control levels or according to protocol. *Never* discontinue heparin without physician's directive.
- Apply pressure dressing over puncture sites. If cardiac catheterization was performed, inspect site at frequent intervals for evidence of hematoma formation. Immobilize extremity for 6-8 hr after catheterization procedure.
- Avoid unnecessary venipunctures, IM injections, or arterial puncture. Obtain laboratory specimens from heparin-lock device.

- Monitor patient for indicators of internal bleeding: back pain; abdominal pain; decreased BP; pallor; and bloody stool or urine. Report significant findings to physician.
- Monitor patient for signs of intracranial bleeding q2h: change in LOC; headache; dizziness; vomiting; and confusion.
- Test all stools, urine, and emesis for occult blood.
- Use care with oral hygiene and when shaving patient. For more information about safety precautions, see "Altered Protection" in Pulmonary Embolus p. 197.

NIC Bleeding Reduction; Bleeding Precautions; Surveillance; Hemorrhage Control; Neurologic Monitoring

Decreased cardiac output (or risk for same) related to alterations in rate, rhythm, and conduction secondary to increased irritability of ischemic tissue during reperfusion (usually occurs within 1-2 hr after initiation of therapy); reocclusion of thrombolysed vessels; negative inotropic changes secondary to cardiac disease

Desired outcomes: Within 12 hr of initiation of thrombolytic therapy, patient has adequate cardiac output as evidenced by normal sinus rhythm on ECG; peripheral pulses >2+ on a 0-4+ scale; warm and dry skin; and hourly urine output ≥0.5 ml/kg/hr. Patient is awake, alert, and oriented without palpitations, chest pain, or dizziness. Within 48 hr of initiation of thrombolytic therapy, patient maintains stability as just described.

> **Note:** Reocclusion occurs in as many as 16% of patients within 24-48 hr after thrombolysis.

- Monitor ECG continuously during thrombolytic therapy for evidence of dysrhythmias. Consult physician for significant dysrhythmias or new or worsening ST segment elevation.
- With any dysrhythmia, check VS and note accompanying signs and symptoms such as dizziness, lightheadedness, syncope, and palpitations.
- Ensure availability of emergency drugs and equipment: atropine; isoproterenol; epinephrine; amiodarone; lidocaine (use cautiously with AMI); defibrillator-cardioverter; and external and transvenous pacemaker.
- Evaluate patient's response to medications and emergency treatment.
- Monitor patient for signs of reocclusion: chest pain; nausea; diaphoresis; and dysrhythmias. Consult physician for any signs of reocclusion.
- Obtain 12/15/18-lead ECG if reocclusion is suspected.
- Anticipate and prepare patient for cardiac catheterization, PTCA with stent, or repeated thrombolytic therapy.

NIC Hemodynamic Regulation; Circulatory Care; Dysrhythmia Management; Cardiac Care: Acute

Risk for injury related to potential for allergic or anaphylactic reaction to streptokinase or anistreplase secondary to antigen/antibody response

Desired outcome: Patient has no symptoms of allergic response as evidenced by normothermia; RR 12-20 breaths/min with normal pattern and depth (eupnea); HR ≤100 beats/min; BP at baseline or within normal limits; natural skin color; and absence of itching, urticaria, headache, muscular and abdominal pain, and nausea.

- Before treatment, question patient about history of previous streptokinase therapy or streptococcal infection. Consult physician for positive findings.
- Administer prophylactic hydrocortisone as prescribed.
- Monitor patient during and for 48-72 hr after infusion for indicators of allergy: hypotension (brief or sustained); urticaria; fever; itching; flushing; nausea; headache; muscular pain; bronchospasm; abdominal pain; dyspnea; or tachycardia. These indicators can appear immediately after or as long as several days after streptokinase therapy.
- If hypotension develops, increase rate of IV infusion/administer volume replacement as prescribed. Prepare for vasopressor administration if there is no response to volume replacement.
- Treat allergic response with diphenhydramine or other antihistamine as prescribed.

NIC Shock Management: Vasogenic; Shock Management

Bibliography

ACC/AHA: Cardiovascular disease (CVD) release guidelines for management of female patients, retrieved from website: http://www.advisory.com, February 13, 2004.

Akhond H, Rahimi AR: *Haemophilus aphrophilus* endocarditis after tongue piercing, *Emerg Infect Dis* 8(8):850-851, 2002.

Alexander RW, Schlant RC, Fuster V, editors: *Hurst the heart,* ed 10 New York, 2002, McGraw-Hill.

American College of Cardiology/American Heart Association: New Guidelines for Evaluating Acute Coronary Syndrome, *Clin Rev* 11:73-86, 2001.

American Heart Association: Prevention of infective endocarditis, *Circulation* 96:358-366, 1997.

American Heart Association: *Textbook of advanced cardiac life support,* Dallas, Tex, 2000, American Heart Association.

American Heart Association: 2003 *Heart and stroke statistical update,* Dallas, Tex, 2003, American Heart Association.

Ammash NM et al: Clinical profile and outcome of idiopathic restrictive cardiomyopathy, *Circulation* 101:2490, 2000.

Anderson J: Acute treatment of atrial fibrillation and flutter, *Am J Cardiol* 78(8A):17-21, 1996.

Angeja BG, Grossman W: Clinician update: Evaluation and management of diastolic heart failure, *Circulation* 107:659, 2003.

Antman EM, Braunwald E: Acute myocardial infarction. In Braunwald E, editor: *Heart disease: a textbook of cardiovascular medicine,* ed 5, Philadelphia, 1997, Saunders.

Argenziano M, Michler RE, Rose EA: Cardiac transplantation for endstage heart disease, *Heart Vessels* 12:23-27, 1997.

Armstrong PW, Collen D: Fibrinolysis for acute myocardial infarction, *Circulation* 106:2987, 2001.

Ashton HA et al for the Multicentre Aneurysm Screening Study Group: The Multicentre Aneurysm Screening Study (MASS) into the effect of abdominal aortic aneurysm screening on mortality in men: a randomised controlled trial. *Lancet* 360:1531-1539, Nov, 2002.

Barron HV et al for the NRMI 2 investigators: Regional variation in the treatment of women with acute myocardial infarction in the United States: data from the National Registry of Myocardial Infarction 2 (NRMI 2), *Circulation* 96:3002A, 1997.

Barron HV et al for the NRMI 2 investigators: Utilization of reperfusion therapy for acute myocardial infarction in the United States: data from the National Registry of Myocardial Infarction 2 (NRMI 2), *Circulation* 97(12):1150-1156, 1998.

Berkowitz SD et al: Incidence and predictors of bleeding after contemporary thrombolytic therapy for myocardial infarction, *Circulation* 95:2508-2516, 1997.

Birnie D et al: Interatrial conduction of atrial tachycardia in heart transplant recipients: potential pathophysiology, *J Heart Lung Transplant* 19(10):1007-1010, 2000.

Blanche C et al: Heart transplantation in patients seventy years of age and older: a comparative analysis of outcome, *J Thorac Cardiovasc Surg* 121:532-541, 2001.

Blanche C et al: Heart transplantation with donors fifty years of age and older, *J Thorac Cardiovasc Surg* 123:810-815, 2002.

Bonow RO et al: ACC/AHA guidelines for the management of patients with valvular heart disease: executive summary, *Circulation* 98:1949-1984, 1998.

Braunwald E: Pathophysiology of heart failure. In Braunwald E, editor: *Heart disease: a textbook of cardiovascular medicine,* ed 6, Philadelphia, 2001, Saunders.

Braunwald E et al: ACC/AHA guidelines for the management of patients with unstable angina and non-ST segment elevation myocardial infarction: a report of the American College of Cardiology/American Heart Association Task Force on Practice Guidelines (Committee on the Management of Patients with Unstable Angina), *J Am Coll Cardiol* 36:970-1062, 2000.

Bridges MEJ, Woods SL: Cardiovascular chronobiology: implications for critical care nursing, *Crit Care Nurs* 18(4):49-64, 1998.

Buckingham TA: Program abstracts: new approaches in the treatment of atrial fibrillation. Medscape's Coverage of the XXIVth Congress of the European Society of Cardiology: August 31, 2002-September 4, 2002, Berlin, Germany, retrieved from website: www.medscape.com.

Buckingham, TA: Program abstracts: evidence-based indications for cardiac pacing. Medscape's Coverage of the XXIVth Congress of the European Society of Cardiology: August 31, 2002-September 4, 2002, Berlin, Germany, retrieved from website: www.medscape.com.

Burger AJ et al: Effect of nesiritide (B-type natriuretic peptide) and dobutamine on ventricular arrhythmias in the treatment of patients with acutely decompensated congestive heart failure: The PRECEDENT Study. *Am Heart J* 144(6):1102-1108, 2002.

Burke L: Securing life through technology acceptance: the first six months after transvenous internal cardioverter defibrillator implantation, *Heart Lung* 25:352-366, 1996.

Casas RE, Marriott HJL, Glancy DL: Value of leads V_7-V_9 in diagnosing posterior wall acute myocardial infarction and other causes of tall R waves in V_1-V_2, *Am J Cardiol* 79:508-509, 1997.

Chase SL: New strategies in the management of patients with heart failure, *Pharmacol Ther,* Feb:84-96, 1999.

Cimato T, Jessup M: Recipient selection in cardiac transplantation: contraindications and risk factors for mortality. *J Heart Lung Transplant* 21(11):1161-1173, 2002.

Cohn JN: The management of chronic heart failure, *N Engl J Med* 335:490-498, 1996.

Cheek C: What's different about heart disease in women? *Nursing* 33(8):36-43, 2003.

Coffee M, Crowder GK, Cheek DJ: Reducing coronary artery disease by decreasing homocysteine levels, *Crit Care Nurse* 23(1):25-30, 1999.

Crawford MH: *Current diagnosis and treatment in cardiology,* ed 2, New York, 2003, McGraw-Hill.

Crystal E et al: Interventions on prevention of postoperative atrial fibrillation in patients undergoing heart surgery: a meta-analysis, *Circulation* 106:75-80, 2002.

Cushman WC et al for the ALLHAT Collaborative Research Group: Success and predictors of blood pressure control in diverse North American settings: the Antihypertensive and Lipid-Lowering Treatment to Prevent Heart Attack Trial (ALLHAT), *J Clin Hypertension* 4:393-404, 2002; also *JAMA* 288:2981, 2002.

Darovic GO: Cardiovascular anatomy and physiology. In Darovic GO: *Hemodynamic monitoring: invasive and non-invasive clinical application,* ed 3, Philadelphia, 2002, Saunders.

Delgado J et al: Impact of mild pulmonary artery pressure profile after heart transplantation, *J Heart Lung Transplant* 20(9):942-948, 2001.

Dressler D et al: Heart transplantation. *Organ Transplantation: Concepts, Issues, Practice, and Outcomes,* 2002-2003, www.medscape.com.

Dracup KA, Cannon C: Combination treatment strategies for management of acute myocardial infarction: new directions with current therapies. *Crit Care Nurs* (4): 3-14, 1999.

Dracup K, Dunbar SB, Baker DW: Rethinking heart failure, *Am J Nurs* 95(7):22-28, 1995.

Futterman LG, Lemberg L: Radiofrequency catheter ablation for supraventricular tachycardias, *Am J Crit Care* 2(6):500-505, 1993.

Garica TB, Holtz NE: *12 lead ECG: The art of interpretation.* Sudbury, MA, 2001, Jones and Bartlett.

Giles WH et al: Association between total homocysteine and the likelihood for a history of acute myocardial infarction by race and ethnicity: results from the Third National Health and Nutrition Examination Survey, *Am Heart J* 139:443-446, 2000.

Giuliano KK, Warren-Sims T: Transplant issues: infections and immunosuppressant drugs, *Dimens Crit Care Nurs* 18(2):16-19, 1999.

Goldman DS, Hogan TT: Nitrate-tolerance update: mechanism and management, *Pharmacol Ther,* Feb:67-73, 1999.

Grady K, Jalowiec A, White-Williams C: Predictors of quality of life in patients at one year after heart transplantation, *J Heart Lung Transplant* 18(3):202-210, 1999.

Harrison TC, Kessler D: Arrhythmogenic right ventricular dysplasia/cardiomyopathy. *Heart Lung* 30(5):360-369, 2001.

Heart Center Online: Cardiomyopathy center: retrieved from World Wide Web April 28, 2003: *www.heartcenteronline.com.*

Heidenreich PA, Lee TT, Massie BM: Effects of β-blockade on mortality in patients with heart failure: a meta-analysis of randomized clinical trials, *J Am Coll Cardiol* 30(1):27-34, 1997.

Hodgson B, Kizior R: *Saunders' nursing drug handbook,* Philadelphia, 1998, Saunders.

Hourigan L et al: Heparin-induced thrombocytopenia: a common complication in cardiac transplant recipients, *J Heart Lung Transplant* 21(12):1283-1289, 2002.

Hunt SA et al: ACC/AHA guidelines for the evaluation and management of chronic heart failure in the adult: executive summary, a report of the American College of Cardiology/American Heart Association Task Force of Practice Guidelines, *Circulation* 104(24):2996-3007, 2001.

Huszar RJ: *Basic dysrhythmias: interpretation and management,* ed 3, St Louis: Mosby, 2001.

Jacobson C. Beside cardiac monitoring, Critical Care Nurs 23(6): 71-73, 2003.

John R., Lietz K., Schuster M., et al: (2003) Immunologic sensitization in recipients of left ventricular assist devices, *J Thorac Cardiovasc Surg* 125:578-591.

Joint National Committee: The seventh report of the Joint National Committee on Prevention, Detection, Evaluation, and Treatment of High Blood Pressure (JNC 7), NIH Pub. No. 03-5231, May, 2003; on the World Wide Web at the National Heart, Lung, and Blood Institute website: (www.nhlbi.nih.gov/guidelines/hypertension/index.htm).

Keen J, Baird M, Allen J: *Mosby's critical care and emergency drug reference,* ed 2, St Louis, 1996, Mosby.

Khan IA, Ajatta FO, Ansari AW: Persistent ST segment elevation: a new ECG finding in hypertropic cardiomyopathy, *Am J Emerg Med* 17(B):296-299, 1999.

Kinney MR et al: *AACN's clinical reference for critical-care nursing,* ed 4, St Louis, 1998, Mosby.

Kirklin JK et al: Evolving trends in risk profiles and causes of death after heart transplantation: a ten-year multi-institutional study, *J Thorac Cardiovasc Surg* 125:881-890, 2003.

Kline-Rogers E, Martin JS, Smith DD: New era of reperfusion in acute myocardial infarction, *Crit Care Nurs* 19(1):21-33, 1999.

Knight L et al: Caring for patients with third generation implantable cardioverter defibrillators: from decision to implant to patient's return home, *Crit Care Nurs* 17(5):46-63, 1997.

Lamas GA et al: Ventricular pacing or dual-chamber pacing for sinus node dysfunction, *New Engl J Med* 346:1854-1862, 2002.

Lange C et al: Morbidity and mortality in diabetic patients following cardiac transplantation, *J Heart Lung Transplant* 22(3), 244-249, 2003.

Markey DW, Brown RJ: An interdisciplinary approach to addressing patient activity and mobility in the medical-surgical patient, *J Nurs Care Qual* 16(4):1-12, 2002.

Maron BJ: Hypertropic cardiomyopathy, *Circulation* 106(19):2419-2421, 2002.

Martensson J et al: Living with heart failure: depression and quality of life in patients and spouses, *J Heart Lung Transplant* 22(4):460-467, 2003.

McBride L et al: Risk analysis in patients bridged to transplantation, *Ann Thorac Surg* 71:1839-1844, 2001.

McCloskey JC, Bulechek GB, editors: *Nursing Interventions Classification* (NIC), ed 3, St Louis, 2000, Mosby.

McKenna D et al: ALA Alloimmunization in patients requiring ventricular assist device support, *J Heart Lung Transplant* 21(11):1218-1224, 2002.

McNamara RL et al: Management of atrial fibrillation: review of the evidence for the role of pharmacologic therapy, electrical cardioversion and echocardiography, *Ann Intern Med* 139:1018-1033, 2003.

Meiser BM et al: Combination therapy with tacrolimus and mycophenolate mofetil following cardiac transplantation: importance of mycophenolic acid therapeutic drug monitoring, *J Heart Lung Transplant* 18(2):143-149, 1999.

Menon V, Fincke R: Cardiogenic shock: a summary of the randomized SHOCK Trial, *Congest Heart Failure* 9(1):35-39, 46, 2003.

Mirsa I, James S, Holt P: Biatrial pacing for paroxysmal atrial fibrillation: a randomized prospective study into the suppression of paroxysmal atrial fibrillation using biatrial pacing, *J Am Coll Cardiol* 40:457-463, 2002.

Moriguchi JD et al: *Pre-transplant panel reactive antibodies are associated with increased risk of transplant coronary artery disease in cardiac transplant recipients,* Presented at Thoracic Transplantation 1999: In the Next Millennium, Vail, Colo, March, 1999.

Mosca L et al: AHA Guidelines: evidence-based guidelines for cardiovascular disease prevention in women, *Circulation* 109:672-693, 2004.

Moustapha A, Anderson HV: Contemporary views of the acute coronary syndromes, *J Invasive Cardiol* 15(2):71-79, 2003.

Murphy MJ, Berding CB: Use of measurements of myoglobin and cardiac troponins in the diagnosis of acute myocardial infarction, *Crit Care Nurs* 19(1):58-66, 1999.

NASA-JSC: *Ventricular assist device,* Retrieved from World Wide Web, 2003: www.jsc.nasagov.

Piano MR et al: The molecular and cellular pathophysiology of heart failure, *Heart Lung* 27:3-19, 1998.

Pratt NG: Pathophysiology of heart failure: neuroendocrine response, *Crit Care Nurs Q* 18(1):22-31, 1995.

Saint Joseph's Hospital of Atlanta: *Policies, procedures, transplant programs and transplant classes,* 2002-03.

Salyer J et al: Lifestyle and quality of life in long term cardiac transplant recipients, *J Heart Lung Transplant* 22(3): 309-21, 2003.

Schwammenthal E et al: Dobutamine echocardiography in patients with aortic stenosis and left ventricular dysfunction: predicting outcome as a function of management strategy, *Chest* 119:1766-1777b, 2001.

Sgarbossa EB, Birnbaum Y, Parrillo JE: Electrographic diagnosis of acute myocardial infarction: current concepts for the clinician, *Am Heart J* 141(4):507-516, 2001.

Siomko, AJ: Demystifying cardiac markers, *Am J Nurs* 100(1):36-41, 2000.

Smith TW et al: Management of heart failure. In Braunwald E, editor: *Heart disease: a textbook of cardiovascular medicine,* ed 5, Philadelphia, 1997, Saunders.

Snow V et al: Management of newly detected atrial fibrillation: a clinical practice guideline from the American Academy of Family Physicians and the American College of Physicians, *Ann Intern Med* ##:1009-1017, 2003.

Society of Critical Care Medicine: Current concepts in dysrhythmia management. In SCCM: *1998 Educational and scientific symposium highlights,* Anaheim, Calif, 1998, Society of Critical Care Medicine.

Tahan HA: Patients waiting for heart transplantation: an analysis of vulnerability, *Crit Care Nurs* 18(24):40-48, 1998.

The Joint European Society of Cardiology/American College of Cardiology Committee: Myocardial infarction redefined—a consensus document of The Joint European Society of Cardiology/American College of Cardiology Committee for the Redefinition of Myocardial Infarction, *J Am Coll Cardiol* 36:959-969, 2000.

Thoratec Corporation: *Heartmate Vented Electric LVAS and Implantable Pneumatic LVAS,* Woburn, Mass, 2002.

United Network of Organ Sharing (UNOS): Policy 3.7, 2002. (*See actual policy for detailed criteria and rules.*)

Update on Adverse Events Following Civilian Smallpox Vaccination—United States, *MMWR* 52(21):492, 2003, website: www.cdc.gov/mmwr/PDF/wk/mm5221.pdf, April 21, 2003.

Wagar S et al: Nonsurgical reduction of the interventricular septum in patients with hypertrophic cardiomyopathy, *N Engl J Med* 347(17):1326-1333, 2002.

Wallace CJ: Dual-chamber pacemakers in the management of severe heart failure, *Crit Care Nurs* 18:57-67, 1998.

Zalenski R et al: Value of posterior and right ventricular leads in comparison to the standard 12-lead electrocardiogram in evaluation of ST segment elevation in suspected acute myocardial infarction, *Am J Cardiol* 79:1579-1585, 1997.

Zamora M: (1999) *Cytomegalovirus prophylaxis following thoracic transplantation: clinical outcomes and cost-efficacy,* Presented at Thoracic Transplantation 1999: In the Next Millennium, Vail, Colo, March, 1999.

CHAPTER 5

Renal-Urinary Dysfunctions

Acute Renal Failure

PATHOPHYSIOLOGY

Acute renal failure (ARF) is a syndrome characterized by an abrupt deterioration of renal function, resulting in the accumulation of metabolic wastes, fluids, and electrolytes, and usually accompanied by a marked decline in urinary output. ARF is one of few types of total organ failure that may be reversible with proper treatment. Formation of urine is a three-step process consisting of (1) ultrafiltration of delivered blood by the glomeruli (renal cortex), (2) internal processing of the ultrafiltrate via tubular secretion and reabsorption (renal parenchyma), and (3) excretion of waste products from the kidneys through the ureters, bladder, and urethra. Corresponding to those steps, ARF is categorized as prerenal, intrarenal, and postrenal (Table 5-1).

Prerenal failure or azotemia is the result of decreased blood flow to the kidneys. The events leading to prerenal insults cause decreased renal vascular perfusion and may be associated with systemic hypoperfusion. If treated promptly, this form of ARF is readily reversible. Chronic heart failure, drugs such as nonsteroidal antiinflammatory drugs (NSAIDs) and angiotensin-converting enzyme (ACE) inhibitors, volume loss, or sequestration and shock states (especially septic shock), may all lead to reduced renal perfusion. If not managed aggressively, parenchymal (intrarenal) involvement or acute tubular necrosis (ATN) can result. Intrarenal damage may result from a mean arterial pressure <75 mm Hg. Autoregulation fails; the sympathetic response increases and, with the action of the renin-angiotensin system, results in severe constriction of the afferent arteriole. Glomerular blood flow and hydrostatic pressure are reduced, and the glomerular filtration rate decreases. The amount of cellular damage depends on the duration of ischemia: mild damage (≤25 min), moderate/severe (40-60 min), and irreversible damage (may occur within 60-90 min).

The most common cause of ARF is ATN. ATN may be the result of nephrotoxic injury, a prolonged reduction in renal perfusion (ischemic injury), or pigmenturia (myoglobinuria and hemoglobinuria). Prolonged renal hypoperfusion due to shock, particularly septic shock, is a common cause of ATN. Renal ischemia may potentiate the injury produced by nephrotoxins. Toxic ATN, caused by nephrotoxic agents (aminoglycoside antibiotics, radiographic contrast agents), is an insult or injury to the tubular cell. Thrombotic occlusion, malignant hypertension, emboli, thrombotic thrombocytopenic purpura (TTP), hemolytic-uremic syndrome (HUS), and vasculitis can all result in ATN.

ATN is characterized by tubular cell necrosis, cast formation, and tubular obstruction caused by casts and cellular debris. Therapy is focused on maintenance of renal perfusion pressure, administering renal vasodilators to restore blood flow, and promoting diuresis to "wash out" the intratubular debris. Sometimes ATN is nonoliguric. Oliguria may occur with both toxic ATN and ischemic ATN. Common nephrotoxic agents are found in Table 5-2.

Postrenal failure is the least common cause of ARF and may be either intrarenal (within the kidney) or extrarenal (outside the kidney in another area of the elimination tract) obstruction. Intrarenal obstruction is often due to crystal deposition caused by medications (e.g., acyclovir, indinavir,

TABLE 5-1   Causes of Acute Renal Failure

Prerenal (decreased renal perfusion)	Intrarenal (parenchymal damage; acute tubular necrosis)	Postrenal (obstruction)
Hypovolemia	*Nephrotoxic Agents*	
• GI losses	• Antibiotics (aminoglycosides,	**Calculi**
• Hemorrhage	sulfonamides, methicillin)	**Tumor**
• Third-space (interstitial)	• Diuretics (e.g., furosemide)	**Benign prostatic**
losses (burns, peritonitis)	• Nonsteroidal antiinflammatory	**hypertrophy**
• Dehydration from diuretic	drugs (e.g., Ibuprofen)	**Necrotizing papillitis**
use	• Contrast media	**Urethral strictures**
Hepatorenal syndrome	• Heavy metals (e.g., lead, gold,	**Blood clots**
Edema-forming conditions	mercury)	**Retroperitoneal fibrosis**
• Right ventricular failure	Organic solvents (e.g., carbon	
• Cirrhosis	tetrachloride, ethylene glycol)	
• Nephrotic syndrome	**Infection (gram-negative**	
Renal vascular disorders	**sepsis), pancreatitis, peritonitis**	
• Renal artery stenosis	**transfusion reaction (hemolysis)**	
• Renal artery thrombosis	• **Rhabdomyolysis with myoglobinuria**	
• Renal vein thrombosis	**(severe muscle injury)**	
	• Trauma	
	• Exertion	
	• Seizures	
	• Drug-related: heroin, barbiturates,	
	IV amphetamines, succinylcholine	
	Glomerular diseases	
	• Poststreptococcal glomerulonephritis	
	• IgA nephropathy (e.g., Berger's	
	disease)	
	• Lupus glomerulonephritis	
	• Serum sickness	
	• **Ischemic injury**	

GI, Gastrointestinal; *IgA,* immunoglobulin A; *IV,* intravenous.

sulfonamides, methotrexate) or endogenous substances (oxalate, uric acid). Extrarenal obstruction may be related to bladder outlet problems (prostate and urethral obstruction) or stones, clots, pus, tumor, fibrosis, or ligation of papilla within the ureters.

Fluid, electrolyte, and acid-base disorders that occur with ARF include hypervolemia, hyperkalemia, hyperphosphatemia, hypocalcemia, hypermagnesemia, and metabolic acidosis (Table 5-3). Phosphate levels rise because of impaired excretion of phosphorus by the renal tubules with continued gastrointestinal (GI) absorption. Hypocalcemia results from the lack of active vitamin D, which would otherwise stimulate absorption of calcium from the GI tract, or high phosphate levels, which inhibit absorption of calcium. Hypocalcemia triggers the parathyroid glands to secrete parathyroid hormone (PTH), which mobilizes calcium from the bone into the blood. Hypermagnesemia is generally moderate (2-4 mg/dl) and is rarely symptomatic unless the patient receives magnesium-containing antacids (e.g., Maalox, Milk of Magnesia).

There are three identifiable stages/phases of ARF:

1. Oliguric phase: a drop in the 24-hr urinary output to ≤400 ml lasting approximately 7-14 days. About 30% of patients have nonoliguric renal failure.
2. Diuretic phase: a doubling of the urinary output from the previous 24-hr total. During this phase the patient may produce as much as 3-5 L of urine in 24 hr.
3. Recovery phase: a return to a normal 24-hr volume (1500-1800 ml). Usually, renal function continues to improve and may take 6 months-1 yr from the initial insult to return to baseline functional status.

T A B L E 5 - 2   Common Nephrotoxic Agents

Drugs	X-ray contrast media
Antineoplastics Methotrexate Cisplatin	*Biologic substances* Myoglobin Tumor products
Antibiotics Cephalosporines Aminoglycosides Tetracycline	*Chemicals* Ethylene glycol Pesticides Organic solvents
Nonsteroidal antiinflammatory drugs Ibuprofen Ketorolac	*Heavy metals* Lead Mercury Gold

T A B L E 5 - 3   Altered Electrolyte Balance in ARF

Condition/cause	Nursing implications

Hyperkalemia
Decreased ability to excrete K^+;
K^+ release with catabolism
	• Monitor ECG for tall and peaked T waves, loss of P waves, prolonged PR interval, widened QRS, and cardiac arrest (more likely seen with K^+ >6.5 mEq/L).
	• Monitor serum K^+ levels for values ≥5 mEq/L.
	• Monitor patient for such indicators as paresthesias, muscle weakness or flaccidity, and HR <60 beats/min.
	• Teach patient and significant others the indicators of hyperkalemia and the importance of notifying nurse promptly if they occur.
	• Provide a list of foods high in potassium (see Table 10-13), and stress the importance of avoiding these foods.
	• Implement the following to help minimize the cellular release of potassium:
	  ❏ Ensure that patient consumes only the amount of protein prescribed by physician; enforce sound infection control techniques to minimize risk of infection; and treat fevers promptly. Catabolism of protein, which occurs in these situations, causes potassium to be released from the tissues.
	  ❏ Ensure that patient consumes the allotted amounts of carbohydrates, and limit strenuous patient activity as prescribed, both of which will spare protein.
	• Be aware that hyperkalemia can be a fatal complication, especially during the oliguric phase of ARF, because of its adverse effect on cardiac status. Keep emergency supplies (i.e., manual resuscitator, crash cart, emergency drug tray) readily available.
	• For more information, see "Hyperkalemia," p. 552.

Continued

TABLE 5-3   Altered Electrolyte Balance in ARF—cont'd

Condition/cause	Nursing implications
Hypokalemia Prolonged, inadequate oral intake; use of potassium-losing diuretics without proper replacement; excessive loss from vomiting, diarrhea, or gastric or intestinal suctioning	• Monitor ECG for prolonged PR interval, flattened or inverted T wave, depressed ST segment, presence of U wave, and ventricular dysrhythmias; ECG changes are more likely to occur at serum K$^+$ levels <3 mEq/L. • Be alert to serum K$^+$ <3.5 mEq/L. • Monitor patient for muscle weakness, soft and flabby muscles, paresthesias, decreased bowel sounds, ileus, weak and irregular pulse, and distant heart sounds. Neuromuscular symptoms are seen at serum levels of approximately 2.5 mEq/L. • Teach patient and significant others the indicators of hypokalemia and the importance of notifying nurse promptly if they occur. • Provide a list of foods high in potassium (see Table 10-13), and assist with planning menus that incorporate them. • Administer potassium-sparing diuretics (e.g., spironolactone, triamterene) as prescribed. • Administer oral or IV potassium supplements as prescribed; for oral route, administer with at least 4 oz water or juice to minimize gastric irritation. • For more information, see "Hypokalemia," p. 549.
Hypernatremia Kidney's inability to excrete excess sodium; decreased water intake; increased water losses via osmotic diuresis; excessive parenteral administration of sodium-containing solutions (e.g., sodium bicarbonate, 3% sodium chloride)	• Monitor serum sodium levels for serum Na$^+$ >147 mEq/L. • Monitor VS and I&O hourly; weigh patient daily. • Be alert to dry mucous membranes, flushed skin, firm and rubbery tissue turgor, hyperthermia, oliguria, or anuria. • Assess sensorium for restlessness and agitation; institute seizure precautions as indicated. • Administer prescribed IV replacement fluids. • Administer diuretics as prescribed. • For more information, see "Hypernatremia," p. 547.
Hyponatremia Loss through vomiting, diarrhea, profuse diaphoresis; use of potent diuretics; salt-losing nephropathies; administration of large amount of sodium-free IV fluids (may be associated with fluid volume excess or postobstructive diuresis)	• Monitor for serum Na$^+$ <137 mEq/L. • Monitor I&O hourly; record weight daily for trend. • Assess patient for abdominal cramps, diarrhea, nausea, dizziness when changing position, postural hypotension, cold and clammy skin, and apprehension. • Provide parenteral replacement therapy as prescribed. • Institute a safe environment for individuals with altered LOC. • For more information, see "Hyponatremia," p. 545.
Hypocalcemia Poor absorption of dietary calcium; precipitation of calcium out of the tissues in the presence of elevated phosphorus level; inadequate absorption and utilization of calcium occurring with lack of conversion of vitamin D to its usable form	• Monitor for serum Ca^{++} <8.5 mg/dl. • Monitor for numbness and tingling around the mouth, muscle twitching, facial twitching, and tonic muscle spasms. Assess for Trousseau's sign (carpopedal spasm) and Chvostek's sign (spasm of lip and cheek). • Administer calcium and vitamin D supplements as prescribed. Reinforce the necessity of taking these medications as prescribed.

TABLE 5-3   Altered Electrolyte Balance in ARF—cont'd

Condition/cause	Nursing implications
Hypocalcemia—cont'd	• Teach patient and significant others the indicators of hypocalcemia. • Teach the importance of continued medical follow-up to check serum Ca^{++} levels. • For more information, see "Hypocalcemia," p. 554.
Hyperphosphatemia Abnormal retention of phosphates caused by the kidneys' inability to excrete excess phosphorus	• Monitor for serum phosphate >4.5 g/dl. • Although most foods contain generous amounts of phosphate, those especially high in phosphate include beef, pork, dried beans, dried mature peas, and dairy products (see Table 10-13). Monitor patient's diet accordingly. • Administer phosphate binders as prescribed. Assess for constipation, which may result from use of phosphate binders. • Teach patient and significant others the relationship between calcium and phosphate levels in the body. • Emphasize that maintaining good phosphate control and calcium balance may help control itching and prevent future problems with bone disease • Reinforce the need for follow-up visits to check serum phosphate levels. • For more information, see "Hyperphosphatemia," p. 560.
Hypermagnesemia Administration of magnesium-containing medications to patients with impaired renal function	• Monitor serum Mg^{++} levels >2.5 mEq/L. • Assess for diaphoresis, flushing, hypotension, drowsiness, weak-to-absent DTRs, bradycardia, lethargy, and respiratory impairment. • Teach the above indicators to patient and significant others. • Avoid giving medications that contain magnesium (see Table 10-16). Emphasize to patient that such medications should not be taken without physician's approval. • For more information, see "Hypermagnesemia," p. 565.
Metabolic acidosis Kidneys' inability to excrete excess acid produced by normal metabolic processes; marked tissue trauma, infection, and diarrhea may contribute to a more rapid development of acidosis (often associated with K^+ >5 mEq/L)	• Monitor for HCO_3^- <22 mEq/L and pH <7.35. • Monitor I&O, LOC, and VS. Be alert to Kussmaul respirations, SOB, anorexia, headache, nausea, vomiting, weakness, apathy, fatigue, and coma. • Institute seizure precautions in the presence of altered LOC. • Administer IV fluids and bicarbonate as prescribed. • Teach patient the importance of dietary restrictions, particularly of protein, and of maintaining adequate carbohydrate intake to prevent worsening acidosis. • Stress that patient should report to physician increased temperature and other signs of infection. • Teach patient the importance of taking sodium bicarbonate as prescribed and of maintaining dialysis schedule (both hemodialysis and peritoneal dialysis help correct acidosis). • For more information, see "Chronic Metabolic Acidosis," p. 578.

Continued

T A B L E 5 - 3 Altered Electrolyte Balance in ARF—cont'd	
Condition/cause	**Nursing implications**

Uremia

Failure of the kidneys to excrete urea, creatinine, uric acid, and other metabolic waste products

- Monitor patient for chronic fatigue, insomnia, anorexia, vomiting, metallic taste in the mouth, pruritus, increased bleeding tendency, muscular twitching, involuntary leg movements, decreasing attention span, anemia, muscle wasting, and weakness.
- Teach patient and significant others that the indicators of uremia develop gradually and are very subtle. Explain the importance of notifying nurse of sudden worsening of the symptoms that may be present.
- Monitor and record dietary intake of protein, potassium, and sodium.
- Use lotions and oils to lubricate patient's skin and relieve drying and cracking.
- Provide oral hygiene at frequent intervals, using a soft-bristle toothbrush and mouthwash, to help combat patient's thirst and the metallic taste caused by uremia. Chewing gum and hard candy also may help alleviate thirst and the unpleasant taste.
- Encourage isometric exercises and short walks, if patient is able, to help maintain patient's muscle strength and tone, especially in the legs.
- Teach significant others that because of patient's decreasing concentration level, they should communicate with patient by using simple and direct statements.
- Teach patient to maintain good nutrition by ingesting the allotted amounts of carbohydrates and high–biologic value protein to support cell rebuilding and decrease waste products from protein breakdown.
- Explain that profuse bleeding can occur with uremia and that knives, scissors, and other sharp instruments should be used with caution.
- Stress that OTC medications such as aspirin and ibuprofen may enhance bleeding tendency.
- Emphasize the importance of follow-up visits to evaluate the progression of uremia.
- Stress the dialysis schedule should be maintained to decrease the symptoms of uremia and correct many of the metabolic abnormalities that occur.

ARF, Acute renal failure; *Ca++,* calcium; *DTR,* deep tendon reflex; *ECG,* electrocardiogram; *HCO_3^-,* bicarbonate; *HR,* heart rate; *I&O,* intake and output; *IV,* intravenous; *K+,* potassium; *LOC,* level of consciousness; *Mg++,* magnesium; *Na+,* sodium; *OTC,* over-the-counter; *SOB,* shortness of breath; *VS,* vital signs.

ASSESSMENT

ARF can dramatically affect fluid, electrolyte, and acid-base balances and may lead to metabolic encephalopathy.

History and risk factors: Chronic illness (e.g., hypertension, diabetes, cardiomyopathy, peripheral vascular disease), recent infections or sepsis (e.g., streptococcal), recent episodes of hypotension (e.g., major bleeding, septic shock, major surgery), exposure to nephrotoxins (e.g., carbon tetrachloride, diuretics, aminoglycoside antibiotics, contrast media), recent blood transfusion, urinary tract disorders, toxemia of pregnancy or abortion, recent severe muscle damage (e.g., rhabdomyolysis with myoglobinuria), crush injury, burn trauma.

T A B L E 5 - 4   Diuretic Use in Acute Renal Failure

Types	Mechanisms of action	Potential fluid and electrolyte abnormalities
Osmotic diuretics		
Mannitol Urea	Increase osmotic pressure of the filtrate, which attracts water and electrolytes and prevents their reabsorption	Hyponatremia Hypokalemia Rebound volume expansion
Loop diuretics		
Furosemide Ethacrynic acid Bumetanide Torsemide	Inhibit reabsorption of Na^+ and Cl^- at the ascending loop of Henle in the medulla; they produce a vasodilatory effect on the renal vasculature	Hypokalemia Hyperuricemia Hypocalcemia Hyperglycemia and impairment of glucose tolerance Dilutional hyponatremia Hypochloremic acidosis
Thiazides		
Bendroflumethiazide Benzthiazide Chlorothiazide sodium Hydrochlorothiazide Hydroflumethiazide Polythiazide Trichlormethiazide	Inhibit Na^+ in the ascending loop of Henle at the beginning of the distal loop	Hypokalemia Dilutional hyponatremia Hypercalcemia Metabolic alkalosis Hypochloremia Hyperuricemia Hyperglycemia and impaired glucose tolerance
Thiazide-like diuretics		
Chlorthalidone Indapamide Metolazone Quinethazone	Action same as thiazides	Same as thiazides
Potassium-sparing diuretics*		
Amiloride HCl Spironolactone Triamterene	Inhibit aldosterone effect on the distal tubule, causing Na^+ excretion and K^+ reabsorption	Hyperkalemia Hyponatremia Dehydration Acidosis Transient increase in BUN
Carbonic anhydrase-inhibitors		
Acetazolamide sodium Dichlorphenamide Methazolamide	Block the action of the enzyme carbonic anhydrase, producing excretion of Na^+, K^+, HCO_3^-, and water	Hyperchloremic acidosis Hypokalemia Hyperuricemia

Note: Loop or osmotic diuretics (or a combination of both) are used in patients with acute renal failure to prevent hypervolemia and to stimulate urinary output.
*Used with caution in patients with oliguria.
BUN, Blood urea nitrogen; *Cl⁻*, chloride; *HCO_3^-*, bicarbonate; *K⁺*, potassium; *NA⁺*, sodium.

T A B L E 5 - 5   Drugs that Require Dosage Modification in Renal Failure

Antimicrobials	Cardiovascular agents	Analgesics	Sedatives	Miscellaneous
Amikacin	ACE inhibitors	Meperidine	Meprobamate	Cimetidine
Amphotericin B	Digitoxin	Methadone	Phenobarbital	Clofibrate
Chloramphenicol	Digoxin			Glycoprotein IIB, IIIA
Ethambutol	Guanethidine			inhibitors
Gentamicin	Procainamide			Insulin
Kanamycin				Neostigmine
Lincomycin				NSAIDs
Penicillins				Platelet inhibitors
Promethazine				Promethazine
Sulfonamides				
Tobramycin				
Vancomycin				

NSAIDs, Nonsteroidal antiinflammatory drugs.

T A B L E 5 - 6   Drugs to Avoid in Renal Failure

Amiloride
Aspirin
Cisplatin
Lithium carbonate
Magnesium-containing medications (see Table 10-16)
Nitrofurantoin
Nonsteroidal antiinflammatory drugs (e.g., ibuprofen)
Phenylbutazone
Spironolactone
Tetracycline

Clinical presentation
Prerenal: Likely oliguric but may be nonoliguric, urinary sodium (Na^+) <20 mEq/L, elevated specific gravity, increased urine osmolality, normal or mildly abnormal sediment with presence of hyaline and granular casts, elevated plasma blood urea nitrogen (BUN)/creatinine ratio (>20:1).
Intrarenal: Likely oliguric but may be nonoliguric, urinary Na^+ >20 mEq/L, low specific gravity, decreased urinary osmolality, markedly abnormal sediment containing red blood cell (RBC) casts and cellular debris in urine, decreased plasma BUN/creatinine ratio (10:1). The most common cause of ARF.
Postrenal:
Urinary chemical indices are ineffective in determining postrenal failure. Likely oliguric but may be nonoliguric, normal or mildly abnormal sediment (hematuria, pyuria, and crystals). Often associated with urinary tract or pelvic cancer or renal/ureteral calculi. The least common cause of ARF.
Fluid volume alterations
Excess: Peripheral edema, jugular vein distention, S_3 and S_4 gallops, crackles, increased BP, oliguria.
Deficit: Decreased blood pressure (BP), poor skin turgor, flushed skin, dry mucous membranes, oliguria.
Electrolyte imbalances: Dysrhythmias, altered mental status, GI disturbances, neuromuscular dysfunction.
Metabolic acidosis: Weakness, disorientation, shortness of breath (SOB), Kussmaul respirations, central nervous system (CNS) depression.
Uremic manifestations: Accumulation of urea, creatinine, uric acid; anemia and bleeding tendencies; fatigue and pallor; increased BP, congestive heart failure, pericarditis with tamponade, pul-

monary edema; anorexia, nausea, vomiting, diarrhea; behavioral changes; decreased wound-healing ability; increased susceptibility to infection.

Physical assessment

Cardiovascular: S$_3$ and S$_4$ gallops, pericardial friction rub, jugular vein distention, tachycardia, dysrhythmias, increased BP, pulsus paradoxus in the presence of fluid volume excess, edema (peripheral, periorbital, sacral), capillary fragility, purpura.

Respiratory: Crackles, hyperventilation.

Neuromuscular: Weakness, lethargy, muscle irritability, muscle tenderness, asterixis.

Cutaneous: Pallor; presence of uremic frost in persons with severe uremia.

DIAGNOSTIC TESTS

Serum blood urea nitrogen (BUN), creatinine, uric acid, and electrolyte levels: Creatinine is the most reliable indicator of renal function but can also be markedly elevated in the presence of massive skeletal muscle injury (e.g., multiple trauma, crush injuries). BUN is influenced by hydration, catabolism, GI bleeding, infection, fever, and corticosteroid therapy. BUN, creatinine, and uric acid levels will be elevated in the presence of ARF, as will potassium, phosphorus, and possibly magnesium.

Creatinine clearance test: For clinical purposes this is the most reliable estimation of glomerular filtration rate. Accuracy depends on complete collection. Creatinine clearance decreases with age. Normal creatinine clearance is 95-125 ml/min. In the presence of ARF it usually is <50 ml/min.

Urinalysis: The presence of sediment-containing tubular epithelial cells, cellular debris, and tubular casts supports a diagnosis of ARF. Large amounts of protein and many RBC casts are common in ARF when it is secondary to parenchymal (intrarenal) disease. Sediment is normal when the causes are categorized as prerenal. Large amounts of myoglobin may be present in the setting of rhabdomyolysis or severe skeletal muscle injury.

Urinary sodium: A prerenal cause is signaled by a sodium count <10 mEq/L.

CBC and coagulation studies (PT, PTT): Complete blood cell count (CBC), prothrombin time (PT), and partial thromboplastin time (PTT) to evaluate for hematologic complications. Baseline hematocrit (Hct) may be low as a result of ARF, and Hct and hemoglobin (Hgb) will fall steadily if the patient has bleeding or hemodilution from fluid overload.

ABG values: Low Paco$_2$ and plasma pH values reflect the metabolic acidosis associated with ARF.

Ultrasonography: Identifies hydronephrosis, fluid collection, and masses.

Intravenous pyelograms (IVP), both retrograde and antegrade: To diagnose partial or complete obstruction.

Renal scan: Provides information about renal perfusion.

Renal angiography and venography: Assess for the presence or absence of thrombotic or stenotic lesions in the main renal vessels.

Renal biopsy: If the cause of renal failure cannot be determined, percutaneous renal biopsy should be considered. Exact indicators for performing renal biopsy have not been established. Can reveal the presence of acute glomerulonephritis, vasculitis or interstitial nephritis, which may respond to corticosteroid or other immunosuppressive therapy.

COLLABORATIVE MANAGEMENT

Prerenal and intrarenal acute renal failure

Volume replacement: Replacement solutions include free water plus electrol͙͙͙t through the urine, wounds, drainage tubes, diarrhea, and vomiting. Usually losses are repl͙͙ a volume-for-volume basis. Maintenance fluids total approximately 1500 ml/24 hr. With a m͙͙ate fluid deficit (5% weight loss), at least 2400 ml is given over a 24-hr period. A severe deficit͙ 5% weight loss) requires a replacement of at least 3000 ml/24h.

Forced alkaline diuresis: Use of mannitol or sodium bicarbonate solution to manage pigmenturia (myoglobinuria, hemoglobinuria) due to rhabdomyolysis or severe crush or skeletal muscle injury, along with aggressive volume replacement to help maintain renal perfusion pressure an͙ reduce cast formation leading to renal tubular obstruction.

Diuretics (furosemide [Lasix], bumetanide [Bumex], torsemide [Demadex], and ethacrynic acid [Edecrin]): Decrease filtrate reabsorption and enhance water excretion. They may be used, only after adequate hydration, to increase urine output or in an attempt to prevent onset of oliguria. If volume overload is present, diuretics are used to prevent pulmonary edema. In hypovolemic patients, if used without adequate hydration, they can be harmful. Osmotic diuretics, such as mannitol, may be used to increase intravascular volume, promote renal blood flow, increase glomerular filtration rate, and stimulate urinary output. See Table 5-4 for additional information on diuretics.

Dopamine: Controversial treatment wherein low doses, usually ≤2 mcg/kg/min, are used to stimulate dopaminergic receptors, encourage renal vasodilation, and promote renal blood flow. A growing number of studies have shown that this approach is ineffective and should be discontinued if the patient remains oliguric. Slightly higher doses (e.g., 3-10 mcg/kg/min) are used to stimulate beta1– (β_1-) receptors, resulting in improved BP and cardiac output. Urine output increases as a result of improved renal perfusion. Doses >10 mcg/kg/min lack renal vasodilatory effects and may cause damaging renal vasoconstriction.

Nesiritide: Synthetic BNP (brain natriuretic peptide) which results in vasodilation, natriuresis, diuresis, and decreased renin angiotensin activity, resulting in lower pulmonary capillary wedge pressure (PCWP), decreased systemic vascular resistance (SVR) and increased cardiac output/cardiac index (CO/CI.) Used to manage heart failure associated with prerenal azotemia. Increased cardiac output augments renal perfusion and may provide adjunctive therapy for ARF.

Management of hyperkalemia: Intravenous calcium gluconate 10% (immediate onset), infusion of glucose-insulin-bicarbonate (20-60 minute onset), inhaled albuterol (30-60 minute onset), sodium polystyrene sulphonate (i.e., Kayexelate) with sorbitol enema (1-4 hour onset), and hemodialysis (1-3 hour onset) may be used for control of elevated potassium. Higher levels of potassium require treatment with the quickest onset.

Removal or discontinuation of toxic agent: Agents such as aminoglycoside antibiotics, angiotension-converting enzyme (ACE) inhibitors used for blood pressure control and heart failure prevention, nonsteroidal antiinflammatory drugs (NSAIDs) used for pain management, must be discontinued or removed.

Prevention of contrast-induced nephropathy: Hydration, intravenous (IV) Corlopam, or oral or inhaled Mucomyst may be used before sending borderline or patients with renal insufficiency for radiologic procedures requiring contrast media. Specific protocols have been developed for each therapy. Aggressive hydration and possibly IV mannitol after the procedure may also assist in clearing contrast from the patient.

Dialytic (renal replacement) therapy: Maintains homeostasis (see discussion, p. 334).

Nutrition therapy: Involves a diet high in carbohydrates and with catabolic patients, essential and nonessential amino acids to prevent endogenous protein catabolism and muscle breakdown; low in sodium for individuals who retain sodium and water; high in sodium for those who have lost large volumes of sodium and water as a result of diuresis or other body drainage; low in potassium if the patient is retaining potassium; and if not catabolic, low in protein to maintain daily requirements while minimizing increases in azotemia. Nutrition is delivered via oral, enteral, or total parenteral nutrition (TPN). (See Table 10-12 for a list of foods high in sodium and Table 10-13 for a list of foods high in potassium.)

Hematologic problems and blood transfusions: Packed RBCs are given if indicated to maintain a stable Hct. There are two major hematologic complications of renal failure:

Anemia: Caused by decreased erythropoietin, low-grade GI bleeding from mucosal ulceration, blood drawing, and shortened life of the RBCs. Erythropoietin (Epogen) is used for primary prevention and treatment of anemia.

Prolonged bleeding time: Caused by decreased platelet adhesiveness. As renal failure progresses, anemia becomes more profound and platelet adhesiveness decreases further.

Pharmacotherapy

Antihypertensives: See Table 4-23.

Phosphaders (aluminum hydroxide antacids, calcium carbonate antacids, and calcium acetate) sphorus and control hyperphosphatemia and hypermagnesemia. They are given with m

Sodium: Controls metabolic acidosis and promotes shift of potassium back into the cells.

Water-sin supplements: For patients receiving dialytic therapy. Water-soluble vitamins are diffused s the membrane and are removed during dialysis.

Recombinant erythropoietin (Epogen, Procrit): Intravenous/subcutaneous (IV/SC) preparation given 3×/wk after dialysis in doses of 50-500 U/kg to correct anemia of chronic renal failure. Maintenance doses are given 3×/wk to maintain Hct levels of 33%-38%. Adverse reactions include development or worsening of hypertension, clotting of vascular access, depletion of iron stores, and slight increases in predialysis levels of BUN, creatinine, and potassium in individuals with Hct <30%.

Note: See Table 5-5 for a list of common medications that require dosage modification for patients with ARF. Drugs that require dosage modification in renal failure are those that are excreted primarily by the kidneys. Dosage must be governed by clinical responses, as well as serum levels, if available. Nephrotoxic drugs should be avoided (Table 5-6). Also avoid drugs that are toxic to other organs if they accumulate, those that aggravate uremic symptoms, and those that contribute to metabolic derangements of renal failure.

Postrenal acute renal failure

Relief of obstruction: Achieved via catheterization with indwelling urinary catheter, nephrostomy tube, or ureteral stent to relieve obstruction before surgical intervention; lithotripsy to disintegrate stones; or prostatectomy if benign prostatic hypertrophy is the cause of the obstruction.

Monitoring of fluid and electrolyte balance: Postobstructive diuresis may result in hypovolemia (see p. 539), hyponatremia (see p. 545), hypokalemia (see p. 549), hypocalcemia (see p. 554), and hypomagnesemia (see p. 562). See Table 5-3 for factors leading to altered electrolyte balance in ARF.

Culturing of urine and administration of antibiotics: If indicated.

NURSING DIAGNOSES AND INTERVENTIONS

Fluid volume excess related to compromised regulatory mechanism secondary to acute renal failure
Desired outcome: Within 24-48 hr of onset, patient becomes normovolemic as evidenced by balanced intake and output (I&O); urinary output ≥0.5 ml/kg/hr; body weight within patient's normal range; BP within patient's normal range; central venous pressure (CVP) 2-6 mm Hg; heart rate (HR) 60-100 beats/min; and absence of edema, crackles, gallop, and other clinical indicators of fluid overload.

> **Note:** Although patient is retaining sodium, his or her serum sodium level may be within normal limits or decreased from baseline because of the dilutional effect of the fluid overload.

- Document I&O hourly. Consult physician if urinary output falls to <0.5 ml/kg/hr.
- Weigh patient daily; consult physician regarding significant weight gain (e.g., 0.5-1.5 kg/24 hr).
- Assess for and document the presence of basilar crackles, jugular vein distention, tachycardia, pericardial friction rub, gallop, increased BP, increased CVP, or SOB, any of which are indicative of fluid volume overload. Chronic heart failure may require additional support measures to help resolve ARF.
- Assess for and document the presence of peripheral, sacral, or periorbital edema.
- Restrict patient's total fluid intake to 1200-1500 ml/24 hr or as prescribed. Measure all output accurately, and replace milliliter for milliliter at intervals of 4-8 hr or as prescribed.
- Provide ice chips, chewing gum, or hard candy to help patient quench thirst and moisten mouth.
- Monitor serum osmolality and serum sodium values. These values may be decreased because of the dilutional effect of fluid overload.
- Recognize that if it is delivered, TPN will provide the largest volume of fluid intake for the patient. If total fluid intake is >2000 ml/day, ultrafiltration (UF) with dialysis (see p. 335) or continuous renal replacement therapy (CRRT): (continuous venovenous hemofiltration [CVVH], continuous venovenous hemodialysis [CVVHD], continuous venovenous hemodiafiltration [CVVHDF], slow continuous ultrafiltration [SCUF], or continuous arteriovenous hemofiltration [CAVH]) may be necessary to maintain fluid and electrolyte balance (see p. 338).
- If patient is retaining sodium, restrict sodium-containing foods (see Table 10-12, p. 544) and avoid diluting IV medications with high-sodium diluents. Also avoid sodium-containing medications such as sodium penicillin.

You may also wish to refer to the following interventions from the Nursing Interventions Classification (NIC):

◀ NIC   Electrolyte Management: Hypokalemia; Electrolyte Management: Hyponatremia; Fluid/Electrolyte Management; Fluid Management; Fluid Monitoring. Additional, optional interventions include Dysrhythmia Management; Hemodialysis Therapy; Hemodynamic Regulation; Invasive Hemodynamic Monitoring; Medication Management; Positioning; Skin Surveillance; and Weight Management.

Fluid volume deficit related to active loss secondary to diuresis, vomiting, diarrhea, and hemorrhage; failure of regulatory mechanism with fluid shift to interstitial compartments
Desired outcomes: Within 24 hr of this diagnosis, patient becomes normovolemic as evidenced by balanced I&O; urinary output ≥0.5 ml/kg/hr; CVP 2-6 mm Hg; HR 60-100 beats/min; BP within patient's normal range; and absence of thirst and other indicators of hypovolemia. Patient's weight stabilizes within 2-3 days.

- Weigh patient daily. Consult physician for weight loss of 1-1.5 kg/24 hr.
- Monitor and document I&O hourly. Consult physician if patient's output is <0.5 ml/kg/hr. With deficit, intake should exceed output by 0.5-1 L (depending on severity of dehydration) q24h.

- Consult physician for increase in losses from vomiting, diarrhea, or wound drainage or sudden onset of diuresis.
- Observe for and document indicators of dehydration and hypovolemia (e.g., poor skin turgor, dry and sticky mucous membranes, thirst, hypotension, tachycardia, decreasing CVP, increasing BUN and creatinine).
- Encourage oral fluids if they are allowed. Ensure that IV fluid rates are maintained as prescribed.
- Approximately 20% of patients with ARF have GI bleeding. Monitor Hgb, Hct, and BUN levels. In the presence of bleeding with ARF, Hgb and Hct values will fall steadily (rapidly if there is massive bleeding).

> **Note:**   A patient with ARF may have an Hct in the range of 20%-30% if prerenal azotemia has occurred over time. Anemia occurs as a result of prolonged renal insufficiency leading to failure. BUN will increase in the presence of GI bleeding without a concomitant rise in serum creatinine level.

- Test all stools, emesis, and peritoneal dialysate drainage for occult blood. Check urine and dialysate drainage at least q8h.
- To minimize the risk of bleeding, keep side rails up, minimize invasive procedures, use small-gauge needles for injections, minimize blood drawing, and promote the use of electric razors and soft-bristle toothbrushes. If possible, avoid intramuscular (IM) or SC injections for 1 hr after hemodialysis. Apply gentle pressure to injection sites for at least 2-3 min.
- Inspect gums, mouth, nose, skin, and perianal and vaginal areas q8h for bleeding. Also inspect hemodialysis insertion and peritoneal access sites for evidence of bleeding q8h. Apply a soft, occlusive, sterile dressing to access sites to protect skin from irritation and bleeding caused by catheter movement.

Altered nutrition: less than body requirements, related to catabolic state and excessive metabolic needs secondary to ARF; anorexia and psychologic aversion to dietary restrictions

Desired outcomes: Within 72 hr of this diagnosis, patient has adequate nutritional intake as evidenced by a caloric intake that ranges from 35-45 calories (cal)/kg normal body weight; a daily protein intake that consists of 50%-75% of high–biologic value proteins; and a nitrogen intake of 4-6 g more than nitrogen loss (calculated from 24-hr urinary urea excretion and protein intake).

- Infuse enteral feedings and TPN as prescribed.
- Assess and document patient's intake of nutrients every shift.
- Weigh patient daily. Consult physician for significant findings (e.g., loss of >1.5 kg/24 h).
- Control nausea and anorexia using small, frequent meals. Present appetizing food in a pleasant atmosphere; eliminate any noxious odors. As indicated, administer medication with prescribed antiemetic ½ hr before meals.
- Control catabolism:
    - ❏ As prescribed, use cooling blanket or antipyretic agents to control fever. Fever increases tissue catabolism, which in turn increases metabolic needs. Critically ill patients are often catabolic and require, careful nutritional management, especially when either hemodialysis, peritoneal dialysis, or CRRT is implemented. Supplementation with 10-20gm/day essential and nonessential amino acids may be needed. The end products of protein metabolism that accumulate in renal failure are reflected by an increase in BUN level. Ensure intake of protein with high biologic value (e.g., eggs, meat, fowl, milk, fish), which contains essential amino acids necessary for cell building.
    - ❏ Provide adequate calories: Be sure that caloric intake ranges from 30-60 cal/kg normal body weight for a critically ill adult in ARF. The exact amount will vary with age, gender, activity, and the degree of preexisting malnutrition. Foods that may be used to increase caloric intake include fats and concentrated carbohydrates.
- Manage electrolytes:
    - ❏ Restrict high-potassium foods such as bananas, citrus fruits, fruit juices, nuts, tea, coffee, legumes, and salt substitute. In ARF the kidneys are unable to excrete potassium effectively.
    - ❏ Assess sodium requirement, since it will vary greatly. If oliguria is present, sodium intake may be restricted in the diet. If diuresis is present, sodium intake may be increased because of excess sodium loss in the urine. Intervene accordingly.
    - ❏ Treat hypocalcemia if present early in ARF as a result of decreased absorption of calcium from the gut and the presence of hyperphosphatemia. Replace calcium orally (e.g., with dairy products) or intravenously and administer phosphate binders as prescribed.

NIC Nutrition Management; Nutritional Monitoring; Fluid Management; Fluid Monitoring. Additional, optional NIC interventions include: Bowel Management; Energy Management; Enteral Tube Feeding; Exercise Promotion; Gastrointestinal Intubation; Hyperglycemia Management; Hypoglycemia Management; Intravenous Insertion; Intravenous Therapy; Medication Management; Mutual Goal Setting; Phlebotomy: Venous Blood Sample; Positioning; Teaching: Individual; Teaching: Prescribed Diet; Total Parenteral Nutrition Administration; and Venous Access Devices Maintenance.

Risk for infection related to inadequate secondary defenses as a result of immunocompromised state associated with ARF; multiple invasive procedures

Desired outcomes: At the time of discharge from intensive care unit (ICU), patient is free of infection as evidenced by normothermia; negative culture results of dialysate and body secretions; and white blood cell (WBC) count ≤11,000/mm^3. NOTE: After the initial insult, infection is the primary cause of death in ARF.

- Monitor and record patient's temperature q8h. If it is elevated (i.e., >37° C [98.6° F]), monitor temperature q4h. Because ARF may be accompanied by hypothermia, even a slight rise in temperature of 1°-2° may be significant.
- Inspect and record the color, odor, and appearance of all body secretions. Be alert to cloudy or blood-tinged peritoneal dialysate return, cloudy and foul-smelling urine, foul-smelling wound exudate, purulent drainage from any catheter site, foul-smelling and watery stools, foul-smelling vaginal discharge, or purulent sputum.
- Be aware that uremia retards wound healing; therefore, it is important that all wounds (including scratches resulting from pruritus) be assessed for indicators of infection. Send sample of any suspicious fluid or drainage for culture and sensitivity (C&S) tests as indicated.
- Monitor WBC count for elevations, and obtain specimens for C&S as prescribed.
- Use aseptic technique when manipulating central lines, peripheral IV lines, and indwelling catheters. Avoid use of indwelling urinary catheter in patients with oliguria and anuria. The presence of a catheter in these patients further increases the risk of infection.
- Be aware that catabolism of protein, which occurs with infection, causes potassium to be released from the tissues.
- Provide oral hygiene q2h to help maintain the integrity of the oral mucous membranes.
- Reposition patient q2-4h to help maintain the barrier of an intact integumentary system. Provide skin care at least q8h.
- Encourage good pulmonary hygiene by having patient practice deep-breathing exercises (and coughing, if indicated) q2-4h.

NIC Infection Control; Infection Protection. Additional, optional interventions include Airway Management; Exercise Promotion and Therapy (all listed); Medication Management; Respiratory Monitoring; Teaching: Disease Process; Tube Care: Urinary; and Vital Signs Monitoring.

Knowledge deficit: biochemical alterations associated with ARF

Desired outcome: Within 72 hr of admission, patient and significant others verbalize accurate information regarding patient's disease state and the measures that can be taken to prevent its occurrence or minimize its effects.

- Determine patient's and significant others' knowledge about patient's disease process and the biochemical alterations (hyperkalemia, hypokalemia, hypernatremia, hyponatremia, hypocalcemia, hyperphosphatemia, hypermagnesemia, metabolic acidosis, and uremia) that can occur.
- Teach patient and significant others the signs and symptoms of the biochemical alterations (see Table 5-3 and "Altered Protection," p. 328).
- Provide lists of foods high in potassium (see Table 10-13), sodium (see Table 10-12), phosphorus (see Table 10-14), and magnesium (see Table 10-15), which patient should add or avoid when planning meals. In addition, provide a list of medications that contain magnesium (see Table 10-16), which should not be taken without physician approval.
- Explain the importance of consuming only the amount of protein prescribed by physician and avoiding exposure to persons with infection or a febrile illness to minimize catabolism of protein, which causes potassium to be released from the tissues. Reinforce that patient should consume the prescribed diet, and limit strenuous activity as prescribed, both of which will spare protein and thus minimize potassium release.
- Teach patient to report to physician an increase in temperature or other signs of infection.
- Reinforce the importance of taking vitamin D and calcium supplements as prescribed.
- Teach the relationship between calcium and phosphate levels. Emphasize that maintaining good phosphate control and calcium balance may help control itching and prevent future problems with bone disease.
- Stress the importance of taking phosphate binders (e.g., Amphojel, Alternagel, PhosLo) as prescribed and to avoid antacids containing magnesium (e.g., Maalox, Milk of Magnesia).

- Teach patient not to take over-the-counter (OTC) medications without first consulting physician. Aspirin, for example, exacerbates the bleeding tendency caused by uremia.
- Instruct patient about the importance of maintaining the prescribed dialysis schedule, inasmuch as dialysis will help correct acidosis, uremia, and many of the metabolic abnormalities that occur.
- Teach patient to use lotions and oils to lubricate skin and relieve drying and cracking.
- Stress the importance of follow-up monitoring of serum electrolyte levels.

NIC Teaching: Disease Process; Teaching: Individual; Teaching: Prescribed Medication. Additional, optional interventions include Discharge Planning; Medication Management; and Weight Management.

Altered protection related to neurosensory changes secondary to electrolyte imbalance, metabolic acidosis, and uremia

Desired outcomes: Within 48-72 hr of onset, patient verbalizes orientation to time, place, and person and maintains his or her normal mobility.

- Monitor patient for the following mentation and motor dysfunctions associated with ARF:
  - ❑ Hyperkalemia (during oliguric phase): muscle weakness, irritability, paresthesias.
  - ❑ Hypokalemia (during diuretic phase): lethargy; muscle weakness, softness, flabbiness; paresthesias.
  - ❑ Hypernatremia: fatigue, restlessness, agitation.
  - ❑ Hyponatremia: dizziness when changing position, apprehension, personality changes, agitation, confusion.
  - ❑ Hypocalcemia: neuromuscular irritability, tonic muscle spasms, paresthesias.
  - ❑ Hyperphosphatemia: excessive itching, muscle weakness, hyperreflexia.
  - ❑ Hypermagnesemia: drowsiness, lethargy, sensation of heat.
  - ❑ Metabolic acidosis: confusion, weakness.
  - ❑ Uremia: confusion, lethargy, itching, metallic taste, muscle twitching.
- Explain to significant others that patient's decreasing attention level necessitates simple and direct communication efforts.
- To alleviate unpleasant metallic taste caused by uremia, provide frequent oral hygiene. Because patient with uremia is at increased risk for bleeding, ensure use of soft-bristle brushes. If appropriate, provide chewing gum or hard candy, which may help alleviate the unpleasant metallic taste.
- Encourage isometric exercises and short walks, if patient is able, to help maintain muscle strength and tone, especially in the legs.
- Decrease environmental stimuli, and use a calm, reassuring manner in caring for patient.
- Encourage establishment of sleep/rest patterns by scheduling daytime activities appropriately and promoting relaxation method (see "Health-Seeking Behavior," p. 259).
- Assess for decreased tactile sensations in the feet and legs, which may occur with peripheral neuropathy. Be alert to the potential for pressure sores and friction burns, which may occur with peripheral neuropathy.
- Use splints and braces to aid in mobility for patients with severe neuropathic effects.

NIC Infection Control; Infection Protection. Additional, optional interventions include Nutrition Management; Nutrition Therapy; Nutritional Counseling; Pressure Management; Pressure Ulcer Prevention; and Teaching: Individual.

Constipation related to immobility; restrictions of fresh fruit and fluids; use of phosphate binders

Desired outcome: Within 48 hr of onset, patient has bowel movements of soft consistency.

- Monitor and record the number and quality of patient's bowel movements.
- Administer prescribed stool softeners and bulking agents, such as psyllium husks.
- If these measures fail, administer oil retention or tap water enemas as prescribed. Because excess fluid can be absorbed from the gut, avoid using large-volume water enemas.
- Encourage moderate exercise on a routine basis.
- Establish a regular schedule for fluid intake within patient's prescribed limits.
- Administer metoclopramide as prescribed to increase motility in the presence of autonomic neuropathy.

NIC Constipation/Impaction Management. Additional optional interventions include Exercise Promotion; Medication Administration: Oral; Medication Management; Pain Management; and Skin Surveillance.

Impaired skin integrity (or risk for same) related to uremia with resulting pruritus and edema

Desired outcome: Patient's skin remains intact.

- Monitor patient for presence of pruritus with resulting frequent and intense scratching. Pruritus decreases with reduced BUN level and control of hyperphosphatemia. Monitor laboratory values of BUN and phosphorus, and report levels outside the optimal range (BUN >20 mg/dl and phosphorus >4.5 mg/dl or 2.6 mEq/L). Pruritus increases in the presence of secondary hyperparathyroidism.

Monitor serum calcium and PTH levels, and report elevations (Ca^{++} >10.5 mg/dl and PTH >30% above the upper limit of the test used).

- Administer phosphate binders (e.g., Alternagel) as prescribed, and if possible reduce patient's dietary intake of phosphorus (see Table 10-14).
- Ensure that patient's fingernails are cut short and that the nail tips are smooth.
- Because uremia retards wound healing, monitor scratches for indicators of infection.
- Because of reduced oil gland activity associated with uremia, the patient's skin may be quite dry. Use skin emollients liberally, and avoid harsh soaps and excessive bathing.
- Advise patient of the potential for bruising because of clotting abnormality and capillary fragility.
- Administer oral antihistamine, such as diphenhydramine, to relieve itching as prescribed.

NIC Skin Surveillance; Pressure Ulcer Prevention. Additional, optional interventions include Bathing; Bleeding Reduction; Cutaneous Stimulation; Exercise Promotion and Therapy (all listed); Electrolyte Monitoring; Exercise Promotion: Stretching; Fluid/Electrolyte Management; Infection Control; Infection Protection; Medication Management; Nail Care; Nutrition Management; Perineal Care; Surveillance; and Vital Signs Monitoring.

ADDITIONAL NURSING DIAGNOSES

For patients undergoing dialytic therapy, see nursing diagnoses and interventions in "Renal Replacement Therapies," p. 334. Also see the following as appropriate: "Nutritional Support," p. 1; "Prolonged Immobility," p. 61; "Psychosocial Support," p. 68; and "Psychosocial Support For the Patient's Family and Significant Others," p. 78.

Renal Transplantation

Renal transplantation, to a large extent a result of advances in the development of immunosuppressive medications in the late 1960s and the 1970s, has become an accepted mode of treatment for end-stage renal disease. Approximately 30%-40% of individuals who need transplantation have chronic renal failure caused by glomerulonephritis; 20%-30% have pyelonephritis or other interstitial disease; 15%-20% have multisystem disease; and approximately 10% have cystic kidney disease. There are two types of transplant donors—living and cadaveric. The 1-yr success rate with live donor transplantation is 90%-95%. The 1-yr success rate with cadaveric transplantation since the advent of calcinuerin inhibitors (cyclosporine and tacrolimus) has improved to 80%-90%. The majority of patients do not have a suitable (medically or psychologically) live donor and therefore are placed on a cadaveric waiting list. The demand exceeds the supply, with approximately 50,000 patients awaiting transplantation in the United States alone.

Rejection and infection remain the major complications after transplantation. Rejection is the phenomenon that represents the recipient's immunologic response to the transplanted kidney. There are two types of lymphocytes involved in the rejection response, and either or both may participate: B lymphocytes, which form antibodies (humoral immunity), and T lymphocytes, which produce cell-mediated immunity. The rejection response can be categorized into four distinct types: hyperacute, accelerated acute, acute, and chronic (Table 5-7).

ASSESSMENT FOR REJECTION

Sudden drop in urine output: Oliguria or anuria may develop.

> **Note:** A sudden drop in output in the first 24 hr after surgery, when a Foley catheter is in place, may signal the presence of clot obstruction, which should be ruled out as the first cause of oliguria.

Elevated temperature: Low-grade, persistent fevers of 37.2°-37.8° C (99°-100° F) can occur with rejection. In the presence of accelerated or acute rejection, the patient may have fevers ranging from 37.8°-40° C (100°-104° F).

Edema: May increase in grade from 1+ (slight indentation over bony areas such as the tibia) to 3+ and 4+, with the degree of indentation increasing significantly.

Hypertension: BP that increases ≥10 mm Hg over baseline.

Weight gain: Increase of 2-3 lb over a 24-hr period.

BUN and creatinine values: Will increase from previous 24-hr levels and continue to rise until rejection is reversed.

24-hr urine collection: Will exhibit a change in components (e.g., decreases in creatinine clearance, total amount of creatinine excreted, and urinary sodium excretion; increase in protein excretion).

TABLE 5-7   Types of Renal Rejection

Type	Mechanism	Clinical presentation	Treatment
Hyperacute	Preformed antibodies against donor antigens	Occurs in the operating room. Kidney turns blue and becomes soft and flabby	Removal of kidney
Accelerated acute	May be mediated by humoral antibody or primed lymphocytes (possible presensitization in the recipient)	Occurs 48-72 hr after transplantation. Abrupt fall in urine output; leukocytosis or leukopenia; tenderness over kidney; decreased flow on renal scan; profound thrombocytopenia	Bolus IV steroids for 3-4 days; antilymphocyte preparations; poor prognosis for reversal
Acute	Cell-mediated T lymphocytes infiltrate renal tissue; humoral-mediated antigen-antibody complexes, platelets, and fibrin aggregates are present in glomerular and peritubular capillaries; may be a combination of cell-mediated and humoral-mediated	Occurs from 1-2 wk to several months after transplantation. Fever, leukocytosis, and enlarged and tender kidney; drop in urine output, weight gain (1-1.5 kg/24 h), hypertension, elevated BUN and creatinine	Bolus steroids, antilymphocyte preparations; and monoclonal antibody treatments most effective in reversing this type of rejection; good prognosis
Chronic	Probably a combined effect of antibody and cell-mediated components	Occurs months to years after transplantation. Slow, progressive decrease in renal function; hypertension; proteinuria	None known; poor prognosis for graft survival

BUN, Blood urea nitrogen; *IV,* intravenous.

Note: In the early postoperative period, the urine may remain bloody for several days, causing urinary protein concentration to be falsely elevated because of Hgb breakdown in the urine.

Renal scan: Will exhibit decreased blood flow.
Kidney assessment: May reveal a firm, large kidney that may be tender on palpation.

DIAGNOSTIC TESTS

Renal scan: Evaluates blood flow to the kidney and rate of excretion of substances into the bladder.
Renal biopsy: Determines presence, type, and severity of rejection.
Renal ultrasound: To rule out possibility of obstruction.

TREATMENT OPTIONS FOR REJECTION

Megadoses of IV methylprednisolone (Solu-Medrol): Block the production of interleukin-(IL-) 2, thereby barring essential factors for activated T cells; prevent transcription of IL-1. The release of IL-1 and IL-2 is part of the process of helper T-cell and cytotoxic T-cell differentiation, which occurs during the immune response that is triggered when foreign antigens are present in the body. Methylprednisolone also is used for its antiinflammatory properties (Table 5-8).
Antithymocyte or antilymphocyte preparations: See Table 5-8.
Monoclonal antibody (Orthoclone OKT3): Reacts with and blocks the function of the T3 complex on the surface of the T lymphocytes, causing their entrapment by cells in the spleen and liver and leading to their destruction. The T3 complex is responsible for the ability of the T lymphocyte to identify a transplanted organ as foreign (see Table 5-8).

T A B L E 5 - 8 Immunosuppressives (Standard Agents and Prophylaxis)

Drug name	Action	Dosage
Azathioprine (e.g., Imuran)	Blocks proliferation of immunocompetent lymphoid cells; affects the rapidly dividing B and T cells	Ranges from 1.5-2 mg/kg/day; IV or PO
Mycophenolate mofetil (e.g., CellCept)	Inhibits the proliferative response of T and B lymphocytes, suppressing the antibody formation by B lymphocytes	Ranges from 1.0-1.5 gm IV or PO q12h
Corticosteroids (prednisone)	Suppress the body's inflammatory and allergic processes	Varies; total dose tapered to 20-30 mg/day by first postoperative month
Cyclosporine (e.g., Sandimmune, Neoral, Gengraf, Eon)	Interferes with helper T lymphocyte function; used in combination with corticosteroids and azathioprine or mycophenolate mofetil	8-14 mg/kg/day PO; 3-4 mg/kg via continuous infusion
Tacrolimus (e.g., Prograf)	Inhibits T lymphocyte activation, used in combination with corticosteroids and azathioprine or mycophenolate mofetil	0.1-0.2 mg/kg/day PO in divided doses q12h 0.03-0.05 mg/kg/day as continuous IV infusion
Sirolimus (e.g., Rapamune)	Inhibits T lymphocyte activation and proliferation. Inhibits antibody formation	Loading dose of 6-10 mg followed by 2-4 mg qd
Antilymphocyte sera (e.g., ATGAM)	Immunoglobulin preparation that coats the T cells, making them susceptible to phagocytosis	Prophylaxis: 10-15 mg/kg IV over 4-5 hr for 5-10 days Rejection: 10-15 mg/kg IV over 4-6 hr for 10-14 days
Antithymocyte globulin (e.g., Thymoglobulin)	Possible actions include T cell clearance and modulation of T cell activation	Prophylaxis: 1.5 mg/kg IV over 4-5 hr for 3-5 days Rejection: 1.5 mg/kg IV over 4-6 hr for 7-14 days
Basiliximab (e.g., Simulect)	Binds to and blocks IL-2 receptor, inhibiting activation of lymphocytes	20 mg IV within 2 hours before transplant and 20 mg IV 4 days after transplant
Daclizumab (e.g., Zenapax)	Inhibits IL-2 binding, preventing mediated activation of lymphocytes	1 mg/kg IV 24 hr before transplant followed by 4 doses of 1 mg/kg IV every 14 days
Monoclonal antibody (Orthoclone OKT3)	Reacts with T3 complex on the surface of the T cells, causing their removal from the circulation	5 mg IV push over 30-60 sec for 10-14 days to treat rejection

Note: Each of these agents, when used individually or in combination, leads to an increased incidence of infection and malignancy secondary to their immunosuppressive properties.
IL, Interleukin; *IV,* intravenous; *PO,* oral.

Graft irradiation: Destroys lymphocytes within the graft. Irradiation is performed with 150 rad for approximately 3 days in succession.

NURSING DIAGNOSES AND INTERVENTIONS

Fear and anxiety related to threat to health status secondary to potential loss of the kidney from rejection
Desired outcomes: Within 48 hr after the transplant, patient verbalizes accurate information about the signs and symptoms of rejection. Patient's fear and anxiety are controlled as evidenced by HR ≤100 beats/min, BP within patient's normal range, and respiratory rate (RR) ≤20 breaths/min. Patient demonstrates ability to relax, discusses anxiety related to the rejection, and exhibits increased involvement in his or her own care.
- Provide opportunities for patient to express fears, concerns, and anxieties about kidney rejection.
- Assess patient's knowledge of the signs and symptoms of rejection. Ensure that patient and significant others can verbalize knowledge of the following indicators of rejection:
  - ❑ Persistent, low-grade fever of 37.2°-37.8° C (99°-100° F).
  - ❑ Increased swelling of feet, ankles, hands, or face.
  - ❑ Weight gain >1 kg/24 hr.
  - ❑ Painful and swollen kidney.
  - ❑ Elevated BP.
  - ❑ Decreased 24-hr urine output.
- Reassure patient that several medication regimens (e.g., corticosteroids, antilymphocyte preparations, monoclonal antibody) are available to treat rejection episodes.
- Reassure patient that rejection does not necessarily mean kidney loss. Under most circumstances, rejection can be reversed.
- Reassure patient that retransplantation is a viable option if kidney loss occurs.

NIC Anxiety Reduction; Coping Enhancement. Additional, optional interventions include Progressive Muscle Relaxation; Self-Esteem Enhancement; Simple Relaxation Therapy; and Support Group.

Knowledge deficit: immunosuppressive medications and their side effects
Desired outcome: Within 72 hr after initiation of medications, patient and significant others verbalize accurate information regarding the prescribed immunosuppressive agents, the side effects that can occur, and precautions that should be taken.
- Provide patient with verbal and written information for the type of immunosuppressive agent that has been prescribed. Discuss the generic name, trade name, purpose, usual dosage, route, side effects, and precautions (see Table 5-8 for purpose, usual dosage, and route) for each medication. Commonly prescribed medications follow:

Azathioprine (Imuran):
- Major side effects include leukopenia and thrombocytopenia, nausea and vomiting, and diarrhea. In addition, it increases the risk of cancer and can contribute to an increased susceptibility to infection and hepatotoxicity.
- Report fever, chills, cough, muscle or joint pain, rapid heartbeat, stomach pain with nausea and vomiting, and sores in mouth and on lips.
- Blood should be tested at frequent intervals for evaluation of WBCs and platelets. Report jaundice promptly to health care provider.
- Hair loss can occur early in the treatment course, but occurs less frequently over time.

Tacrolimus (Prograf):
- Major side effects include nephrotoxicity, hypertension, neurotoxicity, tremors, tingling of the hands and feet, paresthesias, insomnia, headache, tinnitus, hyperglycemia.
- Blood levels of tacrolimus are monitored to ensure maintenance of therapeutic ranges.
- Absorption is increased in a fasting state. Dosing is spaced 12 hr apart.
- Because of the drug's tendency to cause hyperglycemia, monitor blood glucose, and follow a diet low in concentrated carbohydrates.
- Report neurologic symptoms immediately. Report nausea and vomiting. Do not repeat dose unless told to do so by the physician.
- Consult the physician before taking any OTC medications.

Corticosteroids:
- Major side effects include cushingoid features, edema, hypertension, bone disease, muscle wasting, cataracts, steroid-induced diabetes, acne, GI irritation, and capillary fragility.
- Immediately report swelling of ankles, hands, or face; BP >20 mm Hg over baseline; swollen or bleeding gums; night sweats; change in eyesight; or muscle weakness.

Cyclosporine (Sandimmune, Neora, Gengraf, Eon):
- Major side effects include nephrotoxicity, hepatotoxicity, leukopenia, thrombocytopenia, hirsutism, muscle pain, fluid retention, edema, tremors, hypertension, nausea, vomiting, diarrhea, gum hyper-

plasia, anorexia, and anaphylaxis (rare but can occur with IV route). Immediately report these symptoms.
- Blood levels of cyclosporine are monitored at frequent intervals to ensure maximal absorption of oral solution and capsules. This is particularly important for patients experiencing GI malabsorption.
- To make oral solutions more palatable, mix with orange juice or milk and drink immediately. Stir the mixture well, and use a glass container because plastic, foam, or paper will absorb the medication. However, most patients now use the capsule form of cyclosporine.
- Rinse syringe and container with milk or orange juice and drink the remaining solution to ensure that all medication has been taken.
- Take medication 1 hr before or 2 hr after meals; and if taking twice a day, space the doses 12 hr apart.
- Tolerance to the medication, with a decrease in side effects, occurs over time.
- Because of gum hyperplasia, brush teeth with soft-bristle toothbrush and nonabrasive toothpaste after meals and snacks.
- Report nausea and vomiting that occur after dose of cyclosporine, and *do not* repeat dose unless told to do so by physician.
- Report headache, breast enlargement, flushing, and presence of any skin lesions.
- Protect skin from freezing temperatures (e.g., by wearing a mitten when taking foods out of the freezer).
- Consult physician before taking OTC medications.

Mycophenolate mofetil (CellCept):
- Major side effects include GI distress, neutropenia, anemia, thrombocytopenia, and infections.
- Report nausea, vomiting, diarrhea, blood loss in stool, fever, chills, abdominal pain, or sores in the mouth and on the lips.
- Blood should be tested to evaluate WBCs and platelets.

Sirolimus (Rapamune):
- Major side effects include headache, insomnia, diarrhea, nausea, vomiting, hyperlipidemia, rash, mouth sores, and leukopenia and thrombocytopenia.
- Report GI symptoms, rash and mouth sores, and headache.
- Blood should be tested for WBCs and platelets.
- Blood levels are monitored to maintain therapeutic drug levels.

Antilymphocyte sera:
- Major side effects include local phlebitis, thrombocytopenia, pruritus, and serum sickness. Indicators of serum sickness include rashes on the skin or genital area, joint pain and swelling, fever and chills, and night sweats. Consult physician for indicators of serum sickness.

Monoclonal antibody:
- Major side effects include chills and fever, headache, photophobia, nausea, vomiting, diarrhea, dyspnea, and bronchospasm.

Caution: Intensive monitoring is required during the first two doses because of the high frequency of side effects just discussed. In addition, risk of pulmonary edema is increased in the presence of fluid volume excess.
   The patient is premedicated with acetaminophen, diphenhydramine, and hydrocortisone or methylprednisolone to decrease the symptoms just mentioned. A chest x-ray must be clear before the first dose is given.

NIC Teaching: Disease Process; Teaching: Individual; Teaching: Prescribed Medication. Additional, optional interventions include Discharge Planning; Medication Management; and Weight Management.

Risk for infection related to inadequate secondary responses as a result of immunosuppression
Desired outcome: Patient is free of infection as evidenced by normothermia; absence of erythema, swelling, and drainage of catheter and wound sites; absence of adventitious breath sounds or cloudy and foul-smelling urine; negative results of urine, wound drainage, and blood cultures; and WBC count 4,500-11,000/mm^3.
- Assess and record patient's temperature q4h; consult physician for elevations ≥37.8° C (100° F).
- Assess and document condition of indwelling IV sites and other catheter sites q8h. Be alert to swelling, erythema, tenderness, and drainage. Consult physician for any of these findings.
- As prescribed, obtain blood, urine, and wound cultures when infection is suspected.
- Be alert to WBC count >11,000/mm^3 or <4,500/mm^3. A below-normal WBC count with increased band neutrophils on differential (shift to the left) may signal acute infection.

- Inspect graft wound for erythema, swelling, and drainage. Consult physician for significant findings.
- Record volume, appearance, color, and odor of urine. Be alert to foul-smelling or cloudy urine, frequency and urgency of urination, and patient complaints of flank or labial pain, all of which are signs of renal-urinary infection.
- Auscultate lung fields q8h, noting presence of rhonchi, crackles, and decreased breath sounds.
- Use meticulous aseptic technique when dressing and caring for wounds and catheter sites.
- Obtain specimens for urine cultures once a week during patient's hospitalization and once a month after hospital discharge.

NIC Infection Control; Infection Protection. Additional, optional interventions include Airway Management; Exercise Promotion and Therapy (all listed); Medication Management; Respiratory Monitoring; Teaching: Disease Process; Tube Care: Urinary; and Vital Signs Monitoring.

Altered oral mucous membrane related to treatment with immunosuppressive medication

Desired outcomes: Patient's oral mucosa, tongue, and lips are pink, intact, and free of exudate and lesions. Patient states that he or she can swallow without difficulty within 24 hr after treatment for altered oral mucous membrane.

- Inspect the mouth daily for signs of exudate and lesions; consult physician if they are present. Teach patient to perform self-inspection of mouth.
- Teach patient to brush with a soft-bristle toothbrush and nonabrasive toothpaste after meals and snacks.
- To help prevent monilial infection, provide patient with mycostatin prophylactic mouthwash for "swish and swallow" after meals and at bedtime.

NIC Oral Health Maintenance; Oral Health Promotion

Impaired skin integrity (or risk for same): herpetic lesions, skin fungal rashes, pruritus, and capillary fragility, related to treatment with immunosuppressive medications

Desired outcome: Patient's skin is intact and free of open lesions or abrasions.

- Assess for and document daily the presence of erythema, excoriation, rashes, or bruises on patient's skin.
- Assess for and document the presence of rashes or lesions in the perineal area, inasmuch as herpetic lesions are common in the immunosuppressed patient.
- Inspect the trunk area daily for the presence of flat, itchy rashes. Skin fungal rashes are common in the immunosuppressed patient.
- Teach patient the importance of daily skin care with water, nondrying soap, and lubricating lotion.
- Use nonallergenic tape when anchoring IV tubing, catheters, and dressings.
- Assist patient with changing position at least q2h; massage areas that are susceptible to breakdown, particularly areas over bony prominences.

NIC Skin Surveillance; Pressure Ulcer Prevention. Additional, optional interventions include Bathing; Bleeding Precautions; Cutaneous Stimulation; Exercise Promotion and Therapy (all listed); Electrolyte Monitoring; Exercise Promotion: Stretching; Fluid/Electrolyte Management; Infection Control; Infection Prevention; Medication Management; Nail Care; Nutrition Management; Perineal Care; Surveillance; and Vital Signs Monitoring

ADDITIONAL NURSING DIAGNOSES

As indicated, also see "Acute Renal Failure," p. 315. Also see "Powerlessness Related To Actual and Perceived Inability To Control Organ Rejection Episodes" in "Organ Rejection," p. 10. For other nursing diagnoses and interventions, see the following sections, as appropriate: "Nutritional Support," p. 1; "Prolonged Immobility," p. 61; "Psychosocial Support," p. 68; and "Psychosocial Support For the Patient's Family and Significant Others," p. 78.

Renal Replacement Therapies

The patient with renal dysfunction has an increasingly malfunctioning physiologic system. The goal of renal replacement therapy (RRT) is to restore dynamic equilibrium to that system. Renal replacement therapy may be done intermittently or continuously (CRRT). Indications for RRT in a critical care setting include fluid removal, solute removal, and correction of electrolyte and acid-base abnormalities. Both continuous and intermittent RRT use four principles for solute and water removal: diffusion, osmosis, ultrafiltration, and convection.

Diffusion: Movement of solutes from an area of greater concentration to an area of lesser concentration. Diffusion requires a concentration gradient. During dialysis, high concentrations of waste products and excess electrolytes diffuse into the dialysate, which contains much lower concentrations of these solutes.

Osmosis: Passive movement of water from an area of low solute concentration to an area of high solute concentration. Thus the use of high concentrations of glucose in the peritoneal dialysate causes movement of water from the patient's plasma into the dialysate.

Ultrafiltration: Movement of water from an area of higher pressure to an area of lower pressure. In hemodialysis, negative pressure in the dialysate facilitates the rapid removal of excess water from the blood compartment in which positive pressure exists.

Convection: Removal of a substance with fluid across a semipermeable membrane over time.

INDICATIONS FOR RRT/CRRT

- Volume excess
- Hyperkalemia and other electrolyte disturbances
- Metabolic acidosis
- Uremic intoxication
  - ❑ Neurologic (encephalopathy)
  - ❑ Hematologic (bleeding caused by platelet dysfunction)
  - ❑ Gastrointestinal (anorexia, nausea, vomiting)
  - ❑ Cardiovascular (pericarditis)
- Need for removal of dialyzable substances (metabolites, drugs, toxins)

DETERMINING TYPE OF RRT USED

- Availability in the institution of hemodialysis (HD), peritoneal dialysis (PD), and continuous renal replacement (CRRT) including continuous venovenous hemofiltration (CVVH), continuous venovenous hemodialysis (CVVHD), continuous venovenous hemodiafiltration (CVVHDF), slow continuous ultrafiltration (SCUF), and continuous arteriovenous hemo filtration (CAVH). Use of CAVH requires the patient have an average systolic blood pressure of 70 mm Hg. Hypotensive patients will not benefit from CAVH, but can benefit from CVVH (or any other venovenous therapy).
- Type best suited for patient's clinical status. Catabolism, for example, causes rapid rises in BUN, creatinine, and potassium values. The patient needs rapid removal of metabolic wastes (i.e., hemodialysis) (Table 5-9). Advantages and disadvantages of RRT methods are found in Table 5-10. Complications of RRT are found in Table 5-11.
- Blood or peritoneal access route availability.
- Ability to effect safe anticoagulation.

PERITONEAL DIALYSIS

The semipermeable membrane used during peritoneal dialysis is the patient's peritoneum. A special catheter is placed in the peritoneal cavity, and dialysate solution is instilled. Water, electrolytes, and waste products cross between the capillary bed of the peritoneum and the dialysate via osmosis and diffusion.

System components

Catheter: Two types are commonly used:

- *Trocar:* A stiff Silastic catheter inserted at the bedside that provides temporary access.
- *Soft Silastic indwelling catheter* (e.g., Tenckhoff): Inserted in the operating room to provide permanent access.

Dialysate: A premixed, sterile electrolyte solution with a composition similar to that of normal plasma. The concentration of ionized calcium is high to maintain a positive calcium balance. Hypocalcemia tends to occur in patients with renal failure, and the goal is to maintain serum calcium levels at 8.5-10 mg/dl. Glucose concentrations are variable inasmuch as hypertonic solutions are used to increase osmotic load for greater filtration. Potassium is added according to patient need.

Methods of peritoneal dialysis

Intermittent peritoneal dialysis (IPD): Usually involves 3-4 treatments/wk, lasting 8-10 hr each session. Hospitalized patients with acute renal failure may undergo dialysis for 24 hr every other day.

Continuous ambulatory peritoneal dialysis (CAPD): Involves extension of the time the fluid remains in the abdomen (dwell time) to 4 hr during the day and 8 hr during the night, with 4-5 exchanges during a day. Dialysis occurs 7 days a week, 24 hr a day. This method is the most physiologic form of dialysis. Exchanges may be increased to as frequently as every 2 hr if the physician is trying to avoid placing a patient on hemodialysis.

Continuous cycling peritoneal dialysis (CCPD): Dialysis treatments are performed continuously throughout the night using a special cycling machine.

HEMODIALYSIS

With hemodialysis an artificial semipermeable membrane is used to diffuse water, electrolytes, and waste products from the blood. The patient's blood is heparinized, passed through the dialyzer, and

TABLE 5-9　Comparison of Renal Replacement Therapies

Peritoneal dialysis	Hemodialysis	CAVH	CVVH
Access route			
Peritoneal catheter, which may be used immediately	Subclavian or femoral catheter or arteriovenous shunt, which may be used immediately	Arterial and venous catheters or shunt. Patient's mean arterial pressure drives flow rate	Double-lumen venous catheter. Pump used to achieve flow rate
Semipermeable membrane			
Peritoneum; approximately 2.2 m^2 (the total area available for diffusion of solutes)	Cuprophane or cellulose acetate; 1-2 m^2	High-efficiency, high-flux material (polysulfone, polyamide, and polyacrylonitrile)	Same as CAVH
Molecular movement			
Diffusion by a concentration gradient	Diffusion by a concentration gradient	Diffusion and convection	Same as CAVH
Water removal			
Osmotic pressure, using high glucose concentration	Hydrostatic pressure (pressure gradient across the membrane)	Ultrafiltration—hydrostatic pressure	Same as CAVH
Duration			
6-12 cycles/day, intermittent PD (IPD); 3-4 cycles/day, continuous ambulatory (CAPD); nighttime, continuous cycling (CCPD) machine	3 hr, 3/wk; maximum of 3-4 h/day	Continuous	Same as CAVH
Efficiency			
Slow diffusion; less efficient than hemodialysis	High efficiency	High for fluid removal, moderate solute removal	Same as CAVH
Risk of infection			
High	Lower than peritoneal method	High for access infection	Same as CAVH
Major problem			
Development of peritonitis	May not be tolerated by the patient with hemodynamic instability	Dehydration and hypotension	Same as CAVH

CAVH, Continuous arteriovenous hemofiltration; *CVVH*, continuous venovenous hemofiltration; *PD*, peritoneal dialysis.

then returned to the circulation. For acutely ill patients, dialysis may be needed from 3 times/wk to daily.

System components
Dialyzer (artificial kidney): Consists of the blood compartment, dialysate compartment, and the semipermeable membrane. Small molecules, such as electrolytes, water, and waste products, pass through this membrane; RBCs, protein, and bacteria, however, are too large to cross.

TABLE 5-10 Advantages and Disadvantages of Methods of Renal Replacement Therapy

Advantages	Disadvantages
Hemodialysis	
Very efficient; requires short, frequent treatments	Special equipment and trained staff required
As needed, fluid and chemical balance may be altered rapidly	Heparinization usually required
	Possibility of disequilibrium from too-rapid fluid and biochemical shifts
	Possible difficulty in maintaining vascular access
	Risk of blood loss necessitating transfusion
Peritoneal dialysis	
Simple equipment; rapid initiation of treatment	Time-consuming
Systemic anticoagulation not needed	Risk of peritonitis and pneumonia
Slow dialysis; less risk of hypotension and rapid fluid and electrolyte shifts	Desired effects slower to occur
	Protein loss
	Some patient discomfort
Hemofiltration	
Physiologic process	Low-efficiency solute removal unlear CVVHD or CVVHDF
Ideal for the patient who is hemodynamically unstable	Large volume fluid replacement
Allows administration of large volumes (e.g., TPN)	Potential for electrolyte imbalance
Technically simple	Increased responsibilities for ICU nurses
CVVH effective in patients with MAP <70 mm Hg	

CVVH, Continuous venovenous hemofiltration; *CVVHD,* continuous venovenous hemofiltration with dialysis; *CVVHDF,* continuous venovenous hemodiafiltration; *OICU,* intensive care unit; *MAP,* mean arterial pressure; *TPN,* total parenteral nutrition.

TABLE 5-11 Complications of Renal Replacement Therapies

Hemodialysis	Peritoneal dialysis	Hemofiltration
Hypotension	Bowel or bladder perforation	Bleeding
Air embolus	Hyperglycemic hyperosmolar coma	Infection
Angina and dysrhythmias	Hypernatremia	Volume depletion
Blood loss (dialyzer rupture)	Hypovolemia	Blood leakage
Disequilibrium syndrome	Metabolic alkalosis	Decreased ultrafilration
Hemolysis	Peritonitis	Filter clotting
Hemorrhage	**Procedural complications**	Electrolyte disturbances
Septicemia	Abdominal distention: failure to drain dialysate	Air embolus with CVVH
Bleeding	Catheter obstruction from clots or fibrin	
Clotting	Catheter becoming wrapped in omentum	
High-output heart failure	Cuff erosion	
Infection	Catheter malpositioning	
Phlebitis	Tunnel infection	
Venous spasms		

CVVH, Continuous venovenous hemofiltration.

Dialysate: Electrolyte solution similar to normal plasma. The potassium concentration varies according to patient need. Glucose may be necessary to prevent changes in the patient's serum glucose and osmolality values. Although glucose is a large molecule, it can cross the semipermeable membrane, resulting in hypoglycemia. Use of a glucose bath reduces the risk of hypoglycemia.

Vascular access: Method used to deliver blood to the dialyzer at a rate of at least 200-300 ml/min.
- *Subclavian, internal jugular, or femoral catheter:* Temporary access catheter (usually double-lumen) that is placed in a large vein to enhance blood flow (e.g., Tesio, Vascath).
- *Arteriovenous (AV) fistula:* Anastomosis of an artery and vein, resulting in dilated vessels for easy cannulation and increased blood flow.
- *Graft:* Bovine, Gore-Tex, or saphenous vein. The graft connects the artery and vein internally in the arm or thigh.
- *Hemasite:* A T-shaped device inserted into an arterialized vein with a Gore-Tex graft. The T projects out of the skin, resulting in an external entry point.

CONTINUOUS RENAL REPLACEMENT THERAPY (CRRT)

CVVH, CVVHD, CVVHDF, SCUF, and CAVH are types of renal hemofiltration therapy performed to manage fluid and solute overload in critically ill patients. Their advantage over conventional dialytic therapies is that ultrafiltration occurs more gradually, thus avoiding drastic volume changes and rapid fluid shifts. Treatment duration may be 24 hr or several days, depending on the total amount of fluid to be removed.

Principles:
- Use of a highly permeable, hollow-fiber filter.
- Removal of plasma water and unbound substances, such as urea, calcium, sodium, potassium, chloride, vitamins, and unbound drugs, with a molecular weight between 500 and 10,000 daltons.
- Filtration: Movement of fluid across a semipermeable membrane from an area of greater pressure to one of lesser pressure (pressure gradient).
- Convection: Some elements in plasma water (e.g., urea) conveyed across the membrane as a result of the differences in hydrostatic pressure. The removal of large amounts of plasma water results in the removal of large amounts of filterable solutes.
- For ultrafiltration to occur, there must be a pressure gradient across the membrane that favors filtration. In CAVH or CVVH/other venovenous hemofiltration therapies, this is called *transmembrane pressure (TMP)*. Its major determinants are hydrostatic pressure and oncotic pressure. The higher pressure in the blood compartment is a function of the individual's blood pressure when using CAVH. Pressure in the blood compartment is adequate when the systolic pressure is 50-70 mm Hg. Higher pressures enhance ultrafiltration. Venovenous therapies do not rely on the patient's blood pressure for ultrafiltration. Negative pressure for ultrafiltration can be achieved by lowering the collection container 20-40 cm below the hemofilter. The differences in hydrostatic pressure also cause the crossing of some elements, such as glucose and some vitamins. The longer it takes for blood to clear the filter, the more likely that intermediate molecules (vitamins, glucose) will be filtered out of the patient's system. Opposing the hydrostatic pressure is oncotic pressure, which is maintained by plasma proteins that do not pass through the membrane. When hydrostatic pressure exceeds oncotic pressure, filtration of water and solutes occurs.

Indications for CRRT:
- Massive fluid overload: congestive heart failure, acute renal failure, overaggressive fluid resuscitation in multiple trauma.
- Fluid overload in the presence of hemodynamic instability.
- Cardiogenic shock with pulmonary edema.
- Oliguric patient unresponsive to diuretics.
- Patient with anuria who requires large volumes of parenteral fluid: acts as a supplement to hemodialysis to maintain fluid balance.

Method: The hemofilter and lines are primed with normal saline before the treatment is initiated. Blood flows from the "arterial" (usually femoral or radial) limb of the vascular access through the filter and returns through the venous (usually femoral or cephalic) limb of the access. A continuous infusion of heparin prevents clotting in the lines and filter. Blood is driven through the system by the patient's blood pressure with CAVH, so no pump is used. With CVVH/other venovenous therapies, a pump is used to drive the blood flow. As the blood flows through the filter, water, electrolytes, and most drugs not bound to plasma protein diffuse across the membrane and thus become part of the filtrate. If the objective is the removal of large amounts of fluid and solute (i.e., urea, potassium, creatinine), it is necessary to infuse large volumes of filtration replacement fluid (FRF) to maintain electrolyte balance. Nursing responsibilities include initiating treatment, monitoring the patient and the system, and discontinuing treatment. Tables 5-10 and 5-11 discuss the advantages, disadvantages, and complications of RRTs. Table 5-12 discusses troubleshooting major problems with CRRT.

COLLABORATIVE MANAGEMENT

For patients undergoing dialysis

Dietary restrictions

Hemodialysis: Between dialysis treatments the main products of protein metabolism and potassium and sodium will accumulate because of the kidneys' inability to excrete excesses of these products. Therefore it is necessary to restrict the intake of protein to decrease the amount of urea generated, to restrict potassium to prevent hyperkalemia, and to restrict sodium to prevent hypernatremia and curb thirst. Recommended guidelines include protein 1-1.2 g/kg/day; sodium 80-100 mEq/day (individualized); and potassium 40-80 mEq/day (individualized).

Peritoneal dialysis: Patients undergoing peritoneal dialysis tend to lose more protein through the peritoneal membrane. Therefore protein restriction is liberalized to 1.2-1.5 g/kg/day to compensate for the extra loss. If peritonitis develops, protein loss can increase from around 10 g/day to 50 g/day. Patients undergoing CAPD may need calorie restrictions because of the added calories they absorb from the glucose contained in the dialysate. If hypertonic solutions are used several times a day, these patients can absorb as much as 600 calories or more from the dialysate. Potassium may be less restricted in these patients because the dialysate is potassium-free and allows better diffusion of potassium, with less accumulation that would lead to hyperkalemia. Sodium restriction in peritoneal dialysis is approximately 80-100 mEq/day to prevent hypernatremia and control thirst to prevent fluid overload.

Fluid restriction: To prevent fluid overload secondary to the kidneys' inability to excrete excess water. Weight gain between dialysis treatments is usually the result of fluid retention. An attempt is made to limit interdialytic weight gain to 1.5-2 kg by limiting fluid intake to 1500-1800 ml in 24 hr. This restriction is also individualized.

Phosphate binders: To prevent or control hyperphosphatemia, which can occur because of the kidneys' inability to excrete excess dietary phosphates.

Vitamin D analogs (dihydrotachysterol—the active form of vitamin D) and calcium replacement: To prevent hypocalcemia and renal osteodystrophy, which may occur because of the body's inability to absorb calcium and maintain serum levels. If hypocalcemia occurs, the parathyroid glands are activated to release parathormone, which releases calcium from the bone to replenish serum levels. Over time, this can lead to bone demineralization and osteodystrophy.

Water-soluble vitamins and folic acid: Are dialyzable and necessitate replacement after dialysis.

For patients undergoing continuous replacement therapies: venovenous or arteriovenous

The goal is the removal of excess fluid and, with CVVHD/CVVHDF, excess solutes; while maintaining electrolyte balance and adequate fluid intake for homeostasis. In the critically ill adult, catabolic rate is 2-3 times that of normal, and this is balanced with TPN.

TPN: To maintain nutritional requirements.

T A B L E 5 - 12   Troubleshooting Major Problems in Hemofiltration

Problem	Cause	Intervention
Hypotension	Cardiac dysfunction	Cardiotonic and pressor support
	Excessive intravascular volume removal	Fluid replacement
		Recalculate UF rate
Poor ultrafiltration	High Hct	Predilution fluid replacement
	Decreased MAP	Pressor support to increase MAP
	Clotted filter	Flush filter; replace if necessary
Clotted hemofilter	Inadequate anticoagulation	Check ACT or aPPT hourly, and adjust heparin infusion
	Poor blood flow rates	
	Kinks in blood tubing	Pressors or fluid replacement to increase MAP
		Check tubing hourly to guard against kinks
		Change filter and restart therapy

ACT, Activated clotting time; *aPPT,* activated partial thromboplastin time; *Hct,* hematocrit; *MAP,* mean arterial pressure; *UF,* ultrafiltration.

SCUF/CVVH/CAVH: To correct hypervolemic state. A large-bore catheter is used for access.
Predilution fluid replacement: If increased solute removal is required. (See Table 5-13 for differences between predilution and postdilution replacement.)
Filtration replacement fluid: To maintain fluid and electrolyte balance. (See Table 5-14 for calculation of infusion rate of these fluids.) Concentration may vary, depending on the replacement needs of the patient.

Standard fluids infused simultaneously include the following:
1 L 0.9 normal saline (NS) with 7.5 ml 10% CaCl
1 L 0.9 NS with 1.6 ml 50% $MgSO_4$
1 L 0.9 NS
1 L D_5W with 150 mEq $NaHCO_3^-$
Final composition of fluid for typical patient:
Sodium: 150 mEq/L
Chloride: 114 mEq/L
Bicarbonate: 37 mEq/L
Magnesium: 1.6 mEq/L
Calcium: 2.5 mEq/L
Heparin infusion solution: To prevent clotting in the circuit.
Vasopressors—for CAVH only: To maintain arterial pressure, which is necessary for driving the blood through the hemofilter.

NURSING DIAGNOSES AND INTERVENTIONS
For patients undergoing dialysis
Risk for infection related to invasive procedure used to obtain peritoneal or vascular access for dialysis
Desired outcome: Patient is free of infection as evidenced by normothermia; WBC count ≤11,000/mm³; blood and dialysate free of infective organisms; and absence of erythema, purulent drainage, abdominal or access site pain, and cloudy dialysate.
- Assess and document condition of the access site daily. Be alert to the presence of erythema, purulent drainage, or tenderness.
- Peritonitis accounts for a high incidence of failure with peritoneal dialysis. Use strict aseptic technique when cleansing catheter site and connecting and disconnecting dialysate bags. Use an antiseptic solution such as hydrogen peroxide or povidone-iodine to cleanse the access site. Maintain aseptic technique when cleansing and drying the site. Cover the site with a dry, sterile dressing. Because moist surfaces breed bacteria, change the dressing immediately if it becomes wet.
- Keep all external access devices (shunts, subclavian catheters, femoral catheters, peritoneal catheters) covered with a dry, sterile dressing between treatments.
- Document the appearance of peritoneal dialysis effluent. If peritoneal drainage becomes cloudy or contains flecks of material, send specimen for a culture and obtain a cell count to check for increased WBCs in the peritoneal effluent. Consult physician for changes in outflow.

T A B L E 5 - 13 **Approaches to Fluid Replacement**

Predilution: replacement fluid infused proximal to the filter	Postdilution: replacement fluid infused distal to the filter
Patient population: Those with poor blood flow and elevated BUN and Hct levels	*Patient population:* All types
Replacement fluid infused into arterial line	Replacement fluid infused into venous line
Used to enhance urea clearance to ≥18%; decreases oncotic pressure, increasing net TMP; moves urea from erythrocytes into plasma	Used to maintain fluid and electrolyte balance
Increases net fluid removal	Less replacement fluid required
Potentially increases filter life	Simplified clearance determination
*Urea clearance 12.5 ml/min	Urea clearance 10.6 ml/min

BUN, Blood urea nitrogen; *Hct,* hematocrit; *TMP,* transmembrane pressure.
*If increased urea clearance is desired, predilution mode of fluid replacement is used.

TABLE 5-14   Calculation of Filtration Replacement Fluid (FRF) Rate

Infusion rate

Equals ultrafiltrate plus other losses per hour minus all fluid infused minus net removal rate

Example

Ultrafiltrate = 600 ml/hr + Losses (urine, GI) = 100 ml/hr – TPN (total parenteral nutrition) 100 ml/hr; vasopressors 50 ml/hr – Net fluid removal rate 150 ml/hr

FRF rate

= (600 + 100) – (100 + 50 + 150)

700 – 300

FRF rate

= 400 ml/hr

- Report the presence of elevated temperature, malaise, access site drainage, cloudy dialysate, or abdominal pain.
- Teach patient to notify staff members if symptoms of infection occur.

NIC Infection Control; Infection Protection. Additional, optional interventions include Airway Management; Exercise Promotion and Therapy (all listed); Medication Management; Respiratory Monitoring; Teaching: Disease Process; Tube Care: Urinary; and Vital Signs Monitoring.

Altered nutrition less than body requirements, related to dietary restrictions; protein loss occurring with peritoneal dialysis

Desired outcomes: Patient has adequate nutrition as evidenced by stable weekly body weight. Patient's caloric intake ranges from 35-45 calories/kg body weight/day (may not be appropriate for patient with CAPD, who absorbs calories through the dialysate); high–biologic value protein intake is 50%-75% of patient's daily protein intake. Nitrogen intake is 4-6 g more than nitrogen loss (loss calculated from 24-hr urinary urea excretion, and intake estimated from protein intake).

- Document food intake; count calories consumed with each meal. Total caloric intake should be 35-45 calories/kg body weight/24 hr.
- Consult with physician and dietitian regarding use of nutritional supplements for maintaining caloric intake.
- For patient undergoing peritoneal dialysis, encourage intake of protein (e.g., milk shakes with protein supplements, custards).
- Weigh patient daily. Be alert to losses ≥10% of patient's normal body weight over a 1-wk period. Daily fluctuations reflect body fluid changes.
- For the patient receiving hemodialysis, encourage the intake of foods that are high in calories (e.g., butter, honey, hard candy, tapioca, sherbet, corn syrup, ginger ale, jellies, jams, marshmallows). Patients undergoing peritoneal dialysis absorb extra calories from the glucose in the peritoneal dialysate.
- Concentrate protein intake on high–biologic value protein foods (e.g., meats, milk, fish, fowl, eggs).
- Minimize the intake of protein from low–biologic value protein foods (e.g., breads, cereals, pastas, grains, fruits, vegetables).
- For patients receiving hemodialysis in particular, suggest the intake of caloric substances that do not contain protein or electrolytes. Some commercially available products are Cal-Powder, Controlyte, Hycal, and Polycose.
- As appropriate, refer to dietitian, who can teach the patient and significant others meal-planning techniques that will include restrictions while maintaining a high-calorie intake. Many dialysis patients are also diabetic, and careful meal planning is necessary.
- If patient is anorexic or nauseated, provide small, frequent meals. Present appetizing food in a pleasant atmosphere. As indicated, administer prescribed antiemetic ½ hr before meals.

NIC Nutrition Management; Nutritional Monitoring; Fluid Management; Fluid Monitoring. Additional, optional interventions include Bowel Management; Energy Management; Enteral Tube Feeding; Exercise Promotion; Gastrointestinal Intubation; Hyperglycemia Management; Hypoglycemia Management; Intravenous Insertion; Intravenous Therapy; Medication Management; Mutual Goal Setting; Phlebotomy: Venous Blood Sample; Positioning; Teaching: Individual; Teaching: Prescribed Diet; Total Parenteral Nutrition Administration; and Venous Access Devices Maintenance.

Fluid volume excess (or risk for same) related to dietary indiscretions of sodium and fluids; compromised regulatory mechanisms secondary to renal failure

Desired outcome: Within 24-48 hr of admission, patient is normovolemic as evidenced by balanced I&O; stable weight; HR ≤100 beats/min; BP within patient's normal range; RR 12-20 breaths/min; and absence of edema, crackles, and other physical indicators of hypervolemia.
- Monitor and record I&O q4h, and weight daily; report significant findings to physician. Be alert to weight gain of >0.5-1 kg/24 hr.
- Assess and record status of VS, lung sounds, and cardiac rate and rhythm. Be alert to crackles, tachycardia, pericardial friction rub, and pulsus paradoxus.
- Assess for presence of peripheral, periorbital, and sacral edema.
- Maintain fluid restrictions as prescribed.
- Elevate head of bed (HOB) during peritoneal dialysis to relieve pressure of fluid against diaphragm.
- If outflow is poor, change patient's position or irrigate catheter to determine patency.

NIC Electrolyte Management: Hypokalemia; Electrolyte Management: Hyponatremia; Fluid/Electrolyte Management; Fluid Management; Fluid Monitoring. Additional, optional interventions include Dysrhythmia Management; Feeding; Gastrointestinal Intubation; Hemodialysis Therapy; Hemodynamic Regulation; Invasive Hemodynamic Monitoring; Medication Management; Phlebotomy: Arterial and Venous Blood Sample; Positioning; Skin Surveillance; and Weight Management.

Risk for fluid volume deficit related to active loss secondary to excess fluid removal during dialysis; bleeding secondary to heparinization

Desired outcomes: Patient is normovolemic as evidenced by balanced I&O; daily weight within 1-2 lb of calculated dry weight (true body weight without any excess fluid); BP within patient's normal range; CVP ≥2 mm Hg; and HR ≤100 beats/min. Hct is 20%-30% (a range expected for the patient receiving dialysis, inasmuch as anemia is associated with renal failure), and there is no evidence of blood loss caused by line separation or membrane rupture.
- When using hypertonic dialysate for peritoneal dialysis, assess skin turgor, mucous membranes, CVP, BP, and HR for signs of dehydration, which can occur from excessive fluid loss. Be alert to sudden decrease in BP, tachycardia, poor skin turgor, dry mucous membranes, and change in mental status (e.g., restlessness, unresponsiveness).
- When using hypertonic peritoneal dialysate, check finger-stick glucose q4h. Consult physician for blood glucose levels >200 mg/dl.
- Weigh patient daily for trend. Monitor I&O q8h, and consult physician for output >1500 ml over intake.
- Monitor Hct results before each hemodialysis. Notify physician if a >2-point drop occurs.
- If hypotension occurs during peritoneal dialysis, stop the dialysis, consult physician, and encourage oral fluids up to 1000 ml (or per protocol).
- If hypotension occurs during hemodialysis, give normal saline or volume expanders as prescribed and notify physician.
- During hemodialysis, secure lines with tape to prevent disconnection and dislodgment. Consult physician immediately if blood loss occurs because of line separation or dialyzer rupture. As prescribed, send blood sample to laboratory for type and screen. Maintain pressure over any venipuncture sites for at least 5 min after needles have been removed.

NIC Electrolyte Management: Hyperkalemia; Electrolyte Management: Hypermagnesemia; Electrolyte Management: Hypernatremia; Electrolyte Management: Hyperphosphatemia; Fluid Management; Fluid Monitoring; Hypovolemia Management; Intravenous Therapy. Additional, optional interventions include Dysrhythmia Management; Feeding; Fever Treatment; Gastrointestinal Intubation; Hemodynamic Regulation; Invasive Hemodynamic Monitoring; Medication Management; Nutrition Management; Weight Management; and Phlebotomy: Arterial Blood Sample and Venous Blood Sample.

Altered peripheral tissue perfusion (or risk for same) access site, related to interruption of vascular flow secondary to clot formation, pressure, obstruction, or disconnection of vascular access device

Desired outcomes: Patient's access site for dialysis has adequate perfusion as evidenced by palpation of thrill; auscultation of bruit; visualization of blood flow; and warmth of the graftor AV fistula. Warmth and brisk capillary refill (<2 sec) are present in the access extremity.
- Confirm patency of access site by palpating for thrill (vibratory sensation) and auscultating for presence of bruit (buzzing sound) over the graft or AV fistula. Monitor the access extremity for warmth and brisk capillary refill.
- Notify physician promptly if patency cannot be confirmed. Thrombolytic therapy or embolectomy may be indicated to save the fistula or graft.
- Avoid taking BP, drawing blood, or using restrictive clothing, name bands, or restraints on arm with fistula or graft. Teach patient the importance of these restrictions.
- If using a pressure dressing over the access site, make sure it is snug enough to prevent bleeding but not so tight that it could stop blood flow and promote clot formation. Remove the pressure dressing after it has been on the site for 1-2 hr.

- Maintain constant infusion of heparin (e.g., 10 U/ml, or as prescribed, via piggyback) through subclavian internal jugular or femoral line or flush with heparinized saline and cap as prescribed.
- Flush peritoneal catheter before and after dialysis with 30-50 ml normal saline to ensure patency.
- Always check fistula, graft, or shunt for patency after any hypotensive episode.
- If it is suspected that air has entered the vascular access, clamp the line and place the patient in a left side-lying Trendelenburg position, which will trap air at the apex of the right ventricle of the heart, away from the outflow tract. Call physician *stat,* administer oxygen, and monitor VS carefully.
- For more information, see "Pulmonary Embolus," p. 192.

NIC Circulatory Care, Embolus Precautions; Exercise Promotion; Exercise Therapy (all listed); Surveillance

Altered protection (or risk for same) related to neurosensory alterations secondary to endogenous chemical alteration (dialysis disequilibrium syndrome) occurring with rapid removal of metabolic wastes and changes in serum osmolality

Desired outcome: Patient verbalizes orientation to time, place, and person and does not exhibit signs and symptoms of disequilibrium syndrome: headache, nausea, vomiting, restlessness, asterixis, stupor, coma, or seizures.

- Monitor patient for indicators of disequilibrium syndrome.
- Consult physician for changing LOC and other marked signs of disequilibrium.
- Recognize predisposing factors: BUN >150 mg/dl; hypernatremia (serum sodium >147 mEq/L); severe metabolic acidosis; and history of neurologic problems (e.g., seizures). The syndrome often is prevented by short, frequent dialysis exchanges and by increasing the osmolality of dialysate by adding glucose, glycerol, urea, or mannitol, or by giving IV mannitol during treatment.
- Monitor BUN levels before and after dialysis to evaluate for changes occurring along with signs and symptoms of disequilibrium.
- Raise and pad side rails, and keep an appropriately sized airway at the bedside as indicated.

NIC Infection Control; Infection Protection. Additional, optional interventions include Nutrition Management; Nutrition Therapy; Nutritional Counseling; Pressure Management; Pressure Ulcer Prevention; and Teaching: Individual.

Ineffective breathing pattern related to decreased lung expansion secondary to impaired respiratory mechanics occurring with dialysate in the peritoneal cavity

Desired outcome: Patient becomes eupneic within 24 hr of this diagnosis.

- Monitor patient's respiratory rate, depth, and pattern, and assess breath sounds when dialysate is dwelling in the peritoneal cavity.
- Elevate the HOB to reduce pressure of fluid against the diaphragm and increase vital capacity.
- Schedule deep-breathing exercises and incentive spirometry q2-4h.
- Get patient up in a chair 3-4 times/day if possible.

NIC Airway Management. Additional, optional interventions include Acid Base Monitoring; Analgesic Administration; Aspiration Precautions; and Chest Physiotherapy.

For patients undergoing continuous renal replacement therapies: venovenous or arteriovenous

Decreased cardiac output (or risk for same) related to decreased preload and electrical changes secondary to fluid and electrolyte shifts occurring with hemofiltration

Desired outcomes: Patient's cardiac output is adequate as evidenced by systolic BP ≥100 mm Hg (or within patient's normal range); HR 60-100 beats/min; RR 12-20 breaths/min; peripheral pulses >2+ on a 0-4+ scale; brisk capillary refill (<2 sec); and normal sinus rhythm on ECG.

- Assess and document BP, HR, and RR hourly for the first 4 hr of hemofiltration, and then q2h. Be alert to indicators of fluid volume deficit, manifested by a drop in systolic BP to <100 mm Hg, tachycardia, and tachypnea.
- Assess and document peripheral pulses and color, temperature, and capillary refill in the extremities q2h. Be alert to decreased amplitude of peripheral pulses and to coolness, pallor, and delayed capillary refill in the extremities as indicators of decreased perfusion.
- Measure and record I&O hourly. Consult physician for a loss of ≥200 ml/hr over desired loss.
- Monitor cardiac rhythm continuously; notify physician of decrease in BP ≥ 20 mm Hg from baseline, tachycardia, depressed T waves and ST segments, and dysrhythmias, which can occur with hypovolemia, potassium changes, or calcium changes.
- Ensure prescribed rates of ultrafiltration and replacement fluid infusion (see Table 5-14), and adjust if ultrafiltration rate changes. Use an infusion pump for replacement fluids to ensure precise rate of infusion. Also maintain TPN and IV rates, as well as oral intake, within 50 ml of the values used to calculate the filtration fluid replacement rate. If any parameters change >50 ml, recalculate filtration fluid replacement rate and adjust accordingly.

- Monitor serum electrolyte values, being alert to changes in potassium, calcium, phosphorus, and bicarbonate. Compare patient's values with the following normal ranges: potassium 3.5-5 mEq/L; calcium 8.5-10.5 mg/dl; phosphorus 2.5-4.5 mg/dl; and bicarbonate 22-26 mEq/L. (See "Fluid and Electrolyte Disturbances," p. 538, and "Acid-Base Imbalances," p. 566.)

Risk for fluid volume deficit related to active loss secondary to excessive ultrafiltration during CRRT

Desired outcomes: Patient is normovolemic as evidenced by gradual weight loss (<2.5 kg/day) and urinary output ≥0.5 ml/kg/hr in nonoliguric patients. Ultrafiltration rate remains within 50 ml of the desired hourly rate.

- Measure and record I&O q30min for the first 2 hr and then hourly. Ensure that it is within desired limits.
- Weigh patient q8h. Be alert to daily loss ≥2.5 kg.
- Record cumulative ultrafiltrate loss hourly. Measure amount in the ultrafiltrate container. The difference between this value and total hourly intake is the cumulative loss per hr.
- Check replacement fluid rate hourly to ensure that it is within prescribed limits—usually 25 ml of the calculated rate.
- Consult physician for unanticipated fluid loss from vomiting, diarrhea, fever, and wound drainage.
- Consult physician for increased filtration rate, which may occur because of increased BP; or for increased negative pressure, which may be caused by lowering the ultrafiltration collection device.
- Monitor VS hourly; consult physician for increased arterial pressure (≥10 mm Hg above baseline), which would increase flow through the hemofilter, thereby increasing the rate of ultrafiltration.
- Adjust the filtration replacement fluid rate as prescribed when ultrafiltration rate increases.
- Maintain intake (oral, IV, TPN) within 25-50 ml of the value used to calculate fluid replacement rate.

NIC Electrolyte Management: Hyperkalemia; Electrolyte Management: Hypermagnesemia; Electrolyte Management: Hypernatremia; Electrolyte Management: Hyperphosphatemia; Fluid Management; Fluid Monitoring; Hypovolemia Management; Intravenous Therapy. Additional, optional interventions include Dysrhythmia Management; Feeding; Fever Treatment; Gastrointestinal Intubation; Hemodynamic Regulation; Invasive Hemodynamic Monitoring; Medication Management; Nutrition Management; Weight Management; and Phlebotomy: Arterial Blood Sample and Venous Blood Sample.

Fluid volume excess (or risk for same) related to excessive fluid intake associated with decreased ultrafiltration secondary to hypotension, clogged or clotted filter, or kinked lines

Desired outcome: Patient experiences a gradual fluid loss and becomes normovolemic as evidenced by BP remaining at baseline range; activated clotting time (ACT) 2-3 times that of the baseline value; CVP 2-6 mm Hg; HR 60-100 beats/min; RR 12-20 breaths/min; and absence of edema, crackles, and other physical indicators of hypervolemia.

- Monitor BP q30min for the first 2 hr and then hourly. Consult physician for a 10 mm Hg drop in BP, which would decrease the rate of ultrafiltration significantly.
- If ultrafiltration rate is decreased to 50% of the baseline, consult physician and decrease FRF rate as prescribed.
- Check tubes hourly for kinks.
- Maintain constant heparin infusion per infusion pump to maintain ACT at 2-3 times that of the baseline value.
- Monitor clotting time q2h. Use of an activated clotting time device is advisable.
- Inspect vascular access filter and lines for patency hourly. If clotting or clogging with protein is suspected, flush the system with 50 ml normal saline to check patency.
- If clots are present, consult physician. As prescribed, change the filter and recheck ACT/PTT to ensure necessary adjustment in heparin infusion rate.
- On an hourly basis, assess for and document the presence of physical indicators of hypervolemia: CVP >6 mm Hg; BP elevated ≥20 mm Hg over baseline; tachycardia; jugular venous distention; basilar crackles; increasing edema (peripheral, sacral, periorbital); and tachypnea.

NIC Electrolyte Management: Hypokalemia; Electrolyte Management: Hyponatremia; Fluid/Electrolyte Management; Fluid Management; Fluid Monitoring. Additional, optional interventions include Dysrhythmia Management; Feeding; Gastrointestinal Intubation; Hemodialysis Therapy; Hemodynamic Regulation; Invasive Hemodynamic Monitoring; Medication Management; Phlebotomy: Arterial and Venous Blood Samples; Positioning; Skin Surveillance; and Weight Management.

Knowledge deficit: CRRT procedure

Desired outcome: Patient or significant other verbalizes accurate information about the CRRT procedure within 24-48 hr of the instruction.

- Assess patient's knowledge of the procedure, and intervene accordingly.
- Explain necessity of vascular access and the sensations that can be anticipated during cannula insertion.
- Explain importance of and rationale for limited movement of the involved extremity after cannula placement.
- Describe equipment that will be used for the procedure (e.g., CRRT machine, filter, lines, infusion pumps).
- Explain that VS will be assessed and blood tests will be performed at frequent intervals to monitor patient's status during the procedure.
- Explain to patient that his or her blood will be visible in the filter and lines.
- Reinforce that a staff member will be close to patient at all times during the procedure and will explain each step as it occurs.
- Explain that the procedure may require 24 hr or longer to attain fluid balance.
- Teach patient that the typical access sites are the femoral artery and the femoral vein, or the radial artery and the cephalic, the internal jugular, or the subclavian vein.

NIC Teaching: Disease Process; Teaching: Individual; Teaching: Prescribed Medication. Additional, optional interventions include Discharge Planning; Medication Management; and Weight Management.

Impaired physical mobility related to movement restrictions because of access and equipment for hemofiltration

Desired outcomes: Patient exhibits ability to move about in bed with assistance without evidence of disruption of hemofiltration equipment. Patient's skin remains intact, and there is no evidence of muscle atrophy or contracture formation caused by imposed immobility.

- Secure access catheters with gauze wraps (elastic wrap may compress access site and cause clotting) and tape to ensure safe movement of the involved limb without disruption of access cannula.
- Explain to patient the need for care and assistance when moving the involved limb.
- Use soft restraints if movement must be restrained markedly.
- Turn and reposition patient at least q2h, maintaining good body alignment.
- Massage bony prominences during every position change to promote comfort and circulation.
- Support involved extremities with pillows.
- Teach patient assisted ROM exercises on uninvolved extremities. Encourage isometric, isotonic, and quadriceps-setting exercises on uninvolved extremities, especially for patients whose CAVH or CVVH lasts >24 hr.

NIC Exercise Therapy: Ambulation; Exercise Therapy: Joint Mobility. Additional, optional interventions include Activity Therapy; Body Mechanics Promotion; Circulatory Care; Circulatory Precautions; Fall Prevention; Pain Management; Progressive Muscle Relaxation; Skin Surveillance; and Weight Management.

Risk for fluid volume deficit related to potential for blood loss secondary to line disconnection or membrane rupture

Desired outcome: Patient's membrane and line connections remain intact, and ultrafiltrate test results are negative for blood.

- Tape and secure all connections within the system.
- Check connections hourly to ensure that they are secure.
- Avoid concealing lines, filter, or connections with linen.
- Position filter and lines close to the access extremity; secure them with gauze wraps and tape to prevent traction on the connections.
- Inspect ultrafiltrate hourly for any signs of blood. If unsure whether ultrafiltrate contains blood, check the solution for occult blood.
- If the test is positive for blood, clamp the ultrafiltrate port and consult physician for further interventions.

NIC Electrolyte Management: Hyperkalemia; Electrolyte Management: Hypermagnesemia; Electrolyte Management: Hypernatremia; Electrolyte Management: Hyperphosphatemia; Fluid Management; Fluid Monitoring; Hypovolemia Management; Intravenous Therapy. Additional, optional interventions include Dysrhythmia Management; Feeding; Fever Treatment; Gastrointestinal Intubation; Hemodynamic Regulation; Invasive Hemodynamic Monitoring; Medication Management; Nutrition Management; Weight Management; and Phlebotomy: Arterial Blood Sample and Venous Blood Sample.

Research Brief 5-1   The Kidney Early Evaluation Program (KEEP) was started in 1997 to identify persons at high risk for chronic kidney disease (CKD) and encourage those at risk to seek medical evaluation and management. Community screening was conducted using a standardized questionnaire, and test panel administered by local affiliates of the National Kidney Foundation (NKF). High-risk persons were defined as those with history of diabetes or hypertension or a first-order family member with hypertension, diabetes, or kidney disease. Data on the first 11,246 participants were analyzed. Diabetes was present in 2,690 of those screened. Chronic kidney disease was seen in 46.4% of this population. Targeted community screening for kidney disease in a high-risk population can identify persons who may have not otherwise sought medical management.

McGill JB et al: Kidney early evaluation program (KEEP): findings from a community screening program, *Diabetes Educator* 30(2):196-209, 2004.

ADDITIONAL NURSING DIAGNOSES

See "Altered Protection" in "Pulmonary Emboli," p. 192. For more information about fluid and electrolytes, see "Fluid and Electrolyte Disturbances," p. 538. Also see "Prolonged Immobility," p. 61.

Bibliography

Criddle LM: Rhabdomyolysis: pathophysiology, recognition and management, *Crit Care Nurs* 23(6):14-32, December, 2003.

Dipiro J et al: *Pharmacotherapy: a pathophysiologic approach,* Norwalk, Conn, 1997, Appleton & Lange.

Dirkes S: Continuous renal replacement therapy: dialytic therapy for acute renal failure in intensive care, *Nephrol Nurs J* 27(6):581-590, 2000.

Esson M, Schrier R: Diagnosis and treatment of acute tubular necrosis, *Ann Intern Med* 137(9):744-750 2002.

Eknoyan G: Emergence of the concept of acute renal failure, *Am J Nephrol* 22:225-230, 2002.

Gaston R: Maintenancy immunosuppression in the renal transplant recipient: an overview, *Am J Kidney Dis* 38(6):S35, 2001.

Huizinga R: Update in immunosuppression, *Nephrol Nurs J* 29(3):261-267, 2002.

Kaplow R, Barry R: Continuous renal replacement therapies, *Am J Nurs* 102(11):26-33, 2002.

Kim MJ, McFarland GK, McLane AM: *Pocket guide to nursing diagnoses,* ed 7, St Louis, 1997, Mosby.

Lancaster L, editor: *Core curriculum for nephrology nursing,* ed 4, Pitman, NJ, 2001, Anthony J. Janetti.

Metcalfe W et al: Acute renal failure requiring renal replacement therapy: incidence and outcome, *Q J Med* 95:579-583, 2002.

Nowbar S, Anderson RJ: Acute renal failure; Chronic renal failure. In Parrillo JE, Dellinger RP: *Critical care medicine,* ed 2, St Louis, 2002, Mosby.

Pruchnicke M, Dasta J: Acute renal failure in hospitalized patients: part I, *Ann Pharmacother* 36:1261-1266, 2002.

Pruchnicke M, Dasta J: Acute renal failure in hospitalized patients: part II, *Ann Pharmacother* 36:1430-1439, 2002.

Tonelli M et al: Acute renal failure in the intensive care unit: a systematic review of the impact of dialytic modality on mortality and renal recovery, *Am J Kidney Dis* 40(5):875-884, 2002.

Neurologic Dysfunctions

Myasthenia Gravis

PATHOPHYSIOLOGY

Myasthenia gravis (MG) is a chronic, progressive autoimmune disorder causing weakness and abnormal fatigability of the voluntary striated skeletal muscles. Remissions and exacerbations can occur. MG usually affects women between 20 and 40 years of age and men after age 40. The peak incidence for women is during the second and third decades and for men during the sixth decade. The overall ratio of women affected to men is 3:2. The course of the disease depends on the muscle groups involved and the degree of their involvement.

MG causes changes in the structural integrity of the postsynaptic membrane at the neuromuscular junction with a marked reduction in the number of acetylcholine receptors (AChR). Acetylcholine (ACh), a neurotransmitter, is synthesized and stored in the terminal expansion of motor nerve axons. During the several milliseconds of neurotransmission, ACh is released into the synaptic cleft and the attachment of ACh to AChR on the postsynaptic membrane. This activates muscle action potential, with resultant muscle contraction. The process terminates when ACh is removed from the neuromuscular junction by the action of acetylcholinesterase, which deactivates ACh during breakdown. Of patients with MG, 85%-90% have an anti-AChR antibody (immunoglobulin) called AChRIgG, which causes either blockade, decreased synthesis of AChR, or increased degradation of or damage to the postsynaptic membrane. Some patients may have increased proliferative responses of T cells to AChR.

MG is associated with other autoimmune disorders, including rheumatoid arthritis, systemic lupus erythematosus, thyrotoxicosis, Sjögren's syndrome, polymyositis, ulcerative colitis, and pernicious anemia. The thymus gland undergoes pathologic changes in 80% of MG patients, and may produce antiacetylcholine receptor antibodies when exposed to inflammation.

ASSESSMENT

Clinical presentation: Weakness and abnormal fatigability of skeletal muscles which worsens with sustained efforts.

Symptom progression

Ocular muscle group: First muscle group to be affected in 65% of patients. During course of disease, 90% will have ocular involvement. Eye signs include ptosis, diplopia, inability to maintain upward gaze.

Muscles of face and neck, bulbar signs: Second area of involvement. *Bulbar signs* are present, with increased risk of aspiration due to difficulty chewing, dysphagia, dysarthria, inability to close mouth, nasal regurgitation of fluids, mushy and nasal tone to voice, neck-muscle weakness with head bob, inability to raise chin off chest, and loss of facial expression.

Muscles of limbs and trunk: Lastly, there is decreased strength in all extremities, with inability to maintain position without support. Weakness is greater in proximal muscles than distal. Diaphragmatic and intercostal weakness, dyspnea, ineffective cough, and accumulation of secretions, with increased risk for respiratory arrest.

Myasthenic and cholinergic crises: Patients may experience either a myasthenic or cholinergic crisis rapidly or incipiently, ultimately resulting in respiratory failure. Endotracheal (ET) intubation or tracheostomy with mechanical ventilation may be needed. Crisis is dramatic and frightening. The patient is acutely aware of all sensations and may be knowledgeable about the disease. The nurse should listen to and observe the patient closely. Increasing anxiety, apprehension, or insomnia may indicate the onset of crisis.

Although respiratory rate (RR) and arterial blood gas (ABG) values may be normal, the patient may have subtle decreases in chest expansion and air movement. Increased dysphagia, dysarthria, and dysphonia and an accumulation of oropharyngeal secretions increases the risk of aspiration.

Myasthenic crisis: Occurs when the patient needs increased medication as a result of drug tolerance or an exacerbation of the disease. Infection, trauma, surgery, temperature extremes, stress, endocrine imbalance, or intake of medications with neuromuscular-blocking properties, such as sedatives, tranquilizers, opiates, or antibiotics (e.g., neomycin, kanamycin, gentamicin, streptomycin, tetracycline) may prompt crisis.
- *Signs and symptoms:* Increasing muscle weakness despite normal or increased drug dosage, increasing anxiety and apprehension, severe ocular and bulbar weakness, with rapid onset of respiratory muscle weakness, which can lead to respiratory arrest.

Cholinergic crisis: Results from an overdose of anticholinesterase medication, causing a depolarizing neuromuscular blockade.
- *Signs and symptoms:* Increasing muscle weakness, increasing anxiety and apprehension, fasciculations (twitching) around the eyes and mouth, diarrhea and cramping, sweating, pupillary constriction, sialorrhea (excessive salivation), and difficulty breathing and swallowing.

DIAGNOSTIC TESTS

Tensilon test: This test identifies the type of crisis. In myasthenic crisis, the weakness improves with edrophonium chloride (Tensilon), whereas in cholinergic crisis the symptoms worsen. Tensilon is a short-acting anticholinesterase agent that delays hydrolysis of ACh, permitting the ACh released by the nerve to act repeatedly over a longer period. In the patient with MG, weakness and muscle fatigue will improve within 30-60 sec of receiving IV Tensilon injection (2-10 mg), and improvement will last up to 5 min. This test is done by the neurologist who assesses the patient's immediate response.

> **Caution:** Have atropine sulfate at the bedside during Tensilon test to reverse the effects of Tensilon if the patient is in cholinergic crisis.

Serum antibody titer: Elevated serum antibodies against acetylcholine receptors are present in 80%-90% of cases of generalized MG. A correlation between titer level and disease severity and course has not been proven.

Electromyography (EMG): Muscle action potentials are recorded from selected skeletal muscles. The amplitude of the evoked muscle action potentials falls rapidly in persons with MG.

Mediastinal magnetic resonance imaging (MRI) of the thymus gland: To evaluate for thymic abnormalities, present in 80% of patients with MG. Of this group, 65%-90% have thymic hyperplasia, whereas 10%-15% have gross or microscopic thymomas.

Mediastinoscopy: To evaluate for the presence of thymic abnormalities (see preceding section, "Mediastinal MRI").

Thyroid studies: To evaluate for hyperthyroidism. Thyroid abnormalities are often present in young women. MG is also associated with *Hashimoto thyroiditis,* an autoimmune thyroid disorder.

Other laboratory studies: Serum creatine phosphokinase (CPK), erythrocyte sedimentation rate (ESR), and antinuclear antibody levels are studied because of a frequent concurrence of other immunologic disorders with MG.

COLLABORATIVE MANAGEMENT

Emergency interventions for myasthenic or cholinergic crisis: Once the patient is stabilized in the intensive care unit (ICU), the type of crisis is identified, and specific treatment is begun. Anticholinesterase medications may be withheld or reduced temporarily. A "drug holiday" will improve subsequent patient responsiveness to medication. With the resumption of anticholinesterase medications, dosage, timing, and combinations of medications will need readjustment. In severe MG, plasmapheresis (see below) may hasten improvement in signs and symptoms.

Pharmacotherapy during noncrisis periods: Medications must be given on time to maintain therapeutic effects. Drug combinations are patient-specific.

Cholinesterase inhibitors: Pyridostigmine bromide (Mestinon), neostigmine bromide (Prostigmin), and ambenonium chloride (Mytelase) are used to inhibit the hydrolysis of ACh by acetylcholinesterase at the neuromuscular junction. Pyridostigmine is often used, since it has fewer side effects and is longer acting. The patient is given one tablet q3h during the day, and the dose is adjusted based on effects. Sustained-release preparations usually are given at bedtime to maintain the patient's strength throughout the night and early morning hours.

Immunosuppression: glucocorticosteroids (e.g., adrenocorticotropic hormone [ACTH] and prednisone) and other immunosuppressive agents: Glucocorticosteroids are used alone or in conjunction with anticholinesterase drugs. They provide clinical improvement for 70%-100% of patients with MG who refuse surgery and have weakness uncontrolled by anticholinesterase drugs. Although the mechanism of action of steroids is uncertain, studies indicate they directly influence neuromuscular transmission, suppress the action of the immune system by decreasing the size of the thymus gland and lymphatic tissue, decrease circulating lymphocytes, and decrease antireceptor reactivity of peripheral lymphocytes. Treatment is continued indefinitely. Glucocorticosteroids produce favorable results in all patients with muscle involvement, from ocular to severe respiratory impairment. Azathioprine (Imuran) may be used alone or in combination with other therapies in situations in which response to steroids is poor. Side effects include toxic hepatitis, thrombocytopenia, leukopenia, leukemia, lymphoma, infections, vomiting, and teratogenic effects.

Immune globulin: Routine use of human immune globulin (IG) is not recommended, but administration of intravenous immunoglobulin (IVIg) may be considered in patients with severe MG for whom other treatments have been unsuccessful or contraindicated.

Plasmapheresis: A complete exchange of plasma with removal of abnormal circulating antibodies that interfere with acetylcholine receptors. Table 6-1 describes potential complications, nursing assessments and interventions. (For additional information about fluid and electrolyte disturbances, see p. 538.)

Thymectomy: Removal of the thymus gland may prompt clinical improvement in 70% of patients, particularly newly diagnosed females with hyperplasia of thymic tissue. A suprasternal approach, a transsternal approach with sternal splitting, or the minimally invasive technique called video-assisted thoracic surgery (VATS) may be used. Plasmapheresis sometimes is used before surgery to increase strength and allow for a decrease in medication dosage.

Respiratory support: ET intubation or tracheostomy with mechanical ventilation may be necessary, depending on the degree of involvement of the respiratory muscles. (See "Mechanical Ventilation," p. 14.) Bilevel positive pressure ventilation (BiPAP) to permit intubation to be avoided is undergoing clinical trials in MG patients.

Nutritional support: If patient has dysphagia, enteral or parenteral feedings may be needed. (See "Nutritional Support," p.1.)

NURSING DIAGNOSES AND INTERVENTIONS

Impaired gas exchange related to altered oxygen supply associated with decreases in chest expansion and air movement secondary to weakness and abnormal fatigability of pharyngeal, diaphragmatic, intercostal, and accessory muscles of respiration

Desired outcome: Within 12-24 hr of initiation of treatment, patient has adequate gas exchange as evidenced by orientation to time, place, and person; RR ≤20 breaths/min with normal depth and pattern (eupnea); PaO_2 ≥80 mm Hg; $PaCO_2$ ≤45 mm Hg; and oxygen saturation ≥95%.

- Assess patient for indicators of impending respiratory failure or hypoxia: diminished or adventitious breath sounds; changes in rate, rhythm, or depth of respirations; pallor; nasal flaring, use of accessory muscles; and restlessness, irritability, confusion, or somnolence.
- Monitor ventilatory capability via pulmonary function tests. Vital capacity <75% of predicted value, tidal volume <1000 ml (or patient's normal/baseline volume), and RR >34 breaths/min are signals of the need for assisted ventilation.
- Monitor ABG and pulse oximetry results. Falling PaO_2 (<60 mm Hg), rising $PaCO_2$ (>50 mm Hg), and falling oxygen saturation, coupled with changes in vital capacity, tidal volume, and increasing RR, indicate the need for additional respiratory support.
- Provide pulmonary toilet q2h when patient is awake and prn. In addition, turn patient after each physiotherapy session to facilitate lung expansion, decrease risk of atelectasis, and prevent consolidation of secretions.

> **Note:** If mechanical ventilation already is in place, ventilator settings will vary, depending on patient's size and ABG results. Check ventilator settings at set intervals. Consult with anesthesia and/or respiratory therapy staff members regarding setting changes as patient's needs change.

Refer to the following interventions from the Nursing Interventions Classification (NIC):

NIC Respiratory Monitoring; Airway Management; Coping Enhancement; Acid-Base Monitoring; Oxygen Therapy

Ineffective airway clearance related to ineffective cough; decreased energy; abnormal fatigability of diaphragmatic, intercostal, pharyngeal, and accessory muscles of respiration
Desired outcome: Within 24-48 hr of intervention/treatment, patient's airway is clear as evidenced by absence of adventitious breath sounds.

- Assess breath sounds, effectiveness of patient's cough, and the quality, amount, and color of sputum. Consult physician for significant findings, including patient's inability to raise secretions; for secretions that are tenacious, thick, or voluminous.
- Suction secretions as indicated, using hyperoxygenation before and after procedure.

> **Note:** To prevent aspiration of secretions, always suction the trachea and mouth before deflating endotracheal or tracheostomy cuff. Consider use of endotracheal tube (ETT) with continuous supraglottic suction, if available. This is especially important because of the increase in saliva.

- Place patient in semi-Fowler's to high Fowler's position to facilitate chest excursion and decrease risk of aspiration. Fully elevate head of bed (HOB) during feedings.
- Assess vital signs (VS) for indicators of atelectasis and upper respiratory infection (see "Risk for Infection," which follows). Consult physician for significant findings.
- Increase activity as tolerated to minimize stasis of secretions and to facilitate lung expansion.
- Administer or assist with noninvasive positive pressure breathing (BiPAP) as needed..
- Keep a tracheostomy tube and obturator at the bedside in the event of inadvertent extubation.

NIC Airway Management; Artificial Airway Management; Cough Enhancement: Oxygen Therapy; Ventilation Assistance

Risk for infection related to inadequate primary defenses (stasis of secretions); inadequate secondary defenses (suppressed inflammatory response); invasive procedures (e.g., insertion of ETT); chronic disease
Desired outcome: Patient is free of infection as evidenced by normothermia; heart rate (HR) 60-100 beats/min; pulmonary secretions that are clear, thin in consistency, and odorless; and white blood cell (WBC) count $\leq 11,000/mm^3$.

- Monitor for temperature $\geq 37.7°$ (100° F), tachycardia, and diaphoresis.
- Assess color, consistency, amount, and odor of secretions. Report changes in sputum color to the physician. Obtain sputum specimens for culture as indicated.
- Monitor complete blood cell count (CBC) results for elevation of WBC count ($>11,000/mm^3$).
- Administer antibiotics as prescribed.
- Protect patient from persons with infection, particularly upper respiratory infection (URI).
- Turn and reposition patient at least q2h to prevent stasis of secretions.
- See Appendix 8 for more information.

NIC Cough Enhancement; Infection Protection; Surveillance

Impaired swallowing related to decreased or absent gag reflex; decreased strength or excursion of muscles involved in mastication; facial paralysis; mechanical obstruction (tracheostomy tube)
Desired outcome: Before oral foods and fluids are given or reintroduced, patient demonstrates capability for safe and effective swallowing as evidenced by presence of gag reflex and adequate strength and excursion of muscles involved in mastication.

- Assess patient for the presence of the gag reflex, ability to swallow, and strength and excursion of muscles involved in mastication. As indicated, consult with a speech therapist to determine patient's ability to swallow.
- If patient cannot swallow, confer with physician regarding alternate method of nutritional support, such as enteral or parenteral nutrition (see "Nutritional Support," p. 1).
- After patient's gag reflex and ability to swallow return, begin oral feedings cautiously.
  - ❑ When reinstating oral intake, offer a few ice chips to help stimulate the swallowing reflex, progress to semisolid foods (e.g., textured food, applesauce) and then to solid foods. Confer with speech/swallowing therapist regarding a dysphagia diet and teaching swallowing techniques.

❏ Elevate HOB ≥70 degrees to facilitate gravity flow through the pylorus and to minimize regurgitation and aspiration.

❏ Provide small feedings at frequent intervals (e.g., q4h while patient is awake).

❏ Avoid cold foods and beverages, which cause bloating and upward pressure on the diaphragm.

❏ Keep suction equipment at the bedside; suction excess secretions as necessary after each feeding. Inspect the mouth for residual food after meals. Provide for oral hygiene after every meal.

- If patient begins oral feedings with a tracheostomy tube in place, elevate HOB ≥70 degrees. Inflate tracheostomy tube cuff for 30 min before and after feeding to prevent aspiration. Progress the diet slowly, as described in the previous intervention.
- If patient is unable to communicate verbally, be alert to signs of severe aspiration: dyspnea, tachypnea, restlessness, agitation, pallor, and presence of adventitious breath sounds. If these signs occur, discontinue feeding immediately; elevate HOB; and provide oxygen. If a tracheostomy tube is in place, suction to remove food or secretions obstructing the airway.

NIC Aspiration Precautions; Swallowing Therapy; Positioning; Nutrition Management

Sensory/perceptual alterations (visual) related to altered sensory reception associated with diplopia or ptosis

Desired outcome: Within 48-72 hr of this diagnosis, patient relates that vision is adequate to perform activities of daily living (ADLs).

- Assess for and document signs of weakness of the ocular muscles (i.e., diplopia, ptosis, incomplete closure of the eye).
- Provide an eye patch or frosted lens for the patient with diplopia; alternate the patch or lens to the opposite eye q2-3h during patient's waking hours.
- Provide eyelid crutches for the patient with ptosis, or loosely tape eyelids open but *only* when providing direct care.
- Administer artificial tears in each eye at least q4-6h to lubricate and protect corneal tissue.
- As indicated, provide assistance with ADLs and ambulation to protect patient from injury.
- Keep patient's environment consistent to facilitate location of desired objects.

NIC Communication Enhancement: Visual Deficit; Environmental Management; Fall Prevention; Surveillance: Safety

Knowledge deficit: thymectomy procedure, including preoperative and postoperative care

Desired outcome: Before surgery, patient verbalizes understanding of the surgical procedure, including preoperative and postoperative care.

- Explain thymectomy and its relationship to myasthenia gravis.
- Provide information about preoperative routine. Discuss medications, application of antiembolic hose, the potential for postoperative discomfort, and the availability of analgesic agents. Advise patient that medications may change after surgery, as the patient may improve. With a thoracotomy approach, explain postoperative chest tubes. With a transcervical approach, a wound drainage system (e.g., Hemovac) is used.
- Teach coughing and deep-breathing techniques used after surgery.
- Explain that plasmapheresis may be performed preoperatively to improve the patient's clinical state. (See "Knowledge Deficit: Purpose and Procedure for Plasmapheresis," which follows.)
- Explain that pulmonary function and ABG studies will be performed preoperatively and postoperatively to assist in determining the patient's respiratory status.
- Explain the possibility of tracheostomy with assisted ventilation to prevent respiratory problems that can occur from stresses of surgery or myasthenic or cholinergic crisis.
- Explain that results of a thymectomy vary and may not be apparent for several months to years.

Knowledge deficit: purpose and procedure for plasmapheresis

Desired outcome: Before the first plasma exchange, patient verbalizes knowledge of the purpose and procedure for plasmapheresis.

- Assess patient's previous experience with and knowledge of plasmapheresis.
- As appropriate, teach patient the following about plasmapheresis: (1) blood is withdrawn via an arterial catheter, anticoagulated, and then passed through a cell separator; (2) the plasma portion of the blood that contains the AChR antibodies is removed; (3) red blood cells (RBCs), WBCs, and platelets are mixed with saline, potassium, and plasma protein fraction and then are returned to the body.
- Advise patient that plasmapheresis is generally performed to control severe symptoms until other modalities (i.e., medications, thymectomy) take effect, when other treatments have failed, or to increase patient's strength and improve general status before surgery.
- Explain that the nurse will make assessments before, during, and after plasmapheresis (see Table 6-1).
- Advise patient the procedure takes several hours and may be performed daily.

TABLE 6-1   Nursing Interventions for Complications of Plasmapheresis

Hypovolemia

Can result from rapid removal of up to 3 L of body fluid during plasmapheresis with volume replacement that is too slow during the procedure

- Perform a baseline assessment of patient's weight, skin turgor, and VS before the procedure is begun. During plasmapheresis, monitor patient for thirst, poor skin turgor, dizziness, confusion, nausea, and flattened neck veins. Assess VS continuously for evidence of hypovolemia, including decreased BP and increased HR. Monitor Hct for elevation, which occurs with hypovolemia. Weigh patient after procedure. Remember that 1 L of fluid equals 1 kg; thus hypovolemia can be reflected readily in weight changes.
- Provide fluids during plasmapheresis as prescribed, via oral, enteral, or IV access.
- Monitor and record I&O throughout the procedure. Be alert to oliguria (urinary output <30 ml/hr for 2 consecutive hours).
- Protect patients who are dizzy or confused by keeping side rails up and the bed in its lowest position.

Clotting abnormalities

Can result from removal of clotting factors during plasmapheresis

- Assess PT, PTT, and platelet count before and after procedure. Be alert to PT and PTT greater than those of control values and to increased platelet count. Normal ranges are as follows: PT 11-15 sec, PTT 30-40 sec, and platelet count 150,000-400,000/mm^3.
- Be alert to signs of impaired clotting, such as oozing from arterial puncture, venous access, or IV sites. Monitor patient for epistaxis or other signs of hemorrhage, such as elevated pulse rate, decreased BP, or changes in patient's mental status.
- Apply firm, continuous (e.g., for 10 min) pressure to the arterial puncture site once the catheter or needle is removed. A pressure dressing is recommended.
- Check gastric aspirate and stools for occult blood.
- Instruct patient to alert staff to the presence of bleeding from puncture and other sites.

Hypokalemia

Can result from removal of potassium during the plasma exchange

- Assess serum potassium before, during, and after plasma exchange. Be alert to decreasing levels (<3.5 mEq/L).
- Monitor for physical signs of hypokalemia, including bradycardia, fatigue, leg cramps, nausea, and paresthesias.
- Observe cardiac monitor for signs of cardiac dysrhythmias: ST segment depression, flattened T wave, presence of U wave, and ventricular dysrhythmias. Report abnormal cardiac rhythms to physician.
- During reinfusion of blood, administer potassium as prescribed to prevent hypokalemia and dangerous dysrhythmias. If prescribed, administer antidysrhythmic agents.

Hypocalcemia

Can result from binding of calcium to ACD, the anticoagulants used during plasmapheresis

- Assess serum calcium levels before, during, and after plasmapheresis. Be alert to decreasing levels (<8.5 mg/dl).
- Monitor patient for signs of hypocalcemia, such as numbness with tingling of fingers and circumoral area, hyperactive reflexes, muscle cramps, tetany, paresthesia, Chvostek's sign (see p. 554), diffuse irritability, emotional instability, impaired memory, and confusion.
- Observe cardiac monitor for evidence of hypocalcemia: prolonged QT interval caused by elongation of ST segment.
- Encourage patient to drink milk before and during the plasma exchange.
- As prescribed, administer calcium gluconate during plasmapheresis if indicators of hypocalcemia occur.

TABLE 6-1   Nursing Interventions for Complications of Plasmapheresis—cont'd

Myasthenic crisis

Can result from removal of circulating anticholinesterase drugs during plasmapheresis

Cholinergic crisis

Can result from removal of antibodies and decreased need for anticholinesterase drugs after plasmapheresis

- In the event of either crisis, have the following available: IV infusion apparatus, medications (edrophonium chloride [Tensilon], neostigmine bromide, atropine, and pralidoxime chloride [Protopam Chloride]), manual resuscitator, oxygen, suction equipment, and intubation tray if intubation is not already in place.
- Monitor patient for evidence of crisis, such as decreased vital capacity (<1 L), inability to swallow, ptosis, diplopia, dysarthria, dysphonia, dyspnea, muscle weakness, and nasal flaring. Stay with patient if these signs appear, and notify physician promptly.

CAUTION: Patients on prednisone or digitalis therapy are at increased risk for hypokalemia and should be monitored closely for its occurrence.

ACD, Acid-citrate-dextrose; *BP,* blood pressure; *Hct,* hematocrit; *HR,* heart rate; *I&O,* intake and output; *IV,* intravenous; *kg,* kilogram; *L,* liter; *PT,* prothrombin time; *PTT,* partial thromboplastin time; *VS,* vital signs.

- Explain that the degree of weakness may increase during and after the procedure because of the removal of plasma-bound medications (corticosteroids, anticholinesterase agents). Reassure patient that he or she will be monitored closely during the procedure and will receive appropriate medication after plasmapheresis.

Knowledge deficit: signs and symptoms of myasthenic and cholinergic crises

Desired outcome: Within 24 hr of stabilization of respiratory status, patient and significant others verbalize the signs and symptoms of impending myasthenic and cholinergic crises.

- Assess patient's/family's knowledge of myasthenic and cholinergic crises.
- Explain the differences between *myasthenic crisis:* an exacerbation of the myasthenic symptoms, frequently triggered by an infection; and *cholinergic crisis:* an episode triggered by toxic levels of anticholinesterase medication. The crisis, regardless of type, may manifest similar symptoms, including abdominal cramping, diarrhea, generalized weakness, increased pulmonary secretions, and impaired respiratory function.
- Advise patient/family to report immediately indications of crisis.
- Prepare patient for potential discharge when stabilized and consider the use of home health services for follow-up after discharge.
- Recommend that emergency respiratory support equipment (resuscitator bag and suction apparatus) be available in the home if patient has a history of crisis events.
- Advise patient to carry an identification card with diagnosis, medications, medication contraindications, and physician's name and phone number.
- Provide contact information for Myasthenia Gravis Foundation of America, Inc. Address: 222 South Riverside Plaza, Suite 1540, Chicago, IL 60606; phone: 1-800-541-5454, 1-312-258-0522; fax: 1-312-258-0461; website: www.Myasthenia@myasthenia.org.

ADDITIONAL NURSING DIAGNOSES

See also "Nutritional Support," p. 1; "Mechanical Ventilation," p. 14; "Psychosocial Support," p. 68; and "Psychosocial Support for the Patient's Family and Significant Others," p. 78. Also see "Knowledge Deficit: Immunosuppressive Medications and Their Side Effects" in "Renal Transplantation," p. 332.

Guillain-Barré Syndrome (GBS)

PATHOPHYSIOLOGY

Guillain-Barré syndrome (GBS) is an acute inflammatory, immune-mediated, demyelinating polyneuropathy of the peripheral nervous system, affecting 1.5-2 individuals per 100,000 people. GBS affects mainly the Schwann cell, which synthesizes and maintains the peripheral nerve myelin sheath. Studies suggest that macrophages penetrate the basement membrane and strip apparently normal myelin from intact peripheral nerve axons, causing the characteristic signs and symptoms of GBS. The ventral (motor) root axons of the anterior horn cells, which innervate voluntary skeletal muscles, are primarily involved. Dorsal (sensory) root axons of the posterior horn are not as affected. Recovery of neurologic function depends on proliferation of Schwann cells and remyelination of axons. Recovery can be expected in 80%-90% of cases, with minor residual deficits in less than half of the patients, and 2%-5% experiencing recurrence after complete recovery.

ASSESSMENT

History and risk factors: Respiratory or gastrointestinal (GI) illness 10-14 days before onset of the neurologic symptoms, in which (1) a viral agent such as parainfluenza 2 virus, measles, mumps, rubella, varicella, or herpes zoster is present (50% of cases); (2) recent vaccination (15% of cases), such as for influenza; (3) recent surgical procedure (5% of cases). Miller Fisher syndrome, an acute axonal variant of GBS, has been shown to follow infection with *Campylobacter jejuni*.

Clinical presentation: There are several clinical variations of signs and symptoms described as either ascending, descending, the Miller Fisher variant, or pure motor. The disease generally has three phases: (1) acute phase of 1-3 wks after onset of the first symptom; (2) plateau phase beginning with no further clinical deterioration and lasting several days to weeks; and (3) recovery phase, which can last 4 months up to 2 yr and correlates with the remyelination and axonal regrowth process.

Ascending flaccid motor paralysis is the most common presenting sign and is associated with the early loss of deep tendon reflexes (DTRs). Weakness, usually preceding the paralysis, is symmetric, begins in distal muscle groups, and ascends to involve more proximal muscles. Muscles of respiration (intercostals and diaphragm) are frequently involved. Approximately half of all patients will require mechanical ventilation. Complaints of mild sensory symptoms such as distal paresthesias are common. In more serious or prolonged cases, proprioceptive and vibratory dysfunctions are present. Loss of pain and temperature sensations in a glove-and-stocking distribution has been reported. Sensory complaints usually appear first, with muscle weakness developing rapidly over 24-72 hr. About 90% of patients reach the peak of dysfunction within 2 wks.

Autonomic nervous system involvement (a type of autonomic dysreflexia): Occurs in most patients with GBS: sinus tachycardia, bradycardia, orthostatic hypotension, hypertension, excessive diaphoresis, bowel and bladder retention, loss of sphincter control, increased pulmonary secretions, syndrome of inappropriate antidiuretic hormone secretion (SIADH), and cardiac dysrhythmias (a common cause of death).

Cranial nerve involvement: All cranial nerves except I and II may be involved. See Appendix 4.

Physical assessment: Symmetric motor weakness, decreased or absent DTRs, hypotonia or flaccidity of affected muscles, presence of respiratory abnormalities (e.g., nasal flaring, hypoventilation), facial paralysis.

DIAGNOSTIC TESTS

The diagnosis for GBS is based on clinical presentation, history of antecedent illness, and cerebrospinal fluid (CSF) findings. A detailed neurological examination must be done as a baseline to assess for any changes as the disease progresses.

Lumbar puncture (LP) and CSF analysis: CSF analysis usually shows *albuminocytologic dissociation*: an elevated protein, without increase in WBCs. This dissociation may be noted during the course of GBS and is helpful in differentiating GBS from other central nervous system (CNS) disorders. CSF protein, normally between 15-45 mg/dl, may peak 4-6 wks after onset of GBS to levels of several hundred mg/dl. The CSF findings may be due to deposits of immunoglobulins IgG, IgM, and IgA localized to the nerve roots.

Electrodiagnostic studies: Electromyography (EMG) and nerve conduction velocity (NCV) demonstrate profound slowing of motor conduction velocities and conduction blocks several weeks into the illness as a result of the demyelination of peripheral nerves.

Pulmonary function studies: Performed during initial diagnostic evaluation. Vital capacity (VC) of <1 L indicates a possible need for assisted ventilation and should be assessed every 2-4 hr during the early acute phase.

ABG studies: Performed if VC drops below 1 L or if patient demonstrates dyspnea, confusion, restlessness, nasal flaring, use of accessory muscles of respiration, or breathlessness (noted during a count by the patient from 1-10). A decrease in PaO_2 >10-15 mm Hg or an increase in $PaCO_2$ of 10-15 mm Hg over baseline or normal value signals the need for immediate intubation or tracheostomy.

COLLABORATIVE MANAGEMENT

Respiratory support: ET intubation or tracheostomy with assisted mechanical ventilation, as necessary.

Plasmapheresis: Involves a complete exchange of plasma with the removal of abnormal circulating antibodies that affect the peripheral nerve myelin sheath. Removal of these autoantibodies may lessen the duration and severity of GBS. For nursing interventions for complications of plasmapheresis, see Table 6-1.

Intravenous immunoglobulin (IVIg): IVIg given at 0.4 mg/kg/body weight/day for 5 days has been recommended as an alternative to plasma exchange in children and adults with GBS.

Maintenance and monitoring of cardiovascular function: As necessary, cardiac monitoring may be initiated for dysrhythmias; arterial pressure monitoring may be used to evaluate hypertension or hypotension; and antihypertensive agents or vasopressors may be administered to maintain BP within normal levels.

Management of bowel and bladder dysfunction: Nasogastric suction and parenteral infusion may be started for patients with paralytic ileus; an indwelling urinary catheter may be inserted in patients with urinary retention.

Nutritional management: Parenteral feedings are given until return of peristalsis. Tube feedings or gastrostomy feedings are used for patients with severe dysphagia. With recovery of gag reflex and swallowing ability, the diet will progress to semisolid and solid foods, which are more readily swallowed than are liquids.

Rehabilitation: Active and passive range-of-motion (ROM) exercises are performed at frequent intervals during all phases of GBS. Activity must be balanced with caloric intake to prevent muscle wasting. As the patient's condition stabilizes, a physiatrist consultation to plan rehabilitation with physical and occupational therapy should be done while the patient is in critical care. The primary goal is to pace recovery to obtain maximum mobility, promote self-care and adapt to changes in body image. Rehabilitation does not improve nerve regeneration.

Caution: ROM must not be done strenuously during the acute phase because this may exacerbate weakness and possibly accelerate the demyelinating process.

NURSING DIAGNOSES AND INTERVENTIONS

Impaired gas exchange related to altered oxygen supply associated with decreased lung expansion secondary to weakness or paralysis of intercostal and diaphragmatic muscles

Desired outcome: Within 12-24 hr of this diagnosis, patient has adequate gas exchange as evidenced by orientation to time, place, and person; RR 12-20 breaths/min with normal pattern and depth; HR $\leq$100 beats/min; BP within patient's normal range; Pao_2 $\geq$80 mm Hg; $Paco_2$ $\leq$45 mm Hg; and oxygen saturation $\geq$94%.

- Assess neurologic function hourly, or as often as needed. Ascending motor and sensory dysfunctions usually occur rapidly (over 24-72 hr) and can lead to respiratory arrest.
- Monitor for respiratory distress. Report adventitious breath sounds (crackles, rhonchi); decreased or absent breath sounds; temperature $\geq$37.7° C (100° F); increased HR and BP; tidal volume or VC decreased from baseline; decreased Pao_2 or increased $Paco_2$ $\geq$10-15 mm Hg from baseline; abnormal respiratory rate or rhythm; increasing restlessness, anxiety, or confusion.
- Prepare to assist with intubation or tracheotomy for respiratory failure.
- Maintain mechanical ventilation as indicated. (See "Mechanical Ventilation," p. 14.)
- Monitor ABG results and pulse oximetry. Consult physician for continued abnormalities.

NIC Airway Management; Acid-Base Monitoring; Oxygen Therapy; Respiratory Monitoring

Ineffective airway clearance related to ineffective cough; decreased energy; increasing paralysis of respiratory, pharyngeal, and facial muscles; absence of the gag reflex

Desired outcome: Within 12-24 hr of this diagnosis, patient's airway is clear as evidenced by absence of adventitious breath sounds; HR 60-100 beats/min; BP within patient's baseline range; RR 12-20 breaths/min with normal depth and pattern (eupnea); tidal volume within baseline parameters; Pao_2 $\geq$80 mm Hg; $Paco_2$ $\leq$45 mm Hg.

- Monitor for crackles, rhonchi, and decreased or absent breath sounds; increased HR and BP; tidal volume or vital capacity decreased from baseline; abnormal respiratory rate or rhythm; decrease in Pao_2 or increase in $Paco_2$; and increasing restlessness or anxiety.
- Suction the airway as need is determined by auscultation findings. As the paresis or paralysis subsides (usually after 2-4 wks), cranial nerve function will begin to return (i.e., gag reflex, swallowing, coughing). Evaluate patient's ability to cough, whether or not he or she has been placed on mechanical ventilation. Assess for the presence of adventitious sounds to determine effectiveness of patient's cough.
- Deliver oxygen and humidification as prescribed.

- Maintain mechanical ventilation as prescribed. (See "Mechanical Ventilation," p. 14.)
- Maintain adequate hydration to minimize thickening of pulmonary secretions.
- Turn and reposition patient at least q2h to prevent stasis of secretions.

NIC Positioning; Airway Management; Respiratory Monitoring; Cough Enhancement; Airway Suctioning

Risk for disuse syndrome and deep vein thrombus related to ascending flaccid paralysis and paresthesias

Desired outcomes: Patient maintains baseline/optimal ROM of all joints and baseline muscle size and strength; no evidence of deep vein thrombus.

- Assess neurologic function hourly or as often as indicated. Ascending motor and sensory dysfunction usually occurs rapidly (over 24-72 hr). When neurologic dysfunction is progressing in GBS crisis, assess motor and sensory deficits by starting with the lower extremities and working upward.
  - ❏ Assess muscle symmetry by using a side-to-side comparison.
  - ❏ Assess for deep vein thrombus. Monitor for Homan's sign, fever, and calf tenderness. Apply antiembolic stockings as prescribed to help promote tissue perfusion.
  - ❏ Assess muscle strength: *For lower extremities:* have patient pull heel of foot toward the buttocks as you provide resistance by holding onto the foot. *For upper extremities:* have patient extend and flex the wrists and arms against your resistance.
  - ❏ Assess DTRs of the Achilles, patellae, biceps, triceps, and brachioradialis. Normal response is +2; report decreased (+1) or absent (0) response.
  - ❏ Assess for paresthesia, including the location, degree, and whether it is ascending.
  - ❏ Assess position sense by moving patient's big toe or thumb up and down while patient's eyes are closed. Note vibratory sense by placing a vibrating tuning fork over bony prominences.
  - ❏ Assess response to light touch or pinprick by starting at the feet and working upward to determine the level of dysfunction.

> **Note:** Sensory symptoms are usually milder than motor complaints, with vibration and position sensations affected most often. However, about 25% of affected patients will experience pain, requiring analgesia. When light touch, pinprick, and temperature sensations are affected, they most often are found in a glove-and-stocking distribution. Patients frequently experience muscle tenderness and sensitivity to pressure.

  - ❏ Assess for cranial nerve dysfunction (see Appendix 4).
- Record and report sensorimotor deficit, including degree of involvement.
- Turn and reposition patient in correct anatomic alignment q2h or more often if requested by patient. Support patient's position with pillows and other positioning aids.
- To maintain patient's muscle function and prevent contractures, ensure that active or passive ROM exercises are performed q2h during all phases of GBS. Involve significant others in exercises, if appropriate.
- Obtain a physical therapy referral, and begin rehabilitation planning process during the early stages of the disorder.
- As indicated, apply splints to hands-arms and feet-legs to help prevent contracture; alternate splints so that they are on for 2 hr and off for 2 hr.
- Specialty beds may be used to manage the respiratory, integumentary, autonomic, and musculoskeletal problems.

NIC Exercise Therapy (all); Exercise Promotion; Positioning

Autonomic dysreflexia (AD) (or risk for same) related to excessive or inadequate activity of the sympathetic or parasympathetic nervous system

Desired outcome: Patient has no symptoms of autonomic dysreflexia (AD) as evidenced by normal T wave configuration on ECG; HR 60-100 beats/min; BP within patient's normal range; cool and dry skin; patient's normal strength; and absence of headache and chest and abdominal tightness.

- Assess for signs of AD: cardiac dysrhythmias; HR <60 beats/min or >100 beats/min; elevated and sustained BP (e.g., ≥250-300/150 mm Hg); facial flushing; increased sweating, possibly caused by loss of thermal regulation; extreme generalized warmth; profound weakness; and complaints of severe headache or tightening in the chest and abdomen.
- Place patient on cardiac monitor as prescribed.

> **Note:** Because of the risk of fatal cardiac dysrhythmias in GBS, continuous cardiac monitoring is recommended for the first 10-14 days of hospitalization.

- Monitor patient carefully during activities that are known to precipitate AD: position changes, vigorous coughing, straining with bowel movements, and suctioning.
- Be aware of and implement measures to prevent and intervene immediately to remove causes that may precipitate AD such as the following:
  - *Bladder stimuli:* urinary tract infection, cystoscopy, urinary catheter insertion, clogged urinary catheter, urinary calculi.
  - *Bowel stimuli:* fecal impaction, rectal examination, enemas, suppositories.
  - *Sensory stimuli:* pressure caused by tight clothing, dressings, bed covers, thigh straps on urinary drainage bags; prolonged pressure on skin surface or over bony prominences; temperature changes, such as exposure to a cool breeze or draft.
- If indicators of AD are present, implement the following:
  - Elevate HOB or place patient in a sitting position to promote decrease in BP.
  - Monitor BP and HR q3-5min until patient's condition stabilizes.
- Determine and remove offending stimulus:
  - For example, if patient's bladder is distended, catheterize cautiously, using sufficient lubricant.
  - If patient has an indwelling urinary catheter, check for obstruction such as granulation in catheter or kinking of tubing. As indicated, irrigate catheter, using no more than 30 ml normal saline. If infection is suspected, obtain a urine specimen for culture and sensitivity testing once crisis stage has passed.
  - Check for fecal impaction. Perform the rectal examination gently, using an ointment that contains a local anesthetic (e.g., Nupercainal).
  - Check for sensory stimuli, loosen clothing, bed covers, or other constricting fabric as indicated.
- Consult physician if symptoms do not abate within 15-30 min, especially elevated BP. This may lead to: seizures, subarachnoid or intracerebral hemorrhage, or other stroke.
- As prescribed, administer antihypertensive agents and monitor effectiveness.

NIC Dysreflexia Management; Urinary Elimination Management

Decreased cardiac output (or risk for same) related to decreased afterload secondary to reduced peripheral vascular tone

---

Note: Normovolemic patients may have a decreased cardiac output as a result of vasodilation. This is similar to the vascular response seen in distributive (e.g., anaphylactic, septic) shock.

Desired outcome: Patient has adequate cardiac output as evidenced by BP within patient's normal range; HR 60-100 beats/min; urinary output ≥0.5 ml/kg/hr; peripheral pulses >2+ on a 0-4+ scale; orientation to time, place, and person; pulmonary artery wedge pressure (PAWP) 6-12 mm Hg; systemic vascular resistance (SVR) 900-1200 dynes/sec/cm^{-5}; cardiac output (CO) 4-7 L/min; and normal sinus rhythm.

- Monitor patient for indicators of decreased cardiac output: drop in systolic BP >20 mm Hg from baseline, systolic BP <80 mm Hg, or a continuing drop in systolic BP of 5-10 mm Hg with every assessment; HR >100 beats/min; irregular HR; restlessness, confusion, and dizziness; warm and flushed skin; edema; and decreased urinary output <0.5 ml/kg/hr for 2 consecutive hours. Monitor hemodynamic pressures, particularly PAWP, CO, and SVR.
- Assess cardiac rate and rhythm per cardiac monitor; report changes in rate and rhythm.
- Implement measures to prevent decreased cardiac output caused by orthostatic hypotension:
  - Change patient's position slowly.
  - Perform ROM exercises q2h to prevent venous pooling.
  - Apply elastic antiembolic hose as prescribed to promote venous return.
  - Keep patient's legs straight. Do not use pillows or "gatch" the knees on the bed.
  - Collaborate with physical therapist to use a tilt table to help stand the patient.
- As prescribed, administer fluids to treat the hypotension.
- Administer a vasopressor (e.g., norepinephrine) to counteract peripheral vasodilation.

NIC Cardiac Care: Acute; Hemodynamic Regulation; Resuscitation; Shock Prevention

Sensory/perceptual alterations (or risk for same) related to altered sensory transmission secondary to cranial nerve involvement with GBS

Desired outcomes: Patient reports normal vision and exhibits normal pupillary and gag reflexes, intact corneas, ability to masticate, and full ROM of head and shoulders.

- Assess cranial nerve function (see Appendix 4).
  - If patient experiences a deficit, place objects where patient can see them and assist with ADLs.
  - Cover one eye with a patch or frosted lens if patient has diplopia; alternate patch or lens q2-3h during patient's waking hours.
  - Use eyelid crutches for patients with ptosis.

❑ Assess patient for corneal irritation or abrasion. Apply artificial tear drops or ointments as prescribed. Secure the eyelid in a closed position if corneal reflex is diminished or absent.

❑ Suction during oral hygiene. Do not feed patient an oral diet until the gag reflex returns.

❑ Position patient's head in a position of comfort and proper anatomic alignment.

NIC Peripheral Sensation Management; Surveillance: Safety

Constipation, colonic related to hypoperistalsis or paralytic ileus associated with neuromuscular impairment

Desired outcome: Within 3-5 days of this diagnosis, patient has a bowel movement.

- Assess patient's GI status: bowel sounds, abdominal distention, nausea, vomiting, and abdominal discomfort. In the presence of hypoperistalsis or paralytic ileus, patient will exhibit (1) high-pitched, tinkling sounds that will be heard early in obstruction or ileus or (2) a decrease or absence of sounds occurring with complete obstruction or paralytic ileus.

- If patient is having bowel movements, determine the amount, consistency, and frequency. Question patient about his or her usual pattern of bowel elimination.

- Begin bowel training program based on patient's needs and status of dietary intake:
  ❑ Provide a high-fiber diet if patient is able to chew and swallow without difficulty.
  ❑ Give patient prune juice every evening.
  ❑ Establish a regular time for elimination and have a bed pan readily available.
  ❑ Facilitate patient's normal bowel habits; ensure privacy.
  ❑ Administer stool softeners (e.g., docusate sodium) or bulk-building additives such as psyllium.
  ❑ Administer prescribed medicated suppositories.

- Provide 2-3 L/day of fluid to prevent dehydration and constipation. This may be contraindicated for patient with impaired renal or cardiac status.

Caution: Care must be taken to avoid stimulation of autonomic dysreflexia by using generous amounts of anesthetic ointment and ensuring gentle insertion when giving suppository or enema.

NIC Constipation/Impaction Management; Bowel Management; Nutrition Management

- See "Risk for Disuse Syndrome," p. 356, for neuroassessment parameters. Also see Table 6-1 for the following complications: hypovolemia, clotting abnormalities, hypokalemia, and hypocalcemia.

- Resource for education: Guillain-Barré Syndrome Foundation International. Address: PO Box 262, Wynnewood, PA 19096; phone: 1-610-667-0131; fax: 1-610-667-7036; website: www.guillain-barre.com.

ADDITIONAL NURSING DIAGNOSES

See also "Urinary Retention" in "Acute Spinal Cord Injury," p. 146. See "Knowledge Deficit: Immunosuppressive Medications and Their Side Effects" in "Renal Transplantation," p. 332. See "Myasthenia Gravis" for "Risk for Infection," p. 350, and "Impaired Swallowing," p. 350. For other nursing diagnoses and interventions, see the following as appropriate: "Nutritional Support," p. 1; "Mechanical Ventilation," p. 14; "Prolonged Immobility," p. 61; "Psychosocial Support," p. 68; and "Psychosocial Support for the Patient's Family and Significant Others," p. 78.

Cerebral Aneurysm and Subarachnoid Hemorrhage

PATHOPHYSIOLOGY

An aneurysm is a localized dilation of an arterial lumen caused by weakness in the vessel wall. 90% of cerebral aneurysms are berry or saccular, while the other 10% are fusiform, traumatic, septic, dissecting, and Charcot-Bouchard aneurysms. Recent research suggests that cerebral aneurysms result from degenerative vascular diseases complicated by hypertension and atherosclerosis. Aneurysms most often occur at the bifurcation of the blood vessels of the circle of Willis, with 85% in anterior cerebral circulation and 15% in posterior cerebral circulation.

Aneurysms may be asymptomatic, but nearly half of the affected population experience some warning sign or symptom prior to rupture as a result of expansion of the lesion and compression of cerebral tissue. When rupture occurs, a subarachnoid hemorrhage (SAH) into the subarachnoid space (SAS) and basal cisterns results. If the patient survives the initial destruction of brain tissue by the force of arterial blood, intracerebral hemorrhage, and sharply increased intracranial pressure (ICP), the patient is then faced with the possibility of rebleeding and cerebral arterial vasospasm. The greatest incidence of rebleeding is between 3 and 11 days after SAH, with the peak at day 7. Mortality is about 70%. Theories of causation involve the normal process of clot dissolution coupled with fluctuations in arterial pressure.

Cerebral vasospasm, the constriction of the arterial smooth muscle layer of the major cerebral arteries, causes a dramatic decrease in cerebral blood flow, which in turn leads to cerebral ischemia and progressive neurologic deficit. Vasospasm occurs in as many as 60% of patients 4-14 days following SAH, with incidence peaking between 7 and 10 days. The pathogenesis of cerebral vasospasm is poorly understood but may be directly related to the amount of blood in the SAS and basal cisterns. The greater the volume of blood, the more pronounced the vasospasm. As clots in the basal cisterns begin to hemolyze, substances may be released that precipitate vasospasms. Current treatments include careful fluid balance, "triple H" (hypervolemia-hemodilution-hypertension) therapy, calcium antagonists, balloon or chemical angioplasty, and possibly cisternal fibrinolytic drugs. Clinical trials are underway using gene therapy and sustained release cisternal drugs. The patient with a ruptured cerebral aneurysm and SAH is also at risk for communicating hydrocephalus, hypothalamic dysfunction, and hyponatremia.

Communicating hydrocephalus: Communicating hydrocephalus develops in approximately 20% of patients with SAH as a result of the presence of blood in the SAS and ventricular system. The hydrocephalus may be *acute* (lasting <24 hr), *subacute* (lasting >24 h-1 wk), or *delayed* (beginning 10 or more days after SAH). Blood in the SAS and ventricles obstructs flow of CSF, interferes with circulation and resorption of CSF, and causes increased ICP, with concomitant worsening of neurologic status.

Hypothalamic dysfunction: Hypothalamic dysfunction, seen in approximately one third of patients with hydrocephalus after SAH, may result from mechanical pressure on the hypothalamus from a dilated third ventricle. The resultant increase in serum catecholamines leads to overstimulation of the sympathetic nervous system.

Hyponatremia: Hyponatremia may be caused by cerebral salt-wasting syndrome, SIADH, or a combination of factors influencing sodium and water metabolism. Hyponatremia may occur in 10%-50% of patients with SAH. Hyponatremia may lead to intracranial hypertension, cerebral ischemia, seizures, coma, and death. See Table 6-2 for signs and symptoms of cerebral salt-wasting syndrome and SIADH.

> **Note:** Both hypothalamic dysfunction and hyponatremia are seen more frequently in patients with extensive SAH and are positively correlated with the subsequent development of cerebral vasospasm.

ASSESSMENT

Signs and symptoms before and after rupture depend on the size, site, and amount of bleeding.

Warning signs and symptoms (before bleeding): Headaches; occasional ptosis and dilated pupil caused by palsy of cranial nerve III; diplopia, blurred vision, pain above and behind the eye; neck and upper back pain; nausea and vomiting.

T A B L E   6 - 2   Clinical Presentation With Cerebral Salt-Wasting Syndrome and Syndrome of Inappropriate Antidiuretic Hormone (SIADH)

Cerebral salt-wasting syndrome	SIADH
Hypotension	Normotension
Postural hypotension	Normal pulse rate or bradycardia
Tachycardia	Normal or low hematocrit
Elevated hematocrit	Increased glomerular filtration rate
Decreased glomerular filtration rate	Normal or decreased BUN and creatinine
Normal or elevated BUN and creatinine	Normal or low urine output
Normal or low urine output	Normovolemia or hypervolemia
Hypovolemia	Normal hydration
Dehydration	Dilutional hyponatremia
True hyponatremia	Hypoosmolality
Hypoosmolality	Increased body weight
Decreased body weight	

BUN, Blood urea nitrogen.

Clinical presentation after initial bleeding: Meningeal signs (caused by presence of blood in the SAS) include headache, nuchal rigidity, fever, photophobia, lethargy, nausea, and vomiting. Patients report that the headache is the worst they have ever experienced, a sensation of a "bullet going off in the head."

Increased intracranial pressure (IICP): Caused by SAH, intracerebral hemorrhage, or subsequent cerebral edema (Table 6-3; see also "Traumatic Brain Injury," p. 98).

Indicators of hydrocephalus

Acute: Loss of pupillary reflexes, persistent or sudden onset of coma within 24 hr of SAH.

Subacute: Gradual onset of confusion, drowsiness, lethargy, or stupor within 1-7 days of SAH.

Delayed: Gradual onset of confusion, incontinence, or impaired balance, mobility, and gait; intellectual impairment (slowness, mutism); lack of affect; and presence of the grasp and sucking frontal lobe reflexes (abnormal in adults), at about 10 days following SAH.

Hyponatremia: Anxiety, confusion, agitation, disorientation, lethargy, stupor, coma, anorexia, nausea, vomiting, abdominal pain, cold and clammy skin, generalized weakness, and lower extremity muscle cramps. See Table 6-2 for signs and symptoms of cerebral salt-wasting syndrome and SIADH.

Altered hypothalamic regulatory mechanisms: Vomiting, glycosuria, proteinuria, and hyponatremia. Increased circulating catecholamines can cause flushing, diaphoresis, pupillary dilation, decreased gastric motility, increased serum glucose, fever, hypertension, tachycardia, cardiac dysrhythmias, ischemia, and infarction.

Physical assessment: Pathologic reflexes caused by the presence of blood in the SAS.

Kernig's sign: Resistance to full extension of the leg at the knee when the hip is flexed.

Brudzinski's sign: Flexion of the hip and knee with neck flexion.

Funduscopic assessment: May reveal retinal hemorrhage(s) at the side of the optic disc. Hemorrhage is caused by blood from the SAS being forced along the optic nerve sheath under high pressure. The patient may complain of blurred vision or blind spots (scotomata).

Hunt-Hess classification system: Permits objective evaluation of progression of the patient's initial symptoms. Used to predict clinical outcomes and for choosing treatments. Critical care nurses can benefit from using this grading system. Grading is performed according to symptom presentation and level of consciousness (LOC).

> *Grade I:* Asymptomatic, alert, and oriented.
>
> *Grade II:* Alert, oriented, headache, and stiff neck.
>
> *Grade III:* Lethargic or confused; minor focal deficit such as hemiparesis.
>
> *Grade IV:* Stuporous, moderate to severe focal deficits, hemiplegia, possible early decerebrate rigidity, and vegetative disturbances.
>
> *Grade V:* Deep coma, decerebrate rigidity, moribund appearance.

TABLE 6-3 **Indicators of Increased Intracranial Pressure**

Alterations in consciousness: increasing restlessness, confusion, irritability, disorientation, increasing drowsiness, and lethargy

Bradycardia

Increasing systolic BP with a widening pulse pressure

Irregular respiratory patterns (e.g., Cheyne-Stokes, ataxic, apneustic, central neurogenic, hyperventilation)

Hemisensory changes and hemiparesis or hemiplegia: caused by involvement of hemispheric sensory and motor pathways

Worsening headache

Papillary changes

Dysconjugate gaze and inability to move one eye beyond midposition: caused by involvement of cranial nerves III, IV, and VI

Seizures

Involvement of other cranial nerves: depends on the severity of neurologic insult

---

Note: If these indicators of IICP are left untreated, the patient will undergo irreversible brain damage or death. If these indicators occur suddenly, there will be displacement of brain substance (herniation), which will progress rapidly to permanent brain damage or death. For additional information about herniation syndromes, see "Traumatic Brain Injury," p. 98.

BP, Blood pressure.

DIAGNOSTIC TESTS

Computed tomography (CT) brain scan: Usually the first diagnostic procedure for patients with suspicious symptoms. The CT imaging may reveal subarachnoid or intracerebral hemorrhage; size, site, and amount of bleeding; or presence of hydrocephalus caused by blocked CSF resorption. CT results can be negative with small aneurysms, when small hemorrhages are present, or if scan is done 2-3 days following aneurysm rupture.

Four-vessel cerebral angiography: Used to confirm the diagnosis of ruptured aneurysm and SAH. Shows size, location, and vessels involved and if other aneurysms are present. Helps determine the accessibility of the aneurysm and the presence of hematoma, vasospasm, and hydrocephalus. Panangiography of both carotid and vertebral arteries is recommended, since 15%-20% of patients have multiple aneurysms. Aneurysms unable to fill with contrast due to vasospasm, those filled with clotted blood, or those of small size may be missed by angiogram.

3-Dimensional digital subtraction angiography: A new computerized modality that reconstructs the anatomy of the aneurysm to help decide if treatment should be surgical vs. endovascular vs. *no* treatment. The x-ray tube revolves 180 degrees around the patient to create an image of the aneurysm, including its "neck." Visualization of the anatomy and the neck of the aneurysm is vital in choosing the appropriate endovascular treatment option: stents, angioplasty, or coils. Helps to determine risks and benefits of all treatments.

Lumbar puncture (LP) and CSF analysis: Confirms presence of blood in the CSF. CSF pressure, normally 0-15 mm Hg (75-180 mm H_2O), may elevate to 250 mm H_2O. The pressure is proportionate to the amount of bleeding. Protein may increase to 80-130 mg/dl (normal is 15-50 mg/dl). WBC count may be greater than the normal value of $\leq 10/mm^3$; and CSF glucose may be low (<40 mg/dl) in the presence of SAH.

Note: Performance of LP in the patient with SAH and IICP carries substantial risk of herniation and rebleeding. It is performed only when results of the CT are nondiagnostic.

Transcranial Doppler (TCD) ultrasonography: Evaluates arterial blood velocity through cerebral vessels over time to predict the possibility of cerebral vasospasm. A measurable increase in velocity can occur several hours before clinical signs of vasospasm occur. TCD studies can be done at the bedside to allow for timely repeated readings.

ABG analysis: To detect hypoxemia and hypercapnia and to determine appropriate respiratory therapy.

Electrocardiogram (ECG): To detect cardiac changes and dysrhythmias precipitated by hypothalamic dysfunction.

COLLABORATIVE MANAGEMENT

Respiratory support: Maintain patent airway and provide intubation and ventilation if needed. Serial ABG tests are performed to identify hypoxemia (Pao_2 <80 mm Hg) and hypercapnia ($Paco_2$ >45 mm Hg). Hypercapnia is a potent cerebral vasodilator that can increase ICP in patients who are already at risk.

Bed rest, with aneurysm precautions: Try to keep patient quiet and calm in a soothing environment, with lowered lights and noise level. Active ROM and isometric exercises are restricted during acute and preoperative stages to prevent IICP. Passive ROM is prescribed to prevent formation of thrombi, with subsequent pulmonary emboli. Bowel management program is essential to prevent straining at stool.

Intracranial pressure (ICP) monitoring: See "Collaborative Management" in "Traumatic Brain Injury," p. 103.

HOB elevation: A 30- to 45-degree angle facilitates venous outflow from the intracranial cavity and lowers ICP.

Fluid and electrolyte management: Fluid balance is maintained based on CVP, weight, PAWP, and serum osmolality. Electrolytes may be replaced using patient's clinical data and laboratory values. Hyponatremia is treated following careful evaluation for the etiology. Normal saline, packed RBCs, and colloids are recommended to treat true hyponatremia (cerebral salt-wasting.). If the cause is dilutional hyponatremia (SIADH), free water restriction is recommended. Fluid restriction may be 500-800 ml/24 hr to 1000-1500 ml/24 hr. If fluid restriction is not an option, sodium replacement is implemented. All therapies are done cautiously with frequent (at least q4h) assessment of fluid and electrolyte status.

Nutrition therapy: Maintain adequate nutritional intake using parenteral nutrition, lipid emulsions, enteral feedings, or oral intake as indicated by patient's neurologic status. See "Nutritional Support," p. 1.

Pharmacotherapy

Sedatives: Phenobarbital is the drug of choice to reduce increased ICP due to restlessness and irritability.

Antipyretics: Acetaminophen is used to control fever, which increases cerebral metabolism. May be used along with a hypothermia blanket to decrease temperature and with chlorpromazine to control related shivering. Usually aspirin is avoided, since its platelet action impairs clotting and promotes bleeding.

Analgesics: Acetaminophen and codeine sulfate are used for mild-to-moderate pain. Codeine maintains maximal LOC, but should be given with stool softeners to avoid constipation.

Stool softeners: Docusate sodium (Colace) is the drug of choice for preventing straining, which can increase ICP.

Corticosteroids: Dexamethasone (Decadron) is a controversial medication used to relieve cerebral edema and decrease ICP. The patient should be monitored carefully for side effects, including GI tract irritation. Medications that reduce gastric activity reduce the risk of gastritis and ulceration.

Antihypertensives: Hydralazine hydrochloride (Apresoline), reserpine (Serpasil), propranolol (Inderal), labetalol (Normodyne), or sodium nitroprusside (Nipride) may be administered to reduce BP in patients with persistent hypertension. A thiazide diuretic may be used concomitantly with the other medications.

Osmotic diuretics: Mannitol (Osmitrol), urea (Ureaphil), and glycerin (Glycerol) may be used to reduce ICP and treat cerebral edema via diuresis to remove fluid from the brain. Patients should be monitored for electrolyte imbalances, other systemic side effects, and adverse reactions related to fluid shifting.

> **Note:** With the rapid movement of extracellular fluid from brain tissue to plasma with associated decrease in brain volume, potential for rebleeding may be increased after giving mannitol. Mannitol may cause a rebound increase in ICP 8-12 hr after administration, as fluid shifts from cells into the vascular compartment. Furosemide (Lasix) is often used to decrease the rebound effect of mannitol.

Loop diuretics: Furosemide (Lasix) is often used as a sole agent to decrease cerebral edema without causing the rise in intracranial blood volume that occurs with mannitol.

Anticonvulsants: Phenytoin and phenobarbital may be used to control or prevent seizures.

Calcium channel blocker: Nimodipine (Nimotop) inhibits calcium influx across the cell membrane of vascular smooth muscles. The resultant decrease in peripheral vascular resistance and vasodilation have improved outcomes in patients with SAH by increasing perfusion in cerebral vessels. Nimodipine is given as 60 mg enterally every 4 hr for 21 days (the recommended course of therapy).

Triple H therapy: Each of the following therapies may be used singly or in combination.

> **Note:** Although hypervolemic-hypertensive therapy with hemodilution has been proved to be an effective treatment for vasospasm, it carries great risks. The patient's BP, ICP, and neurologic status should be closely monitored. If used preoperatively (rare), this modality may precipitate IICP with rerupture of and rebleeding from the aneurysm. When used postoperatively, the patient may experience cerebral edema with cerebral ischemia and subsequent neurologic deficit.

- *Hypervolemia* (saline, whole blood, packed cells, plasma protein fraction, albumin, or hetastarch): increases circulating volume to prevent ischemia caused by vasospasm.
- *Hemodilution* (albumin and crystalloid fluids): decreases blood viscosity.
- *Hypertension* (dobutamine, phenylephrine, dopamine, isoproterenol, norepinephrine): by increasing BP, cerebral perfusion pressure increases and helps prevent ischemia and infarction.

Treatment of hydrocephalus: Hydrocephalus develops in 20%-25% of patients with subarachnoid hemorrhage from a ruptured cerebral aneurysm. In the acute phase in a patient with decreased LOC and Hunt-Hess classification of II or IV, an external ventriculostomy drain can be placed. For chronic hydrocephalus, one end of a small catheter is positioned into a ventricle, with the other end draining into a body cavity or space (e.g., subarachnoid space, cistern, peritoneum, vena cava, pleura). Major complications include infection and malfunction. If the shunt has a valve for the purpose of controlling drainage or preventing reflux of CSF, the surgeon may request that the valve be pumped periodically to ensure proper functioning. For nursing interventions after shunt placement, see Table 6-4.

Interventions: surgical and endovascular: Based upon the Hunt-Hess classification, location, and size of aneurysm, the decision must be made between treating surgically or performing an endovascular procedure. Recent studies demonstrate improved outcome with surgery during the

TABLE 6-4 **Nursing Interventions After Shunt Placement**

- After the shunting, assess patient for indicators of IICP (see Table 6-3) caused by either the disease itself or shunt malfunction.
- Position patient on side opposite the insertion site, either flat or with head elevated slightly (as prescribed) to prevent pressure on shunt mechanism.
- Assess VS; LOC (orientation to time, place, and person); papillary light reflex; and motor function.
- Monitor I&O, and limit fluids as prescribed.
- Avoid severe head and neck rotation, flexion, or hyperextension to prevent kinking, compression, or twisting of the shunt catheter, which would impede CSF flow.
- If the shunt has a valve for controlling drainage or preventing reflux of CSF, pump the valve to ensure proper functioning, according to surgeon's directive. Usually the valve is located behind or above the ear and is the approximate diameter of a fingertip. Pumping involve gentle, serial compressions of the tissue over the shunt. If the valve is working properly, the emptying and refilling of the valve will be felt with palpation.
- Assess for indicators of meningitis (see p. 385), peritonitis (see p. 152), or septicemia (see p. 502) caused by presence of shunt mechanism.

CSF, Cerebrospinal fluid; *IICP,* increased intracranial pressure; *I&O,* intake and output; *LOC,* level of consciousness; *VS,* vital signs.

first 24-72 hr for patients with grade I or II symptoms. Early surgery may prevent rebleeding, an often fatal complication, and affords time to initiate triple H therapy for vasospasm without risk of rebleeding. Surgery can be delayed until the peak time for vasospasm (7-10 days after SAH) has passed. Patients with grades III-V symptoms are generally considered poor surgical risks, especially in the period immediately after SAH. If these patients are clinically unstable, they may be treated medically until they improve or stabilize enough for endovascular intervention. Surgery is considered for a patient with a large intracranial clot causing life-threatening, intracranial brain shifting. Surgery is delayed for a patient with cerebral vasospasm until the vasospasm subsides.

Repair of a cerebral aneurysm entails a craniotomy with clipping or ligation of the aneurysmal neck, coagulation of the aneurysm, or encasement of the aneurysmal sac in surgical gauze. Surgeons choose a method based on the patient's condition and the size, site, and number of perforating arteries.

Neurovascular interventionalists now offer alternative to surgery using Guglielmi Detachable Coils (GDC coils). The overall size and location of the aneurysm and the aneurysmal neck size are evaluated to decide if this option is feasible. GDC coils are microcoils composed of a soft platinum alloy which are placed with a microcatheter through the femoral artery. The catheter is advanced into the cerebral circulation using radiographic imaging. Low-voltage current is applied to the guidewire to detach the coil(s) placed into the sac of the aneurysm. Placement of one or more coils fills the sac, reduces the pressure inside, and isolates the aneurysm from normal circulation. Average length of stay is 2-4 days unless the aneurysm ruptures, or a high risk of rupture or bleeding is suspected.

Cerebral angioplasty for arterial vasospasm may be used to decrease vascular narrowing and reverse ischemia in patients with new-onset vasospasm within 6-12 hr of onset. Patient selection may be limited to high-risk candidates with surgically difficult or inaccessible aneurysms.

NURSING DIAGNOSES AND INTERVENTIONS

Decreased adaptive capacity: intracranial, related to compromised cerebral circulation secondary to SAS hemorrhage

Desired outcome: Patient has adequate cerebral perfusion within 24-72 hr of treatment, evidenced by findings consistent with baseline or orientation to time, place, and person; equal, normoreactive pupils; BP in patient's usual range; HR 60-100 beats/min; RR 12-20 breaths/min with normal depth and pattern (eupnea); bilaterally equal motor function, with extremity strength and normal tone; ICP 0-15 mm Hg; cerebral perfusion pressure 60-80 mm Hg; and absence of headache, vomiting, or other indicators of IICP.

- Assess hourly for indicators of IICP (see Table 6-3) and herniation (see "Traumatic Brain Injury," p. 100).

- Calculate cerebral perfusion pressure (CPP) by means of the formula:

$$CPP = MAP - ICP$$

when

$$MAP = \frac{\text{Systolic BP} + 2\,(\text{Diastolic BP})}{3}$$

CPP <30 mm Hg causes cerebral anoxia. If ICP monitoring is used, consult physician promptly for ICP ≥15 mm Hg or elevated above patient's baseline (see "Traumatic Brain Injury," p. 103).
- Manage conditions which cause increasing restlessness with concomitant IICP: distended bladder, constipation, hypoxemia, headache, fear, and anxiety.
- Implement measures that help prevent IICP and herniation:
  ❑ Maintain complete bed rest.
  ❑ Keep HOB elevated 15-45 degrees or as prescribed to promote cerebral venous outflow.
  ❑ Avoid hyperflexion, hyperextension, or hyperrotation of the neck to decrease the risk of jugular vein compression, which can impede venous outflow, thereby increasing ICP.
  ❑ Instruct patient to avoid activities using isometric muscle contractions (e.g., pulling or pushing side rails, pushing against the foot board) which raise systolic BP, with resultant increased ICP.
  ❑ Prevent straining with bowel movements. The increased intrathoracic pressure raises ICP.
  ❑ Teach patient to exhale through the mouth to relax when moving or having a bowel movement.
  ❑ Instruct patient to avoid coughing. The increased intrathoracic pressure increases ICP.
  ❑ Teach patient to open the mouth when sneezing to minimize the increase in ICP.
  ❑ Maintain a quiet, relaxed environment; decrease external stimuli in the room such as lights or noise. Limit visitors as needed. Encourage quiet speaking and initiate nonstressful conversations.
  ❑ Minimize vigorous activity by assisting with ADLs (i.e., feeding, bathing, dressing, toileting).
  ❑ Maintain patent airway, adequate oxygen, and ventilation to prevent cerebral hypoxia and hypercapnia. Poor oxygenation causes cerebral vasodilation, cerebral edema, and increased ICP.
  ❑ Monitor ABG values for hypoxemia (Pao_2 <80 mm Hg) or hypercapnia ($Paco_2$ >45 mm Hg).
  ❑ Avoid vigorous, prolonged suctioning, which precipitates hypoxemia and hypercapnia. Preoxygenation with slight hyperventilation using 100% oxygen helps prevent cerebral vasodilation.
  ❑ Limit fluid intake to 1500-1800 ml/24 hr as prescribed.
  ❑ Monitor and record I&O accurately.
- Administer antihypertensive medication as prescribed to keep BP at desired levels.
- Administer stool softeners as ordered, to prevent constipation.
- Administer antitussive agents to prevent coughing and antiemetics to prevent or treat vomiting. Both coughing and vomiting can increase intrathoracic pressure and ICP.
- If IICP occurs suddenly, perform hyperinflation (per agency protocol or medical orders) with a manual resuscitator at a rate of ≥50 breaths/min to decrease $Paco_2$.
- If mannitol is prescribed for acutely increased ICP, administer by bolus (1.5-2 g/kg of 15%-25% solution over 30-60 min). Assess renal status throughout the procedure. The high dose and rapid infusion rate markedly affects the kidneys. Evaluate fluid and electrolyte status (see p. 538), body weight, and total output before and after the infusion. Consult physician if cerebrospinal fluid pressure (i.e., ICP) is not reduced within 15 min of starting the infusion.

■NIC Cerebral Edema Management; Cerebral Perfusion Promotion; Intracranial Pressure (ICP) Monitoring; Neurologic Monitoring; Positioning: Neurologic

Altered protection related to risk of rebleeding from cerebral aneurysm associated with clotting anomaly secondary to normal fibrinolytic response

Desired outcomes: Patient has no symptoms of rebleeding from ruptured cerebral aneurysm, evidenced by orientation to time, place, and person; equal and normoreactive pupils; BP within patient's normal range; HR 60-100 beats/min; RR 12-20 breaths/min with normal depth and pattern (eupnea); bilaterally equal motor function with extremity strength and tone normal for patient; and absence of headache, papilledema, nystagmus, and nausea. ICP is 0-15 mm Hg; CPP is 60-80 mm Hg.

- Assess for signs and symptoms of IICP with herniation, which can signal rerupture with rebleeding from cerebral aneurysm. See following section, "Decreased adaptive capacity."

■NIC Surveillance: Safety; Bleeding Precautions

Decreased adaptive capacity: intracranial, related to compromise of fluid dynamic mechanisms secondary to cerebral vasospasm associated with ruptured cerebral aneurysm

Desired outcomes: Patient has baseline or normal neurologic status, evidenced by orientation to time, place, and person; equal and normoreactive pupils; BP within patient's normal range; HR 60-100 beats/min; RR 12-20 breaths/min with normal depth and pattern (eupnea); bilaterally equal motor function with extremity strength and tone normal for patient; and absence of headache, papilledema, nystagmus, and nausea. ICP is 0-15 mm Hg or at patient's baseline; CPP is 60-80 mm Hg.

- Assess for vasospasm or the potential for it by reviewing and monitoring sequential transcranial Doppler studies done at the bedside.
- Assess for indicators of IICP (see Table 6-3) and herniation (see "Traumatic Brain Injury," p. 100), which may occur either abruptly or gradually. Cerebral vasospasm affects the major cerebral vessels near the ruptured aneurysm and can cause a focal neurologic deficit with or without a major or sudden loss of consciousness. Vasospasm may cause gradual confusion and deteriorating LOC associated with focal motor deficits. A headache that worsens over time and increasing BP may precede the onset of more serious neurologic symptoms.
- If signs of IICP are present, prepare patient for cerebral angiography or CT with contrast medium: the only methods for confirming the presence of vasospasm and ruling out rebleeding.
- Administer prescribed medications (i.e., mannitol, nitroprusside sodium, nimodipine) and intravenous fluids to maximize cerebral circulation and minimize potential cerebral vasospasms.
- If hypervolemic-hemodilution therapy is prescribed, observe for signs and symptoms of fluid overload: imbalanced I&O, tachypnea, crackles, respiratory distress, decreased Hct, hyponatremia , jugular vein distention, peripheral edema, and increased CVP or pulmonary artery pressure (PAP).
- Continue to treat the IICP (see "Decreased Adaptive Capacity: Intracranial, Secondary to Hemorrhage Into the Subarachnoid Space," p. 363).

NIC Cerebral Edema Management; Cerebral Perfusion Promotion; Intracranial Pressure (ICP) Monitoring; Positioning: Neurologic; Neurologic Monitoring

Constipation related to prolonged immobility; decreased fluid intake; inadequate intake of fiber; restriction against Valsalva maneuver for straining

Desired outcome: Patient has bowel movements within his or her normal pattern without straining.

- Obtain data regarding patient's normal bowel pattern and date of last bowel movement.
- Assess for constipation, including abdominal distention, cramping, and complaints of fullness or pressure in the abdomen or rectum. Auscultate for bowel sounds.
- Advise patient to defecate whenever the need arises but to refrain from straining.
- Assist patient into semi-Fowler's or high Fowler's position to facilitate bowel elimination unless this position is contraindicated. Use of a bedside commode is recommended.
- Teach patient to select foods high in fiber to facilitate bowel elimination.
- Unless contraindicated, offer patient a warm drink to stimulate peristalsis.
- Administer stool softeners as prescribed.
- Avoid use of rectal thermometers, suppositories, enemas, or digital evacuation of an impaction. This type of stimulus may cause patient to perform a Valsalva type of maneuver, which in turn may increase intrathoracic and intracranial pressures, resulting in the potential for rerupture and rebleeding from the aneurysm.

NIC Bowel Management; Constipation/Impaction Management

ADDITIONAL NURSING DIAGNOSES

As appropriate, see nursing diagnoses and interventions in "Nutritional Support," p. 1; "Mechanical Ventilation," p. 14; "Alterations in Consciousness," p. 38; "Prolonged Immobility," p. 61; "Psychosocial Support," p. 68; and "Psychosocial Support for the Patient's Family and Significant Others," p. 78. See "Risk for Trauma (Oral and Musculoskeletal)" in "Status Epilepticus," p. 372. See "Pain Related to Headache, Photophobia, and Fever" in "Meningitis," p. 389. Also see "Risk for Fluid Volume Deficit" in "Diabetes Insipidus," p. 400. See "Risk for Injury" in "Syndrome of Inappropriate Antidiuretic Hormone," p. 404.

Care of the Patient After Intracranial Surgery

Cranial surgery is performed to remove a space-occupying lesion such as a tumor, hematoma, or abscess; repair a vascular abnormality such as an aneurysm or arteriovenous malformation (AVM); drain cerebrospinal fluid from the ventricular system; correct skull fractures; obtain tissue for biopsy to confirm a diagnosis and facilitate treatment; control seizures; and reduce pain.

Less invasive intracranial procedures using stereotactic techniques are used for some biopsies and for implantation of deep brain stimulators for control of essential tremors. The type of surgical approach the neurosurgeon takes depends primarily on the location of the pathologic condition. The *supratentorial* approach is used to remove or correct problems in the frontal, temporal, or occipital lobes, as well as in the diencephalic area (i.e., pituitary, hypothalamus). Lesions of the cerebellum and brainstem usually require an *infratentorial* (i.e., suboccipital) approach. The *transsphenoidal* approach gains access to the pituitary gland to remove a tumor, control bone pain associated with metastatic cancer, or attempt to arrest the progression of diabetic retinopathy in a patient with diabetes mellitus.

After intracranial surgery the major goals of treatment are to maintain cerebral function through control of ICP; recognize, prevent, or treat complications; provide supportive care until the patient can resume ADLs; and prepare for rehabilitation.

COMPLICATIONS AFTER INTRACRANIAL SURGERY

Alteration in cerebral tissue perfusion due to increased intracranial pressure with herniation: Cerebral edema, hemorrhage, infection, and surgical trauma can all lead to IICP with herniation (see Table 6-3). Some cerebral edema is expected after intracranial surgery, and usually peaks about 72 hr after surgery (see "Traumatic Brain Injury," p. 100).

Intracranial bleeding: Postoperative bleeding may be intracerebral, intracerebellar, subarachnoid, subdural, epidural, or intraventricular. Coagulation profiles and platelet counts should be monitored closely. Bleeding may be caused by the lengthy and extensive surgical procedure, prolonged anesthesia, preexisting medical problems, or medications. A CT brain scan is often done 24 hr postoperatively. Contusions can develop after evacuation of epidural or subdural hematomas and may create a mass effect.

Hypovolemic shock: May occur as a result of general fluid loss associated with use of osmotic diuretics.

Seizures: Generalized or partial seizures can occur as a result of surgical trauma, irritation of cerebral tissue by the presence of blood, cerebral edema, cerebral hypoxia, hypoglycemia, preexisting seizure disorder, or inadequate anticonvulsant levels.

CNS infection: Meningitis, encephalitis, and ventriculitis may occur as a result of bacterial contamination before, during, or after surgery. For example, organisms introduced at the time of injury (e.g., gunshot wound) or a break in sterile technique may lead to CNS infection. (See "Meningitis," p. 384, and Appendix 8.)

Hydrocephalus: May appear before surgery or occur after surgery as an acute or chronic complication. Usually it is caused by a slowing or complete stoppage of the flow of CSF through the ventricular system secondary to edema, bleeding, scarring, or obstruction. For a discussion of shunt creation, see "Cerebral Aneurysm and Subarachnoid Hemorrhage," p. 363.

Diabetes insipidus (DI) and SIADH: fluid volume deficit or excess: Result from disturbance of the hypothalamus or posterior lobe of the pituitary gland. Antidiuretic hormone (ADH) is produced in the hypothalamus and stored in the posterior pituitary. DI results from decreased ADH production, which leads to excessive urinary output, with potentially serious fluid and electrolyte problems (see "Diabetes Insipidus," p. 400). DI may result from edema, manipulation, or partial or total removal of the gland. SIADH, a less common problem, results from an increase in the release of ADH, which leads to resorption of large amounts of water via the renal tubules with concurrent loss of large amounts of sodium. Like DI, SIADH also can cause serious fluid and electrolyte problems (see "Syndrome of Inappropriate Antidiuretic Hormone," p. 404).

Cardiac dysrhythmias: May occur as a result of cerebral hypoxia or ischemia, manipulation of the brainstem, or the irritating effects of blood in the CSF (see "Dysrhythmias and Conduction Disturbances," p. 231).

Tension pneumocephalus: Occurs as a result of air entering the subdural, extradural, subarachnoid, intracerebral, or intraventricular spaces. May be a complication of infratentorial/posterior fossa craniotomy, burr holes for removal of chronic subdural hematoma, and transsphenoidal hypophysectomy.

CSF leakage: Caused by a channel created between the subarachnoid space (SAS) and the outside from a tear or rupture of the dura mater. A CSF leak may be noted preoperatively after a skull fracture, or it may occur during surgery; the common organisms are gram-negative bacilli. CSF leakage from the ear is *otorrhea*; from the nose it is *rhinorrhea*. The leakage of CSF indicates an open pathway to the SAS, which carries a serious risk of infection. Causes specific to craniotomy include the use of an external ventricular drainage device, remote site infection, and repeat operation.

Respiratory complications: Respiratory complications after intracranial surgery can be particularly serious because any increase in $PaCO_2$ resulting in hypercapnia will lead to cerebral vasodilation with a subsequent increase in intracranial volume, and thus IICP. Respiratory complications include the following:
- Partial or complete airway obstruction caused by accumulation of secretions and improper positioning.
- Neurogenic pulmonary edema caused by a sudden increase in ICP.
- Cerebral edema that causes compression of brainstem respiratory centers.
- Atelectasis and pneumonia.
- Pulmonary embolism.

Gastrointestinal bleeding (Cushing's ulcer) and paralytic ileus: GI bleeding is associated with cerebral trauma and the postoperative period after neurosurgery. Although the cause is unclear, stress from the trauma or the surgery can cause continuous vagal stimulation leading to a hyperacidic state that causes gastric erosion, ulceration, and ultimately hemorrhage. These conditions also result from medications, especially corticosteroids (see "Acute Gastrointestinal Bleeding," p. 459). Paralytic ileus may occur after neurologic surgery. Decreased or absent peristalsis results from prolonged anesthesia, immobility, trauma, electrolyte deficiencies, and mechanical obstruction (e.g., obstipation).

Thrombophlebitis, deep vein thrombosis (DVT), and pulmonary embolism: May result from prolonged bed rest and immobility after intracranial surgery. Other factors such as a prolonged surgical procedure, preexisting coagulopathies, and blood dyscrasias may influence the postoperative complications. Venous thromboembolism is the most frequent complication following craniotomy for removal of brain tumors.

POSTOPERATIVE NEUROLOGIC DEFICITS

Some neurologic deficit(s) may be present before surgery and should be noted and documented. Deficits that occur after surgery may be caused by surgical trauma or the presence of cerebral edema, which interferes with normal brain function. With time, these deficits may improve. The following are some of the neurologic deficits seen in the patient after intracranial surgery.

Diminished LOC: The degree of LOC improvement depends on preoperative damage to cerebral tissue. LOC often improves as anesthesia wears off, cerebral edema subsides, and ICP approaches normal.

Communicative and cognitive deficits: The ability to communicate and understand after surgery depends on the level of preoperative dysfunction, the site of the lesion, extensiveness of the procedure, and the degree of postoperative cerebral edema.

Broca's (expressive, motor, nonfluent) aphasia: Inability to communicate verbally or in writing. Can understand situations, follow commands.

Wernicke's (receptive, sensory, fluent) aphasia: Individual does not understand the situation and cannot follow commands appropriately.

Motor and sensory deficits: Motor deficits (weakness or paralysis) are caused by injury or edema to the primary motor cortex and corticospinal (pyramidal) tracts. Early physical and occupational therapy help to prevent long-term disabilities (foot or wrist drop, contractures, hip rotation.) Assistive devices and splinting techniques help to prevent contractures. Sensory deficits occur when the primary sensory cortex, the sensory association areas of the parietal lobe, or the spinothalamic tracts are injured or edematous. Sensory deficits include inability to distinguish objects according to characteristics (e.g., size, shape, weight) and inability to distinguish overall changes in temperature, touch, pressure, and position. Improvement in both motor and sensory perception may be seen as cerebral edema subsides.

Cranial nerve impairment: The degree of cranial nerve deficit(s) depends on site of the lesion, preoperative deficit, degree of postoperative cerebral edema, and surgical approach. Infratentorial surgery for lesions in the posterior fossa (brainstem and cerebellum) involves significant cranial nerve manipulation with high risk of injury to cranial nerves IX, X and XII, which innervate the pharynx and tongue. Risk of airway obstruction is high. Removal of large tumors (i.e., acoustic neuromas) may injure the facial nerve and result in facial paralysis and loss of corneal reflex. Deficit(s) may improve with decreasing cerebral edema or may be permanent. Nursing assessment of cranial nerve dysfunction is important. For more information about the function of all the cranial nerves, see Appendix 4.

Loss of corneal reflex: May be caused by surgical trauma to frontal lobe motor pathways or brainstem cranial nerve nuclei. Corneal abrasion, ulceration, and blindness may occur if not recognized and treated promptly.

Periocular edema: Seen after supratentorial surgery with manipulation of the scalp and frontal cranial bones or retraction of the frontal lobes.

Hyperthermia: Associated with injury or irritation of the hypothalamic temperature-regulating centers, presence of blood in the CSF, or infection. Elevated temperature increases the metabolic needs of the brain, potentially leading to increased blood flow to the area, with concomitant cerebral edema.

COLLABORATIVE MANAGEMENT AFTER INTRACRANIAL SURGERY

Respiratory support: Supplemental oxygen, intubation, and mechanical ventilation as needed.

Activity restrictions: Activity depends on patient's LOC and general condition.

CSF leak: Treatment of a CSF leak depends upon severity, site, and risk for infection. Interventions include external CSF drainage (i.e., lumbar subarachnoid drain) to divert CSF flow, reduce pressure, and allow the dural tear to heal; surgical intervention to seal the dural leak; or use of epidural blood patch. Symptomatic relief of symptoms such as headache is provided.

Positioning: HOB is most often elevated 30 degrees to promote venous drainage, which reduces ICP.

- In posterior fossa surgery (infratentorial approach), the supporting muscles of the neck are altered. Patients should be turned with the neck in alignment with the head, with the head, neck, and shoulders supported.
- After craniectomy, to avoid injury the patient should not be turned to the side from which bone has been removed. Label head dressing, chart, and bed with location of missing bone.
- After procedures when a large intracranial space is left after extensive surgery, to avoid a sudden shift in intracranial contents, with subsequent hemorrhage or herniation, the patient should not be positioned on operative side immediately after surgery.

Pharmacotherapy: The following may be prescribed after surgery:

Corticosteroids (e.g., dexamethasone): To decrease cerebral edema.

> **Note:**   Research is ongoing to determine whether steroids are effective in the treatment of cerebral edema.

Osmotic diuretics (e.g., mannitol, urea): To control cerebral edema causing IICP.

> **Caution:**   Can cause a hyperosmolar state and dehydration. Monitor serum creatinine and assess fluid status to assess renal status.

Anticonvulsants (e.g., phenytoin, fosphenytoin, phenobarbital): Prevent seizures in the immediate postoperative period caused by cerebral edema and irritation from manipulation of the brain. Anticonvulsants may be continued for a period of 1-2 yr after surgery.

Antibiotics: Prevent/treat postoperative surgical site infection or respiratory or urinary tract infection.

Antipyretics: Treat elevated temperature, which can increase use of oxygen and glucose supplies.

Analgesics: Treat or control headache. Drugs of choice are acetaminophen alone or with codeine sulfate.

Antacids (e.g., Maalox): To prevent the formation of gastric ulceration resulting from steroid use or surgical stress.

Histamine H$_2$-receptor antagonists (e.g., ranitidine [Zantac]): To suppress gastric secretions and thus prevent or facilitate healing of Cushing's ulcer.

Fluid and electrolyte management: To prevent or treat increasing cerebral edema. Usually fluids are limited to 1500-1800 ml/day, depending on patient's body size and overall condition.

Minimize venous thrombosis: Venous imaging techniques such as ultrasonography are used before discharge to detect thrombosis. Enoxaparin 40 mg/day or unfractionated heparin 5000 units bid (if no actual or risk of intracranial bleeding is present) has been used in combination with compression stockings or pneumatic compression devices on the lower extremities.

Nutritional support: The method and type of nutritional support are determined by the patient's condition and may include any of the following: oral feedings, enteral feedings, supplements, or parenteral nutrition (i.e., total parenteral nutrition [TPN], fat emulsion therapy). See "Nutritional Support," p. 1.

Physical medicine consultation: To evaluate patient and plan for rehabilitation: physical, occupational, and speech therapy.

NURSING DIAGNOSES AND INTERVENTIONS

Risk for injury related to possibility of gastric ulcer (Cushing's) or gastritis secondary to hyperacidic state.

Desired outcomes: Patient's gastric pH is >5, and patient has no symptoms of gastric ulcer or gastritis, as evidenced by gastric secretions and stool culture negative for blood; HR ≤100 beats/min; BP within patient's normal range; and absence of midepigastric discomfort.

- Monitor for symptoms of GI bleeding or ulceration: midepigastric discomfort, occult or frank blood in stool or gastric secretions, decreasing BP, or increasing HR. Report positive findings to physician and prepare for insertion of a gastric tube.
- Monitor hematocrit (Hct) or hemoglobin (Hgb) daily; report decreasing values.
- Test gastric drainage pH q4h. Administer H$_2$-receptor antagonists and/or antacids if ordered.
- Implement measures to prevent ulceration and hemorrhage:
  - As prescribed, administer sucralfate (Carafate) and histamine H$_2$-receptor antagonists, antacids to suppress gastric secretions and promote healing.

❏ When administering steroids, aspirin, phenytoin, and other medications that irritate gastric mucosa, administer with a meal or snack.

NIC Surveillance; Bleeding Precautions

ADDITIONAL NURSING DIAGNOSES

See also nursing diagnoses and interventions in "Traumatic Brain Injury," for "Risk for Infection (CNS)," p. 107; "Ineffective Thermoregulation," p. 108; "Risk for Disuse Syndrome," p. 109; and "Impaired Corneal Tissue Integrity," p. 109. See also "Cerebral Aneurysm and Subarachnoid Hemorrhage" for "Decreased Adaptive Capacity Secondary to Hemorrhage into the Subarachnoid Space," p. 363; "Decreased Adaptive Capacity Secondary to Cerebral Vasospasm," p. 364; and "Constipation," p. 365. See "Status Epilepticus" for "Risk for Trauma (Oral and Musculoskeletal)," p. 372. See "Pain Related to Headache, Photophobia, and Fever" in "Meningitis," p. 389. See "Fluid Volume Deficit" in "Diabetes Insipidus," p. 400. See "Risk for Injury" in "Syndrome of Inappropriate Antidiuretic Hormone," p. 404. See "Nutritional Support," p. 1; "Prolonged Immobility," p. 61; "Psychosocial Support," p. 68; and "Psychosocial Support for the Patient's Family and Significant Others," p. 78.

Status Epilepticus

PATHOPHYSIOLOGY

Status epilepticus is a state of recurring or continuous seizures of at least 20- to 30-min duration, in which the patient does not return to full consciousness from the postictal state before another seizure occurs. If possible, treatment should be initiated immediately to prevent neuronal injury, which may begin within 20-30 min. The mortality for status epilepticus is 10%-12%. A practical definition may be revised to include seizures of only 5- or 10-min duration, because of a high likelihood that they will continue. There are two major types, based on the classification of Gastaut and used by Engel. *Generalized status epilepticus* includes convulsive status (generalized tonic-clonic seizures) and absence status (petit mal seizures). Convulsive status is more common and is considered a life-threatening medical emergency, because the hypoxia and neuronal metabolic exhaustion may cause neuronal death. *Partial status epilepticus* includes simple partial status (focal motor or epilepsia partialis continua) and complex partial status (temporal or nontemporal seizures). The term "nonconvulsive status" may be used to describe absence and complex partial status.

Status epilepticus in persons with epilepsy is often due to noncompliance with medications or a drop in anticonvulsant serum levels caused by alcohol abuse or infection. Other causes for individuals with and without preexisting epilepsy include acute metabolic disturbances (e.g., hypoglycemia, hyponatremia, hypocalcemia), stroke, CNS infection (e.g., meningitis, encephalitis), CNS trauma or tumors, and alcohol and drug abuse. Prompt treatment may prevent complications including cardiac dysrhythmias, hyperthermia, aspiration, hypertension, hypotension, anoxia, hyperglycemia, hypoglycemia, dehydration, myoglobinuria, and oral or musculoskeletal injuries.

ASSESSMENT

History and risk factors: Epilepsy, drug or alcohol abuse, recent head injury, infection, headaches. If the patient is taking antiepilepsy medications, note the following: drug name, dosage, time last taken, length of time drug has been taken, and any recent medication changes. Determine if patient is taking any other medications, including name, dose, and time last taken.

Partial status epilepticus

Complex partial status: Manifested as a prolonged confusional state caused by continuous or recurring seizures. Automatisms (e.g., lip smacking, chewing, swallowing) and speech difficulty may occur, followed by a stage of postictal confusion and sleepiness.

Simple partial status: The second most common type, usually manifested as focal motor status (epilepsia partialis continua). Consciousness is typically intact and motor activity is localized to one area of the body (e.g., the face or the hand). It may last for hours or days.

Generalized status epilepticus

Absence status: Characterized by altered consciousness; from a dreamy state to stupor. Automatisms or mild clonic movements (e.g., fluttering of the eyelids) may be present. Clinically, absence status is difficult to differentiate from complex partial status.

Convulsive status: The most common form characterized by generalized tonic-clonic seizures without return to full consciousness. A life-threatening medical emergency.

DIAGNOSTIC TESTS

Serum drug screen: To rule out drug or alcohol intoxication.

Blood chemistry and hematology:

Serum electrolytes, including BUN and glucose, liver enzymes, calcium and magnesium: To rule out electrolyte imbalance or metabolic disturbance.

Complete blood cell count (CBC): To rule out infection and to evaluate other risk factors.

Antiepilepsy serum drug level: To determine the amount of therapeutic drugs in patient's system.

ABG analysis: To obtain baseline levels and determine state of oxygenation.

ECG: To evaluate cardiovascular status, especially during medication administration. Phenytoin and other medications may lead to dysrhythmias and/or hypotension.

Electroencephalogram (EEG): May be monitored continuously or during seizures to evaluate the brain's electrical activity. Information is used to identify type and cause of seizures.

CT brain scan: To rule out presence of a brain lesion.

COLLABORATIVE MANAGEMENT

Support of ventilation and perfusion: Cardiopulmonary function and VS are assessed closely. Measures may be initiated to maintain a patent airway, intubation, and respiratory and cardiovascular support. More extensive evaluation for muscle damage should be done if lengthy seizures continue or occur frequently. Circulation is inadequate for muscles in near continuous contraction. Patients can develop rhabdomyolysis, which can lead to acute renal failure if not appropriately managed.

Establish IV access: For medication administration and to draw needed labwork.

Prevention of Wernicke-Korsakoff syndrome: 100 mg IV thiamine and 50 ml of 50% glucose are administered if chronic alcohol ingestion or hypoglycemia is suspected.

Pharmacotherapy

Administration of fast-acting anticonvulsant: Given to achieve high serum and brain concentrations. Not used as long-acting anticonvulsants.

- *Lorazepam (Ativan):*
  - ❑ Preferred by many epileptologists
  - ❑ 0.1 mg/kg, up to 8 mg, given IV. Do not infuse faster than 2 mg/min.
  - ❑ Monitor respiratory and cardiovascular status continuously.
- *Diazepam (Valium):*
  - ❑ 0.2 mg/kg, up to 20 mg, given IV.
  - ❑ Do not infuse faster than 5 mg/min to avoid respiratory depression, which may occur with faster infusion rate.

Administration of long-acting anticonvulsant

- *Fosphenytoin (Cerebyx):*
  - ❑ Usual IV loading dose is 20 mg/kg PE (phenytoin equivalents). Infusion rate is 100-150 PE/min. Most IV solutions are compatible with fosphenytoin, including dextrose solutions. Phlebitis and soft tissue damage at IV site are not seen as frequently with fosphenytoin.
  - ❑ Monitor VS closely. Hypotension and cardiac dysrhythmias may develop.
  - ❑ If status persists after 20 mg/kg, an additional 5-10 mg/kg may be given, up to a maximal total dose of 30 mg/kg.

OR (if fosphenytoin is **not** used)

- *Phenytoin (Dilantin):*
  - ❑ Usual loading dose is 18-20 mg/kg given IV. Do not infuse faster than 50 mg/min to avoid serious dysrhythmias, including asystole.
  - ❑ Phlebitis and soft tissue damage at IV site may occur
  - ❑ Flush line with normal saline only. Microcrystallization, which occurs when phenytoin is used with dextrose, may also occur when it is used in saline as a continuous drip.
  - ❑ Monitor closely for hypotension and dysrhythmias.

Caution: High doses of phenytoin can cause seizure activity; therefore >30 mg/kg is not recommended.

- ❑ If status persists after 20 mg/kg dose, an additional 5- to 10-mg/kg may be given, up to a maximal total dose of 30 mg/kg.

Administration of IV phenobarbital: Used if patient is allergic to phenytoin.
- ❑ Usual dosage is 20 mg/kg. Do not infuse faster than 50-75 mg/min.

Caution: If given simultaneously with or after lorazepam or diazepam, respiratory depression and hypotension can occur, possibly necessitating ventilatory support.

Aggressive treatment is required for refractory status epilepticus that continues despite administration of benzodiazepines, phenytoin or fosphenytoin, and phenobarbital. Consider deep sedation/general anesthesia using propofol, midazolam, or pentobarbital.

General anesthesia:
- *Pentobarbital coma*
  - ❏ Given only if administration of fast-acting anticonvulsant, long-acting anticonvulsant, or IV phenobarbital is ineffective in stopping the seizure activity.
  - ❏ Loading dose is 5 mg/kg. Maintenance dose is 0.5-3 mg/kg/hr to stop seizures.
  - ❏ Monitor respiratory and cardiovascular activity continuously.
  - ❏ Mechanical ventilation and vasopressors are usually required.
  - ❏ Periodic tapering of pentobarbital is done to see if seizures have remitted.
  - ❏ Patient may be in a coma for days to weeks.
- *Propofol*
  - ❏ Given for refractory status epilepticus.
  - ❏ Loading dose is 1-2 mg/kg given by IV. Initial maintenance dose of 2-10 mg/kg/hr to stop seizure activity. Adjust dose according to EEG findings.
  - ❏ Monitor respiratory and cardiovascular activity continuously.
  - ❏ Mechanical ventilation and vasopressors are required.
  - ❏ Periodic tapering of propofol is done to see if seizures have remitted.
- *Midazolam*
  - ❏ Given for refractory status epilepticus.
  - ❏ Loading dose is 0.2 mg/kg given by IV. Maintenance of 0.75-1 mcg/kg/min to stop seizure activity. Maintenance dose is adjusted according to EEG findings.
  - ❏ Monitor respiratory and cardiovascular activity continuously.
  - ❏ Mechanical ventilation and vasopressors are usually required.
  - ❏ Periodic tapering of midazolam is done to see if seizures have remitted.

Intravenous valproic acid (Depacon), paraldehyde, lidocaine, or neuromuscular blockade: Additional therapies for seizure control. Neuromuscular blockade stops only movements (not brain electrical activity) and should be administered with sedatives.

Nutritional support: Enteral or parenteral nutrition may be necessary, depending on the duration of the status epilepticus and patient's underlying nutritional state.

NURSING DIAGNOSES AND INTERVENTIONS

Impaired gas exchange related to altered oxygen supply associated with hypoventilation and bradypnea secondary to depressant effect of seizures on respiratory center

Desired outcome: Within 1 hr of treatment/intervention, patient has adequate gas exchange as evidenced by Pao_2 >80 mm Hg; $Paco_2$ 35-45 mm Hg; pH 7.35-7.45; and RR 12-20 breaths/min with normal depth and pattern (eupnea).

- Monitor for respiratory distress. Note respiratory rate, depth, and rhythm and skin color. Report use of accessory muscles, rapid or labored respirations, and cyanosis.
- Monitor ABG values to assess oxygenation. Be alert to hypoxemia (Pao_2 <80 mm Hg) and respiratory acidosis ($Paco_2$ >45 mm Hg; pH <7.35).
- Keep intubation equipment ready for airway and ventilation assistance.
- Position an oral airway to help maintain open airway. Suction as necessary.
- Keep patient turned to the side to allow secretions to drain.
- Administer oxygen as prescribed.
- Administer antiepilepsy medications within prescribed criteria to avoid further depression of respiratory center.

NIC Airway Management; Oxygen Therapy; Aspirations Precautions

Altered tissue perfusion: cerebral and cardiopulmonary, related to altered blood flow during continuous seizure activity or vasodilatory effects of specific antiepilepsy medications

Desired outcome: Within 1 hr of treatment/intervention, patient has adequate cerebral and cardiopulmonary perfusion as evidenced by orientation to time, place, and person; normal sinus rhythm on ECG; BP within patient's normal range; RR 12-20 breaths/min with normal depth and pattern (eupnea); and absence of headache, papilledema, and other clinical indicators of IICP.

> **Note:** Metabolic demands of the brain and heart are increased greatly during seizure activity; adequate cerebral perfusion is essential to maintain brain function.

- Support ventilation and perfusion for maximal delivery of oxygen to the brain. Monitor VS q2-4min. Respiratory depression, decreased BP, and dysrhythmias can occur with rapid infusion of diazepam and phenytoin. BP must be maintained within normal limits for optimal brain perfusion.
- Monitor for dysrhythmias, especially during medication administration.
- Ensure safe administration of antiepileptic drugs: diazepam at 5 mg/min; lorazepam at 2 mg/min; phenobarbital at 50-100 mg/min; or phenytoin at 50 mg/min. See "Collaborative Management," p. 370, for details.
- Perform baseline and serial neurologic assessments to determine the presence of focal findings that suggest an expanding lesion (see Table 6-3).

NIC Cerebral Perfusion Promotion; Neurologic Monitoring; Seizure Management; Cardiac Care: Acute

Risk for trauma (oral and musculoskeletal) related to seizure activity

Desired outcome: Patient's mouth and extremities are not injured during the seizure.

- Keep side rails padded and up at all times, with bed in the lowest position.
- Perform protective measures during the seizures:
  - ❑ Put a soft object such as a flat pillow under patient's head.
  - ❑ Move sharp or potentially dangerous objects away from patient.
  - ❑ Loosen any tight clothing.
  - ❑ Avoid restraining patient. The force of tonic-clonic movements may cause strains, strains and fractures of extremities if thrashing occurs with restraints in place.
  - ❑ Avoid forcing airway into patient's mouth when jaws are clenched. Force could break teeth, and patient could swallow or aspirate them.
  - ❑ Avoid use of tongue blade, which could splinter and cut the mouth.
  - ❑ Stay with patient; assess and record seizure type and duration. Record any automatic behavior (e.g., lip smacking, chewing movements), motor activity, incontinence, tongue biting, and postictal state.
- After seizure, reorient and reassure patient.

NIC Environmental Management: Safety; Positioning; Seizure Precautions; Seizure Management

Noncompliance with prescribed medication regimen, related to misunderstanding health care recommendations, not understanding importance of following medication schedule, running out of medication, stopping medication intentionally

Desired outcome: Within the 24-hr period before discharge from the critical care unit, patient verbalizes understanding of the rationale and importance of taking the medication as prescribed, as well as the consequence of noncompliance.

- Once a diagnosis of noncompliance with the medication regimen has been established, determine patient's reason for noncompliance.
- Assess patient's understanding of epilepsy and its treatment.
- Ensure that patient is aware that stopping the antiepilepsy medication can result in serious problems, including status epilepticus. If patient plans to stop the medication for any reason, he or she should consult with the physician.
- Evaluate the effect epilepsy has on patient's lifestyle.
- Once the cause of noncompliance is identified, work to find a solution. If the patient has side effects from the medication, such as gastric upset, suggest that patient try taking the medication after meals. If the gastric upset is a result of increasing the medication, advise patient to increase the dose more slowly.
- Refer patient to regional epilepsy support groups and the Epilepsy Foundation of America (EFA), including regional affiliate and national headquarters.
- As appropriate, refer patient to nurse specialist or social worker at regional center for individual counseling.

NIC Teaching: Prescribed Medication; Decision-Making Support; Coping Enhancement; Values Clarification

Knowledge deficit: disease process, treatment, and lifestyle changes that epilepsy necessitates

Desired outcome: Within the 24-hr period before discharge from the critical care unit, patient verbalizes understanding of epilepsy, including its etiology and pathophysiology and seizure classification, as well as its treatment and the lifestyle changes it necessitates.

- Assess knowledge level and provide necessary information about epilepsy.
- Ask patient to describe seizure(s) in detail, including warning signals (aura) at the beginning of seizures. Explain that the aura or warning signals onset of seizures and that patient should lie down or get into a safe position to prevent injury.
- Assess patient's knowledge of antiepilepsy medications, including name(s), purpose, schedule, dosage, precautions, and side effects. Reinforce importance of maintaining a constant blood level

of medication by taking it as prescribed. Explain if the medication is missed or taken erratically, he or she cannot attain the blood level needed to prevent seizure breakthrough. If a dose of medication is missed, instruct patient to notify his or her physician.
* Emphasize to the patient that a normal life is possible.
* Insure patient knows sleep deprivation can precipitate status epilepticus. Every patient must know his or her own limits. Having epilepsy does not mean it is necessary to get more sleep than do persons who do not have epilepsy.
* Teach patient/significant others the importance of safety measures used during a seizure (see "Risk for Trauma [Oral and Musculoskeletal]" p. 372). Emphasize how to ease patient to the floor and turn him or her to a side-lying position.
* Inform patient of your local driving regulations/laws for persons with epilepsy.
* Teach patient the importance of avoiding dangerous machinery and heights if his or her seizures are not being controlled adequately by medications.

NIC   Teaching: Individual; Support Group

Ineffective individual coping related to frustration secondary to unpredictable nature of the disease
Desired outcome: Within 24-48 hr of this diagnosis, patient verbalizes feelings, identifies strengths and ineffective coping behaviors, and understands responsibility for self-care.
* Assess patient's knowledge of the disease and its treatment. See preceding diagnosis, "Knowledge Deficit."
* Encourage patient to express feelings so areas of major concern are known.
* Involve patient in decisions regarding care so he or she has more sense of control over life (e.g., encourage patient to participate in the decision for scheduling the medications). Problem solve for major concerns.
* Help patient set realistic goals for employment and living arrangements. Refer patient to regional or local EFA as appropriate.
* Encourage patient to educate others in what to do should a seizure occur.
* Encourage involvement in support groups; coping strategies can be learned from other persons with seizures.
* For additional interventions, see "Psychosocial Support," p. 68.

NIC   Coping Enhancement; Crisis Intervention; Emotional Support; Support System Enhancement

ADDITIONAL NURSING DIAGNOSES

For other nursing diagnoses and interventions, see the following as appropriate: "Mechanical Ventilation," p. 14; "Psychosocial Support," p. 68; and "Psychosocial Support for the Patient's Family and Significant Others," p. 78.

Stroke: Ischemic (Acute Ischemic Stroke) and Hemorrhagic (Intracerebral Hematoma)

PATHOPHYSIOLOGY

The term *stroke* refers to an acute vascular injury to the brain. Stroke is the leading cause of adult disability and the third leading cause of death. A stroke has been viewed as a medical emergency since the approval for early use of thrombolytic therapy following ischemic stroke. There are two major stroke types: ischemic and hemorrhagic. Subcategories are shown in Figure 6-1. Each stroke type is defined by the pathophysiologic event. *Acute ischemic stroke (AIS)* and *intracerebral hematoma* (clot that remains after hemorrhage) are discussed here. Other causes of cerebral hemorrhage include subarachnoid hemorrhage (SAH) and arteriovenous malformations (AVM).

AIS caused by thrombi or emboli that interrupt blood flow to the brain accounts for 80% of all strokes. A thrombus is a clot formed in the artery, usually in branches with low flow due to plaque. Cerebral emboli may be formed in the heart and travel to the brain, or be formed in the carotid or other cerebral arteries and migrate to occlude a smaller artery in the brain. Characteristic deficits are produced, depending on the artery involved (Table 6-5).

Low to absent cerebral perfusion leads to *acute ischemic stroke*. Cerebral ischemia disrupts the sodium/potassium (Na^+/K^+) pump, leading to neuronal depolarization and neurotransmitter release, followed by a massive flux of ions and water resulting in brain cell edema. Extracellular K^+ and intracellular calcium (Ca^{++}) increase. Brain cells deprived of oxygen begin anaerobic metabolism. The resulting lactic acidosis and high concentration of intracellular Ca^{++} lead to cellular death.

Lactic acidosis prompts the *CNS ischemic response*: the vasomotor center is stimulated, which causes vasoconstriction with marked elevation in blood pressure. Systolic pressures <220 mm Hg and

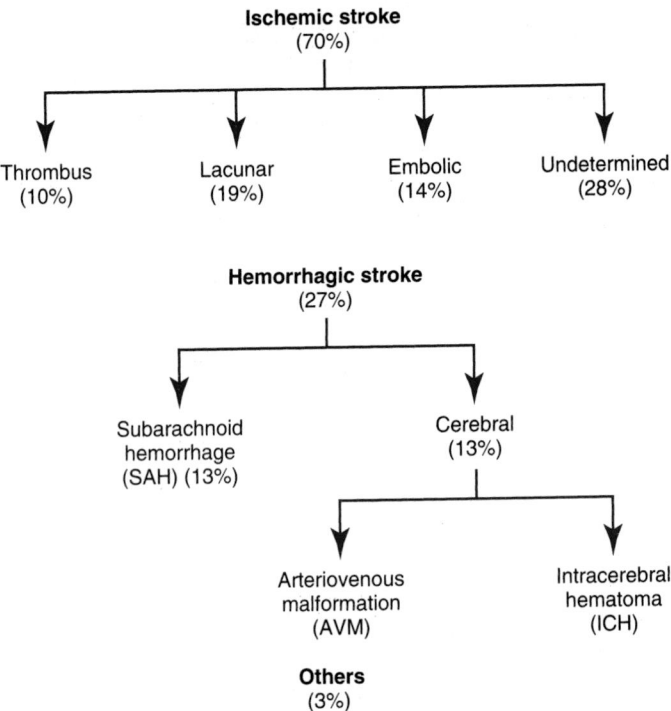

Figure 6-1:   Stroke classification.

diastolic pressures <110 mm Hg are not treated, since this is a natural response to perfuse the ischemic brain. If thrombolytic therapy is to be initiated, the blood pressure is slowly lowered to <185/105 mm Hg. The CNS ischemic response is seen during the acute phase of stroke, but is most pronounced during the Cushing's response before herniation.

Intracerebral hematomas (ICHs) may occur anywhere in the brain (Table 6-6). Although various pathophysiologic events can result in ICH, the most common cause is hypertension, usually resulting in the rupture of a small penetrating artery in the basal ganglia. Damage occurs as accumulated blood destroys and displaces the brain tissue. Disrupted tissue and the ruptured vessel reduce normal blood flow to the area that surrounds the already injured brain tissue, resulting in even greater ischemic injury. Intracerebral blood may rupture into the lateral ventricle, creating risk for communicating hydrocephalus. Lobar hemorrhages are less common and in elderly persons are often caused by cerebral amyloid angiopathy. Other common causes of hemorrhage include vascular malformations, vasculitis, neoplasms, hematologic disorders, and stimulant abuse (e.g., cocaine, amphetamines).

ASSESSMENT

Each stroke type has a unique presentation based on the pathophysiology and the location of the event. A complete and ongoing physical examination is crucial during the initial phase of stroke to detect or help prevent further deterioration.

History and risk factors: Although strokes can occur at any age, most occur in individuals over age 55. Hypertension, smoking, aging, and previous history of transient ischemic attack (TIA) or stroke are the strongest risk factors. Stroke risk factors are classified according to whether they are changeable or unchangeable conditions. Risk factors that cannot be changed are age (higher risk >55 yr); race (risk for blacks is twice that for whites); gender (risk for males is twice that for females); previous history of stroke, TIA, and acute myocardial infarction (AMI increases risk ×10); and family history of stroke or AMI. Risk factors that can be changed include hypertension, heart disease, diabetes mellitus, obesity, hypercholesterolemia, sedentary lifestyle, and smoking.

Cardiac disease is the most common cause of cerebral embolism. Cardiac disorders such as atrial fibrillation, sick sinus syndrome, dilated cardiac myopathy, ventricular thrombus after AMI, and valvular disease are causes of cardioembolic stroke. Thrombotic strokes are usually caused by local

TABLE 6-5 Neuroanatomy Related to Neurologic Deficit

Vessel	Area supplied	Deficit
Internal carotid artery (ICA)	Right or left hemisphere	Contralateral motor or sensory deficit, aphasia with dominant hemisphere, neglect with nondominant hemisphere, contralateral visual field deficit (hemianopia), contralateral eye deviation
Middle cerebral artery (MCA)	Right or left convex surface of the brain, most of the basal ganglia, internal capsule, putamen, and globus pallidus	Contralateral hemiplegia (arm and face >leg), sensory involvement, aphasia of dominant hemisphere, neglect of nondominant hemisphere (denial of weakness), homonymous hemianopia
Anterior cerebral artery (ACA)	Right of left frontal lobe, corpus callosum, caudate nucleus, internal capsule	Weakness or sensory loss of contralateral leg and proximal arm; behavior disturbance: abulia, confusion, memory loss, urinary incontinence
Posterior cerebral artery (PCA)	Midbrain thalamus, choroid plexus, occipital lobe, and medial temporal lobe	Contralateral visual field deficit, color blindness, impaired depth perception, occasional sparing of central vision, memory loss, sensory loss, nystagmus, pupillary abnormalities, ataxia
Vertebral artery	Medulla and/or cerebellum	Face, nose, or eye ipsilateral numbness with contralateral body numbness, facial weakness, vertigo, ataxia, nystagmus, dysphagia, dysarthria
Basilar artery	Pons, midbrain, and/or cerebellum	Quadriplegia or hemiplegia/paresis, locked-in syndrome (pons), dysarthria, dysphagia, ataxia, nystagmus, vertigo, coma

TABLE 6-6 Hemorrhagic Locations and Syndromes

Area	Syndrome
Putamen	Contralateral hemiplegia, hemisensory loss, hemianopia, slurred speech
Thalamic	Contralateral hemiplegia; hemisensory loss; small, poorly reactive pupils; decreased level of consciousness
Pontine	Locked-in syndrome (awake, aware, unable to verbally communicate, quadriplegia), coma
Cerebellar	Occipital headache, ataxia, dizziness, headache, nausea, vomiting
Lobar	Mimics cerebral infarct (e.g., contralateral motor and sensory signs)

atherosclerosis of large vessels (e.g., internal cerebral artery [ICA] or middle cerebral artery [MCA]) related to occlusion of small, perforating vessels (lacunar infarction).

For acute ischemic stroke (AIS)

Clinical presentation: Individuals with ischemic strokes caused by MCA occlusion in the dominant hemisphere usually are awake with hemiparesis, aphasia, visual field cut, and sensory loss. Individuals with AIS stroke usually do not experience pain other than a headache, nor do they have altered LOC unless the stroke causes mass effects as a result of swelling or involves the brainstem or thalamic regions bilaterally. Individuals with acute hemispheric infarction have elevated arterial BP and often appear drowsy even in the absence of swelling. Although both thrombotic and embolic strokes can begin abruptly, the former are more likely to evolve over several hours and may fluctuate over several hours or days. In contrast, the deficit caused by embolic strokes usually is maximal at onset and often occurs during activity.

For intracranial hematoma/intracerebral hemorrhage

Clinical presentation: Depends on the size and location of the hematoma. A relatively small hemorrhage into the brainstem may produce quadriplegia and coma, whereas a hematoma of similar size in the basal ganglia may produce hemiparesis without altered LOC. A larger hematoma (as measured by CT) may indicate a poorer prognosis.

Neurologic findings with ICH are similar to those with AIS. However, individuals with ICH are more likely to have altered LOC, vomiting, headache, very high BP, and IICP. The neurologic deficit may evolve over minutes to a few hours, requiring intubation and ICP monitoring. Neurosurgical intervention is often necessary.

For both stroke types

Physical assessment: The Glasgow coma scale (see Appendix 3) is often used in critical care to evaluate patients with stroke. Because this scale primarily measures LOC, it is not an appropriate scale for stroke patients. The National Institutes of Health (NIH) stroke scale (Table 6-7) provides a better measurement of deficits and is easy to use. It also guides the examiner in evaluating cognitive, language, and motor deficits that are unique to stroke. Comprehensive neurologic assessment assists the critical care nurse in detecting declines in neurologic status and responses to interventions.

Research Brief 6-1 This multicenter national nursing study is collecting data on 800 stroke survivors and the "decision-making partner" to determine the patterns of decision making in obtaining medical care after an acute stroke. This information may help nurses to better educate the public to facilitate more rapid responses to emergent medical care after stroke. Currently half of the patients who have stroke arrive at the hospital within 24 hr. With thrombolytic therapy and other stroke interventions available, the delay to medical care must be reduced.

From O'Donnell L: *Factors related to timing in seeking health care for stroke symptoms,* Grand Rapids, Mich. Manuscript in preparation.

Complications: The most serious are those that affect the CNS and cardiopulmonary systems.
CNS: Increased ICP (IICP) due to extension of the infarct or hematoma and its associated edema. May cause midline shift and herniation; IICP associated with hydrocephalus after ICH; and seizures, which generally occur within the first 24 hr but may present at any time.
Cardiopulmonary: ECG changes: QT prolongation, ST segment depression, T wave inversion, U waves, and ventricular ectopy. Cardiac dysrhythmias after stroke may be caused by release of catecholamines, causing hypertension, cardiac irritability, and/or muscle damage. Individuals with new ECG changes have a less favorable prognosis. ECG monitoring for the first 24-72 hr is recommended, along with evaluation of creatine phosphokinase-myocardial band (CK-MB) isoenzymes.

• • •

Death within the first month after stroke is commonly caused by myocardial infarction (MI), pneumonia, and sepsis. Pulmonary embolism, deep vein thrombosis, skin breakdown, and depression are also common.

DIAGNOSTIC TESTS

CT: Performed within the first 24 hr, primarily as a method of differentiating ischemic from hemorrhagic stroke. Within the first few hours after AIS, the scan appears normal. ICH is easily diagnosed on CT—blood appears as a bright white signal.

TABLE 6-7 NIH Stroke Scale

N I H
STROKE
SCALE

Patient Identification. ___ ___-___ ___ ___-___ ___ ___

Pt. Date of Birth ___ ___/___ ___/___ ___

Hospital _____ (___ ___-___ ___)

Date of Exam ___ ___/___ ___/___ ___

Interval: [ ] Baseline   [ ] 2 hours post treatment   [ ] 24 hours post onset of symptoms ±20 minutes   [ ] 7-10 days
[ ] 3 months   [ ] Other _____ (___ ___)

Time: ___ ___:___ ___   [ ]am [ ]pm

Person Administering Scale _____

Administer stroke scale items in the order listed. Record performance in each category after each subscale exam. Do not go back and change scores. Follow directions provided for each exam technique. Scores should reflect what the patient does, not what the clinician thinks the patient can do. The clinician should record answers while administering the exam and work quickly. Except where indicated, the patient should not be coached (i.e., repeated requests to patient to make a special effort).

Instructions	Scale Definition	Score
1a. Level of Consciousness: The investigator must choose a response if a full evaluation is prevented by such obstacles as an endotracheal tube, language barrier, orotracheal trauma/bandages. A 3 is scored only if the patient makes no movement (other than reflexive posturing) in response to noxious stimulation.	0 = **Alert;** keenly responsive. 1 = **Not alert;** but arousable by minor stimulation to obey, answer, or respond. 2 = **Not alert;** requires repeated stimulation to attend, or is obtunded and requires strong or painful stimulation to make movements (not stereotyped). 3 = Responds only with reflex motor or autonomic effects or totally unresponsive, flaccid, and flexic.	___
1b. LOC Questions: The patient is asked the month and his/her age. The answer must be correct - there is no partial credit for being close. Aphasic and stuporous patients who do not comprehend the questions will score 2. Patients unable to speak because of endotracheal intubation, orotracheal trauma, severe dysarthria from any cause, language barrier, or any other problem not secondary to aphasia are given a 1. It is important that only the initial answer be graded and that the examiner not "help" the patient with verbal or non-verbal cues.	0 = **Answers** both questions correctly. 1 = **Answers** one question correctly. 2 = **Answers** neither question correctly.	___
1c. LOC Commands: The patient is asked to open and close the eyes and then to grip and release the non-paretic hand. Substitute another one step command if the hands cannot be used. Credit is given if an unequivocal attempt is made but not completed due to weakness. If the patient does not respond to command, the task should be demonstrated to him or her (pantomime), and the result scored (i.e., follows none, one or two commands). Patients with trauma, amputation, or other physical impediments should be given suitable one-step commands. Only the first attempt is scored.	0 = **Performs** both tasks correctly. 1 = **Performs** one task correctly. 2 = **Performs** neither task correctly.	___
2. Best Gaze: Only horizontal eye movements will be tested. Voluntary or reflexive (oculocephalic) eye movements will be scored, but caloric testing is not done. If the patient has a conjugate deviation of the eyes that can be overcome by voluntary or reflexive activity, the score will be 1. If a patient has an isolated peripheral nerve paresis (CN III, IV or VI), score a 1. Gaze is testable in all aphasic patients. Patients with ocular trauma, bandages, pre-existing blindness, or other disorder of visual acuity or fields should be tested with reflexive movements, and a choice made by the investigator. Establishing eye contact and then moving about the patient from side to side will occasionally clarify the presence of a partial gaze palsy.	0 = **Normal.** 1 = **Partial gaze palsy;** gaze is abnormal in one or both eyes, but forced deviation or total gaze paresis is not present. 2 = **Forced deviation,** or total gaze paresis not overcome by the oculocephalic maneuver.	___

Rev 10/1/2003

Continued

CT-xenon is a new imaging technique that measures cerebral blood flow (CBF). The measurement provides a regional calculation of actual blood flow. Determination of the CBF guides clinical management of the patient.

A *CTA or CT-angiogram* is done to visualize the vascular system to detect vascular narrowing or occlusion. With new CT imaging techniques, patients can have a comprehensive evaluation of brain tissue (CT), brain blood flow (CT xenon), and venous system (CTA) in a matter of minutes.

Magnetic resonance imaging (MRI) and magnetic resonance arteriogram (MRA): Noninvasive tests that provide detailed information regarding the area of injury or its vascular supply. *Diffusion*

TABLE 6-7   NIH Stroke Scale—cont'd

3. Visual: Visual fields (upper and lower quadrants) are tested by confrontation, using finger counting or visual threat, as appropriate. Patients may be encouraged, but if they look at the side of the moving fingers appropriately, this can be scored as normal. If there is unilateral blindness or enucleation, visual fields in the remaining eye are scored. Score 1 only if a clear-cut asymmetry, including quadrantanopia, is found. If patient is blind from any cause, score 3. Double simultaneous stimulation is performed at this point. If there is extinction, patient receives a 1, and the results are used to respond to item 11.	0 = **No visual loss.** 1 = **Partial hemianopia.** 2 = **Complete hemianopia.** 3 = **Bilateral hemianopia** (blind including cortical blindness).
4. Facial Palsy: Ask – or use pantomime to encourage – the patient to show teeth or raise eyebrows and close eyes. Score symmetry of grimace in response to noxious stimuli in the poorly responsive or non-comprehending patient. If facial trauma/bandages, orotracheal tube, tape or other physical barriers obscure the face, these should be removed to the extent possible.	0 = **Normal symmetrical movements.** 1 = **Minor paralysis** (flattened nasolabial fold, asymmetry on smiling). 2 = **Partial paralysis** (total or near-total paralysis of lower face). 3 = **Complete paralysis** of one or both sides (absence of facial movement in the upper and lower face).
5. Motor Arm: The limb is placed in the appropriate position: extend the arms (palms down) 90 degrees (if sitting) or 45 degrees (if supine). Drift is scored if the arm falls before 10 seconds. The aphasic patient is encouraged using urgency in the voice and pantomime, but not noxious stimulation. Each limb is tested in turn, beginning with the non-paretic arm. Only in the case of amputation or joint fusion at the shoulder, the examiner should record the score as untestable (UN), and clearly write the explanation for this choice.	0 = **No drift;** limb holds 90 (or 45) degrees for full 10 seconds. 1 = **Drift;** limb holds 90 (or 45) degrees, but drifts down before full 10 seconds; does not hit bed or other support. 2 = **Some effort against gravity;** limb cannot get to or maintain (if cued) 90 (or 45) degrees, drifts down to bed, but has some effort against gravity. 3 = **No effort against gravity;** limb falls. 4 = **No movement.** UN = **Amputation** or joint fusion, explain: _____ **5a. Left Arm** **5b. Right Arm**
6. Motor Leg: The limb is placed in the appropriate position: hold the leg at 30 degrees (always tested supine). Drift is scored if the leg falls before 5 seconds. The aphasic patient is encouraged using urgency in the voice and pantomime, but not noxious stimulation. Each limb is tested in turn, beginning with the non-paretic leg. Only in the case of amputation or joint fusion at the hip, the examiner should record the score as untestable (UN), and clearly write the explanation for this choice.	0 = **No drift;** leg holds 30-degree position for full 5 seconds. 1 = **Drift;** leg falls by the end of the 5-second period but does not hit bed. 2 = **Some effort against gravity;** leg falls by 5 seconds, but has some effort against gravity. 3 = **No effort against gravity;** leg falls to bed immediately. 4 = **No movement.** UN = **Amputation** or joint fusion, explain: _____ **6a. Left Leg** **6b. Right Leg**

Rev 10/1/2003

weighted imaging (DWI) and *perfusion weighted imaging (PWI)* are additional tests performed with magnetic resonance to assess CBF. MRI is most useful for ischemic patients in identifying the cause and area involved.

Doppler studies: Include *transthoracic echocardiogram* to evaluate heart structure and function; *transesophageal echocardiogram* and *carotid Doppler or duplex* to evaluate blood flow and presence or degree of stenosis in the extracranial carotid arteries; and *transcranial Doppler* to evaluate the intracranial vessels and assess the velocity of blood flow in the anterior and posterior cerebral circulation. Transcranial Doppler is also used to evaluate vasospasms, to determine brain death via detection of cerebral circulatory arrest, for intraoperative monitoring, and to locate emboli.

Cerebral angiography: Invasive procedure used to visualize the cerebral blood vessels. Provides specific information on the cause of stroke by identifying the blood vessel involved. Interventional radiology is a growing field in the diagnosis and management of cerebral vascular injuries. In comprehensive stroke centers, patients are treated with intraarterial thrombolytic agents to dissolve clots and restore blood flow to the brain. Carotid and cerebral angioplasty with stenting may be done for ischemic events.

T A B L E 6 - 7   NIH Stroke Scale—cont'd

7. Limb Ataxia: This item is aimed at finding evidence of a unilateral cerebellar lesion. Test with eyes open. In case of visual defect, ensure testing is done in intact visual field. The finger-nose-finger and heel-shin tests are performed on both sides, and ataxia is scored only if present out of proportion to weakness. Ataxia is absent in the patient who cannot understand or is paralyzed. Only in the case of amputation or joint fusion, the examiner should record the score as untestable (UN), and clearly write the explanation for this choice. In case of blindness, test by having the patient touch nose from extended arm position.	0 = **Absent.** 1 = **Present in one limb.** 2 = **Present in two limbs.** UN = **Amputation** or joint fusion, explain: _____
8. Sensory: Sensation or grimace to pinprick when tested, or withdrawal from noxious stimulus in the obtunded or aphasic patient. Only sensory loss attributed to stroke is scored as abnormal and the examiner should test as many body areas (arms [not hands], legs, trunk, face) as needed to accurately check for hemisensory loss. A score of 2, "severe or total sensory loss," should only be given when a severe or total loss of sensation can be clearly demonstrated. Stuporous and aphasic patients will, therefore, probably score 1 or 0. The patient with brainstem stroke who has bilateral loss of sensation is scored 2. If the patient does not respond and is quadriplegic, score 2. Patients in a coma (item 1a=3) are automatically given a 2 on this item.	0 = **Normal;** no sensory loss. 1 = **Mild-to-moderate sensory loss;** patient feels pinprick is less sharp or is dull on the affected side; or there is a loss of superficial pain with pinprick, but patient is aware of being touched. 2 = **Severe to total sensory loss;** patient is not aware of being touched in the face, arm, and leg.
9. Best Language: A great deal of information about comprehension will be obtained during the preceding sections of the examination. For this scale item, the patient is asked to describe what is happening in the attached picture, to name the items on the attached naming sheet and to read from the attached list of sentences. Comprehension is judged from responses here, as well as to all of the commands in the preceding general neurological exam. If visual loss interferes with the tests, ask the patient to identify objects placed in the hand, repeat, and produce speech. The intubated patient should be asked to write. The patient in a coma (item 1a=3) will automatically score 3 on this item. The examiner must choose a score for the patient with stupor or limited cooperation, but a score of 3 should be used only if the patient is mute and follows no one-step commands.	0 = **No aphasia;** normal. 1 = **Mild-to-moderate aphasia;** some obvious loss of fluency or facility of comprehension, without significant limitation on ideas expressed or form of expression. Reduction of speech and/or comprehension, however, makes conversation about provided materials difficult or impossible. For example, in conversation about provided materials, examiner can identify picture or naming card content from patient's response. 2 = **Severe aphasia;** all communication is through fragmentary expression; great need for inference, questioning, and guessing by the listener. Range of information that can be exchanged is limited; listener carries burden of communication. Examiner cannot identify materials provided from patient response. 3 = **Mute, global aphasia;** no usable speech or auditory comprehension.
10. Dysarthria: If patient is thought to be normal, an adequate sample of speech must be obtained by asking patient to read or repeat words from the attached list. If the patient has severe aphasia, the clarity of articulation of spontaneous speech can be rated. Only if the patient is intubated or has other physical barriers to producing speech, the examiner should record the score as untestable (UN), and clearly write an explanation for this choice. Do not tell the patient why he or she is being tested.	0 = **Normal.** 1 = **Mild-to-moderate dysarthria;** patient slurs at least some words and, at worst, can be understood with some difficulty. 2 = **Severe dysarthria;** patient's speech is so slurred as to be unintelligible in the absence of or out of proportion to any dysphasia, or is mute/anarthric. UN = **Intubated** or other physical barrier, explain:_____

Rev 10/1/2003

Continued

Laboratory studies: The common lab studies include hematology as well as chemistry, lipid, and coagulation profiles. Less common laboratory tests may include determinations of lupus anticoagulant, anticardiolipin antibody, and hemoglobin electrophoresis (to assess presence of sickle cell disease). A coagulation profile to detect hypercoagulable blood may be done to evaluate levels of proteins C and S and a homocysteine level. These proteins may be deficient in the young (<45 yr) stroke patient, who may have no other risk factors for stroke. Further evaluations may include the following: for syphilis (e.g., Venereal Disease Research Laboratory [VDRL], rapid plasma reagin [RPR], fluorescent treponemal antibody [FTA]); sedimentation rate to assess for infection or vasculitis; and drug screen (e.g., cocaine, amphetamine).

Positron emission tomography (PET) and single photon emission computed tomography (SPECT): To evaluate brain metabolism and blood flow. These tests are performed more commonly in university-affiliated centers.

TABLE 6-7   NIH Stroke Scale—cont'd

11. Extinction and Inattention (formerly Neglect): Sufficient information to identify neglect may be obtained during the prior testing. If the patient has a severe visual loss preventing visual double simultaneous stimulation, and the cutaneous stimuli are normal, the score is normal. If the patient has aphasia but does appear to attend to both sides, the score is normal. The presence of visual spatial neglect or anosagnosia may also be taken as evidence of abnormality. Since the abnormality is scored only if present, the item is never untestable.	0 = **No abnormality.** 1 = **Visual, tactile, auditory, spatial, or personal inattention** or extinction to bilateral simultaneous stimulation in one of the sensory modalities. 2 = **Profound hemi-inattention or extinction to more than one modality;** does not recognize own hand or orients to only one side of space.

Rev 10/1/2003

Lumbar Puncture (LP): To measure CSF pressures and obtain CSF specimen when infection such as meningitis or neurosyphilis is suspected. May be performed when SAH is suspected and CT is normal.

Electroencephalogram (EEG): Although rarely done, may show slowing or low voltage over the infarct except in lacunar infarcts, where results are usually normal.

COLLABORATIVE MANAGEMENT

Goals of management are to prevent secondary neurologic damage and secondary complications, and promote optimal functional outcome. Early detection via accurate neurologic examination and immediate medical or surgical intervention help prevent stroke extension, increased brain edema, and hydrocephalus. Medical and nursing interventions are guided by the findings derived from the physical examination.

Prevention of stroke extension: Depends on adequate perfusion of the penumbra, which is the ischemic brain tissue surrounding the initial infarct that is at immediate risk of infarction. Perfusing the penumbra decreases the potential infarct size and optimizes patient outcome. Controlling arterial BP is essential in limiting the infarct size. Close monitoring and use of potent vasoactive medications achieve BP control. A "normal" BP may be too low, causing further ischemia and infarct by decreasing cerebral perfusion. Arterial BP should not be lowered abruptly in patients with AIS. At times, maintenance of a somewhat elevated BP may be warranted, depending on the underlying vascular and brain pathology. In contrast, with ICH many practitioners believe that an elevated BP should be reduced aggressively. The best approach is unclear, and therefore the treatment of increased BP in ICH requires individual consideration.

ICP monitoring and CPP management: Necessary for patients with increased infarct size, increased edema, and hydrocephalus. Patients with IICP may receive mannitol, which lowers ICP by reducing water within brain cells. Careful monitoring of ICP for rebound effect is necessary after mannitol infusion. Serum osmolality should be assessed to prevent excessive dehydration. Patients with hydrocephalus often require a ventriculostomy. For more information about ICP monitoring and CPP management, see "Traumatic Brain Injury," p. 98.

Optimizing regulatory functions: To prevent secondary complications (Table 6-8). In general, patients with ischemic strokes should be positioned with the HOB flat to increase cerebral perfusion. HOB should be elevated to decrease ICP in patients with hemorrhagic strokes. Patient response determines the best position.

Rehabilitation: Should begin immediately. Consults to physiatrist, physical therapist, occupational therapist, and speech therapist should be made within the first 24 hr.

Pharmacotherapy: Thrombolysis with IV recombinant tissue plasminogen activator (rt-PA) is initiated for *ischemic stroke*, ideally within 3 hr of the onset of symptoms. Intraarterial rt-PA has a 6-hr window. The use of neuroprotective agents and devices to remove cerebral clots, or devices to repair

TABLE 6-8   Maintenance of Normal Regulatory Functions in Stroke

Function	Intervention/goal	Rationale
Temperature	Normothermia	To decrease metabolic demands and ICP
Respiratory	O_2, positioning, respiratory therapy	To optimize O_2 delivery to the brain and prevent atelectasis and pneumonia
Cardiac	Monitor dysrhythmias, fluid, electrolytes	To optimize CO to promote perfusion to the brain
GI	H_2-blockers, bowel program	To prevent stress ulcers, constipation
Nutrition	NPO, enteral, long-term diet	NPO to prevent aspiration; diet to promote healing, meet caloric needs; long-term diet: low-Na+, low-fat, weight reduction if needed
GU	Bladder training ASAP	To prevent unnecessary use of Foley catheter, prevent UTI, and avoid embarrassment and possible retention
Musculoskeletal	ROM, positioning, increasing activity as tolerated, sequential compression stockings, mobility beds	To promote proper alignment and prevent contractures and complications of immobility
Skin	Keep clean and dry, pressure relief	To prevent skin breakdown and dependent edema
Communication	Develop appropriate communication techniques; swallow study within 24 hr	To prevent aspiration and promote meeting patient's needs

CO, Cardiac output; *GI,* gastrointestinal; *GU,* genitourinary; *ICP,* intracranial pressure; *Na+,* sodium; *NPO,* nothing by mouth; *O_2,* oxygen; *ROM,* range of motion; *UTI,* urinary tract infection.

atrial septal defects (ASD), may be attempted if available. Other pharmacotherapy strives to prevent secondary neurologic damage and recurrent stroke.

Anticoagulation: IV heparin may be indicated for patients with progressing stroke or unstable signs and symptoms of stroke such as TIAs and for cardioembolic stroke. If long-term anticoagulation is planned, the patient is converted to oral warfarin (Coumadin) therapy. Newer anticoagulants, including direct thrombin inhibitors, may be used. (see p. 484).

Antiplatelet therapy: Used to reduce risk of stroke and decrease frequency of TIAs. *Aspirin* (30-1300 mg/day dosage range) is the most common agent, usually given 75-325 mg qd. *Aspirin/ extended release dipyridamole* 25/200 mg (Aggrenox) is given bid and has the best stroke risk reduction, but 40% of patients who take it get headaches, and the dose must be titrated to reduce this side effect. *Ticlopidine* (Ticlid) reduces the overall risk for fatal and nonfatal strokes by nearly 25% when compared with aspirin, but is now rarely used due to the side effects. *Clopidogrel* (Plavix) is approved for patients at risk for ischemic events (myocardial, cerebrovascular, peripheral vascular). Plavix 75 mg qd may be given first-line with or without ASA, or as a second-line therapy when ASA has failed.

Antihypertensives: Frequently used in the stroke population to control hypertension (HTN). Agents are selected based on the individual's medical history and race. Long-term therapy may be prescribed based on the National Heart, Lung, and Blood Institute (NHLBI) algorithm (Table 6-9). Systolic BP

T A B L E 6 - 9   Classification and Management of Blood Pressure for Adults[*]

BP Classification	SBP* mm Hg	DBP* mm Hg	Lifestyle modification	Initial drug therapy Without compelling indication	Initial drug therapy With compelling indications (See Table ###)
Normal	<120	and <80	Encourage	No antihypertensive drug indicated.	Drug(s) for compelling indication. [‡]
Prehypertension	120-139	or 80-89	Yes	Thiazide-type diuretics for most. May consider ACEI, ARB, BB, CCB, or combination	Drug(s) for the compelling indications.[‡] Other antihypertensive drugs (diuretics, ACEI, ARB, BB, CCB) as needed.
Stage 1 hypertension	140-159	or 90-99	Yes		
Stage 2 hypertension	≥160	or ≥100	Yes	Two-drug combination for most [†] (usually thiazide-type diuretic and ACEI or ARB or BB or CCB).	

From the Seventh Report of the Joint National Committee on Prevention, Detection, Evaluation, and Treatment of High Blood Pressure (JNC 7) (2003). National High Blood Pressure Education Program; National Heart, Lung, and Blood Institute; U.S. Department of Health and Human Services, National Institutes of Health; NIH Pub No 03-5231, May, 2003.
[*] Treatment determined by highest BP category.
[†] Initial combined therapy should be used cautiously in those at risk for orthostatic hypotension.
[‡] Treat patients with chronic kidney disease or diabetes to BP goal of 130/80 mm Hg.
ACEI, Angiotensin-converting enzyme inhibitor; *ARB,* angiotensin receptor blocker; *BB,* beta-blocker; *BP,* blood pressure; *CCB,* calcium channel blocker; *DBP,* diastolic blood pressure; *SBP,* systolic blood pressure.

is often elevated in the acute phase and requires vasoactive IV medications such as sodium nitroprusside (Nipride) or labetalol (Normodyne). Nicardipine (Cardene IV) is the National Institute of Neurologic Disease Study (NINDS) recommendation for managing HTN in AIS. Hypotension is a concern, especially in the patient with IICP, since MAP is decreased. If MAP is decreased in the presence of a normal or elevated ICP, a decrease in CPP results, further compromising neurologic status. Vasopressors and/or inotropes may be titrated to keep MAP high enough to maintain CPP >60 mm Hg.

Anticonvulsant therapy: Used for seizures in the acute phase. Generally the patient is given a loading dose of phenytoin (Dilantin) or fosphenytoin (Cerebyx), followed by a maintenance dose. Benzodiazepines (e,g., Ativan) may be used initially. Phenobarbital may be used if the patient is in status epilepticus (see p. 370).

Sedation: A thorough neurologic evaluation to rule out organic causes of agitation is indicated. Sedation may be used as adjunctive therapy for patients with IICP. Benzodiazepines, fentanyl (Sublimaze), or morphine sulfate are effective. Pentobarbital coma is occasionally used for patients who experience high ICP that does not respond to other forms of therapy. (see p. 371)

Carotid endarterectomy: Carotid endarterectomies, surgical removal of plaque in the obstructed carotid artery to promote blood supply to the brain, may be performed immediately following stroke. Considered treatment of choice for patients with >70% carotid stenosis.

Craniotomy: May be performed for evacuation of a hematoma or for a young AIS patient with uncontrollable IICP caused by massive edema. A craniotomy with a dural incision or temporal lobectomy is considered. Hematoma evacuation may be performed by aspiration through a burr hole.

NURSING DIAGNOSES AND INTERVENTIONS

Decreased adaptive capacity: intracranial, related to interrupted blood flow secondary to thrombus or embolus

Desired outcome: Within 72 hr of diagnosis, patient has adequate cerebral tissue perfusion, as evidenced by no decrease in LOC; no deterioration in motor function on affected side; and no new or further deterioration of language, cognition, or visual field per NIH Stroke Scale (see Table 6-7).

- Assess for neurologic changes hourly in the acute phase. Use NIH Stroke Scale to record and monitor neurologic changes after stroke.
- Maintain ICP ≤15 mm Hg and CPP >60 mm Hg. CPP = MAP – ICP.
- Position patient to maintain adequate cerebral perfusion. Keep HOB flat as tolerated for patients with ischemic stroke. Keep HOB raised at 30 degrees as tolerated for patients with hemorrhagic stroke. Avoid extreme hip flexion. When positioning, monitor tolerance to position change.
- Consider ICP effects of respiratory care. Suction only if needed. Assess breath sounds frequently. Avoid activities that can increase ICP (e.g., excessive coughing). Avoid hypercapnia and hypoxia.
- Maintain adequate systolic blood pressure (SBP). Higher pressures (140-180 mm Hg) may be necessary to perfuse an area of brain at risk of infarction if ischemia is present. For patients with hemorrhagic stroke, maintain adequate BP. Use vasodilators or vasopressors as necessary to optimize BP and maintain CPP >60 mm Hg for all stroke patients.
- Use sedation as prescribed and monitor response: effects of sedation and changes in ICP.

NIC Cerebral Perfusion Promotion; Positioning: Neurologic; Neurologic Monitoring

Impaired physical mobility related to decreased motor function of upper and/or lower extremities and trunk after stroke

Desired outcome: At time of discharge from ICU, patient has no complications of immobility such as skin breakdown, contracture formation, pneumonia, or constipation.

- Turn and position frequently as tolerated. Transfer toward unaffected side.
- Teach methods for turning and moving using stronger extremity to move weaker extremity.
- Position weaker extremities to avoid contracture formation, frozen shoulder, or foot drop.
- Begin passive ROM within 24 hr of admission. Modify exercises if BP or ICP increases.
- Obtain physical therapy (PT) and occupational therapy (OT) referrals as soon as possible to establish appropriate therapy.
- Have patient cough and breathe deeply as tolerated at scheduled intervals.

NIC Positioning; Exercise Therapy: Joint Mobility; Self-Care Assistance

---

Research Brief 6-2   The study was completed at four university settings to determine if the public could be taught to accurately find the radial pulse and determine if that pulse is regular or irregular. Of the participants, 92% were able to find a radial pulse. Of that group, 86% were able to correctly identify a regular pulse, and 76% were able to correctly identify an irregular pulse. The aim of the project is to teach members of the general public to begin to check their pulses monthly and see a health care provider immediately if the pulse is irregular. More than 80,000 new strokes occur each year as a result of undiagnosed atrial fibrillation. This simple technique may promote early identification and treatment of atrial fibrillation and prevent stroke. "Check Your Pulse America" is a national campaign resulting from this trial. Nurses in every setting should teach this prevention strategy to patients at risk for heart disease and stroke. More information and free brochures can be obtained by contacting the National Stroke Association at 800-STROKES.

From Munschauer R et al: *Screening for atrial fibrillation in the community: a multicenter validation trial,* J Cardiovasc Dis Stroke 8:2, 1999.

Impaired verbal communication related to aphasia secondary to cerebrovascular insult

Desired outcome: At a minimum of 24 hr before discharge from ICU, patient demonstrates improved self-expression and relates decrease in frustration with communication.

- Evaluate for aphasia: partial or complete inability to use or comprehend language and symbols. Assess nature and severity of aphasia: ability to point to and name specific objects, follow simple directions, understand "yes/no" and complex questions, repeat simple and complex words and

sentences, relate purpose or action of the objects, fulfill written request, write request, and read. May occur with dominant (left) hemisphere damage.
- ❏ *Receptive aphasia* (e.g., Wernicke's, sensory): inability to comprehend spoken words. Patient may respond to nonverbal cues.
- ❏ *Expressive aphasia* (e.g., Broca's, motor): difficulty expressing words or naming objects. Gesture, groans, swearing, or nonsense words may be used. Use of a picture or word board may be helpful.
- Assess for dysarthria, which signals risk for aspiration resulting from ineffective swallowing and gag reflexes. Consult with speech therapist to assess ways to promote independence and facilitate swallowing.
- Decrease environmental distractions, such as television or others' conversations. Fatigue affects ability to communicate; plan adequate sleep/rest.
- Communicate frequently as follows: face patient, establish eye contact, speak slowly and clearly, give patient time to process information and give answer, keep messages short and simple, stay with one clearly defined subject, avoid questions with multiple choices, and instead phrase questions that can be answered "yes" or "no," and use the same words each time when repeating a statement or question. If patient does not understand after repetition, try different words. Use gesture, facial expressions, and pantomime to supplement and reinforce message.
- Help patients regain use of symbolic language: start with nouns and progress to more complex statements. Keep a record at the bedside of words to be used (e.g., "pill" rather than "medication"). Treat patient as an adult. Do not speak louder unless patient is hard of hearing. Be respectful.
- Facilitate verbal expression and naming objects: encourage patient to repeat words after you say them to practice verbal expression. Expect labile emotions, because patients are frustrated and emotional about impaired speech. *Patients who cannot monitor their speech may not speak sensible language but may think they are making sense.*
- Avoid labeling patient "belligerent" or "confused" when the problem is aphasia and frustration. *Patients with nondominant (right) hemisphere damage may speak well, but may give overly detailed information, or get off on tangents.* Redirect by saying "Let's go back to what we were talking about."
- Ensure that call light is available and patient knows how to use it. If patient is unable to use call light, check frequently and anticipate needs to ensure safety and trust.

▍NIC Communication Enhancement: Speech, Visual, Hearing Deficits; Active Listening; Anxiety Reduction; Touch

ADDITIONAL NURSING DIAGNOSES

See "Risk for Trauma (Oral and Musculoskeletal)" in "Status Epilepticus," p. 372. See "Traumatic Brain Injury," p. 109, for "Risk for Disuse Syndrome" and "Impaired Corneal Tissue Integrity." See "Prolonged Immobility," p. 61.

Meningitis

PATHOPHYSIOLOGY

Meningitis is an inflammation of the brain and spinal cord (CNS) affecting the meninges (i.e., dura, arachnoid, pia), brain surface, and cranial nerves. There are several types of meningitis, broadly classified as bacterial (pyogenic), tuberculous, fungal, and aseptic.

Bacterial meningitis: The most common form. Can be community-acquired or associated with prior infection, injury (e.g., open/penetrating skull fracture), basilar and facial skull fracture, shunt occlusion/malfunction, craniotomy, otitis media, sinusitis, or bacteremia (e.g., endocarditis, pneumonia).

Streptococcus pneumoniae (S. pneumoniae), a gram-positive coccus, is the leading cause of adult meningitis in the United States. Pneumococcal meningitis occurs in crowded conditions and is spread seasonally (fall and winter). It may follow a recent nasopharyngeal colonization with a pneumococcal strain or upper respiratory tract infection (URI), is seen with pneumococcal disease, is a complication of conditions associated with CSF leaks, and is more prevalent in immunocompromised persons.

Neisseria meningitidis (N. meningitidis), a gram-negative coccus, is the second leading cause of meningitis in adults. Infection is more likely to occur in patients with complement component deficiencies (e.g., congenital or associated with nephrotic syndrome, hepatic failure, systemic lupus erythematosus, multiple myeloma).

Haemophilus influenzae (H. influenzae), the most common cause in children, may affect adults. Predisposing factors include URIs, hypogammaglobulinemia, diabetes mellitus, alcoholism, asplenia, and head trauma. *H. influenzae* vaccine type B has diminished bacterial meningitis substantially in infants and children, making it a disease predominately of adults.

Listeria monocytogenes (L. monocytogenes), a gram-positive rod, is being seen more frequently as a cause of meningitis, especially in immunocompromised patients and those of extreme ages (very young and very old). Outbreaks have been linked to consumption of contaminated dairy products, undercooked chicken, fish, and meats.

Gram-negative species *Escherichia coli, Klebsiella, Proteus,* and *Pseudomonas* are gaining importance, especially in the elderly, the immunocompromised, and in head-injured patients.

Borrelia burgdorferi, the causative agent of Lyme disease, may also cause meningitis.

Acute meningitis may manifest as a community-acquired illness with a negative Gram's stain. The pathogen causing the disease may never be determined. Syphilis, bacteremia, and Lyme disease have been identified in some cases. Variables affecting diagnosis of meningitis include presentation in winter months, age older than 60 yr, and comorbid disease—especially immunodeficiency.

Tuberculous meningitis: *Mycobacterium tuberculosis* is a meningeal infection more common in human immunodeficiency virus (HIV)-infected patients, along with elders and children living among people with tuberculosis.

Fungal meningitis: *Cryptococcus neoformans,* an opportunistic organism seen with acquired immune deficiency syndrome (AIDS), is the leading cause of CNS fungal infection. Other fungi are associated less often.

Aseptic meningitis syndrome: May be drug-induced, related to infection or unrelated to infection. Meningitis has been an adverse drug reaction to nonsteroidal antiinflammatory agents (NSAIDS) and antimicrobials such as trimethoprim-sulfamethoxazole (TMP-SMX). Infectious causes: viral agents, *Mycobacterium pneumoniae, B. burgdorferi* and *Treponema pallidum.* Noninfectious causes: sarcoidosis, leptomeningeal carcinomatosis, systemic lupus erythematosus, Wegener's granulomatosis, and Bechet's disease.

ASSESSMENT

History and risk factors: Time symptoms developed, traumatic injury, exposures to disease, recent surgical procedures.

Clinical presentation

Streptococcus pneumoniae (S. pneumoniae): The classic presentation is fever, headache, meningismus, and altered mental status that progresses quickly to coma. Nuchal rigidity and Kernig's or Brudzinski's sign are present. Nausea, vomiting, profuse sweats, weakness, myalgia, seizures, and cranial nerve palsies also may be present.

Neisseria meningitidis (N. meningitidis): Fever, early macular erythematous rash progressing rapidly to petechial and purpuric states, conjunctival petechiae, and aggressive behavior are typical clinical findings. Dysfunctions of cranial nerves VI, VII, and VIII (see Appendix 4) and aphasia, ventriculitis, subdural empyema, cerebral venous thrombosis, and disseminated intravascular coagulation (DIC) may occur.

Haemophilus influenzae (H. influenzae): The most distinguishing sign is early development of deafness, which can occur within 24-36 hr after onset. A morbilliform or petechial rash may be present.

Listeria monocytogenes (L. monocytogenes): Seizures and focal deficits such as ataxia, cranial nerve palsies, and nystagmus are seen early in the course of infection. Conclusive diagnosis may require serology testing.

Gram-negative species: In elders, fever may be absent or low grade and headache may not be reported. Meningeal signs may be subtle, but confusion, severe mental changes, and pneumonia are commonly reported. Nuchal rigidity in elders must be differentiated from degenerative changes of the cervical spine.

Borrelia burgdorferi (B. burgdorferi): Symptoms of Lyme disease occur in three stages, beginning with a "bull's eye" rash within a few days of the tick bite followed by headache, stiff neck, lethargy, irritability, and changes in mental status, especially memory loss. Stage two, weeks to months after the tick bite, causes persistent headache, nausea, vomiting, malaise, irritability, cranial nerve deficits, mental status changes, peripheral neuropathies, and myalgias. In the last or third stage, arthritic types of symptoms and brain parenchymal changes are apparent.

Acute meningitis with negative Gram's stain: Fever and neck stiffness are the most frequent findings. The Gram's stain for bacteria is negative, but CSF white blood cell count is elevated. Symptoms are similar to other types of meningitis.

Mycobacterium tuberculosis (M. tuberculosis): A slow-onset process that causes neurologic damage before treatment is sought. Symptoms include headache, lethargy, confusion, nuchal rigidity,

cranial nerve abnormalities, SIADH, weight loss, and night sweats. Kernig's and Brudzinski's signs are present. The chest x-ray results may be clear, and purified protein derivative (PPD) may be nonreactive.
Cryptococcus neoformans (C. neoformans): Since the infection is subacute, fever and headache may have a subtle pattern lasting for weeks while other symptoms of meningitis occur, including positive meningeal signs (Table 6-10); alterations in mental status (e.g., hyperactivity, bizarre behavior, emotional lability, poor judgment); photophobia, focal cranial nerve deficits, nausea, vomiting, and (rarely) seizures.
Aseptic meningitis syndrome: Fever, headache, stiff neck, fatigue, anorexia and altered LOC are seen several hours after ingestion of causative drug. Severity varies with amount of drug taken and previous exposures. CSF glucose may be slightly elevated.
Physical assessment: A complete neurologic examination should be performed to establish patient's baseline neurologic function. One or more tests for meningitis usually are positive (see Table 6-10). Examination of associated systems (head, eye, ear, nose, and throat [HEENT] and pulmonary) provide additional data.

DIAGNOSTIC TESTS

CSF analysis: The most important laboratory test for diagnosing meningitis. CSF may be obtained through an intraventricular catheter, ventriculostomy and reservoir via cervical approach, or LP. An LP should not be done following head injury, if focal neurologic deficits or papilledema are present, since these signs indicate IICP (see Table 6-3). Antibiotic therapy should not be delayed if CSF samples cannot be obtained. The CSF is analyzed for cell count with white cell differential, glucose, protein, Gram's stain, acid-fast stain, culture, and sensitivity (Table 6-11). CSF studies include the following:
Cellular study: Cell count with white cell differential, glucose, and protein concentration.
Stains: Gram's stain and acid-fast stain.
Cultures: Bacterial, viral, fungal, *M. tuberculosis* cultures with sensitivities, and aerobic and anaerobic cultures.
Latex agglutination: For bacterial antigens of *N. meningitidis, S. pneumoniae, E. coli,* influenza type B (Hib), group B strep.
Antigen: Cryptococcal and *Histoplasma* polysaccharide antigen (bacterial antigen testing rarely useful).
Antibodies: *Coccidioides immitus* complement fixation antibodies, herpes simplex virus (HSV), and varicella zoster (VZV) antibodies.
Polymerase chain reaction (PCR) assays antibody titers: HSV1, HSV2, VZV, HIV, Epstein-Barr virus (EBV), West Nile virus, cytomegalovirus (CMV), HHV-6.
Other CSF studies: Venereal Disease Research Laboratories (VDRL), FTA-ABS
Clinical studies
Blood, urine, and sputum cultures: Help identify the infecting organisms.
Serum WBC count: Assesses for presence of infection.
CT with contrast and MRI: To rule out hydrocephalus or detect exudate, abscesses, and intracranial pathology (e.g., tumors).

COLLABORATIVE MANAGEMENT

Rapid sterilization of the CSF via appropriate pharmacologic therapy (Table 6-12): Prophylaxis, using appropriate antimicrobials for people exposed to *N. meningitidis* (rifampin or spiramycin) or *H. influenzae* meningitis, is recommended.

T A B L E 6 - 10   Positive Meningeal Signs

Test/description	Positive findings
Stiff neck sign (nuchal rigidity): Raise patient's head by flexing the neck and attempting to make the patient's chin touch the sternum.	Pain and resistance to neck motion
Brudzinski's sign: Assess for nuchal rigidity.	Flexion of the hips and knees when the examiner flexes the patient's neck
Kernig's sign: Flex the patient's leg at the knee and hip when the patient is supine, and then attempt to straighten the leg.	Pain in the lower back and resistance to straightening the leg

T A B L E 6 - 11   Meningitis: Typical CSF Finding

Findings	White cell count	Glucose	Protein
Normal	0-5/mm^3 lymphocytes	40-80 mg/dl	15-50 mg/dl
Bacterial	Predominantly polycytes: 1,000-10,000	<40 mg/dl	100-500 mg/dl
Viral	Predominantly lymphocytes (may see polycytes initially)	Normal	Slightly elevated
Tuberculous	Elevated lymphocytes: 100-400; lymphocyte elevation minimal or absent in immuno-compromised patients	<40 mg/dl or 50% of blood sugar drawn simultaneously	100-500 mg/dl; may increase gradually with progression of disease
Fungal	Predominantly elevated lymphocytes	Slightly decreased	Elevated
Lyme disease	Mildly elevated lymphocytes	Normal	Mildly elevated
Aseptic (nonbacterial)	Elevated lymphocytes	Normal	50-100 mg/dl

CSF, Cerebrospinal fluid.

T A B L E 6 - 12   Common Drug Therapy for the Management of Meningitis

Causative agent	Therapy
Bacterial meningitis	
S. pneumoniae	Penicillin, cefotaxime or ceftriaxone, vancomycin or rifampin + ceftriaxone
H. influenzae	Cefotaxime or ceftriaxone
N. meningitides	Penicillin G—if inadequate response, change to ceftriaxone or cefotaxime
L. monocytogenes	Penicillin, ampicillin + gentamycin
Pseudomonas	Ceftazidime
M. tuberculosis	Isoniazid, rifampin, ethambutol, pyrazinamide
B. burgdorferi	Ceftriaxone or penicillin G
Fungal	
C. neoformans	Amphotericin B + flucytosine, fluconazole, or itraconazole
Cocci	
Gram-positive	Vancomycin + penicillin G + aminoglycosides
Gram-negative	Penicillin G
Bacilli	
Gram-positive	Ampicillin, penicillin + aminoglycosides
Gram-negative	Cephalosporin + aminoglycosides

Adapted from Elmore J et al: Acute meningitis with a negative Gram's stain: Clinical and management outcomes in 171 episodes, *Am J Med* 100(1):78-84, 1996; Quagliarello V, Scheld M: Drug therapy: treatment of bacterial meningitis, *N Engl J Med* 336(10):708-716, 1997; Pacheco T et al: Failure of cefotaxime treatment in an adult with *Streptococcus pneumoniae* meningitis, *Am J Med* 102(3):303-305, 1997; and van der Horst et al: Treatment of cryptococcal meningitis associated with the acquired immunodeficiency syndrome, *N Engl J Med* 337(11):15-21, 1997.

Adjunctive pharmacologic therapies: Dexamethasone may decrease inflammation by reducing cytokines produced by bacterial products. Use is controversial. Steroids are given before or with antimicrobial medications for 2 days total (see Box, below). Monoclonal antibodies have been investigated because they decrease inflammation by deactivating bacterial cell surface components and cytokines produced from leukocyte activation.

Research Box: Use of Steroids in the Treatment of Bacterial Meningitis

Biological basis for effectiveness	Biological basis for potential harm	Effect in adults	Effect in children
Reduces inflammation	Suppresses immune mechanisms	Evidence for use of dexamethasone is not convincing.	Dexamethasone in *H. influenzae* B protects against hearing loss.
Reduces cerebral and spinal cord edema	Masks other infection	Limit use to those with high bacterial concentrations, elevated intracranial pressure, or edema.	Dexamethasone is beneficial in bacterial forms if commenced before antibiotics.
Reduces inflammation of small blood vessels and prevents slow flow to brain tissue	Reduces meningeal inflammation and decreases drug penetration into subarachnoid space Associated with GI hemorrhage, fungal infections, electrolyte imbalance, and hyperglycemia	Randomized trials are needed before recommendations can be made for changes.	Dexamethasone is not associated with adverse effects if use is limited to 2 days. More studies are needed to determine the effect of steroids in other forms of meningitis.

Adapted from Quagliarello V, Scheld M: Drug therapy: treatment of bacterial meningitis, *N Engl J Med* 336(10): 708-716, 1997; Prasad K, Menon G: Steroids in tuberculosis meningitis (Cochrane Review). In The Cochrane Library, Issue 2: Update Software 1998; Updated quarterly.

Nutritional management: Oral feeding should be encouraged when possible. Enteral or parenteral feeding may be initiated. Parenteral nutrition is used if enteral feeding is not tolerated. Hydration should be maintained.

Anticonvulsant therapy: Used prophylactically or if seizures occur. Seizures increase metabolic rate and cerebral blood flow, which may cause deterioration in patients with cerebral edema and intracranial hypertension.

Maintenance of normothermia and fever treatment: Helps prevent intracranial hypertension associated with increased metabolic rate. Fever should be controlled by antipyretics such as acetaminophen or use of other cooling measures such as tepid baths.

Infection prevention: Vaccines are currently available for meningitis prophylaxis, including the following: (1) influenza type B (Hib), given as a childhood immunization; (2) bacillus Calmette-Guérin (BCG), used for tuberculosis, also prevents tuberculosis meningitis; and (3) *N. meningitides* vaccines for specific or combined prophylaxis for five investigational subgroups. The Centers for Disease Control and Prevention (CDC) guidelines recommend Transmission-Based Precautions be implemented until effectiveness of antimicrobial treatment is established. See "Infection Prevention and Control," Appendix 8.

Rehabilitation consults: Physical therapy (PT), occupational therapy (OT), and speech should be initiated as soon as patient is stable, to minimize physical and cognitive complications.

Evaluation of need for support services: Evaluate the need for home health care, support groups, and social services.

NURSING DIAGNOSES AND INTERVENTIONS

Decreased adaptive capacity: intracranial, related to altered fluid dynamics secondary to brain and spinal cord inflammation

Desired outcomes: Within 72 hr of initiation of antimicrobial therapy, patient's ICP returns to normal range as evidenced by orientation to time, place, and person; bilaterally equal and normoreactive pupils; bilaterally equal strength and tone of extremities; absence of cranial nerve palsies; RR 12-20 breaths/min with normal depth and pattern (eupnea); HR 60-100 beats/min; BP within patient's normal range; and absence of headache, vomiting, papilledema, and other clinical indicators of IICP. After instruction, patient verbalizes knowledge of the importance of avoiding Valsalva-like activities.

- Assess neurologic status at least hourly. Monitor pupils, LOC, and motor activity; perform cranial nerve assessments (see Appendix 4). Early indicators of IICP and possible herniation include: decreased LOC, changes in pupillary size and reaction, a decreased motor function (weakness, posturing), and cranial nerve palsies.
- Monitor patient and report physical indicators of IICP (see Table 6-3) to the physician.
- Monitor VS at least every 15 minutes if patient has signs of IICP. Be alert to changes in respiratory pattern, fluctuations in BP and pulse, widening pulse pressure, and slow HR.
- Optimize cerebral oxygenation: maintain a patent airway and provide supplemental oxygen as prescribed. Ensure that patient's neck is not constricted by tracheostomy ties and oxygen tubing.
- Avoid overhydration, which increases cerebral edema. Ensure precise delivery of IV fluids and timely delivery of medications prescribed for the prevention of sudden increases or decreases in ICP, BP, HR, or RR.
- Teach patient to avoid activities that increase ICP: coughing, straining, and bending over.
- If patient shows evidence of IICP, implement measures to decrease ICP (see Table 2-5).

NIC Cerebral Edema Management; Cerebral Perfusion Promotion; Intracranial Pressure (ICP) Monitoring: Neurologic Monitoring; Positioning: Neurologic

Pain related to headache, photophobia, and fever secondary to meningeal irritation

Desired outcome: Within 2 hr of initiating pain treatment, patient reports pain relief, as documented by a pain scale.

- Monitor patient for pain and discomfort. Devise a pain rating scale with patient. Administer analgesics as prescribed. (See p. 52 for additional interventions for pain.)
- Monitor temperature q2h and prn. Administer tepid baths or cooling blanket and prescribed antipyretics/antibiotics to keep temperature within prescribed limits.
- Maintain an environment of comfort for each individual patient.
- Provide care and visiting hours to allow for uninterrupted periods (at least 90 min) of rest. If intracranial pressure is elevated, clustering care is contraindicated.
- Darken patient's room or provide blindfold to minimize the discomfort of photophobia.

Risk for infection related to possible cross-contamination secondary to communicable bacterial and aseptic meningitis

Desired outcome: Other patients, staff members, and patient's significant others do not exhibit evidence of having acquired meningitis: diminished LOC, confusion, fever, headache, nuchal rigidity, and other signs (see previous sections on "Assessment," p. 385, and "Diagnostic Tests," p. 386).

For patients with bacterial meningitis

- Bacterial meningitis is transmitted via droplet contact. Provide patient with a private room.
- Initiate Transmission-Based Precautions: Droplet, on admission, and maintain them for at least 24 hr after start of antimicrobial therapy.
  - ❏ Standard Precautions should be instituted to provide safety and protection regardless if infection is bacterial, fungal, or viral. Be alert for airborne pathogens and those in stool or oral secretions.

ADDITIONAL NURSING DIAGNOSES

See "Risk for Trauma (Oral and Musculoskeletal)" in "Status Epilepticus," p. 372. Because these patients are at risk for SIADH, see "Risk for Injury" in "Syndrome of Inappropriate Antidiuretic Hormone," p. 404. See also appropriate nursing diagnoses and interventions in "Septic Shock," p. 501, inasmuch as these patients are at risk for septic shock. As indicated, see other nursing diagnoses and interventions in "Nutritional Support," p. 1; "Prolonged Immobility," p. 61; "Psychosocial Support," p. 68; and "Psychosocial Support for the Patient's Family and Significant Others," p. 78.

Bibliography

Archives of Neurology, Editorial: Viral infections of the nervous system, *Arch Neurol* 59:712-718, 2002.

Bader MK: The complexity of caring for patients with ruptured cerebral aneurysm: case studies, *AACN Clinical Issues: Adv Prac Acute Crit Care* 8(2):182-195, 1997.

Bader MK et al: New neurointerventional therapies for stroke patients, *Dimens Crit Care Nurs* 16(6):301-311, 1997.

Barch C, issue editor: Stroke, *J Cardiovasc Nurs* 13(1):v-96, 1998.

Barch C et al: Common problems and proven solutions to acute stroke management, *Stroke Interven* 1(3):5-10, 1998.

Bell TE et al: Transcranial Doppler: correlation of blood velocity measurement with clinical status in subarachnoid hemorrhage, *J Neurosci Nurs* 24(4):215-219, 1992.

Bolton CF: The changing concepts of Guillain-Barré syndrome, *N Engl J Med* 333(21):1415-1416, 1995.

Bonthius D, Karacay B: Meningitis and encephalitis in children: an update. *Neurol Clin North Am* 20:1013-1038.

Brott T et al: Measurements of acute cerebral infarction: a clinical examination scale, *Stroke* 20(7):864-870, 1990.

Calder J: Listeria meningitis in adults, *Lancet* 350:307-308, 1997.

Campbell PJ, Edwards SM: Hyperdynamic therapy: the nurse's role in the treatment of cerebral vasospasm, *J Neurosci Nurs* 29(5):318-324, 1997.

Capra C et al: Trimethoprim-sulfamethoxazole-induced aseptic meningitis: case report and literature review. *Intensive Care Med* 26:212-224, 2000.

Carpenito L: *Nursing diagnosis,* ed 9, Philadelphia, 2002, Lippincott.

Davenport RJ et al: Gastrointestinal hemorrhage after acute stroke, *Stroke* 27(3):421-424, 1996.

Elmore J et al: Acute meningitis with a negative Gram's stain: clinical and management outcomes in 171 episodes, *Am J Med* 100(1):78-84, 1996.

Evans V, Barr J: Case study: nursing care of the patient with vertebral artery aneurysm treated by endovascular stenting and coil implantation, *J Neurosci Nurs* 30(5):279-282, 1998.

Fischer P: Acute seizures and status epilepticus: advances in therapy, *Clin Nurs Prac Epilepsy* 4(1):10-12, 1997.

Fowler SB: Neurotrauma family interventions, *J Trauma Nurs* 4(3):68-75, 1997.

Hickey JV: *The clinical practice of neurological and neurosurgical nursing,* ed 4, Philadelphia, 1997, Lippincott.

Huston CJ: Cervical spine injury, *Am J Nurs* 98(6):33, 1998.

Huston CJ, Boelman R: Autonomic dysreflexia, *Am J Nurs* 95(6):55, 1995.

Iowa Outcomes Project. Johnson M, Maas M, editors: *Nursing Outcomes Classification (NOC),* St Louis, 2004, Mosby.

Jolles S, Sewell C, Leighton C: Drug induced aseptic meningitis, *Drug Safety* 22(3):215-226, 2000.

Kaplan S: Management of bacterial meningitis, *Pediatr Infect Dis J* 21:589-592, 2002.

Kelleher J, Raebelm M: Meningococcal vaccine use in college students, *Ann Pharmacother* 36(11):1776-1784, 2002.

Kernich CA, Kaminski HJ: Myths & facts ... about myasthenia gravis, *Nursing '96* 26(7):21, 1996.

Klugman K, Koornhof H: Penicillin-resistant pneumococcal meningitis, *Lancet* 350(9085):1176-1177, 1997.

Lammertse DP: Recovery of neurologic function in spinal cord injury: a review of new and experimental therapies, *Top Spinal Cord Inj Rehabil* 2(3):95-100, 1997.

Larsen R: Treatment of cryptococcal meningitis, *N Engl J Med* 337(21):1557-1558, 1997.

Latov N: Immune-mediated neurological diseases: immunology of neurological diseases, *J Care Manage* 3(5):6-7, 16-18, 1997.

Lowenstein DH, Alldredge BK: Status epilepticus, *N Engl J Med* 338(14):970-976, 1998.

Lucke KT: Pulmonary management following acute spinal cord injury, *J Neurosci Nurs* 30(2):91-104, 1998.

McIntyre P et al.: Dexamethasone as adjunctive therapy in bacterial meningitis: a meta-analysis of randomized clinical trials since 1988, *JAMA* 278(11):925-931, 1997.

McMahon-Parkes K, Cornock MA: Guillain-Barré syndrome: biological basis, treatment and care, *Intensive Crit Care Nurs* 13(1):42-48, 1997.

Memish Z, Alrajhi A: Meningococcal disease, *Saudi Medical Journal* 23(3):259-264, 2002.

Miller L, Choi C: Meningitis in older patients: how to diagnose and treat a deadly infection, *Geriatrics* 52(8):43-55, 1997.

Moore K: Spotting vasospasm is vital for these patients, *RN* 60(6):60, 1997.

Munro R. Meningococcal disease: treatable but still terrifying. *Intern Med J* 32:165-169, 2002.

National High Blood Pressure Education Program, National Institutes of Health, and National Heart, Lung, and Blood Institute: NIH Pub No 93-1088, Jan 1993.

NINDS: *Rapid identification and treatment of acute stroke,* NIH Pub No 97-423, Aug 1997.

NINDS Stroke Study Group: rt-PA stroke treatment, *J Neurosci Nurs* 29(6):349-401, 1997.

O'Donnell L: An elusive weakness: myasthenia gravis, *Med-Surg Nurs* 5(1):44-49, 1996.

O'Donnell LE: Immune-mediated neurological diseases: management of myasthenia gravis—an overview, *J Care Manage* 3(6):4-5, 17-18, 1997.

Pacheco T et al: Failure of cefotaxime treatment in an adult with streptococcus pneumoniae meningitis, *Am J Med* 102(3):303-305, 1997.

Perfect J, Casadevall A: Cryptococcus, *Infect Dis Clin North Am* 16:837-874: 2002.

Pieper DR et al: Surgical management of patients with severe head injuries, *AORN J* 63(5):854-870, 1996.

Plum F, Posner J: *Diagnosis of stupor and coma,* ed 3, Philadelphia, 1980, Davis.

Pope W: External ventriculostomy: a practical application for the acute care nurse, *J Neurosci Nurs* 30(3):185-190, 1998.

Prasad K, Menon G: Steroids in tuberculous meningitis (Cochrane Review). In The Cochrane Library, Issue 2: Update Software 1998. Updated quarterly.

Quagliarello V, Scheld M: Drug therapy: treatment of bacterial meningitis, *N Engl J Med* 336(10):708-716, 1997.

Roos K: What I have learned about infectious diseases with my sleeves rolled up. *Seminars in Neurology,* 22 (1): 9-15: 2002.

Roos K: Mycobacterium tuberculosis meningitis and other etiologies of the aseptic meningitis syndrome, *Semin Neurol* vol 20, no 3: 2000.

Rusy KL: Rebleeding and vasospasm after subarachnoid hemorrhage: a critical care challenge, *Crit Care Nurs* 16(1):41-48, 1996.

Scheld WM, Koedel U, Nathan B, Pfister H: Pathophysiology of bacterial meningitis: mechanism(s) of neuronal injury, *J Infect Dis* 186(Suppl 2):S225-233, 2002.

Segal S, Pollard A: The future of meningitis vaccines, *Hosp Med* 64(3):161-167, 2003.

Schooley Y: *Recommendations for the nursing management of the hyperacute ischemic stroke patient,* American Association of Neuroscience Nurses Clinical Guideline Series, 1998.

Schuchat A et al.: Bacterial meningitis in the United States in 1995, *N Engl J Med* 337:970-976, 1997.

Segatore M: Hyponatremia after aneurysmal subarachnoid hemorrhage, *J Neurosci Nurs* 25(2): 92-99, 1993.

Segreti J, Harris A: Acute bacterial meningitis, *Infect Dis Clin North Am* 10(4):797-809, 1996.

Seybold ME: Update on myasthenia gravis, *Hosp Med* 27(4):71-72, 77-78, 80, 1991.

Stamatos CA et al: Meeting the challenge of the older trauma patient, *Am J Nurs* 96(5):40-48, 1996.

Stephens A: Systems and diseases: the immune system. I. Myasthenia gravis, *Nurs Times* 93(46): 56-59, 1997.

The Italian Guillain-Barré Study Group: The prognosis and main prognostic indicators of Guillain-Barré syndrome: a multicentre prospective study of 297 patients, *Brain* 119:2053-2061, 1996 (Dec, part 6).

Thompson R, Bertram H: Laboratory diagnosis of central nervous system infections, *Infect Dis Clin North Am* 15(4):1047-1071, 2001.

Titler M, Bulechek G, McCloskey J: Use of the nursing intervention classification by critical care nurses, *Crit Care Nurs* 16(4):38-54, 1996.

van der Horst et al: Treatment of cryptococcal meningitis associated with the acquired immunodeficiency syndrome, *N Engl J Med* 337(11):15-21, 1997.

Working Group on Status Epilepticus: Treatment of convulsive status epilepticus: recommendations of the Working Group on Status Epilepticus, *JAMA* 270(7):854-859, 1993.

Zafonte RD, Mann NR: Cerebral salt-wasting syndrome in brain injury patients: a potential cause of hyponatremia, *Arch Phys Med Rehabil* 78(5):540-542, 1997.

CHAPTER 7

Endocrinologic Dysfunctions

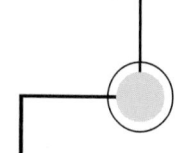

Diabetic Ketoacidosis

PATHOPHYSIOLOGY

Diabetic ketoacidosis (DKA) is a life-threatening complication of diabetes mellitus characterized by hyperglycemia, ketosis, acidosis, hypovolemic shock due to dehydration, and electrolyte imbalance. DKA is seen most often with type 1 diabetes mellitus with acute illness, infection, trauma, or surgery. DKA is somewhat rare with type 2 diabetes mellitus. The absolute insulin deficiency of the type 1 diabetic results from autoimmune destruction of beta-islet pancreatic cells and prevents glucose transport into cells. Type 2 diabetics have both beta-islet pancreatic cells and insulin receptors that are dysfunctional, resulting in low levels of circulating insulin and insulin resistance. Glucose is abundant in the bloodstream and deficient within the cells. With both types of diabetes, the unmet energy requirements of the cells stimulate gluconeogenesis and glycogen conversion in the liver through the release of counterregulatory hormones. The body breaks down fat and protein stores, attempting to provide glucose for the "starving" cells. The rate of breakdown exceeds the body's ability to use these alternate energy sources. Ketones accumulate, causing decreased blood pH: a metabolic acidosis. Hyperglycemia and ketonemia increase serum osmolality, resulting in an osmotic diuresis.

Osmotic diuresis causes loss of sodium, potassium, phosphorus, magnesium, and body water, which leads to dehydration and, possibly, hypovolemic shock. Increased blood viscosity and platelet aggregation can result in thromboembolism. Despite significant loss of potassium in the urine, the patient may initially manifest normal or elevated plasma potassium because of the dramatic shift of potassium out of the cells secondary to insulin deficiency, acidosis, and tissue catabolism. Dehydration lowers blood pressure and decreases tissue perfusion, and cells begin anaerobic metabolism. The resulting lactic acid waste products worsen acidosis. Low pH stimulates the respiratory center, producing deep, rapid, *Kussmaul* respirations. Abundant plasma ketones cause fruity or acetone breath. If not managed, elevated serum osmolality, acidosis, and dehydration depress consciousness to a coma state. Death can result.

ASSESSMENT

History and risk factors: Type 1 or type 2 diabetes mellitus, recent stressor such as illness, infection, trauma, pregnancy, or surgery (most episodes of DKA are precipitated by infection), insufficient or omitted exogenous insulin replacement, severe emotional stress. Vascular events such as myocardial infarction (MI), cerebral vascular accident (CVA) or ischemic bowel may precipitate or worsen DKA.

Clinical presentation: Recent polyuria, polydipsia, polyphagia, weight loss, weakness, fatigue, nausea, vomiting, abdominal pain, altered mental status, and possibly "strokelike" symptoms.

Physical assessment: Dry and flushed skin, dry mucous membranes, poor skin turgor, altered level of consciousness (LOC) (e.g., irritability, lethargy, coma), fruity breath odor, Kussmaul respirations, abdominal pain, nausea, vomiting, and chest discomfort. Presence of hypotension and tachycardia suggests severe volume loss.

Electrocardiogram (ECG) and hemodynamic findings: ECG may show dysrhythmias associated with hyperkalemia: peaked T waves, widened QRS complex, prolonged PR intervals, and flattened-to-absent P wave. After insulin therapy is initiated, hypokalemia is possible (see p. 549).

Note: For additional assessment information, see Table 7-1.

DIAGNOSTIC TESTS
See Table 7-1.

TABLE 7-1 Comparison of Diabetic Ketoacidosis (DKA) and Hyperglycemic Hyperosmolar Nonketotic Syndrome (HHNS)

Criterion	DKA	HHNS
Diabetes type	Type 1	Type 2
Typical age-group	Any age	Usually >50 yr
Signs and symptoms	Polyuria, polydipsia, polyphagia, weakness, orthostatic hypotension, lethargy, changes in LOC, fatigue, nausea, vomiting, abdominal pain	Same as DKA, but slower onset Also, very commonly, neurologic symptoms predominate
Physical assessment	Dry and flushed skin, poor skin turgor, dry mucous membranes, decreased BP, tachycardia, altered LOC (irritability, lethargy, coma), Kussmaul respirations, fruity odor to the breath	Same as DKA, but no Kussmaul respirations or fruity odor to the breath; instead, occurrence of tachypnea with shallow respirations
History and risk factors	Recent stressors such as surgery, trauma, infection, MI; insufficient exogenous insulin; undiagnosed type 1 diabetes mellitus	Undiagnosed type 2 diabetes mellitus; recent stressors such as surgery, trauma, pancreatitis, MI, infection; high-calorie enteral or parenteral feedings in a compromised patient; use of diabetogenic drugs (e.g., phenytoin, thiazide diuretics, thyroid preparations, mannitol, corticosteroids, sympathomimetics)
Monitoring parameters	*ECG:* Dysrhythmias associated with hyperkalemia: peaked T waves, widened QRS complex, prolonged PR interval, flattened or absent P wave. Hypokalemia (K^+ <3 mEq/L), which may produce depressed ST segments, flat or inverted T waves, or increased ventricular dysrhythmias	*ECG* evidence of hypokalemia as listed with DKA *Hemodynamic measurements:* CVP >3 mm Hg below patient's baseline; PADP and PAWP >4 mm Hg below patient's baseline
Diagnostic tests	*Serum glucose:* 200-800 mg/dl *Serum ketones:* positive at >1:2 *Urine glucose:* positive	800-2000 mg/dl Usually absent Positive

TABLE 7-1 Comparison of Diabetic Ketoacidosis (DKA) and Hyperglycemic Hyperosmolar Nonketotic Syndrome (HHNS)—cont'd

Criterion	DKA	HHNS
	Urine acetone: "large"	Negative
	Serum osmolality: 300-350 mOsm/L	> 350 mOsm/L
	Bicarbonate: <15 mEq/L	Normal or slightly decreased if mild acidosis present
	Serum pH: <7.2	Normal or mildly acidotic (pH < 7.4)
	Serum potassium: normal or elevated >5.0 mEq/L initially and then decreased	Normal or <3.5 mEq/L
	Serum sodium: elevated, normal, or low	Elevated, normal, or low
	Serum Hct: elevated because of osmotic diuresis with hemoconcentration	Elevated because of hemoconcentration
	BUN: elevated >20 mg/dl	Elevated
	Serum creatinine: >1.5 mg/dl	Elevated
	Serum phosphorus, magnesium, chloride: decreased	Elevated
	WBC: elevated, even in the absence of infection	Normal unless infection present
Onset	Hours to days	Days to weeks
Mortality	<10%	10%-25% because of age group and complications such as stroke, thrombosis, renal failure

BP, Blood pressure; *BUN,* blood urea nitrogen; *CVP,* central venous pressure; *DKA,* diabetic ketoacidosis; *ECG,* electrocardiogram; *Hct,* hematocrit; HHNS, hyperglycemic hyperosmolar nonketotic syndrome; *LOC,* level of consciousness; *MI,* myocardial infarction; *PADP,* pulmonary artery diastolic pressure; *PAWP,* pulmonary artery wedge pressure; *WBC,* white blood cell count.

COLLABORATIVE MANAGEMENT

Rehydration: Isotonic saline (0.9%) is administered rapidly (1-2 L during the first hour) followed by 200-500 ml/hr as clinically indicated to correct the fluid deficit, which may exceed 6 L. D_5W (5% dextrose intravenous [IV] solution) with saline may be used after the first 1-2 hr if the blood glucose is normalizing. D_5W is used when blood glucose falls to about 250 mg/dl, to prevent hypoglycemia and allow the continued administration of insulin necessary to correct ketoacidosis. As fluid balance normalizes, 0.45% saline with D_5W may be administered prn to facilitate intracellular rehydration.

Rapid-acting insulin/intensive insulin therapy: A loading dose (~10 units) of regular insulin is given, followed by continuous IV insulin infusion at 5-10 units/hr (or 0.1 units/kg/hr can be used.) Insulin protocols may vary. Blood glucose should be lowered gradually to reduce the risk for cerebral edema. Dose is adjusted based on serial glucose measurements. The insulin drip dosage should be decreased and IV 5% dextrose (D_5W) added; or, if patient is hypoglycemic (i.e., the serum glucose drops to <100 mg/dl before correction of acidosis), D50 (50% dextrose) should be given. Studies indicate that blood glucose level should be maintained between 80-110 mg/dl to decrease in-hospital morbidity and mortality. Insulin adheres to plastics. IV tubing should be flushed with 25-50 ml of the insulin solution to saturate the tubing prior to administration.

Restoration of electrolyte balance: Potassium is closely monitored and replaced. As blood glucose is controlled, potassium shifts back into the cells. Potassium replacement corrects the deficit and prevents severe hypokalemia. Deficits may require days to normalize. Hypomagnesemia may not need management unless level is below 1.5 mg/dl, dysrhythmias do not resolve, or potassium replacement is ineffective. Phosphate replacement is used for severe depletion in the presence of acidosis. Phosphate *and* calcium levels are monitored if phosphate replacement is prescribed. Supplemental phosphate may lower calcium levels secondary to calcium-phosphorus binding (see "Hypophosphatemia," p. 558).

Intravenous (IV) bicarbonate: Not routinely given for acidosis correction in DKA because the acidosis of DKA is best corrected by insulin therapy. Bicarbonate may cause paradoxical cerebral spinal fluid acidosis and hypokalemia. May be prescribed for severe acidosis (pH <7.1), if hypotension requires vasopressors. Catecholamines may be ineffective when pH is extremely low. Hyperchloremic acidosis, secondary to DKA or aggressive volume replacement with isotonic saline, usually resolves without treatment.

Vasopressors: May be required if 3-4 L of IV fluid replacement does not correct hypotension. Catecholamines (e.g., norepinephrine, dopamine) are often used. Peripheral circulation must be closely observed to avoid tissue anoxia if the patient is extremely hypovolemic.

Insertion of gastric tube: Used in comatose or obtunded patients when risk is high of vomiting and aspiration from gastric distention or paralytic ileus. Gastroparesis is a common complication of diabetes mellitus.

Management of cerebral edema: Cerebral edema is a rarely seen, but serious complication of fluid resuscitation. Aggressive treatment may prevent respiratory arrest or death. Mannitol infusion (0.5-2 g/kg), other diuretic or ventriculostomy to drain CSF may be used.

Treatment of underlying cause: For example, infection is treated with appropriate antibiotics.

NURSING DIAGNOSES AND INTERVENTIONS

Fluid volume deficit related to decreased circulating volume secondary to hyperglycemia-induced osmotic diuresis

Desired outcomes: Within 12 hr of initiating treatment, patient is euvolemic as evidenced by blood pressure (BP) ≥90/60 mm Hg (or within patient's normal range); mean arterial pressure (MAP) ≥70 mm Hg; heart rate (HR) 60-100 beats/min, central venous pressure (CVP) 2-6 mm Hg, pulmonary artery wedge pressure (PAWP) 6-12 mm Hg, balanced intake and output (I&O), urinary output ≥0.5 ml/kg/hr, firm skin turgor, and pink and moist mucous membranes. ECG exhibits normal sinus rhythm.

- Monitor vital signs (VS) q15min until patient is stable for 1 hr. Monitor CVP, MAP, pulmonary artery pressure (PAP), pulmonary capillary wedge pressure (PCWP), if ordered. Consult physician for the following: HR >140 beats/min or BP <90/60 or decreased ≥20 mm Hg, or MAP decreased ≥10 mm Hg from baseline, CVP <2 mm Hg, and PAWP <6 mm Hg.
- Monitor hydration status: mucous membranes, pulse rate and quality, and blood pressure.
- Monitor I&O. Decreased urine output may indicate inadequate fluid volume or impending renal failure. Consult physician for urine output <0.5 ml/kg/hr for 2 consecutive hours.
- Replace volume with IV fluids. Monitor for fluid overload, which can occur as a result of rapid infusion of fluids: jugular vein distention, dyspnea, crackles (rales), and CVP >6 mm Hg.
- Monitor for abnormal electrolyte levels as ordered.
- Note an increase in anion gap (>14 mEq/L), signaling increased production or decreased excretion of acids. Anion gap should decrease steadily with successful treatment of DKA.
- Monitor for symptomatic cardiac dysrhythmias. (See "Fluid and Electrolytes," p. 538.)
- Observe for clinical signs of electrolyte imbalance associated with DKA and its treatment:
  - ❏ *Hypokalemia:* ventricular dysrhythmias, muscle weakness, anorexia, and hypoactive bowel sounds.
  - ❏ *Hypophosphatemia:* Muscle weakness, malaise, confusion, respiratory failure, decreased oxygen delivery, and decreased cardiac function.
  - ❏ *Hypomagnesemia:* Anorexia, nausea, vomiting, lethargy, weakness, personality changes, tetany, tremor or muscle fasciculations, seizures, confusion, and difficulty managing hypokalemia.
- Weigh patient daily, and monitor trends.

You may also wish to refer to the following interventions from the Nursing Interventions Classification (NIC):

■NIC Hyperglycemia Management; Fluid/Electrolyte Management; Fluid Monitoring; Invasive Hemodynamic Monitoring; Acid-Base Management: Metabolic Acidosis; Electrolyte Management: Hypokalemia

Risk for infection related to inadequate secondary defenses (suppressed inflammatory response) due to protein depletion and hyperglycemia

Desired outcome: Patient is free of infection as evidenced by normothermia; HR ≤100 beats/min; BP within patient's normal range; white blood cell (WBC) count ≤11,000/mm^3, and negative culture results.

* Monitor for signs of infection. Fever may be suppressed secondary to acidosis. Monitor for increased WBC count, which initially may reflect dehydration or the stress response.
* Since patient is at higher risk for bacterial infection, invasive lines should be managed carefully to avoid bloodstream infection (BSI). Central lines should be removed as soon as possible.
* Manage urinary catheters meticulously to prevent urinary tract infection (UTI).
* Maintain skin integrity. Assess for areas of decreased sensation.

NIC Infection Protection; Skin Surveillance

Risk for injury related to altered mental status secondary to hyperosmolality, dehydration, cerebral edema, or hypoglycemia

Desired outcomes: Patient verbalizes orientation to time, place, and person; patient is protected from unnecessary complications and bodily injury.

* Monitor neurological and respiratory status frequently. Have respiratory support equipment readily available. Notify physician of deterioration, and prepare for endotracheal intubation.
* Keep bed in lowest position with side rails raised, if patient is confused.
* Consider gastric tube with suction to decompress comatose patients to decrease likelihood of aspiration.
* Elevate head of bed (HOB) to 45 degrees to minimize the risk of aspiration.
* Monitor blood glucose hourly while on insulin infusion. Consult physician if blood glucose drops faster than 100 mg/dl/hr or if it drops to <250 mg/dl. Obtain prescription for glucose-containing IV solution to prevent hypoglycemia and allow the continued administration of insulin necessary to correct acidosis.

NIC Neurologic Monitoring; Hyperglycemia Management; Hypoglycemia Management

Knowledge deficit: new-onset diabetes or misunderstanding of the causes and prevention of DKA

Desired outcome: By discharge from intensive care unit (ICU), patient verbalizes understanding of causes, symptoms, and prevention of DKA.

* Consider referral to diabetes educator for new-onset diabetes or if patient has not managed condition well in the past. Provide instructions simply, incorporating patient teaching into patient care routines.
* Explain the relationship of DKA to illness and stress. Emphasize importance of adhering to the diabetes regimen, including meal planning, medication, exercise, and monitoring.
* Review illness guidelines for individuals with diabetes (i.e., need for increased fluid and insulin with illness) with patient and significant others.
* Provide hospital and community resources for diabetes education and support.
* Provide address and websites for the American Diabetes Association (ADA): American Diabetes Association, Inc., 18 East 48th St, New York, NY 10017; www.ada.org and www.diabetes.org

NIC Teaching: Disease Process; Teaching: Prescribed Diet; Teaching: Prescribed Medication; Teaching: Prescribed Activity/Exercise; Emotional Support

---

Research Brief 7-1 This prospective, randomized, controlled study involved 1548 adults admitted to a surgical intensive care unit receiving mechanical ventilation. On admission, patients were randomly assigned to receive intensive insulin therapy (blood glucose level maintained at 80-110 mg/dl) or conventional treatment of blood glucose levels >215 mg/dl lowered to target 180-200 mg/dl. After 12 months of study, intensive insulin therapy reduced ICU mortality to 4.6% from 8.0% with conventional therapy (P<0.04 with adjustment for sequential analyses). For patients who remained in the unit >5 days, mortality using intensive insulin therapy was reduced to 10.6% from 20.2% using conventional therapy. Total in-hospital mortality of the study population was reduced by 34%, bloodstream infections by 46%, acute renal failure requiring dialysis or hemofiltration by 41%, the median number of red blood cell transfusions by 50%, and critical illness polyneuropathy by 44%. The greatest reduction in mortality involved deaths due to multiple organ failure with a proven sepsis focus.

From Van den Berghe G et al: Intensive insulin therapy in critically ill patients, *N Engl J Med* 345(19):1359-1367, 2001.

ADDITIONAL NURSING DIAGNOSES

See "Altered Peripheral Tissue Perfusion" in "Hyperglycemic Hyperosmolar Nonketotic Syndrome," p. 399. See also nursing diagnoses and interventions in "Prolonged Immobility," p. 61;

"Psychosocial Support," p. 68; and "Psychosocial Support for the Patient's Family and Significant Others," p. 78.

Hyperglycemic Hyperosmolar Nonketotic Syndrome

PATHOPHYSIOLOGY

Hyperglycemic hyperosmolar nonketotic syndrome (HHNS) is a life-threatening emergency created by a relative insulin deficiency and insulin resistance, resulting in severe hyperglycemia and dehydration. It occurs most commonly in older people with type 2 diabetes. Usually HHNS is precipitated by exacerbation of a chronic disease or another stressor such as trauma or infection. The body's available insulin cannot control blood glucose, but is adequate to prevent lipolysis and formation of ketone bodies, thereby avoiding ketosis. The blood glucose level is higher with HHNS than with DKA, resulting in profound hyperosmolality and osmotic diuresis. Severe dehydration and electrolyte loss occur. Sodium and potassium levels vary at diagnosis, but deficiencies of both are present. Phosphorus and magnesium deficiencies are also common. Those affected may lose from 15%-25% of total body water. Fluids are drawn from cells to dilute the concentrated bloodstream. Significant intracellular dehydration results. Neurologic deficits occur in response to severe dehydration and hyperosmolality. The blood is highly viscous, and flow slows, increasing risk for the formation of thromboemboli. Increased cardiac workload and decreased renal and cerebral blood flow may result in myocardial infarction, renal failure, and stroke.

Unlike DKA, wherein acidosis produces severe symptoms, HHNS develops slowly, and frequently symptoms are nonspecific. Polyuria and polydipsia occur but may be ignored. Neurologic deficits may be mistaken for senility. Similarity of symptoms to other disease processes in elders may delay diagnosis and treatment, allowing the process to progress.

ASSESSMENT

History and risk factors: Type 2 diabetes mellitus; acute exacerbation of a chronic illness, particularly renal or cardiovascular; ingestion of high-caloric enteral or parenteral feedings; stressors such as trauma or infection, which increase insulin need; use of diabetogenic drugs (e.g., glucocorticoids, some diuretics, phenytoin, thyroid preparations).

Clinical presentation: Polyuria, polydipsia, weight loss, weakness, orthostatic hypotension, lethargy, confusion, nausea, abdominal pain, and chest discomfort. Although many patients are seen with altered mental status, only 15% are unresponsive. Seizures may be present.

Physical assessment: Poor skin turgor, dry mucous membranes, tachycardia, tachypnea with shallow respirations.

ECG and hemodynamic findings: Evidence of hypokalemia (increased premature ventricular complexes [PVCs], depressed T waves), CVP >3 mm Hg below patient's baseline, pulmonary artery diastolic (PAD) pressure >4 mm Hg below patient's baseline, and PAWP >4 mm Hg below patient's baseline.

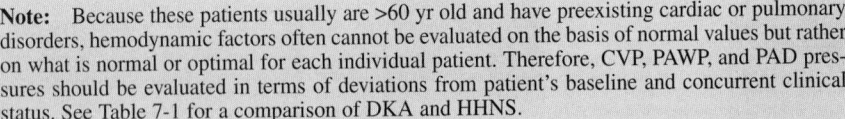

Note: Because these patients usually are >60 yr old and have preexisting cardiac or pulmonary disorders, hemodynamic factors often cannot be evaluated on the basis of normal values but rather on what is normal or optimal for each individual patient. Therefore, CVP, PAWP, and PAD pressures should be evaluated in terms of deviations from patient's baseline and concurrent clinical status. See Table 7-1 for a comparison of DKA and HHNS.

DIAGNOSTIC TESTS

See Table 7-1.

COLLABORATIVE MANAGEMENT

Replacement of electrolytes and extracellular fluid volume: Most often, 0.45% saline or isotonic saline is used; potassium phosphate and magnesium supplements are added on the basis of laboratory values. Usually half of the estimated fluid deficit is replaced during the first 12 hr and the remainder over the next 24 hr. To prevent hypoglycemia, dextrose will be added to the IV solution once the blood glucose falls to 250 mg/dl.

Rapid-acting insulin: A loading dose (~10 units) of regular insulin is given, followed by continuous IV insulin infusion at 5-10 units/hr (or, 0.1 units/kg/hr can be used). Blood glucose should be lowered gradually to reduce the risk for cerebral edema. Dose is adjusted based on serial glucose measurements. The insulin drip dosage should be decreased and IV dextrose added; or, if patient is hypoglycemic (i.e., the serum glucose drops to <100 mg/dl before correction of acidosis), D50 (50% dextrose) should be given. Follow protocol, or consult physician. Studies indicate that blood glucose level should be maintained between 80-110 mg/dl to decrease in-hospital morbidity and mortality. Insulin adheres to plastics. IV tubing should be flushed with 50-100 ml of the insulin solution to saturate the tubing before administration. Despite severe hyperglycemia, HHNS often requires less insulin to correct than does DKA. The condition sometimes can be treated with fluid alone.

Insertion of pulmonary artery (Swan-Ganz) catheter: For continuous assessment fluid and hemodynamic status.

Treatment of underlying cause: The most frequent cause is infection, which is treated with appropriate antibiotics. Omission of prescribed diabetic medications or other concurrent illnesses or events (vascular problems such as MI, CVA, ischemic bowel) may prompt and/or complicate HHNS.

NURSING DIAGNOSES AND INTERVENTIONS

Altered tissue perfusion: peripheral, related to interruption of blood flow (thromboembolism) secondary to increased viscosity of blood, increased platelet aggregation and adhesiveness, and patient immobility

Desired outcome: By the time of hospital discharge, patient has adequate perfusion as evidenced by peripheral pulses >2+ on a 0-4+ scale; brisk capillary refill (<2 sec); warm skin; and absence of swelling, bluish discoloration, erythema, and discomfort in the calves and thighs.

- Maintain adequate hydration to prevent increased blood viscosity. Monitor hematocrit (Hct). With proper fluid replacement, values should return to normal within 24-48 hr. Decreased blood urea nitrogen (BUN) and creatinine are indicators of improved renal perfusion.
- Perform a comprehensive appraisal of peripheral circulation (e.g., check peripheral pulses, edema, capillary refill, color, and temperature of extremities).
- Assess for deep vein thrombosis (i.e., presence of erythema, pain, tenderness, warmth, swelling, bluish discoloration, or prominence of superficial veins in the extremities, especially the lower extremities). Arterial thrombosis produces cyanosis with delayed capillary refill, mottling, and coolness of the extremity. Report significant findings to physician immediately.
- Assist with range-of-motion (ROM) exercises to all extremities q4h to increase blood flow. Apply pneumatic sequential compression stockings or similar devices to the lower extremities as prescribed to help prevent thrombosis.
- Change the patient's position at least q2h as appropriate.
- Administer antiplatelet or anticoagulant medication as prescribed.
- Instruct the patient on the importance of prevention of venous stasis (e.g., not crossing legs, elevating feet without bending knees, exercise).

NIC Hyperglycemia Management; Neurologic Monitoring; Fluid/Electrolyte Management; Fluid Monitoring; Intravenous (IV) Therapy; Invasive Hemodynamic Monitoring; Circulatory Care; Hypoglycemia Management

Knowledge deficit: new-onset diabetes or causes of HHNS

Desired outcome: Before discharge from ICU, patient verbalizes understanding of the basics of diabetes management and prevention of HHNS.

- Teach patient the causes, prevention, and treatment of HHNS. Allow patient to verbalize feelings about the diagnosis; correct any misconceptions. Explain the disease process of diabetes mellitus and HHNS and the common early symptoms of worsening diabetes, including polyuria, polydipsia, polyphagia, dry and flushed skin, and increased irritability.
- Stress the value of testing blood glucose levels as prescribed, or before meals and at bedtime.
- Explain the importance of taking diabetes medication as prescribed. Explain that increased medication may be needed during periods of physical or emotional stress. Blood glucose levels should be monitored closely during these times, as well as during illness or injury.
- Review the importance of regular exercise, consistent dietary intake, preventive measures for avoiding infection, and prompt management of minor injuries.
- Provide information for obtaining medical-alert bracelet or card with patient's diagnosis.
- Stress the necessity for continued medical follow-up.
- Provide booklets or pamphlets about diabetes from the ADA or pharmaceutical companies. Refer patient and significant others to a diabetes education program, if needed.

NIC Teaching: Disease Process; Teaching: Prescribed Diet; Teaching: Prescribed Medication; Teaching: Prescribed Activity/Exercise; Emotional Support

ADDITIONAL NURSING DIAGNOSES

See also "Diabetic Ketoacidosis" for "Fluid Volume Deficit," p. 396; "Risk for Infection," p. 396; and "Risk for injury," p. 397. For other nursing diagnoses and interventions, see the following as appropriate: "Psychosocial Support," p. 68; and "Psychosocial Support for the Patient's Family and Significant Others," p. 78.

Diabetes Insipidus

PATHOPHYSIOLOGY

Diabetes insipidus (DI) is a massive diuresis resulting from a deficiency of antidiuretic hormone (ADH), increased action of vasopressinase (the enzyme that breaks down vasopressin), or decreased renal responsiveness to ADH. Synthesis of ADH in the posterior pituitary gland may be impaired, or the hypothalamus may become dysfunctional (central DI). The hypothalamus stimulates the posterior pituitary to synthesize ADH by releasing hormones. Vasopressinase-induced DI is sometimes seen in the last trimester of pregnancy. DI may be nephrogenic (NDI) secondary to decreased water permeability of the collecting tubules caused by decreased ADH effect. DI is often temporary, occurring suddenly in response to head injury, major trauma, tumor, or inflammation. In some situations the condition may become permanent. Transient DI typically resolves after approximately 5-7 days. If resolution of the problem does not occur within that time frame, the patient usually progresses to permanent polyuria and polydipsia.

The hallmark sign of DI is excretion of large quantities of hypotonic urine, frequently 10-12 L/day or more. As free water is lost, the extracellular fluid volume decreases dramatically, causing plasma osmolality and serum sodium to rise. If individuals cannot respond adequately to the stimulus of thirst, extracellular and intracellular dehydration, hypotension, and hypovolemic shock may ensue. The increased blood viscosity increases the risk of thromboembolus formation. Dehydration, decreased cerebral perfusion, and electrolyte imbalance may produce neurologic symptoms ranging from confusion, restlessness, and irritability to seizures and coma.

ASSESSMENT

History and risk factors

Central DI: Brain tumors, especially in the hypothalamus or pituitary region; neoplasms such as leukemia or breast cancer; surgery in the area of the pituitary gland; intracranial hemorrhage; head injury, especially to the base of the brain; meningitis or encephalitis; any disorder that causes increased intracranial pressure (IICP); cerebral hypoxia.

Vasopressinase-induced DI: Seen in patients during the last trimester of pregnancy who have oligohydramnios, preeclampsia, and/or hepatic dysfunction. These patients break down *only* endogenous vasopressin (antidiuretic hormone/ADH) and can be managed with synthetic vasopressin (desmopressin).

Nephrogenic DI: From medications (e.g., lithium, demeclocycline); chronic hypercalcemia; hypokalemia; osmotic diuresis; congenital disorder of defective expression of renal vasopressin V2 receptors; or patients with pyelonephritis, renal amyloidosis, myeloma, Sjögren's syndrome, or sickle cell anemia.

> **Note:**　As much as 5-12 L/day of urine may be excreted, with specific gravity of 1.000-1.005.

Clinical presentation: Polyuria with dilute urine; extreme thirst.
Physical assessment: Unremarkable if the individual can safely satisfy thirst. If fluid intake is inadequate, patients may become dehydrated, with poor skin turgor, dry mucous membranes, orthostatic hypotension, hypotension, and tachycardia. Altered LOC is seen if serum hyperosmolality and hypernatremia develop. Altered LOC and neurologic changes may also be related to the precipitating event.
Monitoring parameters
Urine output: >200 ml/hr for 2 consecutive hours or >500 ml/hr, especially if risk factors are present.
Hemodynamics: CVP <2 mm Hg; PAWP <6mm Hg.

DIAGNOSTIC TESTS

Urine osmolality: Decreased to <200 mOsm/kg; may be higher if volume depletion is present.
Specific gravity: <1.007.
Serum osmolality: Increased to >300 mOsm/kg.
Serum sodium: Increased to >147 mEq/L.
Plasma ADH: Decreased in central DI.
Water deprivation test: Preliminary measurements of weight, serum and urine osmolality, and urine specific gravity are obtained. Fluid intake is prohibited, and the aforementioned values are measured hourly until urine specific gravity exceeds 1.020 and urine osmolality exceeds 800 mOsm/kg (a negative result) or when 5% of body weight is lost or urine specific gravity does not increase for 3 consecutive hours (a positive result). Less dramatic results may indicate partial DI. To establish a definite diagnosis of DI, it is necessary also to perform the vasopressin test (see next entry).

Caution: The water deprivation test can take up to 16 hr to complete and may produce hypernatremia, severe dehydration, and hypovolemic shock. Patients must be monitored continuously throughout the test. This test may not be necessary in cases of temporary DI in the critical care setting.

Vasopressin test: Vasopressin (exogenous ADH) is administered subcutaneously. Urine specimens are collected q30min for 2 hr and evaluated for quantity and osmolality. Urine osmolality generally will rise significantly in response to the ADH unless the DI has a nephrogenic origin, in which case the response may be minimal.

Caution: This test can induce congestive heart failure secondary to fluid overload in susceptible persons.

COLLABORATIVE MANAGEMENT

Rehydration: Hypotonic IV solutions are frequently used to replace free water lost in the urine. Fluid replacement is very rapid until hemodynamic status becomes stabilized; then it is based on urine output. Hypernatremia, if present, should be corrected slowly, especially if it is chronic. Symptomatic hypernatremia should be corrected more rapidly than asymptomatic hypernatremia.
Exogenous ADH (vasopressin): Several preparations are available, and dosage is adjusted to patient response. Potential side effects related to its vasoconstrictive effects on blood vessels include hypertension, angina, or MI; other side effects include abdominal cramping and increased peristalsis from smooth muscle excitation, and water intoxication. Use of desmopressin has become increasingly popular because it produces fewer side effects (Table 7-2).
Thiazide diuretics in combination with a low-sodium diet: Major form of therapy for nephrogenic DI. This approach reduces the loss of free water in the urine. Amiloride hydrochloride (a potassium-sparing diuretic) is the medication of choice for the treatment of lithium-induced NDI. Nonsteroidal antiinflammatory drugs (NSAIDs) may be used as adjunctive therapy in NDI.
Transsphenoidal hypophysectomy: Although not an appropriate treatment for transient DI that occurs after injury or surgery, this surgical approach to the pituitary gland is the treatment of choice for pituitary tumors of all types, whether or not the pituitary gland itself is removed. It produces immediate results, has a low mortality, and can be effective in the treatment of tumors that are resistant to radiation therapy.

To enter the sella turcica through the sphenoid process, the upper lip is elevated and an incision is made in the gingiva above the maxilla. Because of the site of the incision, patients are at high risk for postoperative infection, particularly of the brain. To minimize this possibility, antibiotic nasal sprays are used preoperatively, and nasal packing impregnated with an antibiotic ointment is kept in place for 24-72 hr after surgery. Complications include pituitary hemorrhage, frontal lobe damage, and hormonal deficiencies after removal of the gland. Tumors occur most often in the anterior pituitary gland; therefore most postoperative hormone deficiencies result from a lack of anterior pituitary hormones. In addition, the patient may have IICP caused by edema or bleeding in the sella turcica and will return from surgery with bilateral periorbital ecchymosis.

TABLE 7 - 2   Vasopressin Preparations

Generic name	Trade name	Route	Onset	Duration	Total daily dose	Comments
Desmopressin acetate	DDAVP Stimate	Intranasal	1-2 hr	8-12 hr	0.1-0.4 ml (10-40 mcg) daily in 1-2 doses	Administered by nasal spray or rhinal tube applicator. Action decreased by nasal congestion/discharge or atrophy of nasal mucosa. Stored in refrigerator. Drug of choice for chronic CDI.
		Subcutaneous	Within ½ hr	1½ - 4 hr	0.5-1 ml (2-4 mcg) daily in 2 divided doses	Keep refrigerated. More potent than intranasal route.
		Intravenous	Within ½ hr	1½ - 4 hr	0.5-1 ml (2-4 mcg) daily in 2 divided doses	Keep refrigerated. More potent than intranasal route.
		Oral tablets	1-2 hr	8-12 hr	0.1-0.8 mg daily in 2-3 divided doses	Simple to use. More consistent absorption and few side effects.
Vasopressin	Pitressin	Subcutaneous Intramuscular	1-2 hr 1-2 hr	2-8 hr 2-8 hr	5-10 units (20 units/ml); given q3-4 hr	Used primarily to confirm the diagnosis, differentiate between CDI and NDI, and treat acute situations.
Lysine vasopressin	Diapid	Intranasal	Within 1 hr	3-8 hr	7-14 mcg in 4 doses (q6h)	Lower cost than DDAVP for patients with partial CDI who require 1-2 daily doses.

CDI, Central diabetes insipidus; *NDI,* nephrogenic diabetes insipidus.

NURSING DIAGNOSES AND INTERVENTIONS

Fluid volume deficit related to failure of regulatory mechanisms (resulting in polyuria) secondary to ADH deficiency or altered ADH action

Desired outcome: Within 12 hr of initiating therapy, patient is normovolemic as evidenced by BP 110-120/70-80 mm Hg (or within patient's normal range); CVP $\geq$2 mm Hg; PAWP $\geq$6 mm Hg; HR 60-100 beats/min; intake equal to output plus insensible losses; and stable weight.

- Keep careful I&O records. Urine output >200 ml/hr for 2 consecutive hours, or 500 ml/hr, in the presence of risk factors (see p. 400), should be reported to physician promptly.
- Give fluids as appropriate. Keep water pitcher full and within easy reach of patient. Administer hyperosmolar tube feedings or solutions with extreme caution. They can worsen fluid losses through the gastrointestinal (GI) tract by inducing osmotic diarrhea.
- Administer hypotonic solutions (e.g., D_5W, $D_5$0.25 or 0.45 NaCl) for intracellular rehydration. Usually, fluids are administered as follows: 1 ml IV fluid for each 1 ml of urine output. In patients with brain injury, moderate diuresis may be permitted to avoid the need for administering osmotic diuretics. Hypernatremia, if present, must be corrected slowly (at a rate no greater than 0.5 mEq/L/hr or 12 mEq/L/day) to prevent cerebral edema, seizures, permanent neurologic damage, or death.
- Administer vasopressin as ordered. Observe for and document effects. Also be alert to side effects of therapy: hypertension, cardiac ischemia, and hyponatremia.
- Weigh patient daily, at the same time and using the same scale and garments to prevent error. Consult physician for weight loss >1 kg/day.
- Observe for indications of dehydration (e.g., poor skin turgor, delayed capillary refill, weak/thready pulse, dry mucous membranes, hypotension).
- Monitor hemodynamic status, including CVP, MAP, PAP, and PCWP, if available.
- Monitor laboratory studies, including serum sodium, serum and urine osmolality, and urine specific gravity; report significant findings to physician. Normal values are as follows: serum sodium 137-147 mEq/L, serum osmolality 275-300 mOsm/kg, urine osmolality 300-900 mOsm/24 hr, and urine specific gravity 1.010-1.030. Monitor urine specific gravity hourly to evaluate response to therapy. Patients may be allowed to develop hypotonic polyuria between doses of vasopressin to demonstrate persistence of DI when transient or triphasic DI is suspected.
- Instruct patients with permanent DI to wear a medical-alert bracelet labeled with diabetes *insipidus*. Immediate family members should be familiar with the patient's current treatment plan in case they are contacted in an emergency.

NIC Fluid/Electrolyte Management; Fluid Monitoring; Hypovolemia Management; Intravenous (IV) Therapy; Invasive Hemodynamic Monitoring; Electrolyte Management: Hypernatremia

Decreased adaptive capacity: intracranial, related to interruption of blood flow secondary to cerebral edema or intracranial bleeding after transsphenoidal hypophysectomy

Desired outcomes: Within 24 hr after initiating treatment, patient has adequate intracranial adaptive capacity as evidenced by ability to verbalize orientation to time, place, and person; respiratory rate (RR) 12-20 breaths/min with a normal pattern and depth (eupnea); equal and normoreactive pupils; and bilaterally equal motor strength and tone that are normal for patient. Patient verbalizes understanding of the importance of avoiding Valsalva types of activities.

- Elevate HOB 30 degrees to minimize intracranial pressure (ICP).
- Perform checks of neurologic status at frequent intervals to assess for signs of IICP, including changes in LOC, respiratory rate or rhythm, and pupillary reflexes (see Table 6-3, p. 360).
- Teach patient to avoid coughing, sneezing, straining, bending, or other Valsalva types of activities because they can increase stress on the operative site, increase ICP, and cause cerebrospinal fluid (CSF) to leak. Tell patient that any necessary coughing or sneezing should be done with the mouth open to minimize the increase in ICP. Administer cathartics, stool softeners, or antiemetics as prescribed to minimize straining and nausea.
- If IICP develops, implement the interventions described in Table 2-6; see also "Care of the Patient After Intracranial Surgery," p. 365.

NIC Neurologic Monitoring; Cerebral Edema Management; Intracranial Pressure (ICP) Monitoring

Risk for infection related to inadequate primary defenses secondary to incisional opening into sella turcica

Desired outcomes: Patient is free of infection as evidenced by normothermia; verbalization of orientation to time, place, and person; and absence of CSF leakage or nuchal rigidity.

- Inspect nasal packing often for frank bleeding or evidence of CSF leak. If glucose is detected in clear nasal drainage (tested using a glucose reagent stick), CSF is leaking. A CSF leak indicates a

flaw in cranial bone integrity. Elevate the HOB to minimize the chance of bacterial migration into the brain. Consult physician promptly for suspected CSF leaks.
* Monitor for infection, including elevated temperature, nuchal rigidity, and altered LOC.
* To prevent injury and contamination of operative site, patients should not brush their teeth until instructed to do so by physician. Provide sponge-tipped applicators for oral hygiene.
* For additional information, see "Care of the Patient after Intracranial Surgery," p. 365.

NIC Incision Site Care; Infection Protection; Neurologic Monitoring

Knowledge deficit: management of permanent DI; care after transsphenoidal hypophysectomy
Desired outcome: Before discharge from ICU, patient verbalizes understanding of the basics of DI management and care after transsphenoidal hypophysectomy, if appropriate.
* Teach patient appropriate administration of exogenous vasopressin and its side effects.
* Explain the importance of weighing daily at the same time of day and in the same clothing and reporting weight gains or losses to physician.
* Demonstrate the method for accurate measurement of urine specific gravity and the importance of keeping accurate records of test results.
* Teach when to seek medical attention, including signs of dehydration and water intoxication.
* Explain the importance of obtaining a medical-alert bracelet and identification (ID) card.
* Stress the importance of continued medical follow-up.

Care after transsphenoidal hypophysectomy
* Explain lifetime exogenous hormone replacement if the anterior pituitary gland was removed or damaged. If the entire pituitary gland was removed, teach the indicators of hormone replacement excess or deficiency.
  ❏ *Adrenal hormone excess:* weight gain, moon face, easy bruising, fatigue, polyuria, polydipsia.
  ❏ *Adrenal hormone deficiency:* weight loss, easy fatigability, abdominal pain, excess pigmentation.
  ❏ *Thyroid hormone excess:* heat intolerance, irritability, tachycardia, weight loss, diaphoresis.
  ❏ *Thyroid hormone deficiency:* bradycardia, cold intolerance, weight gain, slowed mentation.
  ❏ *Androgen replacement deficiency:* some degree of sexual dysfunction, ranging from menstrual irregularities to infertility and impotence.
* For patients with permanent need for hormone replacement, explain the method for obtaining a medical-alert bracelet and ID card outlining diagnosis and appropriate treatment in the event of an emergency.

NIC Teaching: Disease Process; Teaching: Prescribed Medication; Emotional Support

ADDITIONAL NURSING DIAGNOSES

Also see "Risk for Injury" in "Diabetic Ketoacidosis," p. 396. Also see "Altered Peripheral Tissue Perfusion" in "Hyperglycemic Hyperosmolar Nonketotic Syndrome," p. 399. As appropriate, see "Psychosocial Support," p. 68, and "Psychosocial Support for the Patient's Family and Significant Others," p. 78.

Syndrome of Inappropriate Antidiuretic Hormone

PATHOPHYSIOLOGY

Syndrome of inappropriate antidiuretic hormone (SIADH) or "water intoxication" results from excessive levels of circulating ADH. The causes of SIADH are many but typically fall into one of three categories: (1) excessive production or release of ADH; (2) respiratory disorders, which increase the release of ADH by an unknown mechanism; or (3) ectopic ADH secretion by malignant tumors, particularly tumors of the lung. In the presence of increased ADH, water normally excreted in urine is inappropriately reabsorbed and returned to the circulation, diluting the serum sodium and decreasing serum osmolality. Fluid volume expansion increases glomerular filtration and decreases aldosterone release. Both phenomena increase urinary excretion of sodium, further reducing serum sodium level. The hyponatremia creates an osmotic gradient, causing water to move into cells. In the brain, increased water creates cerebral edema and alters neurologic function. Retained water expands both the extracellular and intracellular fluid compartments. Death can result if the problem is not well managed.

ASSESSMENT

History and risk factors: Cancer of the lung, pancreas, duodenum, and prostate may secrete a biologically active form of ADH. Other common causes include head trauma, brain tumor, hemorrhage, and infection; also implicated are positive pressure ventilation, physiologic stress, chronic metabolic illness, pulmonary infections (e.g., tuberculosis, pneumonia, pulmonary abscess), and medications (e.g., thiazide and thiazide-like diuretics, chlorpropamide, carbamazepine, antipsychotics, antidepressants, NSAIDs).

Clinical presentation: Decreased urine output with very concentrated urine. Signs of water intoxication may appear, including lethargy, headache, declining LOC, seizures, nausea, vomiting, and eventually coma.

Despite retention of water, peripheral edema rarely develops. Reduced aldosterone release minimizes fluid volume expansion and edema formation. The primary symptoms of SIADH are neurologic secondary to water movement into the brain cells. The severity of symptoms depends on the degree of cerebral overhydration and how quickly hyponatremia develops. Hyponatremia that develops quickly (<48 hr) is more likely to cause symptoms than hyponatremia that develops chronically.

Physical assessment: Weight gain without edema; slightly elevated BP.

Monitoring parameters: CVP >6 mm Hg; PAWP >12 mm Hg in the absence of underlying cardiac or pulmonary disease; and urine output <0.5 ml/kg/hr with specific gravity >1.030 in the presence of adequate fluid intake.

DIAGNOSTIC TESTS

Serum sodium level: Decreased to <130 mEq/L.
Plasma osmolality: Decreased to <275 mOsm/kg.
Urine osmolality: Elevated disproportionately in relation to plasma osmolality.
Urine sodium level: Increased to >40 mEq/L.
Urine specific gravity: >1.030.
Plasma ADH level: Elevated.

COLLABORATIVE MANAGEMENT

Fluid restriction: Based on urine output. Usually fluids are limited to 1000 ml/day. Once the serum sodium level is normal, fluids may be increased to urine output plus estimated insensible losses.

Isotonic (0.9%) or hypertonic (3%) saline infusion: May be given if the patient has severe hyponatremia. Sodium solutions may be administered with IV furosemide (Lasix) or osmotic diuretics, such as mannitol, to promote water excretion.

Demeclocycline (Declomycin) or lithium: Inhibits action of ADH on the distal renal tubules to promote water excretion.

Treatment of underlying cause: SIADH associated with surgery, trauma, or drugs is usually temporary and self-limiting. If chronic, the focus is to treat the underlying cause.

NURSING DIAGNOSES AND INTERVENTIONS

Risk for injury related to hyponatremia; induced alteration in neurologic function; too-rapid correction of hyponatremia

Desired outcomes: Within 48 hr of initiating treatment, patient verbalizes orientation to time, place, and person. CVP, PAWP, and BP are within patient's normal range. Patient remains free of signs of injury.

- Assess LOC, VS, hemodynamic measurements, and I&O hourly; weigh patient daily. Monitor for decreased LOC; elevated BP, CVP, and PAWP; urine output <0.5 ml/kg/hr; and weight gain.
- Obtain specimens for ordered laboratory analysis of sodium levels (e.g., serum and urine sodium, serum and urine osmolality, urine specific gravity). Monitor for decreased serum sodium and plasma osmolality, urine osmolality that is disproportionately elevated compared to plasma osmolality, and increased urine sodium. Normal values are the following: urine specific gravity 1.010-1.030, serum sodium 137-147 mEq/L, urine osmolality 300-1090 mOsm/kg, and serum osmolality 275-300 mOsm/kg. Consult physician for significant findings.
- Restrict fluids as ordered. Explain treatment to patient and significant others. Do not keep water or ice chips at the bedside. Give IV solutions with an infusion pump.
- Elevate HOB no more than 20 degrees to promote venous return and thus reduce ADH release. Decreased venous return is a stimulus to the release of ADH.
- Administer demeclocycline, lithium, and furosemide as prescribed; carefully observe and document patient's response.
- Administer hypertonic sodium chloride as prescribed. Rate of administration is usually based on serial serum sodium levels. To minimize the risk of too-rapid correction of hyponatremia, ensure that laboratory specimens are drawn on time. *Serum sodium should not be allowed to increase more than 12 mEq/L in 24 hr* because of the risk of neurologic damage (central pontine myelinolysis), particularly if the hyponatremia is of chronic rather than acute type. Monitor for indications of fluid

overload (e.g., crackles, elevated CVP or PCWP, edema) as appropriate. Consult physician promptly for significant findings.
- Institute seizure precautions. These include padded side rails, supplemental oxygen, bite block, and oral airway at the bedside. Side rails should remain up when a staff member is not present.
- Provide care calmly and gently to minimize discomfort, which increases ADH release.

NIC Fluid/Electrolyte Management; Neurologic Monitoring; Electrolyte Management: Hyponatremia; Seizure Precautions

ADDITIONAL NURSING DIAGNOSES
See also "Altered Protection" in "Hyponatremia," p. 545.

Acute Adrenal Insufficiency (Adrenal Crisis)

PATHOPHYSIOLOGY
Acute adrenal insufficiency (adrenal or Addisonian crisis) is a life-threatening condition characterized by severe fluid and electrolyte imbalances related to both mineralocorticoid and glucocorticoid deficiencies. Mineralocorticoid (aldosterone) deficiency results in large urinary losses of sodium and water, with the development of hyponatremia and hypovolemia. Hyperkalemia and metabolic acidosis develop because of decreased urinary excretion of potassium and hydrogen. Glucocorticoid (cortisol) deficiency intensifies the clinical effects of hypovolemia by causing a decrease in vascular tone and decreased vascular response to catecholamines (epinephrine and norepinephrine). Cortisol depletion also may cause hypoglycemia as a result of the body's inability to maintain blood glucose levels in the fasting state. Severe hypotension, shock, and eventually death will occur without intravenous adrenocortical hormone and fluid replacement. In patients with chronic primary adrenal insufficiency or *Addison's disease*, acute crises may be prevented by tripling replacement hormone doses during periods of stress.

Primary adrenal insufficiency is caused by destruction of the adrenal glands by autoimmune process, infection, hemorrhage, bilateral adrenalectomy, tumor invasion, or enzymatic deficiencies. There is decreased production of adrenocortical hormones (both glucocorticoids and mineralocorticoids). Rapid withdrawal of exogenous steroids or inadequate dosage may prompt adrenal crisis. *Secondary adrenal insufficiency* may result from exogenous steroid administration or destruction of the anterior pituitary gland by tumors, infarcts, trauma, surgery, or infection. Mineralocorticoid release is maintained in secondary adrenal insufficiency, since it depends on the action of angiotensin II rather than pituitary release of adrenocorticotropic hormone (ACTH).

ASSESSMENT
History and risk factors: Adrenal crisis may be precipitated by an extreme emotional or physiologic stressor, which increases the need for adrenal hormones. Patients who take exogenous steroids are at risk if physiologic demands increase or doses are withdrawn abruptly. Addisonian crisis is a potential complication of adrenalectomy, hypophysectomy, sepsis, and human immunodeficiency virus (HIV) disease.
Clinical presentation: Hypotension (particularly postural), tachycardia, confusion, weakness, nausea, abdominal pain, hyperthermia (in some individuals).
Physical assessment: Orthostatic hypotension, poor skin turgor, sunken and soft eyeballs, muscle weakness, weight loss. Patients with primary adrenal insufficiency may have a bronze hue to the skin secondary to excess production of ACTH.
ECG findings: Signs of hyperkalemia: peaked T waves, widening QRS complex, lengthened PR interval, and flattened-to-absent P wave. As hyperkalemia worsens, these signs progress and may result in asystole.

DIAGNOSTIC TESTS
Random serum cortisol levels: Decreased.
Corticotropin stimulation test: Adrenal function is considered abnormal if the plasma cortisol level is <18 mcg/dl after an injection of synthetic ACTH (cosyntropin).
Serum sodium levels: Decreased to <137 mEq/L.
Serum aldosterone levels: Depressed in primary Addison's disease.
Serum potassium levels: Increased to >5 mEq/L initially; may decrease dramatically with treatment.
Fasting blood glucose levels: Decreased to <80 mg/dl.
BUN and serum creatinine: Often increased secondary to renal hypoperfusion.

COLLABORATIVE MANAGEMENT

Glucocorticoid replacement: The crisis state necessitates large doses of IV steroids. An immediate IV bolus of hydrocortisone may be administered, followed by repeat doses as needed q6-8h or by continuous infusion. Emergency mineralocorticoid replacement (fludrocortisone) is usually unnecessary. Hydrocortisone has mineralocorticoid effects.

IV fluids: Rapid volume replacement is essential. One liter of D5NS is given over 1 hr, followed by an additional 1-2 L over the next 6-8 hr as needed. Volume expanders may be used if hypotension persists.

Vasopressors: May be used if the patient does not respond to the initial therapy (see Appendix 7). Because these patients have decreased response to catecholamines, most vasopressors and inotropic agents will be less effective than they would be in normal individuals.

IV glucose: Supplemental glucose may be required to correct hypoglycemia.

Supplemental sodium: Normal saline is given during volume replacement. Hypertonic (3%) saline may be required.

Insertion of flow-directed pulmonary artery catheter: To continuously assess volume and overall hemodynamic status.

Treatment of underlying cause

NURSING DIAGNOSES AND INTERVENTIONS

Fluid volume deficit related to failure of regulatory mechanisms secondary to impaired secretion of aldosterone, causing increased sodium excretion with resultant diuresis

Desired outcome: Within 8 hr of initiating treatment, patient is normovolemic as evidenced by BP within patient's normal range; HR 60-100 beats/min; RR 12-20 breaths/min with normal pattern and depth (eupnea); CVP 2-6 mm Hg; PAWP 6-12 mm Hg; normal sinus rhythm on ECG; and orientation to time, place, and person.

- Monitor VS and hemodynamic measurements q15min until they have been stable for 1 hr. Consult physician promptly for deterioration in VS or hemodynamics.
- Measure BP and HR with patient lying and sitting. A drop of ≥20 mm Hg or an increase in HR >20 beats/min lasting for more than 3 min after changing position indicates dehydration.
- Administer IV fluids to replace fluid volume. Initially, rapid fluid replacement is essential.
- Maintain accurate I&O record. Weigh patient daily at the same time using the same scale.
- Monitor for electrolyte imbalance. Imbalances associated with adrenal insufficiency include the following:
  ❏ *Hyponatremia:* headache, malaise, muscle weakness, abdominal cramps.
  ❏ *Hyperkalemia:* lethargy, nausea, hyperactive bowel sounds with diarrhea, numbness or tingling in extremities, muscle weakness.
- Monitor ECG continuously; observe for hypokalemic changes (see "ECG Findings," p. 550).
- Monitor laboratory results. With appropriate treatment, serum sodium levels should rise to normal and serum potassium levels should fall to normal. Prevent rapid correction or overcorrection of hyponatremia. Serum sodium levels should not be allowed to increase more than 12 mEq/L during the first 24 hr of treatment because of the risk of neurologic damage.
- Assess mental and respiratory status at frequent intervals. Institute safety measures as indicated. Reorient and reassure patient as needed.
- Encourage oral fluid intake as patient's condition stabilizes. Add sodium-rich foods (see Table 10-11) as tolerated. Begin oral glucocorticoid replacement therapy as prescribed.
- Consult physician if signs and symptoms of fluid and/or electrolyte imbalance persist or worsen.

NIC Fluid Monitoring; Neurologic Monitoring; Hypovolemia Management; Electrolyte Management: Hyponatremia; Electrolyte Management: Hyperkalemia

Risk for injury related to potential for acute regulatory dysfunction (cortisol and aldosterone deficiency) secondary to increased psychologic, emotional, or physical stressors with increased hormonal demand and inadequate adrenal reserves

Desired outcomes: Patient verbalizes orientation to time, place, and person and has stable weight, urine output <80-125 ml/hr, HR 60-100 beats/min, BP within patient's normal range, and normothermia.

- Monitor and report signs of increasing crisis: urinary output increased from usual amount, changes in LOC, orthostatic hypotension, nausea, vomiting, and tachycardia.
- Provide a quiet, nonstressful environment. Adjust lighting to meet needs of individual activities, avoiding direct light in the eyes. Control noise when possible. Prevent unnecessary interruptions, and allow for rest periods. Limit the number of visitors and the length of time they spend with patient. Speak softly and reassuringly to patient.
- Monitor for and manage hyperthermia using tepid baths, antipyretics, and cooling blankets.

- Maintain a cool environmental temperature. Maintain strict environmental asepsis, and monitor patient carefully for signs of infection. Avoid exposing patient to staff members or visitors who have colds or infections.

NIC Fluid Monitoring; Environmental Management; Infection Protection

Knowledge deficit: prevention of adrenal crisis in patients with chronic adrenal insufficiency or those undergoing steroid therapy

Desired outcome: Before discharge from ICU, patient understands factors that increase the risk of adrenal crisis, how to avoid adrenal crisis, precautions that must be taken, and when to notify physician.

- Teach patient about prescribed medications, including purpose, dosage, route of administration, and potential side effects (Table 7-3). Medication administration should mimic normal diurnal pattern of plasma cortisol levels (e.g., two thirds in the morning and one third in late afternoon).
- Provide dietary instruction: dietary sodium and potassium may need to be adjusted on the basis of the patient's clinical condition and drug therapy (see discussions of sodium and potassium in "Fluid and Electrolyte Disturbances," p. 538).
- Explain the importance of controlling stress, both emotional and physiologic, which increases adrenal demand. Teach patient to seek medical intervention during times of increased stress (e.g., fever, infection), inasmuch as medication dosages may need to be increased.
- Teach indicators of overreplacement and underreplacement of steroids, which require prompt medical attention (see Table 7-3).
- Stress the importance of never abruptly discontinuing use of any steroid preparation. Use must be tapered to avoid precipitation of crisis.
- Remind patient of the importance of continued medical follow-up.
- Explain the procedure for obtaining a medical-alert bracelet or card.

NIC Teaching: Disease Process; Teaching: Prescribed Medication; Emotional Support

ADDITIONAL NURSING DIAGNOSES

See also "Diabetic Ketoacidosis" for "Risk for Infection," p. 396 and "Risk for injury," p. 397. See "Altered Peripheral Tissue Perfusion" in "Hyperglycemic Hyperosmolar Nonketotic Syndrome," p. 399. For other nursing diagnoses and interventions, see "Psychosocial Support," p. 68, and "Psychosocial Support for the Patient's Family and Significant Others," p. 78.

TABLE 7-3 Patient and Family Education Concerning Glucocorticoid and Mineralocorticoid Replacement

Glucocorticoids (e.g., cortisone, acetate, prednisone)
- Take medication in a diurnal pattern to mimic normal secretion (i.e., two thirds of dose in the morning and one third of dose in the afternoon).
- Take steroids with food to decrease gastric irritation.
- Weigh self regularly, and report to physician gains of >2 lb/wk.
- Avoid exposure to infection, and be alert to indicators of infection (e.g., fever, nausea, diarrhea, malaise).
- Contact physician promptly during periods of physical or emotional stress; dosages will require adjustment at these times.
- Indicators of overreplacement: weight gain (moon face, truncal obesity); edema; thin, fragile skin (striae, easy bruising); slow wound healing; chronic fatigue; emotional lability.
- Indicators of underreplacement; weight loss; hyperpigmentation; skin creases; anorexia; nausea; abdominal discomfort; chronic fatigue; depression; irritability.

Mineralocorticoids (e.g., fludrocortisone, desoxycorticosterone acetate)
- As prescribed, modify diet with liberal amounts of sodium (see Table 10-11), protein, and carbohydrates.
- Weigh self regularly, and report to physician sudden gains or losses >2 lb/wk.
- Contact physician promptly during periods of physical or emotional stress; dosages will require adjustment at these times.
- Indicators of overreplacement: edema, muscle weakness, hypertension
- Indicators of underreplacement
- Excessive urination, weight loss, decreased skin turgor

Thyrotoxic Crisis (Thyroid Storm)

Thyroid storm is a *medical emergency* caused by hyperthyroidism. The crisis results from a surge of thyroid hormones into the bloodstream which marked increases body metabolism. Precipitating factors include infection, trauma, labor and delivery, and emotional stress, which increase demands on body metabolism. Thyrotoxic crisis may follow subtotal thyroidectomy because of manipulation of the gland during surgery. The effects of hyperthyroidism are due to excessive circulating thyroid hormone, which exaggerates the functions of all body systems to produce a hypermetabolic state. *Graves' disease* (diffuse toxic goiter) accounts for approximately 85% of reported cases of hyperthyroidism. It is characterized by spontaneous exacerbations and remissions of hypermetabolism that seem unaffected by therapy. Recent diagnostic tests have isolated a long-acting thyroid stimulator, suggesting the disease is an autoimmune response. Hyperthyroidism occurs in 1 in 500 pregnancies and is second in frequency only to diabetes as an endocrine disorder of pregnancy. During pregnancy, thyroid storm is seen most often in patients with undertreated or undiagnosed hyperthyroidism. As many as 20%-30% of cases may result in maternal and fetal mortality.

ASSESSMENT

History and risk factors: Patient with history of hyperthyroidism including Grave's disease, thyroid nodules, or toxic goiter who has undergone a recent stressful experience including pregnancy, labor, and/or delivery.

Clinical presentation: Marked confusion and disorientation, tachycardia, palpitations, widened pulse pressure, hyperpyrexia, chest discomfort in a patient with enlargement of the thyroid gland, muscle weakness, hyperreflexia, fine tremor, fine hair, thin skin, hypercholesterolemia, impaired glucose tolerance, exophthalmos, stare, and/or lid lag. Males often have gynecomastia.

Physical assessment: Confused person with acute exacerbation of tachycardia, hyperpyrexia (fever), central nervous system (CNS) irritability; sometimes coma or heart failure.

DIAGNOSTIC TESTS

Serum TSH (thyroid-stimulating hormone or thyrotropin): Decreased in the presence of disease.
Serum free thyroxine triiodothyronine (free T3): Elevated in the presence of disease.
Radioactive iodine-131 (^{131}I) uptake and thyroid scan: Clarifies size of gland and detects presence of hot or cold nodules.
Radioactive iodine-131 (^{131}I) scintiscan: Defines functional characteristics of the gland.
12-lead ECG: To rule out MI or other acute coronary syndromes.
Echocardiogram: To diagnose ventricular function in diagnosis of congestive heart failure.

COLLABORATIVE MANAGEMENT

Oxygen: Used per nasal cannula or mask as needed to maintain SpO_2 >90%.
Antithyroid agents: Propylthiouracil (PTU) has been the first line of treatment. Can be used on the pregnant patient. If the patient is unable to swallow, the medication is given using a nasogastric tube. Methimazole may also be used. Leukopenia, rash, urticaria, fever, arthralgias, and, rarely, agranulocytosis may result from treatment. Agranulocytosis (complete lack of granulocytes) causes fever and sore throat. If agranulocytosis is confirmed by complete blood count (CBC), the PTU should be stopped. Iodides (potassium iodide or Lugol's solution) are given several hours after PTU to avoid a build-up of hormones stored in the thyroid gland.
Iodides: Sodium or potassium iodide drops may be given to help inhibit the release of thyroid hormone or to help abate accumulation of hormones stored in the thyroid.
Beta (β)-adrenergic blocking agents (e.g., esmolol, metoprolol, propranolol): To relieve tachycardia, anxiety, heat intolerance, and tremor.
Intravenous fluids: Given to help rehydrate the patient. Fever and rapid metabolism can lead to dehydration.
Control of fever: Antipyretic medications (i.e., acetaminophen) or hypothermia blanket is used. Aspirin is contraindicated, as it worsens thyroid crisis.
Correction of electrolyte imbalance: Various imbalances may occur. Replace electrolytes as appropriate.
Glucocorticoids: Administered to help inhibit conversion of thyroxine (T_4) to T_3 and prevent adrenal insufficiency.
Radioactive iodine: Usually reserved for the following indications: (1) failure to respond to antithyroid drugs; (2) relapse after 1-2 yr of therapy; (3) toxic multinodular goiter; (4) solitary toxic nodules; or (5) noncompliant patients. ^{131}I is the most commonly used agent. Use usually results in hypothyroidism, controlled easily with replacement therapy. Cannot be used for the pregnant patient, as the thyroid gland of the fetus may be destroyed.

Mild tranquilizers: To minimize anxiety and promote rest.

Subtotal thyroidectomy: Surgical removal of part of the gland often is the best treatment for patients with extremely enlarged glands or multinodular goiter. Surgery is avoided in the pregnant patient due to risk of miscarriage or preterm delivery. The patient is prepared with antithyroid agents until normal thyroid function is achieved (usually 6-8 wk). The most frequent postoperative complication is hemorrhage at the operative site. The following complications are rare but can be extremely serious: hypoparathyroidism, laryngeal nerve injury, and tetany from damage to the parathyroid glands.

NURSING DIAGNOSES AND INTERVENTIONS

Ineffective protection related to potential for thyrotoxic crisis (thyroid storm) secondary to emotional stress, trauma, infection, pregnancy (especially labor and delivery), or surgical manipulation of the gland

Desired outcomes: Patient is free of symptoms of thyroid storm as evidenced by normothermia; BP ≥90/60 mm Hg (or within patient's baseline range); HR ≤100 beats/min; and orientation to person, place, and time. If thyroid storm occurs, it is noted promptly and reported immediately.

- Measure and report rectal or core temperature >38.3° C (101° F): often the first sign of impending thyroid storm.
- Monitor VS hourly for evidence of hypotension and increasing tachycardia and fever.
- Monitor patient for signs of congestive heart failure, which occurs as an effect of thyroid storm: jugular vein distention, crackles (rales), decreased amplitude of peripheral pulses, peripheral edema, and hypotension. Immediately report any significant findings to physician, and prepare to transfer patient to ICU if they are noted. Maternal and fetal monitoring are initiated on pregnant patients.
- Provide a cool, calm, protected environment to minimize emotional stress if possible. Reassure patient, and explain all procedures. Limit the number of visitors.
- Ensure good hand washing and meticulous aseptic technique for dressing changes and all procedures. Advise visitors who have contracted or been exposed to a communicable disease either not to enter patient's room or to use appropriate infection control precautions.
- Administer acetaminophen to decrease temperature.

> **Caution:**   Aspirin is contraindicated because it releases thyroxine from protein-binding sites and increases free thyroxine levels.

- Provide cool sponge baths or apply ice packs to patient's axilla and groin areas to decrease fever. If high temperature continues, obtain a prescription for a hypothermia blanket.
- Administer PTU as prescribed to prevent further synthesis and release of thyroid hormones.
- Administer β-blockers as prescribed to block sympathetic nervous system (SNS) effects.
- Administer IV fluids as prescribed to provide adequate hydration and prevent vascular collapse. Fluid volume deficit may occur because of increased fluid excretion by the kidneys or excessive diaphoresis. Carefully monitor I&O hourly to prevent fluid overload or inadequate fluid replacement. Decreasing output with normal specific gravity may indicate decreased cardiac output, whereas decreasing output with increased specific gravity can signal dehydration.
- Administer iodides as prescribed, 1 hr after administering PTU.

> **Caution:**   If given before PTU, iodides can exacerbate symptoms in susceptible persons.

- Administer small doses of insulin as prescribed to control hyperglycemia. Hyperglycemia can occur as an effect of thyroid storm because of the hypermetabolic state.
- Administer prescribed supplemental O_2 to support increased metabolism.

NIC Cardiac Care: Acute; Surveillance: Late Pregnancy; Fluid/Electrolyte Management; Hyperglycemia Management; Energy Management; Nutritional Monitoring; Vital Signs Monitoring

Impaired swallowing (or risk for same) related to edema or laryngeal nerve damage resulting from surgical procedure

Desired outcomes: Patient reports swallowing with minimal difficulty, has minimal or absent hoarseness, and is free of symptoms of respiratory dysfunction as evidenced by RR 12-20 breaths/min with

normal depth and pattern (eupnea) and absence of inspiratory stridor. Laryngeal nerve damage, if it occurs, is detected promptly and reported immediately.
- Monitor respiratory status for signs of edema (i.e., dyspnea, choking, inspiratory stridor, inability to swallow). Assess patient's voice. Slight hoarseness is normal after surgery. Persistent hoarseness indicates laryngeal nerve damage. If bilateral nerve damage is present, upper airway obstruction can occur. Report findings to physician promptly.
- Elevate HOB 30-45 degrees to minimize edema and incisional stress. Support patient's head with flat or cervical pillows so that it is in a neutral position.
- Keep tracheostomy set and O_2 equipment at the bedside at all times. Suction upper airway as needed, using gentle suction to avoid stimulating laryngospasm.
- To minimize pain and anxiety and enhance patient's ability to swallow, administer analgesics promptly and as prescribed.

NIC Airway Management; Nutrition Therapy; Respiratory Monitoring; Aspiration Precautions; Swallowing Therapy

Anxiety related to SNS stimulation
Desired outcomes: Within 24 hr of hospital admission, patient is free of harmful anxiety as evidenced by a HR ≤100 beats/min, RR 12-20 breaths/min with normal depth and pattern (eupnea), and absence of or decrease in irritability and restlessness. Patient and significant others verbalize knowledge about the causes of the patient's behavior.
- Assess for anxiety; administer short-acting sedatives (e.g., lorazepam) as prescribed.
- Provide a quiet, stress-free environment away from loud noises or excessive activity.
- Limit number of visitors and the amount of time they spend with patient. Advise significant others to avoid discussing stressful topics and to refrain from arguing with the patient.
- Administer β-blockers as prescribed to reduce anxiety, tachycardia, and heat intolerance.
- Reassure patient that anxiety is related to the disease and that treatment decreases severity.
- Inform significant others patient's agitated behavior should not be taken personally.

NIC Anxiety Reduction; Coping Enhancement; High-Risk Pregnancy Care

Imbalanced nutrition: Less than body requirements related to hypermetabolic state and/or inadequate nutrient absorption
Desired outcomes: By a minimum of 24 hr before hospital discharge, patient has adequate nutrition as evidenced by stable weight and a positive nitrogen balance.
- Provide foods high in calories, protein, carbohydrates, and vitamins.
- Administer vitamin supplements as prescribed, and explain their importance to patient.
- Administer prescribed antidiarrheal medications, which increase absorption of nutrients from the GI tract.
- Weigh patient daily, and report significant losses to physician.

NIC Nutrition Management; Weight Gain Assistance; Nutritional Counseling

Disturbed sleep pattern related to accelerated metabolism
Desired outcome: Within 48 hr of hospital admission, patient relates the attainment of sufficient rest and sleep.
- Adjust care activities to patient's tolerance.
- Provide frequent rest periods of at least 90-min duration. If possible, arrange for patient to have bed rest in a quiet, cool room.
- Administer short-acting sedatives (e.g., lorazepam) as prescribed to promote rest.

NIC Sleep Enhancement; Anxiety Reduction; Meditation Facilitation

Impaired tissue integrity of the cornea related to dryness that can occur with exophthalmos in persons with Graves' disease
Desired outcome: Within 24 hr of admission, patient's corneas are moist and intact.
- Teach patient to wear dark glasses to protect the cornea.
- Administer lubricating eyedrops as prescribed to supplement lubrication and decrease SNS stimulation, which can cause lid retraction.
- If appropriate, apply eye shields or tape the eyes shut at bedtime.
- Administer thioamides as prescribed to maintain normal metabolic state and halt progression of exophthalmos.

NIC Eye Care; Skin Care: Topical Treatments

Knowledge deficit: potential for side effects from iodides and thioamides or stopping thioamides abruptly
Desired outcome: Within the 24-hr period before hospital discharge, patient verbalizes knowledge about potential side effects of prescribed medications, signs and symptoms of hypothyroidism and hyperthyroidism, and the importance of following the prescribed medical regimen.
- Explain importance of taking antithyroid medications daily, as prescribed.
- Teach indicators of hypothyroidism (e.g., early fatigue, weight gain, anorexia, constipation, menstrual irregularities, muscle cramps, lethargy, inability to concentrate, hair loss, cold intolerance,

and hoarseness), which may occur from excessive antithyroid medication, and the signs and symptoms that necessitate medical attention, including cold intolerance, fatigue, lethargy, and peripheral or periorbital edema.
- Teach side effects of thioamides and symptoms that require medical attention: appearance of a rash, fever, or pharyngitis, which can occur in the presence of agranulocytosis.
- Discuss signs of worsening hyperthyroidism including high body temperature, palpitations, rapid HR, irritability, anxiety, and feelings of restlessness or panic.
- Explain importance of continued and frequent medical follow-up.
- Indicators that require medical attention: fever, rash, or sore throat (side effects of thioamides), and symptoms of hypothyroidism or worsening hyperthyroidism.
- For patients receiving radioactive iodine, explain the importance of not holding children to the chest for 72 hr following therapy, since children are more susceptible to the effects of radiation. Explain that there is negligible risk for adults.
- Importance of avoiding physical and emotional stress early in the recuperative stage and maximizing coping mechanisms for dealing with stress.

NIC Learning Facilitation; Health Education; Teaching: Disease Process; Teaching: Prescribed Medication; Teaching: Activity/Exercise

Myxedema Coma

Myxedema coma is a life-threatening condition which occurs when hypothyroidism is untreated, or when a stressor such as infection affects an individual with hypothyroidism. The clinical picture of myxedema coma includes exaggerated hypothyroidism, with decreased mental status or coma, hypoventilation, hypothermia, hypotension, seizures, and shock. Myxedema coma usually develops slowly, has a >50% mortality rate, and requires prompt, aggressive treatment. Hypothyroidism results in inadequate amount of circulating thyroid hormone, causing a decrease in metabolic rate that affects all body systems.

Primary hypothyroidism (90% of cases) is caused by pathologic changes in the thyroid caused by dietary iodine deficiency, thyroiditis, thyroid atrophy or fibrosis of unknown cause, radiation therapy to the neck (e.g., with treatment for hyperthyroidism), surgical removal of all or part of the gland, drugs that suppress thyroid activity including PTU and iodides, or a genetic dysfunction resulting in the inability to produce and secrete thyroid hormone. *Secondary hypothyroidism* is caused by dysfunction of the anterior pituitary gland, which results in decreased release of TSH. It can be caused by pituitary tumors, postpartum necrosis of the pituitary gland, or hypophysectomy. *Tertiary hypothyroidism* is caused by a hypothalamic deficiency in the release of thyrotropin-releasing hormone (TRH).

ASSESSMENT

History and risk factors: Signs and symptoms may be life-threatening in a patient with history of hypothyroidism who has experienced a recent stressful event. Undiagnosed patients may report early fatigue, weight gain, anorexia, lethargy, cold intolerance, menstrual irregularities, depression, and muscle cramps.
Clinical presentation: Hypoventilation, hypoglycemia, hypothermia, hypotension, bradycardia, and shock.
Physical assessment: Possible presence of goiter, bradycardia, hypothermia, deepened voice or hoarseness, hypercholesterolemia, and obesity. The skin may be dry, cool, and coarse, and the hair may be thin, coarse, and brittle. The tongue may be enlarged (macroglossia), and the reflexes may be slowed.

DIAGNOSTIC TESTS

TSH: Elevated unless the disease is long-standing or severe.
Free thyroxine index (FTI) and thyroxine (T_4) levels: Decreased.
^{131}I **scan and uptake:** Will be <10% in a 24-hr period. In secondary hypothyroidism, uptake increases with administration of exogenous TSH.
Thyroperoxidase antibodies: Positive test signals chronic autoimmune thyroiditis.

COLLABORATIVE MANAGEMENT

Intubation and mechanical ventilation: To compensate for decreased ventilatory drive and possibly weakened musculature.

IV thyroid supplements: Rapid IV administration of thyroid hormone with careful monitoring, as this may cause hyperadrenalism. Concomitant administration of IV hydrocortisone helps prevent adrenal problems.

Treatment of hypotension: Administration of IV isotonic fluids (normal saline and lactated Ringer's solution). Hypotonic solutions, such as 5% dextrose in water (D_5W), are contraindicated because they decrease serum Na+ levels further. These patients respond poorly to vasopressors because of altered metabolism.

Treatment of hypoglycemia: IV solutions containing glucose or 50% dextrose (D_{50}).

Treatment of hyponatremia: Fluids are restricted, and/or hypertonic (3%) saline is administered.

Treatment of associated illnesses such as infections

Oral thyroid hormone (i.e., levothyroxine): Given early in treatment for primary hypothyroidism. To prevent hyperthyroidism caused by too much exogenous hormone, patients are started on low doses that are increased gradually, based on serial laboratory tests (TSH and T_4) and adjusted until the TSH is in a normal range. This therapy is continued for the patient's lifetime. For patients with secondary hypothyroidism, thyroid supplements can promote acute symptoms and therefore are contraindicated.

Stool softeners: To minimize constipation owing to decreased gastric secretions and peristalsis.

Avoid barbiturates: Because of alterations in metabolism, patients with hypothyroidism do not tolerate barbiturates and sedatives, and therefore CNS depressants are contraindicated.

Avoid external warming: External warming measures are contraindicated for hypothermia because they can produce vasodilation and vascular collapse.

NURSING DIAGNOSES AND INTERVENTIONS

Ineffective protection (myxedema coma) related to inadequate response to treatment of hypothyroidism or stressors such as infection

Desired outcomes: Patient is free of symptoms of myxedema coma as evidenced by HR ≥ 60 beats/min, BP $\geq 90/60$ mm Hg (or within patient's normal range), RR ≥ 12 breaths/min with normal depth and pattern (eupnea), and orientation to person, place, and time.

- Monitor VS frequently and note bradycardia, hypotension, or decrease in RR. Report systolic BP <90 mm Hg, HR <60 beats/min, or RR <12 breaths/min.
- Monitor patient for hypoxia. Report significant findings to physician.
- Monitor serum electrolytes and glucose levels. Note decreasing Na^+ (<137 mEq/L) and glucose (<60 mg/dl).
- Restrict fluids or administer hypertonic saline as prescribed to correct hyponatremia.
- Administer IV thyroid replacement hormones with IV hydrocortisone and IV glucose to treat hypoglycemia.
- Monitor for heart failure: jugular vein distention, crackles (rales), shortness of breath (SOB), peripheral edema, weakening peripheral pulses, and hypotension. Notify physician of any significant findings.
- Keep an oral airway and manual resuscitator at the bedside in the event of seizure, coma, or the need for ventilatory assistance.

NIC Vital Signs Monitoring; Respiratory Monitoring; Shock Prevention; Cardiac Care: Acute

Ineffective breathing pattern (or risk for same) related to upper airway obstruction occurring with enlarged thyroid gland and/or decreased ventilatory drive caused by greatly decreased metabolism

Desired outcome: Patient maintains effective breathing pattern as evidenced by RR 12-20 breaths/min with normal depth and pattern (eupnea), normal skin color, O_2 saturation $\geq 95\%$, and absence of adventitious breath sounds. If ineffective breathing pattern occurs, it is reported and treated promptly.

- Assess rate, depth, and quality of breath sounds. Monitor for inadequate ventilation: changes in respiratory rate or pattern, falling SpO_2, pallor, or cyanosis. Report findings to physician promptly, including presence of adventitious sounds (e.g., from developing pleural effusion) or decreasing or crowing sounds (e.g., from swollen tongue or glottis).
- Measure SpO_2 intermittently or continuously in patients with decreased ventilatory drive.
- Teach patient coughing, deep breathing, and use of incentive spirometer. For respiratory distress, assist physician with intubation or tracheostomy and maintenance of mechanical ventilatory assistance. Suction upper airway prn.

NIC Respiratory Monitoring; Airway Management

Excess fluid volume related to compromised regulatory mechanisms occurring with associated adrenal insufficiency

Desired outcome: By a minimum of 24 hr before hospital discharge, patient is normovolemic as evidenced by urinary output ≥30 ml/hr, stable weight, nondistended jugular veins, presence of eupnea, and peripheral pulse amplitude ≥2+ on a 0-4+ scale.
- Monitor I&O hourly for evidence of decreasing output.
- Weigh patient at the same time every day, using the same scale. Monitor for the following indicators of heart failure: jugular vein distention, crackles (rales), SOB, dependent edema of extremities, and decreased pulse amplitude. Report significant findings to physician.
- Restrict fluid and Na$^+$ intake as prescribed.

NIC Fluid Management; Electrolyte Monitoring; Hypervolemia Management

Activity intolerance related to weakness and fatigue secondary to slowed metabolism and decreased cardiac output caused by pericardial effusions, atherosclerosis, and decreased adrenergic stimulation
Desired outcome: During activity patient rates perceived exertion at ≤3 on a 0-10 scale and exhibits cardiac tolerance to activity as evidenced by HR ≤20 beats/min over resting HR, systolic BP ≤20 mm Hg over or under resting systolic BP, warm and dry skin, and absence of crackles (rales), murmurs, chest pain, and new dysrhythmias.
- Monitor VS frequently for hypotension, slow pulse, dysrhythmias, complaints of chest pain or discomfort, decreasing urine output, and changes in mentation. Promptly report significant changes to physician.
- Balance activity with adequate rest to decrease workload of the heart.
- Administer IV isotonic solutions such as normal saline to help prevent hypotension.

NIC Energy Management; Activity Therapy; Exercise Promotion: Strength Training

Risk for infection related to compromised immunologic status secondary to alterations in adrenal function
Desired outcome: Patient is free of infection as evidenced by normothermia, absence of adventitious breath sounds, normal urinary pattern and characteristics, and well-healing wounds.
- Monitor for infection: fever, erythema, swelling, or discharge from wounds or IV sites; urinary frequency, urgency, or dysuria; cloudy or malodorous urine; presence of adventitious sounds on auscultation of lung fields; and changes in color, consistency, and amount of sputum. Minimize risk of urinary tract infection (UTI) by providing care of catheters.
- Provide care to maintain skin integrity and prevent pressure ulcers.
- Advise visitors who have contracted or been exposed to a communicable disease not to enter patient's room without appropriate infection control precautions.

NIC Risk Identification; Infection Protection

Risk for imbalanced nutrition: More than body requirements of calories, related to slowed metabolism
Desired outcomes: Patient does not gain weight. Within the 24-hr period before hospital discharge, patient verbalizes understanding of the rationale and measures for the dietary regimen.
- Provide a diet that is high in protein and low in calories and sodium.
- Encourage foods that are high in fiber content (e.g., fruits with skins, vegetables, whole grain breads and cereals, nuts) to improve gastric motility and elimination.
- Administer vitamin supplements as prescribed.

NIC Nutritional Counseling; Nutritional Management; Weight Management

Constipation related to inadequate dietary intake of roughage and fluids, bed rest, and/or decreased peristalsis secondary to slowed metabolism
Desired outcome: Within 48-72 hr of admission, patient resumes normal pattern of bowel elimination.
- Monitor bowel function; report problems to the physician. Note decreasing bowel sounds, distention, and increased abdominal girth (may indicate ileus or an obstruction).
- Encourage patient to maintain a diet with adequate roughage and fluids. Ensure that fluid intake in persons without underlying cardiac or renal disease is at least 2-3 L/day.
- Administer stool softeners and laxatives as prescribed.

Caution: *Suppositories may be contraindicated because of the risk of stimulating the vagus nerve (decreases HR and BP).*

NIC Constipation/Impaction Management; Fluid Management

Knowledge deficit: management of hypothyroidism
Desired outcome: Within the 24-hr period before hospital discharge, patient verbalizes knowledge of potential side effects of prescribed medications, dietary guidelines, signs and symptoms that require medical attention, and importance of following the prescribed medical regimen.
- Provide teaching about medications including drug name, purpose, dosage, schedule, precautions, drug/drug and food/drug interactions, and potential side effects. Remind patient that thioamides,

iodides, and lithium are contraindicated because they decrease thyroid activity. Be sure patient is aware that thyroid replacement medications are to be taken for life.
* Review dietary requirements and restrictions, which may change as hormone replacement therapy takes effect.
* Explain expected changes with hormone replacement therapy: increased energy level, weight loss, and decreased peripheral edema. Neuromuscular problems should improve.
* Stress importance of continued, frequent medical follow-up.
* Discuss importance of avoiding physical and emotional stress, and ways for patient to maximize coping mechanisms for dealing with stress.
* Review signs and symptoms that require medical attention: fever or other symptoms of upper respiratory, urinary, or oral infections and signs and symptoms of hyperthyroidism, which may result from excessive hormone replacement.

▌NIC Medication Management; Exercise Promotion; Teaching: Prescribed Diet; Teaching: Disease Process; Anxiety Reduction

Bibliography

Bailes BK: Hyperthyroidism in elderly patients, *AORN J* 69(1):254-256, 258, 1999.
Bendz H, Aurell M: Drug-induced diabetes insipidus: incidence, prevention and management, *Drug Safety* 21(6):449-456, 1999.
Bell DS, Alele J: Diabetic ketoacidosis: why early detection and aggressive treatment are crucial, *Postgrad Med* 101(4):193-198, 203-204, 1997.
Bolli GB: How to ameliorate the problem of hypoglycemia in intensive as well as non-intensive treatment of type 1 diabetes, *Diabetes Care* (Suppl 2):B43-52, March 1999.
Braithwaite SS: Thyroid disorders. In Parrillo JE, Dellinger RP: *Critical care medicine: principles of diagnosis and management in the adult,* St. Louis, 2002, Mosby.
Carson PP: Emergency: adrenal crisis, *Am J Nurs* 100(7):49-50, 2000.
Chan TYK: Drug-induced syndrome of inappropriate antidiuretic hormone secretion: causes, diagnosis and management, *Drugs Aging* 11(1):27-44, 1997.
Deletter EA et al: Medicolegal implications of hidden thyroid dysfunction: a study of two cases, *Med Sci Law* 40(3):251-257, 2000.
Diehl-Oplinger L, Kaminski MF: Choosing the right fluid to counter hypovolemic shock. *Nursing* 34(3):52-54, 2004.
Ezzone SA: SIADH, *Clin J Oncol Nurs* 3(4):187-188, 1999.
Fain JA: Diabetes update, part 2: unlock the mysteries of insulin therapy. *Nursing* 34(3):41-45, 2004.
Fisken RA: Severe diabetic ketoacidosis: the need for large doses of insulin, *Diabet Med* 16(4):347-350, 1999.
Fitzgerald P: Endocrinology. In Tierney Jr. LM, McPhee SJ, Papadakis MA: *Current medical diagnosis and treatment,* ed 43. New York, 2004, Lange Medical Books/McGraw-Hill.
Freeland BS: Emergency: diabetic ketoacidosis, *Am J Nurs* 98(8):52, 1998.
Funnell MM, Barlage DL: Diabetes update, part 1: managing diabetes with "agent oral," *Nursing* 34(3):36-40, 2004.
Garber AJ, Moghissi ES: Consensus development conference on inpatient diabetes and metabolic control: position statement, American College of Endocrinology, December 16, 2003.
Goldberg RB, Machado R: Atypical ketoacidosis in type 2 diabetes, *Hosp Pract* 33(3):105-108, 111-112, 117-118, 1998.
Goldsmith C: Hypothyroidism, *Am J Nurs* 99(6):42-43, 1999.
Gonzalez-Campoy JM, Robertson RP: Diabetic ketoacidosis and hyperosmolar nonketotic state: gaining control over extreme hyperglycemic complications, *Postgrad Med* 99(6):143-152, 1996.
Grinslade S, Buck EA: Diabetic ketoacidosis: implications for the medical-surgical nurse, *Medsurg Nurs* 8(1):37-45, 1999.
Gross P et al: The treatment of severe hyponatremia, *Kidney Int* 53(64):S6-S11, 1998.
Keenan AM: Syndrome of inappropriate secretion of antidiuretic hormone in malignancy, *Semin Oncol Nurs* 15(3):160-167, 1999.
Konick-McMahan J: Riding out a diabetic emergency, *Nursing* 29(9):34-39, quiz 40, 1999.
Lewis R: Diabetic emergencies part 1: hypoglycemia, *Accid Emerg Nurs* 7(4):190-196, 1999.
Luken KK: Clinical manifestations and management of Addison's disease, *J Am Acad Nurse Pract* 11(4):151-154, 1999.
Matz R: Managing fluid abnormalities in uncontrolled diabetes mellitus, *J Crit Ill* 12(5):278-282, 1997.
Miller J: Management of diabetic ketoacidosis, *J Emerg Nurs* 25(6):514-519, 1999.
Nickolaus MJ: Diabetes insipidus: a current perspective, *Crit Care Nurs* 19(6):18-30, 1999.

Olkers W: Adrenal insufficiency, *N Engl J Med* 335(16):1206-1212, 1996.

Parkar N, Taylor RW: Adrenal insufficiency in the critically ill patient. In Parrillo JE, Dellinger RP: *Critical care medicine: principles of diagnosis and management in the adult*, St Louis, 2002, Mosby.

Singer I, Oster JR, Fishman LM: The management of diabetes insipidus in adults, *Arch Intern Med* 157(12):1293-1301, 1997.

Singh RK, Perros P, Frier BM: Hospital management of diabetic ketoacidosis: are clinical guidelines implemented effectively? *Diabet Med* 14(6):482-486, 1997.

Slover-Zipf J: Hypoglycemia treatment, *Am J Nurs* 99(10):14, 1999.

Stoller WA , Massone T: Acute diabetic emergencies and hypoglycemia. In Parrillo JE, Dellinger RP: *Critical care medicine: principles of diagnosis and management in the adult*, St Louis, 2002, Mosby.

Van den Berghe G et al: Intensive insulin therapy in critically ill patients, *N Engl J Med* 345(19):1359-1367, Nov, 2001.

Waltman PA, Brewer JM, Lobert S: Thyroid storm during pregnancy, *Crit Care Nurs* 24(2):74-80, April 2004.

Williams M: Disorders of the adrenal gland, *Semin Periop Nurs* 7(3):179-185, 1998.

CHAPTER 8

Gastrointestinal Dysfunctions

Gastroesophageal Varices

PATHOPHYSIOLOGY

Liver disease (e.g., cirrhosis) or anatomic obstruction within the venous portal system increases portal pressure, causing gastric and esophageal veins to become tortuous, dilated, and engorged with blood. As resistance to blood flow in the portal venous system increases, portosystemic collateral channels open and divert portal blood into the systemic circulation. These collaterals manifest as varicosities at the lower end of the esophagus, the stomach, the rectum, the umbilicus, and the ovaries, and sometimes in the small bowel or in stomal sites. As venous portal pressure increases, veins dilate beneath the esophageal epithelium. Eventually, the overlying submucosa retreats, leaving the veins unprotected. Further pressure on the venous walls results in rupture, hemorrhage, and hematemesis. Blood loss is influenced by severity of rupture in addition to exacerbating factors such as clotting disorders and thrombocytopenia. The risk of bleeding from varices increases when hepatic venous pressure gradients (HVPG) reach a 10-12 mm Hg threshold. Gastric varices bleed less frequently, but more severely, than esophageal varices. High morbidity and mortality are associated with variceal hemorrhage. Mortality rates can be as high as 50% following the first bleed and 30% after subsequent bleeds. Up to 8% of patients die within 24 hr from uncontrolled bleeding.

In Western countries the most common cause of portal hypertension is cirrhosis. Cirrhosis itself causes loss of hepatocytes, degeneration of the parenchyma, and swelling, and eventually shrinkage of the liver into a hard, fibrotic mass. Life-supporting functions of the liver (i.e., detoxification, hormonal metabolism, vitamin absorption, bilirubin metabolism) gradually decline as blood flow to the liver is shunted via collateral vessels and obstructed by increasing fibrosis.

Large portosystemic shunts result in complications, including hepatic encephalopathy, septicemia, and metabolic abnormalities. In addition, acute blood loss from variceal bleeding results in hypoxic damage to liver cells and may precipitate complications of hepatic insufficiency such as jaundice, ascites, and encephalopathy. Childs classification scores assist in determining the mortality rate from esophageal varices: respectively, Childs class A = 5%, class B = 25%, and class C = 50%. Variceal hemorrhage with subsequent liver failure is a leading cause of death in patients with liver cirrhosis and portal hypertension.

ASSESSMENT

History and risk factors: Portal hypertension may arise from excessive ethanol ingestion (averaging >60 g/day); previously diagnosed cirrhosis, hepatitis, parasitic infection, schistosomiasis, intraabdominal or biliary infection, biliary disease, traumatic portal vein injury, congenital liver disease, and tumor invasion. The following events may precipitate bleeding in patients with gastroesophageal varices: (1) insertion of a gastric tube, (2) coagulopathy and/or heparin therapy, (3) infection, (4) Valsalva maneuver, (5) vigorous coughing, and (6) erosion of mucosa (e.g., erosive gastritis, esophagitis).

Clinical presentation: Massive, painless bleeding, possibly with signs of shock, is usually the first and most common presentation. Blood loss is variable, but a "clinically significant bleed" is one which requires two units of blood within 24 hr with systolic BP <100 mm Hg or a postural change >20 mm Hg. Melena, with or without hematemesis, is another frequent occurrence. Portal hypertensive gastropathy, peptic ulcer disease, and Mallory-Weiss syndrome (see "Acute Gastrointestinal Bleeding," p. 459) may contribute to the usually massive blood loss. Rapid blood loss leads initially to thirst, dizziness, disorientation, and hypovolemic shock, and eventually to coma and death as the hemorrhage continues. High portal venous pressures with massive bleeding (40% of blood volume) result in death within 10-30 min.

Physical assessment: Hematemesis of frank red blood and/or old swallowed blood that resembles coffee grounds, along with cool, pale skin, syncope, vertigo, altered mental status, and restlessness are readily apparent. Pale, dry oral mucosa, cracked lips, poor skin turgor, and "sunken-looking" eyeballs are further evidence of hemorrhage. Yellowing of the skin and the sclera is associated with jaundice, which is frequently present. Mild-to-marked edema generally develops within hours of bleeding onset. This is the result of stimulation of the sympathetic nervous system and baroreceptors, which causes release of antidiuretic hormone (ADH) and results in sodium and water retention. Splenomegaly is commonly associated with portal hypertension. In persons with cirrhosis, the liver usually is small and firm. An enlarged and tender liver is associated with hepatic inflammation. Large hemorrhoids may be present on rectal examination, along with stool that contains occult or frank blood. If aspiration of gastric contents has occurred, coarse crackles and rhonchi may be auscultated.

Vital signs and hemodynamic measurements: Vital signs usually reflect a hypovolemic state: tachycardia, tachypnea, decreased BP with orthostasis. Hemodynamics reflect a hypovolemic or hyperdynamic state. In the presence of a hypovolemic state, central venous pressure (CVP), pulmonary artery pressure (PAP), and pulmonary artery wedge pressure (PAWP) are decreased. Cardiac output (CO) is variable, depending on adequacy of stroke volume and the presence of tachycardia. Systemic vascular resistance (SVR) is increased if sympathetic stimulation predominates, or it is decreased in association with a hyperdynamic state similar to systemic inflammatory response syndrome (SIRS). If hypovolemia is corrected, a hyperdynamic cardiovascular state is present. The CO is elevated, peripheral vascular resistance is lowered, pulses are bounding, and the extremities are warm and flushed.

DIAGNOSTIC TESTS

Hematologic tests: Hematocrit (Hct), hemoglobin (Hgb), and red blood cells (RBCs) will be decreased because of acute large blood volume loss and mild anemia associated with hypersplenism. If a slow bleed is present and equal amounts of plasma and cells are being lost, the Hct and Hgb may not show a decrease for 24 hr. If bleeding continues without fluid replacement, lost volume is compensated for by shifting fluid from the intracellular space.

Reticulocyte counts increase as bone marrow increases production of immature RBCs to replace those lost. Initially platelets increase as the body attempts to form clots. As platelets are depleted by continued bleeding, counts fall. Liver disease and alcoholism cause increases in mean corpuscular volume (MCV). When the MCV is increased, the RBCs are said to be macrocytic and thus anemia may be termed *macrocytic* and *normochromic* (normal Hgb). Platelet and white blood cell (WBC) counts may be decreased initially because of splenic enlargement. As a result of coagulopathies in patients with hepatocellular disease, prothrombin time (PT) is prolonged. The clotting deficiency is usually unresponsive to vitamin K therapy.

Biochemical tests: An elevated blood urea nitrogen (BUN) is caused by elevated blood proteins from the digestion of blood in the gastrointestinal (GI) tract. Hypernatremia is a result of hypovolemia. Urine osmolality is increased because of ADH secretion, increased protein intake (from hemorrhaged blood in the gut), and cirrhosis. The severity of liver damage can be estimated by elevations of values in serum total bilirubin, decreases in albumin (see "Hepatic Failure," p. 427), and prolongation of PT.

Ammonia is an end product of protein metabolism and is formed from the action of bacteria on proteins in the intestinal lumen and from hydrolysis of glutamine in the kidneys. The liver normally removes most of the ammonia from the portal vein and converts it to urea for excretion by the kidneys. When the liver is not functioning properly and blood is shunted from the liver by collateral vessels, ammonia levels build. Large protein loads from gastrointestinal bleeding may result in greatly increased ammonia levels.

Note: A fasting venous blood sample for serum ammonia is obtained, placed on ice, and transported immediately to the laboratory to ensure accuracy of the test. If an arterial line is available, an arterial sample is preferable.

Blood alcohol: Ethyl alcohol levels may be tested on admission to distinguish acute intoxication from encephalopathy.

Occult blood tests: To test for blood in stool or gastric secretions. Occult blood may persist in the stool for as long as one week after a significant GI bleed.

Endoscopy: Endoscopy allows direct visualization of active hemorrhage or evidence of a recent hemorrhage. It is usually performed after stabilizing the patient. Variceal bleeding may be treated by banding or sclerotherapy during the procedure (see "Collaborative Management," p. 421). Aspiration, cardiac dysrhythmias, and severe hemorrhage are serious complications of the procedure. Endotracheal intubation may be performed before the procedure to protect the airway. See Table 8-1 for nursing implications of endoscopy. Erythromycin, a motilin agonist, induces gastric emptying. Giving 250mg IV 20 minutes before endoscopy allows easier visualization, reduces scope time, and reduces the need for repeat procedure.

Liver biopsy: See "Hepatic Failure," p. 435.

COLLABORATIVE MANAGEMENT

Stabilization of the bleeding varices is the immediate concern. The two priorities are restoring blood volume and assessing and monitoring the degree of vascular compromise. Once stabilized, short-term and long-term management of gastroesophageal variceal bleeding depends on the underlying cause of portal hypertension, the severity of the bleeding episode, previous bleeding episodes, and previous response to therapy. Preserving and optimizing liver function is especially important for patients with cirrhosis and underlying hepatocellular disease to reduce the risk of disabling encephalopathy. Preventing complications in the portal hypertensive patient with gastroesophageal bleeding is important and is accomplished through the use of lactulose and oral nonabsorbable antibiotics for 5 days after the acute bleed to decrease the incidence of infections by enteric organisms.

TABLE 8-1   Nursing Care of the Patient Undergoing Gastroesophageal Endoscopy

Before procedure
- Explain procedure to patient and significant others.
- Ensure informed consent form has been signed before sedation is administered.
- Maintain NPO status for 8 hr before procedure.
- Administer premedication as prescribed, usually at a reduced dose if cirrhosis or hepatitis is present, and monitor for side effects.
- Clear stomach of blood and gastric contents immediately before endoscope is passed.
- Verify the patency of at least 1 large-bore (>18 gauge) IV catheter.
- Administer erythromycin intravenously 20 min before start of procedure (if patient not allergic).
- Spray back of throat with local anesthetic within 5 min of the endoscope being passed. Make sure patient does not inhale as spray is administered.

During procedure
- Keep patient in side-lying position to reduce the likelihood of aspiration.
- Have nasopharyngeal suction equipment, as well as a crash cart, readily available.

After procedure
- Maintain side-lying position until patient is fully alert to reduce the likelihood of aspiration.
- Ensure that 2-4 hr after the procedure the gag reflex has returned.
- Note evidence of change in rate of hemorrhage if a banding or sclerotherapy procedure was performed.
- Monitor for the following: aspiration pneumonia (evidenced by difficulty breathing, diminished breath sounds, coarse crackles, and rhonchi); cardiac dysrhythmias; perforation (evidenced by retrosternal pain, bleeding, fever, and dysphagia); and cervical neck perforation (evidenced by crepitus or neck or throat pain).

IV, Intravenous; *NPO,* nothing by mouth.

Fluid resuscitation: Large-bore intravenous (IV) lines are required to infuse isotonic fluids until albumin, packed RBCs, and fresh-frozen plasma are available. To monitor the progress of the resuscitation, a Foley catheter and central venous catheter (preferably a pulmonary artery catheter) should be placed. The central venous catheter will provide hemodynamic monitoring of vital signs (VS), CVP, PAWP, and other parameters, as is essential to prevent hypovolemic shock while avoiding overtransfusion and associated cardiopulmonary problems. Ideally, patients should be underinfused, keeping their hematocrit in the 25%-30% range to prevent edema and increased variceal pressure from overtransfusion, which can cause rebleeding.

D_5W, sodium chloride, and Ringer's lactate (RL) are used for initial resuscitation and volume replacement. Excessive use of saline infusions is avoided because sodium is retained and contributes to ascites. Ringer's lactate is not recommended for patients with significant liver dysfunction because the damaged liver may not be able to convert the lactate to bicarbonate. Serum lactate accumulates and contributes to metabolic acidosis. Packed RBCs are transfused as soon as they are available to maintain an Hct of 25%-30%. This Hct should be higher in patients with an underlying cardiac condition to prevent the complications associated with cardiac ischemia. Platelets are given if the platelet count is markedly reduced or if spontaneous bleeding occurs from sites other than varices. Albumin is administered if the patient continues to be hypovolemic despite an Hct above 28% or if the patient is hypoalbuminemic. Serial Hct evaluations are necessary to estimate ongoing blood loss and need for RBC replacement.

Vasopressin (Pitressin): Vasopressin is a naturally occurring, potent vasoconstrictor that is given IV at 0.1-0.4 units/min, and its actions are dose-dependent. It is used, in conjunction with nitroglycerin, until bleeding has been under control for at least 12 hr. Vasopressin acts by decreasing intrahepatic vascular resistance or by dilation of the portocollateral circulation. Secondarily it causes peripheral vasodilation, which produces reflex splanchnic vasoconstriction and a decrease in blood flow. Vasopressin has systemic vasoconstrictive and cardiotoxic side effects. In 25% of cases its use has to be stopped as a result of system vasoconstriction with increased peripheral vascular resistance and reduced coronary blood blow, decreased heart rate, and reduced cardiac output. Nitroglycerin should be coadministered to potentiate the reduction in portal pressure while reducing the cardiac side effects (Table 8-2).

T A B L E   8 - 2   Adverse Effects of Vasopressin and Nitroglycerin

Vasopressin	Nitroglycerin
Cardiovascular	
Increased cardiac afterload	Reduced preload
Baroreceptor-mediated bradycardia	Reduced afterload
Reduced cardiac output	Orthostatic hypotension
Impaired cardiac contractility	Dilation of peripheral arteries and veins
Dysrhythmias, including premature ventricular complex (PVC) and ventricular tachycardia	Dilation of coronary arteries
Myocardial ischemia and infarction	
Potentially fatal dysrhythmias	
Gastrointestinal	
Splanchnic vasoconstriction resulting in bowel ischemia, mesenteric infarction, and necrosis	Reduction in portal pressures
Increased gut motility resulting in abdominal cramps and diarrhea	Nausea, vomiting, diarrhea
Other	
Increased water resorption by the kidneys, resulting in antidiuresis, fluid overload, hyponatremia, and increasing ascites	Relaxation of smooth muscles
Respiratory arrest	Syncope
Cerebral hemorrhage	Restlessness
Limb ischemia	Cerebral edema
	Daily headache

Nitroglycerin: Nitroglycerin is often given with vasopressin to counteract the vasoconstrictive effects of vasopressin and to allow for higher doses of vasopressin to be administered. Several studies have shown that together they are actually more effective for control of acute gastroesophageal bleeding than either used alone. Nitroglycerin can be given by IV, sublingually, or transdermally. For use in gastroesophageal bleeding it should be given by IV at 1mg/kg/min and titrated to obtain a systolic blood pressure of 110-120 mm Hg.

Beta-(β-) adrenergic blocking agents: Nadolol, a nonselective β-blocker (longer-acting than propranolol) is not metabolized by the liver and has less effect on renal function. The side-effect profile is considerably less than that of propranolol. Doses of nonselective β-blockers are selected by incremental increases to reach an end point of a 25% reduction in resting heart rate (HR).

Octreotide: Is a synthetic analogue of somatostatin (which is not available in the United States). It reduces hepatic blood flow, wedged hepatic venous pressure, and azygous blood flow. Octreotide is safer to use, with less potential for severe side effects, than vasopressin. Octreotide is given prophylactically intravenously for 5 days after acute hemorrhage, because 40% of rebleeding occurs within 5 days of the initial bleed and early rebleeding increases the risk of death considerably within the first 6 weeks after an initial bleed. Octreotide is given as a bolus: 100 mcg/hr and then 50 mcg/hr. Some physicians will use octreotide intravenously for 2 days after a bleed and then give 100 mcg q8h subcutaneously for another 3 days.

Norfloxacin: Forty-six percent of hospitalized patients with cirrhosis have an infection. Up to 35% of these infections are acquired in the hospital and are usually bacterial in nature. Patients who are admitted with a gastroesophageal hemorrhage appear more prone to developing infections, particularly bacteremia and spontaneous bacterial peritonitis (SBP). Infections are associated with a higher mortality and the current antibiotic of choice to administer prophylactically is norfloxacin by mouth (PO) 400 mg bid for 5 days.

Erythromycin: Is a macrolide antibiotic and is primarily used for numerous infections. One of its side effects is useful in patients who have had a gastroesophageal bleed and need endoscopy. It happens to be a motilin agonist, which induces gastric emptying. It has started being used as an IV medication before endoscopy to aid in the clearance of the stomach for better visualization.

Lactulose: A nonabsorbable disaccharide which is given on a daily basis to patients with hepatic encephalopathy. It is titrated based on bowel movements. Desirable effects are usually observed at three to four loose (nondiarrheal) stools per day.

Nasogastric intubation: A nasogastric (NG) tube is placed in the stomach to reduce the risk of tracheobronchial aspirations and prepare the stomach for an endoscope and possible treatment by removing blood. It can also help ascertain the size of the hemorrhage. Iced lavage is not routine anymore and is rarely used, if ever.

Gastroesophageal endoscopy: This procedure is usually carried out once the patient's condition is stabilized. Many times banding (see next section) is also performed at the same time to prevent rebleeding. Patients are usually given IV erythromycin approximately 20 min before the procedure is carried out (see Table 8-1). Clinical complications commonly seen after an acute bleed need to be prevented. Lactulose should be given to control hepatic encephalopathy, as well as prophylactic antibiotics (norfloxacin) for 5-7 days after the bleed to reduce the incidence of enteric organisms causing infections.

Endoscopic variceal ligation (banding): The procedure of choice to prevent a first bleeding episode, also used for patients who rebleed. Many endoscopists feel it is safer and more effective, particularly if used in combination with a β-blocker such as nadolol. Compared to sclerotherapy, banding controls bleeding better, has less mortality, requires fewer sessions to obliterate veins and has fewer local complications. It is also useful to control acute esophageal variceal bleeding. This procedure has no effect on portal hypertension; therefore, the potential for complication(s) from portal hypertension still exists.

Endoscopic sclerotherapy: Works by injecting a sclerosing solution of sodium tetradecyl sulfate, morrhuate sodium, polidocanol, ethanolamine oleate, or ethanol into the varices. The solution causes inflammation, with fibrosis and then obliteration of the varices. Sclerotherapy has a 0.5%-2% mortality rate along with the potential complications of perforation, bleeding, pleural effusion, pulmonary edema, stricture formation, impaired esophageal motility, esophageal ulceration, mediastinitis, and bacteremia, all of which has caused the procedure not be used as first-line therapy for gastroesophageal bleeds. This procedure is not used to prevent a first bleed. It is most effective when used in combination with the pharmacologic therapy octreotide.

Ultrasonography: Endoscopic ultrasonography is useful in aiding visualization, diagnosis and guidance of further treatment in gastric varices and is also useful to predict possible recurrence of varices. It provides a way to observe the stigmata of a recent hemorrhage, and is often the only way to confirm that such a bleed has taken place.

Transjugular intrahepatic portal-systemic shunts (TIPS): This nonsurgical procedure is useful as a "rescue therapy" for patients (especially those awaiting a transplant) with uncontrolled or recurrent variceal bleeding in spite of previous endoscopic therapy. Ninety percent of TIPS procedures are successful. Variceal rebleeding rates are approximately 20%. One and occasionally two vascular stents are placed within the liver to connect the portal and the hepatic veins. Blood from the spleen and bowels bypasses the diseased liver on its way back to the heart. A major disadvantage of TIPS is the 50% stenosis rate within the first year. It is a costly procedure over time, as it requires a monitoring program to prevent complete stenosis and reintervention. TIPS is known to cause encephalopathy to some degree in up to 50% of the patients who have the procedure.

Angiographic studies: The most common procedure is portal venography by indirect angiography. The femoral artery is catheterized, and contrast material is injected into the splenic artery. Contrast material flows through the spleen into the splenic and the portal veins. This procedure is used to establish portal venous anatomy before operations such as TIPS, portal systemic shunt, or hepatic transplantation. In patients with previously constructed surgical shunts, patency may be confirmed. See Table 8-3 for nursing implications of angiographic studies.

Hepatic vein wedge pressure (HVWP) is measured by introducing a double-lumen balloon catheter into the femoral vein and threading it into one of the hepatic veins. This is an accurate measurement of the liver's contribution to resistance to portal venous flow. Normal HVWP is 5-6 mm Hg; values of about 20 mm Hg are typical for patients with cirrhosis.

Direct access to the portal vein may be achieved through transhepatic portography. During this procedure, varices may be obliterated by injection of thrombin or Gelfoam into veins that supply the varices.

> **Note:** Transhepatic portography involves a direct puncture through the liver and has many of the same risks as does liver biopsy. Patients returning from this procedure should be positioned on their right side and monitored closely (see Table 8-7).

Esophageal balloon tamponade: A procedure which is rarely used, and not as first-line hemorrhage control, the multilumen/multiballoon Sengstaken-Blakemore (S-B) tube, the Minnesota tube, or the single-balloon Linton tube is inserted through a nostril or the mouth. It is passed into the stomach, where the gastric balloon is inflated with 250-300 cc of air. It is then pulled snug against the gastroesophageal junction. The esophageal balloon is inflated to 20-40 mm Hg. Esophageal balloon tamponade is useful for control of acute bleeding because of the direct, constant pressure that is applied

---

T A B L E 8 - 3   Nursing Care of the Patient Undergoing Angiographic Studies

Before procedure
- Explain procedure to patient and significant others.
- Ensure an informed consent was signed before sedation was administered.
- Maintain NPO status for 8 hr before procedures.
- Verify patency of IV catheter.
- Note allergies to seafood, iodine, and contrast material.
- Administer sedative as prescribed, usually at a reduced dose if cirrhosis or hepatitis is present.

During procedure
- Assist radiology personnel with positioning and draping patient.
- Monitor vital signs q15min or more often for evidence of anaphylaxis or hemorrhagic shock.

After procedure
- Check vital signs q15min initially and q1-2h once patient's condition has stabilized.
- Maintain patient in supine position with affected leg straight.
- Check dressing often for signs of continued bleeding from puncture site.
- Keep pressure dressing and sandbag over puncture site for 6-8 hr.
- Evaluate distal pulses and perfusion in affected extremity q1-2h for 8 hr. Arterial thrombosis and large hematomas that compromise femoral blood flow may develop as a result of manipulation of the artery and clotting abnormalities associated with liver disease.
- Monitor urine output q1-2h and report volume <0.5 ml/kg/hr.

IV, Intravenous; *NPO,* nothing by mouth.

to the varices. Traction on the tubes, which places constant pressure on the varices, is essential for effective tamponading. This may be used for temporary hemorrhage control because long-term use has been implicated in a higher rate of rebleeding and an increased complication rate. The balloon is not to be left inflated for more than 24 hr. Esophageal necrosis, esophageal rupture, and tissue necrosis are some side effects from tamponade. If bleeding resumes after deflation, surgery is indicated.

Esophageal staple transection: A procedure used rarely before surgery is tried, transection of the distal esophagus with a staple gun is reported to be superior to one session of sclerotherapy. It is effective in patients who have rebled after sclerotherapy. Potential complications are similar to those associated with esophageal band ligation or sclerotherapy (Table 8-4).

Surgical management: Emergency surgery for variceal bleeding is associated with a higher mortality (up to 50%) than other procedures, particularly in patients of Childs class C. Ideally it is best to stabilize the patient and control acute bleeding medically. Surgery can then be performed at a later date with less risk to the patient. Numerous surgical procedures exist that directly control bleeding or indirectly reduce variceal pressure, which will stop bleeding.

Surgeries that are a direct interruption of portosystemic blood flow are as follows: transabdominal, transthoracic, or transthoracoabdominal esophageal transection; gastric devascularization with splenectomy (Suguira procedure); gastric transection; or selective shunts (distal splenorenal and gastric venocaval). Nondecompressive surgery and portocaval shunts may reduce the risk of first bleed. Surgical procedures in many of these high-risk patients is not advisable because of the increased mortality. Many of these procedures bypass the liver completely, which allows for encephalopathy. Combination therapy may be a better option, particularly in those patients in Childs class C (see "Hepatic Failure," p. 427, for additional information on portal hypertension).

Other: Orthotopic liver transplantation (OLT) has a 1-yr survival rate of 85%-90%. The 5-yr survival rate is now 65%-75%. Liver transplant is a last resort, and many patients undergo numerous other procedures first. The main factors affecting survival after OLT are recurrence of immunosuppression-related complications.

NURSING DIAGNOSES AND INTERVENTIONS

Fluid volume deficit related to active loss of circulating blood volume secondary to variceal bleeding
Desired outcomes: Within 12 hr of this diagnosis, patient becomes normovolemic as evidenced by mean arterial pressure (MAP) >70 mm Hg; HR 60-100 beats/min; brisk capillary refill (<2 sec); CVP 2-6 mm Hg; PAWP 6-12 mm Hg; cardiac index (CI) >3 L/min/m^2; urinary output >0.5 ml/kg/hr; and patient is oriented to time, place, and person.
- Administer prescribed fluids at rapid rate (wide open for active, massive bleeding). See "Fluid Resuscitation," p. 420, for types of fluids indicated. Minimize IV infusion of sodium-containing

---

T A B L E   8 - 4   Side Effects and Potential Complications of Esophageal Banding, Sclerotherapy, and Esophageal Stapling

Anticipated mild side effects
    Mild retrosternal pain
    Transient fever
    Diminished breath sounds
    Transient dysphagia
    Local ulceration

Serious side effects/complications
    Bleeding from remaining varices, ulcers, gastric varix, or portal hypertensive gastropathy
    Stricture formation evidenced by prolonged dysphagia
    Perforation evidenced by bleeding, severe substernal pain, or fever
    Pulmonary problems including aspiration pneumonia, pleural effusion, mediastinitis, empyema, atelectasis
    Bronchoesophageal fistula
    Bacteremia/septicemia evidenced by fever, tachycardia, positive blood culture results
    Anaphylaxis
    Gastric wall necrosis
    Chylothorax, pneumothorax, or subcutaneous emphysema

solutions, which can contribute to fluid sequestration (ascites) and precipitate hepatorenal syndrome in susceptible patients (see "Hepatic Failure," p. 427).

- Monitor for distended neck veins, crackles in the lungs, peripheral edema, weight gain, and rebleeding of varices. All of these symptoms signal fluid overload.
- Monitor BP q15min, or more frequently in the presence of brisk bleeding. Be alert to decreases in MAP to >10 mm Hg less than baseline.
- Monitor HR, electrocardiogram (ECG), capillary refill, respiratory rate (RR), and cardiovascular status q15min, or more frequently in the presence of active bleeding or if using vasopressin or similar agents. Be alert to increases in HR, delayed capillary refill, and changes in level of consciousness (LOC), which reflect hypovolemia. Be aware that an altered LOC can be caused by encephalopathy as well as by hypovolemia. Anticipate vasopressin-induced reflex bradycardia; consult physician if bradycardia is severe (HR <60 beats/min) or compromises tissue perfusion.
- Measure central pressures and thermodilution CO/CI q1-2h, or more frequently if the patient is unstable or receiving vasoactive agents. Be alert to low or decreasing CVP and PAWP. Assess for signs of overaggressive fluid resuscitation, including elevated CVP, PAP, and PAWP and aggravation of variceal bleeding in some patients. Anticipate compensatory increases in CO/CI, with CI usually >3. Monitor Svo_2 as possible to evaluate adequacy of tissue oxygenation. Evaluate volume status by noting increases or decreases in PAWP values and urinary output.
- Measure urinary output hourly, as well as urine osmolality levels, color, quantity, and specific gravity of urine. Be alert to output <0.5 ml/kg/hr for 2 consecutive hours. Anticipate decreased urinary output after initial dose of vasopressin. Expect diuresis after vasopressin has been discontinued.
- Measure abdominal girth every shift. A permanent marker should be used to mark a spot on the abdomen where all measurements will be made.
- Monitor for physical indicators of hypovolemia including cool extremities, capillary refill >2 sec, absent or decreased amplitude of distal pulses, and change in LOC.
- Measure and record all GI blood losses from hematemesis, hematochezia (red blood through rectum), and melena. Test all stools and gastric contents for occult blood.
- Administer vasopressin as prescribed. Ensure patency of IV catheter. Monitor for serious side effects such as bradycardia, ventricular irritability, chest pain, abdominal cramping, hyponatremia, water intoxication, and oliguria (see Table 8-2). Administer vasopressin concurrently with IV nitroglycerin to reduce adverse cardiovascular effects and improve efficacy. Consult physician and reduce rate of infusion in the presence of serious adverse effects.
- Be alert to adverse side effects of esophageal banding and/or sclerotherapy: infection, pulmonary complications (i.e., Pao_2 <80 mm Hg, basilar crackles, diminished breath sounds), and esophageal ulceration (i.e., difficulty swallowing, pain, continued bleeding). Anticipate mild retrosternal pain and transient fever after the procedure.
- Avoid use of indwelling gastric tubes for routine gastric drainage because they irritate varices and may prolong or renew bleeding.
- Place all intravenous fluids on pumps, once fluid resuscitation is completed, to avoid fluid overload.

You may also wish to refer to the following interventions from the Nursing Interventions Classification (NIC):

NIC Bleeding Precautions; Blood Product Administration; Fluid/Electrolyte Management; Hypovolemia Management; Shock Management

Decreased cardiac output related to altered rate or rhythm secondary to myocardial ischemia from prolonged, massive bleeding or vasopressin-induced coronary vasoconstriction; decreased preload secondary to acute blood loss; increased afterload secondary to vasoconstrictive effects of shock or vasopressin therapy

Desired outcome: Within 24 hr of this diagnosis, patient's cardiac output is adequate as evidenced by normal sinus rhythm on ECG; CI within normal limits or increased (>3 L/min/m^2); MAP >70 mm Hg; and Svo_2 60%-80%.

- Monitor BP, HR, ECG, and PAP (see first four entries under preceding nursing diagnosis, "Fluid Volume Deficit").
- Monitor arterial blood gas (ABG) values for evidence of hypoxemia. Be alert to and consult physician for Pao_2 <80 mm Hg. Administer oxygen if need for it is indicated by ABG values. Place patient in semi-Fowler's position to optimize oxygenation; keep pulse oximeter on.
- Monitor Hct; consult physician for values <25%-30% (for each unit of packed RBCs transfused, Hct increases approximately 3%).
- Monitor patient for evidence of myocardial ischemia if Hgb is greatly decreased or if the patient is receiving vasopressin (see tenth entry in preceding nursing diagnosis, "Fluid Volume Deficit").

Observe ECG for ventricular dysrhythmias and ST segment changes. Instruct patient to report chest discomfort promptly. Administer prn nitrates as prescribed.

- Minimize patient's activity during acute bleeding episode to reduce myocardial oxygen demands. Explain and encourage adherence to total bed rest regimen. As possible, monitor Svo_2 to evaluate adequacy of tissue oxygenation (see Table 1-16). Patients with baseline cardiopulmonary disease may need to be transfused to achieve an Hct of 30% to prevent cardiac ischemia.
- Measure thermodilution CO/CI q1-2h. Be aware that a "normal" CO may be a low value for the patient with a hyperdynamic circulatory state associated with cirrhosis. Maintain CI >3 L/min/m².
- Maintain MAP >70-80 mm Hg (see preceding nursing diagnosis, "Fluid Volume Deficit") to promote adequate tissue perfusion. Avoid excessive fluids and prevent hypervolemia, which could increase variceal bleeding. Supplemental O_2 via nasal cannula may be necessary to decrease or prevent ischemia in those patients with poor oxygenation.

NIC Cardiac Care: Acute; Hemodynamic Regulation; Oxygen Therapy; Shock Management; Invasive Hemodynamic Monitoring

Ineffective airway clearance related to tracheobronchial obstruction by esophageal balloon device; tracheobronchial obstruction by pharyngeal secretions above the inflated esophageal balloon device; perceptual/cognitive impairment secondary to encephalopathy

Desired outcome: Within 4 hr of this diagnosis, patient's airway becomes clear as evidenced by auscultation of normal breath sounds, absence of adventitious sounds, and RR 12-20 breaths/min with normal depth and pattern (eupnea).

- Position patient in a side-lying position during vomiting episodes unless he or she is fully alert and is more comfortable in an upright position.
- As necessary, suction oropharynx with Yankauer or similar suction device to remove blood and secretions.
- Auscultate lung fields during and after vomiting episodes for presence of rhonchi, which can signal aspiration of gastric contents. Auscultation at frequent intervals is necessary while inflated esophageal balloon device is in place to ensure device is not partially occluding the airway.
- Provide oral care at frequent intervals to assist in mobilizing oropharyngeal secretions. A dilute solution of hydrogen peroxide and normal saline may be helpful in removing dried blood from the teeth and oral mucosa. Use saline to rinse hydrogen peroxide solution from patient's mouth.
- Monitor for early signs of respiratory failure: increasing RR, work of breathing (WOB), and $Paco_2$ and decreasing Spo_2 via continuous pulse oximetry and decreasing Pao_2.
- Implement the following interventions for patients with an S-B or similar tube:
  - ❑ Consult physician regarding possibility of endotracheal (ET) intubation (before S-B tube insertion), particularly if decreased mental status, massive variceal bleed, or massive hematemesis is present.
  - ❑ Verify proper tube placement by means of immediate chest x-ray.
  - ❑ Be certain that oral secretions are suctioned from above the inflated esophageal balloon via a proximal tube or an additional lumen in the tube for this purpose. Label proximal tube or lumen with the warning "Do Not Irrigate."
  - ❑ Ensure patency of gastric and esophageal drainage lumens. Irrigate gastric lumen q1-2h and as necessary to ensure patency.
  - ❑ Be aware that proximal migration of the esophageal balloon or rupture of the gastric balloon may result in total airway obstruction. Auscultate breath sounds q1-2h. Keep a pair of scissors in an obvious place (e.g., taped to the wall above the bed) near the patient at all times to cut and immediately deflate all lumens of the S-B tube should respiratory distress occur.
  - ❑ Check security of tape, tube connections, and traction initially and q2h. Firm traction is established by taping the tube to a helmet or a firm, padded retainer. The traction device should be designed so that it minimizes pressure to facial tissue and prevents tissue necrosis.
  - ❑ Document quantity and characteristics of gastric drainage q4h.

NIC Aspiration Precautions; Artificial Airway Management; Oxygen Therapy; Respiratory Monitoring

Altered tissue perfusion (or risk for same): gastrointestinal, related to interruption of venous and arterial blood flow secondary to pressure on esophageal tissue from balloon tamponade; hypovolemia secondary to variceal hemorrhage

Desired outcomes: Esophageal balloon pressure is maintained within prescribed range (usually 20-40 mm Hg). Patient has no symptoms of esophageal perforation as evidenced by BP within patient's normal range; HR 60-100 beats/min; PAP >20/6; PAWP >6 mm Hg; SVR <1200 dynes/sec/cm⁻⁵; CI >3 L/min/m²; and absence of sudden substernal chest or back pain.

- Check and record the esophageal balloon pressure q2-4h. Maintain within prescribed range (usually 20-40 mm Hg). Release pressure at prescribed intervals.
- Carefully document date and time of balloon inflation and deflation. Tissue necrosis is likely to occur if balloons are left inflated for >24 hr.

- Up to 24 hr after insertion, assist physician in relieving traction and deflating the esophageal balloon. The tube remains in place with the gastric balloon inflated for the next 24 hr, and the patient is closely monitored for rebleeding. If no further rebleeding occurs, the gastric balloon is deflated and the tube removed.
- Promptly consult physician for signs of esophageal perforation: sudden epigastric or substernal pain, back pain, shock state.

NIC Gastrointestinal Intubation; Shock Management

Impaired swallowing (or risk for same) related to mechanical obstruction secondary to edema or stricture formation after sclerotherapy; irritated esophageal tissue secondary to banding, sclerotherapy, esophageal stapling, or balloon tamponade.

Desired outcome: By the time of discharge from intensive care unit (ICU) or hospital, patient swallows food and demonstrates ability to pass food through the lower esophagus into the stomach.

- After banding or sclerotherapy treatments, evaluate patient for subjective complaints of difficulty in swallowing or pain during swallowing. Consult physician for significant findings.
- Plan a soft and bland diet, as tolerated by patient, which can be initiated 24 hr after banding, sclerotherapy, esophageal stapling, or balloon tamponade.
- Instruct patient to avoid mechanically or chemically irritating foods. Initially, foods that are too hot, too cold, or too spicy should be avoided.
- Caution patient that certain foods or substances (e.g., alcohol) may cause a burning sensation during the swallowing process because of esophageal mucosal erosion. Instruct patient to avoid mechanical or chemical irritants.

NIC Swallowing Therapy; Nutrition Management

Ineffective thermoregulation (or risk for same) related to infusions of nonwarmed blood, blood products, and intravenous fluids; too-rapid fluid loss secondary to esophageal variceal bleeding

Desired outcomes: Patient's will not drop body temperature more than 2° F per hour while fluid resuscitation is ongoing nor develop shock from body temperature being too low.

- Use blood warmer for all infusions, particularly blood and blood products, thus allowing body temperature to stay closer to normal.
- Institute active external rewarming measures: provide warm blankets and cover patient's head to decrease heat loss. Do not rewarm faster than 2° F per hour; otherwise rewarming shock may ensue.
- Monitor temperature q1-2h.

Research Brief 8-1   Much controversy exists as to whether endoscopic screening for esophageal varices is useful, let alone cost-effective. Current practice guidelines for patients with Childs class A or B cirrhosis who have never bled is to follow these patients with an endoscopy every 2 years if no varices are present at "first-look" endoscopy. Decision analysis software was used to study a hypothetical cohort of patients with Childs class A or B cirrhosis whose esophageal varices status is unknown. Costs per initial variceal bleed prevented by each of the 18 preventive strategies were analyzed. Costs were estimated based on direct health care costs without cost discounting. The analysis suggests that the current practice guidelines may incur costs over $170,000 per variceal bleed prevented when compared with empiric β-blocker therapy alone. It is suggested that further studies be pursued to reexamine what the "standard of care" for esophageal varices should be in relation to cost-effectiveness.

Spiegel BMR et al: Endoscopic screening for esophageal varices in cirrhotics: is it cost effective: *Hepatology* 37(2):366-377, 2003.

Knowledge deficit: lack of exposure to health care information or cognitive limitation secondary to hepatic encephalopathy

Desired outcome: Within the 24-hr period before hospital discharge, patient states the signs and symptoms of variceal hemorrhage, the importance of medical follow-ups, and the necessity of avoiding activities that increase the risk of variceal bleeding.

- Teach patient the signs and symptoms of actual or impending hemorrhage including nausea, dark stools, lightheadedness, vomiting of blood, or passing of frank blood in stools. Stress importance of seeking medical attention promptly if indicators of hemorrhage appear.
- Stress the importance of medical follow-up for management of variceal bleeding—either chronic sclerotherapy or shunt surgery.
- Teach patient about prescribed medications, including drug name, purpose, dosage, schedule, precautions, and potential side effects.
- Teach patient to carry a current list of medications with current dosages at all times.

- Caution about the necessity of avoiding heavy lifting, straining, and other activities associated with the Valsalva maneuver. Stool softeners, increased oral fluids, and a bulking agent may be necessary daily to prevent straining at stool.
- Teach the importance of avoiding mechanically irritating foods, such as nuts, corn chips, and improperly chewed food. Stress importance of avoiding nonsteroidal antiinflammatory drugs (NSAIDs) and alcohol, which irritate the esophageal and gastric mucosa.
- Teach patient and family members the signs and symptoms of hepatic encephalopathy.
- Teach patient and family members the importance of lactulose titration based on mental status and frequency/consistency of stools.

ADDITIONAL NURSING DIAGNOSES

If portal hypertension is caused by cirrhosis, refer to "Hepatic Failure," p. 427, for additional nursing diagnoses. For other nursing diagnoses and interventions, see "Psychosocial Support," p. 68, and "Psychosocial Support for the Patient's Family and Significant Others," p. 78.

Hepatic Failure

PATHOPHYSIOLOGY

Necrosis of liver parenchyma results in varying degrees of hepatic failure with accompanying sequelae. Worldwide, hepatitis B virus (with or without accompanying hepatitis D) and hepatitis C are the most common causes of hepatic failure, accounting for as many as 60% of all cases. Damage to the hepatocytes and liver structure can be acute or chronic. The amount of destruction to the liver varies with duration of illness, underlying etiology, preexisting conditions, treatment, and lifestyle changes (e.g., eliminating alcohol).

Acute liver failure: Acute liver failure (ALF) is responsible for approximately 2000 deaths a year and about 5% of all liver transplants in the United States. ALF is divided into three types, based on length of time between appearance of jaundice to development of encephalopathy. The three types are *hyperacute, acute,* and *subacute.* Patients with hyperacute liver failure develop encephalopathy within 7-8 days from onset of jaundice. In the United States the most common cause is acetaminophen overdose. Other causes include drug toxicity, Q fever, falciparum malaria, sickle cell crisis, *Amanita* mushroom poisoning, or acute hepatitis A, B, or B with D. Progression from jaundice to encephalopathy occurs within 8-29 days in patients with acute liver failure. Acute alcoholic hepatitis, which can be clinically severe, does not exhibit liver necrosis as massive as the other etiologies. Hepatitis A infection is mostly mild when acquired in childhood but can be very hepatoxic when contracted in adulthood, or when superimposed on another hepatitis infection (i.e., chronic hepatitis B or C). Patients presenting with history of jaundice to encephalopathy of 5- to 26-wk duration may exhibit submassive hepatic necrosis. Many of them arrive to be seen by physicians or emergency departments when damage to the liver parenchyma is extensive, necessitating consideration of immediate orthotopic liver transplantation as the only life-saving treatment. In the absence of preexisting liver disease, ALF is potentially reversible when the condition is treated promptly. These patients are usually young adults and commonly have acetaminophen toxicity as etiology. Overall mortality from all causes of ALF is 50%-80% without liver transplantation.

Chronic hepatic failure: Loss of hepatocytes, abnormal microcirculation, and impaired function of 6-month or longer duration are hallmarks of chronic liver failure. Chronic liver disease is associated with widespread tissue necrosis, fibrosis, nodule formation in the liver, and eventual cirrhosis, ultimately resulting in hepatic failure. The usual causes of chronic liver failure are long-term alcohol ingestion, chronic viral hepatitis, prolonged cholestasis, and metabolic disorders.

Manifestations of liver failure: There are various manifestations of acute and chronic liver failure. Regardless if acute or chronic, liver failure affects the physiologic status of virtually every organ system. It takes a team of experienced healthcare workers to manage the complications of liver failure patients. A delicate balance must be kept to keep identified problems from worsening and new problems from developing, further complicating the management of such ill patients.

Renal complications: Defined by the International Ascites Club, "*Hepatorenal syndrome (HRS)* is a clinical condition that occurs in patients with advanced chronic liver disease, liver failure, and portal hypertension characterized by impaired renal function and marked abnormalities in the arterial circulation and activity of the endogenous vasoactive systems. In the kidney there is marked renal vasoconstriction that results in low glomerular filtration rate (GFR), whereas in the extrarenal circulation there is predominance of arterial vasodilation, which results in reduction of total systemic vascular resistance and arterial hypotension." (Gines, Arroya, and Rodes) Factors that may reduce renal perfusion in persons with chronic liver disease are dehydration, lactulose therapy, NSAIDs use, hemorrhage, and paracentesis.

Sodium retention is the first problem observed in kidney function in patients with liver disease. Renal vasoconstriction is the second problem which, when severe, leads to hepatorenal syndrome. Patients with cirrhosis are the most likely candidates to develop HRS. There are two types of HRS: type 1 and type 2. The precipitating factors for both types are bacterial infections, such as spontaneous bacterial peritonitis (SBP), an episode of GI bleeding, hypovolemic shock, ischemic hepatitis, and diuretic management of ascites. Type 1 (which develops in many patients with type 2), typically seen in alcoholic cirrhosis, is rapid and progressive impairment of renal function as evidenced by doubling of creatinine >2.5 mg/dl or a 50% reduction of the 24-hr creatinine clearance to <20 ml/min in less than 2 wks. It has a low survival rate as a result of more severe liver failure, with patients succumbing after an average of 2 wks. Type 2 is moderate renal failure that remains steady for months. Patients are usually in better clinical condition, with a smaller and more stable reduction in GFR, and their liver disease is usually not as advanced as those with type 1.

Several studies have shown different treatment modalities to be effective: (1) acute administration of ornipressin with intense vasoconstrictor effect in the splanchnic circulation; (2) markedly expanding plasma volume with albumin and giving misoprostol (a prostaglandin analog) on a long-term basis shows marked renal function improvement; (3) albumin and ornipressin together and (4) terlipressin (a vasopressin analog with a prolonged half-life) plus albumin. TIPS is also effective, but pharmacologic therapy, with one of the drugs just mentioned, is the treatment of choice before invasive procedures. Giving albumin to expand plasma volume when infection (such as SBP) is suspected, along with antibiotics, can reduce the chance of developing HRS.

Cardiovascular complications: Circulatory abnormalities often are present and include a hyperdynamic systemic circulation, with increased cardiac output and decreased systemic vascular resistance. There are reduced β-adrenergic receptor signal transduction, defective cardiac excitation-contraction coupling, and conduction abnormalities. Increased nitric oxide activity plays a large role in the vasodilated state. In the final stages of ALF, profound peripheral vasodilation causes hemodynamic collapse. Patients may arrive to be seen with low blood pressure, tachycardia, a cardiac flow murmur, warm extremities, an active precordial impulse, palmar erythema, and/or spider angioma. The hyperdynamic circulatory state actually worsens for 1 to 3 months after TIPS and therefore, TIPS is a procedure to be used only with caution in carefully selected patients.

Pulmonary complications: Up to 70% of patients with chronic liver disease have some type of pulmonary symptom. Many patients will have either microvascular dilation leading to hepatopulmonary syndrome (HPS) or arteriolar vasoconstriction leading to portopulmonary hypertension (PPH). Both of these conditions can make a patient ineligible for a liver transplant. In HPS, spider angioma, platypnea (orthostatic dyspnea), digital clubbing, and cyanosis are common findings. These patients progressively worsen; intrapulmonary vasodilation develops and gas exchange deteriorates. Numerous therapies have been tried, with liver transplantation being the only one proven to be effective. Although a significant improvement in gas exchange is observed after transplantation, it may take up to 1 year for arterial hypoxemia to normalize.

Portopulmonary hypertension (PPH) is defined by the National Institutes of Health Patient Registry for the Characterization of Primary Pulmonary Hypertension as mean pulmonary artery pressure greater than 25 mm Hg and a pulmonary capillary wedge pressure lower than 15 mm Hg in the setting of portal hypertension. Symptoms include fatigue, dyspnea, peripheral edema, syncope, chest pain, and on exam a systolic murmur. ECG abnormalities are common (90%) and usually show a right bundle branch block, right axis deviation, or a right ventricular hypertrophy. These patients are controversial liver transplant patients because there is a 40% mortality postoperatively and PPH is irreversible with transplantation. Therefore the treatment focus is palliative; several different approaches are being tried. Calcium channel blockers, oral vasodilators, and chronic IV use of epoprostenol and isosorbide mononitrate have prolonged survival up to 5 yr.

Other: Fluid retention and ascites are attributed to several factors, including (1) intrahepatic vascular obstruction with transudation of fluid into the peritoneum; (2) defective albumin synthesis, resulting in decreased colloid osmotic pressure with failure to retain intravascular fluid; and (3) disturbances of various hormones, including renin, aldosterone, and renal prostaglandins, resulting in sodium and water retention. Ascites and edema are associated with chronic and acute hepatic failure, although massive ascites is usually the result of cirrhosis.

ASSESSMENT

History and risk factors: Worldwide, viral hepatitis accounts for the most cases of acute liver failure. Other causes include metabolic liver diseases (Wilson's disease, alpha$_1$-[α_1-] antitrypsin deficiency), liver ischemia from cardiovascular disease, hypotension, autoimmune hepatitis, and acute fatty liver in pregnancy. Exposure to hepatotoxic agents such as halothane, monoamine oxidase inhibitors (MAOIs), herbal preparations, isoniazid, acetaminophen (>10 g—less if cirrhosis, malnutrition, alcohol ingestion or a fasting state is present), carbon tetrachloride, the street drug "ecstasy," and bacterial agents is an additional factor.

Clinical presentation: One or more of the following are present: cerebral dysfunction, jaundice, portal hypertension, variceal bleeding, elevated aminotransferases, elevated bilirubin, and increased PT. Ascites and edema are also common findings. In the later stages of hepatic failure, deep coma, seizures, and decerebrate posturing are possible. In the absence of jaundice, laboratory evaluation of PT and liver function tests is necessary to prevent a misdiagnosis of septicemia, drug overdose, or a psychotic episode.

Physical assessment

Encephalopathy: An element of hepatic encephalopathy must be present for the diagnosis of fulminant hepatic failure (FHF). Encephalopathy is a marker signaling the beginning of a life-threatening condition: acute liver failure. Grade I encephalopathy includes lethargy, depression, slurred speech, subtle personality changes, euphoria, and sleep disturbances. In grade II, the patient experiences inappropriate behavior, disorientation, and restlessness and is more drowsy than in grade I. In grade III, patients experience somnolence but are arousable by gentle stimulation. They respond inappropriately to questions and may stare blankly as if catatonic. In grade IV, the patient is in a coma and may be able to respond to pain with deep stimulus. It is during grade III that patients are sedated, intubated, and placed on a ventilator to protect the airway and reduce the risk of cerebral edema. *Metabolic encephalopathy*, with varying degrees of consciousness and mental function, is attributed to ammonia toxicity and other metabolic derangements. Increased intracranial pressure (ICP) and cerebral edema are present with acute hepatic failure but are not usually seen in chronic hepatic failure. Cerebral edema is present in as many as 80% of patients with FHF and is a frequent cause of death. In patients with cirrhosis, diversion of portal blood flow via large collateral vessels contributes to encephalopathy.

Jaundice: Usually present first in the sclera and, as bilirubin increases in the serum, generalized yellowing of the skin occurs. Jaundice associated with hepatic failure occurs when the failing liver is unable to metabolize bilirubin. Those with jaundice may have abdominal pain, nausea, vomiting, and change in stool and urine color. Fluid sequestration (noted as edema, ascites, and weight gain), weight loss, and muscle wasting are also seen in patients with chronic hepatic failure. Small, bright red vascular spider veins (spider telangiectasis, spider angioma) are frequently found on the abdomen, face, neck, and arms of a patient with cirrhosis. In FHF, they are usually absent. In acute or chronic hepatic failure, asterixis, a flapping tremor of the hands when the arms are extended, may be present.

Fetor hepaticus: A foul odor detectable on a patient's breath with severe liver disease. Coagulopathies are responsible for multiple ecchymotic areas, purpura, and bleeding of the oral and nasal mucosa. Bleeding tendencies are caused by inadequate vitamin K absorption, failure of the liver to synthesize clotting factors or to clear activated clotting factors, and thrombocytopenia. Infections, including sepsis, are common as a result of a generalized state of debilitation and failure of the liver to produce immune-related proteins and filter blood from the intestines.

Metabolic abnormalities: Include severe hypoglycemia because of a loss of hepatic glycogen stores and impaired degradation of insulin. Dilutional hyponatremia is caused by secondary hyperaldosteronism. Hypokalemia occurs frequently because of hyperaldosteronism, excessive renal losses prompted by alkalosis, and use of loop diuretics. Hypokalemia increases renal production of ammonia, which contributes to hepatic encephalopathy.

King's College Hospital criteria: Widely used to assess prognosis of patients with acute liver failure not only from acetaminophen overdose, but other causes as well (Table 8-5).

In chronic liver disease, the liver is usually small and hard. Individuals with fulminant hepatic failure often have a small, nonpalpable liver. Patients with chronic failure usually have an enlarged spleen. Distended abdomen with shifting dullness to percussion and positive fluid wave are present because of ascites. With severe ascites, hernias are common and the umbilicus is frequently everted. Usually, jugular vein distention is the result of increased right atrial pressure (RAP) caused by increased intrapleural pressures from diaphragmatic elevation. Hormonal changes that result in gynecomastia, testicular atrophy, and scant body hair are common in men with chronic hepatic disease.

Vital signs and hemodynamic monitoring: Elevated temperature caused by infection; normal to bounding pulses; low to normal blood pressure (BP); elevated cardiac output associated with decreased peripheral vascular resistance and expanded total blood volume. In the presence of tense ascites, which increases intraabdominal pressure, the patient will exhibit impaired right ventricular filling with decreased stroke volume and decreased cardiac output. With massive variceal hemorrhage or late septic shock, pulses will be diminished and BP will be low, reflecting circulatory collapse.

TABLE 8-5   King's College Hospital Criteria

ALF from acetaminophen:

PH < 7.30 (24 hours after ingestion and after adequate fluid resuscitation)—irrespective of encephalopathy grade

PT* > 100 seconds or INR > 6.5 **with**

Serum creatinine > 3.4 mg/dl in stage 3 or 4 encephalopathy

ALF from other causes:

PT > 100 seconds, (INR > 6.5)—regardless of encephalopathy grade **or** any three of the following regardless of encephalopathy grade:

1. Age < 10 years
2. Age > 40 years
3. Non-A, non-B hepatitis
4. Duration of jaundice before onset of encephalopathy of more than 7 days
5. PT > 50 seconds (INR > 3.5)
6. Serum bilirubin > 17.5 mg/dl

---

*PT is the most sensitive prognostic marker.
INR, International normalized ratio.

DIAGNOSTIC TESTS

Virologic markers: See Table 8-6.

Liver-related serum biochemical tests

Alanine aminotransferase (ALT—formerly, serum glutamic pyruvic transaminase [SGPT]): This enzyme is found primarily in the liver, and its measurement is used as a marker of hepatocellular damage and to monitor potentially hepatotoxic drugs, treatment for hepatitis, and progression of postnecrotic cirrhosis. It is useful in determining whether jaundice is caused by liver disease or has a hemolytic cause. Increased levels are found in hepatocellular injury, hepatitis, pancreatitis, obstructive jaundice/biliary obstruction, active cirrhosis, metastatic liver tumor, liver congestion, and liver injury in myocardial infarction. Values over 300 units/L are present with acute hepatic failure.

Aspartate aminotransferase (aspartate aminotransferase [AST]/serum glutamic-oxaloacetic acid transaminase [SGOT]): This enzyme is present in organs with high metabolic activity such as the heart, liver, skeletal muscle, kidney, brain, pancreas, spleen, and lungs. Damage to the cells of these organs will cause a rise in the AST approximately 12 hr after injury, and levels remain elevated for 4-6 days. In liver disease, elevations 10-100 times normal are not unusual, especially in acute hepatitis, active cirrhosis, and hepatic necrosis.

Alkaline phosphatase (ALK phos): ALK phos is found in almost all tissue. Most elevations of ALK phos can be localized to an origin in the liver or bone. ALK phos is elevated to varying degrees in liver diseases such as obstructive jaundice, hepatocellular carcinoma, biliary cirrhosis, hepatitis, and cirrhosis of the liver.

Gamma-glutamyl transpeptidase (GGT/GGTP): This enzyme is present in numerous tissues, but levels are highest in liver disorders. This test can be used to confirm that ALK phos is elevated due to a hepatic related condition. Elevations occur in metastasis to the liver, cholestatic diseases, and secreted primarily through bile. cirrhosis of the liver, and alcoholic liver disease.

Bilirubin: Total bilirubin is a by-product of hemolysis. Elevations occur with excessive RBC destruction or when the liver is unable to process normal amounts of bilirubin. Elevations occur in viral hepatitis and cirrhosis. Conjugated (direct) bilirubin circulates until it reaches the liver, joins glucuronide, and is excreted into the bile. Unconjugated (indirect) bilirubin is protein-bound. An elevation of both occurs in hepatitis, cirrhosis, and hepatic metastasis. A persistently elevated level of bilirubin is a poor prognostic sign (see Table 8-6).

Albumin: Synthesized by the liver, maintains blood oncotic pressure and coagulation proteins needed to form a fibrin clot. Low levels are a signal to altered synthetic liver function. Decreased levels seen with ascites and severe liver disease. Persistently low levels suggest a poor prognosis.

Prothrombin Time (PT): A useful prognostic indicator in liver disease, PT measures the rate of conversion of prothrombin to thrombin in the presence of a tissue extract (thomboplastin) and calcium ions. The PT is prolonged when factors I, II, V, VII, and X are deficient alone or in any combination.

Other serum biochemical tests

Sodium: Fluid is retained in greater quantity than sodium, resulting in hyponatremia. Patients with cirrhosis, tense ascites, hepatorenal syndrome, and end-stage liver disease are often hyponatremic.

Text continued on p. 435

TABLE 8 - 6 Types and Characteristics of Viral Hepatitis

	Hepatitis A	Hepatitis B	Hepatitis C	Hepatitis D	Hepatitis E	Hepatitis G
Likely modes of transmission	Enteric; fecal-oral; usually through food or drinking contaminated water	Contact with blood, body fluids (seminal fluid, vaginal secretions, saliva, open sores; found also in tears, urine, breast milk)	Contact with blood, serum, or body fluids; perinatal transmission, blood transfusions, sexual contact	Similar to HBV; but an incomplete virus that can cause infection only in the presence of HBV	Enteric; fecal-oral; is foodborne or waterborne	Contact with blood, body fluids, or serum
Population most often affected	Varies, based on hygienic and sanitary conditions; children, employees in daycare centers, international travelers, household contacts, sexual and possibly injection drug users	Sexually active young adults, injection drug users, hemophiliacs, hemodialysis patients, prisoners or prison personnel, international travelers, those with multiple sexual partners	Injection drug-users, health care workers, U.S. transfusion recipients before 1991	Infects individuals only with HBV infection, so risk factors same as HB	After flooding in countries with poor sanitation; in 20% of pregnant women, infection is fatal; countries with the most outbreaks: Nepal, North Africa, Mexico, and countries of the former Soviet Union	As for HBV and HCV
Measures for reducing exposure	Hand washing, good personal hygiene, sanitation, Standard Precautions (see Appendix 8)	Standard Precautions (see Appendix 8), hand washing, good personal hygiene, condom use, sterilization of nondisposable items, avoiding used needles, carefully handling needles and sharps, use of safety engineered devices	As for HBV	As for HBV	As for HBV	As for HBV

Continued

TABLE 8-6 Types and Characteristics of Viral Hepatitis—cont'd

	Hepatitis A	Hepatitis B	Hepatitis C	Hepatitis D	Hepatitis E	Hepatitis G
Prophylaxis	Immunization with HBV vaccine is not prophylactic for HAV virus; patients with HBV or HCV virus should receive HAV vaccine, especially if traveling outside the United States	Immunization of all health care workers with blood and body fluid exposure, as well as high-risk groups; routine immunization of children; screening of all blood products; barrier precautions during sexual activity	Screening all donated blood/blood products; protective devices for health care workers; use of Standard Precautions; no vaccine available; "cure" in up to 80% of patients; based on genotype	Immunization against HBV	Gamma-globulin manufactured from sources in endemic countries has shown little protective effect against HEV; the best prophylaxis to date is use of sanitary measures	Screening of donated blood; protective devices for health care workers, Standard Precautions; no vaccine or cure available
Incubation	2-6 wk	1-6 months	18-180 days (45-55 days average)	Variable; not well established	Range is 15-65 days; average is 40 days	Believed to be 2-6 wk
Serum markers	Antibody to HAV (anti-HAV) of the IgM class in the acute state; when recovered, anti-HAV of the IgG class; if vaccinated, anti-HAV IgG is present in serum	In the acute stage, anti-HB_cIgM, HB_sAg, and HB_eAg; in the chronic stage, anti-HB_c Total HB_sAg, HB_eAg (during increased replication), HB_eAb (during low replication); when recovered, anti-HB_c total will be present along with anti-HB_sAg; if vaccinated, anti-HB_sAb is present	HCV antibody indicates exposure but does not differentiate between acute and chronic exposure; HCV-RNA quantitative measures virus circulating in the serum and is a measure of treatment effectiveness	RIA test for total antibody (anti-HD) to D-antigen; with this test, both IgG and IgM antibodies are measured; D-antigen (HDAg), IgM antibody to HDAg (IgM anti-HD), and HDV-RNA	Immune electron microscopy (IEM) identifies HEV antigen and antibody; IgG anti-HEV is detectable over years; IgM antibodies are usually detectable only up to 7 months; HEV-RNA can be used to diagnose non-A, non-B, non-C cases	HGV antibody

Treatment	Symptomatic					
		Supportive measures and monitoring for progression toward chronic disease or fulminant hepatitis (rare); for chronic cases, Lamivudine 100 mg PO daily, adefovir dipiroxil 10 mg PO daily, or interferon-alpha 5 million units injected subcutaneously daily for 4 to 6 months, or 10 million units injected every other day for 4-6 months	When state is acute, patient should be monitored for progression to chronic or fulminant state; most patients are diagnosed in the chronic state, years after contracting the virus; for chronic disease: pegylated interferon-alpha injected once weekly with ribavirin PO daily. If acute HCV, studies have shown that interferon monotherapy 3 million units every other day for 6 months eradicated the virus	Interferon products may be tried	Supportive	Chronic liver disease not associated with this virus; no treatment is recommended at this time

Continued

TABLE 8-6 Types and Characteristics of Viral Hepatitis—cont'd

	Hepatitis A	Hepatitis B	Hepatitis C	Hepatitis D	Hepatitis E	Hepatitis G
Comments	Can cause FHF if superimposed on chronic HCV	Chronic hepatitis may develop; FHF may ensue, especially if coinfected with HDV	Chronic hepatitis develops in 85% of those infected; HAV and HBV vaccination is important; HAV or HBV superimposed on HCV can cause FHF; 50% of all liver transplants in the United States are the result of liver failure related to HCV infection	Fulminant hepatitis occurs 10 times more often in HDV and HBV coinfection; HDV acquired after chronic HBV infection is termed *superinfection*; superinfection of HDV with chronic HBV infection can cause acute hepatitis	During epidemics, the case fatality rate for HEV is 1%-2%; coinfection with HAV and HEV is possible; not endemic to the United States, Canada, or western Europe	Many with HCV also have HGV; may not cause a disease state; more HGV is detectable in serum versus the liver; as many as 4% of U.S. blood donors are HGV-positive

FHF, Fulminant hepatic failure; *HAV,* hepatitis A virus; *HB_c,* hepatitis B core (antigen); *HB_cAb,* hepatitis B_c antibody: a marker for hepatitis B infection; *HB_eAg,* hepatitis B_e antigen; *HB_sAb,* hepatitis B surface antibody; *HB_sAg,* hepatitis B surface (antigen); *HBV,* hepatitis B virus; *HCV,* hepatitis C virus; *HD,* hepatitis D; *HDAg,* hepatitis D-antigen; *HDV,* hepatitis D virus; *HEV,* hepatitis E virus; *HGV,* hepatitis G virus; *IgG,* immunoglobulin G; *IgM,* immunoglobulin M; *RIA,* radioimmunoassay; *RNA,* ribonucleic acid.

Potassium: Hypokalemia is observed in those with liver disease accompanied by ascites and in those with chronic alcoholic liver disease. If the patient has hepatorenal syndrome, hyperkalemia is observed.

Glucose: Hypoglycemia is usually present in severe or terminal liver dysfunction, causing altered mentation and lethargy. This is the result of impaired gluconeogenesis and glycogen depletion in the cirrhotic liver.

BUN: In liver failure the BUN is decreased. If the patient is bleeding and has renal insufficiency, the BUN may be elevated.

Ammonia: Increased because of the failing liver's inability to clear nitrogenous and other waste products. GI bleeding or an increase in intestinal protein from dietary intake will also increase ammonia levels (see "Gastroesophageal Varices," p. 417).

Hematologic tests: As many as 70% of patients have platelet counts < 100,000/mm^3 because of platelet destruction and malfunctioning hepatic synthesis of platelets. An increase in mean corpuscular volume (MCV) may be present, causing the RBCs to be macrocytic. The anemia present in hepatic failure is then termed *macrocytic* and *normochromic* (normal Hgb). Elevated thrombin-antithrombin III complex is present, which can cause intravascular coagulation. On rare occasions, disseminated intravascular coagulation (DIC) results. If GI bleeding is present, a decreased Hgb and Hct are evident. Leukocytes are usually normal unless sepsis is present, causing an elevation. The PT measures factors I, II, V, VII, and X. PT prolongation indicates disease progression and a worsening prognosis. Vitamin K does not cause a response when administered unless the prolongation of the PT is the result of a vitamin K deficiency.

Liver biopsy: After ultrasound localization and a local anesthetic agent is administered, a Trucut or Menghini needle is inserted into the eighth or ninth intercostal space in the midaxillary line to obtain a specimen of liver tissue (percutaneous liver biopsy). If a percutaneous biopsy is not feasible because of prolonged PT or a platelet count < 50,000/mm^3, a transvenous biopsy may be performed via the jugular and hepatic veins. Before biopsy, laboratory tests should include a complete blood cell count (CBC), platelet count, a PT/partial thromboplastin time (PTT), and a type and cross-match. Patients are instructed to exhale and stop breathing while the needle is inserted during the biopsy. Patient movement during the procedure may cause puncture of an abdominal organ or a lung. (See Table 8-7 for nursing care of the patient undergoing liver biopsy.)

Electroencephalogram (EEG): Often abnormal in hepatic encephalopathy. The grade of hepatic encephalopathy does not correlate well with the findings on the EEG. None of the findings are specific since many metabolic disorders produce abnormal EEGs.

Cerebral computed tomography (CCT): In some cirrhotic patients, regardless of the cause of liver disease, CCT shows cortical and subcortical atrophy. While not useful in diagnosing hepatic encephalopathy, CCT is a good test to perform if the differential diagnosis includes subdural hematoma, or there is doubt about the etiology of altered consciousness.

Brain flow studies: If patient is in a hepatic coma, brain death cannot be confirmed by EEG. Therefore brain blood-flow study (technetium scan) is required if an assessment of brain function is needed.

Neuropsychological testing: A battery of six tests, called PHES (Psychometric Hepatic Encephalopathy Score), which can be completed in less than 10 minutes. Normal subjects score 0.5 ± 1.83 with those scoring beyond –4 considered abnormal. Tests include serial dotting, line drawing, and number connection.

Abdominal paracentesis: Patients with severe ascites are managed with diuretics and large-volume (>5L) paracentesis with or without infusion of albumin or another plasma volume expander. An increase in cardiac output is noted immediately after the procedure. Vital signs including temperature should be checked often, along with intake and output (I&O). Creatinine should be monitored closely as it trends upward 24-48 hr after the procedure. Peritonitis, hyponatremia, hyperkalemia, GI bleeding, bacteremia, encephalopathy, and renal insufficiency are complications. See "Fluid Volume Deficit," p. 439, and "Infection," p. 444, for nursing implications.

Urinalysis: Urine sodium excretion (< 10 mEq/day) with normal urinary sediment is a sign of hepatorenal syndrome, which may be observed in fulminant hepatic failure. Another disorder, acute tubular necrosis, is usually diagnosed if urine sodium excretion is > 20 mEq/day and urinary sediment shows cellular casts. Gross inspection may reveal dark urine that produces a yellow foam when shaken. Increased urobilinogen and bilirubin will be present. In the presence of ascites, the 24-hr urine volume will be decreased and the 24-hr sodium value will be reduced (< 5 mEq/day in severe cases).

Radioisotope liver scan: A radioactive labeled compound that is easily absorbed by the Kupffer cells of the liver is injected into the patient. The radiation that is emitted can be photographed with a scintillation camera or an x-ray, and the lesions appear as areas of "hot spots." This test is best used to determine the presence of three-dimensional lesions, hepatocellular carcinomas, melanomas,

---

T A B L E   8 - 7   **Nursing Care of the Patient Undergoing Percutaneous Liver Biopsy**

Before biopsy
- Explain the procedure to patient and significant others.
- Patient should sign informed consent for procedure before sedation is administered.
- Ensure that values are known for patient's prothrombin time and platelet count which are less than 1 month old.
- Ensure that patient has not had any salicylates or NSAIDs for 7 days before the biopsy.
- If patient is on an anticoagulant, it should have been stopped 72 hours before the biopsy.

During biopsy
- Assist patient with proper positioning and with remaining motionless during procedure.
- Coach patient in sustaining exhalation during procedure (or manually ventilate intubated patient to prevent lung inflation during puncture) to avoid pneumothorax.

After biopsy
- Apply pressure dressing.
- Position patient on the right side for a minimum of 2 hours after the biopsy to tamponade the puncture site.
- Auscultate breath sounds immediately after the procedure and at 1- to 2-hour intervals until patient discharge to detect pneumothorax or hemothorax (unlikely but serious complications). Diminished sounds on the right side and tachypnea suggest one of these conditions.
- Enforce bed rest for 2 hours after biopsy to minimize the risk of hemorrhage from the puncture site.
- Monitor patient for indicators of peritonitis or intraperitoneal bleeding: severe abdominal pain, abdominal distention and rigidity, rebound tenderness, nausea, vomiting, tachycardia, tachypnea, pallor, decreased BP, and rising temperature.
- If bleeding is suspected, contact physician and obtain an ultrasound study of the abdomen, to include the liver.
- Right shoulder pain may persist for 24-48 hours after biopsy of the liver.

Hodgkin's, and some non-Hodgkin's lymphomas, and to visualize the anatomy and function of the liver and biliary system.

Computed tomography (CT): Lesions as small as 1 cm can be identified with CT scanning without obesity and intestinal factors affecting the results. Oral and intravenous contrast agents can be administered to help distinguish the bowel lumen and blood vessels and tissues respectively. Portal hypertension, splenomegaly, and changes consistent with steatosis and hemochromotosis can also be identified.

Magnetic resonance imaging (MRI) and magnetic resonance arteriogram (MRA): MRIs produce sharp contrast between tissues and water and/or fat. Since there is lack of ionizing radiation, MRI can image in transverse, longitudinal, coronal, or oblique planes. MRI is as good as a contrast CT to detect mass lesions in the liver. MRA is commonly used in the potential living liver donor candidate work-up to visualize the hepatic ducts and the hepatic arteries and veins for the liver transplant surgeons.

Ultrasound (US): Can aid in determining the size of the liver and the presence of abnormal tissue. Ultrasound is also useful for biopsy to mark the correct spot for a liver biopsy or when "blind" methods have been attempted without success.

Electrocardiogram (ECG): Factors such as hypokalemia, acidosis, or hypoxia may cause cardiac dysrhythmias. The heart should be monitored continuously, as should oximetry.

COLLABORATIVE MANAGEMENT

Correction of precipitating factors: Hepatic failure may develop suddenly in a patient with compensated liver disease. Sustained hypoxia or hypotension from any cause can aggravate hepatocellular failure and must be corrected promptly. Ethanol, hepatotoxic drugs, and hepatotoxic alternative therapies are eliminated. Sedatives and tranquilizers may contribute to hepatic encephalopathy and should be discontinued.

Fluid and electrolyte management: Free water clearance is affected in FHF, causing hyponatremia even though increased total body sodium is present. If hyponatremia is profound, sodium-containing fluids are avoided because they contribute to ascites and peripheral edema and may potentiate renal insufficiency. D_5W generally is used for fluid resuscitation to prevent hypernatremia. Mannitol or albumin is given to increase intravascular oncotic pressure and maintain intravascular volume.

Potassium is decreased with the use of mannitol. Hypokalemic alkalosis can worsen encephalopathy and precipitate dysrhythmias. Fresh frozen plasma may be used if clotting factors are deficient, but infusions of large amounts can lead to hypernatremia. Packed RBCs are given if there is brisk bleeding or a low Hct. CVP or PAP monitoring along with ICP monitoring may be initiated to ensure adequate tissue perfusion without fluid overload. A hyperdynamic circulatory state is supported by fluid administration and sympathomimetic agents (e.g., dopamine) as necessary.

Note: Accurate measurements and careful interpretation of hemodynamic parameters are essential because fluid balance is delicate in critically ill patients with hepatic failure; also, hemodynamic measurements can be difficult to interpret because of the hyperdynamic circulatory state. SVO_2 monitoring is helpful in evaluating the adequacy of tissue oxygenation.

Bed rest: Necessary to reduce metabolic demands placed on the liver during normal daily activity.
Nutritional therapy: The catabolic rate in acute liver failure increases 4 times over normal and is associated with negative nitrogen balance. Therefore, to ensure tissue repair, a high-calorie, 80- to 100-g protein-containing diet of dairy products and vegetables is indicated for patients without evidence of encephalopathy, inasmuch as the liver is capable of significant regeneration under optimal circumstances. Sodium is moderately restricted unless significant ascites and peripheral edema are present. Then a 500-mg or less sodium-restricted diet is prescribed. If GI function is impaired and the patient is unable to tolerate enteral feedings, parenteral nutrition is initiated. Total caloric intake should be 2500-3000/day.

For the patient with acute hepatic encephalopathy, protein is eliminated from the diet until recovery. During recovery, vegetable protein (preferred over animal protein) is gradually reintroduced at 10-20 g every 48-72 hr. It is gradually increased to 40 g/day. This dose at this rate prevents tissue catabolism. Some advocate use of enteral or parenteral branched-chain amino acid supplements in an attempt to correct the amino acid imbalance that is common among patients with an encephalopathic condition, but their effectiveness is controversial. Potassium loss must be replaced by potassium-rich foods or supplements. Blood sugar levels should be kept above 80 mg/dl and monitored every 2-4 hr. Parenteral lipid replacement should be used with caution as fatty liver (steatosis) has been reported to have developed after their use.
Pharmacotherapy: Some commonly used drugs are hepatotoxic (Table 8-8).
Sedatives: Avoided if at all possible because they can precipitate or contribute to encephalopathy. If sedative use is necessary, oxazepam (Serax) is an acceptable choice because it can be eliminated

---

TABLE 8-8   Drugs With Hepatotoxic Potential

Acetaminophen	Methyldopa
Ampicillin	Monoamine oxidase (MAO) inhibitors
Antidepressants	Nonsteroidal antiinflammatory drugs (NSAIDs)
Carbamazepine	Oral contraceptives
Carbenicillin	Penicillin
Carbon tetrachloride	Phenytoin
Chloramphenicol	Propylthiouracil
Chlorpromazine	Pyrazinamide
Clindamycin	Rifampin
Cocaine	Salicylates
Dantrolene	Sulfonamides
Ethanol	Tetracyclines (especially parenteral)
FUDR (intraarterial)	Valproic acid
Halothane	Yellow phosphorus
Hydrochlorothiazide	Numerous complementary and alternative (CAM) medications
Isonazide	
Ketoconazole	
Methotrexate	

FUDR, 5-Flourouracil deoxyribonucleoside.

safely by patients with hepatic disease. Other sedatives may be used cautiously and in reduced dosages.

Histamine H₂-receptor antagonists: Prophylactic H_2-receptor antagonists are prescribed to block acid secretion and prevent gastric erosions, which are common in patients with chronic or severe hepatic failure. Famotidine, ranitidine hydrochloride, and nizatidine are competitive blockers of histamine, and thereby inhibit all phases of gastric acid secretion.

Sucralfate (Carafate): Binds to gastric erosions, aiding in healing established ulcers, and coats the gastric/duodenal mucosa, thereby preventing stress ulcers.

Dextrose: Moderate to severe hypoglycemia can occur because of impaired gluconeogenesis and impaired insulin degradation. Checks of blood sugar levels q6-8h are necessary to detect hypoglycemia. In the event of hypoglycemia, a bolus of 50% dextrose or continual infusion of a 10% solution is indicated.

N-acetylcysteine (NAC): Administering NAC protects the liver against free-radical injury and is useful in acetaminophen overdose and carbon tetrachloride or trichloroethylene exposure. NAC helps replace glutathione stores in the liver, protecting hepatocytes. It can be administered orally at 140 mg/kg or parenterally 140 mg/kg in 5% dextrose with subsequent doses at 70 mg/kg. Careful observation is necessary during IV administration, as an anaphylaxis-like reaction has been observed.

Penicillin/silibinin: Used commonly as an antidote in Europe for *Amanita phalloides* poisoning, penicillin 300,000-1,000,000 units/kg/day and silibinin 20-50 mg/kg/day given intravenously is alleged to be hepatocyte-protective. This combination protects as-yet-unaffected hepatocytes, thereby preventing further hepatocyte necrosis.

Zinc: In malnourished individuals it is useful not only as mineral replacement therapy, but also to reduce the chance for, or severity of, encephalopathy as it increases hepatic urea synthesis. In other countries, the use of ornithine-aspartate is advocated to improve hepatic and muscular ammonia elimination.

Protection of health care workers: Health care workers whose jobs involve potential exposure to blood or other body fluids should be vaccinated with the hepatitis B vaccine. Health care workers must protect themselves from potential infection by consistent use of appropriate infection control measures (see Appendix 8).

Management of bleeding complications: Fresh-frozen plasma and platelets are administered to correct defects in clotting factors and thrombocytopenia. Vitamin K may be prescribed to help correct bleeding tendencies. Serious coagulopathies that require specialized component therapy may develop (see "Disseminated Intravascular Coagulation," p. 489).

Management of respiratory failure: Intubation or mechanical ventilation may be indicated in the following instances: impaired gag reflex caused by advanced encephalopathy, aspiration of gastric contents, or impairment of ventilation secondary to ascites. Continuous pulse oximetry is used for patients with respiratory failure or those at high risk for same. The need for adequate tissue oxygenation is crucial inasmuch as hepatic hypoxia significantly contributes to hepatic failure.

Management of ascites
Restriction of fluid intake
Restriction of physical activity
Sodium: If ascites causes discomfort, pain, or dyspnea, sodium is limited to <500 mg/day.

Diuretics: If more conservative measures are ineffective in controlling ascites, spironolactone (Aldactone), an aldosterone antagonist with weak diuretic action and potassium conservation, may be used. Another potassium-sparing diuretic, amiloride, may be used as well. If these are ineffective, more potent diuretics such as furosemide (Lasix) or thiazides are added with concurrent use of potassium supplement. For severe ascites, mannitol may be added to the regimen.

Paracentesis: Therapeutic paracentesis is the treatment of choice in patients with refractory ascites. Repeated daily removal of 4-6 L/day of ascitic fluid may be attempted as a temporary measure to relieve refractory ascites. Once discharged from the ICU, if patients cannot make frequent trips to the hospital, TIPS or peritoneal-venous shunt (PVS) is indicated unless the Childs score is 12 or more, in which case PVS is a better option.

Peritoneal-venous shunt: First introduced in 1974, peritoneal-venous shunt (PVS) (e.g., Le Veen, Denver) may be placed surgically in patients with refractory or life-threatening ascites. PVS helps to expand the circulating volume, improve the response to diuretics, and improve circulatory and renal function, thereby helping to prevent hepatorenal syndrome (HRS). The peritoneal cavity is drained by a long, perforated catheter, which is connected to a pressure-sensitive valve. The valve attaches to a subcutaneous catheter that drains into the intrathoracic superior vena cava. The device is designed so that fluid can flow in only one direction, from the peritoneum into the bloodstream. The most common complication is frequent obstruction, which requires reoperation; others include fluid overload, infection, DIC, peritonitis, and shunt occlusion. A rapid increase in intravascular volume may precipitate variceal hemorrhage in susceptible persons. Patients on the waiting list for liver transplantation should not undergo this procedure. See Table 8-9 and "Fluid Volume Excess," p. 440, for nursing implications.

Management of encephalopathy

Elimination or correction of precipitating factors: As many as 80% of patients with cirrhosis and liver failure have some degree of cerebral dysfunction or encephalopathy as a result of metabolic causes or hepatic decompensation. The causes and precipitating factors are now known to be many: changes in the permeability of the blood-brain barrier, an increase in endogenous benzodiazepines, impairment of neuronal membrane sodium-potassium adenosinetriphosphatase (ATPase), abnormal neurotransmitter balance, GI bleed, increased dietary protein, and electrolyte disturbance.

Restriction of physical activity: Permits less stress on all the organs of the body, including those that may be affected by chronic liver disease. Less activity reduces the number of metabolites that must be processed by the liver.

Restriction or elimination of dietary protein: Can be reintroduced if symptoms improve—preferably dairy and vegetable proteins.

Early and thorough catharsis by magnesium citrate or tap water enema: Very helpful to eliminate blood in intestines from GI bleeding. Also useful in eliminating protein if it is lingering in the bowel from ileus, constipation, or other causes.

Administration of antibiotics: Bacterial translocation is problematic in the chronic hepatic failure patient as a result of preexisting cirrhosis. Patients who develop infections have a higher mortality rate. It is recommended that a 5-7 day course of broad-spectrum antibiotics (i.e., from the fluoroquinolone class) be given prophylactically.

Administration of lactulose: A partially absorbed, synthetic disaccharide that contains both galactose and lactose. It decreases the pH of the colon by its conversion into lactic, acetic, and formic acids. The unmetabolized lactulose left in the colon produces osmotic diarrhea and causes ammonia

---

Caution: Lactulose may worsen hypernatremia and promote cerebral edema. It should be used with caution.

---

to migrate from the blood to the colon. Ideally, the dose is adjusted to produce two to three semiformed stools/day.

ICP monitoring: Brain damage may occur when ICP is about 25 mm Hg. This can occur quickly and without obvious accompanying signs/symptoms. It is advisable to use CP monitoring on the most critically ill patients awaiting orthotopic liver transplant to detect cerebral edema and guide pharmacologic management (e.g., mannitol, furosemide) and other therapeutic measures. See discussion in "Traumatic Brain Injury," p. 98.

Hepatic transplantation: The orthotopic liver transplant survival rate is more than 90% for the first year after transplant. In cases of chronic progressive or acute hepatocyte damage, it is the only treatment available. Because organs are in such limited supply, adult living donor liver transplantation is being used in those recipients whose diagnosis necessitates a liver, but whose model for end-stage liver disease (MELD) scores are not high enough to place them at the top of the list. New methods are being sought to extend the life of the native liver until a donor liver becomes available. Auxiliary liver transplantation allows the native liver to remain in the recipient, which will allow it to regenerate. This procedure is only used in potentially reversible conditions. Hepatocyte transplantation, bioartificial liver support, extracorporeal whole-organ perfusion, and other methods such as xenotransplantation are being explored as tools to increase waiting time to transplantation.

NURSING DIAGNOSES AND INTERVENTIONS

Fluid volume deficit related to decreased intake secondary to medically prescribed restrictions; decreased circulating volume secondary to hypoalbuminemia, altered hemodynamics, fluid sequestration, diuretic therapy, diarrhea from lactulose, bleeding varices

Desired outcomes: Within 24 hr of this diagnosis, patient becomes normovolemic as evidenced by MAP >70 mm Hg; HR 60-100 beats/min; brisk capillary refill (<2 sec); distal pulses >2+ on a 0-4+ scale; CVP 2-6 mm Hg; PAP 20-30/8-15 mm Hg; PAWP 6-12 mm Hg; CI >3 L/min/m^2; SVR 900-1200 dynes/sec/cm^{-5}; urinary output >0.5 ml/kg/hr; and orientation to person, place, and time.

- Monitor and document BP hourly, or q15min in the presence of unstable VS. Be alert to MAP decreases >10 mm Hg from previous measurement.
- Monitor and document HR, ECG, and cardiovascular status hourly, or more frequently in the presence of unstable VS. Be alert to increases in HR suggestive of hypovolemia or circulatory decompensation. Be aware that HR increases may also be caused by fever related to infection or cerebral

edema, and monitor for dysrhythmias from electrolyte imbalances secondary to diarrhea, gastric suctioning, or diuretic therapy.

- Measure central pressures and thermodilution CO q1-4h. Be alert to low or decreasing CVP, PAWP, and CO. Calculate SVR q4-8h, or more frequently in unstable patients. An elevated HR, decreased PAWP, CO less than baseline, or CI <3, along with decreased urinary output, suggest hypovolemia. Because of altered vascular responsiveness, the SVR may not be increased in patients with hypovolemic hepatic failure. Be aware that a "normal" CO value may actually be too low for these patients. A hyperdynamic circulatory state should be supported. Monitor Svo_2 as possible to evaluate the adequacy of tissue oxygenation.
- Measure and record urinary output hourly. Be alert to output <0.5 ml/kg/hr for 2 consecutive hours. Estimate volume status and adequacy of cardiovascular function by evaluating BP, HR, CVP, PAP, PAWP, urinary output, distal pulse amplitude, capillary refill, and level of consciousness. Consider cautious increases in fluid intake (e.g., 50-100 ml/hr), and then reevaluate volume status as already described. Use extreme caution in administering potent diuretics, inasmuch as they may precipitate encephalopathy or renal disease by causing rapid diuresis and electrolyte changes.
- Estimate ongoing fluid losses. Weigh patient daily. Measure all drainage from peritoneal or other catheters q2-4h. Compare 24-hr intake with output, and record the difference. Weight loss should not exceed 0.5 kg/day because more rapid diuresis can lead to intravascular volume depletion and impair renal function.
- Monitor serum albumin and total protein, and consult physician if levels are reduced. Administer albumin replacements as prescribed.
- If fluid volume deficit is related to variceal hemorrhage, see this nursing diagnosis in "Gastroesophageal Varices," p. 423.

NIC Cerebral Edema Management; Electrolyte Management; Fluid Management; Electrolyte Management: Hypokalemia

Fluid volume excess: interstitial or intracellular, related to compromised regulatory mechanisms secondary to acute or chronic hepatic failure

Desired outcomes: Within 48 hr of this diagnosis, patient becomes normovolemic as evidenced by CVP 2-6 mm Hg; PAWP 6-12 mm Hg; HR 60-100 beats/min; RR 12-20 breaths/min with normal depth and pattern (eupnea); decreasing or stable abdominal girth; and absence of crackles, edema, uncomfortable ascites, and other clinical indicators of fluid volume excess.

- Monitor VS, hemodynamic parameters, and cardiovascular status q1-2h, more frequently if patient is undergoing ultrafiltration therapy, and immediately after peritoneal-venous shunt surgery. Be alert to CVP values >6 mm Hg or PAWP >12 mm Hg. Consult physician for elevated values.
- Monitor for peripheral edema. Note severity and location. Jugular vein distention at a 45-degree head-of-bed (HOB) elevation may indicate fluid overload or decreased cardiac output.
- Monitor patient for evidence of fluid overload. Note presence of dyspnea, tachypnea, rhonchi, orthopnea, basilar crackles that do not clear with coughing, labored and/or shallow breathing, elevated BP, or S_3 heart sound. Consult physician if these signs develop.
- Use minimal amounts of fluids necessary to administer IV medications and maintain IV catheter patency.
- If fluids are restricted, offer mouth care and/or ice chips (included as part of oral fluid measurement).
- Measure and record abdominal girth daily. Be aware that abdominal girth measurements are subject to error and great care is necessary to ensure accuracy. Measure at the widest point, and mark this level for subsequent measurements with a permanent marker. If tolerated by the patient, measure him or her in the supine position. If the supine position is not possible, measure patient in the same position each time. Weigh daily at the same time, in the same clothing, using the same scale and method.
- Monitor serum electrolyte levels, especially sodium and potassium, and consult physician for significant deviations from normal. Normal values are serum sodium 137-147 mEq/L and serum potassium 3.5-5.0 mEq/L.
- Ensure proper functioning of peritoneal-venous shunt and TIPS in patients after surgery (Table 8-9).

NIC Electrolyte Management: Hypernatremia; Fluid Management; Invasive Hemodynamic Monitoring

Altered nutrition: less than body requirements, related to inability to digest food secondary to anorexia, nausea, and medically prescribed dietary restriction; decreased absorption of nutrients secondary to decreased intestinal motility, altered portal blood flow, decreased intestinal absorption of vitamins and minerals, altered protein metabolism; the diseased liver's inability to utilize nutrients

Desired outcomes: Within 3-4 days of this diagnosis, patient has adequate nutrition as evidenced by a state of nitrogen balance as shown by daily fecal excretion of 2-3 g of nitrogen and 13-20 g of urinary nitrogen, thyroxine-binding prealbumin 200-300 mcg/ml, and retinol-binding protein 40-50 mcg/ml. Blood glucose levels remain within an acceptable range of 100-160 mg/dl.

T A B L E 8 - 9 Nursing Care After Peritoneal Venous Shunt Surgery

- Measure urinary output hourly and CVP or PAP q1-2h.
  - ❑ Anticipate rapid fluid mobilization, as evidenced by increased CVP and increased urinary output.
  - ❑ Notify physician of abnormal CVP or PAP or lack of diuresis. Failure to mobilize ascitic fluid may signal shunt occlusion or failure.
  - ❑ Report lessening of urinary output, since renal function may diminish after this procedure.
- Administer IV diuretics as prescribed; monitor K^+ levels; and administer K^+ supplements as prescribed.
  - ❑ Anticipate prescribed K^+ supplements during the first 24 hr after surgery.
  - ❑ Be aware that furosemide (Lasix), which is frequently prescribed, may cause K^+ depletion. Likewise, the anticipated diuresis depletes K^+.
- Instruct and coach patient in the use of the incentive spirometer or similar hyperinflation device.
  - ❑ Devices that create inspiratory resistance and encourage deep inspiration promote negative inspiratory pressure and facilitate flow of ascitic fluid.
  - ❑ Encourage patient to cough hourly.
- Apply elastic abdominal binder.
  - ❑ This intervention facilitates the flow of ascitic fluid by increasing the pressure gradient externally.
- Monitor for evidence of variceal bleeding; report evidence of bleeding to physician.
  - ❑ Expanded blood volume may increase variceal pressure, resulting in bleeding. Bleeding is evidenced by a sudden decrease in Hct (a mild dilutional decrease is anticipated in the immediate postoperative period), unexplained nausea, lightheadedness, dark stools, or hematemesis. (See "Gastroesophageal Varices," p. 417)
- Monitor for evidence of peritonitis, endocarditis, or other infection.
  - ❑ Infection occurs frequently. Anticipate antibiotic coverage during the immediate postsurgical period. Assess abdominal incision for leakage of peritoneal fluid, which commonly occurs. Change the dressing immediately if leakage is detected.
- Monitor for evidence of postshunt coagulopathy.
  - ❑ See "Altered Protection," p. 444, for details.
  - ❑ Monitor for other postshunt complications.
  - ❑ Assess for lower extremity edema. After some shunting procedures, none of the venous blood passes through the liver and protein end products are not completely detoxified. These patients are usually placed on a low-protein diet.

CVP, Central venous pressure; *Hct,* hematocrit; *IV,* intravenous; *K^+,* potassium; *PAP,* pulmonary artery pressure.

- Confer with physician, dietitian, and pharmacist (if parenteral feedings are necessary) to estimate patient's current nutritional and metabolic needs, based on anthropometric data, creatinine excretion, albumin, and transferrin, as well as presence of encephalopathy, chronic hepatic disease, infection, and nutritional status before hospitalization. For general information, see "Nutritional Support," p. 1.
- In the absence of adequate bowel functioning or with poor oral intake, consult physician regarding administration of parenteral (preferred) or enteral nutrients. If insertion of a feeding tube becomes necessary, use caution to minimize the risk of rupturing gastroesophageal varices. If parenteral feedings are being administered, monitor IV site for infection and other complications.
- Note, monitor, and record food/fluid ingested and daily caloric intake. Note all sources of food (including meals not prepared in the hospital), paying particular attention to foods that contain sodium and significant amounts of protein.
- Administer vitamin supplements as prescribed, particularly the fat-soluble ones.
- Encourage food to be brought from home if desired by patient, and make sure it meets prescribed dietary restrictions.
- Encourage bed rest to reduce metabolic demands on the liver and to promote hepatic regeneration. Increase patient's activity levels gradually as condition improves.
- Monitor blood glucose levels q8h or as prescribed. Monitor patient for clinical indicators of hypoglycemia: altered mentation, irritability, diaphoresis, anxiety, weakness, and tachycardia. Consult physician for blood glucose levels <65 mg/dl. Administer D_{10} or D_{50} as prescribed for hypoglycemia. Clinical signs of hypoglycemia can be confused with hepatic encephalopathy. Be sure to

validate clinical signs with blood glucose levels. Be aware that mild elevations in blood sugar are anticipated in some patients with chronic liver disease. Administer hypoglycemic agents as prescribed for blood glucose levels >160 mg/dl.

NIC Nutrition Management; Hypoglycemia Management; Energy Management

Impaired gas exchange related to altered oxygen supply secondary to arteriovenous shunting, ventilation-perfusion mismatch, and diaphragmatic limitation associated with ascites, hydrothorax, or central respiratory depression occurring with encephalopathy

Desired outcomes: Within 4 hr of this diagnosis, patient has adequate gas exchange as evidenced by Pao_2 >80 mm Hg; $Paco_2$ <45 mm Hg; RR 12-20 breaths/min with normal depth and pattern (eupnea); oxygen saturation >92% with or without oxygen supplementation or mechanical ventilation; and orientation to person, place, and time.

> **Note:**   Level of consciousness is difficult to evaluate in the presence of moderate to severe hepatic encephalopathy, and obtaining a baseline level of consciousness is imperative.

* Monitor and document respiratory rate q1-4h. Note pattern, excursion, depth, and effort.
* Administer supplemental oxygen as prescribed to enhance cerebral and hepatic oxygenation.
* Maintain body positions that optimize ventilation. Elevate HOB 30 degrees or higher, depending on patient comfort and hemodynamic status. If patient has increased ICP, the HOB should not be elevated above 20 degrees. If patient has a unilateral lung problem, position him or her with the unaffected lung dependent. Correlate body position with blood gas and oximetry results.
* Standing will increase intrapulmonary shunting through the lower part of the lungs, thereby enhancing detection of arterial deoxygenation. If possible, obtain an arterial blood gas with the patient standing.
* Monitor Pao_2, $Paco_2$, and oxygen saturation; consult physician for abnormalities. Continuous pulse oximetry should be in use. Monitor ABGs and electrolytes as available.
* Assess patient q4-8h for indicators of atelectasis (e.g., diminished breath sounds, basilar crackles, difficulty breathing), hydrothorax (e.g., diminished breath sounds, dullness to percussion), and pulmonary infection (e.g., yellow, green, or thick sputum, rhonchi, fever). Consult physician if physical assessment findings suggest respiratory complications.
* Evaluate obtunded patient for presence of gag reflex. Consult physician regarding need for ET intubation if the gag reflex is depressed. Suction mouth frequently; offer/assist with frequent mouth care.

NIC Oxygen Therapy; Aspiration Precautions

Altered thought processes related to endogenous chemical alteration (accumulation of ammonia or other central nervous system [CNS] toxins occurring with hepatic dysfunction), therapeutically restricted environment, sleep deprivation, hypoxia, sensory overload (noise, personnel) in ICU, and medication (side effects, toxic levels from liver's inability to detoxify appropriately)

Desired outcomes: By the time of hospital discharge, patient exhibits stable personality pattern, age-appropriate behavior, intact intellect appropriate for level of education, distinct speech, and coordinated gross and fine motor movements. Handwriting is legible, and psychometric test scores are improved from baseline range.

* Avoid or minimize precipitating factors for hepatic encephalopathy (Table 8-10).
  * ❑ Help patient keep circadian rhythms in sync (e.g., keep lighting in room appropriate for the time of day, correlate activities of daily living [ADLs] to the correct time of day).
  * ❑ Check gastric secretions, vomitus, and stools for occult blood. Consult physician promptly if test results are positive for blood or if GI bleeding is obvious.
  * ❑ Evaluate Hct and Hgb for evidence of bleeding. Consult physician for very low values or values that deviate from baseline. Anticipate mild-to-moderate anemia.
  * ❑ Consult physician promptly for indicators of infection (see "Risk for Infection," p. 444).
  * ❑ Evaluate serum ammonia levels (normal levels are 40-110 mg/dl). Report significant elevations from baseline. Ammonia values and their measurement vary greatly and do not always correlate directly with encephalopathy. To help ensure accurate results, place specimens for ammonia analysis on ice and transport immediately to laboratory.
  * ❑ Be alert to potential sources of electrolyte imbalance (e.g., diarrhea, vomiting, occult bleeding).
  * ❑ Avoid use of sedative or tranquilizing agents. If sedatives are necessary, oxazepam (Serax) and antihistamines (e.g., Benadryl) are the safest.

T A B L E 8 - 10   Factors That Contribute to Hepatic Encephalopathy

Chronic factors

Portal-systemic shunting (entry of portal blood into systemic veins without being metabolized
   by the liver): may occur via damaged liver, collateral vessels, or surgically created portacaval
   anastomosis

Dietary protein intake

Intestinal bacteria

Acid-base imbalance

Progressive hepatic insufficiency

Precipitating factors

Dehydration/electrolyte imbalance: may occur with overdiuresis, diarrhea, vomiting, or other factors

Excessive paracentesis

Surgery in a cirrhotic patient

Excessive alcohol ingestion

Sedatives/hypnotics

Infection

Constipation

Extrahepatic bile duct obstruction

Acute hepatocellular damage

Viral hepatitis

Alcoholic hepatitis

Drug/chemical reactions (see Table 8-8)

Drug overdose

- ❏ If patient is pulling out tubes, apply mitts rather than restraints.
- ❏ Avoid use of conventional and alternative drugs that are hepatotoxic (see Table 8-8).
- ❏ Correct hypoxemia; administer supplemental oxygen as necessary (see "Impaired Gas Exchange," p. 442).
- Evaluate patient for CNS effects such as personality changes, childish behavior, intellectual impairment, slurred speech, ataxia, and asterixis.
- Administer daily handwriting or psychometric tests (if appropriate for patient's level of consciousness) to evaluate mild or subclinical encephalopathy. Report significant deterioration in handwriting or in test scores.
- Consult physician for abnormal EEG reports.
- Eliminate dietary protein for patients with severe encephalopathy. As prescribed, reintroduce protein gradually as tolerated after patient's clinical symptoms improve (i.e., patient becomes more alert; neuromuscular coordination improves).
- Administer enemas as prescribed to clear the colon of intestinal contents that contribute to encephalopathy. Repeat enemas as necessary to ensure thorough cleansing of the colon.
- Administer neomycin as prescribed to reduce intestinal bacteria, which contribute to the production of cerebral intoxicants. Monitor patient for evidence of ototoxic effects (i.e., decreased hearing) and nephrotoxic effects (e.g., urinary output < 0.5 ml/kg/hr, increased creatinine levels) of neomycin use. Avoid neomycin administration for patients with renal insufficiency.
- Administer lactulose as prescribed to reduce ammonia formation in the intestine. Consult physician to adjust dose to produce two to three semiformed stools daily. Avoid lactulose-related diarrhea because it may cause dangerous dehydration and electrolyte imbalance.
- Protect the confused or unconscious patient from injury.
  - ❏ Enlist the aid of family or friends to watch patient during confused or restless periods.
  - ❏ Have call light within patient's reach at all times.
  - ❏ Tape all catheters and tubes securely to prevent dislodgment.
- Consider possibility of seizures in the patient with severe encephalopathy; have airway management equipment readily available.
- Minimize unnecessary noise, lights, and other environmental stimuli. For more information, see "Psychosocial Support" for "Sensory/Perceptual Alterations," p. 70, and "Sleep Pattern Disturbance," p. 471.

- Monitor ICP and cerebral perfusion pressure (CPP). For patients with increased intracranial pressure (IICP), position carefully (HOB <20 degrees) and avoid fluid overload, hypercarbia, and hypoxemia. Administer mannitol and furosemide (Lasix) as prescribed. Sedation or coma induction may be indicated if cerebral edema does not respond to the measures just mentioned.

NIC Environmental Management; Delirium Management; Intracranial Pressure Monitoring

Risk for infection related to inadequate secondary defenses (impaired reticuloendothelial system phagocytic activity and portal-systemic shunting); multiple invasive procedures; chronic malnutrition in the individual with cirrhosis

Desired outcome: Patient is free of infection as evidenced by normothermia; HR <100 beats/min; RR <20 breaths/min; negative culture results; WBC count <11,000/mm^3; clear urine; and clear, thin sputum.

- Monitor VS for evidence of infection (e.g., increases in heart and respiratory rates). Check rectal or core temperature q4h for increases. Avoid measuring temperatures rectally in the patient with rectal varices.
- If temperature elevation is sudden, obtain specimens for blood, sputum, and urine cultures or from other sites as prescribed. Consult physician for positive culture results.
- Monitor CBC, and consult physician for significant increases in WBCs. Be aware that a normal or mildly elevated leukocyte count may signify infection in patients with hepatic failure inasmuch as patients with chronic liver disease often have leukopenia, with WBC counts <3000/mm^3.
- Evaluate secretions and drainage for evidence of infection (e.g., sputum changes, cloudy urine).
- Evaluate IV, central line, and paracentesis site(s) for evidence of infection (erythema, warmth, unusual drainage). It is normal for a paracentesis puncture site to have a small amount of drainage immediately after the procedure. Prolonged or foul-smelling drainage can signal infection.
- Prevent transmission of infectious agents by washing hands well before and after caring for patient and by wearing gloves when contact with blood or other body substances is possible. Dispose of all needles and other sharp instruments in puncture-resistant, rigid containers. Keep containers in each patient room and in other convenient locations. Avoid recapping and manipulating needles before disposal. Teach significant others and visitors proper hand-washing technique. Restrict visitors with evidence of communicable disease.
- Administer antibiotics as prescribed. Use caution and reduced dosage when administering antibiotics (especially aminoglycosides) to patients with low urinary output or renal insufficiency.

NIC Infection Protection; Surveillance

Altered protection related to clotting anomaly; thrombocytopenia; itching; disorientation

Desired outcomes: Patient's bleeding, if it occurs, is not prolonged. Patient's skin is not damaged from scratching. Patient's confusion (if present) and level of consciousness will not lead to injury (see "Altered Thought Processes," p. 442).

- Avoid giving intramuscular (IM) injections. If they are necessary, use small-gauge needles and maintain firm pressure over injection sites for several minutes. Avoid massaging IM injection sites.
- Maintain pressure for several minutes over venipuncture sites. Inform laboratory personnel of patient's bleeding tendencies.
- Avoid arterial punctures. If it is necessary to obtain ABG values, consult physician regarding use of an indwelling arterial line. If this is not possible, be certain to maintain pressure over the arterial puncture site and elevation for at least 10 min.
- Monitor PT levels and platelet counts daily. Consult physician for significant prolongation of the PT or for significant reduction in the platelet count.
- Assess patient for signs of bleeding. Note oral and nasal mucosal bleeding and ecchymotic areas, and test stools, emesis, urine, and gastric drainage for occult blood. Be alert to prolonged bleeding or oozing of blood from venipuncture sites and incisions. Consult physician for positive findings.
- Use electric rather than safety razor for patient shaving. Provide soft-bristle toothbrush or sponge-tipped applicator and mouthwash for oral hygiene.
- Avoid indwelling gastric drainage tubes if possible, because they may irritate gastric mucosa or varices, causing bleeding to occur.
- Administer fresh-frozen plasma and platelets as prescribed. Monitor carefully for fluid volume overload (see "Fluid Volume Excess," p. 440).
- Administer vitamin K as prescribed.
- A postshunt coagulopathy may develop in some patients after peritoneal-venous shunt surgery. Monitor these patients closely (see fifth intervention of this diagnosis).
- If fibrin split products (FSP) are present in the blood and thrombocytopenia is significant, the patient may have DIC (see "Disseminated Intravascular Coagulation," p. 489).
- When moving patient, avoid applying shearing forces to skin.

- Keep sheets free of wrinkles. Keep clothing from bunching against patient's skin.
- Dry skin well after morning care. Provide adequate lotion to skin, avoid massaging it in deeply, and rub gently.
- Use paper tape if it is necessary to place tape directly on skin. If possible, use gauze to secure a dressing or IV line, and tape over the gauze to prevent it from unwrapping.

Altered tissue perfusion: renal, related to risk of diminished arterial flow secondary to increased preglomerular vascular resistance (see Table 8-10 for other contributing factors).

Desired outcome: By the time of transfer from ICU, patient has adequate renal perfusion as evidenced by urinary output > 0.5 ml/kg/hr.

- Monitor CVP, PAWP, and SVR q1-4h to ensure optimal filling pressures (see "Fluid Volume Deficit," p. 439). Monitor filling pressures hourly immediately after paracentesis or if patient is dehydrated or hemorrhaging.
- Monitor serum and urine sodium levels. Serum sodium < 120 mEq/L and urine sodium < 10 mEq/L are associated with the development of hepatorenal syndrome. Consult physician for significant alterations in serum and urine sodium levels. Normal values are 135-147 mEq/L for serum and > 10 mEq/L for urine.
- Monitor creatinine and potassium values, and consult physician for significant increases. Be aware that BUN level is not an accurate indicator of renal function, especially in the patient with hepatic failure, because alterations in hepatic function can cause decreased BUN values and GI bleeding results in increased BUN values. Normal serum creatinine is 0.7-1.5 mg/dl, and normal serum potassium is 3.5-5 mEq/L.
- Minimize infusion of sodium-containing fluids because they contribute to ascites and peripheral edema and may potentiate functional renal failure.
- Monitor for hypophosphatemia (normal values 2.5-4.8 mg/dl) as evidenced by mental confusion, metabolic acidosis, anorexia, cardiac dysrhythmias, hemolytic anemia, lethargy, and bone pain. Administer replacement therapy as ordered.
- Monitor for hypomagnesemia (1.8-3 mg/dl) as evidenced by muscle weakness, nausea, vomiting, tremors, tetany, and lethargy. Administer replacement therapy as ordered.
- For patients receiving lactulose, adjust dosage so that patient has two to three soft stools/day.
- For additional information, see nursing diagnoses and interventions in "Acute Renal Failure," p. 315.

Impaired tissue integrity related to chemical irritants (bile salts), impaired mobility, and fluid excess (tissue edema)

Desired outcomes: Patient's tissue remains intact; pruritus is relieved or reduced within 12 hr of this diagnosis.

- Bathe patient with a nonsoap cleanser such as Cetaphil. Follow baths with unscented lotion, which should be applied while the skin is still moist.
- Use a low-pressure mattress to minimize pressure on fragile tissues.
- Turn, reposition (at least q2h), and provide appropriate support to body and over bony prominences to prevent pressure sores.
- If patient is confused or obtunded, place his or her hands in soft gloves or mitts to minimize damage from scratching, and keep nails short.
- Administer cholestyramine (e.g., Questran, LoCholest, Cholestid) as prescribed to reduce bile acids in the serum and skin and thereby relieve itching. Avoid administration of other oral medications within 2 hr of cholestyramine administration because they may bind with it in the intestine and reduce its absorption.
- Also see last four interventions under "Altered Protection," p. 444.

Knowledge deficit: Lack of exposure to health care information; cognitive limitation secondary to hepatic encephalopathy

Desired outcome: Within the 24-hr period before hospital discharge, patient states signs and symptoms of early hepatic encephalopathy; the importance of medical follow-up; the need to adhere to the prescribed diet; the importance of rest; infection control measures; availability of alcohol and drug treatment programs; medication instructions; and signs and symptoms of other complications.

- Stress importance of sufficient rest and adherence to prescribed diet.
- Infection control: if hepatic failure is related to hepatitis B virus (HBV) infection, HBV prophylaxis should be considered for sexual partners and household members with possible exposure to HBV (e.g., those who unknowingly shared a toothbrush or razor). Teach patient and exposure contacts practices that reduce the risk of exposure (e.g., condom use, having own personal grooming items). Prescreening for the presence of hepatitis B (HB) antibodies is encouraged if it does not delay treatment for more than 14 days after last exposure. A dose of hepatitis B immune globulin (HBIG) is recommended immediately for sexual contacts and household contacts with possible blood and body fluid exposure. A second administration of HBIG vaccine should follow 1 month

later. The HB vaccine series should be initiated for sexual and household contacts at risk. The first and second vaccines can be given at the same time the two HBIG vaccines are given. Make sure both vaccines are given in separate areas. The HB vaccines are to be given deltoid IM only. Stress importance of not sharing intimate items (e.g., razors, toothbrush, nail clippers).

- If hepatic failure is related to hepatitis C virus (HCV), no prophylaxis is available to exposed persons. Therefore baseline hepatitis C (HC) antibodies should be measured, and 1 month later a second sample should be drawn and tested. Based on results, an infectious disease consult may be indicated, along with possible treatment. It is important to note, however, that those with sexual exposure have less than a 5% chance of seroconversion. Those with exposure to blood, particularly through hollow-bore needles, have the greatest chance of seroconversion.
- Inform patient about the availability of alcohol-treatment and drug-treatment programs if alcohol- and drug-related hepatic failure has occurred.
- Explain the availability of support groups (i.e., Alcoholics Anonymous, Al-Anon) for patients and family members when hepatic failure is related to chronic alcohol ingestion.
- Caution about the importance of avoiding over-the-counter (OTC) medications without first consulting physician. Advise patient to confer with physician regarding use of NSAIDs, aspirin (ASA), and other medications that contain salicylates for minor aches and pains after hospital discharge.
- Provide a list of patient's prescribed medications, including drug name, dosage, purpose, schedule, precautions, and potential side effects.
- Teach the signs and symptoms of infection: fever; unusual drainage from paracentesis or other invasive procedure sites; warmth and erythema surrounding the invasive sites; or abdominal pain. Have patient demonstrate technique for measuring oral temperature with type of thermometer used at home.
- Teach the signs and symptoms of unusual bleeding, including prolonged mucosal bleeding, very large or painful bruises, and dark stools. Caution patient that, if possible, major dental procedures should be postponed until bleeding times normalize.
- Inform patient about sodium restriction if ascites developed during the course of the illness.
- Advise protein restriction if the patient has residual or chronic encephalopathy. Instruct patient to avoid constipation by increasing bulk in the diet or by using agents prescribed by physician.
- Caution about the necessity of alcohol cessation for at least several months after complete recovery from the acute episode. After full recovery, one or two glasses of beer or wine a week are usually allowed if hepatic failure was not related to alcohol ingestion.
- Instruct patient to weigh him- or herself daily and to report weight loss or gain of >5 lb.

Research Brief 8-2 Psychometric tests or neurophysiologic techniques are used to diagnose subclinical hepatic encephalopathy (SHE). A large number of normal-appearing patients with cirrhosis are affected by SHE. Many hepatologists believe that these particular patients have subtle motor and cognitive deficits that can impair activities of daily living. Critical Flicker Frequency (CFF) may be useful for the detection and monitoring of SHE. Intrafoveal stimulation with CFF uses stepwise increases of light frequency (fusion threshold) to determine at which frequency the flickering light is perceived as fused light; in the stepwise decreasing frequency (flicker threshold), the point at which fused light flickers is measured.

CFF is a test that reflects the functional efficiency of the cerebral cortex and has shown moderate correlations with psychometric tests, Childs score, and plasma ammonia levels in patients with SHE. CFF is a standard test used in such conditions as multiple sclerosis, Alzheimer's disease, and cerebro-organic syndromes. Advantages of its use in SHE is in its ease of use, reproducibility, ability to be administered in the office, and length of time required to administer the test.

From Kircheis G et al: Critical flicker frequency for quantification of low-grade hepatic encephalopathy, *Hepatology* 35(2):357-366, 2002.

Potential risk for injury related to invasive procedures
Desired outcome: Patient does not sustain an injury related to liver biopsy, ICP monitoring, or other invasive procedures.

- Ensure that patient fully understands procedure and signs informed consent for it before any sedation has been given.
- Fully prepare patient emotionally and physically for the procedure.
- Monitor patient closely after procedure; observe changes in VS that correlate with observations of patient.

- Monitor dressing over puncture wounds for bleeding. Document amount, frequency of dressing changes, what types of dressings are applied, what the drainage looks like/smells like (if applicable), and what the wound looks like.
- Monitor for fever.
- Check for drug allergies prior to procedure.
- If subject is encephalopathic, ensure airway is clear, and ensure that someone will accompany patient to and from procedure. Also ensure that a nurse will be with the patient when he or she is undergoing the procedure.
- Ensure that IV access is established and works in case of an emergency necessitating its use.

ADDITIONAL NURSING DIAGNOSES

As appropriate, see the following for additional nursing diagnoses and interventions: "Nutritional Support," p. 1; "Mechanical Ventilation," p. 14; "Prolonged Immobility," p. 61; "Psychosocial Support," p. 68; and "Psychosocial Support for the Patient's Family and Significant Others," p. 78.

Acute Pancreatitis

PATHOPHYSIOLOGY

Pancreatitis is an autodigestive process of pancreatic tissue by its own enzymes. Chronic pancreatitis is an ongoing inflammatory disorder characterized by irreversible damage and ultimate organ destruction. With acute pancreatitis (AP), injury to pancreatic acinar cells (where pancreatic enzymes are normally stored in their inactive form), and premature activation of the enzyme trypsin is recognized as the initiating event, resulting in necrosis or autodigestion of the organ. Episodes may recur, but the gland remains relatively normal before and after the attack. Although gallstone disease (38%) and alcohol ingestion (35%) account for the majority of cases, several other factors are believed to cause acute pancreatitis, such as endoscopic retrograde cholangiopancreatography (ERCP) (4%), trauma (1.5%), and certain drugs (1.4%) (Table 8-11).

AP may be clinically classified as mild or severe. In cases of mild acute pancreatitis, there is local inflammation, minimal interstitial edema with sporadic acinar cell damage, and no infection or organ system failure. Patients usually improve in 48-72 hr with supportive care. This form accounts for the majority of cases with mortality being <1%. *Severe acute pancreatitis (SAP)* is a life-threatening condition that is accompanied by necrosis and infection, with mortality rates between 30% and 50%. Inflammatory mediators released at the site of tissue damage cause severe vascular damage with major capillary leakage, resulting in hypovolemia and tissue hypoxemia. Locally this causes severe organ edema, which frequently leads to rupture of the pancreatic ducts and spillage of pancreatic enzymes into the peritoneum, resulting in a chemical peritonitis. The spread of inflammatory mediators to distant sites results in systemic inflammation and eventual multiple organ failure.

It is important to identify those patients with SAP to rapidly implement appropriate recourses. Ranson's criteria provides a scale of severity for acute pancreatitis based on age and laboratory studies. Pancreatitis is classified as severe when three or more of Ranson's criteria are met during the first 48 hr following presentation (Table 8-12). Mortality is approximately 16%-20% with 3-5 positive signs, and near 50% with six positive signs. The acute physiology and chronic health evaluation (APACHE) II scoring system is another tool to determine severity, but it is complex and time-consuming. This section discusses the severe form of acute pancreatitis.

Complications: Marked depletion of intravascular plasma volume is the result of fluid sequestration into the interstitium and retroperitoneum. Massive, life-threatening hemorrhage from rupture of necrotic tissue results in serious blood volume depletion. Hypoalbuminemia is frequently present and contributes to hypovolemia. Hypotension persists in some patients despite volume repletion. If hypovolemia is not detected and treated promptly, acute renal failure becomes likely. Mild-to-severe respiratory failure with hypoxemia is common. Respiratory insufficiency is related to right-to-left vascular shunting within the lung and alveolar-capillary leakage caused by circulating proteolytic enzymes, vasoactive amines, and other inflammatory mediators. In addition, elevation of the diaphragm, atelectasis, and pleural effusion caused by subdiaphragmatic inflammation can compromise ventilation further. Intravascular coagulopathy develops in some patients, which can lead to life-threatening complications such as the formation of pulmonary emboli. Hypocalcemia, which is common, is attributed to calcium-binding in areas of fat necrosis within the pancreas and small intestine. The formation of pancreatic pseudocysts or abscesses as a result of necrosis and the collection of purulent

TABLE 8-11 Precipitating Factors for Acute Pancreatitis

Mechanical blockage of pancreatic ducts
- Biliary tract disease (e.g., gallstones)
- Structural abnormalities (e.g., pancreas divisum)
- Preceding ERCP

Toxic/metabolic factors
- Alcohol
- Hypertriglyceridemia
- Hypercalcemia (e.g., hyperparathyroidism)

Infection

Trauma
- External
- Surgical
- Iatrogenic

Ischemia
- Prolonged/severe shock
- Vasculitis

Tumors

Drugs
- NSAIDs
- Estrogens
- Corticosteroids
- Thiazides
- Tetracycline
- Sufonamides

ERCP, Endoscopic retrograde cholangiopancreatography; *NSAIDs,* nonsteroidal antiinflammatory drugs.

TABLE 8-12 Ranson's Criteria for Classifying the Severity of Pancreatitis

At presentation
- Age >55 yr
- WBCs >16,000
- Glucose >2000
- AST >250
- LDH >350

During initial 48 hours
- Base deficit >4 mEq/L
- BUN increased >5 mg mg/dl
- Fluid sequestration >6 L
- Serum Ca^{++} <8
- Hematocrit decrease >10%
- Po$_2$ (from ABG) <60 mm Hg

ABG, Arterial blood gas; *AST,* aspartate aminotransferase; *BUN,* blood urea nitrogen; *Ca^{++},* calcium; *LDH,* lactate dehydrogenase; *PO$_2$,* partial pressure of oxygen; *WBCs,* white blood cells.

material within the tissue can lead to rupture, which in turn can cause sepsis. The ensuing circulatory and respiratory failure often leads to death.

ASSESSMENT

History and risk factors: Excessive alcohol ingestion; biliary tract disease; recent ERCP, high cholesterol levels; use of drugs such as steroids, furosemide, thiazides, and NSAIDs; viral infections (especially mumps and hepatitis); penetrating and blunt injuries to the pancreas. Pregnancy, primary hyperparathyroidism, uremia, and renal transplantation have been implicated as causes.

Clinical presentation: Sudden onset of pain (often after excessive food or alcohol ingestion) lasting 12-48 hr, described as mild discomfort to severe distress, and located from the midepigastria to the right upper quadrant (RUQ). The pain may radiate to the back. Nausea, vomiting, and restlessness typically accompany the pain; diarrhea, melena, and hematemesis may also be present. Abdominal tenderness is common. Dyspnea and cyanosis, which are signs of acute respiratory distress syndrome (ARDS) (see p. 189), may occur as serious complications of acute pancreatitis. With biliary tract disease, jaundice may be present. Grey Turner's sign (a blue-red-purple or green-brown discoloration of the flank) and Cullen's sign (faint, blue-tinged discoloration around the umbilicus) occur in about 1% of cases and are associated with a poor prognosis. Urine output decreases as the body attempts to conserve intravascular volume. Hypocalcemia manifests as numbness or tingling in the extremities that can progress to tetany if calcium is severely depleted.

Physical assessment: Diminished or absent bowel sounds reflective of GI dysfunction and ileus. Palpation will reveal localized tenderness in the RUQ or diffuse discomfort over the upper portion of the abdomen. Mild-to-moderate ascites is present. Breath sounds may be decreased or absent, suggesting focal atelectasis or pleural effusion. Effusions are usually left-sided but can be bilateral. Auscultation of crackles reflects hypoventilation caused by pain, early ARDS, or microemboli. In the presence of hemorrhage or severe hypovolemia, the hands will be cool and sweaty, capillary refill will be delayed, and peripheral pulses will be diminished. With severe hypocalcemia, Chvostek's sign (facial twitching after a tap over the facial nerve) or Trousseau's sign (spasm of the hand that occurs when the arm is constricted with a BP cuff) may be elicited.

Vital signs and hemodynamic measurements: Increased temperature associated with tachycardia and increased BP. Tachycardia, decreased BP, decreased PAP, and decreased CO are present with hemorrhage, shock, or dehydration. Increase in pulmonary vascular resistance (PVR) suggests the presence of ARDS or pulmonary emboli. If systemic inflammation or sepsis is present, CO may be elevated and SVR decreased initially.

DIAGNOSTIC TESTS

Hematologic studies: Leukocytosis with a WBC count of $11,000\text{-}20,000/mm^3$ is reflective of the inflammatory process. Hct and Hgb levels vary, depending on the presence of hemorrhage (decreased) or dehydration (increased).

Chemistry studies: Serum amylase level is usually elevated to 3-5 times that of normal for the first several days. As damage subsides, the level decreases. Amylase may be normal or even decreased in patients with necrotizing AP because of severe pancreatic damage and decreased amylase secretion. Serum lipase levels parallel amylase levels and are more specific for pancreatitis. Serum lipase may remain elevated for up to 14 days. Generally, urine amylase is elevated for 1-2 wks. The amylase/creatinine clearance ratio usually is elevated with obvious pancreatitis. Hypocalcemia is a frequent finding, and values < 8 mg/dl are not uncommon. Because part of the calcium is protein-bound, serum levels depend on albumin levels. As serum albumin levels decrease, reductions in serum calcium levels are anticipated. Hyperglycemia and glycosuria are consequences of glucagon release. Blood glucose values are commonly > 200 mg/dl. Persistent elevation of liver enzymes suggests hepatic inflammation caused by alcohol ingestion or viral hepatitis. Increased serum bicarbonate and hypokalemia values reflect metabolic alkalosis, usually the result of vomiting or gastric suctioning. C-reactive protein is a nonspecific acute-phase reactant that is suggestive of severe acute pancreatitis at levels >10 mg/dl within the first 48 hr of presentation.

Coagulation studies: Decreases in platelets and fibrinogen will be present. Elevations in circulating levels of fibrin are associated with microthrombi in the pancreas and other tissues.

ABG values: Decreased arterial oxygen tension is a common finding and may be present without other symptoms of pulmonary insufficiency. Early hypoxia produces a mild respiratory alkalosis. Arterial oxygen saturation may be diminished.

ECG: ST segment depression and T wave inversion may be seen as a result of the shock state, the severe pain that causes coronary artery spasm, or the effect of trypsin and bradykinins on the myocardium. Hypocalcemia results in widening of the ST segment.

Radiologic procedures: Abdominal x-ray may show dilation of the bowel and ileus. Chest x-ray findings are helpful in distinguishing effusions from atelectasis and in diagnosing ARDS.

CT: Estimates size of the pancreas; identifies fluid collection, cystic lesions, abscesses, and masses; visualizes biliary tract abnormalities; and monitors inflammatory swelling of the pancreas. Now widely available, the spiral CT scan can determine the presence or extent of necrosis, thus can serve as an indicator of disease severity.

Endoscopic retrograde cholangiopancreatography (ERCP): Used to relieve obstruction caused by stone impaction. Not indicated for diagnosis as it may aggravate inflammation.

Endoscopic ultrasonography: Employed to visualize the opening to the pancreas when a biliary cause of AP is suspected, to observe for swelling, ductal abnormalities, and presence of tumors or stones. If these conditions are present, ERCP should not be employed as it may worsen the condition.

COLLABORATIVE MANAGEMENT

Treatment is aimed at aggressive support and prevention of complications. Efforts are directed at pain relief and resting the pancreas until the autodigestive process subsides.

Analgesia: Opioid analgesics are administered for relief of severe pain. Continuous or intermittent IV routes are used, depending on the severity of the pain. Patient-controlled analgesia (PCA) is a helpful mode of delivery. Many opioid analgesics including morphine, fentanyl, and meperidine (Demerol) cause spasm of pancreatic and biliary ducts, which increases pressure and may impede ductal flow. Some authorities believe that meperidine produces less spasm than morphine and therefore recommend it for analgesia in patients with AP. However, the link between spasm of the sphincter of Oddi and abdominal pain is unproven. Meperidine is shorter-acting than morphine, has an active metabolite that may cause seizures, and is more likely to cause muscle fibrosis. Thus, other authorities believe that there is more risk to using meperidine because of its complications. More research is needed in this area. Currently the decision to use morphine or meperidine is of individual choice.

Fluid and electrolyte management: The inflammatory process results in fluid sequestration and extensive intravascular volume loss. Nausea, vomiting, gastric suctioning, and hemorrhage contribute to the hypovolemic state. Colloids and crystalloids are administered to replace volume losses and minimize interstitial edema. Crystalloids alone may be used initially if serum protein levels are adequate. Fluid sequestration in the peritoneum and interstitium continues until the acute phase is arrested; therefore, continual volume replacement is essential. If serum potassium and calcium levels are decreased, replacement therapy is necessary. Because hypercalcemia has been implicated in the genesis of pancreatitis, calcium replacement is prescribed cautiously.

Suppression of pancreatic secretions: Accomplished by withholding oral feedings including water and aspirating gastric secretions via gastric suction; reducing gastric acidity by administering histamine H_2-receptor antagonists and antacids; and reducing physical activity. Gastric suction has not been shown to offer any clear advantage and should be used only for patients with severe nausea and vomiting, abdominal distention, or pain not relieved by analgesia.

Respiratory support: Pulmonary congestion, pleural effusion, and atelectasis result in respiratory insufficiency. Abdominal distention and retroperitoneal fluid sequestration cause diaphragmatic elevation and ventilatory restriction. Early respiratory failure is detected by a decrease in oxygen tension or oxygen saturation. Frequent or continuous pulse oximetry is performed during the first 2-3 days of therapy to detect early hypoxemia. Oxygen administration is initiated if hypoxemia is present. If severe pulmonary insufficiency develops, patient requires ET intubation and positive pressure ventilation. IV fluids are given cautiously to prevent cardiopulmonary compromise.

Nutritional support: Parenteral feedings that provide the nutrients necessary for tissue healing are initiated for patients with severe pancreatitis. High-glucose parenteral regimens compound the hyperglycemia that is commonly present in pancreatitis. For this reason it may be preferable to give a higher percentage of calories as fats. Use of long-chain fatty acids for patients with AP is controversial because there is concern that fatty-acid administration may exacerbate the pancreatitis. Oral feedings are not indicated during the acute episode because they result in pancreatic inflammation by stimulating glandular secretions. Enteral nutrition has been added as a treatment option for the SAP patient. Studies show that there is a trend toward reduction in adverse outcomes with postpyloric (jejunal) enteral feedings, but the data is insufficient to draw firm conclusions. Agents that suppress pancreatic secretions such as somatostatin and octreotide have generally produced disappointing results in human studies. Low-fat oral feedings are begun after the initial episode subsides and bowel function returns.

Surgical management: In general, nonsurgical management of acute pancreatitis is most effective. Because acute pancreatitis is easily confused with acute abdominal emergencies that require urgent surgery, exploratory laparotomy is necessary for some patients. More aggressive surgical procedures, such as pancreatic drainage or débridement, may be necessary for the patient with significant pancreatic necrosis. *Peritoneal lavage* removes toxic factors present in peritoneal exudates. This procedure has not been shown to improve outcomes in the patient with SAP. See Table 8-13 for the nursing interventions related to peritoneal lavage.

Antibiotic coverage: Prophylactic antibiotic use is necessary for gut decontamination in SAP to reduce the chances of septic complications and improve the chances for survival.

NURSING DIAGNOSES AND INTERVENTIONS

Fluid volume deficit related to active loss secondary to fluid sequestration within the peritoneum and hemorrhage associated with tissue necrosis; insufficient oral intake

T A B L E 8 - 13   Nursing Interventions for the Patient Undergoing Peritoneal Lavage for Acute Pancreatitis

- Ensure sterile technique throughout all phases of lavage to prevent serious complications caused by infection.
- Warm lavage fluid to patient's body temperature to prevent cramping, hypothermia, and discomfort.
- Measure lavage infusion fluid loss/retention. Document input and output throughout entire procedure. Document and report daily fluid balance—either excess or deficit.
- Turn patient gently from side to side as needed to promote drainage.
- Monitor patient carefully for decrease in ventilatory excursion caused by pressure from lavage fluid. Drain fluid and consult physician promptly if signs and symptoms of respiratory distress develop.
- Maintain head of bed at 30 degrees or higher.
- Check urine for glucose, and monitor blood glucose levels. Glucose in the lavage fluids can contribute to the glucose intolerance that frequently occurs in patients with pancreatitis. Insulin administration may be required in some instances.
- Note and document characteristics (color, odor, clarity, amount) of lavage return. Documents and report changes.

Desired outcome: Within 24 hr of this diagnosis, patient becomes normovolemic as evidenced by MAP >70 mm Hg; HR 60-100 beats/min; normal sinus rhythm on ECG; CVP 2-6 mm Hg; PAWP 6-12 mm Hg; CO $\geq$ 4-6 L/min; CI $\geq$ 3 L/min/m^2; SVR 900-1200 dynes/sec/cm^{-5}; PVR 60-100 dynes/sec/cm^{-5}; brisk capillary refill (< 2 sec); peripheral pulses > 2+ on a 0-4+ scale; urinary output $\geq$ 0.5 ml/kg/hr; and stable weight.
- Administer crystalloids, colloids, or a combination of both as prescribed.
- Monitor BP q1-4h if losses are caused by fluid sequestration, inadequate intake, or slow bleeding. Monitor BP q15min if patient has active blood loss or unstable VS. Be alert to MAP decreases of $\geq$ 10 mm Hg from previous BP.
- Monitor HR, ECG, and cardiovascular status hourly. Monitor these parameters q15min, or more frequently in the presence of active bleeding or unstable VS. Be alert to increases in HR, which suggest hypovolemia.

Note: Increases in HR also may be caused by fever or hypermetabolic state.

- Measure hemodynamic parameters (i.e., CVP, PAWP, CO) and thermodilution CO q1-4h. Be alert to low or decreasing CVP, PAWP, and CO. Calculate SVR and PVR q4-8h, or more frequently in unstable patients. An elevated HR, decreased PAWP, decreased CO (CI < 3 L/min/m^2), and increased SVR suggest hypovolemia. As available, monitor Svo$_2$ to evaluate adequacy of tissue oxygenation. Pulmonary hypertension is anticipated in patients with ARDS. Assess for signs of overaggressive fluid resuscitation (see "Fluid Volume Excess," p. 452).
- Measure urinary output hourly. Be alert to output < 0.5 ml/kg/hr for 2 consecutive hours. Evaluate intravascular volume and cardiovascular function, and increase fluid intake promptly if decreased urinary output is caused by hypovolemia and hypoperfusion.
- Monitor for physical indicators of hypovolemia, including cool extremities, delayed capillary refill (> 2 sec), and decreased amplitude of or absent distal pulses.
- Estimate ongoing fluid losses. Measure all drainage from tubes, catheters, and drains. Note the frequency of dressing changes because of saturation with fluid or blood. Weigh patient daily, using the same scales and method. Compare 24-hr urine output with 24-hr fluid intake, and record the difference.
- Evaluate character of all fluids lost. Note color and odor. Be alert to the presence of particulate matter, fibrin, and clots. Test GI aspirate, drainage, and excretions (including stool) for the presence of occult blood.

NIC Fluid/Electrolyte Management; Fluid Monitoring; Hemodynamic Regulation; Hypovolemia Management; Invasive Hemodynamic Monitoring; Shock Prevention; Bleeding Precautions; Bleeding Reduction; Hypervolemia Management

Decreased cardiac output related to myocardial depression secondary to circulating vasoactive amines or hypocalcemia; decreased preload secondary to hypovolemia

Desired outcome: Within 12 hr of this diagnosis, cardiac output becomes adequate as evidenced by CI $\geq$ 2.5 L/min/m^2; brisk capillary refill (< 2 sec); peripheral pulses > 2+ on a 0-4+ scale; urinary output $\geq$ 0.5 ml/kg/hr; and warm skin.

- Restore acceptable preload by correcting hypovolemia (see preceding nursing diagnosis, "Fluid Volume Deficit").
- Administer inotropic agents as prescribed. Monitor hemodynamic parameters carefully to minimize adverse affects of inotropic therapy (see Appendix 7).
- Provide patient with frequent rest periods. Space out procedures and treatments to allow long periods (at least 90 min) of uninterrupted rest.
- Minimize anxiety-producing situations, and assist patient with reducing anxiety (see "Health-Seeking Behavior," p. 259, and "Anxiety," p. 69).

NIC Cardiac Care: Acute; Hemodynamic Regulation; Shock Management: Cardiac; Dysrhythmia Management; Anxiety Reduction; Energy Management

Fluid volume excess related to excessive intake secondary to overaggressive fluid resuscitation and peritoneal lavage.

Desired outcome: Within 24 hr of this diagnosis, patient becomes normovolemic as evidenced by MAP 70-95 mm Hg; HR 60-100 beats/min; RR 12-20 breaths/min with normal pattern and depth (eupnea); CVP 2-6 mm Hg; PAWP 6-12 mm Hg; CI ≥ 2.5 L/min/m^2; and absence of adventitious breath sounds and S$_3$ gallop.

- Evaluate patient q1-4h for clinical indicators of fluid volume excess: dyspnea, orthopnea, increased respiratory rate and effort, S$_3$ gallop, or crackles. Document and report changes and new findings.
- Measure hemodynamic parameters (i.e., BP, HR, CVP, PAWP) hourly in patients undergoing peritoneal lavage or in patients with evidence of hypervolemia (i.e., CVP or PAWP increased from baseline or above normal or presence of clinical indicators of fluid volume excess).
- As prescribed, administer inotropic agents to augment myocardial contractility. Evaluate effectiveness by measuring CO and calculating CI q1-2h and by measuring urine output q1-2h. Document and report CI < 2.5 L/min/m^2 and urine output < 0.5 ml/kg/hr for 2 consecutive hours.
- Administer furosemide (Lasix) or other diuretic as prescribed to promote diuresis. Document response to diuretic therapy by noting onset and amount of diuresis.
- Carefully implement peritoneal lavage as prescribed (see "Peritoneal Lavage," p. 450, and Table 8-13).

Pain related to chemical injury to the peritoneum and surrounding tissue secondary to release of pancreatic enzymes

Desired outcomes: Within 2-4 hr of this diagnosis, patient's subjective evaluation of discomfort improves, as documented by a pain scale. Ventilation and hemodynamic status are uncompromised as evidenced by MAP 70-95 mm Hg; HR 60-100 beats/min; and RR 12-20 breaths/min with normal depth and pattern (eupnea).

- As prescribed, administer IV opiate analgesic before pain becomes severe. Be aware that fentanyl, morphine, meperidine, and other opioid analgesics have been linked with biliary spasm and symptoms of biliary colic.

Note: Opioid analgesics decrease intestinal motility and delay return to normal bowel function.

- Pancreatitis can be very painful. Prepare significant others for personality changes and behavioral alterations associated with extreme pain and opiate analgesia. Family members sometimes misinterpret patient's lethargy or unpleasant disposition and may even blame themselves. Reassure them

NIC that these are normal responses.
- Supplement analgesics with nonpharmacologic maneuvers to aid in pain reduction. Modify patient's body position to optimize comfort. Many patients with abdominal pain find a dorsal recumbent or lateral decubitus bent-knee position most comfortable.
- Because anxiety reduction contributes to pain relief, ensure consistency and promptness in delivering analgesic.
- Patients and family members sometimes are distressed at the health team members' inability to relieve pain. Provide continual reassurance that all possible measures are being implemented.
- Monitor respiratory pattern and LOC closely because both may be depressed by the large amounts of opiate analgesics usually required to control pain.
- Monitor HR and BP q1-4h. Monitor CVP and PAWP q4h, or more frequently in patients whose condition is unstable. Consult physician for significant deviations from baseline. Be aware that opiates cause vasodilation and can result in serious hypotension, especially in patients with volume depletion.
- Evaluate effectiveness of medication, and consult physician for dose and drug manipulation. If medications are not effective, prepare patient for splanchnic block or other pain-relieving procedure.

NIC Analgesic Administration; Pain Management; Patient-Controlled Analgesia (PCA) Assistance; Environmental Management: Comfort; Coping Enhancement; Teaching: Prescribed Medication; Simple Guided Imagery; Respiratory Monitoring

- For additional interventions for pain, see p. 51.

Impaired gas exchange related to alveolar-capillary membrane changes secondary to microatelectasis and pulmonary fluid accumulation

Desired outcome: Within 4 hr of this diagnosis, patient has adequate gas exchange as evidenced by $SaO_2 \geq 92\%$; $PaO_2 \geq 80$ mm Hg; $PaCO_2$ 35-45 mm Hg; RR 12-20 breaths/min with normal depth and pattern (eupnea); orientation to time, place, and person; and clear and audible breath sounds.

- Monitor and document respiratory rate q1-4h as indicated. Note pattern, degree of excursion, and whether patient uses accessory muscles of respiration. Consult physician for significant deviations from baseline.
- Auscultate both lung fields q4-8h. Note presence of abnormal sounds (crackles, rhonchi, wheezes) or diminished sounds.
- Be alert to early signs of hypoxia, such as restlessness, agitation, and alterations in mentation.
- Monitor SaO_2 via continuous pulse oximetry or frequent ABG values during the first 48 hr. Many patients with pancreatitis do not have obvious clinical symptoms of respiratory failure, and a decreased arterial oxygen tension may be the first sign of failure. Consult physician if PaO_2 is <60-70 mm Hg or if oxygen saturation falls below 92%.
- Administer oxygen as prescribed. Check oxygen delivery system at frequent intervals to ensure proper delivery, because oxygen is critical to these patients.
- Maintain a body position that optimizes ventilation and oxygenation. Elevate HOB 30 degrees or higher, depending on patient's comfort. If pleural effusion or other defect is present on one side, position patient with the unaffected lung dependent to maximize the ventilation-perfusion relationship.
- Avoid overaggressive fluid resuscitation (see "Fluid Volume Excess," p. 452).

NIC Acid-Base Management; Airway Management; Oxygen Therapy; Respiratory Monitoring; Positioning; Fluid Monitoring; Hypervolemia Management

- See "Acute Respiratory Distress Syndrome," p. 189, for additional information.

Risk for infection related to tissue destruction with resulting necrosis secondary to release of pancreatic enzymes and multiple invasive procedures.

Desired outcome: Patient remains free of infection as evidenced by core or rectal temperature $\leq 37.8°$ C ($\leq 100°$ F); negative culture results; HR 60-100 beats/min; RR 12-20 breaths/min; BP within patient's normal range; CI ≤ 4 L/min/m^2; SVR 900-1200 dynes/sec/cm^{-5}; and orientation to time, place, and person.

- Check rectal or core temperature q4h for increases. Be aware that hypothermia may precede hyperthermia in some patients.
- If temperature suddenly rises, obtain specimens for culture of blood, sputum, urine, and other sites as prescribed. Monitor culture reports, and report positive findings promptly.
- Evaluate orientation and LOC q2-4h. Document and report significant deviations from baseline.
- Monitor BP, HR, RR, CO, and SVR q1-4h. Be alert to increases in HR and RR associated with temperature elevations. An elevated CO (CI > 4 L/min/m^2) and decreased SVR (<900 dynes/sec/cm^{-5}) suggest systemic inflammatory response or sepsis.
- Administer parenteral antibiotics in a timely fashion. Reschedule antibiotics if a dose is delayed for more than 1 hr. Recognize that failure to administer antibiotics on schedule can result in inadequate blood levels and treatment failure. Monitor peak and trough levels for patients receiving aminoglycoside antibiotics. Aminoglycosides; used frequently, require that patient be monitored for hearing loss. Older adults are especially susceptible to the ototoxic and nephrotoxic effects of aminoglycosides. Monitor levels of BUN, creatinine, and urinary output, which are indicators of renal function.

NIC Medication Management; Vital Signs Monitoring; Temperature Regulation; Intravenous (IV) Therapy

Impaired tissue integrity: GI tract, related to release of chemical irritants into the pancreatic parenchyma and surrounding tissue, including the peritoneum

Desired outcomes: By the time of hospital discharge, patient exhibits no further GI tissue destruction as evidenced by reduction in pain; GI aspirate, stools, drainage, and vomitus negative for blood; and return of bowel sounds and bowel function. Gastric pH value remains >5.

- Withhold oral feedings to avoid stimulation of pancreatic enzymes.
- Ensure patency of gastric sump tube to provide continual gastric drainage and prevent pancreatic stimulation. Do not occlude the air vent of double-lumen tube because this may result in vacuum occlusion. Check placement of gastric tube at least q8h, and reposition as necessary.
- Administer antacids and histamine H_2-receptor antagonists as prescribed to decrease gastric and pancreatic secretions and to reduce gastric pH. Monitor gastric pH, and administer antacids to maintain pH value >5.
- Because increased activity can stimulate gastric secretions, limit patient's physical activity during the acute phase.

- Test GI aspirate, drainage, and excretions for the presence of occult blood q12-24h.
- Initiate peritoneal lavage as prescribed (see Table 8-13) to remove irritants from the peritoneum.

NIC Oral Health Maintenance; Acid-Base Management; Gastrointestinal Intubation; Bleeding Precautions

Altered nutrition: less than body requirements, related to decreased oral intake secondary to nausea, vomiting, and nothing by mouth (NPO) status; increased need secondary to tissue destruction or infection

Desired outcomes: Patient maintains baseline body weight and demonstrates a state of nitrogen balance on nitrogen studies.

- Collaborate with physician, dietitian, and pharmacist to estimate patient's individual metabolic needs, based on activity level, presence of infection or other stressor, and nutritional status before hospitalization. Overuse of calcium supplements can cause AP. Develop a plan of care accordingly.
- As prescribed, provide parenteral nutrition during acute phase of pancreatitis. Monitor closely for evidence of hyperglycemia (e.g., Kussmaul respirations; rapid respirations; fruity, acetone breath odor; flushed, dry skin; deteriorating LOC), which commonly is associated with pancreatitis. Administer insulin as prescribed.
- Administer postpyloric, elemental, and enteral feedings via naso-jejunal (NJ) feeding tube or jejunostomy as prescribed for patients with intestinal peristalsis.
- Monitor bowel sounds q4h. Document and report deviations from baseline. Withhold oral or jejunal feedings if bowel sounds are absent unless elemental feedings are used.
- Monitor blood or urine glucose levels q4-8h or as prescribed. Consult physician for blood levels > 200 mg/dl.
- Begin low-fat oral feedings when acute episode has subsided and bowel function has returned. This may take several weeks in some patients.

NIC Nutrition Management; Nutritional Monitoring; Enteral Tube Feeding; Aspiration Precautions; Total Parenteral Nutrition (TPN) Administration; Venous Access Devices (VAD) Maintenance; Hyperglycemia Management; Hypoglycemia Management
- For additional detail, see "Nutritional Support," p. 1.

Knowledge deficit: lack of exposure to health care information

Desired outcome: Within the 24-hr period before hospital discharge, patient verbalizes knowledge regarding availability of alcohol rehabilitation programs, prescribed medications, importance of a low-fat diet, indicators of actual or impending GI hemorrhage, indicators of infection, and the importance of seeking medical attention promptly if signs of recurring pancreatitis appear.

- Inform patients whose pancreatitis is caused by excessive alcohol intake about the availability of alcohol rehabilitation programs.
- Teach patient about prescribed medications including drug name, dosage, purpose, schedule, precautions, and side effects.
- Advise patient about the importance of adhering to a low-fat diet if prescribed.
- Instruct patient about the indicators of actual or impending GI hemorrhage: nausea, vomiting blood, dark stools, lightheadedness, passing frank blood in stools.
- Teach the indicators of infection: fever, unusual drainage from surgical incisions or peritoneal lavage site, warmth or erythema surrounding surgical sites, and abdominal pain. Have patient demonstrate oral temperature-taking technique using the type of thermometer that will be used at home.
- Stress the importance of seeking medical attention promptly if signs of recurrent pancreatitis (i.e., pain, change in bowel habits, passing blood in the stools, or vomiting blood) or infection (see "Risk for Infection," p. 453) appear.

NIC Teaching: Disease Process, Individual, Prescribed Activity Exercise, Prescribed Diet, Prescribed Procedure/Treatment, Prescribed Medication; Behavior Modification

ADDITIONAL NURSING DIAGNOSES

As appropriate, see nursing diagnoses and interventions in the following: "Acute Respiratory Distress Syndrome," p. 189; "Acute Renal Failure," p. 315; "Enterocutaneous Fistulas," p. 465; "Disseminated Intravascular Coagulation," p. 489; and "Septic Shock," p. 501. Also see "Prolonged Immobility," p. 61; "Psychosocial Support," p. 68, and "Psychosocial Support for the Patient's Family and Significant Others," p. 78.

Peritonitis

PATHOPHYSIOLOGY

Peritonitis can be classified as either *primary* or *secondary*. Primary peritonitis is a bacterial infection that occurs spontaneously without any apparent source of contamination. It occurs most commonly in conjunction with cirrhosis of the liver and is associated with a 30%-50% mortality rate. Secondary peritonitis, also called surgical peritonitis, is an inflammation of all or part of the peritoneal cavity and is caused by diffuse microbial proliferation or chemical irritation from leakage of corrosive gastric or intestinal contents into the peritoneum. Ruptured appendix, perforated peptic ulcer, bowel rupture related to ulcerative colitis or Crohn's disease, pancreatitis, abdominal trauma, and ruptured abdominal abscesses are among the many etiologic factors associated with peritonitis. Indwelling tubes and catheters, such as those used for postoperative drainage and continuous ambulatory peritoneal dialysis (CAPD), are foreign bodies that compromise peritoneal integrity and permit the entry of infective organisms that can trigger peritonitis.

Regardless of the initiating factor, the inflammatory process is similar in every case. The initial reactions, which usually are triggered by histamine release, include hyperemia, edema, and vascular congestion. Fluid shifts from intravascular to interstitial spaces as a result of increased vascular permeability. The circulating blood volume is depleted, and hypovolemic shock may ensue. The transudated fluid contains high levels of fibrinogen and thromboplastin. The fibrinogen is converted to fibrin by the thromboplastin. Under normal conditions the peritoneum has fibrinolytic abilities to stop the fibrin formation. When the peritoneum is weakened or injured, however, this ability is hampered and fibrin adhesions form around the damaged area. The fibrin deposits form a barrier that harbors and protects bacteria from the body's defenses, resulting in multiple pockets of infection, which can lead to recurrent infection or septicemia. In most cases the fibrin deposits dissolve, but prolonged or severe inflammation can result in the continuing presence of fibrin, leading to adhesions and potential bowel obstruction.

ASSESSMENT

History and risk factors: Inflammatory processes such as diverticulitis, appendicitis, or Crohn's disease; obstructive events in the small bowel and colon; vascular events such as ischemic colitis, mesenteric thrombosis, or embolic phenomena; blunt or penetrating trauma, especially to hollow viscera; severe hepatobiliary disease; and CAPD. General risk factors include those related to poor tissue healing and infection (e.g., advanced age, diabetes, vascular disease, advanced liver disease, malignancy, malnutrition, debilitation).

Clinical presentation: The primary symptom is pain, which may be quite severe, causing the patient to maintain a fetal position and resist any movement that aggravates the pain. Its onset can be sudden or insidious, with the location varying according to the underlying pathology. Fever and restlessness are common findings in many patients. Nausea, vomiting, anorexia, and changes in bowel habits also may be present and are reflective of GI dysfunction.

Physical assessment: Auscultation of all four quadrants usually reveals diminished or absent bowel sounds. The complete absence of bowel sounds suggests an ileus—a frequent complication of peritonitis. Palpation of the abdomen elicits tenderness that can be generalized or localized, depending on the nature and extent of infection. Rebound tenderness, guarding, and involuntary rigidity also may be present. Occasionally, mild-to-moderate ascites is observed, depending on the cause of the peritonitis. RR is rapid, and the patient usually has a shallow ventilatory pattern to minimize abdominal movement and pain; as a consequence, breath sounds may be diminished. Fluid shifts and hypovolemia can cause restlessness and confusion because of impaired cerebral perfusion.

Vital signs and hemodynamic measurements: Usually fever of $>38°$ C ($100°$-$101°$ F) is present, accompanied by tachypnea and tachycardia that result from increased metabolic demands. During the acute phase the cardiovascular system may be compromised by large fluid shifts from the intravascular space into the abdominal interstitium and peritoneum. This disruption of intravascular volume can lead to hypovolemia with marked tachycardia, hypotension, low CO, decreased PA pressures, and decreased urine output. Depending on disease progression, the patient may exhibit signs of septic shock. Endotoxemic vasodilation is manifested by a low SVR, with an initial increase in HR and CO. This state complicates the initial hypovolemia and may result in a dangerously low MAP, thus impairing renal, cardiac, and cerebral perfusion. See Table 4-24 for a comparison of the hemodynamic profiles for persons with hypovolemic and septic shock.

DIAGNOSTIC TESTS

Hematologic studies: Leukocytosis will be present, with the WBC count usually $>20,000/mm^3$. A low WBC count may indicate an exhausted bone marrow, with a poor prognosis. Initially the Hgb and Hct values may be increased because of hemoconcentration, but they will decrease to baseline levels as normal intravascular volume is restored.

Blood chemistry studies: Depending on the severity of the patient's condition, blood electrolyte levels may be abnormal. If nausea and vomiting are persistent, metabolic alkalosis is expected. This state is reflected by high CO_2 and low Cl^- values. Serum albumin levels are often decreased, especially with bacterial peritonitis. The underlying disease process affects chemistry studies (e.g., patients with pancreatitis usually have elevated amylase levels).

Radiologic procedures: The abdominal x-ray study usually reveals dilation of the large and small bowel, with edema of the small bowel wall. Free air in the abdomen suggests visceral perforation. With CT, abscesses can be visualized and sometimes drained during the procedure, thus avoiding surgery.

Ultrasonography: Useful in locating small amounts of loculated fluid, as well as in differentiating fluid collections in the abdomen. Also helpful in identifying abscesses, bile duct dilation and pancreatitis.

Diagnostic paracentesis: Abdominal paracentesis involves the insertion of a catheter or trocar into the abdomen to obtain a specimen. Sterile saline is infused through the catheter, and the return fluid is analyzed for RBC, WBC, amylase, and bacteria content. If ascites is present, it may not be necessary to infuse saline because fluid can be removed directly for analysis. Paracentesis may be repeated 48 hr after the initiation of treatment to assess patient response. Peritoneal lavage with 1 L of saline may be used to detect peritonitis in patients with suspected secondary or surgical peritonitis (see Table 8-13).

COLLABORATIVE MANAGEMENT

Because peritonitis is usually a complication of another condition, the ultimate aim of therapy is to treat the underlying disease process. Fluid resuscitation and antimicrobial therapy are the mainstay of immediate treatment. Laparotomy is required for the patient with surgical peritonitis. The following are some of the general therapies that apply to the management of peritonitis.

Antimicrobial therapy: Most commonly, both aerobic and anaerobic organisms are found within the abdomen. The availability of broad-spectrum β-lactams and third- and fourth-generation cephalosporins have allowed for a significant reduction in the use of aminoglycosides, thus reducing the risk of nephrotoxicity. For patients undergoing CAPD, vancomycin (Vancocin) may be added if indicated by culture growth. Therapeutic levels are drawn to guide therapy. Refer to Table 8-18 for nursing implications for aminoglycoside therapy.

Pain management: The degree of discomfort caused by peritonitis varies greatly. Opiate analgesics are used to ensure patient comfort but are given cautiously to avoid compromise of abdominal and respiratory function. These analgesics usually require frequent administration, with the dose titrated for each individual.

Fluid and electrolyte management: With bacterial peritonitis a significant intravascular volume depletion may occur. In most cases crystalloids are used initially unless there is evidence of decreased intravascular proteins, in which event colloids such as albumin are indicated. If peritonitis is complicated by hemorrhage, packed RBCs may be given. Electrolyte replacement, typically potassium, is implemented according to laboratory findings. See "Septic Shock," p. 501, for additional information.

Nutritional therapy: Because of the inflammatory process, GI function is compromised and motility is minimal or absent. An enteric tube (nasogastric [NG] tube) is inserted to reduce or prevent distention and promote function. Initially, the patient is placed on NPO status until some GI function is regained. Total parenteral nutrition is crucial for healing and survival until another feeding strategy, such as jejunal feeding, can be tolerated. Elemental feedings can be administered with or without bowel sounds present. When resumption of bowel sounds or passage of flatus signals the return of GI motility, enteral nutrition with conventional tube feedings is begun.

Surgical management: Surgical laparotomy is often necessary, depending on the cause of the peritonitis. All intraabdominal foreign material is removed, and nonviable tissue is débrided. Leaky anastomoses are identified and repaired. If present, bowel perforations and obstructions are corrected and abscesses are drained. This should remove the source of infection and prevent reinfection. Drains are also being successfully placed laparoscopically. Open wound management of the abdomen with scheduled reoperations is often advocated for severe disease, showing good quality of life for survivors. Peritoneal lavage (see Table 8-13) may still be employed, but its benefit as a treatment is unproven.

NURSING DIAGNOSES AND INTERVENTIONS

Fluid volume deficit related to active loss secondary to fluid sequestration within the peritoneum
Desired outcome: Within 8 hr of this diagnosis, patient becomes normovolemic as evidenced by the following parameters: MAP 70-105 mm Hg; HR 60-100 beats/min; normal sinus rhythm on ECG; CVP 2-6 mm Hg; PAWP 6-12 mm Hg; CI 2.5-4 L/min/m^2; urinary output ≥0.5 ml/kg/hr; warm extremities; peripheral pulses >2+ on a 0-4+ scale; brisk capillary refill (<2 sec); orientation to time, place, and person; and stable weight.

- Monitor BP q1-4h, depending on patient stability. Be alert to MAP decreases of ≥10 mm Hg from previous BP reading.
- Monitor HR and ECG q1-4h, or more often if VS are unstable. Be alert to increases in HR, which suggest hypovolemia. Usually the ECG will show sinus tachycardia. In the presence of hypokalemia caused by prolonged vomiting or gastric suction, ECG may show ventricular ectopy, prominent U wave, and depression of the ST segment.

Note: HR increases also may be caused by fever.

- Measure CVP, PAWP, and thermodilution CO q1-4h, depending on stability of patient's condition. Be alert to low or decreasing CVP, PAWP, and CO. Calculate SVR q4-8h, or more frequently in patients whose condition is unstable. A decreased CVP and PAWP, decreased CO (CI < 2.5 L/min/m^2), and increased SVR (>1200 dynes/sec/cm^{-5}) suggest hypovolemia.
- Measure urinary output hourly. Be alert to output < 0.5 ml/kg/hr for 2 consecutive hours, which may signal intravascular volume depletion. Consult physician and increase fluid intake promptly if decreased urinary output is caused by hypovolemia and hypoperfusion.
- Monitor patient for physical indicators of hypovolemia, including cool extremities, capillary refill > 2 sec, decreased amplitude of peripheral pulses, and neurologic changes such as restlessness and confusion.
- Estimate ongoing fluid losses. Measure all drainage from tubes, catheters, and drains. Note the frequency of dressing changes as a result of saturation with fluid or blood. Weigh the patient daily, using the same scales and method. Compare 24-hr body fluid output with 24-hr fluid intake, and record the difference.

NIC Fluid/Electrolyte Management; Fluid Monitoring; Hemodynamic Regulation; Hypovolemia Management; Invasive Hemodynamic Monitoring; Shock Prevention; Dysrhythmia Management

Pain related to biologic or chemical agents causing injury to the peritoneum and intraperitoneal organs

Desired outcomes: Within 2 hr of this diagnosis, patient's subjective evaluation of discomfort improves, as documented by a pain scale. Nonverbal indicators of discomfort, such as grimacing, are absent.

- Monitor patient for the presence of discomfort. Devise a pain scale with the patient, such as rating discomfort from 0 (no pain) to 10. Administer analgesics promptly, before pain becomes severe. Consistency and promptness in delivering analgesics also may help to decrease patient's anxiety, which can contribute to the severity of the pain. Rate the degree of pain relief obtained by using the pain scale. Be aware that opiate analgesics decrease GI motility and may delay the return of normal bowel function.
- Modify patient's body position to optimize comfort. Many patients with severe abdominal pain find a dorsal recumbent or lateral decubitus bent-knee position more comfortable than other positions.
- Monitor respiratory pattern and LOC hourly, because both may be depressed if large amounts of opiates are required to control the pain.
- Monitor HR and BP q1-4h. Monitor CVP and PAWP q4h, or more frequently in patients whose condition is unstable. Consult physician for significant deviations. Be aware that many opiates cause vasodilation and can result in serious hypotension, especially in patients with volume depletion.
- Evaluate effectiveness of the medication on an ongoing basis. On the basis of the patient's clinical response, discuss dose and drug manipulation with physician.
- Avoid administering analgesics to newly admitted patients before they have been fully evaluated by a surgeon, because analgesics can mask important diagnostic clues.

NIC Analgesic Administration; Pain Management; Environmental Management: Comfort; Coping Enhancement; Simple Guided Imagery; Respiratory Monitoring

- See Collaborative Management, p. 52 for additional interventions for patients with pain.

Altered nutrition: less than body requirements, related to decreased intake secondary to impaired GI function

Desired outcomes: Patient maintains baseline body weight, and nitrogen studies show a state of nitrogen balance within 5-7 days of this diagnosis.

- Monitor bowel sounds q1-8h; report significant changes (i.e., sudden absence or return).
- Maintain NPO status during the acute phase of peritonitis with stomach decompression via NG tube.
- Initiate total parenteral nutrition (TPN) with the first 24-48 hr. Evaluate patient for postpyloric (jejunal) elemental feedings. Gradually increase oral or enteral intake with conventional feedings when gastric motility returns.
- If patient has abdominal distention, measure and document abdominal girth q8h. Distention can signal complications such as ileus or ascites.

- Administer histamine H_2-receptor antagonists, antacids, and sucralfate as prescribed to reduce corrosiveness of gastric acid and prevent complications such as stress ulcers.
- Administer prescribed antiemetic medications as indicated.
- Ensure that gastric, intestinal, and other GI drainage tubes are functioning properly. Evaluate character of the drainage (see Table 2-15). Irrigate or reposition tubes as necessary. Patency and proper position of decompression tubes, such as the Miller-Abbott type, are essential for proper function.

NIC   Nutrition Management; Nutritional Monitoring; Gastrointestinal Intubation; Total Parenteral Nutrition (TPN) Administration; Enteral Tube Feeding; Aspiration Precautions; Tube Care: Gastrointestinal
- For additional information, see "Nutritional Support," p. 1.

Risk for infection related to inadequate primary defenses (traumatized tissue, altered perfusion); tissue destruction; environmental exposure to pathogens.

Desired outcome: Septicemia does not develop as evidenced by HR 60-100 beats/min; RR 12-20 breaths/min; SVR 900-1200 dynes/sec/cm^{-5}; CI 2.5-4 L/min/m^2; normothermia; negative culture results; and orientation to time, place, and person.
- Monitor VS and hemodynamic measurements for evidence of septicemia: increases in HR, RR, and CO (CI > 4 L/min/m^2) and a decrease in SVR (< 900 dynes/sec/cm^{-5}). Check rectal or core temperature q4h for increases. Be aware that hypothermia may precede hyperthermia in some patients. Also note that older adults and those who are immunocompromised may not demonstrate a fever, even with severe sepsis.
- If the patient has a sudden temperature elevation, obtain culture specimens of blood, sputum, urine, and other sites as prescribed. Monitor culture reports, and report positive findings promptly.
- Administer parenteral antibiotics in a timely fashion. Reschedule antibiotics if a dosage is delayed for more than 1 hr. Recognize that failure to administer antibiotics on schedule may result in inadequate drug blood levels and treatment failure. Although aminoglycosides in combination with a β-lactam has been accepted therapy, monotherapy with a β-lactam has been shown to be just as effective. See Table 8-18 for aminoglycoside nursing interventions.
- To minimize microbial growth, facilitate drainage of pus, GI secretions, old blood, necrotic tissue, foreign material such as feces, and other body fluids from wounds (see Table 2-14).
- Evaluate wounds for evidence of infection (e.g., erythema, warmth, swelling, unusual drainage). Culture any unusual drainage (see Table 2-14 for a description of normal drainage).
- Evaluate patient's orientation to time, place, and person and LOC q2-4h. Document and report significant deviations from baseline.

NIC   Medication Management; Hemodynamic Regulation; Vital Signs Monitoring; Temperature Regulation; Intravenous (IV) Therapy; Wound Care
- See discussion of sepsis in "Septic Shock," p. 501, for additional information.

Hyperthermia related to infectious process, increased metabolic rate, and dehydration secondary to peritonitis

Desired outcomes: Patient's temperature remains within acceptable limits (36°-38.9° C [97°-102° F]) or returns to acceptable limits within 4-6 hr of this diagnosis. An open airway is secured in the event of hyperthermic seizures.
- Monitor rectal or core temperature q2-4h.
- If a hypothermia blanket is required, perform the following interventions:
  - ❏ Protect the skin that is in contact with the blanket by placing a sheet between the blanket and patient.
  - ❏ Inspect patient's skin q2h for evidence of tissue damage caused by local vasoconstriction. Massage patient's skin q2h to promote circulation and minimize tissue damage.
  - ❏ Check patient's temperature at frequent intervals to ensure that sudden decreases (along with shivering) do not occur, which could increase metabolic demand.
- If patient has a high fever (i.e., $>38.9°$ C [102° F]), administer tepid baths, which may be helpful in reducing the fever.
- Administer antipyretics as prescribed.
- Keep an appropriate-size oral airway and suction equipment in the patient's room for use in the event of seizure activity.

NIC   Fever Treatment; Temperature Regulation; Vital Signs Monitoring

ADDITIONAL NURSING DIAGNOSES

For other nursing diagnoses and interventions, see the following as appropriate: "Hemodynamic Monitoring," p. 23; "Prolonged Immobility," p. 61; "Psychosocial Support," p. 68; "Psychosocial Support for the Patient's Family and Significant Others," p. 78; and "Septic Shock," p. 501.

Acute Gastrointestinal Bleeding

PATHOPHYSIOLOGY

Bleeding can occur at any point along the alimentary tract; however, an upper GI bleed is 5 times more common than a lower one. Together they account for significant morbidity, with a mortality rate around 7%-10%. For an acute upper GI bleed, mortality can be greater than 40% in patients with liver disease or other serious illness. The following overview presents common GI bleeding sites or occurrences.

Esophagus: Gastnsesophageal varices (see p. 417) are the most common cause of massive esophageal hemorrhage. Esophagitis and esophageal ulcers and tumors also can cause acute bleeding, but they occur less frequently. Maneuvers that increase intraabdominal pressure (e.g., retching, vomiting, straining, coughing) can lead to Mallory-Weiss syndrome, a laceration at the esophagogastric junction that results in massive bleeding.

Stomach and duodenum: The most common causes of hematemesis and melena are duodenal and gastric ulcers, accounting for half of massive upper GI bleeding disorders. Stress ulceration is a common and potentially life-threatening phenomenon that occurs in > 85% of critically ill patients. Stress ulcers, also known as *erosive gastritis*, tend to be multiple, shallow lesions located in the proximal stomach. Cushing's ulcer is a related condition occurring in patients who have sustained serious injury, major surgery, or critical CNS disorders. Curling ulcers occur in the esophagus, stomach, and duodenum and are associated with deeper mucosal invasion than stress ulcers. Curling ulcers are seen in patients with major burn injury. They are located in the duodenum and tend to be single, deep ulcers. Gastritis, another common cause of GI bleeding, usually occurs as slow, diffuse oozing that is difficult to control. Benign or malignant gastric tumors may initiate severe bleeding episodes, especially tumors located in the vascular system that supplies the GI tract.

Small intestine: This area of the alimentary tract accounts for only a small portion of GI bleeding episodes. Diverticular disease, arteriovenous malformation, intussusception of the small bowel, acute superior mesenteric artery occlusion, and Crohn's disease are some of the possible causes for bleeding.

Large intestine: Arteriovenous malformation of the ascending colon and the cecum is the usual cause of massive colonic bleeding. Inflammatory bowel diseases such as ulcerative colitis and Crohn's disease result in friable intestinal mucosa, which can lead to massive hemorrhage and other serious complications, including bowel obstruction and perforation. In addition, diverticular disease can cause serious, intermittent bleeding episodes. Other causes include benign or malignant neoplasms and congenital malformation such as hemangioma or telangiectasia.

Neighboring organs: Acute pancreatitis (see p. 447) and pancreatic pseudocyst are disorders associated with hemorrhage. Persons with intraabdominal vascular grafts are at risk for the development of aortoenteric fistulas with massive GI hemorrhage.

Systemic organ diseases: Hypoperfusion associated with decreased cardiac output or volume depletion can lead to GI ischemia, resulting in necrosis and hemorrhage. A high incidence of GI bleeding is associated with uremia because of platelet dysfunction. Collagen diseases can result in thrombosis of small vessels in the small intestine, eventually leading to ulceration. Many blood dyscrasias (e.g., DIC, thrombocytopenia) are associated with hematemesis and melena caused by decreased clotting.

Medications: Long-standing use of ASA, NSAIDs (even at low doses), steroids, or anticoagulants are sometimes associated with serious GI bleeding.

Other trauma: In addition to major abdominal trauma (see p. 149), foreign bodies (e.g., razors, screws, nails) may lacerate gastric or intestinal mucosa, causing bleeding.

ASSESSMENT

History and risk factors: Critical illness, especially that caused by major injury, surgery, CNS disorder, or burns; prolonged shock or hypoperfusion; organ failure; excessive alcohol, NSAIDs, or steroid ingestion; inflammatory bowel disease; foreign body ingestion; hiatal hernia; hepatic, pancreatic, or biliary tract disease; blood dyscrasias; penetrating or blunt trauma; familial cancer; recent abdominal surgery; and the presence of *Heliobacter pylori*, which is found in > 90% of patients with duodenal ulcers and 70% of those with gastric ulcers. Identification of patients who are at risk for recurrent bleeding is essential to guide therapy and prevent poor outcomes. Risk factors associated with rebleeding are listed in Table 8-14.

Clinical presentation: Varies, depending on the amount of blood lost, rate of bleeding, and its effects on cardiovascular and other body systems. Adults can lose up to 500 ml of blood in 15 min and remain free of associated symptoms. A loss of 1000 ml in 15 min usually produces tachycardia, hypotension, nausea, weakness, and diaphoresis. Massive hemorrhage generally is defined as loss of > 30% of total blood volume, or a bleeding episode that requires transfusion of 6 units of blood in

---

T A B L E 8 - 14   Risk Factors To Predict Recurrent Bleeding

- Large volume blood loss on admission without transfusion of >6 units
- Shock
- Age > 60 yr
- Hematemesis as the initial sign of hemorrhage
- Presence of stigmata of recent hemorrhage as identified endoscopically
- Bleeding that occurs while hospitalized for another problem

---

24 hr. Syncope associated with hypotension also may occur. In addition to GI blood loss, sequestration of fluid into the peritoneum and interstitium further depletes intravascular volume. Hematemesis, melena (passage of black, shiny, fetid stools containing blood), and hematochezia (passage of bloody stools) are usually present. Blood can irritate the bowels, thereby increasing transit time and causing diarrhea. Mild to severe pain is often associated with ulcerative or erosive disease. As blood covers and protects the eroded tissue, pain may disappear. Severe hypovolemic shock and decreased cardiac output can lead to ischemia of various organs, especially the brain and kidneys. Alterations in LOC and diminished urinary output will result.

Physical assessment: With profuse, active bleeding, a fast assessment can determine if a shock state is present: the presence of tachycardia, hypotension, cool and diaphoretic extremities, decreased peripheral pulses, delayed capillary refill (> 2 sec), pallor or cyanosis, restlessness, confusion, decreased urine output, and obvious bleeding. Auscultation of the abdomen may reveal hyperactive bowel sounds caused by mucosal irritation by blood, or it may reveal a silent abdomen, which suggests serious complications such as ileus, perforation, or vascular occlusion. Palpation may reveal epigastric tenderness, which is expected in peptic ulceration, or an epigastric mass or enlarged lymph nodes, which indicate gastric malignant disease. Jaundice, vascular spiders, ascites, and hepatosplenomegaly suggest liver disease. A careful digital rectal examination should be performed, along with testing vomitus and stool for occult blood. With upper GI bleeding, emesis or gastric aspirate contains obvious whole blood or old blood that resembles coffee grounds. Stools are usually black and tarry (melena), with a distinctive fetid odor. With lower GI bleeding, stools may be dark or contain fresh blood. Massive lower GI bleeding is associated with dark red "currant jelly" stools or passing fresh blood with clots (hematochezia). Bleeding below the level of the duodenum is not associated with hematemesis.

Vital signs and hemodynamic measurements: HR and BP are quick indicators of a hypovolemic state. Systolic BP < 100 mm Hg with an HR > 100 beats/min in a previously normotensive individual signals a 20% or greater reduction in blood volume. In addition, postural VS should be measured. A decrease in systolic BP > 10 mm Hg or an increase in HR of 10 beats/min indicates a recent blood loss of at least 1000 ml in the adult. Hemodynamic measurements usually reveal a decreased PAP and CO and an increased SVR. After major abdominal surgery a hyperdynamic state may exist similar to that seen in early septic shock, with an increased CO and decreased SVR (see "Septic Shock," p. 593). RR will be mildly elevated as a response to the diminished oxygen-carrying capacity of the blood. If abdominal pain is present, ventilatory excursion may be limited.

DIAGNOSTIC TESTS

Hematologic tests: Serial Hgb and Hct values will reflect the amount of blood lost. Because the ratio of blood cells to plasma remains unchanged initially, the first Hct value may be near normal. However, the Hct is expected to fall dramatically as volume is restored and extravascular fluid mobilizes into the vascular space (hemodilution). Platelet count rises within 1 hr of hemorrhage, and leukocytosis follows.

Chemistry studies: Excessive vomiting or gastric suction may cause a hypochloremic, hypokalemic state accompanied by a rise in the serum bicarbonate level. Increases in BUN without corresponding creatinine increases occur because of excess intestinal protein from the digestion of RBCs. BUN increases are not seen with bleeding from the colon or the lower portion of the small intestine inasmuch as protein digestion occurs higher, in the upper portion. Dehydration and renal insufficiency contribute to an elevated BUN level in affected patients. Plasma protein levels may rise in response to increased hepatic production. Mild hyperglycemia is the result of the body's compensatory response to a stressful stimulus. Hyperbilirubinemia is caused by the breakdown of reabsorbed blood and its pigments. Ammonia levels are usually elevated in patients with hepatic disease.

ABG values: If the shock state is severe, lactic acidosis occurs, reflected by low arterial pH and serum bicarbonate levels and the presence of an anion gap. With a low perfusion state, hypoxemia may be present.

Coagulation studies: Depending on preexisting disease, hypocoagulability may be present. Elevation of fibrinogen levels, fibrin split products (FSP), PT, and PTT may be seen.

12/18-lead ECG: May reflect severe cardiac ischemia as a result of hypoperfusion. Ischemic changes include T wave depression or inversion.

Esophagogastroduodenoscopy (EGD, panendoscopy): The most accurate means of determining source of upper GI bleeding. The esophagus, stomach, and duodenum are visualized directly with a fiberoptic endoscope, which is passed through the mouth. Attempts are made to identify the exact source and characteristics of the ulcer. Findings indicative of bleeding ulcers or ulcers at risk for rebleeding are referred to as stigmata of recent hemorrhage (SRH) (Table 8-15). EGD is usually performed within the first 12 hr after the patient's admission. The procedure provides both critical diagnostic and prognostic information necessary to direct therapy and to identify patients at risk for recurrent bleeding (see Table 8-15). It may be necessary to clear the stomach of blood and clots by lavage before the procedure. Antacids and sucralfate should be withheld until after the procedure, because they alter the appearance of the lesions. Electrocautery, laser, and other therapeutic techniques may be employed during this procedure.

Proctosigmoidoscopy: The rectum and sigmoid colon are visualized directly through an endoscope, which is passed through the anus into the lower GI tract. Mucosal bleeding, polyps, hemorrhoids, and other lesions may be seen. Biopsy specimens may be obtained during this procedure.

Radiologic procedures: Flat-plate abdominal x-ray study may reveal free air under the diaphragm, which suggests perforation. A chest x-ray is taken to establish baseline pulmonary status. Barium studies usually are reserved for nonemergent situations to verify the presence of tumors or other large GI lesions.

Angiography: If the bleeding is rapid and suspected of being arterial or from a large vein, selective angiography of various GI arterial systems may aid in the visualization of bleeding site(s). If the bleeding site is clearly identified, therapeutic embolization may be attempted during angiography.

COLLABORATIVE MANAGEMENT

The overall goal of management is to stop bleeding and prevent rebleeding.

Fluid and electrolyte management: Volume replacement in acute GI bleeding must be performed as quickly as possible. Two large-bore IV lines (14- or 16-gauge) are inserted, and rapid fluid resuscitation is initiated. Crystalloid replacement therapy is initiated with normal saline or lactated Ringer's. Almost all patients with unstable VS and poor tissue oxygenation should be transfused. Packed cells and fresh-frozen plasma should be balanced to provide replacement of cells and clotting components. Generally, fresh-frozen plasma is required after 10 units of packed RBCs are infused. All blood components should be warmed to prevent hypothermia. Large transfusions will cause Ca^{++} to bind with the citrate (the preservative in stored blood) and deplete free Ca^{++} levels. In addition, large-volume blood transfusions can lead to coagulopathy disorders. Vasopressors and inotropic agents should be used *only* if tissue perfusion remains compromised despite adequate intravascular volume replacement. Hemodynamic monitoring is essential for continuous evaluation of the patient's volume status, especially in patients > 50 yr of age or those with chronic illnesses such as cardiovascular, pulmonary, renal, or hepatic disease. Overaggressive volume resuscitation results in fluid volume excess with complications of cardiac failure and pulmonary edema. Electrolyte levels are closely monitored, especially in patients with renal or hepatic disease.

Respiratory support: Because of a decrease in the oxygen-carrying capacity of the RBCs in massive blood loss, oxygen therapy by nasal cannula or face mask is initiated. Continuous or frequent pulse oximetry monitoring is recommended in actively bleeding patients to ensure adequate oxygenation. More aggressive ventilatory support may be required for patients with persistent hypoxemia and other evidence of early respiratory failure or impending ARDS (see p. 189).

T A B L E 8 - 15   Stigmata of Recent Hemorrhage (SRH)

Characteristic endoscopic findings of recent upper gastrointestinal, nonvariceal hemorrhage:
- Active bleeding
- Nonbleeding visible vessel or pigmented protuberance (red, blue, purple, or white elevated mound protruding from the base of the ulcer)
- Adherent or overlying clot without oozing
- Flat, dark slough or spot on the ulcer base

These findings are indicative of high risk for rebleed, requiring more aggressive therapy. For patients who do not exhibit these findings, the risk of rebleeding is significantly lower.

Nutritional support: As soon as the patient's hemodynamic status stabilizes, nutritional support must be considered. TPN is started for patients whose status is likely to remain NPO for days to weeks. Enteral or oral feedings are started when there is no further evidence of GI hemorrhage and bowel function has returned.

Gastric intubation: Gastric intubation is often necessary, especially with upper GI bleeding. Gastric lavage is performed using room-temperature saline to clear blood and clots from the stomach and to allow for estimation of ongoing blood loss. A lavage free of blood suggests a lower GI source of bleeding. There is no evidence that lavage stops the bleeding. Gastric intubation is avoided if esophageal varices are the suspected bleeding source.

Endoscopic therapies: Endoscopic modalities including laser, heater probe, and injection therapy are generally effective in stopping bleeding. Early endoscopy increases diagnostic accuracy, reduces the risk of rebleeding, and decreases the length of hospitalization. Complications include perforation and Mallory-Weiss syndrome. Sigmoendoscopy and colonoscopy may be useful for lower GI bleed.

Pharmacotherapy: Of the pharmacologic agents used to treat active ulcer bleeding and to prevent rebleed, including H_2-receptor agonists, proton-pump inhibitors, prostaglandins, vasopressin, octreotide, only proton pump inhibitors show sufficient evidence of efficacy.

Gastric alkalization with antacids, histamine H_2-receptor antagonists, and other agents is marginally effective in preventing and controlling ulceration, but may contribute to nosocomial pneumonia as a result of increased gastric bacterial counts and the possibility of aspiration. Some recommend sucralfate therapy to coat over gastric alkalization because it does not affect gastric pH.

Antacids: Raise the gastric pH level and decrease the corrosiveness of gastric acid. May help control pain.

Histamine H_2-receptor antagonists (e.g., famotidine, ranitidine): Block gastric acid and pepsin secretion and are employed in the treatment of erosive and ulcerative disease. Cimetidine is avoided in critically ill patients because it inhibits certain liver enzymes, resulting in potential drug interactions.

Sucralfate (Carafate): Oral sucralfate may be prescribed for patients with gastric erosions. The sucralfate combines with gastric acid and forms an adhesive protective coating over damaged mucosa. Frequently causes constipation.

Misoprostol (Cytotec): Synthetic prostaglandin E_1 that enhances the body's normal mucosal protective mechanisms and decreases acid secretion.

Omeprazole (Prilosec): A proton pump inhibitor; deactivates the enzyme system that pumps hydrogen ions from the parietal cells, thus inhibiting gastric acid secretion.

Vasopressin and octreotide: Decrease splanchnic blood flow via vasoconstriction.

Gastric pH monitoring: Performed to assess the pH of gastric contents (intraluminal pH) or of gastric mucosal tissue (intramural pH). The goal of therapy is to maintain gastric pH within a given range, usually 4.0-5.0. Intraluminal pH is measured by aspirating gastric secretions and testing the aspirate with a pH indicator paper. Some gastric tubes have an electronic pH meter attached to the distal end that permits continuous monitoring of intraluminal pH. A more sophisticated device is the gastrointestinal tonometer and sump tube, which measures gastric mucosal pH. Because the gut is especially vulnerable to ischemia associated with hypoperfusion and septic shock states, the intramural pH is a valuable early predictor of intestinal ischemia, sepsis, and multisystem organ dysfunction.

Surgical management: Many surgical techniques are used, depending on the location and severity of the lesion. Ulcerative disease requires surgery if the lesions continue to bleed despite aggressive medical therapy, or if complications such as perforation or obstruction develop. Oversewing of the bleeding vessel usually is followed by an acid-reducing procedure. In the patient whose condition is unstable, vagotomy and pyloroplasty are performed. Antrectomy or parietal cell vagotomy may be performed in patients whose condition is more stable. A common procedure for duodenal ulcers is gastrojejunostomy (Billroth II procedure). Massive lower GI bleeding is difficult to control and may require aggressive surgical procedures such as a colectomy with the creation of a permanent ileostomy or internal ileal pouch. If GI bleeding is caused by Gastroesophageal Varices, see p. 417.

NURSING DIAGNOSES AND INTERVENTIONS

Fluid volume deficit related to active loss secondary to hemorrhage from the GI tract
Desired outcome: Within 8 hr of this diagnosis, patient becomes normovolemic as evidenced by MAP ≥ 70 mm Hg; HR 60-100 beats/min; CVP 2-6 mm Hg; PAWP 6-12 mm Hg; CI ≥ 2.5 L/min/m^2; Hgb approximately 10 g/dl or greater, and urinary output ≥ 0.5 ml/kg/hr.

• Monitor BP q15min during episodes of rapid, active blood loss or unstable VS. Be alert to MAP decreases of > 10 mm Hg from previous reading.
• Monitor postural VS on patient's admission, q4-8h, and more frequently if recurrence of active bleeding is suspected: measure BP and HR with patient in a supine position, followed immediately by measurement of BP and HR with patient in a sitting position (as tolerated). A decrease

in systolic BP >10 mm Hg or an increase in HR of 10 beats/min with patient in a sitting position suggests a significant intravascular volume deficit, with approximately 15%-20% loss of volume.

> **Note:** Increases in HR may be caused by other factors, such as pain and anxiety.

- Monitor HR, ECG, and cardiovascular status hourly, or more frequently in the presence of active bleeding or unstable VS. Be alert to a sudden increase in HR, which suggests hypovolemia.
- Measure central pressures and thermodilution CO q1-4h. Be alert to low or decreasing CVP, PAWP, and CO. Calculate SVR q4-8h, or more frequently in patients whose condition is unstable. An elevated HR, decreased PAWP, decreased CO (CI <2.5 L/min/m^2), and increased SVR suggest hypovolemia and the need for volume restoration.
- Replace volume with prescribed fluids (usually a combination of crystalloid and blood products) via large-bore IV (18-gauge or larger) catheter. If blood transfusion is required see following interventions:
  - ❑ Monitor Hct; consult physician for values <28%-30%. Assess Hct 15 min after transfusion completion.
  - ❑ Monitor international normalized ratio (INR) values; administer fresh-frozen plasma (FFP) to maintain INR near 1.3.
  - ❑ Monitor serum calcium levels closely because of tendency to bind with citrate.
  - ❑ Prepare for platelet transfusion if platelets fall below 50,000 or following 10 units of packed RBCs.
- Measure urinary output hourly. Be alert to output <0.5 ml/kg/hr for 2 consecutive hours. Increase fluid intake if decreased output is caused by hypovolemia and hypoperfusion.
- Measure and record all GI blood losses from hematemesis, hematochezia, and melena.
- Check all stools and gastric contents for occult blood.
- Ensure proper function and patency of gastric tubes. Do not occlude the air vent of double-lumen tubes, because this may result in vacuum occlusion. Confirm placement of gastric tube at least q8h, and reposition as necessary.
- Teach patient signs and symptoms of actual or impending GI hemorrhage: pain, nausea, vomiting of blood, dark stools, lightheadedness, and passage of frank blood in stools. Reinforce the importance of seeking medical attention promptly if signs of bleeding occur.
- Teach patient the importance of avoiding medications/agents with the potential for gastric irritation: aspirin, NSAIDs, ethanol.

NIC Bleeding Reduction: Gastrointestinal; Blood Products Administration; Fluid/Electrolyte Management; Shock Management: Volume; Hemodynamic Regulation; Gastrointestinal Intubation; Bleeding Precautions; Teaching: Individual; Surgical Preparation

Decreased cardiac output related to decreased preload secondary to acute blood loss

Desired outcome: Within 8 hr of this diagnosis, cardiac output returns to or approaches normal limits as evidenced by CI ≥2.5 L/min/m^2; MAP ≥70 mm Hg; urinary output ≥0.5 ml/kg/hr; normal sinus rhythm on ECG; distal pulses >2+ on a 0-4+ scale; and brisk capillary refill (<2 sec).

- Administer oxygen as prescribed to facilitate maximal oxygen delivery to the tissues.
- Monitor continuous or frequent pulse oximetry and ABG values for hypoxemia. Consult physician if arterial Pao$_2$ is <80 mm Hg or if oxygen saturation falls below 92%.
- Monitor ECG for evidence of myocardial ischemia (i.e., T wave depression, QT prolongation, ventricular dysrhythmias).
- Monitor for physical indicators of diminished cardiac output, including pallor, cool extremities, capillary refill delayed for >2-3 sec, and decreased or absent amplitude of distal pulses.
- Monitor VS and thermodilution CO, and replace volume as indicated (see the first five entries under "Fluid Volume Deficit" in preceding nursing diagnosis).
- Monitor urine output hourly; document and report urine output <0.5 ml/kg/hr for 2 consecutive hours.

NIC Cardiac Care: Acute; Oxygen Therapy; Respiratory Monitoring; Invasive Hemodynamic Monitoring; Dysrhythmia Management

Pain related to chemical or physical injury of GI mucosal surfaces caused by digestive juices and enzymes or tissue trauma

Desired outcomes: Within 2 hr of this diagnosis, patient's subjective evaluation of discomfort improves, as documented by a pain scale. Nonverbal indicators of discomfort, such as grimacing, are absent.

- Monitor and document presence of abdominal pain or discomfort. Devise a pain scale with patient, rating discomfort from 0 (no pain) to 10 (severe). Be aware that pain may disappear concomitantly with a bleeding episode inasmuch as blood covers and protects eroded tissue.
- Administer gastric alkalizing agents and sucralfate as prescribed to relieve pain caused by upper GI disorders.

- Measure gastric pH q2-4h or continuously. If measuring by gastric aspirate, be sure to use a clean syringe and discard the first aspirate to ensure accurate results. Adjust gastric alkalizing therapy to maintain pH of 4.0-5.0 or other prescribed range. Avoid excessive alkalization, which has been associated with increased risk of nosocomial pneumonia. As available, use NG tonometer to measure gastric mucosal pH.
- If opiate analgesics are prescribed for postoperative or severe pain, administer with caution. Many opiate analgesics cause vasodilation, thereby decreasing preload and afterload. For patients with GI bleeding and markedly reduced preload, opiate administration can result in dramatic hypotension.
- Monitor respiratory rate and depth to avoid opiate-induced respiratory depression.
- Because anxiety reduction contributes to pain relief, ensure consistency and promptness in delivering analgesic.
- Supplement analgesics with nonpharmacologic maneuvers to aid in pain reduction. Modify patient's body position to optimize comfort. Patients who have pain associated with gastric reflux may be more comfortable with HOB elevated, if this position does not compromise hemodynamic status.

▌NIC Analgesic Administration; Pain Management; Distraction; Environmental Management; Vital Signs Monitoring
- See "Pain," p. 51, for additional interventions.

Altered nutrition: less than body requirements, related to inability to ingest or digest food secondary to vomiting, medically prescribed restrictions, or disease process
Desired outcome: Within 7 days of this diagnosis (or by the time of hospital discharge) patient has adequate nutrition as evidenced by stable weight, thyroxine-binding prealbumin 20-30 mg/dl, and a state of nitrogen balance on nitrogen studies.
- Collaborate with physician, dietitian, and pharmacist to estimate patient's individual metabolic needs on the basis of activity level, underlying disease process, and nutritional status before hospitalization.
- Provide parenteral nutrition during acute phase of the bleeding, as prescribed.
- Begin enteral therapy when acute hemorrhagic episode has subsided and bowel function has returned. This may take several weeks in some patients.
- Monitor thyroxine-binding prealbumin, and report decreasing levels.
- Weigh patient daily at the same time of day, using the same scale. Weight can be a practical indicator of nutritional status if patient's weight changes are interpreted on the basis of the following factors: fluid shifts (edema, diuresis, third spacing), surgical resection, and weight of dressings and equipment.

▌NIC Nutrition Management; Nutritional Monitoring; Total Parenteral Nutrition (TPN) Administration; Enteral Tube Feeding; Aspiration Precautions
- For additional information, see "Nutritional Support," p. 1.

Diarrhea related to irritation and increased motility secondary to the presence of blood in the GI tract
Desired outcome: By the time of hospital discharge, patient's stools are normal in consistency and frequency and negative for occult blood.
- Monitor and record the amount, frequency, and character of patient's stools.
- Provide or have bedpan or bedside commode (only for hemodynamically stable patients) readily available.
- Minimize embarrassing odor by removing stool promptly and using room deodorizers.
- Use matter-of-fact approach when assisting patient with frequent bowel elimination. Reassure patient that frequent elimination is a common problem for most patients with GI bleeding.
- Evaluate bowel sounds q4-8h. Anticipate normal to hyperdynamic bowel sounds. Absence of bowel sounds (especially in association with severe pain or abdominal distention) may signal serious complications such as ileus or perforation.
- Monitor serum sodium, potassium, and calcium levels, and consult physician for abnormalities. Normal values are serum sodium 137-147 mEq/L, serum potassium 3.5-5.0 mEq/L, and serum calcium 8.5-10.5 mg/dl.
- Keep patient on NPO status until diarrhea episodes have subsided.

▌NIC Diarrhea Management; Electrolyte Monitoring; Fluid/Electrolyte Management

ADDITIONAL NURSING DIAGNOSES

See other nursing diagnoses and interventions as appropriate: "Hemodynamic Monitoring," p. 23; "Prolonged Immobility," p. 61; "Psychosocial Support," p. 68; and "Psychosocial Support for the Patient's Family and Significant Others," p. 78.

Enterocutaneous Fistulas

PATHOPHYSIOLOGY

Enterocutaneous fistulas are formed when trauma, surgery, infection, neoplastic disease, or other pathologic condition results in a gastrointestinal-cutaneous communication. The incidence is often underreported or reported with poorly collected data. High-output proximal small bowel fistulas, which are generally defined as having an output > 500 ml/24 hr, are the most difficult to manage. Drainage from proximal fistulas is hypertonic; rich in enzymes, electrolytes, and proteins; thin in consistency; and tends to be copious. Losses as high as 2 L/24 hr are not uncommon. Extensive skin and tissue breakdown often occur because of the presence of activated pancreatic enzymes in fistula drainage. Electrolyte and protein loss is great with high-output proximal fistulas. Drainage from distal sites, such as the ileum and colon, is thick and of less volume than is proximal fistula drainage.

Three factors are associated with mortality in patients with enterocutaneous fistulas: (1) fluid and electrolyte imbalance, (2) malnutrition, and (3) sepsis. Fluid, potassium, sodium, and bicarbonate may be lost in great quantities. Replacement by enteral or parenteral nutrition is complex, and proper balance often is difficult to achieve. Sepsis is frequently associated with bowel fistulization, as either a cause or a result of anastomotic breakdown or as a result of local wound contamination or inadequate drainage. Hypercatabolism and malnutrition are associated with both sepsis and fistulization, creating a great demand for calories and protein. Aggressive nutritional support and meticulous local wound management are critical to patient survival.

ASSESSMENT

History and risk factors: Direct trauma to the GI system, especially to the bowel; infection of surgical wound, drainage tract, or peritoneum; prolonged catabolic state in association with bowel injury, GI neoplasm, GI abscess, or severely inflammatory bowel disease; and complex GI surgical procedures, such as lysis of adhesions for intestinal obstruction or complicated intestinal anastomosis.

Clinical presentation: Varies, according to cause and location of fistula. Discharge of obvious bile, enteric contents, or gas through a surgical incision is an obvious sign of fistulization, as is a sudden increase in the amount of drainage from a surgical incision or drainage catheter. A change in the nature of drainage from serous or serosanguineous to yellow, green, brown, or foul-smelling may indicate a fistula. With pancreatic drainage, a change to milky white suggests a pancreatic fistula. Mental confusion is often present as a result of electrolyte imbalance, dehydration, or early sepsis. Dry mouth, loss of tissue turgor, sunken eyes, and a decreasing urinary output with increasing specific gravity are expected if excessive fluid loss results in dehydration. Erythema, maceration, and edema may be present because of irritating fistula drainage. With persistent fistulization, loss of weight and muscle mass is anticipated because of protein loss and hypercatabolism.

Physical assessment: Sunken eyes, poor skin turgor, and dry oral mucosa, which are associated with dehydration; peripheral edema and muscle wasting related to protein loss; diminished or absent bowel sounds if peritonitis or ileus is present; discomfort and guarding on abdominal palpation over an abdominal mass (abscess) or near a drain site or surgical incision; tenderness, erythema, and possibly pain at the incision/fistula site caused by irritation from fistula output or infection; and muscle weakness and irregular HR if hypokalemia is present. Other assessment findings related to the underlying disease state (e.g., trauma, neoplasm, infection, pancreatitis) may be present.

Vital signs and hemodynamic monitoring: Increased temperature and tachycardia due to infection or dehydration; and decreased BP, PAP, and CO if dehydration is present. If early sepsis is present, expect elevated CO and decreased SVR. Oxygen demand is increased and may exceed supply. Svo_2 will fall without aggressive pulmonary and cardiovascular support. The patient will exhibit general hemodynamic instability until fluid balance, inflammation, and infection are controlled.

DIAGNOSTIC TESTS

Radiography: Water-soluble contrast medium may be injected into the suspected fistula (fistulography) to identify the tract. An upper GI series may be indicated if the suspected fistula is proximal. CT may be used to identify and direct the drainage of abscesses associated with fistulization. An external fistula can be simply confirmed without radiology by the oral administration of methylene blue or charcoal. The visible presence of dye in the drainage confirms the presence of a fistula.

Biopsy: In patients with neoplastic disease a biopsy specimen of the fistula tract may be obtained to determine the presence of malignancy within the tract.

Culture: Fistula effluent from the stomach, duodenum, biliary tree, and pancreas may be cultured for evidence of infection. Small and large bowel fistulas are generally not cultured because of the expected presence of bacteria.

COLLABORATIVE MANAGEMENT

Nutritional support: With distal small bowel and colonic fistulas, enteral elemental diets may be infused into the proximal small bowel (postpyloric or jejunal feedings) if the patient is capable of proximal absorption. Enteral diets are sometimes used if the fistula is extremely proximal. In these patients the feeding is infused distal to the fistula into the jejunum via a fine, weighted intestinal feeding tube. Enteral feedings are slowed or discontinued if fistula output increases after initiation of feedings. Patients with proximal small bowel fistulas, prolonged adynamic ileus, or extensive intraabdominal sepsis usually require TPN. Providing sufficient calories, protein, electrolytes, and fluids for patients with high-output fistulas can be challenging (see "Nutritional Support," p. 1).

Fluid and electrolyte replacement: Normal saline IV solutions, usually with added potassium, are administered to maintain fluid and electrolyte balance. Often the amount to be delivered is prescribed in direct relation to fistula output, especially when the output is widely variable. Effluent from each fistula is measured separately for accurate estimation of specific electrolyte and fluid losses. In general, fistulas that are more proximal result in greater fluid, electrolyte, and protein losses than those that are distal.

Local fistula management: Ideally, drainage from each fistula is collected separately to assess individual fistula activity and healing. Individualized systems of gravity or gentle suction drainage and barrier skin protection are devised for each patient. Good local management reduces the incidence of wound-related bacteremias and increases the rate of wound healing.

Antibiotics: Indicated for infection, which is frequently present. Administration of aminoglycosides requires careful monitoring of peak and trough plasma levels to achieve adequate therapeutic results.

Surgery: A large percentage of patients with gastrocutaneous fistulas require surgery. Surgery is indicated in the following instances: (1) to close fistulas that continue to drain significant amounts despite absence of infection and appropriate nutritional support; (2) to explore and drain fistula tracts that could not be identified or drained by less invasive techniques; and (3) if overwhelming sepsis fails to respond to antibiotics and supportive therapy. In these cases immediate surgery is planned as a life-saving measure. The usual operation to close persistently draining fistulas is resection with end-to-end anastomosis. Postoperatively, parenteral nutrition and antibiotic coverage are continued. A gastrostomy usually is created to allow for prolonged intestinal decompression and drainage. The patient is expected to remain on NPO status for 1-2 wk after surgery, depending on the rate of healing and the return of bowel function.

NURSING DIAGNOSES AND INTERVENTIONS

Impaired tissue integrity related to chemical trauma, infection, or malnutrition
Desired outcome: Within 72 hr of this diagnosis, patient's tissue adjacent to the fistula is free of erythema, excoriation, and edema.
- Assess the extent of the local problem (Table 8-16). Consult physician for signs of extensive damage to the tissue adjacent to the fistula (i.e., severe local erythema, excoriation, edema, maceration).
- Establish drainage and collection system for each fistula (Table 8-17). Consult physician regarding use of continuous wound suction device(s).
- Note character, color, odor, and volume of output from each fistula. Consult physician for significant changes in any of these indicators.
- If increased fistula output results from oral or enteral feedings, eliminate or modify the feedings as prescribed.

T A B L E 8 - 16   Nursing Assessment of the Enterocutaneous Fistula

- Evaluate size, shape, and location of the fistula. Reposition or lift skin folds as necessary.
- Identify any potential leakage tracks created by skin folds or body hollows.
- Examine the condition of adjacent skin and tissue. Note the presence and spread of both erythema and excoriation, which suggest leakage tracks.
- Note the consistency and character of fistula output.
- Assess each fistula separately.
- Document all findings, and compare them with baseline assessment made at the time of initial evaluation.

T A B L E 8 - 17   Recommendations for Containing Fistula Drainage

- Clean the intact skin surrounding the fistula with a nonirritating antibacterial cleanser.
- Clip body hair (if present) around the fistula.
- Remove pooled drainage from the wound and surrounding area by using sterile absorbent pads or gentle suction. The help of an assistant may be necessary to maintain a dry field during application of the collection device.
- Apply a barrier powder (e.g., karaya or Orahesive) to an excoriated skin. A flexible transparent dressing (e.g., Op-Site) can be used to protect intact skin.
- Use a skin paste (e.g., Stomahesive or karaya) to fill in any grooves surrounding recessed fistulas.
- Apply a sized barrier sheet (e.g., Stomahesive, HolliHesive) to the surrounding skin, being careful not to overlap the fistula.
- Attach a collecting bag to the barrier sheet base. For high-output fistulas, a urostomy bag and collecting system may be necessary. Transparent appliances enable observation of drainage. Devices that have a drainage opening permit emptying and measurement of output.
- Reposition the patient frequently to optimize gravity of fistula output. For example, it sometimes is necessary to use a rotating bed frame or a bed modified with foam blocks to facilitate prone positioning.

- Consult ostomy nurse or enterostomal therapist for recommendations in pouching complex or multiple fistulas.

NIC Wound Care; Dressing; Ostomy Care; Tube Care; Fluid/Electrolyte Management
- See "Altered Nutrition," which follows, and "Risk for Infection," immediately after, for interventions that optimize nutrition and prevent infection.

Altered nutrition: less than body requirements, related to protein loss via fistula output, disruption of GI tract continuity, or absorptive disorder

Desired outcome: By the time of hospital discharge, patient has adequate nutrition as evidenced by food intake that increases to his or her recommended daily allowance, and body weight that returns to baseline or within 10% of patient's ideal weight.

- Collaborate with physician, dietitian, and pharmacist to estimate patient's metabolic needs on the basis of activity level, estimated metabolic rate, and baseline nutritional status.
- Monitor for the presence of bowel sounds q8h. If bowel sounds are absent, withhold oral or enteral feedings.
- If fistula output increases in response to enteral feedings, slow the rate of infusion or reduce the strength of the feeding. If the patient tolerates oral feedings but they increase fistula output, increase the frequency of the feedings and decrease the amount consumed at each feeding.
- Be aware that when the entire intestine is not available for normal absorption, elemental feeding formulas (see Table 1-2) may be more readily absorbed.
- Prepare patient for parenteral feedings if oral/enteral feedings are inadequate for patient's requirements.

NIC Nutrition Management; Nutritional Monitoring; Fluid/Electrolyte Management; Total Parenteral Nutrition (TPN) Administration; Enteral Tube Feeding
- For additional information, see "Nutritional Support," p. 1.

Risk for infection related to inadequate primary defenses (altered integumentary system, disruption in continuity of GI system), hypercatabolic state, presence of invasive lines, and protein loss/malnutrition

Desired outcome: Patient remains free of infection as evidenced by core or rectal temperature <37.8° C (100° F); negative culture results; HR 60-100 beats/min; RR 12-20 breaths/min; BP within patient's normal range; and orientation to time, place, and person.

- Check rectal or core temperature q4h for increases.
- If temperature suddenly rises, assess patient for potential sources, noting presence of purulent secretions; erythema around wound, drain, or fistula site; and pain, tenderness, or masses with abdominal palpation. Consult physician for temperature elevation and assessment findings. Obtain specimens for culture of likely sites for infection as prescribed by physician or unit protocol.
- Evaluate orientation and LOC q4h. Document and report significant deviations from baseline values.
- Monitor BP, HR, RR, CO, and SVR q4h. Be alert to increases in HR and RR associated with temperature elevations. As available, monitor Svo_2 continuously or at scheduled intervals. An elevated

CO and a decreased SVR suggest early septic shock (see Table 4-24, p. 292, for a complete hemodynamic profile; also see "Septic Shock," p. 501).
- Administer parenteral antibiotics in a timely fashion. Reschedule antibiotics if a dosage is delayed for more than 1 hr. Recognize that failure to administer antibiotics on schedule can result in inadequate blood levels and treatment failure. Aminoglycosides are used frequently; administer agents promptly, and monitor patient for potential complications (Table 8-18).
- Optimize gravity drainage of fistula by prone or upright positioning as tolerated by patient.
- Wear gloves when contact with drainage is possible. Prevent transmission of potentially infectious agents by washing hands thoroughly before and after caring for patient and carefully disposing of dressings and drainage.

NIC Medication Management; Hemodynamic Regulation; Vital Signs Monitoring; Temperature Regulation; Intravenous (IV) Therapy; Wound Care

Fluid volume deficit related to active loss secondary to fistula drainage

Desired outcome: Within 8 hr of this diagnosis, patient becomes normovolemic as evidenced by balanced daily I&O; urinary output ≥0.5 ml/kg/hr; moist mucous membranes; good skin turgor; HR ≤100 beats/min; CVP 2-6 mm Hg; and PAWP 6-12 mm Hg.
- Evaluate patient's fluid balance by calculating and comparing daily I&O. In patients with high-output fistulas, evaluate total I&O q8h. Record all sources of output, including drainage from each fistula. Replace fistula output with prescribed fluid (usually a balanced salt solution containing potassium) q2-8h.
- Measure urine output q1-4h. Consult physician if urine output is <0.5 ml/kg/hr or if specific gravity increases and urine volume decreases.
- Assess and document condition of mucous membranes and skin turgor. Dry membranes and inelastic skin indicate inadequate fluid volume and the need for increase in fluid intake (PO or IV route).
- Measure and evaluate VS, CVP, and PAP (when available) q1-4h, depending on hemodynamic stability. Be alert to increasing HR, decreasing CVP, and decreasing PAP, which indicate inadequate intravascular volume. Encourage increased oral intake (if possible), or consult with physician regarding increase in IV fluid intake.
- Control sources of insensible fluid loss by humidifying oxygen, maintaining comfortable environment, and controlling fever (if present) with antipyretics such as acetaminophen.

NIC Fluid/Electrolyte Management; Fluid Monitoring; Hemodynamic Regulation; Hypovolemia Management; Invasive Hemodynamic Monitoring; Shock Prevention

Body image disturbance related to biophysical change secondary to presence of external fistula

Desired outcome: By the time of hospital discharge, patient acknowledges body changes as evidenced by viewing fistula and not exhibiting preoccupation with or depersonalization of fistula.
- Evaluate the patient's reaction to the fistula by observing and noting evidence of body image disturbance (see Table 1-40).
- Anticipate feelings of shock and repulsion initially. Be aware that the development of an external fistula usually is an unanticipated complication and patients are not emotionally prepared for the disfigurement.
- Anticipate and acknowledge normalcy of feelings of rejection, isolation, and uncleanliness (because of odor and possible presence of feces).
- Offer patient opportunity to view fistula/wound as desired. Use mirrors if necessary.
- Encourage patient and significant others to verbalize feelings regarding fistula/wound.

T A B L E 8 - 18   *Aminoglycoside Antibodies: Nursing Applications*

- Administer prepared solution over 30-60 min, according to recommendations for specific agent. Too-rapid administration increases the risk of toxicity.
- Reschedule if dosage is delayed >1 hr.
- Obtain serum specimen in a timely fashion so that peak and trough levels can be evaluated adequately.
- Monitor patient for evidence of hearing loss.
- Monitor BUN and creatinine levels and urinary output, which are indicators of renal function.
- Be aware that older adults are especially susceptible to ototoxic and nephrotoxic effects of these medications.
- To avoid potential incompatibilities/interactions, administer to separate sites and stagger schedules when penicillin and cephalosporins are also prescribed.

- If possible, offer the patient an opportunity to participate in wound care. Patient may be able to perform simple tasks, such as holding the bag into which you will deposit the soiled dressing or applying the pouch that collects drainage.
- Convey an accepting attitude toward the patient. Many fistulas that require critical care involve open and infected wounds. If the attending nurse is inexperienced in dressing these complex wounds, another, more experienced nurse should be present during the initial dressing change.
- Reassure patient that the fistula is not permanent. Acknowledge that a scar will be visible but the fistula will close with appropriate care.

NIC Body Image Enhancement; Coping Enhancement; Self-Care Assistance; Support System Enhancement

Altered oral mucous membrane related to prolonged NPO status

Desired outcome: Within 24 hr of this diagnosis, patient's oral mucosa is intact, moist, and free of pain and oral lesions.

- Inspect the patient's oral cavity, noting the degree of moisture, inflammation, bleeding, or lesions. Consult physician for open lesions and bleeding.
- Assist patient with brushing teeth with a soft-bristle toothbrush. Irrigate the oral cavity with a solution of 500 ml normal saline and 15 ml sodium bicarbonate. Provide mouth care q4h.
- For patients with altered LOC, massage gums and teeth with saline-moistened, sponge-tipped applicator and brush teeth gently if there is no evidence of bleeding. Place patient in a side-lying position, and irrigate the mouth with small amounts of a saline and bicarbonate solution (per second entry). Carefully suction the solution from the oral cavity throughout the procedure with a Yankauer tonsil suction device.
- Keep the lips moist with emollients such as lanolin or Eucerin cream. Take care to apply emollient to external tissue only. Oil-containing emollients are harmful if aspirated or otherwise introduced into the respiratory tract.

NIC Oral Health Promotion; Oral Health Maintenance

ADDITIONAL NURSING DIAGNOSES

See "Nutritional Support," p. 1, for additional information about the patient with extra nutritional needs. See "Psychosocial Support," p. 68, for psychosocial nursing diagnoses and interventions. Also see nursing diagnoses and interventions related to sepsis under "Septic Shock," p. 501.

Reference

Gines P, Arroya V, Rodes J: Renal function in cirrhosis: pathophysiology and clinical features. In Zakim D, Boyer TD, editors: *Hepatology: a textbook of liver diseases,* ed 4, Philadelphia, 2003, Saunders.

Bibliography

Afdhal NH: Diagnosing fibrosis in hepatitis C: is the pendulum swinging from biopsy to blood tests? *Hepatology* 37(5):72-974, 2003.

Al-Omran M, Groof A, Wilke D: Enteral versus parenteral nutrition for acute pancreatitis (Cochrane Review). In The Cochrane Library, Issue 4, Chichester, UK, 2003, John Wiley & Sons.

Al-Saden PC: Cirrhosis. In Daly-Gawenda D, editor: *Manual of medical-surgical nursing: med-surg fact finder,* Boston, 1997, Little, Brown.

Al-Saden PC et al: Hepatitis C: an emerging dilemma, *Am Assoc Occupat Health Nurses* 47:217-222, 1999.

Alter H et al: Viral hepatitis. In *Advances in therapeutic hepatology: a world view,* Chicago, 1998, Course booklet at the International Association for the Study of Liver Diseases.

Arguedas MR: The critically ill liver patient: the variceal bleeder, *Semin Gastrointest Dis* 14(1):34-38, 2003.

Arroyo V: Refractory ascites and hepatorenal syndrome (HRS). In *Complications of cirrhosis: pathogenesis, consequences and therapy* (Postgraduate course book), 2001, American Association for the Study of Liver Diseases.

Arroyo V & Jimenez W: Clinical need for antidiuretic hormone antagonists in cirrhosis, *Hepatology* 37(1):13-15, 2003.

Balthazar, EJ: Staging of acute pancreatitis, *Radiol Clin North Am* 40(6):1199-1209, 2002.

Bernard B et al: Antibiotic prophylaxis for the prevention of bacterial infections in cirrhotic patients with gastrointestinal bleeding: a meta-analysis, *Hepatology* 29(6):1655-1661, 1999.

Blei AT: Hepatic encephalopathy. In *Complications of cirrhosis: pathogenesis, consequences and therapy* (Postgraduate course book), 2001, American Association for the Study of Liver Diseases.

Blendis L & Wong F: Prevention of varices rebleeding: are drugs better after all? From "Selected Summaries" in *Gastroenterology* 122(3):832-833, 2002.

Bosch J, Abraldes JG, Groszmann R: Current management of portal hypertension, *J Hepatol* 38: S54-S68, 2003.

Bosscha K et al: Quality of life after severe bacterial peritonitis and infected necrotizing pancreatitis treated with open management of the abdomen and planned re-operations, *Crit Care Med* 29(8):1539-1543, 2001.

Burch J: The nursing care of a patient with enterocutaneous faecal fistulae, *Br J Nurs* 12(12): 736-740, 2003.

Bureau C et al: "A la carte" treatment of portal hypertension: adapting medical therapy to hemodynamic response for the prevention of bleeding, *Hepatology* 36(6):1361-1366, 2002.

Chase SL: Even low doses of NSAIDs pose a GI threat, *RN* 61(3):78, 1998.

Dargan PI, Jones AL: Acetaminophen poisoning: an update for the intensivist, *Crit Care* 6(2): 108-110, 2002.

de Franchis R: Risk of bleeding from esophageal and gastric varices and gastropathy. In *Complications of cirrhosis: pathogenesis, consequences and therapy* (Postgraduate course book), 2001, American Association for the Study of Liver Diseases.

de Franchis R: Evaluation and follow-up of patients with cirrhosis and oesophageal varices, *J Hepatol* 38:361-363, 2003.

de Franchis R, Primignani M: Natural history of portal hypertension in patients with cirrhosis, *Clin Liver Dis* 5(3):645-663, 2001.

DiMango EP, Suresh C: Acute pancreatitis. In Feldman M, Freidman LS, Sleisenger MH, editors: *Gastrointestinal and liver disease pathophysiology/diagnosis/management,* Philidelphia, 2002, Saunders.

Dochterman JM, Bulechek GM, editors: *Nursing interventions classification (NIC),* ed 4, St Louis, 2004, Mosby.

Dupont H, Carbon C, Carlet J: Monotherapy with a broad spectrum beta-lactams as effective as its combination with an aminoglycoside in treatment of severe generalized pancreatitis: a multicenter randomized controlled trail, *Antimicrob Agent Chemother* 44:2028, 2000.

Fallon MB: Hepatopulmonary syndrome and portopulmonary hypertension. In *Complications of cirrhosis: pathogenesis, consequences and therapy* (Postgraduate course book), 2001, American Association for the Study of Liver Diseases.

Farrell JJ, Freidman LS: Evaluating and managing GI bleeding in the elderly: atypical presentations can complicate the workup, *J Crit Illness* 18(5):227-236, 2003.

Ferenci P et al and the members of the Working Party: Hepatic encephalopathy-definition, nomenclature, diagnosis, and quantification: Final report of the working party at the 11th World Congresses of Gastroenterology, Vienna, 1998, *Hepatology* 35(3):716-721, 2002.

Forsmark CE: Chronic pancreatitis. In Feldman M., Freidman LS, Sleisenger MH, editors: *Gastrointestinal and liver disease pathophysiology/diagnosis/management,* Philadelphia, 2002, Saunders.

Frossard JL et al: Erythromycin intravenous bolus infusion in acute upper gastrointestinal bleeding: a randomized, controlled, double-blind trial, *Gastroenterology* 123 (1):17-23, 2002.

Ganger DR: Liver failure. In Parrillo JP, Dellinger RP: *Critical care medicine,* ed 2, St. Louis, 2002, Mosby.

Garcia-Pagan JC: Pharmacological therapy of acute bleeding. In *Complications of cirrhosis: pathogenesis, consequences and therapy* (Postgraduate course book), 2001, American Association for the Study of Liver Diseases.

Garcia-Tsao G: Antibiotic prophylaxis in variceal bleeding. In *Complications of cirrhosis: pathogenesis, consequences and therapy* (Postgraduate course book), 2001, American Association for the Study of Liver Diseases.

Gines P, Ortega R: Role of large-volume paracentesis and importance of albumin. In *Complications of cirrhosis: pathogenesis, consequences and Therapy* (Postgraduate course book), 2001, American Association for the Study of Liver Diseases.

Grace ND: Diagnosis and treatment of gastrointestinal bleeding secondary to portal hypertension, *Gastroenterology* 92(7), 1997.

Grace ND: Pharmacological prevention of first and recurrent variceal bleeding. In *Complications of cirrhosis: pathogenesis, consequences and therapy* (Postgraduate course book), 2001, American Association for the Study of Liver Diseases.

Grace ND et al.: Portal hypertension and variceal bleeding: an AASLD single topic symposium, *Hepatology* 28(3):868-880, 1998.

Grap MJ et al: Oral care in the adult intensive care unit, *Am J Crit Care* 12:113-119, 2003.

Green RM, Flamm S: AGA technical review on the evaluation of liver chemistry tests, *Gastroenterology* 123(4):1367-1384, 2002.

Hashizume M et al: Laparoscopic gastric devascularization and splenectomy for sclerotherapy-resistant esophagogastric varices with hypersplenism, *J Am Coll Surg* 187(3):263-270, 1998.

Henderson JM: Surgical management: shunts vs. liver transplant. In *Complications of cirrhosis: pathogenesis, consequences and therapy* (Postgraduate course book), 2001, American Association for the Study of Liver Diseases:169-173, Nov 9-10, 2001.

Henriksen JH, Moller S, Bendtsen F: The heart, arterial compliance and vascular resistance in cirrhosis, In *Complications of cirrhosis: pathogenesis, consequences and therapy* (Postgraduate course book), 2001, American Association for the Study of Liver Diseases.

Hoofnagle JH: Chronic viral hepatitis. In *Clinical and pathological correlations in liver disease: approaching the next millennium* (Post-graduate course book), Chicago, at the American Association for the Study of Liver Diseases, 1998.

Katerndahl D: In reply: Meperine or morphine in acute pancreatitis (Letter to the editor), *Am Fam Physician* July 15, 2001: www.aafp.org.

Kircheis G et al: Critical flicker frequency for quantification of low-grade hepatic encephalopathy, *Hepatology* 35(2):357-366, 2002.

LaBerge JM: TIPS: initial therapy or last resort? In *Complications of cirrhosis: pathogenesis, consequences and therapy* (Postgraduate course book), 2001, American Association for the Study of Liver Diseases.

Lee F, Cundiff D: Meperidine vs morphine in pancreatitis and cholecystitis, *Arch Intern Med* 158(21):2399, 1998.

Lichenstein GR: American Gastroenterological Association medical position statement: Evaluation of liver chemistry tests; *Gastroenterology* 123(4):1364-1366.

Lindor KO, Dickson ER, editors: Pbc, psc, and adult cholangiopathies, *Clin Liver Dis* 2(2):217-449, 1998.

Meguid MM, Campos ACL: Nutritional management of gastrointestinal fistulas, *Surg Clin North Am* 76(5):1035-1080, 1996.

Mergenger K, Baillic J: Fortnightly review: acute pancreatitis, *Br Med J* 316(7124):44-48, 1998.

Merli M et al.: Incidence and natural history of small esophageal varices in cirrhotic patients, *J Hepatol* 38:266-272, 2003.

Minei JP, Champine JG: Abdominal abscesses and gastrointestinal fistulas. In Feldman M, Freidman LS, Sleisenger MH, editors: *Gastrointestinal and liver disease pathophysiology/diagnosis/management,* Philadelphia, 2002, Saunders.

Mizock BA: Nutritional support. In Parrillo JE, Dellinger RP: *Critical care medicine,* ed 2, St Louis, 2002, Mosby.

Munro CL, Grap MJ: Oral health and care in the intensive care unit: state of the science, *Crit Care Nurse* 13(1):25-33, 2004.

Pessoa MG et al: Quantitation of hepatitis G and C virus in the liver: evidence that hepatitis G virus is not hepatotropic, *Hepatology* 27:877-880, 1998.

Pianka JD, Affronti J: Management principles of gastrointestinal bleeding, *Prim Care* 28(3):557-574, 2001.

Podnos YD et al: Failure of the King's College Hospital criteria to predict outcome in a patient with acetaminophen toxicity and fulminant hepatic failure, *Hosp Physician* Sept:53-56, 2001.

Powers J, Chance R, Bortenschlager L: Bedside placement of small bowel feeding tubes in the intensive care unit, *Crit Care Nurse* 23(1):16-24, 2003.

Qadir MT et al: Penicillium peritonitis in a patient receiving continuous ambulatory peritoneal dialysis, *Heart Lung* 27(1):67-68, 1998.

Quillen SM: Identification of acute pancreatitis in the ambulatory setting, *Gastroenterol Nurs* 24(1): 20-22, 2001.

Schwartz SI et al, editors: *Principles of surgery,* ed 7, New York, 1999, McGraw-Hill.

Schaffner JA, Gastrointestinal bleeding; acute pancreatitis. In Parrillo JE , Dellinger RP: *Critical care medicine* ed 2, St Louis, 2002, Mosby.

Selvey LA et al: Is there evidence for vector transmission of GBV-C? *Lancet* 351:1104-1105, 1998.

Shakil AO, Mazariegos GV, Kramer DJ: Fulminant hepatic failure. In Fung JJ, Rakela J, editors: *Surg Clin North Am* 79:77-108, 1999.

Sharara AI, Rockey DC: Therapy for primary prophylaxis of varices: and the winner is....? From Hepatology Elsewhere in *Hepatology* 37(2):473-475, 2003.

Stacy KM: Gastrointestinal disorders and therapeutic management. In Urden LD, Stacy KM, Lough ME, editors: *Thelan's critical care nursing diagnosis and management,* St. Louis, 2002, Mosby.

Sung JC: Update on treatment of variceal hemorrhage, *Dig Dis* 20(2):134-144, 2002.

Thuluvath PJ, Morss S, Thompson R: Spontaneous bacterial peritonitis—in-hospital mortality, predictors of survival, and health care costs from 1988 to 1998, *Am J Gastroenterol* 96:1232–1236, 2001.

Trujillo EB, Robinson MK, Jacobs DO: Feeding critically ill patients: current concepts, *Crit Care Nurse* 21:131-134, 2001.

Trupp R: Case presentation: a gastroventricular fistula resulting from peptic ulcer disease, *Heart Lung* 27(1):71-73, 1998.

Van Stiegmann G: Endoscopic therapy: banding vs. sclerotherapy and other treatments. In *Complications of cirrhosis: pathogenesis, consequences and therapy* (Postgraduate course book), 2001, American Association for the Study of Liver Diseases.

Vaquero J, Blei AT: Fulminant hepatic failure; etiology and management in 2003; *Curr Gastroenterol Reports* 5:39-47, 2003.

Wright JA: Seven abdominal assessment signs every emergency nurse should know, *J Emerg Nurs* 23(5):446-450, 1997.

Zakim D, Boyer TD, editors: *Hepatology: a textbook of liver diseases,* ed 4, Philadelphia, 2003, Saunders.

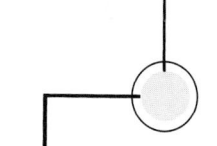

CHAPTER 9

Hematologic Dysfunctions

The hematologic or hematopoietic system involves the blood, the lymph, and components that form and circulate blood and lymph. Blood-forming organs include the bone marrow, the thymus gland, the liver, the spleen, and the lymph nodes. Lymph is derived from the interstitial fluid passing into the lymphatic capillaries. The primary functions of the hematologic system are the following:
• Respiratory gas exchange (oxygen [O_2] and carbon dioxide [CO_2])
• Delivery of nutrients to the body cells
• Elimination of wastes from the body cells
In addition, blood also has a role in these functions:
• Protection from foreign antigens and infectious organisms
• Temperature regulation
• Delivery of hormones
• Fluid and electrolyte balance
• Acid-base balance
Blood is composed of plasma, erythrocytes (red blood cells [RBCs]), leukocytes (white blood cells [WBCs]), and thrombocytes (platelets). Dysfunctions in the hematologic system lead to problems performing the eight functions listed above. The hematologic dysfunctions addressed in this chapter are anemias, bleeding, and thrombotic disorders.

Profound Anemias/Hemolytic Crisis

PATHOPHYSIOLOGY
For anemias
Anemia reflects a reduction in total body hemoglobin concentration and is common in critically ill patients. By the third day in an intensive care unit (ICU), 95% of patients have reduced hemoglobin concentrations. Anemia may be classified under one of three functional classes after initial evaluation of the complete blood count (CBC) and reticulocyte index. (See Table 9-1 for functional classification.)

As the hemoglobin decreases, the oxygen-carrying capacity of the blood is reduced, resulting in tissue hypoxia unless compensatory mechanisms are adequate to assist the body with oxygen delivery. Examples of anemias under each functional class are as follows:
❑ *Hemolysis/blood loss:* Hemolytic anemias caused by abnormal hemoglobin (i.e., hemoglobin S, C, D, and E), RBC membrane anomalies (e.g., spherocytosis, hemolytic uremic syndrome), physical trauma to blood (e.g., extracorporeal "bypass" circulation, balloon counterpulsation, prosthetic heart valves), abnormal RBC-related antibodies (e.g., drug-induced hemolysis), and presence of bacterial endotoxins (e.g., malaria, clostridia). Acute or chronic blood loss may be

TABLE 9-1   Functional Classes of Anemia

Blood loss/hemolysis	Decreased RBC production	Maturation disorders
Autoimmune diseases	Damaged bone marrow	Abnormal RBC cytoplasm
Abnormal hemoglobin	Iron deficiency	Abnormal RBC nucleus
Abnormal RBC membranes	Erythropoietin deficiency	Iron deficiency
Bleeding/hemorrhage	Inflammation/infection	
Excessive phlebotomies	Metabolic disturbance	

due to chronic gastrointestinal (GI) bleeding, excessive menstruation, trauma, ruptured blood vessel(s), multiple phlebotomies to obtain laboratory samples for diagnosis/monitoring, and other disorders.

❑ Decreased RBC/erythrocyte production: Iron deficiency, lead poisoning, thalassemias, megaloblastic/pernicious anemia, renal failure, aplastic/hypoplastic anemia, anemia of chronic inflammatory disease, anemia associated with critical illness.

❑ Maturation disorders: Iron deficiency

For hemolytic crisis

Hemolytic crisis is an acute disorder that frequently accompanies hemolytic anemias. It is characterized by premature pathologic destruction (hemolysis) of RBCs. As RBC destruction accelerates, the oxygen-carrying capacity of the blood decreases, which results in a reduction in the amount of oxygen delivered to the tissues. This hypoxic state produces tissue ischemia and can progress to tissue infarction. Hemolytic episodes can be triggered by both emotional and physiologic states, including stress, trauma, surgery, acute infectious processes, and abnormal immune responses.

ASSESSMENT

For anemias

Clinical presentation (chronic indicators): Pallor, melena, hematochezia, fatigue, weight loss, dyspnea on exertion, uremia, sensitivity to cold, intermittent dizziness, excessive menstruation, paresthesias, and history of iron deficiency, folic acid deficiency, and vitamin B_{12} deficiency.

❑ *Chronic hemolytic anemia:* Jaundice, renal failure, hematuria, arthritis, increased incidence of gallstones, skin ulcers.

Clinical presentation (acute indicators): Fever, chest pain, acute heart failure, confusion, irritability, tachycardia, orthostatic hypotension, dyspnea, tachypnea, frank bleeding, critical illness for >3 days.

Physical assessment: Inspection may reveal tachypnea, orthopnea, tachycardia, weight loss, altered mental status, spider angiomas, electrocardiogram (ECG) changes, unusual fatigue or weakness, smooth tongue, unusual bleeding (i.e., stool, urine, emesis), monoarticular or polyarticular arthritis, and skin ulcers. Palpation may detect bone tenderness (especially sternal), enlargement of the liver and/or spleen, and joint tenderness. Auscultation may reveal crackles associated with heart failure.

For hemolytic crisis

Risk factors: Individuals with mild or chronic hemolytic anemia may be asymptomatic until they are exposed to a severe stressor, such as an acute infectious process, profound emotional upset, critical illness, surgery, or trauma. With added stress, hemolysis can accelerate to a crisis state wherein patients experience organ congestion from massive amounts of hemolyzed blood cells, precipitating multiple organ dysfunction syndrome (MODS) and shock.

Clinical presentation (acute): Fever; abdominal, chest, joint, and back pain; jaundice; headache; dizziness; palpitations; shortness of breath (SOB); hemoglobinuria; lymphadenopathy; splenomegaly; and signs of peripheral nerve damage including paresthesias, paralysis, chills, and vomiting.

Clinical presentation (chronic): Anemia; pallor; fatigue; dyspnea on exertion; icterus; bone infarctions; monoarticular and polyarticular arthritis; hematuria; renal failure; increased gallstone formation; and skin ulcers.

Physical assessment: Depending on severity and duration of the anemia, the patient may exhibit impaired growth and development. Inspection may reveal the presence of jaundice, SOB, monoarticular or polyarticular arthritis, retinal detachment and associated vitreous hemorrhage, and hemiplegia. Palpation may demonstrate splenomegaly, lymphadenopathy, hepatomegaly, or abdominal guarding. Chronic skin ulcers may be seen, particularly in the ankle area.

DIAGNOSTIC TESTS FOR ANEMIA

RBCs: Reduced; in hemolytic crisis an increased number of premature RBCs will be present.

Reticulocyte count: RBC precursors; elevated because of increased bone marrow production of RBCs.

Hemoglobin (Hgb) and hematocrit (Hct): Decreased.

Morphologic classification of RBCs: Mean corpuscular volume (MCV).
- Macrocytic: MCV >100 mcg^3
- Microcytic: MCV <80 mcg^3
- Normocytic: MCV 80-100 mcg^3

Sickle cell test: Screens for the presence of hemoglobin S, which is indicative of sickle cell anemia.

Hemoglobin electrophoresis: Screens for abnormal hemoglobins often present in hemolytic anemias:
- *Hemoglobins A$_1$, A$_2$, and F:* Normally found in the body.
- *Hemoglobin C:* Causes RBCs to sickle.
- *Hemoglobins D and E:* Rarely occur "singly"; sometimes present with sickle cell disease or thalassemias.
- *Hemoglobin H:* Causes premature destruction of RBCs and abnormal binding of O_2 to the RBC.
- *Hemoglobin S:* Most common abnormal hemoglobin, occurring in 10% of the African American population; causes sickle cell disease or seen with sickle cell trait.

Erythrocyte sedimentation rate (ESR): Elevated in hemolytic anemia more often than in other anemias.

C$_3$ proactivator: Increased in hemolytic anemia.

Total iron-binding capacity (TIBC): Normal or reduced, depending on the type of anemia.

Ferritin: Reduced in patients with iron deficiency anemia; normal or elevated with anemia of critical illness.

Transferrin: Reduced with anemia of chronic inflammation, anemia of critical illness.

Transferrin saturation: Reduced with anemia of chronic inflammation, anemia of critical illness.

Serum iron: Reduced with iron deficiency anemia, anemia of chronic inflammation, anemia of critical illness.

Folate: Reduced with nutritional deficiency leading to megaloblastic anemia.

Erythropoietin (EP): Reduced in patients with renal disease and normal in those who are critically ill who should have an elevated level if anemia of any cause is present. Reticulocyte response to EP has been shown to be reduced in many critically ill patients with elevated EP levels.

Vitamin B$_{12}$: Reduced in patients with pernicious anemia.

Unconjugated bilirubin: Elevated in hemolytic anemia as a result of the liver's inability to process increasing bilirubin released during hemolysis.

Serum lactic dehydrogenase isoenzymes (LDH$_1$ and LDH$_2$): Elevated in hemolytic anemia because of the release of these enzymes when an RBC is destroyed.

Haptoglobin level: Decreased in hemolytic anemia as a result of increased binding of haptoglobin (a plasma protein) to facilitate removal of increased amounts of hemoglobin from the bloodstream.

Peripheral blood smear: May reveal abnormally shaped RBCs, such as spherocytes. Red cell hyperplasia is present in nearly all cases of chronic hemolysis with intact bone marrow.

Bone marrow aspiration: May reveal abnormal size, shape, or amounts of erythrocytes or reticulocytes in various anemias.

Coombs test: Positive in antibody-mediated/immunologic hemolysis.

Immunoglobulin levels: Frequently elevated with sickle cell disease.

Glucose-6-phosphate dehydrogenase (G6PD) levels: Decreased in G6PD deficiency, but cannot be tested while hemolysis is active.

Radiologic examinations/tests
- *X-rays and bone scans:* May reveal increased density or aseptic necrosis of the bones.
- *Liver/spleen scans:* May reveal disease or dysfunction of either organ, which may contribute to anemia.

COLLABORATIVE MANAGEMENT

All anemias

Volume replacement: If patient is hypovolemic, aggressive fluid and/or blood replacement is mandatory to prevent profound hypotension and shock. Fluid challenges/boluses also assist in prevention of deposition of hemolyzed RBCs in the microvasculature.

Transfusions/blood component replacement: Packed RBCs may be necessary in the management of profound anemia to help increase the blood's oxygen-carrying capacity. For patients who refuse blood transfusions, aggressive strategies to augment RBC production such as intravenous iron therapy and subcutaneous administration of erythropoietin may be implemented. These therapies may take up to 7 days to promote significant improvement in the reticulocyte count and hemoglobin and hematocrit levels. The oxygen-carrying capacity of banked blood is best when used within 14 days of collection. Blood >21 days after collection has been linked to increased mortality rates in the critically ill, especially HIV patients. Benefits must be weighed against risks, particularly in immunosuppressed patients.

Research Brief 9-1   This multi-center, prospective study of 284 ICUs in 213 United States hospitals enrolled 4892 patients to quantify the incidence of anemia and red blood cell (RBC) transfusions incritically ill patients and to evaluate clinical outcomes in anemic patients related to RBC transfusions. Anemia was found to be common in the critically ill. While in ICU, 44% of patients received at least one transfusion. Transfusion practice has remained almost unchanged in the past 10 years. Patients who received transfusions had more total complications, and those with multiple transfusions had longer hospital and ICU length-of-stay, with increased mortality. The number of RBC transfusions was an independent predictor of worse clinical outcome.

From Corwin HL et al: The CRIT study: anemia and blood transfusion in the critically ill—current clinical practice in the United States, *Crit Care Med* 32(1):39-52, 2004.

Oxygen therapy: To relieve SOB or dyspnea. Methods of oxygen delivery range from nasal cannulas, to various face masks, to mechanical ventilation in severe cases.

Selected anemias
Vitamin B$_{12}$: Injections or intravenous (IV) infusion is necessary for management of pernicious anemia, a type of megaloblastic anemia caused by failure of the gastric mucosa to absorb vitamin B$_{12}$.
Iron supplements: For iron-deficiency states to help increase production of normal-size RBCs. May be given intravenously or enterally. Iron levels must be normal to facilitate the action of erythropoietin injections.
Folic acid supplement: Necessary for RBC production. Supplements of 1 mg/day are used to treat megaloblastic anemia and, theoretically, to prevent hemolytic crisis in patients with hemolytic anemia. It is not effective in all patients with hemolytic anemia.
Epoetin alfa: erythropoietin, recombinant (Epogen/Procrit): Stimulates production of RBCs in patients with bone marrow hypofunction/lack of production of RBCs, particularly when related to renal failure. Has been used as an alternative strategy in patients who refuse blood transfusions (in conjunction with intravenous iron, if needed) and in anemia associated with critical illness. Critically ill patients may or may not respond to erythropoietin.
Bone marrow transplantation: Recommended for some patients with sickle cell disease or aplastic anemia to provide a mechanism for regenerating normal RBC production.
Elimination of causative factor: Certain drugs and chemicals, cold temperatures, and stress can worsen many anemias, but most profoundly hemolytic and aplastic anemias. Identifying and removing the causative agent can prevent life-threatening crisis. If the patient is bleeding, the cause of the bleeding must be addressed and the bleeding controlled.

Hemolytic anemias only
Red cell exchange therapy for sickle cell crisis: Cytapheresis procedure for patients who are unresponsive to other treatments for sickle cell disease.
Thrombocytapheresis: Cytapheresis procedure for patients experiencing symptoms of excessive thrombosis, to reduce platelets rapidly in an attempt to decrease clotting before onset of MODS.
Corticosteroids: Therapy used with limited success in management of hemolytic anemia.
Pain management: Aspirin, acetaminophen, nonsteroidal antiinflammatory drugs (NSAIDs), narcotics, and sedatives may be necessary for relief of pain and anxiety associated with hemolytic anemia, particularly during hemolytic crisis.
Splenectomy: Sometimes recommended for patients suspected of having splenic sequestration crisis related to hemolytic anemia.
Antisickling agents: Some clinical trials are underway to evaluate the efficacy of these agents in ablating the sickling phenomenon.

NURSING DIAGNOSES AND INTERVENTIONS

Impaired gas exchange related to lack of RBCs; hemoglobin abnormalities

Desired outcome: Within 3-24 hr of onset of treatment, patient has adequate gas exchange as evidenced by heart rate (HR) and respiratory rate (RR) within 10% of patient's baseline (or HR 60-100 beats/min and RR 12-20 breaths/min); Hgb and Hct returned to patient's baseline (or Hgb >12 mg/dl and Hct >37%); oxygen saturation >90%; and blood pressure (BP) returned to patient's baseline (or >90 mm Hg systolic within 24 hr of initiation of treatment).

- Administer supplemental oxygen as needed, using appropriate device (i.e., nasal cannula, face mask/shield, or mechanical ventilation as necessary).
- Monitor rate, rhythm, and depth of respirations.
- Monitor for increased restlessness, anxiety, and air hunger.
- Monitor oxygen saturation using pulse oximeter continuously. Consult with physician for persistent values <90% or, if oxygen saturation is chronically decreased, a sustained drop of >10% of baseline.
- Note changes in Sao_2, Svo_2, end-tidal CO_2 and changes in arterial blood gas (ABG) values, as appropriate.
- Monitor oxygen liter flow. Provide for oxygen when patient is transported.
- Maintain large-bore (18-gauge) intravenous (IV) catheter(s) in case transfusion or rapid volume expansion is necessary.
- Transfuse with packed cells (RBCs) (Table 9-2) as prescribed to facilitate oxygen delivery and assist in volume expansion, and/or implement aggressive strategy to augment RBC production.
- Describe the purpose of blood product transfusion therapy to the patient and significant others.
- Carefully evaluate dyspnea and chest pain in patients with sickle cell disease because of the possibility of pulmonary infarction.

You may also wish to refer to the following interventions from the Nursing Interventions Classification (NIC):

NIC Airway Management; Oxygen Therapy; Respiratory Monitoring; Circulatory Precautions; Cardiac Precautions

Activity intolerance related to anemia/lack of oxygen-carrying capacity of the blood

Desired outcomes: Within 24 hr of onset of treatment, patient's activity tolerance improves as evidenced by HR and RR returning to within 10% of baseline (or HR 60-100 beats/min and RR 12-20 breaths/min) and BP returning to within 10% of patient's baseline (or systolic BP >90% mm Hg). Within 24 hr of initiation of treatment patient is able to assist minimally with self-care activities.

- Alternate periods of rest and activity to avoid stress that increases oxygen demand.
- Collaborate with occupational therapy (OT), physical therapy (PT), and/or recreational therapy personnel in planning and monitoring an activity program as appropriate.
- Determine patient's physical limitations. Focus on what patient can do, rather than on deficits.
- Reposition patient slowly while monitoring effects on myocardial and cerebral perfusion.
- Reduce fear, pain, and anxiety to decrease oxygen demand.
- Determine causes of fatigue (e.g., treatments, pain, medications).
- Monitor nutritional intake to ensure adequate energy resources.
- Teach patient to avoid stressful situations, which can exacerbate symptoms of anemia and precipitate hemolytic crisis in patients with hemolytic anemia.
- Teach signs of hypoxemia: altered mental status, activity intolerance, SOB, chest pain, and weakness.
- Teach patient and significant others about the specific anemia affecting the patient.
- See this diagnosis in "Prolonged Immobility," p. 61.

NIC Activity Therapy; Energy Management; Teaching: Prescribed Activity/Exercise

Risk for impaired skin integrity related to impaired oxygen transport secondary to chronic anemia

Desired outcome: Patient's skin remains intact during hospitalization.

- Keep extremities warm to promote circulation and help prevent tissue hypoxia.
- Perform a comprehensive appraisal of peripheral circulation (e.g., check peripheral pulses, edema, capillary refill, color and temperature of extremity).
- Monitor for sources of pressure and friction.
- Monitor for infection, especially of edematous areas.
- Use a bed cradle to reduce pressure of covers on extremities.
- Monitor skin and mucous membranes for areas of discoloration and bruising.
- Monitor skin for rashes, abrasions, excessive dryness, and moisture.
- Provide adequate nutrition and nutritional supplements as appropriate. Negative nitrogen state or low serum protein or albumin increases the risk for skin breakdown.
- Teach patient the signs of skin breakdown, since it can occur at any time with chronic anemia.
- Instruct the patient on the importance of preventing venous stasis.
- Teach patient about appropriate nutrition as discussed in "Nutritional Support," p. 1.

TABLE 9 - 2 Blood and Blood Products*

Product	Volume	Infusion time	Contents	Possible complications
Whole blood (rarely used)	500 ml/unit	2-4 hr or <1 hr in emergency	All blood components. If fresh, processed with citrate-phosphate-dextrose (CPD)	Hepatitis, transmission of HIV (human immunodeficiency virus), CMV (cytomegalovirus), EBV (Epstein-Barr virus), and other organisms; transfusion reactions; all types
Packed red blood cells	200-250 ml/unit	1-4 hr or <1 hr in emergency	Red blood cells	See whole blood
Fresh-frozen plasma	200-250 ml/unit	20 min to thaw ½ to 1 hr or <½ hr in emergency	All clotting factors except platelets	See whole blood
Platelets	35-50 ml/unit	Direct IV push at 30-50 ml/min; may combine or "pool" several bags into one; given in multiple units	Platelets	Transfusion reaction: febrile or mild allergic; may need to premedicate with acetaminophen (Tylenol) or diphenhydramine HCl (Benadryl); rare instance of septic reaction
Cryoprecipitate	10-20 ml/unit	May need 10-30 units infused at 1 unit/min or 10-20 ml/min	Factor VIII: factor XIII and fibrinogen	Small possibility of febrile or mild allergic reaction; rare instance of septic reaction
Granulocytes	300 ml/unit	1-2 hr; administer slowly for 5 min as test dose	White blood cells (WBC) extracted from 1 unit of whole blood	Transfusion reactions: all types; often ineffective in elevating WBC count
Leukocyte-poor and washed, frozen red blood cells	250-300 ml/unit	2 hr or 1-2 hr in emergency	Red cells washed with saline (and possibly irradiated) to remove WBCs and protein from RBCs	Markedly reduced possibility of transfusion reactions: all types
Factor VIII concentrate	10-20 ml/unit	May need >10 units infused at 1 unit/min	Factor VIII (pooled from possibly thousands of donors)	Small possibility of febrile or mild allergic reaction; rare instance of septic reaction
Factor IX concentrate	20-30 ml/unit	May need >10 units infused at 1 unit/min	Factor IX (pooled from possibly thousands of donors)	Small possibility of febrile or mild allergic reaction; rare instance of septic reaction
Volume expanders Albumin (5% or 25%) Plasma protein fraction (PPF) Salt-poor albumin	Varies with each product	1 ml/min or as rapidly as tolerated in shock states	Reconstituted from human blood, plasma, or serum	Possible hypervolemia with rapid infusions, particularly with 25% albumin

*Use correct filter with each blood product; most filters can be used to administer 2-4 units; either piggyback or flush products with normal saline solution *only.*

- Apply appropriate skin-saving dressing (e.g., Duoderm) or initiate aggressive skin care regimen to areas of breakdown.
- For additional interventions, see "Wound and Skin Care," p. 45.

NIC Pressure Management; Pressure Ulcer Prevention; Skin Surveillance; Nutrition Management; Circulatory Precautions

For hemolytic crisis

Altered tissue perfusion: peripheral, cardiopulmonary, gastrointestinal, renal, and cerebral, related to interruption of arterial or venous blood flow secondary to formation of microthrombi

Desired outcome: Within 24 hr of onset of treatment, patient has adequate perfusion as evidenced by warm extremities; pink nail beds; peripheral pulses at least 2+ on a scale of 0-4+ or patient's baseline; capillary refill <2 sec; BP within 10% of patient's normal range (or systolic BP >90 mm Hg); HR and RR within 10% of patient's baseline (or HR 60-100 beats/min, RR 12-20 breaths/min with a normal depth and pattern [eupnea]); oxygen saturation >90%; urinary output ≥0.5 ml/kg/hr; and orientation to time, place, and person.

- Initiate aggressive IV fluid volume replacement as prescribed to prevent deposition of hemolyzed RBCs in the microvasculature.
- Assess extremities for inadequate peripheral perfusion: amplitude of peripheral pulses, coolness, pallor, and prolonged capillary refill. Use Doppler if unable to palpate pulses.
- Evaluate chest pain. Note cardiac dysrhythmias and symptoms of decreased cardiac output. Monitor respiratory status for symptoms of heart failure.
- Monitor vital signs frequently for signs of impending shock: increased HR and RR, increased restlessness and anxiety, and cool and clammy skin, followed by a decrease in BP.
- Monitor abdomen for signs of decreased perfusion.
- Keep lower extremities elevated slightly to promote venous blood flow.
- Monitor ventilation and perfusion: assess ABG values for acidosis (i.e., pH <7.35, hypercarbia/CO_2 retention [$Paco_2$ >45 mm Hg]), indicating hypoperfusion, and respiratory insufficiency. Assess for hypoxemia using continuous pulse oximetry to detect decreased oxygen saturation. Consult physician for sustained deterioration in status.
- Monitor urinary output for decrease, which can signal decreased renal perfusion. Consult physician for urine output <0.5 ml/kg/hr for 2 consecutive hours.
- Monitor neurologic status q2-4h, using the Glasgow Coma Scale (see Appendix 3).
- Teach patient and significant others about hemolytic anemia, including the signs of impending hemolytic crisis, rendering information on the following:
  - ❏ *Indicators of impending hemolytic crisis:* Fever, abnormal pain, headache, blurred vision, dizziness, unsteady gait, palpitations, paresthesias, and paralysis.
  - ❏ *Support groups:* Names, phone numbers, and addresses of other persons/groups that can assist with support of people with hemolytic anemias.
  - ❏ *Smoking cessation:* Support groups and programs that assist in stopping cigarette smoking to decrease vasoconstriction associated with nicotine intake.
  - ❏ *Medications:* Drug name, dosage, frequency, and possible side effects, especially related to steroids: increased appetite, weight gain, "moon face," "buffalo hump," increased possibility of infection, headaches, and increased BP. Explain possible steroid-induced diabetes mellitus.
  - ❏ *Prevention of infection*: Important if patient is on long-term steroid therapy or had a splenectomy. The patient should obtain an annual flu vaccine; practice good personal hygiene; obtain regular dental check-ups; and get adequate rest, sleep, and relaxation. For splenectomy, patients should have a pneumococcal vaccine and wear a medical-alert identification bracelet.

NIC Cardiac Care: Acute; Circulatory Care: Arterial Insufficiency; Circulatory Care: Venous Insufficiency; Respiratory Monitoring; Shock Management: Cardiac; Cerebral Perfusion Promotion; Neurologic Monitoring; Peripheral Sensation Management; Fluid/Electrolyte Management; Fluid Management; Vital Signs Monitoring

Pain related to tissue ischemia secondary to vessel occlusion; inflammation/injury secondary to blood within the joints

Desired outcomes: Within 1-2 hr of initiating treatment, patient's subjective evaluation of discomfort improves as documented by a pain scale; nonverbal indicators of discomfort are reduced or absent.

- Monitor patient for signs of discomfort, including increases in HR, BP, and RR. Devise a pain scale with patient, rating discomfort from 0 (no pain) to 10.
- Perform a comprehensive assessment of pain to include location, characteristics, onset/duration, frequency, quality, intensity or severity of pain, and precipitating factors.
- Medicate for pain as prescribed. Assess effectiveness of medication using the pain scale. Confer with physician if pain relief is ineffective; devise an alternate plan for analgesia.

- If pain medication injections are frequent, consider an IV rather than an intramuscular (IM) route, when possible.
- Administer adjuvant analgesics and/or medications when needed to potentiate analgesia.
- Consider continuous infusion (alone or with bolus opioids) to maintain serum levels.
- Collaborate with the physician if drug, dose, route of administration, or interval changes are indicated, making specific recommendations based on equianalgesic principles.
- Consider alternate method of pain control such as relaxation techniques: guided imagery, controlled breathing, meditation, and listening to soft, soothing music. Use therapeutic/healing touch to relieve pain if practitioner is trained and patient agrees to participate. Alternatively, consult trained practitioner.
- Control environmental factors that may add to discomfort (e.g., room temperature, light, noise).
- Apply warm compresses to joints to increase circulation and thereby improve tissue oxygenation.
- Apply elastic stockings to promote venous return and enhance circulation.
- Teach patient to perform isometric or range-of-motion (ROM) exercises to promote circulation.
- Help allay fears by reassuring patient that pain will decrease as the crisis subsides.
- Provide emotional support to patient during the crisis episode. Reassure patient that the crisis is time-limited, and enable significant others to be with patient, if possible, during the crisis.
- Teach patient to assess extremities daily for evidence of tissue breakdown or blood sequestration (i.e., swelling, erythema, tenderness) so that early interventions can be implemented in an attempt to prevent severe pain.

NIC Analgesic Administration; Pain Management; Medication Administration; Medication Administration: Intravenous (IV); Heat/Cold Application; Anxiety Reduction; Therapeutic Touch; Music Therapy; Meditation Facilitation

Risk for fluid volume deficit or excess related to failure of renal regulatory mechanisms of fluid and electrolyte balance secondary to microthrombi occluding the nephrons

Desired outcome: Patient's volume status returns to normal/baseline as evidenced by urinary output ≥0.5 ml/kg/hr; stable weight; BP within patient's normal range; HR 60-100 beats/min; RR 12-20 breaths/min; good skin turgor; moist mucous membranes; urine specific gravity 1.005-1.025; pulmonary artery wedge pressure (PAWP) 6-12 mm Hg (or patient's baseline); pulmonary artery diastolic (PAD) 8-15 mm Hg (or patient's baseline); and central venous pressure (CVP) 2-6 mm Hg (5-12 cm H_2O).

- Monitor intake and output (I&O) hourly. Consult physician for a urinary output <0.5 ml/kg/hr for 4 consecutive hours. Insert urinary catheter if appropriate.
- Monitor and document heart rate, rhythm, pulses, and blood pressure.
- Evaluate efficacy of volume expansion by closely comparing CVP, PAWP, and PAD. Overzealous volume expansion can lead to heart failure and pulmonary edema, with CVP >20%-25% normal values and PAD and/or PAWP >16 mm Hg.
- Administer diuretics as prescribed in the well-hydrated patient with urine output <0.5 ml/kg/hr.
- Assess patient for volume depletion, including poor skin turgor; dry mucous membranes; hypotension; tachycardia; and decreasing urine output, PAWP, PAD, and CVP.
- Monitor electrolytes and serum osmolality. A universal increase in electrolytes and osmolality is indicative of dehydration. A universal decrease signals fluid overload.
- Assess pH (normal range is 7.35-7.45) before replacing electrolytes. Acidosis and alkalosis alter electrolyte values. Replace potassium if the pH is outside the normal range.

NIC Electrolyte Monitoring; Fluid Management; Fluid Monitoring; Intravenous (IV) Therapy; Hypervolemia Management; Shock Management: Volume

ADDITIONAL NURSING DIAGNOSES

Uncontrolled bleeding and complications of hemolysis can be terrifying to the patient and significant others, who may fear that the patient will die. See "Psychosocial Support," p. 68 and "Psychosocial Support for the Patient's Family and Significant Others," p. 78, accordingly.

Bleeding and Thrombotic Disorders

Bleeding can result from qualitative (dysfunctional) or quantitative (lack of) abnormalities of platelets and/or coagulation factors, including proteins, in the plasma. Thrombocytopenia is common in the critically ill and, like anemia, necessitates differential diagnosis. The *cause* of thrombocytopenia, rather than simply the decreased platelets, poses the greatest threat to the critically ill patient. The four main causes of thrombocytopenia are as follows:

1. *Hemodilution:* related to administration of large amounts of retained fluids, IV fluids, multiple medications given in 50-100-ml "piggybacks," or blood/blood products.

2. *Increased platelet destruction or consumption:* includes heparin-induced thrombocytopenia (HIT); antiphospholipid antibody syndrome (APAS) or lupus anticoagulant syndrome; idiopathic thrombocytopenic purpura (ITP); thrombotic thrombocytopenic purpura (TTP); hemolytic-uremic syndrome (HUS); severe sepsis; and hemolysis, elevated liver enzymes, and low platelet count (HELLP) syndrome. Disseminated intravascular coagulation (DIC) presents with a combined coagulopathy and platelet consumption.
3. *Platelet sequestration:* related to hypersplenism and hypothermia.
4. *Decreased production of platelets:* caused by alcohol (ETOH) abuse, bone marrow irradiation, bone marrow/stem cell disease, graft vs. host disease, aplastic anemia, vitamin B_{12} or folate deficiencies, metastatic carcinoma, some renal diseases, leukemia, and myeloproliferative disorders.

Platelet destruction may be mediated by either congenital autoimmune or alloimmune disorders, or by acquired immunologic or nonimmunologic mechanisms. Causative or related factors include septicemia, systemic inflammatory response syndrome (SIRS), pulmonary hypertension, extracorporeal circulation, thrombotic disorders, acute transplant rejection, severe allergic reactions, rheumatic disorders, intravascular catheters and prosthetics, fat emboli, acute respiratory distress syndrome (ARDS), and human immunodeficiency virus (HIV) infection. The most diagnostic finding associated with severe thrombocytopenia is presence of petechiae in dependent areas (i.e., back, posterior thighs of bedridden patients). Larger purpura such as ecchymoses and hematomas may also be present but are nonspecific for diagnosis of platelet disorders. Patients must be assessed for risk of bleeding with thrombocytopenia, considering the severity and cause along with comorbid factors.

Coagulopathies leading to bleeding (with/without associated thrombi) may be caused by liver disease, vitamin K deficiency, pregnancy-induced hypertension associated with HELLP syndrome, or other defects of blood coagulation factors, such as hemophilia, von Willebrand's disease, and DIC.

Patients prone to thromboembolic conditions include those with *platelet abnormalities* including thrombocytosis, diabetes mellitus, hyperlipidemia, heparin-induced thrombocytopenia, systemic lupus erythematosus; *blood vessel defects* including venous disease/stasis, roughened surface of vascular endothelium (seen with arteriosclerosis, trauma, severe sepsis, SIRS, or infection), atrial fibrillation, grafts or other devices in place, hyperviscosity, TTP, hemolytic uremic syndrome, vasculitis; and those with *systemic illness and conditions,* including long bone fractures, orthopedic surgery, abdominal surgery, malignancy, pregnancy or postpartum (risk of venous thromboembolism is five times higher than for nonpregnant women), oral contraceptives, nephrotic syndrome, inflammatory bowel disease, slow/stagnant blood flow through the vessels (e.g., shock states, severe peripheral vascular disease), infusion of prothrombin complex, and sickle cell disease.

When patients are evaluated for a bleeding disorder, the process should include evaluation of platelets, deficiency of a single coagulation factor (factors VII, VIII, IX, X, or XI) or multiple coagulation factors, for endogenous or exogenous antibiotics in the circulation, and consumptive coagulopathy (e.g., ITP, TTP, vasculitis, hemolytic uremic syndrome, obstetric complication, trauma, liver disease).

Those suspected of having thromboembolic disease may require evaluation of coagulation factors, circulating antibodies, abnormal proteins (deficient protein C or S), and other endogenous chemicals.

Normal blood coagulation is activated most often as a result of injury to blood vessels, causing the following series of events:
1. *Reflex vasoconstriction:* Vascular spasm that decreases blood flow to the site of injury.
2. *Platelet aggregation:* Leads to formation of a platelet plug to help repair the injury. If the damage to the vessel is small, the plug is sufficient to seal the injury. If the hole is large, a blood clot is necessary to stop the bleeding.
3. *Activation of plasma clotting factors:* Leads to the formation of a fibrin clot. The pathways that initiate clotting factors (Figure 9-1) include the following:
   a. *Intrinsic system:* Initiated by "contact activation" subsequent to an endothelial injury. The problem is "intrinsic" to the circulation, or begins with an injury to the blood or circulatory system.
   b. *Extrinsic system:* Initiated by tissue thromboplastin released from injured tissue. The problem is "extrinsic" to the circulation, or begins with an injury to tissue rather than within the blood system.
   c. *Common pathway:* The final part of the coagulation system, which completes the clot formation process begun by either the intrinsic or extrinsic pathway.
   d. *Clot retraction:* Several minutes after its formation, the clot contracts for 30-60 min to express most of the fluid from within the clot. The expressed fluid is called *serum,* because most of the clotting factors have been used/removed by the clot formation process. Serum is unable to clot. The absence of clotting factors differentiates *serum* from *plasma.*

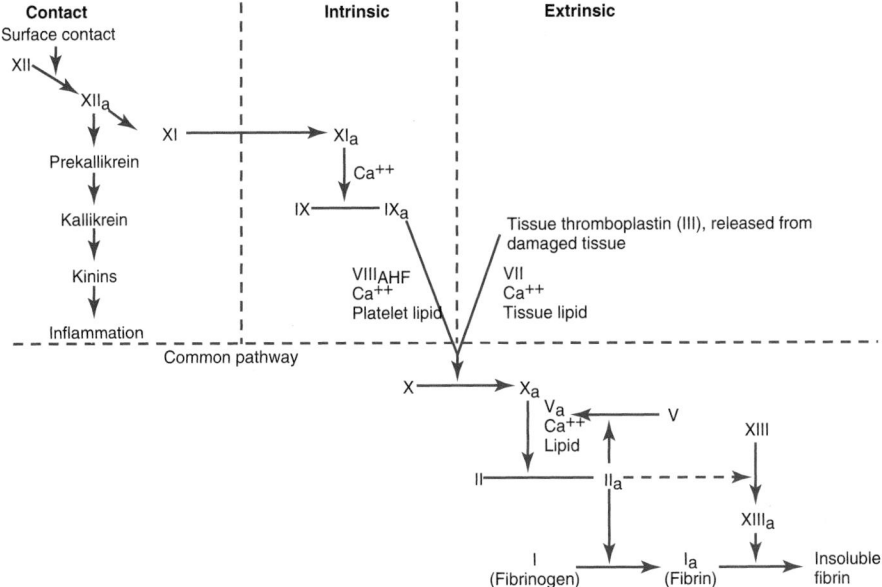

Figure 9-1: Coagulation pathway.
From Hamilton GC, Janz TG: Disorders of hemostasis. In Rosen P et al: *Emergency medicine: concepts and clinical practice,* ed 4, St Louis, 1998, Mosby.

4. *Growth of fibrous tissue:* Tissue which completes the clot within approximately 7-10 days after injury. This process results in permanent closure of the vessel injury. Both the intrinsic and extrinsic pathways are activated after rupture of a blood vessel. Tissue thromboplastin from the vessel initiates the extrinsic pathway, while contact of factor XII and platelets with the injured vessel wall traumatizes the blood, which initiates the intrinsic pathway. The extrinsic pathway is able to form clots in as little as 15 sec with severe trauma, whereas the intrinsic pathway requires 2-6 min for clot formation.

HEPARIN-INDUCED THROMBOCYTOPENIA

PATHOPHYSIOLOGY

Heparin is the most widely used IV anticoagulant and one of the most frequently prescribed drugs in the United States. Heparin prevents the conversion of fibrinogen to fibrin. Incidence of heparin-induced thrombocytopenia (HIT), also called *heparin-induced thrombocytopenic thrombosis (HITT), white clot syndrome,* or *heparin-associated thrombocytopenia (HAT) types I and II,* results when heparin therapy causes either a mild to moderate (i.e., HAT type I) or severe (i.e., HAT type II) decrease in the number of freely circulating platelets. Platelets in affected patients manifest unusual aggregation, which can result in heparin resistance, arterial and venous thrombosis, and subsequent emboli in extreme cases (Figure 9-2). Depending on the source of the heparin received, incidence of HIT is reported in about 5% of all patients receiving heparin. Bovine (beef-based) heparin has been associated with HIT more frequently than other heparins. It is estimated that as many as 50% of patients on heparin may be asymptomatic, but generate antibodies to heparin-platelet factor 4 (H-PF4), which increases the risk of HIT on their next exposure to heparin. Incidence of HIT is not related to the heparin dosage and has been seen in patients receiving low-dose SC heparin, as well as in patients receiving simple heparin "flushes" to maintain patency of IV lines.

   Two types of HIT have been described:

Mild to moderate, low morbidity: Generally occurs 1-2 days after initiation of heparin. It may resolve within 5 days after symptoms begin. Platelets may decrease to levels as low as 100,000/mm^3 or may remain in the low-normal range. No treatment is required, and heparin therapy may be continued if the patient is asymptomatic.

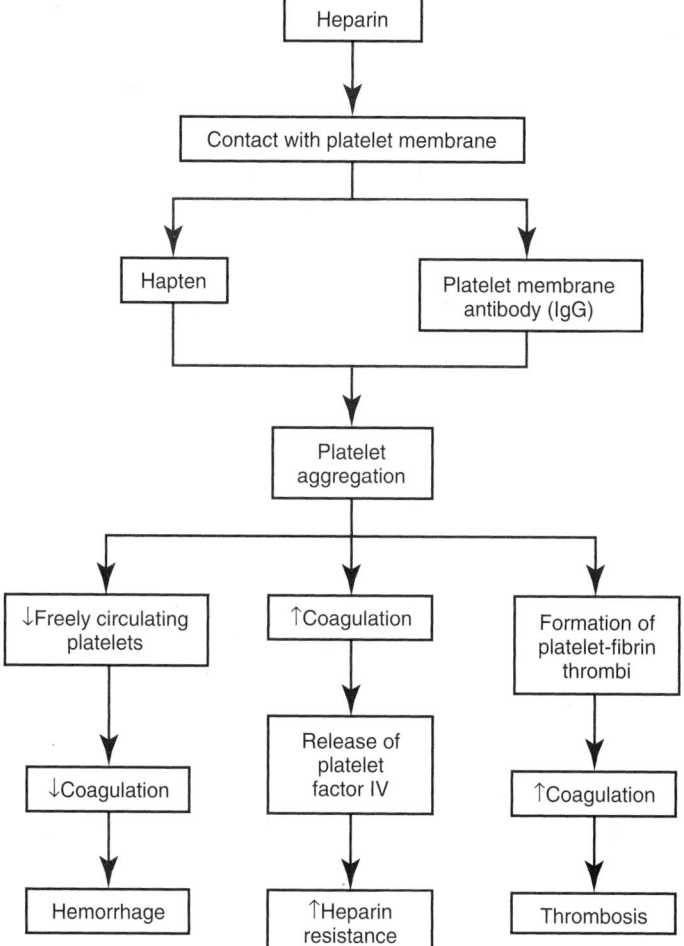

Figure 9-2: Heparin-induced thrombocytopenia. *IgG,* Immunoglobulin G.

High morbidity (immune-mediated): Generally begins 5-7 days after initiation of heparin. Symptoms persist until heparin is discontinued. Platelets decrease to <100,000/mm³. Thrombosis with subsequent embolization and bleeding is apparent. Complications include pulmonary emboli, myocardial infarction, cerebral infarction, and circulatory impairment resulting in limb amputations. Mortality rate is 29%. Overall, 0.6% of all patients receiving heparin therapy develop thrombo-embolization.

ASSESSMENT

Risk factors: Prior drug-induced immunologic thrombocytopenia.
Clinical presentation
Mild to moderate, low morbidity: Slight decrease in platelet count without clinical symptoms.
Severe, high morbidity (immune-mediated): Hemorrhage, ecchymosis, gingival bleeding, hemopty-sis, epistaxis, and possible chest pain, SOB, and strokelike symptoms. Extreme cases: arterial throm-bosis of the distal aorta and proximal lower limb arteries.
Physical assessment (severe, immune-mediated): Presence of petechiae, purpura, bruising from mucosal surfaces or wounds. The patient may also manifest signs of arterial occlusion: cold, pulse-less extremities; severe chest pain and SOB, indicative of myocardial ischemia; paresthesias; paraly-sis; and diminished level of consciousness (LOC), indicative of cerebral ischemia.

DIAGNOSTIC TESTS

Platelet count: Mild to moderate: 100,000-150,000/mm^3; severe: <100,000/mm^3 caused by severe clumping or aggregation of platelets.

Bleeding time: Prolonged if platelets are <100,000/mm^3.

Platelet antibody screen: Positive findings because of the presence of immunoglobulin G (IgG) platelet antibodies.

Coagulation screening (prothrombin time [PT]; partial thromboplastin time [PTT], thromboplastin time): Normal, inasmuch as the clotting factors that govern these test results are normal.

Fibrinogen: May be low-normal or low because of increased consumption. Normal is 200-400 mg/dl.

Fibrin degradation products: Elevated to ≥40 mcg/ml because of fibrinolysis of platelet-fibrin thrombi. Normal is <10 mcg/ml.

Platelet aggregation: Results will be >100% (or high value of specific laboratory) because of release of platelet membrane antibody.

Heparin-induced platelet aggregation: Reflects abnormal aggregation curve with decrease in the optical density in the aggregometer.

Serotonin release testing and ELISA heparin PF4: Help in the differential diagnosis of HIT.

Bone marrow aspiration: Normal or increased number of megakaryocytes (platelet precursors), indicative of normal bone marrow production of platelets.

COLLABORATIVE MANAGEMENT

Heparin therapy: If the platelet count is >100,000/mm^3 and the patient is symptom-free, heparin is sometimes continued, but an alternate thrombin inhibitor may be recommended. Oral anticoagulation should begin immediately, if possible. If the platelet count is <100,000/mm^3 and the patient develops bleeding or thrombosis: *heparin must be discontinued immediately (including heparin flushes), alternate anticoagulant initiated,* and subsequent complications managed as they occur. Use of low–molecular weight heparins is contraindicated.

Monitoring heparin therapy: A preheparin platelet count is done to establish baseline values. Daily platelet counts should be done for at least the first 4 days of heparin therapy. Subsequent counts are done q2days. If increasing amounts of heparin are needed to maintain therapeutic levels (i.e., PTT 40-60 sec), heparin resistance should be suspected, which sometimes precedes HIT (see Figure 9-2).

Administration of defibrinogenating agents: Ancrod (Arvin) may be given to reduce the possibility of thrombosis.

Administration of direct thrombin inhibitors: Argatroban and hirudin, direct thrombin inhibitors, block thrombin generation needed for fibrin formation. They may be used alone or in combination with warfarin, as an alternate anticoagulation strategy. Ximelagatran is the first orally available thrombin inhibitor. Bivalirudin is not licensed for use with HIT, but can be used in patients undergoing percutaneous coronary interventions.

Vena caval filter: If patient experiences thrombosis with decrease or loss of perfusion to an extremity, the physician may consider surgical insertion of a vena caval filter to reduce the risk of pulmonary emboli caused by clot migration from an extremity. See "Pulmonary Emboli," p. 192.

Platelet transfusions: May be initiated after heparin therapy is discontinued if bleeding fails to subside.

Plasma exchange: In severe cases, 2-3 L of plasma is removed and replaced with albumin, crystalloids, or fresh-frozen plasma to assist in decreasing bleeding by removing bound heparin from the body.

Warfarin, thrombolytics, and platelet inhibitors: If the patient needs further anticoagulation, warfarin sodium (Coumadin) should be considered. Streptokinase, urokinase, and alteplase (rt-PA) have been used successfully to manage pulmonary emboli in HIT. Platelet inhibitors are contraindicated, due to platelet dysfunction already present.

New anticoagulants: New medications using recombinant DNA technology focus on each step of the coagulation process; many are under development. These agents are grouped into three stages of coagulation: initiation, propagation, and fibrin formation. Tissue factor pathway inhibitor (TFPI), nematode anticoagulant peptide, and factor VIIai target initiation of coagulation. Soluble thrombomodulin, drotrecogin alfa (activated Protein C), protein C concentrate, fondaparinux, and idraparinux inhibit clot propagation. Direct thrombin inhibitors (antithrombins) block fibrin formation for clot completion.

Research Brief 9-2 A meta-analysis of 29 randomized controlled trials and four prospective cohort studies (studies performed in outpatient settings) was done to determine the risk of bleeding in patients receiving warfarin for thromboembolism. The investigators limited the search to English-language articles done during or after 1989, when the INR (international normalized ratio) was implemented. After combining data, analysis revealed that major bleeding (requiring transfusion or hospitalization) was either intracranial/into a body cavity or fatal and occurred in 1 in 14 patients per year (7.22 per 100 patient years; 95% CI 7.19-7.24). To account for different lengths of treatment, the authors converted all outcomes into event rate per year.

From Linkins LA, Choi PT, Douketis JD: Clinical impact of bleeding in patients taking oral anticoagulant therapy for venous thromboembolism, *Ann Intern Med* 139:893-900, 2003.

NURSING DIAGNOSES AND INTERVENTIONS

Altered protection related to decreased platelet count with risk of bleeding and thromboembolization
Desired outcome: Within 24 hr of discontinuing heparin therapy, patient exhibits no signs of new bleeding, bruising, or thrombosis as evidenced by HR 60-100 beats/min or within 10% of patient's baseline; RR 12-20 breaths/min with normal depth and pattern (eupnea); systolic BP ≥90 mm Hg; and all peripheral pulses at patient's baseline or >2+ on a 0-4+ scale.

- Assess patient at least q2h for signs of bleeding, including hemoptysis, GI bleeding, hematuria, and bleeding from invasive procedure sites or mucous membranes.
- Monitor the patient closely for hemorrhage.
- Note Hgb and Hct levels before and after blood loss, as indicated.
- Monitor for signs of persistent bleeding (e.g., check all secretions for frank or occult blood).
- Assess patient at least q2h for signs of thrombosis, including decreased peripheral pulses, altered sensation in extremities (i.e., paresthesias, numbness), pallor, coolness, cyanosis, or capillary refill time >2 sec.
- Perform a comprehensive assessment of peripheral circulation (e.g., check peripheral pulses, edema, capillary refill, and color and temperature of extremities).
- Monitor extremities for areas of heat, pain, redness, or swelling.
- Maintain adequate hydration to prevent increased blood viscosity.
- Avoid IM injections and venous and arterial punctures as possible until bleeding time normalizes.
- Protect the patient from trauma that may cause bleeding. Avoid taking rectal temperatures.
- Monitor platelet count daily for significant changes. Consult physician for values that remain <150,000/mm^3 or below patient's baseline.
- Assess ECG for heart rate and rhythm, and assess respiratory rate and pattern and BP for evidence of active bleeding. Be alert to sustained increase in HR and RR or ECG changes, such as ST segment depression or elevation, since these indicators may precede hypotension.
- Monitor heparin dosage carefully. If increasing doses are required to maintain a therapeutic level (PTT 40-60 sec or 2-2 ½ times patient's baseline), consult physician for possible heparin resistance, an early indicator of HIT. If heparin has been discontinued and new anticoagulants initiated, monitor appropriate values. If a direct thrombin inhibitor (e.g., Argatroban) is used alone, or in combination with warfarin, monitor PT and international normalized ratio (INR).
- Monitor Hgb and Hct values daily in patients with recent or active bleeding.
- Assess patient's neurologic status hourly if platelets continue dropping and fall to <30,000.
- Monitor for signs of multiple organ dysfunction syndrome (MODS) secondary to thrombosis or prolonged hypotension, if patient has hemorrhaged.
- Teach patient and significant others basic pathophysiology of HIT, and instruct them to report this problem to all subsequent health care providers. Teach patient to wear a medical-alert bracelet to alert health care providers if patient becomes unable to speak.

NIC Surveillance: Safety; Bleeding Precautions

Fluid volume deficit (or risk for same) related to active blood loss
Desired outcomes: Patient becomes normovolemic within 24 hr of onset of treatment as evidenced by HR within patient's normal range or 60-100 beats/min; RR 12-20 breaths/min with normal depth and pattern (eupnea); and urinary output ≥0.5 ml/kg/hr; absence of abdominal discomfort, back pain, or pain from invasive procedure sites.

- Monitor patient for signs of hypovolemia, including increased HR and RR, decreased BP, increased restlessness or fatigue, and decreased urine output.
- Maintain accurate I&O record. Weigh daily and monitor trends.

- Administer supplemental oxygen if patient is actively bleeding.
- Assess for intraabdominal bleeding: note any abdominal pain, tenderness, guarding, or back pain.
- Check excretions for occult blood, and observe for blood in emesis, sputum, feces, urine, nasogastric (NG) drainage, and wound drainage as appropriate.
- Instruct the patient and/or family on the need for blood replacement as appropriate.
- Replace lost volume with plasma expanders (e.g., albumin, hetastarch) or blood products as indicated. See Table 9-2 for more information.

NIC Electrolyte Management; Fluid Management; Fluid Monitoring; Hypovolemia Management; Intravenous (IV) Therapy; Shock Management: Volume; Blood Products Administration

ADDITIONAL NURSING DIAGNOSES

Uncontrolled bleeding or thrombotic complications can be terrifying for the patient and significant others, who may fear that the patient will die. See nursing diagnoses and interventions in "Psychosocial Support," p. 68, and "Psychosocial Support for the Patient's Family and Significant Others," p. 78, accordingly.

IMMUNE THROMBOCYTOPENIC PURPURA (ITP)

PATHOPHYSIOLOGY

Immune thrombocytopenic purpura (ITP) is a disorder characterized by premature platelet destruction, resulting in a decrease in the platelet count to below 100,000/mm^3. Normal platelet life span averages 1-3 wk, whereas in ITP the platelet life span averages 1-3 days because of the presence of antiplatelet IgG and IgM antibodies, which destroy platelets in the reticuloendothelial system of the spleen. The coagulopathy is believed to be an autoimmune response and manifests as both an acute and a chronic problem.

Acute ITP is primarily a childhood disease, characterized by an abrupt onset of severe thrombocytopenia with evident purpura. Usually it occurs <21 days after a viral infection. At the onset, platelets decrease to <20,000/mm^3. The chronic form is typically a disease of adults ages 20-50 yr, but it has occurred in a small percentage of children and elders. The chronic disease rarely resolves spontaneously, sometimes responds to treatment of the underlying disorder, and usually is not associated with infection but can be related to autoimmune disorders (e.g., systemic lupus erythematosus, rheumatoid arthritis) and neoplastic disorders (e.g., chronic lymphocytic leukemia, Hodgkin's/non-Hodgkin's lymphoma). Women are affected three times more often than are men. Petechiae and purpura are commonly seen on the distal upper and lower extremities. Patients may feel symptom-free until actual bleeding begins. Intracranial hemorrhage is a potential complication. Platelet counts decrease to as low as 5,000/mm^3 in some patients but may be as high as 75,000/mm^3 in others.

ASSESSMENT

Risk factors: In acute ITP there usually is a history of antecedent viral infection occurring about 3 wk before the hemorrhagic episode. The chronic form usually is insidious and sometimes is seen in association with autoimmune hemolytic anemia, HIV disease, hemophilia, Hodgkin's lymphoma, chronic lymphocytic leukemia, systemic lupus erythematosus, sarcoidosis, high-titer anticardiolipin antibodies, and thyrotoxicosis.

Clinical presentation: Petechiae, purpura, and prolonged bleeding are commonly seen. Occasionally, epistaxis, GI and gingival bleeding, and increased menstrual flow are present. The rarest complication is intracranial hemorrhage, occurring in <1% of patients. Signs of an autoimmune process such as fever, splenomegaly, or lymphadenopathy may occur, but because they are not specific to ITP, they require further evaluation.

Physical assessment: Presence of petechiae and purpura anywhere on the skin or mucous membranes, most commonly on the distal upper and lower extremities. Ecchymosis is apparent in traumatized areas, along with generalized bruising. Neurologic signs should be monitored closely in patients with acute ITP. Joint tenderness and visual (retinal) disturbances may be noted because of bleeding into these areas.

DIAGNOSTIC TESTS

Platelet count: Decreased to 5,000-75,000/mm^3 because of premature destruction. Normal range is 150,000-400,000/mm^3.
Bleeding time: Prolonged when platelet count is <100,000/mm^3.

Screening coagulation tests (PT, PTT, thrombin time): Normal, because these tests measure non-platelet components of the coagulation pathway.

Platelet antibody screen: Positive findings because of the presence of IgG and IgM antiplatelet antibodies.

Complete blood cell count (CBC) with differential: Hgb and Hct may be decreased because of insidious blood loss or simultaneous hemolytic anemia (Evans's syndrome); WBC count will be normal unless the ITP is associated with another disease that alters the differential leukocyte count.

Bone marrow aspiration: Biopsy will reveal megakaryocytes (platelet precursors) in normal or increased numbers with a "nonbudding" appearance, possibly indicating defective maturation or failure of platelet production.

Capillary fragility test: Will show >1+, which signals that more than 11 petechiae were present in a 2.5-cm radial area on the skin after prolonged application of a BP cuff. Normal is 1+ or <10 petechiae.

COLLABORATIVE MANAGEMENT

Platelet transfusions: Platelets are given only in cases of life-threatening hemorrhage. The shortened platelet life span renders prophylactic transfusions ineffective.

Glucocorticoid therapy: Adrenocorticosteroids (e.g., prednisone 0.25-1 mg/kg/day) are effective in increasing the platelet count in 1-3 wk after initiation of treatment. Effectiveness is attributed to suppression of phagocytic activity of the macrophage system (particularly the spleen), which increases the life span of the antibody-coated platelets. If improvement does not occur within 2-3 wk, excessive doses of steroids are required, or patient cannot tolerate tapering of steroids, splenectomy should be considered. "Normal" responders are able to have steroid dosage tapered over several weeks until platelets reach a sustained value of 50,000/mm³. Relapse during or after tapering prednisone is a common occurrence.

Splenectomy: Treatment of choice in cases refractory to glucocorticoid therapy. The condition stabilizes in 70%-90% of patients who undergo splenectomy. The positive results are attributed to the removal of the site of destruction of the antibody-sensitized platelets. Prospective splenectomy candidates should have pneumococcal, meningococcal, and possibly *Haemophilus influenzae* type b vaccinations before a planned splenectomy, to reduce the risk of postoperative infection with these organisms.

IV infusions of gamma globulin: Given 400 mg/kg/day for 5 days, resulting in increased platelet count in 60%-70% of patients. It is less effective in patients with long-standing chronic ITP. The platelet level at initiation of treatment is unrelated to the patient's response. Duration of response may be longest in individuals who achieve the highest initial platelet increases.

Anti-Rh immunoglobulin: Low dose (200-1000 mcg) given IV for 1-5 days has been effective in limited studies. Success of treatment is attributed to sensitization of recipient RBCs, which results in low-grade hemolysis and blockade of the platelet destruction by the reticuloendothelial system.

Immunosuppression: Various immunosuppressive drugs including azathioprine, cyclophosphamide, vincristine, and cyclosporine, given alone or in combination with prednisone, have been used successfully in limited situations. A trial of immunosuppression therapy may be indicated in patients who fail to respond to splenectomy or in those who are too unstable to be surgical candidates.

Vinca "alkaloid-loaded" platelets: Transfusions of platelets "loaded" with vinblastine may reduce the phagocytic destruction of platelets in patients who fail to respond to other treatments.

Colchicine: A small percentage of patients refractory to other treatments may improve with 1.2 mg colchicine daily for ≥2 wk. The drug has been used successfully in limited studies.

Danazol: 400-800 mg/day has resulted in complete remission or partial improvement in 60%-70% of patients in several studies. Use is controversial because other researchers have reported poor results and many untoward side effects.

Plasmapheresis: Several days of machine-assisted plasma exchange to remove approximately 1-1½ times the patient's total plasma volume per procedure and replace it with a suitable solution (e.g., colloids, crystalloids, plasma). Therapy is reserved for patients with life-threatening hemorrhage unresponsive to other measures. It is costly and of marginal benefit.

NURSING DIAGNOSES AND INTERVENTIONS

Altered protection related to decreased platelet count, resulting in increased risk of bleeding

Desired outcomes: Within 72 hr of onset of treatment, patient exhibits no clinical signs of new bleeding or bruising episodes. Secretions and excretions are negative for blood, and vital signs (VS) are within 10% of patient's normal range. Within the 24-hr period before discharge from intensive care, patient and significant others verbalize understanding of the indicators of impending bleeding.

- Monitor patient for bleeding and hemorrhage, including elevated HR and RR, decreasing BP, oozing from invasive procedure sites, bleeding mucous membranes, hematuria, and GI bleeding. Note Hgb and Hct levels before and after blood loss, as indicated.
- Protect the patient from trauma that may cause bleeding. Avoid taking rectal temperatures.
- Monitor skin or mucous membranes for discoloration, bruising, breakdown, redness.
- Monitor coagulation studies, including PT, PTT, fibrinogen, fibrin degradation products (FDP), fibrin split products (FSP), and platelet counts as appropriate.
- Consult physician for sustained low platelet values (<100,000/mm^3).
- Avoid administering NSAIDs (e.g., aspirin, ibuprofen). Teach patient to avoid all medications that potentially decrease platelet aggregation, especially aspirin.
- For severe menorrhagia, confer with physician regarding need for progestational hormones for suppression of menses. Assess blood loss by weighing perineal pads or tampons.
- During the acute (bleeding) phase of ITP, teach patient to perform oral hygiene using sponge-tipped applicators soaked in water or dilute mouthwash to help prevent gum bleeding.
- Teach patient that it is always safer to use an electric razor for shaving.
- Instruct family member/caregiver about signs of skin breakdown, as appropriate.
- Teach patient and significant others to recognize the signs of impending hemorrhage: more rapid pulse and breathing, easy bruising, painful joints, and blood in sputum, urine, or stool.

NIC Bleeding Precautions; Skin Surveillance

Decreased adaptive capacity: intracranial (or risk for same), related to potential for intracranial hemorrhage (<1% of patients) secondary to decreased platelet level

Desired outcomes: Throughout the hospitalization, patient remains free of symptoms of intracranial hemorrhage as evidenced by orientation to time, place, and person; normoreactive pupils and reflexes; patient's normal visual acuity, motor strength, and coordination; and absence of headache and other clinical indicators of increased intracranial pressure (IICP).

- Assess patient for initial signs of IICP, including diminished LOC, headaches, pupillary responses (e.g., unequal; sluggish/absent response to light), visual disturbances, weakness and paralysis, slow HR, and change in respiratory rate and pattern.
- Monitor trend of Glasgow Coma Scale, ICP, and cerebral perfusion pressure (CPP).
- Increase frequency of neurologic monitoring as appropriate.
- Avoid activities that increase intracranial pressure.
- If initial signs of IICP are noted, consult physician immediately. Severe intracranial bleeding can lead to herniation. ICP can increase rapidly with severe bleeding, sometimes causing death within 1 hr of onset. Signs of impending herniation include unconsciousness, failure to respond to deeply painful stimuli, decorticate or decerebrate posturing, Cushing's triad (i.e., bradycardia, increased systolic BP, widening pulse pressure), nonreactive/fixed pupils, unequal pupils, or fixed and dilated pupils. See p. 100 for more information about herniation.
- Consult with physician regarding management of IICP (see p. 103 for collaborative interventions for IICP). For additional interventions for IICP, see Table 2-5.
- Teach patient to avoid Valsalva maneuver (e.g., straining at stool or when lifting; forceful and sustained coughing or nose blowing), which could cause intracranial bleeding.
- Teach the importance of avoiding tobacco products (particularly cigarettes) and excessive caffeine, which may cause vasoconstriction. Constricted vessels may prevent platelets from circulating through portions of the capillary network.
- Confer with physician regarding use of stool softeners or cough suppressants as necessary.

NIC Cerebral Edema Management; Cerebral Perfusion Promotion; Intracranial Pressure (ICP) Monitoring; Neurologic Monitoring

Risk for fluid volume deficit related to active loss secondary to intraabdominal bleeding or postsplenectomy intraabdominal bleeding

Desired outcome: Patient remains normovolemic as evidenced by HR, RR, and BP within 10% of patient's normal range (or HR 60-100 beats/min, RR 12-20 breaths/min with normal depth and pattern [eupnea], systolic BP ≥90 mm Hg); urinary output ≥0.5 ml/kg/hr; and absence of abdominal pain or tenderness, back pain, and frank bleeding from the splenectomy incision.

- Monitor fluid status, including I&O, and signs of hypovolemia, including increases in HR and RR and decreases in BP, and urinary output, restlessness, fatigue, and orthostatic vital signs.
- Inspect for bleeding from mucous membranes, bruising after minimal trauma, oozing from puncture sites, and presence of petechiae. Maintain patent IV access.
- Administer supplemental oxygen as necessary for postoperative status or active bleeding.
- Replace lost volume with plasma expanders (e.g., albumin, hetastarch) and/or blood products as indicated. See Table 9-2 for information about blood products.

- Inform patient of the importance of wearing a medical-alert bracelet and obtaining a pneumococcal vaccination if a splenectomy has been performed.

NIC Bleeding Precautions; Electrolyte Management; Fluid Management; Fluid Monitoring; Hypovolemia Management; Intravenous (IV) Therapy; Shock Management: Volume; Blood Products Administration

Pain related to joint inflammation and injury secondary to bleeding into the synovial cavity of the joint(s); postsplenectomy pain

Desired outcomes: Within 4 hr of initiating treatment, patient's subjective evaluation of discomfort improves as documented by a pain scale; nonverbal indicators of discomfort are absent or decreased. HR, RR, and BP are within 10% of patient's baseline.

- Devise a pain scale with patient, rating discomfort from 0 (no pain) to 10. Perform a comprehensive assessment of pain to include location, characteristics, onset/duration, frequency, quality, intensity or severity, and precipitating factors.
- Ensure that patient receives appropriate analgesic care. Consult with physician regularly until patient's pain is controlled. Avoid use of meperidine for pain relief in elders because adverse effects are common.
- Teach patient causes of the pain, how long it may last, and about discomforts from procedures.
- Elevate patient's legs to decrease joint pain in the lower extremities. Avoid knee flexion. Support extremities with pillows, making sure bed is not "gatched" at the knee.
- Teach patient to splint abdomen when coughing after splenectomy.
- Evaluate patient's anxiety level, and provide emotional support to control fear and anxiety. If patient becomes agitated, evaluate potential causes including hypoxemia, poor pain or anxiety control, fluid and electrolyte imbalance, and alcohol or drug withdrawal, and intervene appropriately.
- See p. 51 for additional pain interventions. Also see "Prolonged Immobility," p. 61, for patients who are unable to move or who have limited movement.

NIC Analgesic Administration; Pain Management; Coping Enhancement; Anxiety Reduction

ADDITIONAL NURSING DIAGNOSES

Uncontrolled bleeding can be terrifying for the patient and significant others, who may fear that the patient will die. Refer to nursing diagnoses in "Psychosocial Support," p. 68, and "Psychosocial Support for the Patient's Family and Significant Others," p. 78, for appropriate interventions.

DISSEMINATED INTRAVASCULAR COAGULATION

PATHOPHYSIOLOGY

Disseminated intravascular coagulation (DIC) is a syndrome characterized by overstimulation of the normal coagulation cascade, often related to severe sepsis or shock. DIC is a coagulopathy with potential to cause both profuse bleeding and widespread thrombosis leading to MODS. Inherent bodily control of bleeding requires a balance between procoagulants and thrombus formation, along with anticoagulants, inhibitors, and thrombolysis (see Figure 9-1, Table 9-3). The delicate balance may be upset by disease processes (Table 9-4), resulting in a cascade of uncontrolled coagulation and fibrinolysis. The abnormal clotting cascade that develops during DIC is as follows:

- Platelets and coagulation factors are activated by a disease stimulus and are rapidly consumed, particularly factors V and XIII and fibrinogen.
- Thrombin is formed very rapidly, and inherent inhibitors cannot stop the formation of the vast amounts of thrombin generated. Thrombin directly activates fibrinogen.
- Fibrin is deposited throughout the capillary beds of organs and tissues.
- The fibrinolytic system lyses fibrin and impairs thrombin formation.
- FDPs (or FSPs) result from fibrinolysis, which changes platelet aggregation and inhibits fibrin polymerization. See Figure 9-1 for the normal coagulation pathway.

A predisposing event that damages the vascular endothelium initiates the clotting cascade. Studies reflect that both the intrinsic and extrinsic pathways are activated initially, resulting in an abnormal acceleration of the clotting process. Thrombocytopenia occurs because of thrombin production and microvascular thrombus formation.

ASSESSMENT

Risk factors: Any clinical state or pharmacologic therapy (e.g., chemotherapy) that inhibits the removal of activated clotting factors, FDPs, and thromboplastin by the reticuloendothelial system. Any patient is at high risk following severe trauma or with systemic inflammatory response syndrome

T A B L E 9 - 3   Clotting Factors: Primary Actions

Coagulation factor	Thrombin-sensitive/ promotes vasoconstriction	Vitamin K-sensitive	Sites of heparin activity
I Fibrinogen	✓		
II Prothrombin		✓	✓ IIa
III Tissue thromboplastin (tissue factor)			
IV Calcium			
V Proaccelerin (AC globulin [AC-g])	✓		
VI Not assigned			
VII Proconvertin stable factor (prothrombin accelerator)		✓	
VIII Antihemophilic factor A (antihemophilic factor [AHF], antihemophilic globulin [AHG])	✓		
IX Antihemophilic factor B (plasma thromboplastin component [PTC], Christmas factor)		✓	✓ IXa
X Stuart-Prower factor (Stuart factor)		✓	✓ Xa
XI Plasma thromboplastin antecedent (antihemophilic factor C)			✓ XIa
XII Hageman factor (contact factor)			
XIII Fibrin stabilizing factor	✓		
Other factors:			
Prekallikrein (Fletcher factor)			
High-molecular-weight kininogen (HMWK-Fitzgerald factor)			
Platelets			

(SIRS), a severe infection, sepsis, severe sepsis, or septic shock. Obstetrics patients with abruptio placenta, amniotic fluid embolism, or eclampsia release procoagulation factors, placing them at risk. DIC may manifest as a profound bleeding/clotting disorder in the *acute* phase or as a less symptomatic *chronic* disorder.

In chronic (compensated) DIC, activation of coagulation and fibrinolysis does not occur rapidly enough to exceed the rate of production of clotting factors or inhibitors. The course of DIC depends on the intensity of the stimulus, coupled with the status of the liver, bone marrow, and vascular endothelium. Whether DIC leads to bleeding or to thrombosis is profoundly affected by the underlying disease process.

Clinical presentation: *Abrupt onset of bleeding* or oozing of blood from all invasive procedure sites and mucosal surfaces (e.g., oral, nasal, tracheal, gastric, urethral, vaginal, rectal). In addition, the patient may have hematuria, petechiae, stools or gastric aspirate positive for occult blood, pallor, tachycardia, tachypnea, vertigo, hypotension, ecchymoses (e.g., on palate, gums, skin, conjunctivae), lethargy, irritability, or feeling of impending doom, and possible back pain and abdominal tenderness.

Abnormal thrombosis may manifest with extremity pain, diminished pulses, oliguria or anuria, diminished or absent bowel sounds, severe chest pain with SOB (indicative of either myocardial infarction or pulmonary embolism), or paresis or paralysis (indicative of cerebral thrombus).

Physical assessment: Bleeding from invasive procedure sites and mucosal surfaces, petechiae, ecchymoses, acrocyanosis, bruising, mottling, SOB, tachypnea, possible Grey Turner's sign (flank ecchymosis), purpura, diminished or absent bowel sounds, weakened or absent peripheral pulses, confusion, decreased responsiveness, abdominal tenderness, weakness, ST segment elevation or depression, and T wave inversion.

DIAGNOSTIC TESTS

Also see Table 9-5.

FDP or FSP: Increased (>10 mcg/ml) because of widespread fibrinolysis, which produces FDPs as the end product of clot lysis. Critical value: >40 ng/ml.

TABLE 9-4 Clinical Conditions That Can Activate Disseminated Intravascular Coagulation (DIC)

Obstetric	GI disorders	Tissue damage	Infections	Hemolytic processes	Vascular disorders	Miscellaneous
Abruption placentae	Cirrhosis	Surgery	Viral	Transfusion reaction	Shock	Fat or pulmonary embolism
Toxemia	Hepatic necrosis	Trauma	Bacterial	Acute hemolysis secondary to infection or immunologic disorder	Aneurysm	Snake bite
Amniotic fluid embolism	Acute fulminant hepatitis	Burns	Rickettsial		Giant hemangioma	Neoplastic disorder
Septic abortion	Pancreatitis	Prolonged extracorporeal circulation	Protozoal			Acute anoxia
Retained dead fetus	Peritoneovenous shunts	Transplant rejection	Fungal			
Hydatid mole	Necrotizing enterocolitis	Heat stroke				

T A B L E   9 - 5　**Blood Coagulation Screen in Disseminated Intravascular Coagulation (DIC)**

Parameter	Normal	Acute DIC	Chronic DIC
Fibrinogen	150-400 mg/dl (adult)	Decreased	Normal or increased
Fibrin degradation	<10 mcg/ml	Positive (increased)	Positive (increased)
Platelet count	150,000-400,000/mm^3 (adult)	Decreased	Normal or increased
Partial thromboplastin time (PTT); also known as activated partial thromboplastin time (aPTT)	25-35 sec	Increased	Normal
Prothrombin time (PT)	11-15 sec	Increased	Normal
Thrombin time	1.5 × Control value	Increased	Increased

D-dimer assay: Increased to >500 because of increased thrombin and plasmin generation. This is a rapid measurement technique, less sensitive than FDPs, and not recommended as a substitute for FDPs and fibrinogen determinations.

Fibrinogen levels: May remain normal or decrease in the early acute phase. As the process continues, fibrinogen levels will decrease. Normal range is 150-400 mg/dl.

PTT or activated partial thromboplastin time (aPTT): Prolonged (>40 sec) because of activation of the intrinsic pathway, causing consumption of coagulation factors. Critical value: >70 sec. In chronic DIC the value may be normal (25-35 sec) or less than normal.

PT: Prolonged (>15 sec) because of activation of the extrinsic pathway, causing consumption of the extrinsic clotting factors. Critical value: >40 sec.

Thrombin time: Prolonged (>1.5 times the control value or >2 sec in excess of a 9- to 13-sec control value) because of rapid conversion of fibrinogen into fibrin.

Antithrombin III (AT-III): Decreased (<50% of control value using a plasma sample, or <80% using functional values) because of rapid consumption of this thrombin inhibitor. The action of AT-III is catalyzed by heparin.

Euglobulin clot lysis time: This test measures fibrinogen activity via measurement of plasminogen and plasminogen activator, which assist in prevention of fibrin clot formations. Decreased time is seen with DIC. Normal: lysis in 2-4 hr. Critical value: 100% lysis in 1 hr.

Platelet count: Decreased (<140,000/mm^3) because of rapid rate of platelet aggregation to form clots during DIC. Aggregation decreases the freely circulating platelets.

Alpha$_2$-(α_2-) antiplasmin: Decreased because of rapid consumption of same in response to large amounts of plasmin generated. When all α_2-antiplasmin is depleted, excessive hyperfibrinolysis (massive, rapid clot lysis) occurs.

Protamine sulfate test, FSP: Results are positive (normal: negative), indicative of presence of fibrin strands. It is associated with the formation of excessive amounts of thrombin and secondary fibrinolysis.

Peripheral blood smear: For visualization during microscopic examination of schistocytes and burr cells, which indicate the deposition of fibrin in the small blood vessels.

COLLABORATIVE MANAGEMENT

Treatment of the underlying disease process often corrects the secondary DIC. Other treatments may vary in effectiveness, depending on the underlying disease. Use of heparin and antifibrinolytic agents in DIC is controversial, inasmuch as these agents have not improved survival in DIC and may exacerbate bleeding (heparin) or thrombosis (antifibrinolytic agent).

Treatment of the primary pathology: Aggressively treat the underlying cause. A primary disease promotes the development of DIC. If treatment of the disease fails, the mortality rate of DIC is high. When DIC occurs without apparent cause, the possibility of undiagnosed malignancy (e.g., prostate cancer), a large abdominal aortic aneurysm, a progressive gram-negative bacterial infection, or hepatic cirrhosis should be explored. If the diagnosis is by laboratory tests alone, conservative management is appropriate. Other conditions and medication side effects should be considered (Table 9-6).

Continuous IV heparin therapy: There are three conditions associated with DIC in which heparin may be effective:

TABLE 9-6 Causes of Thrombocytopenia (Decreased Platelets) in Critical Care

Increased destruction or consumption	Decreased production	Splenic sequestration	Medications
DIC	HIV	Malignancy	Chemotherapy
ITP and TTP	Malignancy	Portal hypertension	Thiazides
Sepsis	Malnutrition		Heparin
Burns	Nutritional deficit		Quinidine
Viral infection	(B_{12} or folate deficiency)		Furosemide
Massive bleeding with	Radiation therapy		Sulfonamides
blood transfusions	Ethanol abuse		Penicillin
			Cimetidine
			Ranitidine
			Digoxin

1. Underlying malignancy/carcinoma.
2. Acute promyelocytic leukemia (APML).
3. Purpura fulminans/extreme purpura, often seen with severe sepsis.

If used, the patient should have clinically obvious thrombosis. Low-dose therapy (5-10 units/kg/hr) is considered. Heparin binds to antithrombin, which then inhibits proteases involved in both the intrinsic and common coagulation pathways, resulting in a strong anticoagulant effect. Use of higher-dose heparin in DIC is associated with a high risk of bleeding, and greater efficacy has not been documented. Heparin may be considered for serious bleeding or clotting when the condition underlying the DIC is not rapidly reversible and the patient's vascular system is surgically intact.

Note: APML patients with DIC often experience accelerated symptoms of fibrinolysis (declotting) when receiving chemotherapy. If these individuals receive heparin, an antifibrinolytic agent such as epsilon- (ε-) aminocaproic acid (Amicar) may be added to decrease bleeding.

Antifibrinolytic agents: ε-Aminocaproic acid (Amicar) and tranexamic acid (Cyklokapron) are used to inhibit fibrinolysis in patients who are bleeding as a result of a variety of causes. In patients with DIC, these agents should be used with extreme caution because they may convert a bleeding disorder into a thrombotic problem. When used in DIC, these agents are used in combination with heparin to minimize the potential for thrombosis. Failure rates with use are high.

Thrombolytic agents: Use of streptokinase, urokinase, and tissue plasminogen activator (TPA) is not indicated for patients with thrombosis because these agents may facilitate excessive bleeding.

Blood component replacement: Clotting factors and inhibitors are replaced in the form of fresh-frozen plasma. The PT/INR may be the most accurate parameter(s) for guiding plasma replacement. Patients with markedly decreased fibrinogen levels may be given cryoprecipitate, which contains 5-10 times more fibrinogen than plasma contains. Thrombocytopenia in DIC may not be severe. The platelet count is usually >50,000/mm³. General replacement therapy guidelines indicate approximately 10 units of cryoprecipitate should be given for every 2-3 units of plasma. Platelet transfusions are used if the patient has impaired platelet production and profuse bleeding. AT-III concentrate has been used on a limited basis (see Table 9-1). More recently, DIC is being managed with antithrombin concentrate, activated protein C (APC) (drotrecogin alfa), tissue factor pathway inhibitor (TFPI), and synthetic serine protease inhibitors (e.g., aprotinin).

Red blood cell replacement: Packed RBCs may be administered to increase oxygen-carrying capacity with a hemoglobin value <9 mg/dl or >20% below the patient's baseline if the patient is chronically anemic.

Vitamin K_1 (phytonadione) and folate: Patients with DIC are at high risk for deficiency of these substances, and administration of both vitamins is recommended for most patients.

Protease inhibitors: Gabexate, nafamostat, and trasylol have been used.

Vasoactive drugs: If patient becomes severely hypotensive due to heart failure, the following drugs may be considered: milrinone, dobutamine, dopamine, epinephrine, and nitroprusside (see Appendix 7).

NURSING DIAGNOSES AND INTERVENTIONS

Altered protection related to bleeding resulting from overstimulation of the clotting cascade and rapid consumption of clotting factors
Desired outcome: Within 48-72 hr of initiation of treatment, patient is free of symptoms of bleeding as evidenced by absence of frank bleeding from invasive procedure sites and mucosal surfaces; secretions and excretions that are negative for blood; absence of large or increasing ecchymoses; decreasing purpura; and HR, RR, and BP within 10% of patient's baseline (or HR 60-100 beats/min, RR 12-20 breaths/min, systolic BP >90 mm Hg).

- Discuss bleeding history with patient or significant others. Assess prior incidences of bleeding from gums, skin, or urine; tarry/bloody stools; bleeding from muscles or into joints; hemoptysis, vomiting of blood, epistaxis, or prolonged bleeding from small wounds or after tooth extraction; or unusual bruising or tendency to bruise easily.
- Question patients about current medications, including over-the-counter (OTC) preparations, since many medications promote bleeding (Table 9-7).
- Monitor coagulation tests daily. Consult physician for abnormal values (see Table 9-5).
- Monitor closely for increased bleeding, bruising, petechiae, and purpura. Assess for internal bleeding by testing suspicious secretions (i.e., sputum, urine, stool, emesis, gastric drainage) for the presence of blood. Monitor for hemorrhage.
- Monitor neurologic status (see Glasgow Coma Scale, Appendix 3) q2h by assessing LOC, orientation, pupillary reaction, and movement and strength of extremities. Changes in status can indicate intracranial bleeding.
- Use alcohol-free mouthwash and swabs for oral care to minimize gingival/gum injury. Use normal saline solution (NSS) or solution of NSS and sodium bicarbonate (500 ml NSS with 15 ml bicarbonate) to irrigate the oral cavity if irritated. Massage gums gently with a sponge-tipped applicator to help remove debris. Do not attempt to remove large clots from the mouth, to avoid profuse bleeding.
- Use electric rather than safety razor for shaving patient.
- Refrain from inserting objects into a bleeding orifice. Avoid taking rectal temperatures.
- Protect the patient from trauma. Avoid unnecessary venipunctures and IM injections.
- If patient undergoes an invasive procedure, manually hold pressure over the insertion site for 3-5 min for IV catheters and 10-15 min for arterial catheters or until bleeding subsides.
- Instruct the patient and/or family on signs of bleeding and appropriate actions.
- Teach patient the importance of avoiding vitamin K-inhibiting and platelet aggregation-inhibiting medications (see Table 9-7), which promote bleeding.

NIC Infection Control; Infection Protection; Bleeding Precautions; Surveillance: Safety

Risk for fluid volume deficit related to bleeding/hemorrhage
Desired outcomes: Patient remains normovolemic as evidenced by HR and RR within 10% of patient's baseline (or HR 60-100 beats/min and RR 12-20 breaths/min with normal depth and pattern [eupnea]); BP within patient's baseline (or systolic BP >90 mm Hg); warm extremities; distal pulses >2+ on a 0-4+ scale; urinary output ≥0.5 ml/kg/hr; and capillary refill <2 sec. Within 24 hr of initiating treatment, patient verbalizes orientation to time, place, person, and self.

- Monitor every 2 hrs for increases in HR and RR, decreased BP, and decreasing pulse pressure.
- Measure urinary output q2-4h. Consult physician for output <0.5 ml/kg/hr.
- Maintain accurate I&O record. Weigh daily, and monitor trends.
- Increase measurement of VS and urine output to at least q30min for active bleeding. For profuse bleeding, check VS at least q15min. Inspect invasive procedure sites and dressings for bleeding.
- Monitor CBC daily for significant alterations in Hct, Hgb, and platelets (Table 9-8).
- Ensure that patient has typed and cross-matched blood available for transfusion.
- Monitor coagulation studies (PT, PTT, fibrinogen, FDP/FSP, platelet counts), as appropriate.
- Assess for signs of impending shock if the following signs are noted: increased HR and RR; decreased BP; or pallor, diaphoresis, cool extremities, delayed capillary refill, decreased pulse amplitude, restlessness, or disorientation.
- Maintain at least one 18-gauge or larger IV catheter for use during shock management, at which time rapid infusion of blood products or IV fluids may be necessary. For more information, see Advanced Cardiac Life Support (ACLS) algorithms, Appendix 1.
- Evaluate the effects of fluid therapy.

NIC Electrolyte Management; Fluid Management; Fluid Monitoring; Hypovolemia Management; Intravenous (IV) Therapy; Shock Management: Volume

TABLE 9-7 Medications That May Promote Bleeding

Medications that inhibit platelets or cause thrombocytopenia		Medications that inhibit vitamin K
Analgesics	*Diuretic agents*	*Salicylates*
Nonsteroidal antiinflammatory agents (NSAIDs)	Sulfonamide derivatives	Aspirin and aspirin-combination drugs
Aspirin	Acetazolamide	Other salicylates
Acetaminophen	Chlorpropamide	**Coumarins**
Antipyrine	Chlorothiazide	Anisindione
Ibuprofen	Chlorthalidone	Dicumarol
Indomethacin	Clopamide	Warfarin
Fenoprofen	Diazoxide	**Broad-spectrum antibiotics**
Sodium salicylate	Furosemide	Sulfonamides
Antirheumatic agents	Bumetanide	Triple sulfa
Oxyphenbutazone	Hydrochlorothiazide	Sulfamethoxazole
Phenylbutazone	Tolbutamide	Sulfasalazine
Hydroxychloroquine	Spironolactone	Sulfisoxazole
Gold salts	Mercurial diuretics	Sulfamethoxazole-trimethoprim
Antimicrobials	**Glycoprotein IIB IIIA inhibitors**	Clindamycin
Ampicillin	Abciximab	Gentamicin
Cephalothin	Eptifibatide	Neomycin
Methicillin	Tirofiban	Tobramycin
Penicillin	**Phenothiazines**	Vancomycin
Pentamidine	Chlorpromazine	Imipenem
Streptomycin	Promethazine	Cefamandole
Sulfonamides (antibiotics)	Trifluoperazine	Cefoxitin
Chloramphenicol	**Phosphodiesterase inhibitors**	**Vitamins**
Isoniazid	Caffeine	A
	Dipyridamole	E
Other		
Antihistamines		
Ethanol		
Heparin		
Beta-adrenergic blocking agents		
General anesthetics		
Local anesthetics		
Chemotherapeutic agents		
Vitamin E		
Estrogens		
Digitoxin		
Cimetidine		
Levodopa		
Propylthiouracil		

Continued

TABLE 9 - 7   **Medications That May Promote Bleeding—cont'd**

Medications that inhibit platelets or cause thrombocytopenia	Medications that inhibit vitamin K
Nitrofurantoin	
Rifampin	
Trimethoprim	
Anticoagulants	
Heparin	
Enoxaparin	
Dalteparin	
Thrombolytics	
Alteplase	
Reteplase	
Streptokinase	
Urokinase	
Anisoylated plasminogen streptokinase	
Tenecteplase	
Theophyllines	
Antiplatelet drugs	
Aspirin	
Ticlopidine	
Clopidogrel	
Prostaglandins	
I_2	
D_2	
E	
Sedative-hypnotics	
Benzodiazepines	
Clonazepam	
Diazepam	
Vasodilators	
Nitroglycerin	
Nitroprusside	

T A B L E   9 - 8   Complete Blood Count Values

Parameters	Common measurement value	Population
Red blood cells (RBCs)	4-5.5 million/mm^3	Adult females
	4.5-6.2 million/mm^3	Adult males
Hemoglobin (Hgb)	12-16 g/dl	Adult females
	14-18 g/dl	Adult males
Hematocrit (Hct)	37%-47%	Adult females
Mean corpuscular volume (MCV)	83-93 mcg^3	Adults
Mean cell hemoglobin (MCH)	26-34 pg	Adults
Mean cell hemoglobin concentration (MCHC)	31%-38%	Adults
White blood cells (WBCs)	4,500-11,000/mm^3	Adults
Differential white blood cells		
Granulocytes		
Segmented neutrophils (Segs)	54%-62%	Adults
Band neutrophils (Bands)	3%-5%	Adults
Eosinophils (Eos)	1%-3%	Adults
Basophils (Basos)	0-0.75%	Adults
Monocytes (Monos)	3%-7%	Adults
Lymphocytes (Lymphs)	25%-33%	Adults
Platelets	150,000-400,000/mm^3	Adults

Altered tissue perfusion (or risk for same): peripheral, cardiopulmonary, cerebral, gastrointestinal, and renal, related to blood loss or presence of microthrombi
Desired outcomes: Patient has adequate perfusion as evidenced by peripheral pulses >2+ on a scale of 0-4+; brisk capillary refill (<2 sec); BP within patient's normal range; CVP ≥5 cm H_2O or ≥2 mm Hg; PAWP 6-12 mm Hg; and HR regular and ≤100 beats/min. Patient is oriented to time, place, person, and self and has urinary output ≥30 ml/hr (0.5 ml/kg/hr) and oxygen saturation >90%.
- Assess and document peripheral perfusion q2h, including temperature, sensation, pulses, and movement in extremities. Perform a comprehensive assessment of peripheral circulation (i.e., check peripheral pulses, edema, capillary refill, and color and temperature of extremities).
- Monitor VS frequently. Evaluate chest pain. Document cardiac dysrhythmias.
- Monitor BP and assess for early signs of perfusion deficit at least q2h, including dizziness, confusion, and decreased urinary output.
- Monitor for decreased myocardial or pulmonary perfusion as evidenced by chest pain, ST segment depression or elevation, T wave inversion, SOB, dyspnea, and decreased oxygen saturation using continuous pulse oximetry.
- Monitor PAWP, observing for both high and low readings. Decreased pressures are indicative of hypovolemia/hemorrhage. Elevated PAD pressures may signal pulmonary embolus.
- Monitor cardiac output (CO), and calculate systemic vascular resistance (SVR), pulmonary vascular resistance (PVR), and cardiac index (CI). Anticipate vasoconstriction with hypovolemia: SVR will be elevated >1400 dynes/sec/cm^{-5}. CO may increase or decrease from normal range of 4-7 L/min, depending on cardiac contractility. PVR may be elevated >240 dynes/sec/cm^{-5} in the presence of pulmonary emboli.
- Monitor GI status by observing tolerance to diet or tube feedings, bowel habits (e.g., constipation, diarrhea), character of stool (e.g., tarry, bloody), and presence or absence of bowel sounds.

NIC Cardiac Care: Acute; Circulatory Care: Arterial Insufficiency; Circulatory Care: Venous Insufficiency; Respiratory Monitoring; Shock Management: Cardiac; Cerebral Perfusion Promotion; Neurologic Monitoring; Peripheral Sensation Management; Fluid/Electrolyte Management; Fluid Management; Vital Signs Monitoring

Impaired gas exchange (or risk for same) related to loss of oxygen-carrying capacity through hemorrhage or pulmonary microembolus formation
Desired outcome: Patient's gas exchange is adequate as evidenced by Pao_2 ≥80 mm Hg; $Paco_2$ 35-45 mm Hg; pH 7.35-7.45; RR 12-20 breaths/min with normal depth and pattern (eupnea); oxygen saturation >90%; HR 60-100 beats/min; Svo_2 >60%; and orientation to time, place, and person.

- Assess respiratory status q2h, noting rate, rhythm, depth, and regularity of respirations.
- Monitor for signs of respiratory failure: restlessness, anxiety, and air hunger indicative of hypoxemia; ABG values for increased $Paco_2$ and decreased pH indicative of hypoventilation; or oxygen saturation <90% via pulse oximetry indicative of decreased ventilation. Consult physician if signs of respiratory insufficiency are present.
- Monitor Svo_2: steady increase or decrease from patient's normal level may indicate deterioration.
- Assess lungs for bibasilar crackles (rales), indicative of pulmonary edema.
- Monitor patient's respiratory secretions. Institute respiratory therapy treatments as needed.
- Monitor for pulmonary embolus, including sharp, stabbing chest pain, dyspnea, pallor, cyanosis, pupillary dilation, rapid or irregular pulse, profuse diaphoresis, and anxiety. Assess need for supplemental oxygen, and consult physician immediately. Patients with severe pulmonary emboli may require mechanical ventilation. See "Pulmonary Emboli," p. 192.
- Assess patient for changes in sensorium (i.e., confusion, lethargy, somnolence), indicative of inadequate cerebral oxygenation or CO_2 retention (respiratory insufficiency).

NIC Airway Management; Oxygen Therapy; Respiratory Monitoring

Risk for injury related to blood product administration

Desired outcome: Throughout transfusion and up to 8 hr after transfusion, patient does not exhibit signs of a blood transfusion reaction as evidenced by absence of fever and chills; normal appearance of skin (i.e., no flushing, rash, lesions); and baseline RR, BP, and HR.

- Check blood to be transfused with another professional to ensure the patient receives the correct blood. Verify the following: patient's name and hospital number, blood unit number, blood expiration date, blood group, and blood type.
- When blood products are being infused, check VS q15min for the first hour. Check patient frequently throughout the first 15 min of the transfusion to observe for signs of an acute hemolytic transfusion reaction, including fever, chills, dyspnea, hypotension, flushing, tachycardia, back pain, hematuria, and shock.
- Observe for transfusion reactions throughout the transfusion and during the 8-hr period afterward. If a transfusion reaction (Table 9-9) occurs, implement the following:
  1. If the transfusion is in progress, stop the infusion immediately.
  2. Maintain IV access with NSS.
  3. Maintain BP with a combination of volume infusion and vasoactive drugs, if indicated. See ACLS algorithms, Appendix 1, accordingly.
  4. Monitor HR and ECG for changes. Treat symptomatic dysrhythmias as prescribed by a physician.
  5. Administer ordered diuretics and fluids to promote diuresis (urine output approximately 100 ml/hr).
  6. Obtain blood and urine for a transfusion workup per institution blood bank protocol.
  7. Perform blood cultures if patient exhibits signs of sepsis.
- If an intravascular hemolytic reaction is confirmed, implement the following:
  1. Monitor coagulation studies, including PT, PTT, and fibrinogen levels (see Table 9-5).
  2. Monitor renal status by measuring the following: blood urea nitrogen (BUN), creatinine, potassium, and phosphate levels.

T A B L E   9 - 9 **Acute Transfusion Reactions**

Type	Symptoms	Time frame
Acute intravascular hemolytic	Fever, chills, dyspnea, tachycardia, hypotension, back pain, flushing, hematuria, shock	After start of transfusion within 5-30 min
Acute extravascular hemolytic	Fever, elevated bilirubin, unusually low posttransfusion hematocrit and hemoglobin	Usually within 8 hr Delayed: 7-10 days
Allergic (mild)	Rash, hives pruritus	Within 1 hr
Anaphylactic	Dyspnea, shortness of breath, bronchospasms, tachycardia, flushing, hypotension, shock	Within 30 min-1 hr
Febrile	Fever, chills	Within 4 hr
Hypervolemic	Dyspnea, tachycardia, bibasilar crackles, jugular jugular venous distention, possible hypertension, headache	Within 1-2 hr
Septic	Fever, chills, tachycardia, hypotension, vomiting, shock, muscle pain, cardiac arrest	Within 5 min-4 hr

3. Monitor lab values for hemolysis: increased lactate dehydrogenase (LDH), bilirubin, and haptoglobin.
- With massive transfusion for severe bleeding, manage hypocalcemia caused by citrated blood; hyperkalemia of uncertain etiology; hypothermia from refrigerated blood; ARDS; coagulopathy; and hemochromatosis (iron overload).

NIC Bleeding Precautions; Bleeding Reduction; Blood Products Administration

ADDITIONAL NURSING DIAGNOSES

The uncontrolled bleeding related to DIC can be terrifying to the patient and significant others, who may fear that the patient will die. Refer to nursing diagnoses in "Psychosocial Support," p. 68, and "Psychosocial Support for the Patient's Family and Significant Others," p. 78. For patients who manifest activity intolerance, see that nursing diagnosis in "Prolonged Immobility," p. 61. For patients with sepsis or septic shock, refer to p. 593.

Bibliography

Aster RH: Heparin-induced thrombocytopenia and thrombosis, *N Engl J Med* 332(20):1374-1376, 1995 (editorial).

Balk R et al: Therapeutic use of antithrombin concentrate in sepsis, *Semin Thromb Hemost* 24(2):183-194, 1998.

Colvin BT: Management of disseminated intravascular coagulation, *Br J Haematol* 101(suppl 1):15-17, 1998.

Corwin HL et al: The CRIT study: anemia and blood transfusion in the critically ill—current clinical practice in the United States, *Crit Care Med* 32 (1):39-52, 2004.

Esmon CT et al: The protein C pathway: new insights, *Thromb Hemost* 78(1):70-74, 1997.

Fahey VA: Heparin-induced thrombocytopenia, *J Vasc Nurs* 13(4):112-116, 1995.

Francis JL et al: Comparison of bovine and porcine heparin in heparin antibody formation after cardiac surgery, *Ann Thorac Surg* 75:17-22, 2003.

George JN: For low platelets, how low is dangerous? *Cleve Clin J Med* 71(4):277-278, 2004.

Griffiths E, Dzik WH: Assays for heparin-induced thrombocytopenia, *Transfus Med* 7(1):1-11, 1997.

Guzzi L: The incidence and impact of heparin-induced thrombocytopenia (HIT) in the critical care setting, *Critical Care Express Report*: based on data presented in the CME symposium "The Incidence and Impact of Heparin-induced Thrombocytopenia (HIT) in the Critical Care Setting" held during the 33rd Congress of the Society of Critical Care Medicine, February 22, 2004 in Orlando, Fla, 2004, Millenium Medical Communications.

Haas S: Venous thromboembolism in medical patients—the scope of the problem, *Semin Thromb Hemost* 29 (Suppl 1):17-21, 2003.

Harenberg J et al: Dosage, anticoagulant and antithrombotic effects of heparin and low-molecular-weight heparin in the treatment of deep vein thrombosis, *Semin Thromb Hemost* 23(1):83-90, 1997.

Horne MK, Fu C-L: Hemorrhagic and thrombotic disorders. In Parrillo JE Dellinger RP: *Critical care medicine: principles of diagnosis and management in adults,* ed 2, St Louis, 2002, Mosby.

Kelton, JG, Warkentin TE: Heparin-induced thrombocytopenia: diagnosis, natural history and treatment options, *Postgrad Med* 103(2):169-171, 175-178, 1998.

Klein HG, Higgins MJ: Use of blood components in the intensive care unit. In Parrillo JE, Dellinger RP: *Critical care medicine: principles of diagnosis and management in adults,* ed 2, St Louis, 2002, Mosby.

Lechner DL: A standardized weight-based heparin protocol: improving clinical outcomes, *Nurs Manage* 28(4):29-32, 1997.

Linkins L, Weitz JI: New anticoagulants, *Semin Thromb Hemost* 29(6):619-631, 2003.

Muhlberg AH, Ruth-Sahd L: Holistic care: treatment and interventions for hypovolemic shock secondary to hemorrhage, *Dimensions Crit Care Nurs* 23(2):55-59, March/April, 2004.

Pablinger I, Grafenhofer H: Anticoagulation during pregnancy, *Semin Thromb Hemost* 29(6): 633-638, 2003.

Pechet L: The hemolytic anemias. In Rippe JM et al: *Intensive care medicine,* ed 3, Boston, 1996, Little, Brown.

Penner JA: Disseminated intravascular coagulation in patients with multiple organ failure of non-septic origin, *Semin Thromb Hemost* 24(1):45-52, 1998.

Ray MJ, Marsh NA: Aprotinin reduces blood loss after cardiopulmonary bypass by direct inhibition of plasmin, *Semin Thromb Hemost* 78(3):1021-1026, 1997.

Rice L et al: Delayed-onset heparin-induced thrombocytopenia, *Ann Intern Med* 136:210-215, 2002.

Riewald M, Reiss H: Treatment options for clinically recognized disseminated intravascular coagulation, *Semin Thromb Hemost* 24(1):53-59, 1998.

Simko LC, Lockhart JS: Action STAT: heparin-induced thrombocytopenia and thrombosis, *Nursing* 26(3):33, 1996.

Warkentin TE: Platelet count monitoring and laboratory testing for heparin-induced thrombocytopenia, *Arch Pathol Lab Med* 126:1415-1423, 2002.

Williams RT et al : Anti-platelet factor 4/heparin antibodies: an independent predictor of 30-day myocardial infarction after acute coronary ischemic syndromes, *Circulation* 107:2307-2312, 2003.

CHAPTER 10

Multisystem Stressors

Systemic Inflammatory Response Syndrome (SIRS), Sepsis, and Septic Shock

PATHOPHYSIOLOGY

Systemic inflammatory response syndrome (SIRS) is a state of generalized, uncontrolled inflammation. Inflammation is a complex response initiated by mechanical, ischemic, chemical, or microbial sources. SIRS is characterized by signs of systemic inflammation such as fever and leukocytosis. The purpose of the inflammatory response of immunity is to protect the body from further injury and promote rapid healing. Vasodilation occurs, along with increased microvascular permeability, neutrophil activation and adhesion, and enhanced coagulation. The vascular response is initiated at the cellular level by histamine, prostaglandins, bradykinin, and numerous other mediators. In some instances, regulatory mechanisms fail and uncontrolled systemic inflammation overwhelms the body's normal protective response. This leads to systemic vasodilation, hypotension, a generalized increase in vascular permeability, extravascular fluid sequestration, increased cellular aggregation with microvascular obstruction, and greatly accelerated coagulation.

The term *sepsis* implies an infectious process: when infection is the underlying cause of SIRS. Most septic events require antibiotic management and generally resolve without the need for hospitalization. Microorganisms commonly seen in infections of critically ill patients include gram-negative enteric pathogens (e.g., *Escherichia coli, Klebsiella* spp., *Enterobacter* spp., *Pseudomonas aeruginosa*), *Staphylococcus aureus,* coagulase-negative staphylococci, *Enterococcus* spp., and *Candida* spp. Antibiotic-resistant bacteria (e.g., *methicillin-resistant staphylococcus aureus* [MRSA]) are also commonly seen.

Severe sepsis is the compounding of sepsis by comorbid conditions. Severe sepsis accompanied by hypotension that does not respond to volume infusion is called *septic shock.* Impaired perfusion may cause lactic acidosis, oliguria, or acute alterations in mental status. Genetic predisposition and other factors compound severe sepsis, leading to *multiple organ dysfunction syndrome (MODS),* multiple organ failure (MOF) and may be terminal. MODS is diagnosed when two or more vital organ systems fail.

A new view of severe sepsis is evolving. Severe sepsis has recently been viewed as endothelial dysfunction resulting from overwhelming inflammatory mediation, in conjunction with profound, unopposed coagulation. When infection causes a generalized inflammatory response, or SIRS, the normally smooth surface of microvascular (capillary) endothelium is damaged by the initial response. Systemic mediators are released to facilitate healing of the endothelium. Since endothelial damage is widespread, the *hyperinflammatory* response leads to accelerated microcoagulation as *microclots* form on the roughened capillary endothelium, consuming platelets and inhibiting clot lysis (fibrinolysis). This progresses to uncontrolled alterations in the vascular tone with vasodilation in the large vessels (where blood pressure is measured.) Both vasodilation and constriction occurs in capillaries, where oxygen delivery takes place. Coupled with microvascular clotting, the process limits oxygen delivery and may lead to organ ischemia.

Problems of severe sepsis and septic shock include the following:
- Hyperinflammation
- Hypercoagulatiion
- Microvascular obstruction
- Endothelial permeability
  See Figure 10-1 for a depiction of the pathophysiologic process of sepsis.

Research Brief 10-1   Microvascular circulatory impairment due to damage of the vascular endothelium had been proposed for 10 years as the cause of the cascade of events leading to multiple organ dysfunction syndrome, but little evidence existed that this damage occurred. Inflammatory mediators are largely responsible for endothelial damage. The authors confirmed that an increased level of circulating endothelial cells was present in patients with sepsis and septic shock, compared to a group of normal, healthy volunteers. This was one of the first studies to obtain measurable evidence to confirm that the endothelium was damaged in human sepsis.

Mutunga M et al: Circulating endothelial cells in patients with septic shock. *Am J Resp Crit Care Med* 163:195-200, 2001.

ASSESSMENT

History and risk factors: Infection, malnutrition, immunosuppression, chronic health problems (e.g., liver or renal disease), bone marrow suppression, advanced age, recent traumatic injuries, or surgical or invasive procedures; sequential infections. Underlying diseases or conditions such as splenectomy, intravenous (IV) substance abuse, and rheumatic heart disease are other risk factors.

Clinical presentation: May present with tachycardia unresponsive to fluid bolus; tachypnea, hyperthermia or hypothermia, and hyperglycemia. Criteria for diagnosis of sepsis are evolving. In 1992 the American College of Chest Physicians (ACCP) and Society of Critical Care Medicine (SCCM) stated that diagnosis of SIRS was based on the following: tachypnea (respiratory rate [RR] >20 breaths/min); hypocarbia (<32 mm Hg); tachycardia (heart rate [HR] >90 beats/min); temperature >38° C (100.4° F) or <36° C (96.8° F); white blood cell count [WBC] >12,000/mm^3 or <4000/mm^3; or >10% immature (band) forms. In 2004 the SCCM developed the following *definition of sepsis: a documented or suspected infection with one or more of the following*: fever, hypothermia, HR >90 or >2 standard deviations (SD) above the normal for age; tachypnea, altered mental status, hyperglycemia >120mg/dl in absence of diabetes, leukocytosis, leucopenia, normal WBC with > 10% immature forms (bands), plasma C-reactive protein >2 SD above normal, and decreased protein C level.

Physical assessment: See Tables 10-1 and 10-2.

Hemodynamic measurements: *Early stages:* Increased respiratory rate (RR) and heart rate (HR); decreased blood pressure (BP). Temperature >38.3° C (101° F) but sometimes normal or even decreased, especially in elders. The hemodynamic presentation varies with fluid balance and cardiac function of the patient. Cardiac output/cardiac index (CO/CI) are often elevated, pulmonary artery wedge (PAWP) and central venous pressures (CVP), which depend on the compliance of the ventricles, may be normal to low, and the Svo_2 (reflecting tissue use of oxygen) in early stages may be low to normal. Adequacy of tissue oxygenation should be measured by serum lactate levels to assess for the degree of anaerobic metabolism present. Lactate is produced when poor circulation and oxygenation prompt cells to initiate anaerobic metabolism.

Late stages: Terminal heart failure, with decreasing heart rate and blood pressure, pump failure exhibited by an increase in PAWP and CVP with normal to high (60%-80%) Svo_2. Occlusion of the capillaries (microcirculation) limits oxygen utilization at the cellular level, causing Svo_2 to increase.

DIAGNOSTIC TESTS

Complete blood cell count (CBC): White blood cell count may be normal, elevated, or decreased. The presence of more than 10% of bands indicates an inflammatory response.

Blood chemistry: In physiologic stress states (e.g., infection, trauma, hypoxia), hormones are released to increase generation of additional glucose from nonglucose products (gluconeogenesis). These hormones create insulin resistance, and glucose uptake by the cells is impaired. Hyperglycemia is common but may improve as the liver fails, since the liver has a key role in gluconeogenesis. If catecholamines (e.g., norepinephrine, phenylephrine) are given to increase blood pressure, this may prolong hyperglycemia, since catecholamines create insulin resistance.

Blood cultures and antibiotic sensitivity testing of isolates: Identify causative organism(s).

Culture and antibiotic sensitivity testing of suspect infection sites (e.g., urine, sputum, blood, intravenous [IV] lines, incisions): Correlate with blood cultures to identify source(s) of the sepsis.

Arterial blood gas (ABG) values: When metabolic acidosis (low HCO_3^- or base deficit more negative than −2) is present, a serum lactate (normal is <2 mMol/L) should be drawn to assess severity of tissue hypoxia. Initially, patients may compensate by hyperventilating to lower CO_2. Later, respiratory failure with respiratory acidosis may ensue.

Clotting studies: May reflect decreased platelets (>50% drop over 3 days is an indicator of severe sepsis), increased prothrombin time (PT), increased partial thromboplastin time (PTT), increased international normalized ratio (INR), and increased fibrin split products. These results all reflect activation of the clotting cascade and may signal development of disseminated intravascular coagulation (DIC).

X-rays: Chest x-ray to check for pneumonia or acute respiratory distress syndrome (ARDS) prior to computed tomography (CT) scanning of the lung. Other x-rays are done to assess underlying condition.

Computed tomography (CT): Lung CT is more reflective of changes in the pulmonary microcirculation, and most accurately depicts extravascular lung water. Also used to assess for abnormalities such as intraabdominal abscess or perforated viscus.

COLLABORATIVE MANAGEMENT

Treatment: Recommended to be done according to the following sepsis bundles:

4-Hour sepsis bundle without shock (severe sepsis)
- Presumptive diagnosis is made within 2 hr.
- Serum lactate should be measured with severe sepsis.
- Antibiotics are administered within 1 hr of a presumptive diagnosis of severe sepsis
- Glucose control <140 mg/dl (intensive insulin therapy may be used to reduce glucose to 80-110 mg/dl)
- Plateau pressure should be on average <30 cm H_2O for ventilated patients.
- Activated protein C (drotrecogin alfa) is considered for severe sepsis using local guidelines.

4-Hour sepsis bundle with septic shock
- Immediate fluid resuscitation should be performed.
- Antibiotics should be administered within 1 hr of presumptive diagnosis.
- Obtain CVP if BP not responsive to fluids or serum lactate elevated.
- Vasopressors are administered for mean arterial pressure (MAP) less than 65 mm Hg during fluid resuscitation and after adequate fluid resuscitation.
- Inotropes and/or packed red blood cells (PRBCs) (when appropriate) are used for central venous oxygen saturation <70% after fluid replacement.
- Glucose levels <140 mg/dl are controlled (intensive insulin therapy may be used to reduce glucose to 80-110 mg/dl)
- Plateau pressure is kept at an average of <30 cm H_2O for ventilated patients.
- Activated protein C (drotrecogin alpha) use is considered, using local guidelines.
- Steroids are given for septic shock requiring continued use of vasopressors.

Supplemental oxygen: Administered to support ventilation and oxygen delivery to the tissues. The amount and method of oxygen administered are guided by ABG results. Intubation and mechanical ventilation may be necessary.

Fluid administration: Intravenous volume expansion is implemented to maintain adequate ventricular filling pressures and volume, which are compromised with increased capillary permeability and vasodilation. Lactated Ringer's solution, normal saline, albumin, and fresh-frozen plasma are used.

Positive inotropic drugs (e.g., dopamine, dobutamine, epinephrine): May be given to augment cardiac contractility and cardiac output. In the late stages of sepsis, positive inotropic drugs may be given with *vasodilators* such as nitroprusside and nitroglycerin, which decrease preload and afterload by dilating veins and arteries, if this strategy for heart failure improves blood pressure.

Vasopressors (e.g., dopamine, norepinephrine, phenylephrine): May be administered in cases when optimal left ventricular preload fails to restore adequate tissue perfusion (i.e., the initial mean arterial pressure [MAP] is very low or MAP is persistently <60 mm Hg). Goal of therapy is to optimize CI.

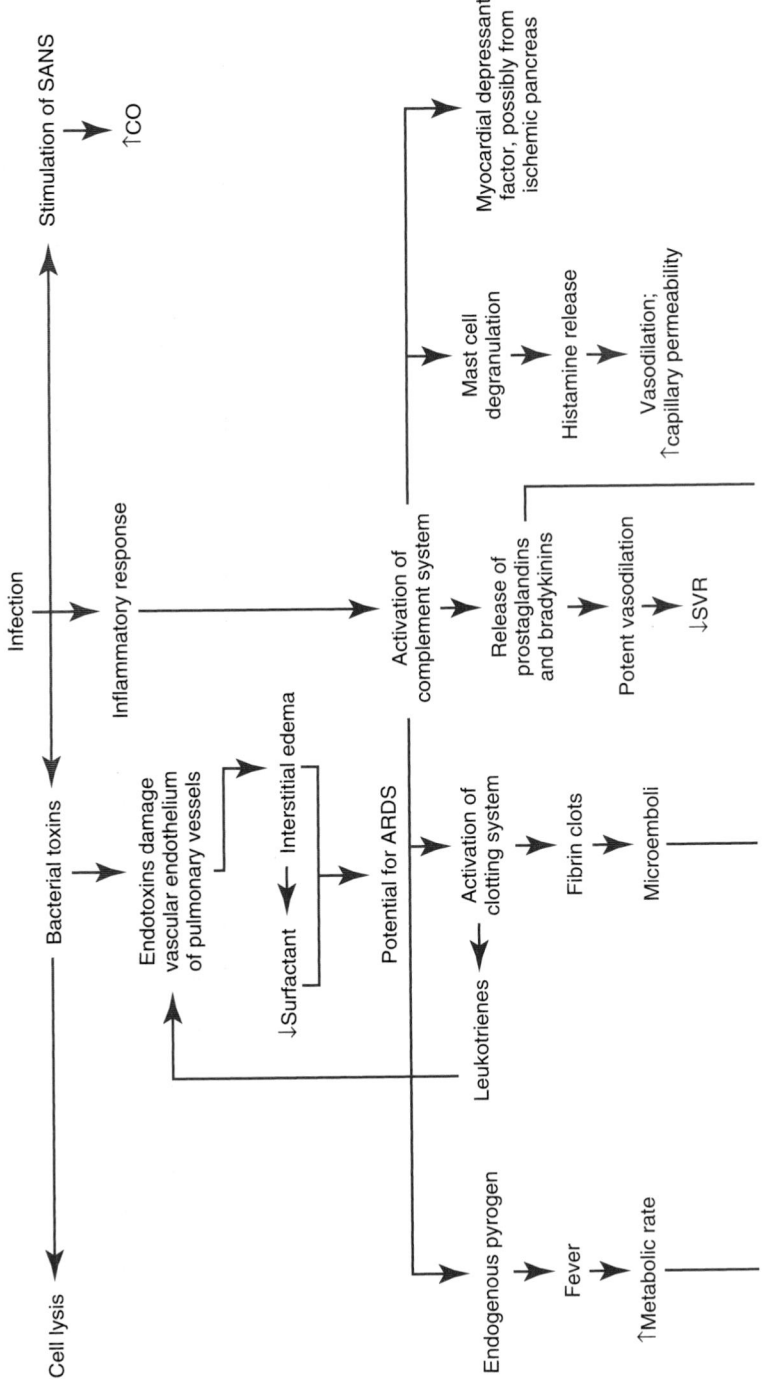

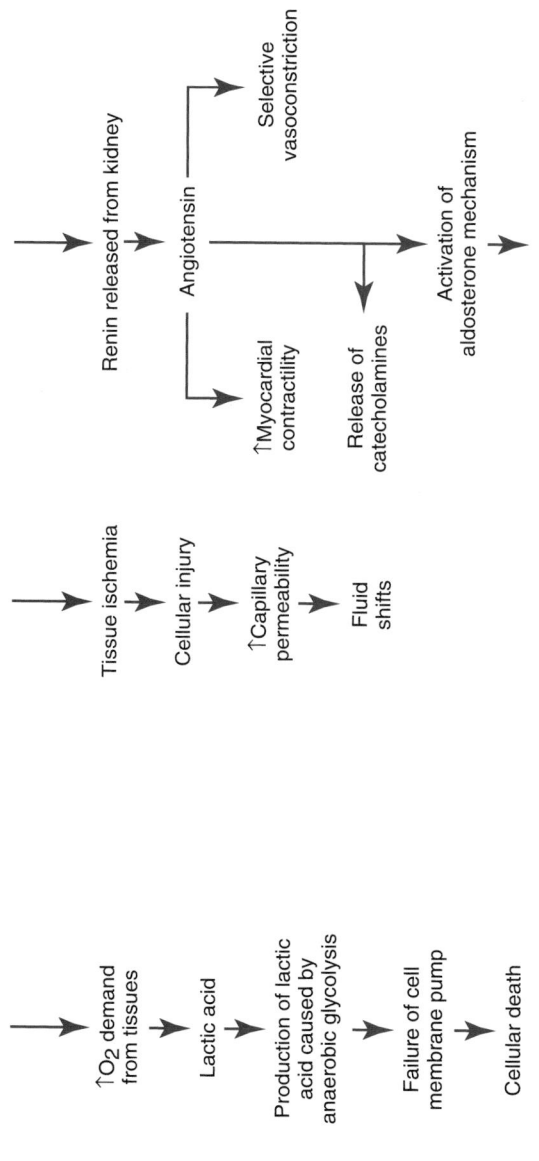

Figure 10-1: Pathophysiologic process of sepsis. *SANS,* Sympathetic/autonomic nervous system; *CO,* cardiac output; *ARDS,* acute respiratory distress syndrome; *SVR,* systemic vascular resistance.

T A B L E 10 - 1 Assessment Guidelines for the Patient with Sepsis in the Early Hyperdynamic Stage

Clinical indicator	Cause
Cardiovascular	
Increased HR (>100 beats/min)	Sympathetic/autonomic nervous system (SANS) stimulation
Decreased BP (<90 mm Hg systolic)	Vasodilation
CO >7 L/min; CI >4 L/min/m^2	Hyperdynamic state secondary to SANS stimulation
Svo$_2$>80%	Decreased utilization of oxygen by cells
PAWP usually <6 mm Hg	Venous dilation; decreased preload
SVR <900 dynes/sec/cm^{-5}	Vasodilation
Strong, bounding peripheral pulses	Hyperdynamic cardiovascular system
Respiratory	
Tachypnea (>20 breaths/min) and hyperventilation	Decreases in cerebrospinal fluid pH that stimulate the central respiratory center
Crackles	Interstitial edema occurring with increased vascular permeability
Paco$_2$ <35 mm Hg	Tachypnea and hyperventilation
Dyspnea	Increased respiratory muscle work
Renal	
Decreased urine output (<0.5 ml/kg/hr)	Decreased renal perfusion
Increased specific gravity (1.025-1.035)	Decreased glomerular filtration rate
Cutaneous	
Flushed and warm skin	Vasodilation
Metabolic	
Increasing body temperature (usually >38.3° C [100.9° F])	Increased metabolic activity; release of pyrogens secondary to invading microorganisms; release of interleukin-I by macrophages
pH <7.35	Metabolic acidosis occurring with accumulation of lactic acid
↑ Blood sugar	Release of glucagons; insulin depletion
Neurologic	
Changes in LOC	Decreased cerebral perfusion and brain hypoxia
Fluid	
↑Fluid retention	↑ ADH, ↑ aldosterone

ADH, Antidiuretic hormone; *beats/min,* beats per minute; *BP,* blood pressure; *CO,* cardiac output; *CI,* cardiac index; *HR,* heart rate; *LOC,* level of consciousness; *PAWP,* pulmonary artery wedge pressure; *SVR,* systemic vascular resistance.

Nutritional support: Short- and medium-chain fatty acids and branched-chain amino acids are administered to stop protein catabolism. The short- and medium-chain fatty acids are absorbed more readily and metabolized more easily than long-chain fatty acids. They may be given orally (e.g., MCT Oil, which is a proprietary name for triglycerides of medium-chain fatty acids), or by IV route (e.g., intralipid solutions). Branched-chain amino acid solutions are used in sepsis, as they are metabolized by muscle rather than the liver and can therefore be used in the presence of organ failure.

Antipyretic agents, cooled IV fluid, or cooling blanket: To normalize temperature.

Glucose-potassium-insulin (GKI): This combination may be given to increase cardiac performance during sepsis.

NURSING DIAGNOSES AND INTERVENTIONS

Fluid volume deficit related to active loss from vascular compartment secondary to increased capillary permeability and shift of intravascular volume into interstitial spaces

T A B L E 10 - 2   Assessment Guidelines for the Patient with Sepsis in the Late Stage

Clinical indicator	Cause
Cardiovascular	
Extreme tachycardia with S_3 sound	Compensatory attempt by sympathetic nervous system to maintain CO
Profound hypotension	Decreased stroke volume. Diastolic BP may remain high because of vasoconstriction
CO <4 L/min; CI <2.5 L/min/m^2	Failure of compensatory mechanisms
PAWP usually >12 mm Hg	Increased left ventricular end-diastolic pressure (LVEDP) because of increased residual volume from decreased stroke volume
SVR >1200 dynes/sec/cm^{-5}	Vasoconstriction
Weak or absent peripheral pulses	Decreased peripheral perfusion because of decreased CO
Svo_2 ≤60%	Decreased oxygen binding to hemoglobin because of acidosis
Respiratory	
Decreased respiratory rate (<12 breaths/min) and depth	Central respiratory center depression
Crackles, rhonchi, wheezes	Accumulation of lung secretions
Increased Fio_2 required to maintain Pao_2 (possible ARDS)	Ventilation/perfusion mismatch and decreased lung compliance
Renal	
Decreased urine output progressing to anuria	Decreased renal perfusion and tubular ischemia
Decreased fractional excretion of sodium	Activation of the aldosterone mechanism and release of ADH, which stimulate sodium and water retention
Cutaneous	
Cool, pale skin or cyanosis	Sustained vasoconstriction
Neurologic	
Decreased LOC, coma	Severe hypoxia
Hematologic	
Oozing from previous venipuncture sites	Development of DIC caused by stimulation of coagulation process, and fibrinolysis
Acid-base status	
pH <7.35; $Paco_2$ >45 mm Hg; HCO_3^- <22 mEq/L (or less than expected)	Mixed acid-base disorder: respiratory acidosis and metabolic acidosis

ARDS, Acute respiratory distress syndrome; *ADH,* antidiuretic hormone; *CI,* cardiac index; *CO,* cardiac output; *DIC,* disseminated intravascular coagulation; *LOC,* level of consciousness; *PAWP,* pulmonary artery wedge pressure; *SVR,* systemic vascular resistance.

Desired outcomes: Within 4 hr of initiation of therapy, patient is normovolemic as evidenced by peripheral pulses >2+ on a 0-4+ scale; stable body weight; urine output ≥0.5 ml/kg/hr; systolic BP ≥90 mm Hg or within patient's normal range; and absence of edema and adventitious lung sounds. PAWP is 6-12 mm Hg, CO is 4-7 L/min, and systemic vascular resistance (SVR) is 900-1200 dynes/sec/cm^{-5}.

- Monitor hemodynamic pressures, particularly PAWP, CO, and SVR. During the early stage of sepsis, filling pressures (PAWP and CVP) may be normal to low, but as biventricular dysfunction occurs, these pressures may increase. If the patient manifests a compensatory increase in cardiac output, the calculated SVR may initially be low, and rise as the cardiac output drops.
- Administer crystalloid and colloid fluid replacement as prescribed. Often fluid replacement therapy will be given to maintain a PAWP of 6-12 mm Hg. Assess PAWP and lung sounds at frequent

intervals during fluid replacement to detect evidence of fluid overload: crackles and increasing PAWP.
- Administer positive inotropic agents as prescribed to maintain adequate cardiac output in the presence of massive vasodilation.
- Assess fluid volume by monitoring BP and peripheral pulses hourly. Report systolic BP <90 mm Hg (or 20-30 mm Hg less than presepsis level) and decreasing amplitude of peripheral pulses.
- Weigh patient daily; monitor intake and output (I&O) every shift, noting 24-hr trends. Report urine output <0.5 ml/kg/hr. The patient's weight may actually increase with fluid volume deficit because of a shift of intravascular volume into interstitial spaces.
- Monitor specific gravity, being alert to increases >1.030, which indicate a dehydration state, or a fixed specific gravity of 1.010, which may signal inadequate glomerular filtration.
- Assess for interstitial edema as evidenced by pretibial, sacral, ankle, and hand edema, as well as crackles on auscultation of lung fields.
- As prescribed, administer vasopressor agents to help maintain perfusion.
- Position patient supine with the legs elevated to increase venous return and preload.

You may also wish to refer to the following interventions from the Nursing Interventions Classification (NIC):

NIC Invasive Hemodynamic Regulation; Fluid/Electrolyte Management; Hypovolemia Management; Fluid Management; Shock Management: Volume

Decreased cardiac output related to negative inotropic changes in the heart (late stage) secondary to effects of tissue hypoxia, worsening during late septic shock

Desired outcome: Within 8 hr of initiation of therapy, patient has adequate cardiac output as evidenced by systolic BP ≥90 mm Hg (or within patient's normal range); HR ≤100 beats/min; peripheral pulses >2+ (on a scale of 0-4+); urine output ≥0.5 ml/kg/hr; PAWP ≤12 mm Hg; CO ≥4 L/min; CI ≥2.5 L/min/m^2; and Svo$_2$ 60%-80%.
- Assess patient for signs of decreased cardiac output: decreasing BP, increasing HR, decreasing amplitude of peripheral pulses, restlessness, decreasing urinary output, and increasing PAWP.
- Administer positive inotropic agents as prescribed to augment cardiac contractility.
- Position patient supine with the legs elevated to optimize preload and enhance stroke volume.
- Assess CO at least q4h. Optimally, CO will be ≥4 L/min and CI will be ≥2.5 L/min/m^2.
- Monitor cardiac rhythm per monitor at frequent intervals. Observe for development of dysrhythmias, such as premature ventricular complexes (PVCs), which may occur with hypoxia, and extreme tachycardia. Dysrhythmias and hypoxia may further reduce cardiac output.
- Minimize myocardial oxygen demand by assisting patient with activities of daily living (ADLs) and ensuring uninterrupted periods of rest.
- Monitor Svo$_2$ continuously; report values outside of normal range.

NIC Cardiac Care: Acute; Hemodynamic Regulation; Invasive Hemodynamic Monitoring; Fluid/Electrolyte Management

Altered tissue perfusion: cerebral, renal, and gastrointestinal, related to hypovolemia secondary to mixed vasodilation and constriction interruption of arterial and venous blood flow secondary to vasoconstriction and thrombus obstruction.

Desired outcomes: Within 24 hr of initiating therapy, patient has adequate perfusion as evidenced by orientation to time, place, and person; peripheral pulses >2+ (on a scale of 0-4+); brisk capillary refill (<2 sec); urine output ≥0.5 ml/kg/hr; and ≥5 bowel sounds/min. BP is 110-120/70-80 mm Hg (or within patient's normal range); Svo$_2$ is 60%-80%; SVR is 900-1200 dynes/sec/cm^{-5}; CO is 4-7 L/min; and CI is 2.5-4 L/min/m^2.
- Assess for changes in level of consciousness (LOC) as an indicator of decreasing cerebral perfusion.
- Assess for the following signs of decreasing renal perfusion: urine output <0.5 ml/kg/hr and increased blood urea nitrogen (BUN), serum creatinine, and serum potassium levels. Normal laboratory values are as follows: BUN ≤20 mg/dl; serum creatinine ≤1.5 mg/dl; and serum potassium ≤5 mEq/L.
- Monitor arterial BP continuously. Be alert to decreased systolic BP, normal or increased diastolic BP, and decreased pulse pressures, which occur in the presence of decreasing perfusion.

Note: Systolic BP will be decreased because of decreased cardiac output, and the diastolic BP may be high secondary to compensatory vasoconstriction.

- Assess peripheral pulses, temperature, color of skin, and capillary refill. With hypoperfusion, pulse amplitude decreases, extremities are cool because of vasoconstriction, skin color is pale or mottled because of decreased perfusion, and capillary refill is delayed.
- Monitor cellular oxygen consumption (Vo_2) as an indicator of tissue perfusion. With sepsis, cellular oxygen delivery is decreased (precapillary vasoconstriction), and thus cellular oxygen use is decreased. Mixed venous blood oxygen saturation (SvO_2) is elevated.
- Administer vasoactive drugs as prescribed. Assess SVR and CO to determine the drug effects. Optimally, SVR will increase to ≥ 900 dynes/sec/cm^{-5}, CO will be 4-7 L/min, and CI will be 2.5-4 L/min/m^2.

Note: Vasoactive drugs used may include vasopressors (e.g., norepinephrine) early in sepsis and vasodilators (e.g., nitroprusside) late in sepsis. Vasopressors are always accompanied by fluid resuscitation as needed.

- Assess for evidence of decreasing splanchnic (visceral) circulation, including decreased or absent bowel sounds, elevated serum amylase level, and decreased platelet count. Normal values are as follows: serum amylase ≤ 180 Somogyi units/dl; platelet count $=150,000$/mm^3.

NIC Cerebral Perfusion Promotion; Circulatory Care; Fluid/Electrolyte Management; Oxygen Therapy; Hemodynamic Regulation; Shock Management; Nutrition Management; Hemodialysis Therapy

Impaired gas exchange related to alveolar-capillary membrane changes secondary to interstitial edema, alveolar destruction, and endotoxin release with activation of histamine and kinins

Desired outcomes: Within 4 hr of initiation of therapy, patient's Pao_2 is >80 mm Hg; $Paco_2$ is <45 mm Hg; pH is 7.35-7.45, and the lungs are clear.

- Assess for and maintain a patent airway by assisting patient with coughing, or suctioning trachea as necessary.
- Assess all ABG values. Be alert to decreasing Pao_2, increasing $Paco_2$, and acidosis (decreasing pH). Monitor patient for the presence of dyspnea, shortness of breath (SOB), and restlessness.
- Listen to breath sounds hourly. The presence of crackles may indicate fluid accumulation.
- If patient exhibits evidence of inadequate gas exchange (e.g., Pao_2 <60 mm Hg while patient is on 100% oxygen via nonrebreather mask), prepare for the probability of endotracheal intubation.
- If patient has been placed on mechanical ventilation, monitor inspiratory peak pressures for increasing trends, which may signal decreasing compliance and development of ARDS. Assess for and document mode of ventilation, tidal volume, Fio_2, RR, and level of positive end-expiratory pressure (PEEP). As ARDS develops, an increasing Fio_2 (>0.50) and increasing levels of PEEP are required to maintain adequate Pao_2 (>60 mm Hg). Consult physician if inspiratory peak pressures increase with each breath or if the following signs of hypoxia occur at the prescribed Fio_2 and level of PEEP: increased HR (≥ 100 beats/min), anxiety, cool extremities, change in mentation, or skin color changes (pallor or cyanosis). (See "Mechanical Ventilation," p. 14.)
- Turn patient q2h to maintain optimal ventilation-perfusion ratios and to prevent atelectasis.

NIC Acid-Base Management: Metabolic Acidosis; Oxygen Therapy; Respiratory Monitoring; Artificial Airway Management; Invasive Hemodynamic Regulation

Ineffective breathing pattern related to decreased lung expansion secondary to central respiratory depression occurring in late shock

Desired outcome: Within 2 hr of treatment/intervention, patient has an effective breathing pattern as evidenced by normal limits of inspiratory-expiratory ratio (1:1-1:2); tidal volume (=4ml/kg); and maximal inspiratory pressures (=20 cm H_2O).

- Monitor for decreasing respiratory rate, depth, and air movement. Ensure that patient demonstrates adequate air movement by noting presence of breath sounds over all lung fields.
- Assist patient into a comfortable position to facilitate respirations. Depending on patient's hemodynamic stability, the optimal position may be a 15-30 degree HOB elevation.
- Assess/measure tidal volume and inspiratory force. Be alert to tidal volume <4-5 ml/kg and inspiratory force <20 cm H_2O as indicators of an ineffective breathing pattern.
- If patient exhibits respiratory depression/ineffective breathing pattern, prepare for the probability of endotracheal intubation.

NIC Respiratory Monitoring; Oxygen Therapy; Mechanical Ventilation

Ineffective thermoregulation related to illness with concomitant endotoxin effect on hypothalamic temperature-regulating center

Desired outcome: Within 24 hr of initiation of treatment, patient becomes normothermic.

- Monitor patient's temperature continuously or at frequent intervals. Use temperature probe (rectal or tympanic) for continuous monitoring of core temperature. Body temperature can range from 38.3°-40.6° C (101°-105° F) in the early stage of sepsis and can be <35.6° C (96° F) in the late stage. Be alert to shaking chills early in sepsis as temperature increases, and to profuse diaphoresis as temperature decreases late in sepsis. Temperatures up to 103° F may be allowed in the septic patient, as increased temperature may help control bacteremia. The following are weighed for each patient to determine the extent of treatment that should be employed to decrease fever (e.g., acetaminophen administration):
  - ❑ Useful effects of a fever: decreased viral and bacterial replication.
  - ❑ Harmful effects of a fever: increased cardiac workload and increased oxygen consumption.
- Administer antimicrobials as prescribed. Observe for untoward effects, including renal toxicity, ototoxicity, allergic reactions, anaphylaxis, pseudomembranous colitis, overgrowth of normal flora, and superimposed infectious processes of the skin, urinary tract, or respiratory tract. Large doses of antibiotics may cause the release of endotoxins from dying bacteria, which may potentiate the progression of septic shock.
- Administer antipyretic agents as prescribed.
- For patients with hyperthermia, use tepid baths, which decrease body temperature by releasing internal heat. Cooled IV fluids also may decrease core temperature. In addition, a cooling blanket may be prescribed to reduce the metabolic rate, thereby decreasing myocardial oxygen demand. Avoid "chilling," which will cause shivering and thus increase myocardial oxygen demand and cardiac workload.
- In the presence of hypothermia, use warm blankets to increase body temperature. Heating devices can damage ischemic cells in peripheral tissues and usually are avoided.

NIC Fever Treatment; Temperature Regulation; Environmental Management

Altered nutrition: less than body requirements, related to increased need secondary to increased metabolic rate

Desired outcome: Within 48 hr of initiation of treatment, patient has adequate nutrition as evidenced by stable weight; serum albumin 3.5 g/dl; thyroxine-binding prealbumin 20-30 mg/dl; retinol-binding protein 4-5 mg/dl; urine urea nitrogen 10-20 mg/dl; and a state of nitrogen balance as determined by nitrogen studies.

- Administer nutritional supplements as prescribed.

Note: Standard total parenteral nutrition (TPN) solutions are not metabolized well in the septic state. Branched-chain amino acid solutions and short- to medium-chain fatty acid solutions may be used (e.g., MCT Oil or FreAmine HBC).

- Observe for and document areas of tissue breakdown, which can indicate a negative nitrogen state.
- Monitor laboratory findings for serum albumin, thyroxine-binding prealbumin, retinol-binding protein, and nitrogen studies.
- Assess and record weight and nutritional intake daily. Consult with nutritional services for calorie count.
- If patient is receiving oral feedings, assess for the presence of bowel sounds at least q2h. Paralytic ileus can occur secondary to an ischemic bowel.
- If the patient is receiving continuous gastric tube feedings, assess for residual feeding q2h. Assess for residual before intermittent tube feedings. If residual is ≥100 ml (or 1½ times the hourly rate of infusion), hold the feeding and consult with physician.

NIC TPN Administration; Enteral Tube Feeding

ADDITIONAL NURSING DIAGNOSES

Also see nursing diagnoses and interventions in "Hemodynamic Monitoring," p. 23; "Psychosocial Support," p. 68; "Psychosocial Support for the Patient's Family and Significant Others," p. 78; and "Acute Lung Injury and Respiratory Distress Syndrome," p. 189. See "Disseminated Intravascular Coagulation" for "Altered Protection," p. 494, and "Altered Tissue Perfusion," p. 497. Also see "SIRS/Sepsis," p. 501.

Multiple Organ Dysfunction Syndrome (MODS)

PATHOPHYSIOLOGY

MODS is defined as impaired functioning of two or more vital organ systems. Often SIRS or septic shock causes MODS, but any shock state may cause tissue hypoxia to the degree that initiates MODS.

Mortality increases as additional organ systems fail. When four or more organ systems fail, the mortality exceeds 80%. MODS is characterized by ARDS, DIC, acute tubular necrosis (ATN), liver failure, hyperdynamic circulatory failure, and metabolic encephalopathy.

History and risk factors: MODS is a systemic manifestation of an event causing massive endothelial dysfunction. SIRS, a common cause of MODS, may be initiated by infection, ischemia, reperfusion injury, intestinal endotoxin, thermal injury, pancreatitis, shock state, trauma, and multisystem injury. Patients with immunosuppression are more susceptible to SIRS/MODS. Factors such as chronic illness, sequential infections, steroid therapy, human immunodeficiency virus (HIV) infection, bone marrow depression, and advanced age contribute to immunosuppression.

Early MODS: Following an initiating event, findings may reflect a hypermetabolic state: restlessness, confusion, fever, SOB, tachypnea, tachycardia, and hyperglycemia.

Late MODS: Findings are consistent with impaired perfusion: diminished LOC, coma, respiratory failure requiring mechanical ventilation, heart failure refractory to inotropes, jaundice, hypoglycemia, oliguria/anuria, bruising, and uncontrolled bleeding.

ASSESSMENT

Physical assessment

Neurologic: Decreased cerebral blood flow with central nervous system (CNS) depression and stupor, progressing to coma.

Respiratory: Tachypnea, hyperventilation, to compensate for metabolic acidosis (early); later, crackles and respiratory depression/acidosis caused by CNS depression, increased lung water indicative of ARDS.

Gastrointestinal (GI): Decreased or absent bowel sounds; jaundice. Digestion ceases.

Genitourinary (GU): Oliguria, anuria. Acute renal failure ensues. May progress to polyuria.

Vital signs/hemodynamics: Early stages characterized by a hyperdynamic hypotension with venous pooling. In advanced stages there is transudation of fluid ("third spacing"), vasoconstriction, reduced blood flow, and a generalized hypodynamic state.

Temperature: Increased to >38° C (100.4° F) or decreased to <36° C (96.8° F); fever (early); thermoregulatory failure and hypothermia (late).

Central venous pressure (CVP): Decreased, caused by relative fluid deficit or false hypovolemia.

Pulmonary artery pressure (PAP): Decreased initially; later increased, as a result of pulmonary vasoconstriction occurring with hypoxemia, pulmonary edema.

PAWP: Decreased initially because of relative fluid deficit; later increased if heart failure present.

SVR: Decreased because of inflammatory mediator-induced vasodilation, but depends on the cardiac output (resistance/flow). Inflammation ensues when perfusion changes following endothelial injury and dysfunction.

CO/CI: Initially increased as a compensatory response to tissue demand; later decreased as heart failure progresses. Initially elevated cardiac output is not reflective of enhanced cardiac performance, but rather reflects low resistance to ejection created by the reduced SVR.

Cerebral perfusion pressure (CPP): Decreased as a direct effect of chemical mediators and decreased cerebral blood flow.

DIAGNOSTIC TESTS

CBC: WBC usually increases early, with increased bands (left shift). WBC may decrease as a result of sequestration within organs and bone marrow exhaustion. Anemia, if present, contributes to tachycardia, hyperdynamic state, and impaired tissue oxygenation.

Chemistries: Early increase in serum glucose results from gluconeogenesis; later, a decrease results from hepatic failure. Venous lactate levels increase if tissue perfusion is inadequate. Renal, cardiac, pulmonary, hepatic, or other organ failure is reflected in electrolyte, enzyme abnormalities.

Culture and sensitivities (C&S): Blood, sputum, urine, surgical, or other site; obtained if infection suspected.

ABGs: Usually show pH <7.35 and hypocarbia (<32 mm Hg) because of the compensatory response to metabolic acidosis.

Imaging: Chest x-ray to check for pulmonary edema, ARDS; other x-rays as indicated according to underlying condition.

COLLABORATIVE MANAGEMENT

Effective resuscitation following the initiating event and the hypermetabolic phase that follows largely determine the degree of organ dysfunction. The more quickly and aggressively the patient is managed for the initiating event, the better the chances of preserving tissues and avoiding permanent organ failure. See "SIRS" for further information regarding strategies to control endothelial damage and the inflammatory response.

Oxygenation: Mechanical ventilation may be necessary if pulmonary edema, ARDS, or other ventilatory impairment is present.

Fluids: Crystalloids, colloids administered to sustain adequate intravascular volume; hyperdynamic state supported until patient stabilizes. Goal is CVP 8-10 mm Hg; or pulmonary capillary wedge pressure (PCWP) 16-18 mm Hg. Ranges may be higher or lower for specific patients.

Hemodynamic monitoring and oxygen transport: To maximize Do_2, Vo_2, and CI. Goal is to maintain Vo_2 above 100 ml/min/m^2. Some literature supports the maintenance of supranormal levels of Do_2, Vo_2. Fluid adjustment, inotropes, vasopressors, and ensuring adequacy of oxygen-carrying capacity via optimal hematocrit (Hct) and oxygen administration are mainstays of management.

Urinary drainage: To monitor hourly urinary output.

Pharmacotherapy

Inotropes and vasopressors: Inotropes such as dopamine, dobutamine, or epinephrine help increase CO. High-dose dopamine, phenylephrine, and norepinephrine stimulate α-receptors and may be used for refractory hypotension. Intramucosal gastric monitoring is recommended, if available, to evaluate tissue oxygenation during vasopressor therapy.

Antibiotics: Broad-spectrum antibiotics if infection suspected.

Analgesia, sedation: To relieve pain and agitation, which increase oxygen consumption.

Hemofiltration and hemodialysis: To provide therapy for acute renal failure. Either intermittent hemodialysis or continuous renal replacement therapy (CRRT) may be initiated. Modes of dialysis remove waste products and excess fluid and may help to remove mediators of the inflammatory response.

Nutritional support: Enteral nutrition (i.e., nasogastric, nasojejunal elemental feedings) is optimal but often not possible. Short- and medium-chain fatty acids (absorbed more readily and metabolized more easily than long-chain fatty acids) are given parenterally. Branched-chain amino acids, metabolized by muscle rather than by the liver, may be used if there is evidence of hepatic failure.

NURSING DIAGNOSES AND INTERVENTIONS

Altered tissue perfusion: cerebral, renal, GI, related to hypovolemia secondary to vasodilation (early) or interrupted arterial/venous blood flow secondary to microvascular obstruction (late)

Desired outcomes: Within 24 hr of initiating therapy, patient has adequate perfusion as evidenced by orientation to time, place, and person; peripheral pulses >2+ on 0-4+ scale; brisk capillary refill (<2 sec); urinary output ≥0.5 ml/kg/hr; and ≥5 bowel sounds/min. BP 110-120/70-80 mm Hg (or within normal level for patient); Svo_2 60% to 80%; SVR 900-1200 dynes/sec/cm^{-5}; CO 4-7 L/min; and CI 2.5-4.0 L/min/m^2.

- Assess for signs of decreased cerebral perfusion: decreased LOC, restlessness.
- Assess for signs of decreased renal perfusion: urinary output <0.5 ml/kg/hr; increased BUN, creatinine, and serum potassium levels. Consider use of continuous renal replacement therapy (CRRT) (e.g., continuous veno-venous hemofiltration [CVVH], continuous veno-venous hemofiltration with dialysis [CVVHD]) for management of acute renal failure.
- Monitor continuously for decreased systolic BP, normal or increased diastolic BP, and decreased pulse pressures indicating decreased perfusion.
- Assess for signs of hypoperfusion: decreased pulse amplitude, cool extremities, pallor or mottling, delayed capillary refill.
- Monitor Svo_2 to assess tissue perfusion. Cellular oxygen delivery may be decreased as a result of precapillary vasoconstriction. Cellular oxygen use is decreased (shunting). High Svo_2 does not indicate adequate tissue oxygenation.
- Administer fluids, inotropes, and/or vasodilators or vasopressors to optimize SVR and CO/CI. Increased filling pressures may help increase cardiac output.
- Assess for decreased splanchnic (visceral) circulation, including decreased or absent bowel sounds, increased amylase, increased liver enzymes, and decreased platelet count.
- Consult physician for failure to respond to therapy as evidenced by signs and symptoms of inadequate tissue perfusion: altered mental status, restlessness; decreased BP, peripheral pulses; urinary output <0.5 ml/kg/hr; Svo_2 <60 or >80%; decreased or absent bowel sounds.
- Consider, with physicians, whether patient may benefit from use of activated protein C (drotrecogin alfa) or steroids to reduce the inflammatory response associated with MODS.
- Treat underlying infection with appropriate antimicrobial therapy, being certain to administer precisely as scheduled to optimize blood levels.

▉NIC Cerebral Perfusion Promotion; Circulatory Care; Fluid/Electrolyte Management; Oxygen Therapy; Hemodynamic Regulation; Shock Management; Nutrition Management; Hemodialysis Therapy

Fluid volume deficit related to loss from vascular compartment secondary to increased capillary permeability and shift of intravascular volume into interstitial spaces.

Desired outcomes: Within 96 hr of therapy initiation, patient is normovolemic, as evidenced by peripheral pulses >2+ on 0-4+ scale; stable body weight; urinary output ≥.0.5 ml/kg/hr; systolic BP ≥90 mm Hg or within normal limits for patient; and absence of edema and adventitious lung sounds. PAWP is 6-12 mm Hg, CO 4-7 L/min, and SVR 900-1200 dynes/sec/cm^{-5}.

- Assess fluid volume by monitoring BP, HR, and peripheral perfusion hourly or more often if unstable. Continuous direct arterial pressure monitoring is optimal.
- During acute hypotension, position patient supine with the legs elevated to optimize preload.
- Give crystalloids and colloids to maintain PAWP of 6-12 mm Hg, or <18 mm Hg with left ventricular (LV) failure. Assess PAWP and lung sounds frequently during fluid replacement to detect signs of overload: crackles and increased PAWP. As indicated, administer PRBCs to increase oxygen-carrying capacity of the blood.
- Monitor hemodynamic pressures and Svo$_2$ as available.
- In early stage, anticipate decreased BP, PAWP, and SVR, and increased CO/CI. Give fluids and inotropes as necessary.
- In late stage, decreased BP may occur, as well as increased PAWP and SVR, and decreased CO/CI. In general, use vasodilators if MAP >100 mm Hg, or use vasopressors if MAP <70 mm Hg. Fluids, inotropes, vasopressors, and vasodilators all may be needed because of MODS and desensitization to endogenous catecholamines. Titrate carefully to optimize CI and maintain Svo$_2$ of at least 60% to 80%.
- Weigh patient daily; monitor I&O every shift and urinary output hourly, noting 24-h trends. Weight may increase despite actual fluid volume deficit as a result of a shift of intravascular volume into interstitial spaces.
- Assess for interstitial edema as evidenced by pretibial, sacral, ankle, and hand edema, and lung crackles. Take measures to protect skin integrity.

NIC Invasive Hemodynamic Regulation; Fluid/Electrolyte Management; Hypovolemia Management; Fluid Management; Shock Management: Volume

Impaired gas exchange related to alveolar-capillary membrane changes secondary to interstitial edema, alveolar destruction, and endothelial damage

Desired outcomes: Within 12 hr of therapy initiation, patient's Pao$_2$ is >80 mm Hg; Paco$_2$ is <45 mm Hg; pH is 7.35-7.45.

- Administer supplemental oxygen to maximize oxygen available to tissues.
- If patient exhibits inadequate gas exchange (e.g., Pao$_2$ is <60 mm Hg on 100% oxygen via nonrebreather mask), endotracheally intubate.
- Maintain patent airway: assist with coughing or suctioning as necessary.
- Assess ABGs for decreased Pao$_2$, increased Paco$_2$, and acidosis. Monitor for dyspnea, SOB, crackles, and restlessness. Adjust supplemental oxygen and ventilator settings as indicated.
- Closely monitor PAWP; keep as low as possible to avoid contributing to excess lung water but high enough to maintain cardiac output. A narrow range of optimal PAWP exists with the intravascular fluid volume deficit, increased capillary permeability, and possible LV failure.
- If patient is on mechanical ventilation, monitor for evidence of ARDS: increased peak inspiratory pressures (e.g., decreased lung compliance); Fio$_2$ >0.50; increased PEEP necessary to maintain adequate Pao$_2$; and diffuse, bilateral pulmonary infiltrates ("white-out") on chest x-ray.
- Turn q2h to maintain optimal ventilation-perfusion (V/Q) ratios and prevent atelectasis.

NIC Acid-Base Management: Metabolic Acidosis; Oxygen Therapy; Respiratory Monitoring; Artificial Airway Management; Invasive Hemodynamic Regulation

ADDITIONAL NURSING DIAGNOSES

See also nursing diagnoses and interventions in "Sepsis and Septic Shock," p. 501; "Hemodynamic Monitoring," p. 23; "Psychosocial Support," p. 68; "Psychosocial Support for the Patient's Family and Significant Others," p. 78; and "Acute Respiratory Distress Syndrome," p. 189. See "Disseminated Intravascular Coagulation" for "Altered Protection," p. 494, "Altered Tissue Perfusion," p. 497, "Mechanical Ventilation," p. 14, "Acute Respiratory Failure," p. 201, "Acute Renal Failure," p. 315, and "Hepatic Failure," p. 427.

Anaphylactic Shock

PATHOPHYSIOLOGY

Systemic anaphylactic shock (anaphylaxis) is a potentially life-threatening situation resulting from an exaggerated or a hypersensitivity response to an antigen (or allergen). The classic form occurs in a sensitized person (i.e., someone who has been exposed previously to the same antigen), 1-20 min after exposure to the antigenic substance. Anaphylaxis is most often caused by drugs, foods, insect stings or bites, antisera, and blood products.

The hypersensitivity response occurs on the surface of the mast cells, located primarily in the lungs, in small blood vessels, and in connective tissue. The antigen combines with sensitized antibodies from previous exposure (usually immunoglobulin E [IgE] type) and attaches to basophils circulating in the blood. Inflammatory mediators are then released from the granules within the cells, including histamine, serotonin, kinins, and eosinophil and neutrophil chemotactic factors. The antigen-antibody complexes activate production of prostaglandins and leukotrienes, which are termed *slow-reacting substances of anaphylaxis (SRSA)*: chemical mediators that produce systemic effects with potentially deleterious results, including profound shock.

Histamine is the primary mediator in an anaphylactic response. Activation of histamine receptors causes increased capillary permeability, increased pulmonary secretions, bronchoconstriction, and systemic vasodilation. The *leukotrienes* produce severe bronchoconstriction and cause venule dilation and increased vascular permeability. The *prostaglandins* exaggerate bronchoconstriction and potentiate the effects of histamine on vascular permeability and pulmonary secretions. *Kinins* contribute to bronchoconstriction, vasodilation, and increased vascular permeability. The combined effects of these substances cause airway obstruction and respiratory distress, which can lead to respiratory arrest, with a relative hypovolemia caused by massive vasodilation. Fluids shift from the vasculature into interstitial spaces, creating vasogenic (vasodilated) shock progressing to end-organ dysfunction secondary to tissue hypoxia from poor perfusion. Eosinophilic chemotactic factor of anaphylaxis (ECFA) is then released to attract eosinophils, which work to neutralize mediators such as histamine. This response cannot reverse the anaphylaxis. (See Figure 10-2 for a depiction of the pathophysiologic process of anaphylaxis.)

ASSESSMENT

History and risk factors: Recent exposure to pharmacologic agents (e.g., penicillin, anesthetics, vaccines), contrast medium, commonly allergenic food (e.g., seafood, shellfish, nuts, grains, dairy products), insect bites or stings (e.g., wasps, hornets, bees, fire ants), or latex; recent blood transfusions.

Clinical presentation: Varies with the means of antigen entry, the amount absorbed, rate of absorption, and the degree of hypersensitivity. Dramatic symptoms usually develop within minutes and progress rapidly. More rapid onset correlates with more severe symptoms. *General early indicators* (occuring within seconds to minutes) include uneasiness, lightheadedness, tingling feeling, flushing, and pruritus. *General late indicators* (occuring within minutes) include rapid progression of urticaria involving large areas of skin; angioedema (tissue swelling; more commonly the eyes, lips, tongue, hands, feet, and genitalia); cough, hoarseness, dyspnea, and respiratory distress; lightheadedness or syncope; and abdominal cramps, diarrhea, and vomiting. Symptoms vary with means of antigen entry:

Ingestion: Cramping, diarrhea, nausea, and vomiting may precede systemic shock symptoms.

Inhalation: Cough, hoarseness, wheezing, dyspnea.

Allergic: Edema, urticaria, itching at the site of a bee sting or drug injection.

Physical assessment: See Table 10-3.

Hemodynamic measurements: As vasogenic shock evolves, decreased arterial BP, MAP, CO (<4 L/min), CI (<2.5 L/min), SVR (<900 dynes/sec/cm^{-5}), and PAWP (<6 mm Hg) are present from worsening vasodilation, progressive shifting of intravascular fluid to interstitial spaces, and decreasing venous return.

DIAGNOSTIC TESTS

The diagnosis of anaphylaxis is based on presenting signs and symptoms. Treatment should be initiated before laboratory results are available. Tryptase, a chemical mediator released by mast cells following anaphylaxis, increases ≤1 hr following anaphylaxis and remains elevated for 4-6 hr. IgE levels may confirm allergic origin. ABG values are reviewed to evaluate respiratory status.

COLLABORATIVE MANAGEMENT (See Figure 10-3)

Airway maintenance: Early, rapid endotracheal intubation should be done to manage rapidly progressing laryngeal edema. Severe laryngeal edema may cause complete airway obstruction in minutes. A tracheostomy or emergency cricothyroidotomy is necessary if endotracheal intubation is not possible.

Epinephrine: Epinephrine reverses anaphylaxis by increasing myocardial contractility, dilating bronchioles, constricting blood vessels, inhibiting histamine release, and counteracting histamine. Dosage and route vary. Suggested guidelines:

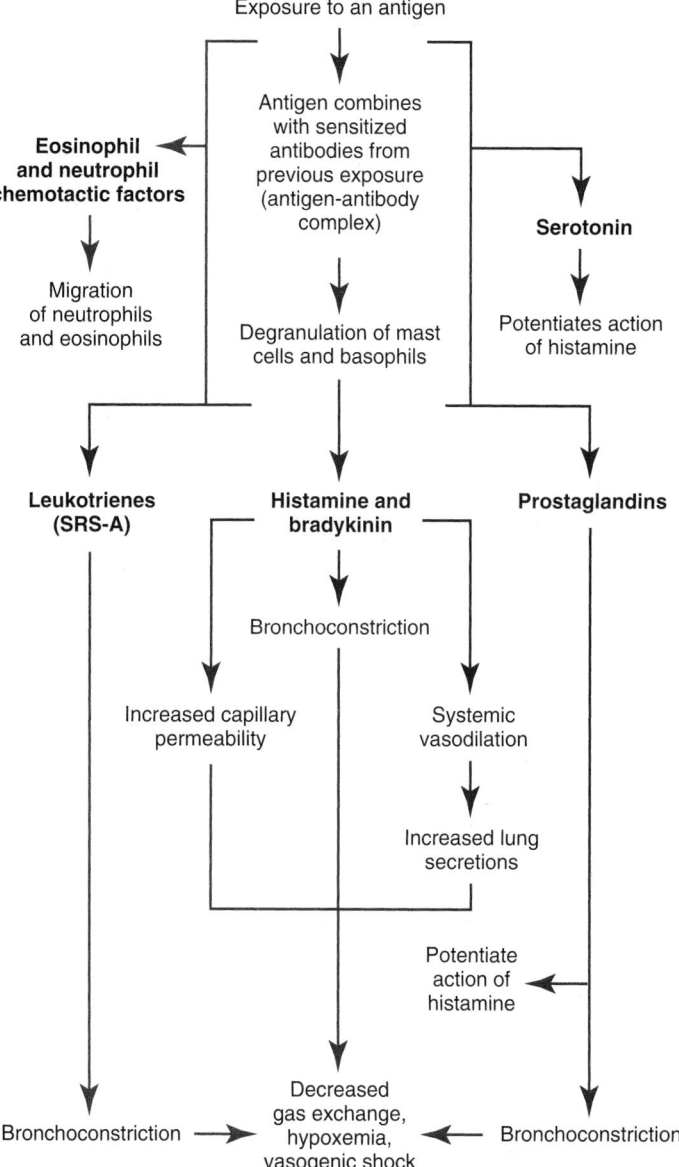

Figure 10-2:   Pathophysiologic process of anaphylaxis. (Major chemical mediators are in boldface print.) *SRS-A,* Slow-reacting substance of anaphylaxis.

Note: Individuals taking β-adrenergic blocking agents such as propranolol may not respond as rapidly as expected to epinephrine and may require higher or additional dosing. Glucagon may help to counteract the effects of β-blocking drugs.

- *Standard adult dose*: 0.2-0.5 mg (0.2-0.5 ml of a 1:1000 solution) given by intramuscularly (IM) or subcutaneously (SC).

TABLE 10-3   Systemic Effects of Anaphylaxis

System	Effects	Cause
Neurologic	Apprehension; headache; confusion; decreased LOC progressing to coma	Vasodilation; hypoperfusion; cerebral hypoxia or cerebral edema occurring with interstitial fluid shifts
Respiratory	Dyspnea progressing to air hunger and complete respiratory obstruction; hoarseness; noisy breathing; high-pitched, "barking" cough; increased pulmonary wheezes; crackles; rhonchi; decreasing breath sounds; pulmonary edema (some patients)	Laryngeal edema; bronchoconstriction; increased pulmonary secretions
Cardiovascular	Decreased BP leading to profound hypotension; increased HR; decreased amplitude of peripheral pulses; palpitations and dysrhythmias (atrial tachycardias, premature atrial beats, atrial fibrillation, premature ventricular beats progressing to ventricular tachycardia, or ventricular fibrillation); lymphadenopathy	Increased vascular permeability; systemic vasodilation; decreased cardiac output with decreased circulating volume; reflex increase in HR; vasogenic shock
Renal	Decreased urine output; incontinence	Decreased renal perfusion; smooth muscle contraction of urinary tract
Gastrointestinal	Nausea, vomiting, diarrhea, abdominal cramping	Smooth muscle contraction of GI tract; increased mucus secretion
Cutaneous	Urticaria; angioedema (hands, lips, face, feet, genitalia); itching; erythema; flushing; cyanosis	Histamine-induced disruption of cutaneous vasculature; vasodilation, increased capillary permeability; decreased oxygen saturation

BP, Blood pressure; *HR*, heart rate; *GI*, gastrointestinal; *LOC*, level of consciousness.

- *Alternate initial dose*: 0.1 mg (0.1 ml of a 1:1000 solution) may be administered.
- *Repeat dosage*: may be repeated q10-15min prn.
- *IV dosage:* preferred if patient is in shock and/or has severe airway obstruction: Initial dose of 0.1-0.25 mg (1.0-2.5 ml of 1:10,000 solution) over 5-10 min. The dose may be increased to 0.3-0.5 mg. Repeat q5-15min as needed.
- *IV infusion:* after initial dose, an IV drip of epinephrine 1.0 mg in 250 ml D$_5$W may be infused at 1 mcg/min, and increased to 4 mcg/min (or more) as needed to achieve desired response.
- *Endotracheal (ET) tube:* 1.0-2.5 ml of 1:10,000 solution (1 mg epinephrine in 10-ml solution) into ET tube, followed by use of manual resuscitation (Ambu) bag. May repeat if needed.

Supplemental oxygen: Administered to support ventilation and aerobic metabolism. Amount and method of oxygen administration are guided by ABG results. Often initiated at 6 L/min via nasal cannula or oxygen mask.

Fluid resuscitation: IV crystalloids (e.g., lactated Ringer's, 0.9% normal saline) and/or colloids (e.g., albumin and plasma protein fraction) to increase intravascular volume. Colloids increase colloid osmotic pressure to help retain fluid in the blood vessels. May require rapid infusion of 2-3 L of fluids.

Vasopressors: Used if fluid replacement does not increase blood pressure. Drugs are titrated for the desired response. (See Appendix 7.) Usual dosages are as follows:

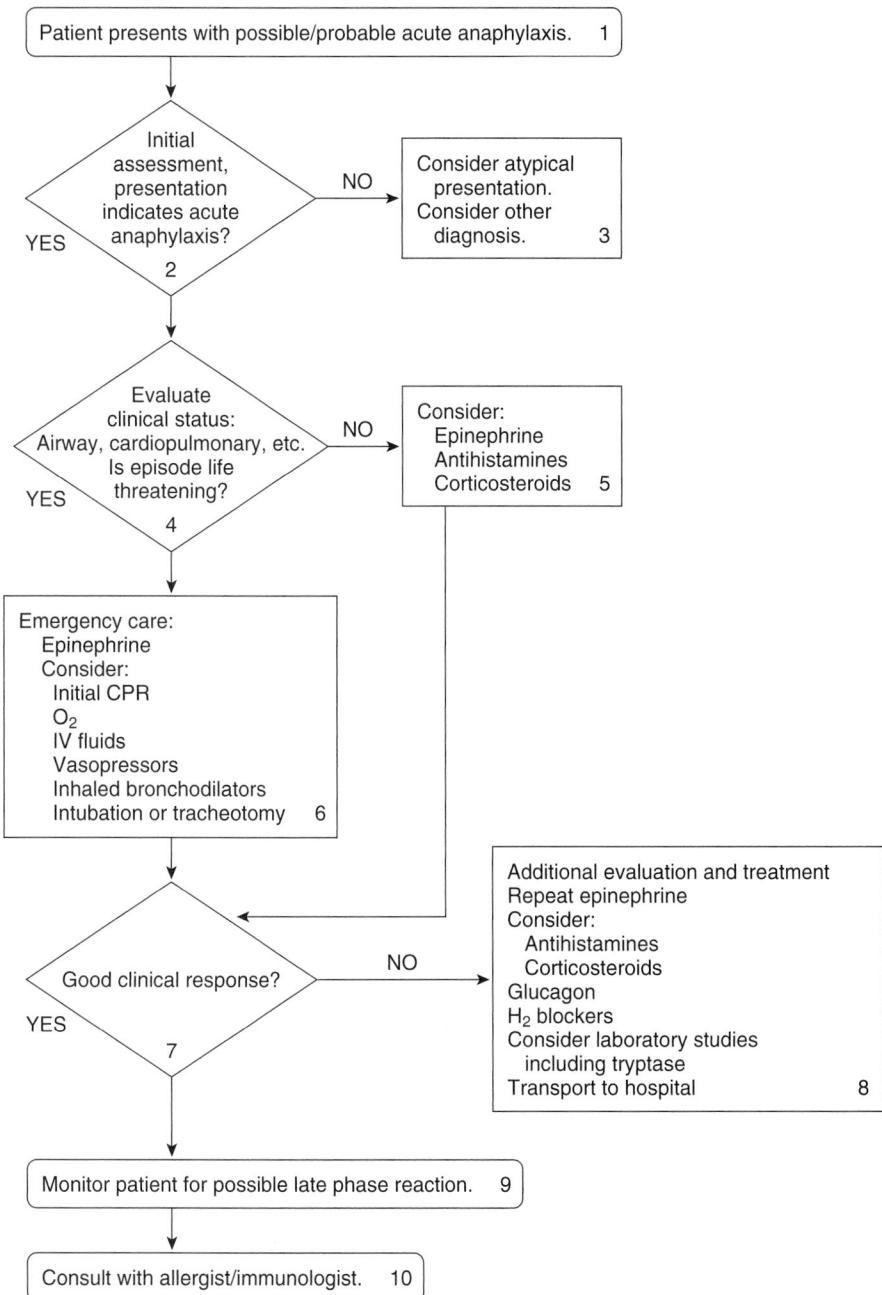

Figure 10-3: Algorithm for the treatment of acute anaphylaxis.
From Nicklas RA et al: The diagnosis and management of anaphylaxis. *J Allergy Clin Immunol*
101(6 Pt 2):S465-S528, 1998.

- *Dopamine hydrochloride:* Effects are dose-dependent. Increases cardiac contractility at 5-10 mcg/kg/min and systemic vascular resistance at 10-20 mcg/kg/min. Consider switching to norepinephrine if dose exceeds 20 mcg/kg/min.
- *Norepinephrine:* Initial dosage is 2-8 mcg/min and can be increased to achieve the necessary BP.
- *Phenylephrine:* Usual dosage is 40-60 mcg/min. Doses exceeding 200 mcg/min have been used.

Antihistamines: *Diphenhydramine*: Usual dose is 20-50 mg, but 50-100 mg may be given IV or IM to relieve urticaria and abdominal cramping. IV *H_2-antagonists* (e.g., cimetidine, ranitidine) are also used.

Aminophylline (theophylline ethylenediamine): 2-4 mg/min (0.5 mg/kg) given by IV infusion stimulates bronchodilation and relieves bronchospasm.

Corticosteroids: Used to help decrease release of chemical mediators that increase capillary permeability. *Hydrocortisone sodium succinate*: loading dose is 100-1000 mg IV; or *methylprednisolone sodium succinate:* loading dose is 125-250 mg IV. Followed by IV or oral (PO) corticosteroids for several days.

Inhaled bronchodilators (e.g., albuterol): May be given for continued bronchospasm.

Glucagon IV bolus: Use is controversial for counteracting effects of β-blocking drugs or for other patients who have limited response to treatment. Relaxes smooth muscle and increases HR and force of contraction.

Electrocardiogram (ECG) monitoring: To detect dysrhythmias.

NURSING DIAGNOSES AND INTERVENTIONS

Ineffective airway clearance related to airway obstruction secondary to bronchoconstriction, increased secretions from the histamine response, and presence of leukotrienes and prostaglandins.
Desired outcome: Within 20 min of treatment/intervention, patient has adequate spontaneous tidal and expiratory volumes as evidenced by easier breathing; audible breath sounds in expected range, and no adventitious breath sounds.

- Assess continuously for obstructed airway and increased respiratory effort. Note increased pulmonary secretions, cough, expiratory wheezing, SOB, and dyspnea. Suction prn.

> **Note:**   As bronchoconstriction and obstruction progress, wheezing may decrease; therefore it is important to note decreasing air movement—not just adventitious sounds.

- Administer epinephrine as prescribed.
- Identify patient requiring actual/potential airway insertion. Consult physician and prepare for ET intubation if lingual edema is present and/or respiratory distress continues.

> **Caution:**   An oral airway provides airway support only as far as the posterior pharynx. If laryngeal edema is present, the oral airway cannot relieve symptoms because the obstruction is below the oral airway.

- If ET intubation is attempted and is not possible due to laryngeal edema, prepare for tracheostomy or cricothyroidotomy.
- Administer IV and inhaled bronchodilators as appropriate. May cause dysrhythmias.
- Monitor and report ABG values with increasing Pa_{CO_2} (>50 mm Hg) or decreasing Pa_{O_2} (<60 mm Hg) indicative of impending respiratory failure.

■ NIC Airway Insertion and Stabilization; Airway Management; Anaphylaxis Management; Medication Administration, Medication Management, Respiratory Monitoring

Impaired gas exchange related to alveolar-capillary membrane changes secondary to increased capillary permeability associated with histamine response
Desired outcome: Within 20 min of initiation of treatment/intervention, patient has adequate alveolar exchange of CO_2 or O_2 as evidenced by easier breathing; Pa_{O_2} ≥80 mm Hg; and Sp_{O_2} ≥90%.

- Monitor patient for signs and symptoms of respiratory failure.
- Administer supplemental oxygen as ordered.
- Monitor patient by continuous pulse oximetry. Report levels <90% to the physician.
- Administer antihistamines as prescribed.
- Administer glucocorticoids as prescribed.
- Position patient to alleviate dyspnea (assist patient to sitting position if BP is stable).
- Stay with patient to promote safety and reduce fear. Use calm, reassuring approach.

NIC Anaphylaxis Management; Emotional Support; Medication Administration, Medicatio.. Management, Respiratory Monitoring

Decreased cardiac output related to decreased preload and afterload secondary to vasodilation and increased capillary permeability

Desired outcome: Within 4 hr of initiation of treatment, patient has adequate cardiac output as evidenced by BP ≥90/60 mm Hg; strong peripheral pulses; CO ≥4 L/min; CI ≥2.5 L/min/m^2; SVR ≥900 dynes/sec/cm^{-5}; urinary output ≥0.5 ml/kg/hr; and normal sinus rhythm on ECG.

- Assess for physical and hemodynamic indicators of decreased cardiac output:
  - ❑ Palpate peripheral pulses for decreasing amplitude.
  - ❑ Assess arterial BP for any decrease, an indicator of failed compensatory mechanisms.
  - ❑ Monitor SVR. A decrease (<800 dynes/sec/cm^{-5}) is associated with decreased afterload (vasodilation) and may precipitate decreased CO.
  - ❑ Monitor CO and CI if available. A CI of <2.0 L/min/m^2 is usually associated with hypoperfusion.
- Monitor for dysrhythmias, such as atrial tachycardias, PVCs, ventricular tachycardia, and ventricular fibrillation, which may signal hypoxemia or occur as side effects of drugs such as aminophylline or epinephrine.
- Monitor for increases and decreases in edema.

Note: Continued swelling, despite treatment, may indicate ineffective treatment, overaggressive fluid therapy, or heart or kidney failure.

- Administer epinephrine as prescribed. Observe for therapeutic effects as evidenced by increased SVR, increased CO/CI, increased arterial BP and MAP, stronger peripheral pulses, warming of extremities, and increased urine output.
- Administer fluid replacement therapy as prescribed, using a large-bore IV catheter. Colloids and crystalloids may be given together.

Note: During fluid resuscitation, assess patient for indicators of fluid volume excess, including crackles with chest auscultation, presence of S$_3$ heart sounds, and jugular venous distention. If hemodynamic monitoring lines are present, be alert to increasing PAP, PAWP, and right atrial pressure (RAP).

- Prepare for possible vasopressor infusion if hypotension persists after fluid resuscitation and epinephrine administration.

NIC Anaphylaxis Management; Hemodynamic Regulation; Hypovolemia Management; Medication Administration, Medication Management, Cardiac Care: Acute

Altered tissue perfusion: peripheral, renal, and cerebral, related to hypovolemia secondary to fluid shift from the vascular space to the interstitial space

Desired outcome: Within 4 hr of initiation of treatment, patient has adequate perfusion as evidenced by strong proximal peripheral pulses; brisk capillary refill; warm extremities temperature; urinary output ≥0.5 ml/kg/hr; uncompromised neurologic status; and no restlessness, listlessness, and unexplained anxiety.

- Assess peripheral pulses. Report decreased amplitude of pulses.
- Assess capillary refill. Delayed capillary refill (>2 sec) is likely with edema and decreased vascular volume.
- Assess degree of peripheral edema.
- Assess color and warmth of extremities. Report presence of coolness and pallor.
- Monitor BP at frequent intervals. Be alert for indicators of hypotension such as BP readings >20 mm Hg below patient's normal pressure, dizziness, restlessness, altered mentation, and decreased urinary output.
- Monitor urine output hourly. Swan-Ganz catheter may be needed to guide fluid resuscitation.
- Observe for indicators of decreased cerebral perfusion such as anxiety, restlessness, confusion, and decreased LOC.

Note: Changes in LOC may signal either decreased cerebral perfusion (tissue hypoxia) or increasing intracranial pressure (ICP) caused by interstitial swelling from capillary permeability.

- Administer fluid and pharmacologic agents as prescribed (see previous nursing diagnosis).

NIC Anaphylaxis Management; Hemodynamic Regulation; Hypovolemia Management; Medication Administration, Medication Management

Impaired skin integrity related to urticaria and angioedema secondary to allergic response

Desired outcomes: Within 4 hr of initiation of treatment, patient states urticaria is controlled. Skin remains intact.

- Assess patient for urticaria (hives) and itching of hands, feet, neck, and genitalia.
- Administer antihistamines as prescribed to relieve itching.
- Discourage patient from scratching the skin. If unavoidable, teach patient to use pads of fingertips rather than nails.
- Apply cool washcloths or covered ice as a soothing measure to irritated and edematous areas.

NIC Environmental Management: Comfort; Medication Administration; Pruritis Management

Knowledge deficit: severe hypersensitivity reaction, its causes, and its symptoms, related to no prior exposure or incomplete understanding

Desired outcome: By the time of discharge from the critical care unit, patient demonstrates increased knowledge of severe hypersensitivity reactions as evidenced by verbalization of potential causative factors, symptoms of allergic reaction, need to inform health care providers of allergies, importance of wearing medical-alert identification, prescribed treatment modalities when in contact with allergen, and the necessity of informing primary health care provider immediately of any allergic symptoms.

- Provide information about the antigenic agent that caused the anaphylaxis, including ways to avoid it in the future.
- Explain need for wearing a medical-alert identification tag or bracelet to identify the allergy.
- Give information about anaphylaxis emergency treatment kits. Teach patient self-administration technique and the importance of prompt treatment.
- Stress the importance of seeking treatment immediately if symptoms of allergy occur, including flushing, warmth, itching, anxiety, and hives.
- Explain the importance of identifying and checking all over-the-counter (OTC) medications for the presence of potential allergens.

NIC Health Education; Risk Identification; Teaching: Prescribed Medication

ADDITIONAL NURSING DIAGNOSES

Also see nursing diagnoses and interventions in "Hemodynamic Monitoring," p. 23; "Psychosocial Support," p. 68; "Psychosocial Support for the Patient's Family and Significant Others," p. 78; and "Mechanical Ventilation," p. 14. See also "Hypovolemia" for "Altered Cerebral, Renal, and Peripheral Tissue Perfusion," p. 542.

Organ Rejection

PATHOPHYSIOLOGY

Graft or organ rejection is the main problem with transplantation. A transplanted organ originates from a donor who is genetically different from the recipient (the exception is a kidney from an identical twin). The organ contains foreign antigens that trigger an immune response in the recipient, which leads to organ rejection. Historically, rejection has been classified as hyperacute, accelerated acute, acute, and chronic (Table 10-4). An untreated rejection response results in complete destruction of the organ. Table 10-5 describes the clinical presentation for various types of acute organ rejection.

When the body detects the presence of a foreign substance, the immune system mounts a defense with nonspecific inflammation and phagocytosis. Antibody-mediated (humoral) and cell-mediated immunity work together to defend after exposure to an antigen. *Antibody-mediated immune response* stimulates B-lymphocyte activity. When an antigen is encountered, the B lymphocyte enlarges, divides, and differentiates into a plasma cell that produces and secretes antigen-specific immunoglobulins, or antibodies. The formation of this antigen-antibody complex triggers events that augment the nonspecific responses of inflammation and phagocytosis. *Cell-mediated immune response* involves T lymphocytes. T lymphocytes recognize a foreign antigen on the surface of the macrophage, bind to the antigen, enlarge, and produce a sensitized clone, which migrates through the body to the site of the antigen. When the sensitized T cell combines with the antigen, chemicals are released that kill foreign cells directly, and facilitate phagocytosis and the inflammatory response. (See Figure 10-4 for a delineation of this process.)

TABLE 10-4   Characteristics of Organ Rejection by Category

Type of rejection	Characteristics	Outcome
Hyperacute	Described in "Renal Transplantation," p. 329 Occurs immediately Antibody-mediated Result of preformed circulatory antibodies	Irreversible and untreatable
Accelerated acute	Occurs 3-5 days after transplant Antibody-mediated Rapid loss of function Fever and oliguria	Irreversible and untreatable
Acute	Primarily T cell–mediated Possible presence of humoral component Occurs weeks, months, or years after transplant	Treatable and reversible multiple episodes affect long-term graft survival
Chronic	Develops slowly over months to years Probably a combination of cellular- and humoral-mediated processes	Untreatable; eventually leads to graft loss

TABLE 10-5   Clinical Presentation with Acute Organ Rejection

Organ	Clinical presentation	Treatment options
Heart	10-14 days after transplantation. Indicators include fever, anxiety, lethargy, low back pain, atrial or ventricular dysrhythmias, gallop, pericardial friction rub, jugular venous distention, hypotension, and decreased CO late in rejection.	Methylprednisolone sodium succinate (500 mg-1 g) daily for 2-4 days. Antilymphocyte sera (rabbit, horse, goat) IV for 6-14 days. Monoclonal antibody for 10-14 days. Retransplantation necessary for intractable acute rejection.
Liver	4-10 days after transplantation. Indicators include malaise; fever; abdominal discomfort; swollen, hard, tender graft; tachycardia; RUQ or flank pain; cessation of bile flow; change in bile fluid from golden to colorless; jaundice; elevated PT, bilirubin, transaminase, and alkaline phosphatase.	Methylprednisolone sodium succinate (500 mg-1 g) daily for 2-4 days. Antilymphocyte sera (rabbit, horse, goat) IV for 6-14 days. Monoclonal antibody for 10-14 days. Retransplantation necessary for recurrent unresponsive rejection.
Pancreas	Time of rejection occurrence varies. Patient may have hyperglycemia, pancreatitis, pain over graft. Open biopsy may be necessary to diagnose rejection.	Methylprednisolone sodium succinate (250 mg-1 g) daily for 2-4 days. Antilymphocyte sera (rabbit, horse, goat) IV for 6-14 days. Monoclonal antibody for 10-14 days. Retransplantation for unresponsive rejection.

Continued

TABLE 10-5   Clinical Presentation with Acute Organ Rejection—cont'd

Organ	Clinical presentation	Treatment options
Lung	Expected during the first 21 days after surgery, with increased frequency and severity 6-8 wks after transplantation. Classic rejection: decreased lung ventilation and perfusion alveolar exudate containing desquamated pneumocytes and inflammatory cells Atypical rejection: decreased ventilation without blood flow reduction; ventilation-perfusion imbalances, and respiratory insufficiency with shunting Vascular rejection: increased vascular resistance; decreased blood flow to graft	Methylprednisolone sodium succinate (250 mg-1 g) daily for 2-4 days. Antilymphocyte sera (rabbit, horse, goat) IV for 6-14 days. Retransplantation for unresponsive rejection

CO, Cardiac output; *IV,* intravenous; *RUQ,* right upper quadrant; *PT,* prothrombin time.

DIAGNOSIS AND ASSESSMENT OF REJECTION

Biopsy of the transplanted organ provides the means of diagnosing rejection, its severity, and the possibility of response to antirejection therapy. The following diagnostic tests are also performed:

Cardiac
Chest x-ray: Will reveal increased dimensions of the heart late in rejection.
ECG: Will show presence of atrial and ventricular dysrhythmias and decreased QRS voltage.
CBC: Will show increased total lymphocyte count.
VS and heart sounds: May reveal decreased stroke volume, cardiac output, cardiac tones, and BP; and presence of S_3 and S_4 sounds, pericardial friction rub, extrasystole, and crackles.

Liver
Serum bilirubin level: Total bilirubin will rise in relation to baseline postoperative level.
Transaminase level: Will increase from baseline; may be markedly elevated early in rejection.
Alkaline phosphatase level: Will increase from baseline.
Prothrombin time: Will be prolonged.
CBC: May reveal decreased platelet count and increased total lymphocyte count.

Pancreas
Open biopsy is the only means by which a definitive diagnosis can be made.
Fasting and 2-hr postprandial plasma glucose: Levels will be increased above normal ranges.
Serum amylase: Levels may be elevated, indicating presence of pancreatitis, an inconsistent marker of rejection.
C peptide (serum and urine): Levels may be decreased.
Pancreas radioisotope flow scan: Determines organ viability. Decreased flow may indicate rejection.

Lung
Transbronchial biopsy is not helpful in detecting rejection; the morbidity risk increases with open biopsy.
Leukocyte and absolute lymphocyte counts: Rise during rejection.
VS and hemodynamics: Can change suddenly with increases in the following: pulmonary vascular resistance (PVR), HR, BP, SVR, and CO.
ABG values: Decrease in Pao_2 and increase in $Paco_2$ occur with rejection.

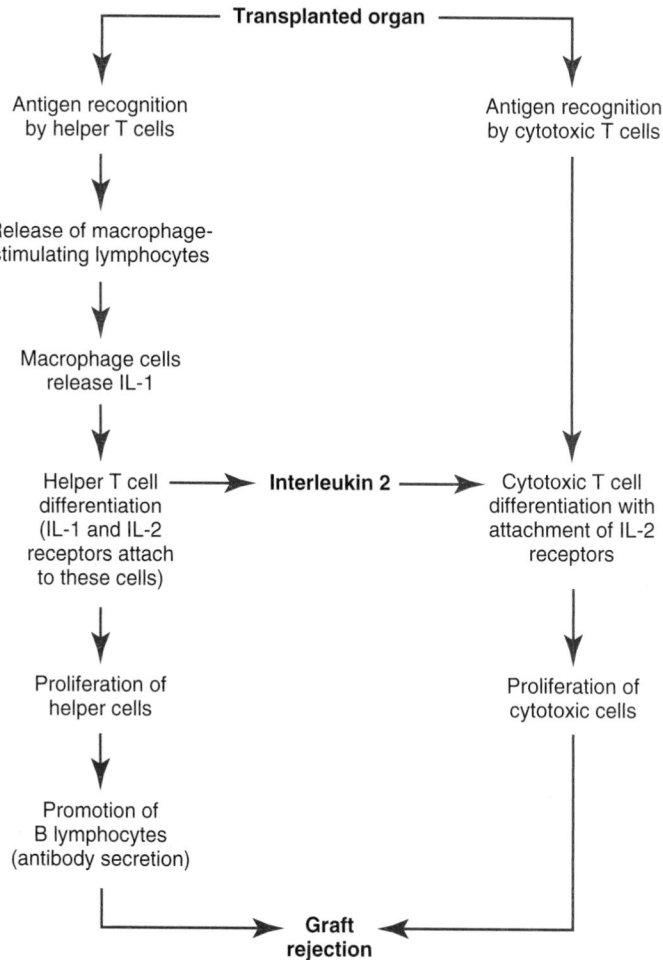

Figure 10-4. Immune response with organ transplantation. *IL-1*, Interleukin-1; *IL-2*, interleukin 2.

Renal
See "Renal Transplantation," p. 329.

MECHANISMS OF IMMUNOSUPPRESSIVE AGENTS

The following drugs may be used in various combinations for additive effect in preventing or modifying the rejection response. The goal of therapy is to achieve enough immunosuppression to prevent graft rejection but not so much as to leave the patient unable to defend against infections.

Azathioprine (Imuran): Interferes with deoxyribonucleic acid (DNA) synthesis and inhibits mitosis of immunologically competent cells. Cell division and proliferation occur in response to antigenic stimulation. Azathioprine affects rapidly replicating cells at an early stage of lymphocyte activation and is believed to block proliferation of helper T cells and cytotoxic T cells. Azathioprine is converted to mercaptopurine (6-MP) and further metabolized in the liver by xanthine oxidase.

Note: Allopurinol inhibits xanthine oxidase-mediated metabolism and may potentiate or cause toxicity of azathioprine. If allopurinol is used with azathioprine, the dose of azathioprine may be reduced by one fourth to one third.

Mycophenolate mofetil: Inhibits denovo purine biosynthesis during cell division. It inhibits the proliferation of T and B lymphocytes, the production of antibodies, and the generation of cytotoxic T cells.

Corticosteroids: Suppress production of cytotoxic T lymphocytes from noncytotoxic precursor cells. Evidence indicates that steroids may prevent release of interleukin-(IL-) 1 and IL-2. IL-1 is released by the macrophages and promotes differentiation of helper T cells. The release of IL-2 promotes differentiation of cytotoxic cells.

Antilymphocyte sera (antilymphocytic globulin [ALG] or antithymocyte gamma-globulin [ATGAM or thymoglobulin]): The antilymphocyte antibodies in the sera are useful in the treatment of steroid-resistant rejection and are potent suppressors of cell-mediated immunity. They are directed against many different antigens on the surface of human lymphocytes and affect immunity via reduction of T lymphocytes.

Monoclonal antibody (Orthoclone OKT3): This homologous antibody reacts with and blocks the function of the chemical (T3) complex on the surface of the T lymphocytes. The T3 complex is responsible for the T lymphocyte's identification of a transplanted organ as foreign and the attempts to reject it. OKT3 binds to the T3 antigen on the surface of the T cells, enhancing phagocytosis and entrapment of the cells in the spleen and liver. The lymphocytes are removed from the circulation by this process in approximately 10-15 min.

Cyclosporine (Sandimmune or Neoral): Inhibits production and release of lymphokines and generation of cytotoxic and plasma cells by blocking the response of cytotoxic T lymphocytes to IL-2. Cyclosporine is metabolized by the cytochrome P-450 enzyme system in the liver. Careful monitoring of cyclosporine drug levels, with concomitant dose adjustments, is necessary when cyclosporine is used with other drugs (Table 10-6).

Tacrolimus (Prograf): Blocks T-cell activation genes by a similar mechanism to cyclosporine. It is also metabolized by the cytochrome P-450 enzyme system in the liver. Careful drug level monitoring and awareness of the interactions of concomitant medications and the potential for dose adjustment are imperative.

Sirolimus (Rapamune): Inhibits T-lymphocyte activation and proliferation. Inhibits antibody formation.

NURSING DIAGNOSES AND INTERVENTIONS

Anxiety/fear related to threat of change in health status secondary to potential loss of transplanted organ because of rejection

Desired outcomes: Patient expresses anxieties and fears regarding possibility of organ loss and verbalizes accurate information about the signs and symptoms of organ rejection. Within 12 hr of this

---

T A B L E   10 - 6   Calcineurin Inhibitor Drug Interactions

Drugs causing decreased blood levels of CyA* and Prograf	Drugs causing increased blood levels of CyA[†] and Prograf
Carbamazepine	Cimetidine
Isoniazid	Danazol
Phenobarbital	Diltiazem
Phenytoin	Erythromycin
Rifampin	High-dose corticosteroids
Sulfamethoxazole	Ketoconazole
Trimethoprim	Methyltestosterone
	Nicardipine
	Oral contraceptives
	Ranitidine

NOTE: Careful monitoring of CyA and Prograf blood levels and adjusting dosage as indicated are necessary when these drugs are used in patients taking cyclosporine or Prograf.
*Decreased blood levels may precipitate organ rejection.
[†]Increased blood levels may cause nephrotoxicity.
CyA, Cyclosporine.

diagnosis, patient's fear and anxiety are controlled as evidenced by BP within patient's normal range; HR ≤100 beats/min; and RR ≤20 breaths/min with normal depth and pattern (eupnea).
- Encourage patient to discuss concerns and fears.
- Assess patient's knowledge about the rejection process and the signs and symptoms that occur.
- Use short, simple sentences to explain patient's current organ function and the signs and symptoms of organ rejection (see Table 10-5).
- Discuss appropriate medications being given to prevent ongoing rejection (see p. 523).
- Explain that rejection does not always cause organ loss. Under most circumstances, rejection can be reversed.
- Reassure patient that retransplantation is a viable option if organ loss occurs.

NIC Anxiety Reduction; Coping Enhancement; Teaching: Individual; Teaching: Disease Process

Fluid volume excess (or risk for same) related to compromised regulatory mechanism secondary to diminished organ function with rejection episode

Desired outcome: Patient is normovolemic as evidenced by stable weight; urine output ≥0.5 ml/kg/hr; BP within patient's normal range; HR 60-100 beats/min; RR 12-20 breaths/min with normal depth and pattern (eupnea); and absence of edema, crackles, and other clinical indicators of fluid overload.
- Measure weight daily. Remember that a 1-kg weight gain can signal approximately 1 L of fluid retention.
- Measure I&O q1-2h; note 24-hr trends. Assess for increased BP, tachycardia, and tachypnea, which are indicators of fluid overload.
- Auscultate for presence of crackles (rales) and pericardial friction rub at least q8h.
- Assess and document the presence of peripheral, sacral, and periorbital edema on a scale of 0-4+.
- Consult physician promptly for any significant findings from the aforementioned assessments.

NIC Fluid Monitoring; Hypervolemia Management; Electrolyte Monitoring

Powerlessness related to actual and perceived helplessness with controlling organ rejection episodes

Desired outcome: Within 72 hr of this diagnosis, patient relates that he or she can control aspects of daily care, as well as assume responsibility for taking medications appropriately and obtaining follow-up care.
- Encourage patient to express feelings of frustration and powerlessness regarding organ rejection.
- Enable and encourage patient to participate in decisions about care routines. Help patient identify areas of the care plan that he or she can control, such as timing of morning care or initiating rest periods.
- Reinforce that taking medications appropriately and keeping appointments for follow-up care *are* within patient's control and are significant in the prevention of rejection and organ destruction.
- Solicit comments and opinions from patient. Honor patient's opinions and preferences.

NIC Self-Esteem Enhancement; Self-Responsibility Facilitation; Mutual Goal Setting

Body image disturbance related to biophysical changes secondary to side effects from immunosuppressive medications

Desired outcome: Within 48-72 hr of this diagnosis, patient verbalizes understanding of body changes that may occur with immunosuppression medications, along with interventions to minimize their effect on body image.
- Identify body changes associated with steroid therapy: profuse diaphoresis, changes in fat distribution, "moon face," acne, bruising.
  - ❏ Suggest that patient try different brands of deodorants or talcs to help counteract the odor from profuse diaphoresis and wear cotton clothing, which absorbs perspiration.
  - ❏ If patient usually wears makeup, suggest that to minimize the effects of facial swelling, patient apply makeup that highlights the eyes.
  - ❏ Suggest that patient refrain from wearing prints and stripes, which may increase attention to fat distribution in the trunk area.
  - ❏ Advise patient to use facial astringents to keep skin clean and to minimize acne.
  - ❏ Suggest that patient wear long sleeves and slacks to cover bruised arms and legs.
  - ❏ Suggest that patient participate in a support group for transplant patients.
- Teach patient about body changes that are associated with cyclosporine: hirsutism and gum hyperplasia.
  - ❏ Suggest that female patient use facial depilatories.
  - ❏ Teach patient to use a soft-bristle toothbrush and mouthwash for frequent, gentle mouth care.

NIC Body Image Enhancement; Emotional Support; Self-Awareness Enhancement; Support Group

ADDITIONAL NURSING DIAGNOSES

See "Renal Transplantation" for "Knowledge Deficit: Immunosuppressive Medications and Their Side Effects," p. 332; "Risk for Infection," p. 333; "Altered Oral Mucous Membrane," p. 334; and "Impaired Skin Integrity," p. 334. For other nursing diagnoses and interventions, see the following, as appropriate: "Prolonged Immobility," p. 61; "Psychosocial Support," p. 68; and "Psychosocial Support for the Patient's Family and Significant Others," p. 78.

Drug Overdose

OVERVIEW/ EPIDEMIOLOGY

Drug overdose and accidental poisonings are common events, varying widely with respect to drug class, victim profile, and clinical scenario. Over two million human toxic exposure cases are reported to poison control centers annually. The 5 million total reported cases at all sites is probably an underestimation due to underreporting and misdiagnosing.

Type, amount, and route of use of the drug determine the effects, management, outcome, prognosis, and physical presentation. Every drug has a threshold for occurrence of serious toxic effects. Drugs of abuse are more dangerous, as they are uncontrolled and unregulated, with a haphazard nature of administration. The patient's history is often unavailable or of poor quality. Time is critical to successful treatment. A thoughtful and stepwise approach to laboratory testing, medical and nursing interventions, pharmacologic support, and general supportive measures is essential. No organ or body system is protected from the detrimental effects of drug overdose.

TREATMENT OPTIONS

Gastric decontamination: Gastric decontamination is a general term referring to interventions used to prevent absorption of a toxin. Timely administration is essential for success. Best results are obtained if done within an hour of ingestion. Five interventions are discussed:

Activated charcoal: A fine, insoluble, nonabsorbable powder which binds with many toxic drugs to enhance their elimination. Activated charcoal *does not bind* with lithium, potassium, potassium chloride, ethanol, iron, acidic or alkaline corrosives, or hydrocarbons. Use is common, well-researched and has proven efficacy in the pre- and postabsorption phases. The dose is 1 g/kg initially, followed by repeat doses of 0.5 to 1 g/kg every 2 to 4 hr. Combining the first dose with sorbitol increases the tolerability of charcoal, but has not been proven to enhance drug elimination. Contraindicated in cases of bowel obstruction or perforation and in patients with depressed mental status unless intubated.

Ipecac: Ipecac syrup is a drug used to induce vomiting as part of treatment of drug overdoses and in certain poisonings. Effectiveness diminishes rapidly with time, so it should be given within 60 min of ingestion of a toxin. It is most often used in the home after a witnessed ingestion. It should not be given if the patient has depressed mental status and is at risk to aspirate. Thus, if the patient has taken a central nervous system depressant which may lead to progressive deterioration in mental status, ipecac should not be used; nor should it be given for ingestion of a corrosive or low-viscosity hydrocarbon. Ipecac may cause bradycardia, which combined with vomiting may cause hemodynamic compromise; particularly if cardiotoxic drugs such as digoxin or cyclic antidepressants are involved.

Gastric lavage: Commonly known as "pumping the stomach," insertion of nasogastric tube with vigorous enteral irrigation is a decreasingly important adjunct for treatment of ingested overdose; no longer recommended as routine management by the American and European toxicology associations. If used, it must be done as soon as possible and has little benefit if more than 60 min has passed since ingestion. When using lavage, the airway must be protected and lavage should continue until the fluid is clear of fragments (usually requires about 5 L of fluid). Neither gastric lavage nor ipecac should be attempted if they delay or interfere with activated charcoal administration in appropriate patients.

Large, life-threatening amounts of ingested toxin (which may be poorly bound to activated charcoal used prior to lavage) may justify use. The contraindications to ipecac apply to this intervention. Additionally, patients at risk for esophageal hemorrhage or perforation should not be lavaged.

Whole bowel irrigation: The administration of a polyethylene glycol balanced electrolyte solution to rapidly cleanse the bowel may be useful in cases where activated charcoal is ineffective, such as with ingestions of iron, lithium, and sustained released tablets. It may diminish the effectiveness of activated charcoal, should not be done concurrently, and is contraindicated when ileus, gastrointestinal (GI) bleeding, bowel obstruction, or bowel perforation is present.

Cathartics: Although often mixed with activated charcoal, cathartics such as sorbitol have not been proven effective in enhancing the elimination of toxins from the GI tract. May help avoid constipation induced by activated charcoal.

INGESTION OF UNKNOWN SUBSTANCES

Many patients with drug overdose first arrive to be seen with altered mental status and without a useful or reliable history. Identification of the ingested substance is difficult. Lab screening is done for common drugs of abuse including amphetamines, barbiturates, benzodiazepines, cocaine, opioids, phencyclidine, and cannabinoids. Specific drug levels are available for salicylates, acetaminophen, digoxin, theophylline, iron, and lithium. When one of these drugs is not the offending agent, a number of signs and symptoms should be noted and tests done to determine the list of potential offending agents. It is beyond the scope of this chapter to include all the drugs and toxins leading to common presenting symptoms, but important clues to the poison may be gleaned from answering the following questions:

- Heart rate and rhythm: is the patient bradycardic or tachycardic? Is a dysrhythmia present?
- Mental status: is the patient overall depressed or agitated? Is delirium present?
- Temperature: is hypothermia or hyperthermia present?
- Is the patient having seizures?
- Eyes: are pupils showing miosis or mydriasis? Is nystagmus present?
- Muscle tone: is the patient flaccid or rigid? Are dyskinesias present?
- Lungs: if respiratory failure is occurring, is it related to depression, aspiration, edema, hemorrhage, bronchospasm, or cardiac failure?
- Is pH from the arterial blood gas acidotic or alkalotic?
- Anion gap abnormality: if present, is it elevated or decreased?
- Blood glucose: is the patient hyperglycemic or hypoglycemic?
- Psychosocial: does the patient have a history of psychiatric disorders, of drug abuse, or of depression? Is the patient on any drugs with narrow therapeutic windows, and is a list of current medications (including OTC) available?

Specific antidotes for common drug overdoses/toxicities: Table 10-7 gives specific drug treatments for a few of the more common and critical drug overdoses:

ACETAMINOPHEN (APAP)

One of the most commonly ingested drugs in overdose. Most patients admit taking this drug.

Routes of administration
Oral (most common); rectal per suppository.

T A B L E   10 - 7   Management of Drug Overdose

Target (toxic) drug or class	Treatment or antidote
Acetaminophen	N-Acetylcysteine
Benzodiazepines	Flumezanil
Beta-(β-) blockers	Glucagon; beta-(β-) agonists
Calcium channel blockers	Calcium IV, glucagon
Cyclic antidepressants	Sodium bicarbonate
Digitalis glycosides	Digoxin immune fab
Heparin	Protamine
Insulin	Glucagon, dextrose, octreotide
Iron	Deferoxamine
Lead, arsenic, mercury, or other heavy metals	Edetate calcium disodium (EDTA), dimercaptol injection, penicillamine
Methanol	Ethanol, folinic acid
Opiates	Naloxone
Organophosphate insecticides	Atropine, pralidoxime
Warfarin	Vitamin K (IV or PO)

Effects on body systems
Cardiovascular: Hepatic damage may prompt cardiac complications including dysrhythmias, ischemia and injury (chest pain/pressure, nausea, SOB, T wave inversion and ST segment elevation on ECG).
Respiratory: Bronchospasm (wheezes and difficulty breathing) and tachypnea have been reported as a hypersensitivity reaction or as a side effect of *N*-acetylcysteine. See "Collaborative Management" section that follows.
Neurologic: Coma and seizures.
Hepatic: Acute ingestion will cause hepatic necrosis, which can lead to liver failure. Hypoglycemia, right-sided abdominal pain, and nausea with vomiting may be noted; usually 1-2 days after ingestion.
Renal: Acute tubular necrosis with renal failure is seen in some cases but often resolves.
Associated findings: Hypophosphatemia, metabolic acidosis, hypothermia, thrombocytopenia, and hemorrhagic pancreatitis.

Diagnostic tests
Serum blood levels (therapeutic levels: 10-20 mcg/ml): The first serum blood levels are drawn 4 hr after ingestion, if possible. Subsequent levels are drawn periodically (e.g., q4h) until levels are below the predicted hepatotoxic range.
Additional tests: Serum Na^+, K^+, CO_2, BUN, blood glucose, creatinine, liver enzymes, bilirubin; PT, coagulation studies; CBC; protein; amylase; and ABGs may be done.

Collaborative management
Support of cardiovascular and respiratory systems: Supplemental oxygen should be given if ABG values indicate a trend toward respiratory failure. If the patient has an ineffective or absent breathing effort, mechanical ventilation is provided. Serial ECGs monitor for dysrhythmias. Symptomatic ventricular dysrhythmias and bradyarrhythmias are treated per ACLS guidelines (see Appendix 1.)
Removing acetaminophen from the patient: A combination of activated charcoal and *N*-acetylcysteine (Mucomyst, NAC) administered orally or via a gastric tube is the preferred treatment. Activated charcoal effectively adsorbs APAP if given within 4 hr. Mucomyst prevents systemic toxicity; especially if given 8-10 hr after ingestion. Lavage and ipecac are used only if <1 hr has elapsed since ingestion. Administration of the activated charcoal and NAC *should not be delayed* to give ipecac and perform lavage.
Treatment of nausea and vomiting: Fluid replacement therapy with lactated Ringer's solution or D_5NS; antiemetics, such as promethazine hydrochloride (Phenergan).
Rewarming: A heating blanket is applied if patient has hypothermia.
Treatment of hypoglycemia: Usually done with a bolus of D_{50} and continuous infusion of D_5W, based on serum glucose results. Hypoglycemia occurs because of the potent hepatotoxic effects of acetaminophen.

ALCOHOL
Route of administration
Oral.

Effects on body systems
Cardiovascular: Tachycardia, atrial fibrillation, cardiac arrest.
Respiratory: Hypoventilation with acute intoxication, respiratory failure, aspiration.
Neurologic: Confusion, aggressive behavior, irritability, tremors, hallucinations (especially auditory), memory loss, stupor, coma, seizures, loss of deep tendon reflexes (DTRs).
Renal: May have significant output initially; will demonstrate dehydration with acute intoxication.
Associated findings: Dry oral mucosa, odor of alcohol on breath, hypoglycemia, hypothermia, lactic acidosis, hypokalemia.

Diagnostic tests
Blood alcohol level and a urine drug screen are performed, along with serum K^+, Na^+, CO_2, BUN, glucose, creatinine. CBC, liver function studies, and blood gas values may be done.

Collaborative management
Support of cardiovascular and respiratory systems to prevent collapse: Oxygen supplementation; treatment of ventricular dysrhythmias and bradyarrhythmias per ACLS. (See Appendix 1.)
Fluid/potassium replacement: See discussions, pp. 541 and 550.
Removing alcohol from the patient: Alcohol is usually metabolized by the patient. Blood alcohol level decreases 20-30 mg/dl/hr (legal limit for driving is <100 mg/dl). Coma may occur if

the level is >300 mg/dl, but this is influenced by each individual's metabolic process and tolerance. When extreme amounts of alcohol have been absorbed into the system, the liver and kidneys may not be able to break down and excrete the alcohol. Hemodialysis (see p. 335) may be used for a life-threatening intoxication.

Prevention of emesis: Antiemetics are given, and a gastric tube is inserted and maintained at low continuous suction.

Anticipation and treatment of withdrawal: Benzodiazepines are the drugs of choice for treating alcohol withdrawal. Lorazepam, which can be given IV, IM, PO, or sublingually (SL), is the preferred agent on most alcohol withdrawal protocols. Longer-acting agents (chlodiazepoxide and diazepam) are also used, because of the decreased risk of recurrent withdrawal and/or seizures. Oxazepam and lorazepam have a mechanism of metabolism that is less liver-dependent and are useful in cases involving cirrhosis. Medications are given as needed for withdrawal symptoms. In patients at high risk for severe withdrawal symptoms, or if withdrawal would be dangerous, benzodiazepines may be given on a schedule.

Treatment of hypoglycemia: A bolus of D_{50} and continuous infusion of D_5W, based on serum glucose. Thiamine should be given before glucose to avoid sudden onset of heart failure and worsening neurologic impairment.

Treatment of delirium tremens (DTs): The most severe manifestation of withdrawal, which can result in death. Symptoms develop 48-96 hr after cessation of drinking and include confusion, disorientation, delirium, agitation, severe diaphoresis, tachycardia, fever, and hypotension. DTs generally resolve within 3-5 days. Patients are sedated with benzodiazepines, allowed to rest and sleep, and oriented frequently to reality.

Treatment/prevention of seizures: Alcohol withdrawal seizures may occur in a range from the first 6-48 hr to late onset at 10 days after abstinence. Benzodiazepines are given to raise the seizure threshold during the withdrawal period. Additional seizure management should reflect institution protocol. If the patient has a history of a primary seizure disorder, an anticonvulsant agent may also be indicated.

Prevention of Wernicke-Korsakoff syndrome: Caused by thiamine deficiency and manifested by diplopia (the first real diagnostic clue), confusion, excitation, peripheral neuropathy, severe recent memory loss, impaired thought processes, and confabulation. Prophylactic administration of thiamine is recommended: IM thiamine on admission; supplemental oral thiamine; and multivitamins and multiminerals high in C, B complex, zinc, and magnesium. Multivitamins and minerals are given to prevent malnutrition related to inadequate food intake and malabsorption caused by alcohol's irritating effect on the GI tract.

Caution: Ingestion of carbohydrates, either orally or parenterally, increases the body's demand for thiamine. For patients with a history of chronic alcohol ingestion, administration of thiamine should precede administration of glucose to prevent sudden profound thiamine deficiency and irreversible neurologic impairment.

AMPHETAMINES

Street names
Methamphetamine, speed, crystal meth, white crosses, ice, crank, ecstasy.

Routes of administration
Oral, IV, IM, smoked.

Effects on body systems
Cardiovascular: Tachycardia, atrial and ventricular dysrhythmias, hypertension, myocardial ischemia and infarction, cardiovascular collapse.
Respiratory: Hyperventilation and respiratory failure related to cardiovascular collapse.
Neurologic: Confusion, aggressive behavior, hyperactivity, convulsions, delusions, irritability, tremors, hallucinations, memory loss, stupor, stroke, coma.
Renal: Renal failure related to dehydration and rhabdomyolysis.
Associated findings: Mydriasis, fasciculations, hyperthermia, thrombocytopenic purpura.

Diagnostic tests
Blood and urine are tested for substances of abuse. Serum K^+, Na^+, CO_2, BUN, glucose, creatinine, CBC, liver studies, and cardiac enzyme levels with isoenzyme fractionations are monitored.

Collaborative management

Support of cardiovascular and respiratory systems to prevent collapse: Antidysrhythmic agents are given per ACLS guidelines to manage tachycardias. Ischemia is treated with nitrates; myocardial infarction is treated per ACLS guidelines for acute coronary syndromes (see Appendix 1).

Removing amphetamines from the patient: For oral ingestion, activated charcoal is administered orally or via gastric tube. Ipecac is not recommended. Acidification of the urine with ammonium chloride helps clear amphetamine.

Treatment of hypertension: Antihypertensives such as nitroprusside (Nipride) or labetalol may be needed to decrease BP.

Prevention/treatment of seizures: IV diazepam 0.1-0.2 mg/kg is administered slowly and repeated q5min until sedation is achieved. Lorazepam is an alternative benzodiazepine.

Psychosis: Haldol 5 mg is given IM or IV. Repeat dose may be required to control behavior.

Treatment of hyperthermia: A cooling blanket, antipyretics, and iced intravenous fluids are used.

Treatment of dehydration: Done by fluid replacement, such as lactated Ringer's solution and D_5NS.

Anticipation and treatment of rhabdomyolysis: Usually treated with sodium bicarbonate infusion, mannitol, or furosemide (Lasix).

BARBITURATES

See Table 10-8.

Street names
Yellow jackets, reds, barbs.

Routes of administration
Oral, IV, IM.

Effects on body systems

Cardiovascular: Hypotension, bradycardia, cardiac arrest.

Respiratory: Hypoventilation leading to respiratory failure and respiratory arrest.

Neurologic: Symptoms may include headache, vertigo, dizziness, lethargy, ataxia, stupor, flaccidity, seizures, absent doll's-eye reflex, coma, loss of DTRs, and nystagmus (see coma scale, which follows under "Classification of Barbiturate Intoxication").

Renal: Acute renal failure is possible.

Associated findings: Hypothermia, nausea, vomiting. Patient may experience opposite reactions of euphoria and excitability before the normal sedative effects occur. Withdrawal symptoms (tremors and convulsions) may occur.

Classification of barbiturate intoxication

Alert: No signs of CNS depression.

Drowsy: CNS depression from alert to stuporous.

Stuporous: Markedly sedated; responsive to verbal and tactile stimuli.

T A B L E 10 - 8   Common Barbiturates

Generic name	Common brand name	Half-life (hr)
Amobarbital	Amytal	8-42
Secobarbital	Seconal	19-34
Pentobarbital	Nembutal	15-48
Phenobarbital	Luminal and others	24-140
Butabarbital	Butisol	34-42
Secobarbital/amobarbital	Tuinal	8-42

NOTE: Withdrawal symptoms can be correlated with the half-life of the drug that was used. Withdrawal from drugs with shorter half-lives produces more intense symptoms that last for shorter periods, whereas withdrawal from drugs with longer half-lives produces less intense symptoms that can be prolonged. Moreover, the severity of the withdrawal is directly related to the drug's dosage.

Coma 1: Responsive to painful but not to verbal and tactile stimuli; no change in respirations or BP.
Coma 2: Unconscious; unresponsive to pain; no change in respirations or BP.
Coma 3: Unresponsive to pain; slow, shallow, or rapid spontaneous respirations; low but adequate BP.
Coma 4: Unresponsive to pain; apnea or inadequate BP, or both.

Diagnostic tests
Serum drug screen is analyzed. In addition to serum K^+, Na^+, CO_2, BUN, glucose, and creatinine, the CBC, ABGs, and liver function studies are evaluated.

Collaborative management
Support of cardiovascular and respiratory systems to prevent collapse: Electrical rhythm is monitored; bradyarrhythmias are treated per ACLS guidelines (see Appendix 1). After fluids are replaced, vasopressor therapy (see Appendix 7), including dopamine and norepinephrine bitartrate (Levophed), may be initiated for hypotension. Mechanical ventilation may be required, depending on the degree of hypoxia and CO_2 retention.
Removing barbiturates from the patient: If less than 1 hour since ingestion, ipecac is given to promote vomiting, or gastric lavage (provided there is no delay in the administration of activated charcoal). Activated charcoal is administered orally or via gastric tube to bind with the substance in the stomach; hemodialysis may be used if patient is in stage 4 coma. Sufficient sodium bicarbonate should be given to alkalinize the urine to a pH of 7.5.
Prevention/treatment of seizures: Phenytoin or diazepam may be given.
Sedation for withdrawal symptoms: Typically the barbiturate that was ingested is tapered gradually to zero.
Prevention of aspiration: A gastric tube is inserted, which is then connected to low suction.
Treatment of nausea and vomiting: Antiemetics are administered, usually IV promethazine hydrochloride.
Treatment of hypothermia: A warming blanket is used.

BENZODIAZEPINES
See Table 10-9.

Routes of administration
Oral, IM, IV.

Effects on body systems
Cardiovascular: Hypotension, tachycardia.

T A B L E 1 0 - 9   Common Benzodiazepines

Generic name	Common brand name	Half-Life (hr)
Chlordiazepoxide	Librium and others	7-28
Diazepam	Valium and others	20-90
Lorazepam	Ativan	10-20
Oxazepam	Serax	3-21
Prazepam	Centrax	24-200[*]
Flurazepam	Dalmane	24-100[*]
Chlorazepate	Tranxene	30-100
Temazepam	Restoril	9.5-12.4
Clonazepam	Klonopin	18.5-50
Alprazolam	Xanax	12-15
Halazepam	Paxipam	14

[*]Includes half-life of major metabolites.
NOTE: Withdrawal symptoms can be correlated with the half-life of the drug that was used. Withdrawal from drugs with shorter half-lives produces more intense symptoms that last for shorter periods, whereas withdrawal from drugs with longer half-lives produces less intense symptoms that can be prolonged. Moreover, the severity of the withdrawal is directly related to the drug's dosage.

Respiratory: Respiratory arrest.
Neurologic: Drowsiness, ataxia, slurred speech, coma. Withdrawal may be manifested by seizures.
Renal: Renal failure because of rhabdomyolysis.
Associated findings: Hypothermia.

Diagnostic tests
Serum and urine drug screens are analyzed. Serum K^+, Na^+, CO_2, BUN, glucose, creatinine, CBC, and liver studies are evaluated.

Collaborative management
Support of cardiovascular system to prevent collapse: Electrical rhythm is monitored. Atrial fibrillation or flutter may be treated with digoxin or amiodarone, with initial rate control using diltiazem or β-blockers. Severe supraventricular tachyarrhythmias may be treated with adenosine. Verapamil is an alternative agent, provided there are no contraindications such as heart failure, hypotension, or Wolff-Parkinson-White syndrome. Hypotension is treated with fluid replacement, followed by dopamine or norepinephrine (Levophed).
Support of respiratory system: Apnea monitoring and mechanical ventilation (see p. 14) may be indicated.
Removing benzodiazepines from the patient: Ipecac is indicated to induce vomiting if less than 60 min after ingestion; gastric lavage within the same time frame, activated charcoal to bind with the substance in the stomach.
Prevention of seizures: Phenytoin is administered.
Prevention of aspiration: Gastric tube is inserted, which is then connected to low intermittent suction.
Identification of rhabdomyolysis: Seizure activity and breakdown of muscle cause protein to precipitate in the kidneys, leading to renal failure. Increased BUN, creatinine, and urine protein values are noted. Prevention of seizures is the best treatment for prevention of rhabdomyolysis.
Treatment of hypothermia: A warming blanket is used if indicated.
Flumazenil administration: Sedative and respiratory depressant effects may be reversed by flumazenil (Romazicon). Repeat doses may be necessary, since the duration of action of many benzodiazepines exceeds that of flumazenil. Use with caution, especially in patients with possible multiple drug overdose. Flumazenil may precipitate seizures in benzodiazepine-dependent patients and causes arrhythmias in patients who also have high levels of cyclic antidepressants.

COCAINE
Street names
Crack, rock, freebase, snow.

Routes of administration
Nasal or IV (cocaine, snow); smoked (crack, rock, freebase).

Effects on body systems
Cardiovascular: Hypertension; sinus tachycardia and sinus bradycardia; ventricular dysrhythmias such as PVCs, ventricular tachycardia, and ventricular fibrillation; myocardial infarction; heart failure; cardiomyopathy; acute endocarditis; and aortic dissection. Acute intoxication may result in profound hypotension and shock.
Respiratory: Sharp pleuritic pain, hemoptysis, pneumothorax, bronchospasm, pulmonary edema, and respiratory failure. Both lactic acidosis and metabolic acidosis have been seen.
Neurologic: The degree of CNS stimulation depends on the route and amount of drug taken. Headache, hyperexcitation, paranoia, delirium, hallucinations, tremors, and aggression may be seen. Mentation may vary from stimulated, euphoric, and excited states to delirium, stupor, and coma. Seizures are common, usually tonic-clonic, and may last for hours. Initially patients may seem well-coordinated, but later may show tremors and fasciculations as their condition deteriorates.
Renal: Renal failure can occur and has been related to profound hypotension and rhabdomyolysis.
Associated findings: Hyperthermia is common, and rectal temperatures may be elevated to as high as 43° C (109.4° F). Perforated nasal septum, track marks related to IV use, and mydriasis (dilated pupils) occur.
Indicators of withdrawal: Poor concentration, anergia, anhedonia, bradykinesis, sleep disturbance, decreased libido, intense cocaine craving, depression, and suicidal tendencies.
Indicators of cocaine psychosis: Tactile and visual hallucination and paranoia.

Peak action
Intranasal 20-60 min.
Oral 60-90 min.
IV 5 min.
Smoked <5 min.

Cutting agents
Cutting agents are substances mixed with pure cocaine to increase bulk and include procaine, phencyclidine (angel dust), amphetamine, quinine, talc, and strychnine. Agents used in the preparation of crack include powdered cocaine, water, baking soda, and lidocaine. Cutting agents can become emboli that shower into cerebral and pulmonary circulation, with subsequent effects.

Diagnostic tests
Assessing blood levels of cocaine is usually of little diagnostic value. Urinalysis provides a quantitative method for identifying the presence of a cocaine metabolite. Serum K^+, Na^+, CO_2, BUN, glucose, creatinine, CBC, and liver function studies may be done.

Collaborative management
Support of cardiovascular system to prevent collapse: Electrical rhythm is monitored. Supraventricular tachycardia and ventricular dysrhythmias are managed per ACLS guidelines (see Appendix 1). Monitor ECG for ischemic changes or infarction pattern (T wave inversion or ST segment elevation or depression).
Support of respiratory system: Comatose patients are placed on mechanical ventilation (see p. 14).
Identification of route of administration and removing cocaine following oral ingestion: An x-ray of the GI tract may reveal a cocaine-filled condom. Surgery may be performed to remove it. Activated charcoal may be administered to bind with cocaine in the stomach, or a laxative or suppository may be given to facilitate rectal excretion. An approach under investigation is to flush cocaine from the circulation using IV ammonium chloride.
Treatment of hypotension or hypertension: Antihypertensives or vasopressors are administered as indicated.
Treatment of volume deficiency: IV fluid replacement is done, such as with lactated Ringer's solution or D_5NS.
Prevention/treatment of seizures: Diazepam, phenytoin, or phenobarbital is administered.
Treatment of hyperthermia: A cooling blanket, ice, and/or acetaminophen is used. Core temperature is the most accurate measurement.
Prevention of aspiration: A gastric tube is inserted, then connected to low continuous suction.

HALLUCINOGENS
Common agents
Lysergic acid diethylamide (LSD), mescaline, morning glory seeds, nutmeg.

Routes of administration
Oral, IV, nasal, smoked.

Effects on body systems
Effects will depend on the amount and type of drug ingested.
Respiratory: Apnea, respiratory arrest.
Neurologic: Hallucinations and paranoid behavior patterns, tremors, seizures, coma.
LSD: Patient may describe tasting or hearing colors or exhibit mental dissociation.
Mescaline: Sense of being followed by moving geometric shapes.
Associated findings: Hyperthermia and diaphoresis. In addition, visual hallucinations may occur.

Diagnostic tests
Serum plasma is analyzed for the presence of the drug. Serum K^+, Na^+, CO_2, BUN, glucose, and creatinine, CBC, and liver studies are evaluated.

Collaborative management
Support of cardiovascular system to prevent collapse: Manage blood pressure and heart rate/rhythm per ACLS guidelines (see Appendix 1).

Removing hallucinogens from patient: If oral ingestion is recent (<1 hr), ipecac is administered to induce vomiting or gastric lavage may be attempted, as long as activated charcoal therapy is not delayed. Activated charcoal is administered orally or via gastric tube to bind with the substance in the stomach.

Prevention of seizures: Anticonvulsants such as phenytoin or diazepam are administered.

OPIOIDS

Examples of opioids include codeine, fentanyl, heroin, hydrocodone, hydromorphone hydrochloride (Dilaudid), levorphanol tartrate (Levo-Dromoran), meperidine hydrochloride (Demerol), methadone (Dolophine), morphine, opium, oxycodone hydrochloride (Percocet-5, Tylox, Oxycontin), and oxymorphone (Numorphan).

Routes of administration
Oral, IV, IM, smoked.

Effects on body systems
Cardiovascular: Profound hypotension, bradycardia, cardiovascular collapse, sudden death.
Respiratory: Atelectasis, acute pulmonary edema, infiltrates related to aspiration complications, respiratory depression, apnea, hypoventilation, and bronchospasm.
Neurologic: Range from decreased mental alertness to stupor and coma; pinpoint pupils, seizures.
Renal: Renal failure has been associated with profound hypotension and rhabdomyolysis.
Associated findings: Track marks and scarring on arms and in hidden locations of the body, including between the toes and in the vessels underneath the tongue.

Diagnostic tests
Urine sampling for drug detection is the best way to identify the drug. Serum K^+, Na^+, CO_2, BUN, glucose, creatinine, CBC, and liver studies are evaluated.

Collaborative management
Support of cardiovascular system to prevent collapse: Electrical rhythm is monitored; bradyarrhythmias are treated per ACLS guidelines (Appendix 1). Vasopressor therapy is initiated for hypotension after fluids have been replaced.
Removal of orally ingested opioids from patient: If oral ingestion within the last 60 min is suspected, ipecac is used to induce vomiting; activated charcoal is administered orally or via gastric tube to bind with the substance in the stomach.
Reversal of opioid effects: Administration of naloxone hydrochloride (Narcan). After the initial dose of naloxone, the patient must be monitored closely, since additional doses may be required. Respiratory depression and coma may occur when the effects of naloxone wear off and the opiate effects predominate. The half-life of naloxone is 60-90 min, and effects last 2-3 hr. If the narcotic effects last longer than the effects of the naloxone, the patient may slip into coma once the naloxone wears off. In this case, a continuous naloxone infusion may be considered.
Treatment of drug withdrawal symptoms: Hallucinations are treated with haloperidol (Haldol).
Support of respiratory system: Pulmonary edema is treated with diuretics and restriction of IV fluid intake. An individual whose respiratory system is deteriorating is placed on apnea monitoring or mechanical ventilation (see p. 14).
Prevention of aspiration: A gastric tube is inserted, then connected to low continuous suction.
Prevention/treatment of seizure activity: Anticonvulsant therapy is done, such as phenytoin administration.
Prevention of rhabdomyolysis: See discussion, p. 532.

PHENCYCLIDINE
Street names
PCP, angel dust, mist, peep, hog, crystal.

Routes of administration
Oral, nasal, smoked.

Effects on body systems
Cardiovascular: Hypertension, hypertensive crisis, tachycardia.
Respiratory: Respiratory depression, respiratory arrest, laryngeal stridor, bronchospasm.

Neurologic: Ranges from hyperexcitability, hyperreflexia, muscle rigidity, and paranoid and psychotic behavior to stupor, seizures, and coma. Coma: eyes may be open in a blank stare, nystagmus, and pinpoint pupils.
Renal: Renal failure precipitated by rhabdomyolysis and myoglobinuria.
Associated findings: Hypothermia or hyperthermia, hypoglycemia.

Diagnostic tests
Blood and urine samples are tested for the presence of the drug. Serum K^+, Na^+, CO_2, BUN, glucose, creatinine, CBC, and liver studies may be evaluated.

Collaborative management
Support of cardiovascular system to prevent collapse: Electrical rhythm is monitored and tachydysrhythmias are treated as previously discussed. Nitroprusside is used for antihypertensive therapy. Nitroglycerin may be given to treat ischemia.
Removal of phencyclidine from the patient: No specific antidote is available, although multiple administrations of charcoal to bind with the ingested substance in the stomach are standard practice. The first dose of charcoal may be accompanied with sorbitol. After ruling out the possibility of rhabdomyolysis, acidification of the urine with ammonium chloride or ascorbic acid to a pH around 5.5 is done.
Prevention/treatment of seizure activity: Phenytoin and diazepam are given. Diazepam is administered IV at an initial dose of 2-5 mg. May be repeated q30min until sedation is achieved. Haldol may be given 5-10 mg IV to control psychosis. The effects of Haldol usually occur within 5-10 min of administration.
Respiratory support: Pulmonary edema is treated with diuretics and restriction of IV fluid intake. Persons with hypoxia and respiratory distress require monitoring of pulse oximetry and may require mechanical ventilation.
Prevention of aspiration: A gastric tube is inserted, then connected to intermittent low suction.
Prevention of rhabdomyolysis: See discussion, p. 532.
Treatment of hypothermia or hyperthermia: A warming or cooling blanket is used as appropriate.

SALICYLATES
Examples include aspirin, bismuth subsalicylate, fendosal.

Routes of administration
Oral, rectal (suppository).

Effects on body systems
Respiratory: Hyperventilation, hyperpnea, pulmonary edema.
Neurologic: Coma, cerebral edema (manifested by indicators of increased intracranial pressure [IICP] [see Table 6-3]).
Renal: Renal failure secondary to rhabdomyolysis.
Hepatic: Liver dysfunction, hepatitis.
Associated findings: Hyperthermia, bleeding, anemia, thrombocytopenia, hypokalemia, and tinnitus.

Diagnostic tests
Blood plasma is analyzed for the presence and amount of the salicylate and repeated q4-6h. Repeat testing is helpful, especially if the patient ingested sustained-release salicylates. Serum K^+, Na^+, CO_2, BUN, glucose, creatinine, CBC, and liver studies are evaluated.

Collaborative management
Support of cardiovascular system to prevent collapse: Electrical rhythm is monitored. Ventricular dysrhythmias and bradyarrhythmias are treated per ACLS guidelines (see Appendix 1).
Removal of salicylates from the patient: Ipecac is administered to induce vomiting (<60 min after ingestion); activated charcoal is administered orally or via gastric tube to bind with the substance in the stomach; several doses of activated charcoal may be necessary to achieve a 10:1 ratio of charcoal to salicylate. Hemodialysis may be necessary if the substance has been absorbed into the system. Charcoal hemoperfusion may clear salicylates somewhat, but cannot correct acid/base, electrolyte, and fluid problems associated with severe poisoning.
Fluid replacement: Replace fluids with lactated Ringer's solution or D_5NS 20 ml/kg over 1-2 hr. Sodium bicarbonate may be added at a rate of 1 mEq/kg/hr to promote forced alkaline diuresis.

Potassium replacement: See discussion, p. 550.
Treatment of hyperthermia: A cooling blanket or applications of ice is used.
Treatment of cerebral edema: Hyperventilation (via mechanical ventilation) or mannitol are used.
Respiratory support: Mechanical ventilation (p. 14) is used as indicated.
Treatment of pulmonary edema: Nitrates, morphine, diuretics, potassium replacement, and intermittent positive pressure breathing (IPPB) are possible. See discussion, p. 223.
Prevention of aspiration: A gastric tube is inserted, then connected to low suction.
Replacement of blood loss: Done by delivery of blood and blood products.

CYCLIC ANTIDEPRESSANTS

Examples include amitriptyline hydrochloride (Elavil), doxepin hydrochloride (Sinequan), imipramine hydrochloride (Presamine, Tofranil), trimipramine maleate (Surmontil), nortriptyline (Pamelor, Aventyl), and desipramine (Norpramin).

Route of administration
Oral.

Effects on body systems
Cardiovascular: Hypotension, sinus tachycardia, supraventricular tachycardia, ventricular dysrhythmias, conduction defects, myocardial infarction, cardiopulmonary arrest. Hypertension has been noted. Monitor ECG for widening QRS complex. Progressive QRS widening signals worsening toxicity.
Respiratory: Respiratory arrest, pulmonary edema, ARDS. Hyperventilation also has been noted.
Neurologic: Central nervous system depression, coma, seizures, delirium, hallucinations.
Renal: Acute tubular necrosis; renal failure secondary to rhabdomyolysis.
Pancreatic: Pancreatitis.
Associated findings: Hyperthermia or hypothermia.

Diagnostic tests
Blood plasma, urine, and gastric contents are analyzed to determine the presence and amount of the drug. Serum K^+, Na^+, CO_2, BUN, glucose, creatinine, CBC, and liver studies are evaluated. Cardiac enzymes and isoenzyme fractionations are assessed for presence and degree of myocardial damage.

Collaborative management
If the patient is symptom-free, monitor for a minimum of 6-8 hr, noting VS and width of QRS complex.
Support of cardiovascular system to prevent collapse: Electrical rhythm is monitored for at least 6 hr to enable assessment for a widening QRS complex, which is a signal of worsening toxicity. Supraventricular tachycardias are treated with adenosine or verapamil; ventricular dysrhythmias are treated with antidysrhythmics such as lidocaine or amiodarone. Atropine and pacing may be indicated in the presence of symptomatic conduction defects.
Removing cyclic antidepressants from the patient: Activated charcoal is administered via gastric tube to bind with the ingested substance in the stomach. Ipecac to promote vomiting is not recommended.
Reversal of the effects of the drugs: IV sodium bicarbonate is used. An alternative approach is to promote a state of respiratory alkalosis by increasing respiratory rate via mechanical ventilation.
Prevention/treatment of seizures: Phenytoin and diazepam are administered.
Respiratory support: Mechanical ventilation is used (see p. 14). Pulmonary edema is treated with nitrates, morphine, diuretics, potassium replacement, and IPPB treatments.
Treatment of hypotension: Fluid replacement is carried out, followed by administration of dopamine and norepinephrine bitartrate (Levophed) as indicated.
Treatment of hyperthermia or hypothermia: A cooling or a warming blanket is used as indicated.
Prevention of aspiration: A gastric tube is inserted, then connected to low intermittent suction.

FOR ALL DRUG OVERDOSES

Nursing diagnoses, interventions, and outcomes
Airway clearance, ineffective related to presence of tracheobronchial secretions or obstruction; decreased sensorium
Desired outcomes: Chest x-ray is clear. Within 2-24 hr of intervention/treatment, patient has a clear airway as evidenced by clear breath sounds over the upper airways and lung fields; RR 12-20

breaths/min with normal depth and pattern (eupnea); Pao_2 ≥80 mm Hg; $Paco_2$ 35-45 mm Hg; pH 7.35-7.45; and Spo_2 ≥92%.
- Assess for respiratory distress hourly and prn. Note secretions; stridor; gurgling; shallow, irregular, or labored respirations; use of accessory muscles of respiration; restlessness and confusion; and cyanosis (a late sign of respiratory distress).
- Suction oropharynx, or use suction via ET tube prn.
- Administer bronchodilators as appropriate.
- Monitor ABG values for evidence of hypoxia (Pao_2 <80 mm Hg) and respiratory acidosis ($Paco_2$ >45 mm Hg; pH <7.35).
- Monitor respiratory patterns; provide continuous apnea monitoring if available.
- If patient has been placed on mechanical ventilation, monitor for indicators of airway obstruction (see "Mechanical Ventilation," p. 14).
- Monitor oxygen saturation continuously. Be alert to values <92% with response depending on patient's baseline and clinical presentation.
- Monitor for nausea and vomiting. Evaluate effects of antiemetics.

NIC Respiratory Monitoring, Airway Management, Aspiration Precautions

Hyperthermia related to overdose of cocaine, hallucinogens, phencyclidine, salicylates, or cyclic antidepressants

Desired outcome: Optimally, within 24-72 hr of intervention, patient becomes normothermic.

> **Note:** With massive overdose, temperature regulation may never be achieved.

- Monitor for hyperthermia: temperature >38.3° C (>101° F), pallor, absence of perspiration, and torso that is warm to the touch. If means are available, provide continuous monitoring of temperature. Otherwise, measure rectal, core, or tympanic temperature hourly and prn.
- Monitor effects of cooling blanket, cooling baths, and ice packs to the axillae and groin.
- Maintain fluid replacement as prescribed. Monitor hydration status and trend of I&O.
- Monitor neurologic status hourly and prn until stabilized.
- Monitor VS continuously or hourly and prn until stabilized.
- Administer and evaluate effects of antipyretic medications.

NIC Fever Treatment; Temperature Regulation; Vital Signs Monitoring; Medication Prescribing

Fluid volume, deficient related to low intake or losses secondary to vomiting or diaphoresis and shock conditions

Desired outcome: Patient remains normovolemic as evidenced by urine output >0.5 ml/kg/hr; moist mucous membranes; balanced I&O; BP within patient's normal range; HR <100 beats/min; stable weight; CVP 2-6 mm Hg; and PAWP 6-12 mm Hg.
- Monitor hydration status. Note signs of continuing dehydration: poor skin turgor, dry mucous membranes, thirst, weight loss >0.5 kg/day, urine specific gravity >1.020, weak pulse with tachycardia, and postural hypotension.
- If the patient has a Swan-Ganz catheter:
  ❑ Monitor systemic and pulmonary vascular resistance as appropriate.
  ❑ Monitor cardiac output as appropriate.
  ❑ Monitor pulmonary capillary/artery wedge pressure and central venous/right atrial pressure.
  ❑ Administer positive inotropic/contractility medications.
- Evaluate the effects of fluid therapy.
- Assess for indicators of electrolyte imbalance, especially the presence of hypokalemia. Be alert to irregular pulse, cardiac dysrhythmias, and serum potassium level <3.5 mEq/L.
- Monitor I&O hourly; assess for output elevated disproportionately to intake, bearing in mind the insensible losses.
- Monitor laboratory values, including serum electrolyte levels and serum and urine osmolality. Note BUN values elevated disproportionately to the serum creatinine (indicator of dehydration rather than renal disease), high urine specific gravity, low urine sodium, and rising Hct and serum protein concentration. Optimal values are the following: serum osmolality 275-300 mOsm/kg; urine osmolality 300-1090 mOsm/kg; BUN 10-20 mg/dl; serum creatinine 0.7-1.5 mg/dl; urine sodium 40-180 mEq/24 hr (diet dependent); Hct 37%-47% (female), or 40%-54% (male); and serum protein 6-8.3 g/dl.
- Maintain fluid intake as prescribed; administer prescribed electrolyte supplements.

NIC Fluid/Electrolyte Management; Fluid Monitoring; Surveillance; Hypovolemia Management

Sensory/perceptual: visual, tactile, auditory, kinesthetic, disturbed related to chemical alterations secondary to ingestion of mind-altering drugs

Desired outcome: Within 48 hr of intervention, patient verbalizes orientation to time, place, and person.
- Establish and maintain a calm, quiet environment to minimize patient's sensory overload.
- Assess patient's orientation to time, place, and person. Reorient as necessary.
- Explain procedures before performing them. Include significant others in orientation process.
- Do not leave patient alone if agitated or confused.
- Administer antianxiety agents as prescribed.
- If patient is hallucinating, intervene in the following ways:
  - ❏ Be reassuring. Explain that hallucinations may be very real to patient but that they are not real, that they are caused by the substance that patient consumed, and that they will go away eventually.
  - ❏ Try to involve family and significant others, because patient may have more trust in them.
  - ❏ Explain that restraints are necessary to prevent harm to patient and others. Reassure patient that restraints will be used only as long as they are needed.
  - ❏ Tell patient that you will check on him or her at frequent intervals (e.g., q5-10min) or that you will stay at patient's side.

▌NIC Delusion Management; Environmental Management; Fall Prevention; Surveillance: Safety

Violence: self-directed (or risk for same) related to mind-altering drugs or depressed state
Desired outcome: Patient, staff, and patient's significant others are free of injury.
- If patient's condition is stable, provide auxiliary staff member, such as orderly or nursing assistant, to watch patient when awake.
- Speak with patient in a quiet and calm voice, using short sentences.
- Establish a therapeutic relationship with patient.
- Encourage patient to take control over his or her own behavior.
- Facilitate support by significant others.
- Limit interventions.
- Administer and evaluate effectiveness of sedation to calm patient.
- Keep all sharp instruments out of patient's room. Follow agency protocol accordingly.
- Develop appropriate behavior expectations and consequences, given the patient's level of cognitive functioning and capacity for self-control.

▌NIC Behavior Management: Self-Harm; Substance Use Treatment: Alcohol Withdrawal; Substance Use Treatment: Overdose, Suicide Prevention

ADDITIONAL NURSING DIAGNOSES

See nursing diagnoses and interventions in the following as appropriate: "Nutritional Support," p. 1; "Mechanical Ventilation," p. 14; "Hemodynamic Monitoring," p. 23; "Prolonged Immobility," p. 61; "Psychosocial Support," p. 68; "Psychosocial Support for the Patient's Family and Significant Others," p. 78; "Acute Respiratory Distress Syndrome," p. 189; "Acute Respiratory Failure," p. 201; "Acute Coronary Syndromes," p. 205; "Heart Failure/Pulmonary Edema," p. 220; "Cardiomyopathy," p. 226; "Dysrhythmias and Conduction Disturbances," p. 231; "Aortic Aneurysm/Dissection," p. 288; "Acute Renal Failure," p. 315; "Renal Replacement Therapies," p. 334; "Status Epilepticus," p. 369; "Hepatic Failure," p. 427; "Acute Pancreatitis," p. 447; "Fluid and Electrolyte Disturbances," p. 538; and "Acid-Base Imbalances," p. 566. In addition, see "Traumatic Brain Injury" for "Impaired Corneal Tissue Integrity," p. 109.

Fluid and Electrolyte Disturbances

The volume and composition of body fluids and electrolytes is affected by hormonal, renal, vascular, and exogenous factors. An understanding the complexity of chemical currents, cellular function, and distribution of water between the cells and vessels provides the information used to facilitate the best patient outcome.

Water is the major constituent of the human body, comprising 55%-72% of body mass. Body water decreases with both age and increasing body fat. The average male adult is approximately 60% water by weight, while the average female adult is 55% water by weight. *Two thirds* of body fluid is within the *intracellular fluid compartment (ICF)*. ICF contains a high concentration of potassium (K^+), magnesium (Mg^+), phosphates (PO_4^-), proteins and sulfates. The *extracellular fluid (ECF) compartment* is composed of *interstitial fluid,* which surrounds the cells and *intravascular fluid,* contained within blood vessels. ECF contains the remaining *one third* of body fluid and has a high concentration of the plasma ions sodium (Na^+), chloride (Cl^-), and bicarbonate (HCO_3^-).

The composition and concentration of ECF is primarily regulated by the concentration of Na^+, which defines the relative relationship of sodium and water. Although ECF is altered and then modified as the body reacts with its surrounding environment, ICF remains relatively stable. Intracellular stability is important for maintaining normal cellular function.

In addition to water, body fluids contain two types of dissolved substances: electrolytes and non-electrolytes. *Electrolytes* are substances which carry an electrical current and can dissociate into ions, which have either a positive or negative charge. They are measured by their capacity to combine (milliequivalents/liter [mEq/L]) or by the molecular weight in milligrams (millimoles/liter [mmol/L]). *Nonelectrolytes* are substances such as glucose and urea that do not dissociate in solution and are measured by weight (milligrams per 100 milliliters, or mg/dl). The body fluid compartments are separated by a semipermeable membrane, which allows movement of dissolved substances/particles between compartments, while maintaining the unique composition of each compartment (Table 10-10).

OSMOLALITY

Osmolality is the number of particles in solution. This concentration of particles determines the relationship of fluid between the ICF and ECF. Normal osmolality is regulated by a wide variety of mechanisms, which include arterial blood pressure, sympathetic stimulation, renal regulation, and hormonal outflow.

$$\text{Osmolality} = 2(Na^+) + \text{Glucose}/18 + \text{BUN}/2.8 \quad \text{Normal 265 to 285 mOsm/L}$$

HORMONAL INFLUENCE

Antidiuretic hormone (ADH) or vasopressin is a hormone released by the posterior pituitary in response to a reduction in intravascular volume (hypovolemia) or an increase in extracellular osmolality. It acts on the kidney at both the glomerulus and the tubules to conserve water by increasing urine concentration. The hormone regulates the electrolyte and fluid balance to keep serum in "perfect" concentration (osmolality). Thirst is stimulated by hypovolemia and increased osmolality.

Aldosterone is another regulator of fluid volume. It is released by the adrenal cortex in response to an increased plasma renin level, acts on the kidney to conserve sodium (along with water), and increases potassium and hydrogen excretion.

Atrial natriuretic peptide (ANP) is a hormone released by the cardiac atria in response to increased atrial pressure (e.g., acute volume expansion). ANP reduces blood pressure and vascular volume by increasing excretion of sodium and water by the kidneys, decreasing release of aldosterone and ADH, and by direct vasodilation.

FLUID DISTURBANCES

Fluid changes affect the volume status, regulation, and the composition of body fluids. Fluid loss or gain changes the concentration of particles in fluid compartments.

HYPOVOLEMIA

Pathophysiology

Extracellar fluid (ECF) volume depletion or *hypovolemia* may be caused by abnormal skin losses, gastrointestinal losses, polyuria/diuresis, bleeding, decreased intake, and movement of fluid into a third space (e.g., pleura, peritoneum, interstitium). Depending on the type of fluid lost or "third-spaced,"

T A B L E 10 - 10   Primary Constituents of Body Water Compartments*

Element	Intravascular	Interstitial	Intracellular (skeletal muscle cell)
Na^+	142 mEq/L	145 mEq/L	12 mEq/L
Cl^-	104 mEq/L	117 mEq/L	4 mEq/L
HCO_3^-	24 mEq/L	27 mEq/L	12 mEq/L
K^+	4.5 mEq/L	4.5 mEq/L	150 mEq/L
HPO_4^-	2 mEq/L	2 mEq/L	40 mEq/L

*This is a partial list. Other constituents include calcium (Ca^{++}), magnesium (Mg^{++}), and proteins.
Cl^-, Chloride; HCO_3^-, bicarbonate; HPO_4^-, phosphate; K^+, potassium; Na^+, sodium.

hypovolemia may be accompanied by acid-base, osmolar, or electrolyte imbalances. Severe ECF volume depletion can lead to *hypovolemic shock* and cellular dehydration, which causes alterations in electric potentials (the ability to conduct impulse) throughout the body.

Compensatory mechanisms in hypovolemia include increased sympathetic nervous system stimulation: increased HR, increased force of cardiac contraction (positive inotropic effect), vasoconstriction to maintain perfusion to oxygen-dependent organs (i.e., heart, lungs, brain), increased thirst, and increased release of aldosterone and ADH (vasopressin). Reduced perfusion to high-flow, low oxygen–consuming organs (i.e., kidney, mesenteric bed, skeletal muscles) may lead to acute renal failure, ischemic bowel, and skeletal muscle cell rupture.

Hypovolemic shock develops when the intravascular volume decreases to the point where compensatory mechanisms can no longer maintain the perfusion needed for normal, aerobic cellular function. Without normal levels of oxygen, cellular metabolism becomes anaerobic, resulting in acidosis, cardiac depression, intravascular coagulation, increased capillary permeability, and release of toxins. If shock is not adequately treated, it may become irreversible, leading to death.

Assessment
History and risk factors
Abnormal GI losses: Vomiting, nasogastric (NG) suctioning, diarrhea, intestinal drainage.
Abnormal skin losses: Excessive diaphoresis secondary to fever or exercise; burns.
Abnormal renal losses: Diuretic therapy, polyuria/osmotic diuresis (seen with diabetic ketoacidosis [DKA], hyperglycemic hyperosmolar nonketotic syndrome [HHNS], nephrotoxicity, and rhabdomyolysis), diabetes insipidus, acute renal failure (diuretic phase), adrenal insufficiency.
Third spacing or plasma-to-interstitial fluid shift: Peritonitis, intestinal obstruction, burns, ascites, severe sepsis.
Hemorrhage: Major trauma, GI bleeding, obstetric complications, postoperative bleeding, high dosage of anticoagulants or antiplatelet medications.
Altered intake: Coma, fluid deprivation.
Clinical presentation: Dizziness, weakness, fatigue, syncope, anorexia, nausea, vomiting, thirst, confusion, constipation, possibly chest and abdominal pain, occasionally strokelike symptoms.
Physical assessment: Decreased BP, especially when standing (orthostatic hypotension); increased HR; decreased urine output; poor skin turgor; dry, furrowed tongue; dry mucous membranes; sunken eyeballs; flat neck veins; increased temperature; possibly pallor (if hemorrhage occurred), acute weight loss (Table 10-11) unless third spacing is occurring.
Hemodynamic measurements: Tachycardia, narrowed pulse pressure, hypotension, urine output <0.5 ml/kg/hr, low CVP (<2 mm Hg), low PAWP (<3 mm Hg).

Note: Early hypovolemic shock is often missed. As the heart rate increases and arteries constrict, BP may be compensated and remain normal or slightly elevated. Widening of pulse pressure (systolic BP–diastolic BP = pulse pressure) is a more accurate tool in early shock. A pulse pressure of 40 mm Hg may indicate shock. Cardiac output and mean arterial pressure may be compensated by HR and vasoconstriction consecutively.

Note: As shock progresses, heart rate decreases, ventricular compliance and filling time decreases, resulting in ↓CVP, ↓ PAP. Volume status may be underestimated.

T A B L E 10 - 11   Weight Loss As an Indicator of ECF Deficit in the Adult

Acute weight loss	Severity of deficit
2%-5%	Mild
5%-10%	Moderate
10%-15%	Severe
15%-20%	Fatal

ECF, Extracellular fluid.

Diagnostic tests
BUN values: May be elevated because of dehydration, decreased renal perfusion, or decreased renal function. BUN/creatinine ratio of >20:1 suggests hypovolemia.
Hematocrit (Hct) levels: Elevated with dehydration; decreased with bleeding. If patient has lost fluid and blood, the amount of bleeding may be underestimated as a result of hemoconcentration.
Serum electrolyte levels: Variable, depending on type of fluid lost. Hypokalemia often occurs with abnormal GI or renal losses. Hyperkalemia occurs with adrenal insufficiency. Hypernatremia may be seen with increased insensible or sweat losses and diabetes insipidus. Hyponatremia occurs in most types of hypovolemia because of increased thirst and ADH release, which lead to increased water intake and retention, thus diluting the serum sodium. (See individual electrolyte imbalances, p. 545.)
Serum total CO_2 (CO_2 content): Decreased with metabolic acidosis and increased with metabolic alkalosis (see ABG values).
ABG values: Metabolic acidosis (pH <7.35 and HCO_3^- <22 mEq/L) may occur with lower GI losses, shock, or diabetic ketoacidosis. Metabolic alkalosis (pH >7.45 and HCO_3^- >26 mEq/L) may occur with upper GI losses and diuretic therapy.
Urine specific gravity: Increased because of kidneys' attempt to conserve water; may be fixed at approximately 1.010 in the presence of renal disease.
Urine sodium: Demonstrates kidneys' ability to conserve sodium in response to an increased aldosterone level. In the absence of renal disease, osmotic diuresis, or diuretic therapy, value should be <20 mEq/L.
Serum osmolality: Variable, depending on the type of fluid lost and the body's ability to compensate with thirst and ADH.
Urine osmolality: Indicates kidneys' ability to produce concentrated urine. Level should be increased >450 mOsm/kg as the kidneys attempt to conserve water. Comparing urine osmolality to serum osmolality assists in the diagnosis of renal insufficiency. The role of urine production and concentration is to keep serum osmolality "perfect." If serum is concentrated, urine should be more concentrated.

Collaborative management
Restoration of normal fluid volume and correction of acid-base and electrolyte disturbances: The type of fluid replacement depends on the type of fluid lost and the severity of the deficit, and on serum electrolytes, serum osmolality, and acid-base status. IV fluids are provided to expand intravascular volume or to correct an underlying imbalance in fluids or electrolytes. Fluid should be infused at a rate resulting in a positive fluid balance (e.g., 50-100 ml *in excess* of the sum of all hourly losses).
Isotonic solutions: Expand ECF only; do not enter ICF. Appropriate for rapid volume replacement, especially in shock. Example: normal saline (0.9%).
Hypotonic saline solutions: Expand the ECF and provide some free water to the cells. Used in the management of the patient who is both volume-depleted and hyperosmolar (e.g., in cases of hypernatremia or hyperglycemia). Example: 0.45% saline (*half-normal saline*).
Dextrose and water: Provides free water only and will be distributed evenly through both ICF and ECF; used to treat water deficit. Example: D_5W (*5% dextrose in water*).
Mixed isotonic saline/electrolyte solutions: Provide additional electrolytes (e.g., potassium and calcium) and a buffer (e.g., lactate or acetate). Example: *lactated Ringer's solution (Ringer's lactate)*: isotonic solution containing a small amount of K^+ and lactate which metabolizes to bicarbonate in the liver to assist blood buffering.
Blood and albumin: Expand only the intravascular portion of the ECF. Both packed red blood cells and fresh-frozen plasma expand the intravascular volume.
Dextran or hetastarch, hypertonic saline, Hextend: Synthetic colloidal solutions used to expand the intravascular volume.
Restoration of tissue perfusion (hypovolemic shock):
Rapid Volume Replacement With Crystalloids: Fluids may be given rapidly as long as cardiac filling pressures and BP remain low. Overaggressive fluid resuscitation in uncontrolled hemorrhage can increase the risk of secondary hemorrhage as the intravascular hydrostatic pressure increases.
Volume Replacement With Colloids: Use of volume replacement with colloids to prevent the development of pulmonary edema secondary to rapid volume replacement remains controversial. Solutions include albumin and synthetics such as hetastarch.
Blood: Administered only if necessary to maintain oxygen-carrying capacity. Hct should not be raised >35%.
Vasopressors: Used to reduce the size of blood vessels while volume infusions continue to increase blood pressure. Effective for false hypovolemia induced by vasogenic (septic, anaphylactic, neurogenic) shock to control severe vasodilation.

Treatment of underlying cause.

Nursing diagnoses and interventions

Fluid volume deficit related to abnormal loss of body fluids; reduced intake, capillary leak

Desired outcome: Within 24 hr of starting fluid therapy, patient becomes normovolemic as evidenced by urine output ≥0.5 ml/kg/hr; specific gravity 1.010-1.030; stable weight; no clinical evidence of hypovolemia (e.g., furrowed tongue); BP within patient's normal range; HR and pulse pressure normalized, CVP 2-6 mm Hg; PAP 20-30/8-15 mm Hg; CO 4-7 L/min; MAP 70-105 mm Hg; HR 60-100 beats/min; and SVR 900-1200 dynes/sec/cm^{-5}.

- Monitor I&O hourly. During initial therapy, intake should exceed output. Consult physician for urine output <0.5 ml/kg/hr for 2 consecutive hours. Measure urine specific gravity q4h as available. Normal range is 1.010-1.030. Expect it to decrease with therapy.
- Monitor VS and hemodynamic pressures for continued hypovolemia. Be alert to decreased BP, CVP, PAP, CO, and MAP and to increased HR and SVR.
- Place hypotensive patients in supine position with the legs elevated to 45 degrees to increase venous return. Avoid Trendelenburg position: causes abdominal organs to lean on the diaphragm, thereby impairing ventilation.
- Weigh patient daily. *Daily weight measurements are the single most important indicator of fluid status, because acute weight changes usually indicate fluid changes.* A decrease in daily weight of 1 kg is equal to the loss of 1 L of fluid. The adult who is not eating or receiving enteral or parenteral nutrition may lose 0.25 kg of nonfluid weight daily as body tissues are used for glucose production. Weigh patient at the same time of day (preferably before breakfast) on a balanced scale, with patient wearing approximately the same clothing. Document type of scale used (i.e., standing, bed, chair).
- Administer PO and IV fluids as prescribed. Ensure adequate intake, especially in older adults, a population at higher risk for volume depletion. Give water with enteral feedings and supplements. Monitor for signs of fluid overload or too-rapid fluid administration: crackles (rales), decreased oxygen saturation (pulse oximetry/SpO$_2$), SOB, tachypnea, tachycardia, increased CVP, increased PA pressures, neck vein distention, and edema.
- Ensure a patent IV access and availability of blood products if needed.
- Monitor patient for hidden fluid losses. Measure/record abdominal girth or limb size if indicated.
- Monitor for signs of abdominal compartment syndrome: an acute increase in ventilator pressures and a decrease in SpO$_2$.
- Monitor for signs of bleeding: decreased Hct, Hgb, tachycardia. Remember that Hct, serum Na$^+$, and BUN may decrease in dehydrated patients as rehydration progresses.
- Monitor for hypocalcemia: may develop in rapidly transfused patients due to the citrate used in banked blood (citrate binds calcium, making it unavailable for cellular uptake). Sudden symptoms may include refractory hypotension (see p. 554). Calcium chloride or gluconate may be prescribed.

You may also wish to refer to the following interventions from the Nursing Interventions Classification (NIC):

NIC Fluid Monitoring; Hypovolemia Management; Fluid Resuscitation; Intravenous (IV) Therapy; Invasive Hemodynamic Monitoring; Shock Management: Volume

Altered tissue perfusion: cerebral, renal, and peripheral, related to hypovolemia

Desired outcome: Within 12 hr after initiation of volume resuscitation, patient has adequate perfusion as evidenced by alertness; warm and dry skin; BP within patient's normal range; HR ≤100 beats/min; urinary output ≥0.5 ml/kg/hr; and capillary refill <2 sec.

- Monitor for signs of decreased cerebral perfusion: vertigo, syncope, confusion, restlessness, anxiety, agitation, excitability, weakness, nausea, and cool and clammy skin. Consult physician for worsening symptoms.
- Protect patients who are at high risk for falling: those who are confused, dizzy, or weak. Keep side rails up and bed in lowest position with wheels locked. Assist with ambulation. Raise patient to sitting or standing positions slowly. Monitor for orthostatic hypotension: decreased BP, increased HR, dizziness, and diaphoresis. If symptoms occur, return patient to supine position.
- To avoid unnecessary vasodilation, treat fevers promptly.
- Cover patient with a light blanket to maintain body temperature.
- Palpate peripheral pulses bilaterally in arms and legs (radial, brachial, dorsalis pedis, posterior tibial). Use a Doppler ultrasonic device if unable to palpate pulses. Rate pulses (0-4+ scale). Consult physician for weak/absent pulses.

Note: Abnormal pulses also may be caused by a local vascular disorder.

- Consult physician for urinary output <0.5 ml/kg/hr for 2 consecutive hours.

NIC Neurologic Monitoring; Circulatory Care

Additional Nursing Diagnoses
For additional nursing diagnoses, see specific medical disorder, electrolyte imbalance, or acid-base disturbance.

HYPERVOLEMIA

Pathophysiology
Hypervolemia is a state of higher-than-normal intravascular volume that occurs in four situations: (1) excessive retention of sodium and water caused by a chronic renal stimulus to conserve sodium and water; (2) abnormal renal functioning causing reduced excretion of sodium and water; (3) excessive administration of IV fluids; (4) interstitial-to-plasma fluid shifting. Hypervolemia may lead to heart failure and pulmonary edema, especially in the patient with cardiovascular dysfunction.

Assessment
History and risk factors
Retention of sodium and water: Heart failure, hepatic failure, nephrotic syndrome, excessive administration of glucocorticosteroids, syndrome of inappropriate antidiuretic hormone (SIADH).
Abnormal renal function: Acute or chronic renal failure with oliguria or anuria.
Excessive administration of IV fluids.
Interstitial-to-plasma fluid shifting: Remobilization of fluid after treatment of burns, excessive administration of hypertonic solutions (i.e., mannitol, hypertonic saline) or colloid oncotic solutions (i.e., albumin).
Clinical presentation: SOB, orthopnea, possible peripheral edema.
Physical assessment: Edema, weight gain, increased BP (decreased BP as the heart fails), bounding pulses, ascites, crackles, rhonchi, wheezes, distended neck veins, moist skin, tachycardia, gallop rhythm, tachypnea, decreased oxygen saturation.
Hemodynamic measurements: Increased CVP, PAP, PAWP. MAP is increased unless heart failure is present.

Diagnostic tests
Laboratory findings are variable and usually nonspecific.
Hct levels: Decreased because of hemodilution by excess fluids in the vasculature.
BUN levels: Decreased in pure hypervolemia. Increased with renal failure (nitrogenous waste products are unable to be excreted).
ABG values: May reveal hypoxemia (decreased PaO_2) and alkalosis (decreased $PaCO_2$) if early pulmonary edema is present, due to tachypnea. Respiratory acidosis (increased $PaCO_2$) may be present in severe pulmonary edema. Diffusion of oxygen is difficult across the alveolar capillary membrane with increased interstitial volume load.
Serum sodium and serum osmolality: Decreased if hypervolemia is from water retention (i.e., chronic renal failure.)
Urinary sodium: Elevated if the kidney is excreting excess sodium. Sodium excretion prompts fluid excretion. Urinary sodium is not elevated with secondary hyperaldosteronism (e.g., heart failure, cirrhosis, nephrotic syndrome) because hypervolemia occurs secondary to a chronic renal stimulus (aldosterone increases resorption of Na^+).
Urine specific gravity: Decreased if the kidney is excreting excess volume. May be fixed at 1.010 in acute renal failure.
Chest x-ray: May reveal signs of pulmonary vascular congestion.

Collaborative management
The goal of therapy is to treat the cause and return ECF to normal.
Restriction of sodium and water: Oral, enteral, or parenteral. Table 10-12 lists foods high in sodium.
Diuretics: May be given IV or PO. Loop diuretics (i.e., furosemide) are indicated for severe hypervolemia or heart failure. Diuresis may prompt profound electrolyte loss.
Dialysis or continuous renal replacement therapy (CRRT): In renal failure or life-threatening fluid overload (see "Renal Replacement Therapies," p. 334).

Note: Also see specific discussions under "Burns," p. 159; "Acute Lung Injury and Respiratory Distress Syndrome," p. 189; and "Acute Renal Failure," p. 315.

T A B L E 10 - 12 **Foods High in Sodium**	
Bouillon	Olives
Celery	Pickles
Cheeses	Preserved meat
Dried fruits	Salad dressings and prepared sauces
Frozen, canned, or packaged foods	Sauerkraut
Monosodium glutamate (MSG)	Snack foods (e.g., crackers, chips, pretzels)
Mustard	Soy sauce

Nursing diagnoses and interventions

Fluid volume excess related to excessive fluid intake; excessive sodium intake; compromised regulatory mechanism

Desired outcome: Within 24 hr of starting treatment, patient is normovolemic as evidenced by absence of edema; BP within patient's normal range; HR 60-100 beats/min; CVP 2-6 mm Hg; PAP 20-30/8-15 mm Hg; MAP 70-105 mm Hg; and CO 4-7 L/min.

- Monitor I&O hourly. With the exception of oliguric renal failure, urine output should be $\geq$0.5 ml/kg/hr. Measure urine specific gravity or urine osmolality q4h. If patient is receiving diuretic therapy, specific gravity should be <1.010-1.020 or <500 mOsm/L.
- Monitor and manage edema (pretibial, sacral, periorbital); rate on a 0-4+ scale.
- Weigh patient daily. *Daily weight measurements are the single most important indicator of fluid status.*
- Limit oral, enteral, and parenteral sodium intake as prescribed. Be aware that medications may contain sodium (e.g., penicillins, bicarbonate). See Table 10-12 for some foods high in sodium.
- Limit fluids as prescribed. Offer a portion of allotted fluids as ice chips to minimize patient's thirst. Teach patient and significant others the importance of fluid restriction and how to measure fluid volume.
- Provide oral hygiene at frequent intervals to keep oral mucous membrane moist and intact.
- Document response to diuretic therapy (e.g., increased urine output, decreased CVP/PAP, decreased adventitious breath sounds, decreased edema). Many diuretics (e.g., furosemide, thiazides) cause hypokalemia. Observe for indicators of hypokalemia: muscle weakness, dysrhythmias (especially PVCs and ECG changes such as flattened T wave, presence of U waves). See "Hypokalemia," p. 549. Potassium-sparing diuretics (e.g., spironolactone, triamterene) may cause hyperkalemia: signs include weakness, ECG changes (e.g., peaked T wave, prolonged PR interval, widened QRS complex). See "Hyperkalemia," p. 552. Consult physician for significant findings.
- Observe for indicators of overcorrection and dangerous volume depletion: vertigo, weakness, syncope, thirst, confusion, poor skin turgor, flat neck veins, and acute weight loss.
- Monitor VS and hemodynamic parameters for volume depletion occurring with therapy: decreased BP, CVP, PAP, MAP, and CO; increased HR. Consult physician for significant changes or findings.
- Monitor appropriate laboratory tests (e.g., BUN and creatinine in renal failure). Consult physician for abnormal trends.

NIC Fluid Monitoring; Hypervolemia Management; Fluid/Electrolyte Management; Invasive Hemodynamic Monitoring; Hemodialysis Therapy

Impaired gas exchange (or risk for same) related to alveolar-capillary membrane changes secondary to pulmonary vascular congestion occurring with ECF expansion

Desired outcomes: Within 12 hr of initiating treatment, patient has adequate gas exchange as evidenced by RR $\leq$20 breaths/min with normal depth and pattern (eupnea); HR $\leq$100 beats/min; Pao_2 $\geq$80 mm Hg; pH 7.35-7.45; $Paco_2$ 35-45 mm Hg; and Spo_2 $\geq$92%. Patient does not exhibit crackles, gallops, or other clinical indicators of pulmonary edema. PAP is $\leq$30/15 mm Hg and PAWP is $\leq$12 mm Hg.

- Monitor patient for signs of acute pulmonary edema, a potentially life-threatening complication of hypervolemia: air hunger, decreased pulse oximetry, anxiety, cough with production of frothy sputum, crackles, rhonchi, tachypnea, increasing ventilator pressures, tachycardia, gallop rhythm, and elevation of PAP and PAWP. Administer diuretics and other medications to reduce venous return to the heart as prescribed.

- Monitor ABG values for hypoxemia and respiratory alkalosis. Monitor oxygen saturation. Administer oxygen to maintain $SpO_2 \geq 92\%$. Increased oxygen requirements may signal increased pulmonary vascular congestion.
- Keep patient in semi-Fowler's position or position of comfort to minimize dyspnea.

NIC Respiratory Monitoring

Impaired skin and tissue integrity (or risk for same) related to edema secondary to fluid volume excess

Desired outcome: Patient's skin and tissue remain intact.

- Assess and document circulation to extremities at least each shift. Note color, temperature, capillary refill, and peripheral pulses. Consult physician if capillary refill is delayed or if pulses are diminished or absent.
- Turn and reposition patient at least q2h to minimize tissue pressure.
- Check tissue areas at risk with each position change (e.g., heels, sacrum, areas over bony prominences).
- Use pressure-relief mattress as indicated.
- Support arms and hands on pillows and elevate legs to decrease dependent edema. Do not elevate legs in the presence of pulmonary congestion.
- Treat pressure ulcers per unit protocol. Consult physician if sores, ulcers, or areas of tissue breakdown are present; especially with patients who are at high risk for infection (i.e., those with diabetes mellitus or renal failure or who are immunosuppressed).
- Consult a skin/wound care nurse specialist for advanced tissue breakdown or any alteration in tissue integrity in high-risk patients.

NIC Circulatory Care; Skin Surveillance

ELECTROLYTE DISTURBANCES

SODIUM IMBALANCE (NORMAL SERUM LEVEL NA⁺: 137-147 mEq/L)

Sodium is the main cation ($^+$ or positive ion) of ECF and is the major determinant of ECF osmolality and fluid status. Under normal conditions *ECF osmolality is estimated by doubling the serum sodium value.* Sodium imbalances are associated with parallel changes in osmolality. *As serum osmolality decreases,* the osmotic gradient allows water to move into cells, creating high pressures in the abdominal, cerebral, and musculoskeletal compartments. *As serum osmolality increases,* the osmotic gradient pulls water out of cells, since very little sodium is intracellular. This alters the depolarization gradient and causes intracellular dehydration.

Sodium is regulated mainly by the kidneys, and controlled by hormones from the posterior pituitary and adrenal cortex. Renal tubules tightly regulate Na^+ excretion and resorption with, or without, fluid. ***ADH*** *prompts the kidneys to conserve* ***water***. The adrenal cortical hormone, aldosterone, is another important regulator of sodium and ECF volume. *Release of* ***aldosterone*** *causes the kidneys to conserve* ***sodium and water*** to increase ECF volume. Because changes in serum sodium levels often reflect changes in water balance, gains or losses of total body sodium may not be accurately reflected by the serum sodium level.

Sodium (Na^+) and water are both filtered by the kidney, but their regulation is independent. If serum Na^+ concentration decreases (*hyponatremia*), the kidneys respond by excreting water. If serum sodium concentration increases (*hypernatremia*), serum osmolality increases, stimulating the thirst center and causing an increased release of ADH by the posterior pituitary gland.

HYPONATREMIA (SERUM SODIUM <135 mEq/L)

Pathophysiology

Hyponatremia occurs from a net gain of water or a loss of sodium-rich fluids that have been replaced by water (net gain fluid > net gain Na^+). The most common cause of hyponatremia is water gain from renal dysfunction. The kidneys should increase output if intake increases. As serum osmolality decreases, fluid shifts into cells, causing swelling and sometimes compartment syndromes.

There are three types of hyponatremia: *hypovolemic, hypervolemic,* and *euvolemic.* Dilutional states are the most frequent cause of hyponatremia in the critically ill. Clinical indicators and treatments depend on the cause of hyponatremia and whether or not it is associated with normal, decreased, or increased ECF volume. For more information, see "Burns," p. 159; "Heart Failure," p. 220; "Acute Renal Failure," p. 315; and "Syndrome of Inappropriate Antidiuretic Hormone," p. 404.

Assessment
History and risk factors
Decreased ECF volume
- GI losses: diarrhea, vomiting, fistulas, NG suction.
- Renal losses: diuretics, salt-wasting kidney disease, and adrenal insufficiency.
- Skin losses: burns, wound drainage, excessive diaphoresis.

Normal/increased ECF volume
- Hypothyroidism or syndrome of inappropriate antidiuretic hormone (SIADH).
- Edematous states: heart failure, cirrhosis, and nephrotic syndrome.
- Vigorous administration of hypotonic IV fluids or very dilute enteral feedings.
- Oliguric renal failure.
- Primary polydipsia.
- Any patient with impaired ability to excrete free water (e.g., those being treated with thiazide diuretics) is at risk for hyponatremia if given hypotonic fluids.

Note: Hyperlipidemia, hyperproteinemia, and hyperglycemia may cause a pseudohyponatremia. Pseudohyponatremia reduces the Na^+ content, but also causes a reduction in volume. Actual osmolality may be normal or high. If blood glucose, lipids, or proteins are elevated, an osmolality calculation or laboratory determination should be performed. Hyperlipidemia and hyperproteinemia reduce the percentage of plasma water. With hyperglycemia, the osmotic action of elevated glucose causes water to shift out of the cells into the ECF, thus diluting the serum sodium. For every 100 mg/dl that glucose is elevated, sodium is diluted by 1.6 mEq/L. The sodium-to-water ratio of plasma is unchanged, but the amount of sodium in the plasma is reduced.

Clinical presentation: Neurologic symptoms usually do not occur until the serum sodium level has decreased to 120-125 mEq/L, and are more likely to begin with a sudden decrease than a gradual decrease. Seizures, coma, and permanent neurologic damage may occur when the plasma sodium level is <115 mEq/L.
Hyponatremia with decreased ECF volume: Irritability, apprehension, dizziness, personality changes, poor skin turgor, postural hypotension, dry mucous membranes, cold and clammy skin, tremors, seizures, coma.
Hyponatremia with normal or increased ECF volume: Headache, lassitude, apathy, confusion, weakness, edema, weight gain, elevated BP, hyperreflexia, muscle spasms, convulsions, coma.
Hemodynamic measurements
Decreased ECF volume: Evidence of hypovolemia: decreased CVP, PAP, CO, MAP; increased SVR.
Increased ECF volume: Evidence of hypervolemia: increased CVP, PAP, MAP.

Diagnostic tests
Serum sodium: Will be <135 mEq/L.
Serum osmolality: Decreased, except in cases of pseudohyponatremia.
Urine specific osmolality: Usually >100 mOsm/kg H_2O, but less than the plasma level. In SIADH, the urine will be inappropriately concentrated (more concentrated than expected).
Urine sodium: Decreased (usually <20 mEq/L) except in SIADH, salt-wasting kidney disease, adrenal insufficiency, or excessive diuretic therapy.

Collaborative management
The goals of therapy are to raise the serum sodium at a safe rate, correct any volume abnormality, and treat the underlying cause. The presence of acute, symptomatic hyponatremia requires more aggressive treatment than chronic, asymptomatic hyponatremia.

Caution: Overly rapid correction of chronic hyponatremia may result in permanent neurologic damage.

Hyponatremia with reduced ECF volume
Replacement of sodium and fluid losses: Adequate replacement of fluid volume is essential to *turn off* the physiologic stimulus to ADH release and enable the kidneys to restore the balance between sodium and water.
Replacement of other electrolyte losses: For example, potassium, bicarbonate.

IV hypertonic saline (3% NaCl): Used if serum sodium is dangerously low or the patient has extreme symptoms. The therapeutic goal is to slowly shrink the cerebral cells. The goal is to give enough 3% NaCl to correct symptoms—*not* to return the sodium level to normal.
- *Increase serum Na⁺ 0.5 to 1 mmol/L/hr* if patient is not symptomatic or has mild symptoms
- *Increase serum Na⁺ 3-6 mmol/L/hr* if patient is convulsing.

Hyponatremia with expanded ECF volume
Removal or treatment of underlying cause.
Diuretics.
Water restriction: Restricting fluid intake to 1000 ml/day will establish negative water balance and increase serum sodium levels in most adults.

> **Note:** See "Syndrome of Inappropriate Antidiuretic Hormone," p. 404, for specific treatment.

Nursing diagnoses and interventions
Fluid volume deficit related to active fluid loss; excessive intake of hypotonic solutions; compromised regulatory mechanisms
Desired outcome: Within 24 hr of initiating treatment, patient becomes normovolemic as evidenced by HR 60-100 beats/min; RR 12-20 breaths/min; BP within patient's normal range; CVP 2-6 mm Hg; and PAP 20-30/8-15 mm Hg.
- If patient is receiving hypertonic saline, assess carefully for signs of intravascular fluid overload: tachypnea, tachycardia, acute SOB, crackles (rales), rhonchi, increased CVP and PAP, gallop rhythm, and increased BP.
- For other interventions, see "Hypovolemia," p. 542, for "Fluid Volume Deficit."

NIC Fluid Monitoring; Electrolyte Management: Hyponatremia; Fluid/Electrolyte Management; Intravenous (IV) Therapy; Invasive Hemodynamic Monitoring

Altered protection related to neurosensory alterations secondary to sodium level <120-125 mEq/L
Desired outcomes: Within 48 hr of treatment, patient verbalizes orientation to time, place, and person and does not exhibit signs of physical injury caused by altered sensorium. Serum sodium level increases to >125 mEq/L in the first 48 hr after treatment.
- Assess and document LOC, orientation, and neurologic status with each VS check. Reorient patient as necessary. Consult physician for significant changes.
- Inform patient and significant others that altered sensorium is temporary and will improve with treatment.
- Keep side rails up and bed in lowest position with wheels locked.
- Use reality therapy such as clocks, calendars, and familiar objects; keep these items at the bedside within patient's visual field.

If seizures are expected, pad side rails and keep an appropriate-size airway at the bedside.
- Monitor serum sodium levels closely. Permanent neurologic damage may occur with untreated, severely symptomatic hyponatremia secondary to cerebral edema.

> **Caution:** Overly aggressive or inappropriate treatment of hyponatremia can also cause permanent neurologic damage secondary to osmotic demyelination syndrome.

- Osmotic demyelination is poorly understood but should always be suspected after hypertonic resuscitation when patients display bilateral neurologic deficits, flaccidity, and quadriparesis. Initially, sodium levels should not increase at a level >0.5-1.0 mEq/L/hr in patients being treated for symptomatic hyponatremia with hypertonic NaCl. After an initial 6-8 mEq/L increase in the serum sodium level, the rate of increase should not be >0.5 mEq/L/hr. Levels should not increase at an average rate of >0.5 mEq/L/hr in patients without symptoms. The total increase in the first 24 hr of treatment should not exceed 12 mEq/L.

NIC Neurologic Monitoring; Electrolyte Management: Hyponatremia; Seizure Precautions

HYPERNATREMIA (SERUM SODIUM LEVEL >145 mEq/L)
Pathophysiology
Hypernatremia may occur with either free water loss or sodium gain. Hypernatremia always causes hypertonicity because sodium is the major determinant of ECF osmolality. Hypertonicity causes a shift of water out of the cells, which leads to intracellular dehydration. Hypernatremia usually results from volume depletion (hypovolemia) and is rarely caused by increased sodium intake.

Assessment
History and risk factors
Water (volume) loss: Increased diaphoresis, respiratory infection, mechanical ventilation, diabetes insipidus, osmotic diuresis (e.g., hyperglycemia), osmotic diarrhea.
Sodium gain: IV administration of hypertonic saline or sodium bicarbonate, increased oral intake, primary aldosteronism, drugs such as sodium polystyrene sulfonate (Kayexalate).
Clinical presentation: Intense thirst, fatigue, restlessness, agitation, coma. Symptoms of hypernatremia occur only in individuals who do not have access to water or who have an altered thirst mechanism (e.g., infants, older adults, those who are comatose).

Note: Symptoms are most likely to develop with a sudden increase in plasma sodium. After 24 hr, brain cells adjust to ECF hypertonicity by increasing intracellular osmolality. The mechanism of action is unclear, but the increased osmolality helps to rehydrate the cells. Individuals with chronic hypernatremia exhibit few symptoms. This adaptive mechanism plays a key role in treatment of hypernatremia. *Overly aggressive water administration may cause rapid movement of water into the cells, which can result in dangerous cerebral edema due to a too-rapid reduction of sodium.*

Physical assessment: Low-grade fever, flushed skin, peripheral and pulmonary edema (sodium gain); postural hypotension (water loss)—usually mild.
Hemodynamic measurement: Variable.
Sodium excess: Increased CVP and PAP.
Water loss: Decreased CVP and PAP, although these changes may be minimized by the extracellular shift of fluid that occurs with hypernatremia.

Diagnostic tests
Serum sodium: Will be >145 mEq/L.
Serum osmolality: Increased because of elevated serum sodium.
Urine specific gravity: Increased because of kidneys' attempt to retain water; will be lower than expected in diabetes insipidus and too dilute in early osmotic diuresis (e.g., hyperglycemia).

Collaborative management
IV or PO water replacement: Used for water loss. If sodium is >160 mEq/L, IV D_5W or hypotonic (0.45%) saline is given to replace pure water deficit. (See "Diabetes Insipidus," p. 400.)
Diuretics and PO or IV water replacement: Used for sodium gain.

Note: Hypernatremia is corrected slowly, over approximately 2 days, to avoid too great a shift of water into brain cells.

Nursing diagnoses and interventions
Protection, ineffective related to neurosensory alterations secondary to primary hypernatremia or cerebral edema occurring with too-rapid correction of hypernatremia
Desired outcomes: Within 48 hr after treatment, patient verbalizes orientation to time, place, and person and does not exhibit evidence of injury caused by altered sensorium or seizures. Serum sodium level is ≤145 mEq/L.
- Monitor serial serum sodium levels (sodium should not decrease at a rate greater than 0.5-1.0 mEq/L/hr); consult physician for rapid decreases. *Cerebral edema may occur if hypernatremia is corrected too rapidly.*
- Assess patient for signs of cerebral edema: lethargy, headache, nausea, vomiting, increased BP, widening pulse pressure, decreased HR, altered sensorium, and seizures.
- Assess and document LOC, orientation, and neurologic status with each VS check. Reorient patient as necessary. Consult physician for deterioration.
- Inform patient and significant others that altered sensorium is temporary and will improve with treatment.
- Keep side rails up and bed in lowest position with wheels locked.
- Use reality therapy such as clocks, calendars, and familiar objects; keep these items at the bedside within patient's visual field.
If seizures are anticipated, pad side rails and keep an appropriate-size airway at the bedside.
- Provide comfort measures to decrease thirst.

▌NIC Neurologic Monitoring; Electrolyte Management: Hypernatremia; Seizure Precautions; Surveillance: Safety

Additional Nursing Diagnoses
See "Hypovolemia" for "Fluid Volume Deficit," p. 542; and "Hypervolemia" for "Fluid Volume Excess," p. 544.

POTASSIUM IMBALANCE (NORMAL SERUM K⁺ LEVEL: (3.5-5 mEq/dl)

Potassium is the primary intracellular cation ($^+$ or positive ion), with normal levels inside cells of 150 mEq/dL. Of total potassium. 98% is inside the cell and markedly affects cell metabolism. Abnormal serum K^+ levels may adversely affect neuromuscular and cardiac function, because it affects resting membrane potential and conduction velocity of nerve and cardiac cells. A relatively small amount of potassium is present in ECF, and concentrations are maintained within a narrow range. Potassium is constantly moving into and out of the cell. Distribution of potassium between ECF and ICF is maintained by the sodium-potassium pump located in the membrane of all body cells and is affected by ECF pH, glucose and protein metabolism, insulin levels, and stimulation of β_2-adrenergic receptors. Acute changes in serum pH are accompanied by reciprocal changes in serum potassium concentration as the exchange of K^+ and H^+ takes place.

The body gains potassium through foods (primarily meats, fruits, and vegetables) and medications. ECF also gains potassium from breakdown or death of cells, when a large amount of intracellular K^+ is released from the cell contents. Potassium is eliminated from the body through the kidneys, the GI tract, and the skin. The potassium level may decrease in the serum (ECF) when K^+ shifts inside the cells. The serum potassium level increases when renal function decreases, when circulation is reduced to a large amount of cells causing cell death, with cellular lysis, and with rhabdomyolysis. Changes in insulin production, insulin and other receptor activity, and catecholamine level affect the movement of K^+ across the cell wall. The kidneys are the primary regulators of potassium balance.

Note: Disorders of potassium balance are potentially life-threatening because of the effects of altered potassium levels on neuromuscular and cardiac function. Suspected alterations in potassium balance require prompt consultation with the physician.

HYPOKALEMIA (SERUM POTASSIUM LEVEL <3.5 mEq/L)
Pathophysiology
Hypokalemia occurs because of a loss of potassium from the body or a movement of potassium into the cells. Serum K^+ levels are an inadequate measure of intracellular K^+, but intracellular measurement is not clinically available.

Note: Changes in serum potassium levels reflect changes in ECF potassium—not necessarily changes in total body levels.

Assessment
History and risk factors
Reduction in total body potassium
• Hyperaldosteronism.
• Diuretic therapy or abnormal urinary losses (e.g., hypomagnesemia).
• Increased GI losses.
• Increased loss through diaphoresis.
• Decreased intake.
• Dialysis.

Note: An inadequate diet may contribute to but will rarely cause hypokalemia. Large amounts of potassium are contained in many common foods. Hypokalemia sometimes develops when patients are maintained on parenteral fluid therapy with inadequate replacement of potassium, or when increased losses occur when oral intake is poor.

Intracellular shift (increased uptake of K+, reduced serum level)
• Increased insulin (e.g., from TPN or aggressive IV insulin use)
• Acute alkalosis: K^+ moves into cells in exchange for H^+ to electrically and pH balance the serum.
Stress: Conditions causing physical or emotional stress may result in hypokalemia because of increased loss of potassium in the urine secondary to increased release of aldosterone; or an intracellular shift of potassium secondary to increased stimulation of β_2-adrenergic receptors.
Clinical presentation: Muscle weakness and cramps, soft and flabby muscles, nausea, vomiting, ileus, paresthesias, enhanced digitalis effect.
Physical assessment: Decreased bowel sounds, weak and irregular pulse, decreased reflexes, and decreased muscle tone.

Diagnostic tests
Serum potassium levels: Values will be <3.5 mEq/L.
ABG values: May show metabolic alkalosis (increased pH and HCO_3^-) because hypokalemia usually is associated with this condition.
ECG findings: ST segment depression, flattened T wave, presence of U wave, ventricular dysrhythmias. With severe hypokalemia, P wave amplitude is increased, PR interval is prolonged, and the QRS and QT complexes widen. Patient is at risk for torsades de pointe and ventricular tachycardia. May cause premature ventricular beats, as hypokalemia increases irritability of the myocardium. Cardiac muscle returns more slowly to full resting or repolarized state. During this slow return to resting, weak impulses from an irritable myocardium may initiate abnormal beats.

> **Note:** Hypokalemia potentiates the effect of digitalis. ECG may reveal signs of digitalis toxicity in spite of a normal serum digitalis level.

Collaborative management
Treatment of underlying cause.
Replacement of potassium: May be done by increasing dietary intake, using K^+ supplements, or with IV infusion. 40-80 mEq/L/day is given in divided doses. IV potassium is necessary if hypokalemia is severe or if the patient is unable to take potassium orally. Table 10-13 lists some foods high in potassium.
IV potassium: Potassium is never administered by IV push. Too-rapid administration can result in life-threatening hyperkalemia. It must be appropriately diluted and administered at rates ≤10-20 mEq/hr or in concentrations ≤30-40 mEq/L (when added to IV solutions) unless hypokalemia is severe.

> **Caution:** Patients receiving 10-20 mEq/hr should be on a continuous cardiac monitor.

If potassium is administered via a peripheral line, the rate of administration may require reduction to prevent irritation of vessels. The development of tall, peaked T waves suggests the presence of hyperkalemia and should be reported to a physician. IV potassium may be administered as potassium chloride or potassium phosphate. Table 10-13 lists some foods high in potassium.
Potassium-sparing diuretics: May be given in place of "potassium-losing" diuretics (thiazides or loop diuretics) with potassium supplements. Spironolactone (e.g., Aldactone) is a potassium-sparing diuretic, whereas furosemide (e.g., Lasix) is a loop diuretic and hydrochlorothiazide (e.g., HCTZ, HydroDiuril) is a thiazide diuretic.

Nursing diagnoses and interventions
Decreased cardiac output (or risk for same) related to altered conduction secondary to hypokalemia or too-rapid correction of hypokalemia, with resulting hyperkalemia.
Desired outcome: Within 2 hr of treatment, patient has normal cardiac conduction as evidenced by normal T wave configuration and normal sinus rhythm without ectopy on ECG.
• Administer potassium supplement as prescribed. Avoid giving IV potassium chloride at a rate faster than recommended, inasmuch as this can lead to life-threatening hyperkalemia. K^+ supplements for symptomatic hypokalemia may be given in isotonic saline, as sometimes D_5W increases insulin-induced intracellular shift of potassium. Concentrated solutions of potassium may be administered in limited volumes (i.e., 20 mEq in 100 ml of isotonic NaCl), administered at <20 mEq/hour. Concentrated solutions are used only with severe hypokalemia.

T A B L E 10 - 13   Foods High in Potassium

Apricots	Nuts
Artichokes	Oranges, orange juice
Avocados	Peanuts
Bananas	Potatoes
Cantaloupes	Prune juice
Carrots	Pumpkins
Cauliflower	Spinach
Chocolate	Swiss chard
Dried beans, peas	Sweet potatoes
Dried fruit	Tomatoes, tomato juice, tomato sauce
Mushrooms	

Note: Potassium chloride should not be added to IV bags while they are hanging on a pole, to avoid accumulation of K^+ at the bottom of the IV bag. The solution container should be inverted before adding the medication and mixed well.

- Be aware that IV potassium chloride (KCl) can cause local irritation of veins and chemical phlebitis. Assess IV insertion site for erythema, heat, or pain. Irritation may be relieved by applying an ice bag, giving mild sedation, or numbing insertion site with a small amount of local anesthetic. Phlebitis may necessitate changing of IV site.
- Oral supplements may cause GI irritation. Administer with a full glass of water or fruit juice; encourage patient to sip slowly. Consult physician for symptoms of abdominal pain, distention, nausea, or vomiting. Do not switch potassium supplements without physician prescription.
- Monitor I&O hourly. Consult physician for urine output <0.5 ml/kg/hr. Unless severe symptoms of hypokalemia are present, potassium supplements should not be given to patients with low urine output; hyperkalemia may develop in patients with oliguria (output <15-20 ml/hr). High urine output (diuresis or polyuria) increases the risk of hypokalemia.
- Monitor ECG for signs of continuing *hypokalemia* (i.e., ST segment depression, flattened T wave, presence of U wave, ventricular dysrhythmias) or *hyperkalemia* during potassium replacement (i.e., tall, thin T waves; prolonged PR interval; ST depression; widened QRS complex; loss of P wave).
- Monitor serum potassium levels in patients at risk for hypokalemia, such as patients taking diuretics or undergoing gastric suction.
- Administer potassium cautiously in patients at risk to develop hyperkalemia: those receiving potassium-sparing diuretics (e.g., spironolactone or triamterene) or angiotensin converting enzyme– (ACE-) inhibitors (e.g., captopril).
- Monitor patients on digitalis, because hypokalemia potentiates the effects. Signs of increased digitalis effect include the following: multifocal or bigeminal PVCs, paroxysmal atrial tachycardia with AV block, and other heart blocks.

NIC Electrolyte Management: Hypokalemia; Medication Administration; Dysrhythmia Management

Ineffective breathing pattern (or risk for same) related to weakness or paralysis of respiratory muscles secondary to sudden, *severe* hypokalemia (potassium <2-2.5 mEq/L)

Desired outcome: Within 2 hr of treatment, patient has effective breathing pattern as evidenced by normal respiratory depth and pattern (eupnea) and rate of 12-20 breaths/min.

- If patient has worsening hypokalemia, note if respirations become rapid and shallow; if so, notify physician. Severe hypokalemia causes respiratory muscle weakness. Shallow respirations, apnea, and respiratory arrest may occur.
- Keep manual resuscitator at patient's bedside when severe hypokalemia is present. Reposition patient q2h to prevent stasis of secretions; suction airway as needed.
- Encourage deep breathing (and coughing if indicated) q2h.

NIC Respiratory Monitoring

HYPERKALEMIA (SERUM POTASSIUM LEVEL >5 mEq/L)

Pathophysiology

Hyperkalemia results from increased intake of potassium, decreased urinary excretion of K^+, or sudden movement of K^+ out of cells. The rate of change in serum K^+ is as important as the level. Rapid increases do not allow time to compensate.

> **Note:** Changes in serum potassium levels reflect changes in ECF potassium—not necessarily changes in total body levels of potassium.

Assessment

History and risk factors

Inappropriately high intake of potassium: May be associated with IV potassium delivery or aggressive red blood cell administration. Symptomatic hyperkalemia may develop when appropriate doses of IV potassium chloride (KCl) are administered too rapidly.

Decreased excretion of potassium
- Renal disease, especially acute and chronic renal failure.
- Potassium-sparing diuretics, ACE inhibitors.
- Addison's disease (hypoaldosteronism).

Movement of potassium out of the cells
- Acidosis.
- Insulin deficiency, particularly in dialysis patients.
- Tissue catabolism (e.g., with fever, sepsis, trauma, surgery).

Clinical presentation: Irritability, abdominal cramping, diarrhea, ascending weakness, paresthesias.

Physical assessment: Irregular pulse, abdominal distention, cardiac standstill at levels >8.5 mEq/L.

Diagnostic tests

Serum potassium: Will be >5 mEq/L.

> **Note:** Pseudohyperkalemia may occur with mechanical trauma during venipuncture or incorrect handling of the laboratory specimen. If RBCs hemolyze (are injured), potassium is released from damaged cells while or after specimen has been drawn.

ABG values: May show metabolic acidosis (decreased pH and HCO_3^-) because hyperkalemia often occurs with acidosis.

Diagnostic ECG: Progressive changes include tall, thin T waves; prolonged PR interval; ST depression; widened QRS complex; loss of P wave. Eventually, QRS complex becomes widened further and cardiac arrest occurs.

Collaborative management

Treat the underlying cause and return the serum potassium level to normal.

Acute management

Cation exchange resins (e.g., Kayexalate): Given either orally or via retention enema to exchange sodium for potassium in the gut. Oral Kayexalate is usually combined with sorbitol to promote rapid transit through the gut and induce diarrhea, and thus increase potassium loss in the bowels. The recommended rectal dose for adults is 30-50 g q6h.

Emergency management

IV calcium gluconate: To counteract the neuromuscular and cardiac effects of hyperkalemia. Serum potassium levels will remain elevated.

IV glucose and insulin: To shift potassium into the cells. This reduces serum potassium temporarily.

Sodium bicarbonate: To shift potassium into the cells. Reduces serum potassium temporarily.

β_2-Adrenergic agonists (albuterol): To shift potassium into the cells. This reduces serum potassium temporarily.

> **Note:** The effects of calcium, glucose and insulin, sodium bicarbonate, and ß₂-adrenergic agonists are temporary, lasting only a few hours. These medications should be followed by therapy to remove potassium from the body (i.e., hemodialysis or administration of cation exchange resins).

Hemodialysis: For rapid removal of potassium from the body.

Nursing diagnoses and interventions

Decreased cardiac output (or risk for same) related to electrical factors (ventricular dysrhythmias) secondary to severe hyperkalemia or overcorrection of hyperkalemia, with resulting hypokalemia

Desired outcomes: Within 6 hr after initiation of treatment, patient's cardiac output is adequate as evidenced by PAP 20-30/8-15 mm Hg; CVP ≤6 mm Hg; CO 4-7 L/min; HR ≤100 beats/min; BP within patient's normal range; and absence of the clinical signs of heart failure or pulmonary edema (e.g., crackles, SOB). ECG shows normal sinus rhythm without ectopy or other electrical disturbances. Serum K$^+$ levels normalize.

- Monitor I&O. Consult physician for urine output <0.5 ml/kg/hr. Oliguria increases the risk for development of hyperkalemia.
- Monitor for signs of hyperkalemia: irritability, anxiety, abdominal cramping, diarrhea, ascending weakness, paresthesias, irregular pulse. Assess for hidden sources of potassium: medications (e.g., potassium penicillin G), banked blood, salt substitute, GI bleeding, or catabolic conditions (i.e., infection or trauma).
- Monitor for signs of hypokalemia after treatment: muscle weakness, cramps, nausea, vomiting, decreased bowel sounds, paresthesias, weak and irregular pulse.
- Monitor serum potassium levels, especially in high-risk patients (i.e., those with renal failure). Monitor other lab values associated with conditions that alter potassium levels (e.g., BUN, creatinine, ABGs, glucose). Consult physician for abnormal values.
- Monitor ECG for signs of hypokalemia (i.e., ST segment depression, flattened T waves, presence of U wave, ventricular dysrhythmias), or continuing hyperkalemia (i.e., tall, thin T waves, prolonged PR interval, ST depression, widened QRS complex, loss of P wave). Report changes to physician as soon as possible.
- Administer insulin and glucose in the order prescribed.
- Administer calcium gluconate as prescribed. Use caution in patients receiving digitalis. Monitor for digitalis toxicity. Do not add calcium gluconate to solutions containing sodium bicarbonate, because precipitates may form. For more information about calcium administration, see "Hypocalcemia," p. 554.
- If administering cation exchange resins by enema, encourage patient to retain the solution for at least 30-60 min to ensure therapeutic effects. Administer Kayexalate (without sorbitol) via a Foley catheter inserted into the rectum. The balloon is filled with sterile water to keep the catheter in place, and the catheter is clamped. Cleansing enemas may be done prior to administering Kayexelate to enhance absorption, and afterward to reduce the risk of bowel complications.

NIC Electrolyte Management: Hyperkalemia; Dysrhythmia Management; Hemodialysis Therapy

CALCIUM IMBALANCE (NORMAL SERUM CA^{++} LEVEL: 8.5-10.5 mg/dl, IONIZED 4.5-5.5 mEq/L)

Calcium, one of the body's most abundant ions, combines with phosphorus to form the mineral salts of the bones and teeth. Calcium exerts a sedative effect on nerve cells and has important intracellular functions, including development of the cardiac action potential and contraction of muscles. Only 1% of the body's calcium is contained within ECF, yet this concentration is regulated carefully by the hormones *parathyroid hormone (PTH)* and *calcitonin.*

Slightly less than half of the calcium in the plasma is *free* or *ionized calcium.* The percentage of ionized calcium is affected by plasma pH and the albumin level. About 40% of calcium is bound to protein, primarily albumin. Calcium bound to albumin is not ionized and cannot be used. Albumin releases calcium to the ionized state when needed. Only the ionized calcium exerts physiologic effects and combines with non–protein anions such as phosphate, citrate, and carbonate. Patients with alkalosis may show signs of hypocalcemia because of increased calcium binding. Changes in the plasma albumin level will affect the total serum calcium level without changing the level of ionized calcium.

Note: To determine the "true calcium level" or calcium correction factor: for every gram of albumin <4, add 0.8 to the serum calcium value.

PTH is released by the parathyroid gland in response to low serum Ca^{++} levels to increase movement of Ca^{++} and phosphorus out of the bone (resorption of bone); to activate vitamin D (increases the absorption of calcium from the GI tract); and to stimulate the kidneys to conserve calcium and excrete phosphorus. *Calcitonin* is produced by the thyroid gland when serum Ca^{++} increases to inhibit bone resorption.

Calcium regulates skeletal and cardiac muscle contractions, is part of the clotting cascade, and has other essential functions. It is imperative to maintain the Ca^{++} balance.

HYPOCALCEMIA (SERUM CALCIUM <8.5 mg.dl, IONIZED <4.5 mEq/L)

Pathophysiology

Symptoms of hypocalcemia result from decreased total body calcium or a decreased percentage of ionized calcium. Low total calcium levels may be caused by increased calcium loss, reduced intake secondary to altered intestinal absorption, altered regulation (i.e., hypoparathyroidism); aggressive infusion of citrated blood and renal replacement therapy (CRRT) if citrate is in dialysate. *Elevated phosphorus levels and decreased magnesium levels may precipitate hypocalcemia.*

Assessment

History and risk factors

Decreased ionized calcium

- Alkalosis.
- Rapid administration of citrated blood. Citrate added to the blood to prevent clotting may bind with calcium, causing hypocalcemia.
- Hemodilution (e.g., occurring with volume replacement with normal saline after massive hemorrhage).

Increased calcium loss in body fluids: Occurs when patient experiences large volume diuresis after receiving loop diuretics.

Decreased intestinal absorption

- Decreased intake.
- Impaired vitamin D metabolism.
- Chronic diarrhea.
- After gastrectomy.

Acute and chronic renal failure: See p. 315.

Hypoparathyroidism: Sometimes seen with chronic renal failure patients.

Hyperphosphatemia: Common with renal failure.

Hypomagnesemia: Caused by decreased action of PTH.

Acute pancreatitis: See p. 447.

Clinical presentation: Numbness with tingling of fingers and circumoral region, hyperactive reflexes, muscle cramps, tetany, convulsions. Alterations in mental status may include anxiety, depression, and frank psychosis. In chronic hypocalcemia, fractures may be present because of increased bone porosity. Sudden precipitous drops in plasma calcium levels may cause hypotension secondary to vasodilation and heart failure secondary to decreased myocardial contractility.

Physical assessment

Significant hypotension and coagulopathy: Seen with severe hypocalcemia. Correction at this point is critical.

Positive Trousseau's sign: Ischemia-induced carpopedal spasm. It is elicited by applying a BP cuff to the upper arm and inflating it past systolic BP for 2 min.

Positive Chvostek's sign: Unilateral contraction of facial and eyelid muscles. It is elicited by stimulating the facial nerve·during percussion of the face just in front of the ear.

ECG changes: Prolonged QT interval caused by elongation and elevation of ST segment.

Diagnostic tests

Total serum calcium level: Will be <8.5 mg/dl. Serum calcium levels should be evaluated with serum albumin. For every 1 g/dl drop in the serum albumin level, there is a 0.8-1-mg/dl drop in the total calcium level. Symptomatic hypocalcemia can occur with normal total calcium levels when there is a sudden rise in serum pH.

Ionized serum calcium level: Will be <4.5 mg/dl.

PTH level: Decreased levels occur in hypoparathyroidism; increased levels may occur with other causes of hypocalcemia. Normal range is 150-350 pg/ml (varies among laboratories).

Magnesium and phosphorus levels: May be checked to identify potential causes of hypocalcemia.

Collaborative management

Treatment of underlying cause.

Calcium replacement: Hypocalcemia is treated with PO or IV calcium. Tetany is treated with 10-20 ml of 10% calcium gluconate administered IV or by continuous drip of 100 ml of 10% calcium gluconate in 1000 ml D_5W, infused over at least 4-6 hr. *Magnesium replacement should be for magnesium depletion; hypomagnesemia-induced hypocalcemia is often refractory to calcium therapy alone.*

Vitamin D therapy (e.g., dihydrotachysterol, calcitriol): To increase calcium absorption from the GI tract.

Phosphorus-binding antacids: To reduce elevated phosphorus before treating hypocalcemia. Used primarily in renal failure.

Nursing diagnoses and interventions

Altered protection (risk of tetany and seizures) related to neurosensory alterations secondary to severe hypocalcemia

Desired outcome: Patient does not exhibit evidence of injury caused by severe hypocalcemia.

- Monitor patient for worsening hypocalcemia and consult physician promptly for symptoms that occur before overt tetany: numbness and tingling of fingers and circumoral region, hyperactive reflexes, and muscle cramps. Positive Trousseau's or Chvostek's sign also signals latent tetany. Monitor total and ionized calcium levels as available.

Caution: *Administer IV calcium slowly.* IV calcium should not be given faster than 0.5-1 ml/min. *Rapid administration can cause hypotension.* Observe IV insertion site for infiltration; calcium will slough tissue. *Concentrated calcium solutions (calcium chloride) should be administered through a central line.* Do not add calcium to solutions containing sodium bicarbonate or sodium phosphate to avoid dangerous precipitates. Digitalis toxicity may develop, because calcium potentiates digitalis. Monitor for hypercalcemia: lethargy, confusion, irritability, nausea, and vomiting.

Note: Always clarify type of IV calcium to be given. Both calcium chloride and calcium gluconate come in 10-ml ampules. One ampule of calcium chloride contains 13.6 mEq of calcium, whereas one ampule of calcium gluconate contains 4.5 mEq of calcium.

- For patients with chronic hypocalcemia, administer oral calcium supplements and vitamin D preparations as prescribed. Administer oral calcium 30 min before meals or at bedtime for maximal absorption. Administer phosphorus-binding antacids with meals. If calcium carbonate is being administered primarily to bind phosphorus, administer with food.
- Consult physician if response to calcium therapy is ineffective. Tetany that does not respond to IV calcium may be caused by hypomagnesemia.
- Maintain seizure precautions for affected patients.
- Avoid hyperventilation if hypocalcemia is suspected. Respiratory alkalosis may cause tetany if pH increases when ionized calcium is low.
- Monitor for calcium loss (e.g., with loop diuretics, renal tubular dysfunction) or conditions that place the patient at risk for it (e.g., acute pancreatitis).
- Inform patient and significant others that the neuropsychiatric symptoms of hypocalcemia will improve with treatment.

NIC Neurologic Monitoring; Electrolyte Management: Hypocalcemia; Seizure Precautions; Medication Administration

Decreased cardiac output related to altered conduction or negative inotropy secondary to hypocalcemia or digitalis toxicity occurring with calcium replacement therapy

Desired outcomes: Within 12 hr of initiation of treatment, patient's cardiac output is adequate as evidenced by PAP 20-30/8-15 mm Hg; CVP <6 mm Hg; CO 4-7 L/min; HR =100; BP within patient's normal range; and absence of the clinical signs of heart failure or pulmonary edema (e.g., crackles, SOB). ECG shows normal sinus rhythm without ectopy or other electrical disturbances.

- Monitor ECG for signs of worsening hypocalcemia (e.g., prolonged QT interval) or of digitalis toxicity with calcium replacement: multifocal or bigeminal PVCs; paroxysmal atrial tachycardia with AV block; other heart blocks.
- Hypocalcemia may decrease cardiac contractility. Monitor patient for signs of heart failure or pulmonary edema: crackles, rhonchi, SOB, decreased BP, increased HR, increased PAP, or increased CVP.

NIC Dysrhythmia Management; Cardiac Care

Ineffective breathing pattern related to laryngeal spasm occurring with severe hypocalcemia

Desired outcome: Within 1 hr of initiation of treatment, patient has an effective breathing pattern as evidenced by eupnea; RR 12-20 breaths/min; and absence of the indicators of laryngeal spasm: laryngeal stridor, dyspnea, or crowing.

- Assess patient's respiratory rate, character, and rhythm. Be alert to laryngeal stridor, dyspnea, and crowing, which occur with laryngeal spasm, a life-threatening complication of hypocalcemia.
- Keep an emergency tracheostomy tray at the bedside of all patients with symptoms of hypocalcemia.

NIC Respiratory Monitoring

HYPERCALCEMIA (SERUM CALCIUM LEVEL >10.5, IONIZED >5.5)

Pathophysiology
Hypercalcemia is caused by increased total serum calcium or increased percentage of free, ionized calcium. If hypercalcemia is accompanied by a normal or elevated serum phosphorus level, calcium phosphate crystals may precipitate in the serum and deposit throughout the body. Soft tissue calcifications usually occur when the product of the serum calcium and serum phosphorus (i.e., calcium × phosphorus) exceeds 70 mg/dl.

Assessment
History and risk factors: Hypercalcemia is often caused by hyperparathyroidism (may be stress-related in critical illness), and lymphoproliferative disorders (which cause parathyroid proteins to be produced).
Increased intake of calcium: Excessive administration during cardiopulmonary arrest, milk-alkali syndrome.
Increased intestinal absorption: With vitamin D overdose or hyperparathyroidism.
Increased release of calcium from bone: Hyperparathyroidism, malignancies, prolonged immobilization, Paget's disease.
Decreased urinary excretion: Renal failure, medications (e.g., thiazide diuretics), hyperparathyroidism.
Increased ionized calcium: Acidosis.
Clinical presentation: Symptoms are usually absent unless the serum calcium concentration is >11 mg/dl. They include lethargy, weakness, anorexia, nausea, vomiting, polyuria, itching, bone pain, fractures, calculi, constipation, depression, confusion, paresthesias, personality changes, stupor, and coma. Cardiovascular effects include hypertension, heart block, digitalis sensitivity, and cardiac arrest.
ECG findings: Shortening of ST segment and QT interval. PR interval is sometimes prolonged. Ventricular dysrhythmias can occur with severe hypercalcemia.

Diagnostic tests
Total serum calcium level: Will be >10.5 mg/dl. Serum calcium level should be evaluated with serum albumin level. For every 1 g/dl drop in serum albumin level, total calcium will drop 0.8-1 mg/dl; it is possible that the measured value underpredicts the ionized level.
Ionized calcium level: Will be >5.5 mg/dl.
Parathyroid hormone level: Increased levels occur in primary or secondary hyperparathyroidism.
X-ray findings: May reveal presence of osteoporosis, bone cavitations, or urinary calculi.

Collaborative management
Treatment of underlying cause or contributing factor: May include antitumor chemotherapy for malignancy, partial parathyroidectomy for hyperparathyroidism; discontinuation of calcium supplements, vitamins A and D, and thiazide diuretics.
IV isotonic saline: Administered rapidly to increase urinary calcium excretion. Concomitant administration of furosemide prevents the development of fluid volume excess and further increases in urinary calcium excretion.
Low-calcium diet and cortisone: To reduce intestinal absorption of calcium. Steroids compete with vitamin D, thereby reducing intestinal absorption of calcium.
Decreased bone resorption: Accomplished via increased activity level or administration of biphosphonates or mithramycin. Etidronate and pamidronate are biphosphonates that act directly on bone to reduce decalcification and are used primarily to treat hypercalcemia associated with neoplastic disease. Biphosphonates take several days to work, but the effects may last for days to weeks. Mithramycin is a cytotoxic antibiotic that also decreases bones resorption. Compressional loads (e.g., weight bearing) stimulate bone deposition; thus increased activity decreases bone resorption.
Calcitonin: To reduce bone resorption, increase bone deposition of calcium and phosphorus, and increase urinary calcium and phosphate excretion.
Gallium nitrate: Inhibits osteoclasts and increases bone calcium. Used in the treatment of malignancy-induced hypercalcemia.

Nursing diagnoses and interventions

Altered protection related to neurosensory alterations secondary to hypercalcemia

Desired Outcomes: Within 24-48 hr of initiating treatment, patient verbalizes orientation to time, place, and person. Patient does not exhibit evidence of injury caused by neurosensory changes.

- Monitor patient for worsening hypercalcemia: disorientation to time, place, and person; and deterioration in neurologic status.
- Note personality changes, hallucinations, paranoia, and memory loss. Inform patient and significant others that altered sensorium is temporary and will improve with treatment. Use reality therapy: clocks, calendars, and familiar objects; keep them at the bedside within patient's visual field.
- Administer fluids and diuretics as prescribed. Evaluate response to therapy. Monitor serum calcium levels and albumin levels. Observe for signs of fluid volume excess that develop with treatment.
- Hypercalcemia causes neuromuscular depression with poor coordination, weakness, and altered gait. Provide a safe environment. Keep side rails up and bed in lowest position with wheels locked. Assist with ambulation.
- Monitor for signs of digitalis toxicity (hypercalcemia potentiates digitalis): multifocal or bigeminal PVCs, paroxysmal atrial tachycardia with AV block, other heart blocks.
- Monitor serum electrolytes: calcium, potassium, and phosphorus (normal range is 2.5-4.5 mg/dl). Note changes that result from therapy. Consult physician for abnormal values.
- Encourage increased mobility to reduce bone resorption. Ideally patient should be out of bed and up in a chair at least 6 hr/day.

NIC Fluid Monitoring; Neurologic Monitoring; Electrolyte Management: Hypercalcemia; Dysrhythmia Management; Fluid Management

Altered urinary elimination related to dysuria, urgency, frequency, and polyuria secondary to administration of diuretics, calcium stone formation, or changes in renal function occurring with hypercalcemia

Desired outcome: Within 24 hr of initiation of treatment, patient exhibits voiding pattern and urine characteristics that are normal for patient.

- Monitor I&O hourly. Consult physician for unusual changes in urine volume (e.g., oliguria alternating with polyuria, which may signal urinary tract obstruction, or continuous polyuria). Increased urinary calcium concentrations decrease the kidneys' ability to concentrate the urine, leading to polyuria and potentially to fluid volume deficit. This is a type of nephrogenic diabetes insipidus (see p. 400). Also monitor for signs of volume depletion when giving diuretics: decreased BP, CVP, PAP; increased HR.
- Because hypercalcemia can impair renal function, monitor patient's renal function carefully: urine output, BUN, creatinine values (see "Acute Renal Failure," p. 315).
- Provide patient with a low-calcium diet, and avoid use of calcium-containing medications (e.g., antacids such as Tums). Encourage intake of fruits (e.g., cranberries, prunes, plums) that leave an acid ash in the urine. Acidic urine reduces the risk of calcium stone formation. Also increase fluid intake (at least 3 L in nonrestricted patients) to reduce the risk of renal stone formation.
- Assess patient for indicators of kidney stone formation: intermittent pain, nausea, vomiting, and hematuria.

NIC Fluid Monitoring; Urinary Elimination Management; Electrolyte Management: Hypercalcemia

PHOSPHORUS IMBALANCE (NORMAL SERUM LEVEL 2.5-4.5 mg/dl (1.7-2.6 mEq/L)

Phosphorus, the primary anion ($^-$ or negative ion) of the ICF, has a wide variety of vital functions: formation of energy-storing substances (e.g., adenosine triphosphate [ATP]); formation of red blood cell 2,3-diphosphoglycerate (DPG) (facilitates the release of oxygen from the hemoglobin to be used by the cells); metabolism of carbohydrates, protein, and fat; and maintenance of acid-base balance. In addition, phosphorus is critical to normal nerve and muscle function and provides structural support to bones and teeth.

Plasma phosphorus levels vary with diet and acid-base balance. Glucose, insulin, or sugar-containing foods cause a temporary drop in phosphorus because of a shift of serum phosphorus into the cells. Phosphorous and calcium have an interdependent effect on each other, and share many of the common causes of abnormalities. Alkalosis, particularly respiratory alkalosis, may cause hypophosphatemia as a result of an intracellular shift of phosphorus. Although the exact mechanism for this shift is not fully understood, it may be related to an alkalosis-induced cellular glycolysis, with increased formation of phosphorus-containing metabolic intermediates. Respiratory acidosis may cause a shift of phosphorus out of the cells and contribute to hyperphosphatemia.

Although the level of ECF phosphate is affected by a combination of factors, including dietary intake, intestinal absorption, and hormonally regulated bone resorption and deposition, phosphorus balance depends largely on renal excretion.

HYPOPHOSPHATEMIA (SERUM PHOSPHATE LEVEL <2.5mg/dl OR <1.7mEq/L)

Pathophysiology

Hypophosphatemia (serum phosphorus <2.5 mg/dl) may occur because of transient intracellular shifts, increased urinary losses (most common), decreased intestinal absorption, or increased utilization (see "Assessment" in the next section for history and risk factors). Severe phosphorus deficiency also may develop because of a combination of factors in conditions such as chronic alcohol abuse and diabetic ketoacidosis (DKA).

Assessment

History and risk factors

Intracellular shifts: Carbohydrate load, respiratory alkalosis, treatment of DKA.

Increased utilization because of increased tissue repair: Total parenteral nutrition (TPN) with inadequate phosphorus content; recovery from protein-calorie malnutrition. Hypophosphatemia is common in the critical care patient largely because of nutritional deficiency.

Increased urinary losses: Hypomagnesemia, ECF volume expansion, hyperparathyroidism, use of thiazide diuretics, diuretic phase of acute tubular necrosis (ATN), glucosuria.

Reduced intestinal absorption or increased intestinal loss: Use of phosphorus-binding medications (e.g., aluminum-, magnesium-, or calcium-containing antacids; sucralfate); vomiting and diarrhea; malabsorption disorders such as vitamin D deficiency; prolonged gastric suction.

Mixed causes: Chronic alcohol abuse, DKA, severe burns, artificially ventilated patients, postsurgery status, postrenal transplant status, and sepsis.

Clinical presentation: Patients may have acute symptoms caused by sudden decreases in serum phosphorus, or symptoms may develop gradually because of chronic phosphorus deficiency. The majority of symptoms are secondary to decreases in ATP and 2,3-DPG; therefore, the patient will become acutely hypoxic at the cellular level, producing a high lactate and metabolic acid load.

Acute: Confusion, seizures, coma, chest pain caused by poor oxygenation of the myocardium, muscle pain and weakness, increased susceptibility to infection, numbness and tingling of the fingers and circumoral region, poor coordination, difficulty weaning from mechanical ventilation, respiratory failure.

Chronic: Memory loss, lethargy, weakness, bone pain.

Physical assessment

Acute: Decreased strength as evidenced by difficulty with speaking, weakness of respiratory muscles, and weakening hand grasp. Bruising and bleeding may occur because of platelet dysfunction. Rhabdomyolysis, hemolysis, and myocardial depression may occur in severe hypophosphatemia. Hypoxia may cause an increased RR and respiratory alkalosis because of hyperventilation.

> **Note:** Respiratory alkalosis causes phosphorus to move intracellularly, aggravating the existing hypophosphatemia.

Chronic: Joint stiffness, arthralgia, osteomalacia, cyanosis, and pseudofractures may occur.

Hemodynamic measurements: Severely depleted patients may show signs of decreased myocardial function, including increased PAWP, decreased CO, and decreased BP with decreased response to pressor agents.

Diagnostic tests

Serum phosphorus level: Will be <2.5 mg/dl (1.7 mEq/L).

Mild hypophosphatemia: 1-2.5 mg/dl.

Severe hypophosphatemia: <1 mg/dl.

Parathyroid hormone level: Will be elevated in hyperparathyroidism.

Serum magnesium level: May be decreased because of increased urinary excretion of magnesium in hypophosphatemia.

X-ray findings: May reveal skeletal changes of osteomalacia.

Collaborative management

Identification and elimination of the cause: May include avoiding use of phosphorus-binding antacids (e.g., aluminum, magnesium, or calcium gels or antacids); correction of respiratory alkalosis.

Phosphorus supplementation: Mild hypophosphatemia may be treated by increasing intake of foods high in phosphorus, especially milk (Table 10-14). Moderate hypophosphatemia usually can be treated with oral phosphate supplements such as Neutra-Phos (sodium and potassium phosphate) or

T A B L E 10 - 14   Foods High in Phosphorus

Dried beans and peas
Eggs and egg products (e.g., eggnog, soufflés)
Fish
Meats, especially organ meats (e.g., brain, liver, kidney)
Milk and milk products (e.g., cheese, ice cream, cottage cheese)
Nuts (e.g., Brazil, peanuts)
Poultry
Seeds (e.g., pumpkin, sesame, sunflower)
Whole grains (e.g., oatmeal, bran, barley)

Phospho-Soda (sodium phosphate). Administration of IV sodium phosphate or potassium phosphate is necessary in cases of severe hypophosphatemia or when the GI tract is nonfunctional.

Nursing diagnoses and interventions
Altered protection related to neurosensory alterations secondary to hypophosphatemia
Desired outcomes: Within 24 hr of initiation of treatment, patient verbalizes orientation to time, place, and person. Patient does not exhibit evidence of injury caused by neurosensory changes.
- Monitor serum phosphorus levels in patients at increased risk. Consult physician for decreased levels. Monitor for signs of associated electrolyte and acid-base imbalances: hypokalemia, hypomagnesemia, respiratory alkalosis, and metabolic acidosis.
- Apprehension, confusion, and paresthesias are signals of developing hypophosphatemia. Assess and document LOC, orientation, and neurologic status with each VS check. Reorient patient as necessary. Alert physician to significant changes.
- Inform patient and significant others that altered sensorium is temporary and will improve with treatment.
- When IV phosphorus is administered as potassium phosphate, the infusion rate should not exceed 10 mEq/hr. Monitor IV site for signs of infiltration, because potassium phosphate can cause necrosis and sloughing of tissue.

> **Caution:** *Do not administer IV phosphate at a rate greater than that recommended by the manufacturer.* Potential complications of IV phosphorus administration include *tetany* as a result of hypocalcemia (serum calcium levels may drop suddenly if serum phosphorus levels increase suddenly; see "Calcium Imbalance," p. 554, for additional information); *soft tissue calcification* (if hyperphosphatemia develops, the calcium and phosphorus in the ECF may combine and form deposits in tissue); and *hypotension,* caused by a too-rapid delivery.

- Keep the side rails up and the bed in its lowest position with wheels locked.
- Use reality therapy: clocks, calendars, and familiar objects. Keep these articles at the bedside within patient's visual field.
- If patient is at risk for seizures, pad the side rails and keep an appropriate-size airway at the bedside.

NIC Neurologic Monitoring; Electrolyte Management: Hypophosphatemia; Medication Administration
Impaired gas exchange related to altered oxygen-carrying capacity of the blood secondary to decreased 2,3-DPG

> **Note:** With decreased 2,3-DPG levels, the oxyhemoglobin dissociation curve will shift to the left (i.e., at a given PaO_2 level, more oxygen will be bound to Hgb and less will be available to the tissues).

Desired outcome: Within 12 hr of initiation of treatment, patient has adequate gas exchange as evidenced by RR 12-20 breaths/min with normal depth and pattern (eupnea); orientation to time, place, and person; SpO_2 ≥92%; and absence of the indicators of hypoxia (e.g., restlessness, somnolence).

- Assess patient for signs of hypoxia: restlessness, confusion, increased RR, complaints of chest pain, and cyanosis (a late sign).
- Monitor SpO_2 as available. Administer oxygen as prescribed to maintain SpO_2 at ≥92%.

NIC Respiratory Monitoring

Ineffective breathing pattern related to decreased strength of respiratory muscles secondary to hypophosphatemia

Desired outcome: Within 8 hr of initiation of treatment, the nonventilated patient becomes eupneic. Optimally, for the ventilated patient, improved weaning is noted within 24 hr of initiation of treatment.

- Monitor rate and depth of respirations in patients with severe hypophosphatemia. Assess for decreased tidal volume or decreased minute ventilation. Consult physician for changes.
- Monitor ABG values for evidence of hypoxemia or hypercapnia. Consult physician for significant changes.
- Monitor serum phosphate levels in mechanically ventilated patients; they exhibit a high incidence of hypophosphatemia. Hypophosphatemia may contribute to difficulty in weaning patients from ventilators.
- Administer IV phosphorus as prescribed.

NIC Respiratory Monitoring

Impaired physical mobility related to musculoskeletal impairment (osteomalacia with bone pain and fractures) associated with movement of phosphorus out of the bone secondary to chronic hypophosphatemia; muscle weakness and acute rhabdomyolysis (breakdown of striated muscle) secondary to severe hypophosphatemia.

Desired outcome: Within 24 hr of initiation of therapy, patient is able to move purposefully and has full or baseline range of motion (ROM) and muscle strength.

- Monitor all patients with suspected hypophosphatemia for decreasing muscle strength. Perform serial assessments of hand grasp strength and clarity of speech. Consult physician for changes.
- Monitor serum phosphorus levels for worsening hypophosphatemia. Consult physician for changes.
- Assist the patient with ambulation and activities of daily living (ADLs).
- Encourage intake of foods high in phosphorus (see Table 10-14). Teach patient and significant others the importance of using phosphorus-binding antacids only as prescribed.
- Medicate for pain as prescribed.

NIC Neurologic Monitoring; Electrolyte Management: Hypophosphatemia

Decreased cardiac output related to negative inotropic changes associated with reduced myocardial functioning secondary to severe phosphorus depletion

Desired outcome: Within 12 hr of initiation of treatment, patient's cardiac output is adequate as evidenced by CO ≥4 L/min; CI ≥2.5 L/min/m²; CVP <6 mm Hg; PAP 20-30/8-15 mm Hg; HR ≤100 beats/min; BP within patient's normal range; and absence of the clinical signs of heart failure or pulmonary edema.

- Monitor patient for signs of heart failure or pulmonary edema: crackles, rhonchi, SOB, decreased BP, increased HR, increased PAP, or increased CVP.
- Prevent patient from hyperventilating. Metabolic alkalosis causes increased movement of phosphorus into cells, which will reduce cardiac output.
- For additional interventions if decreased cardiac output develops, see "Cardiomyopathy," p. 226.

NIC Invasive Hemodynamic Monitoring; Cardiac Care

Risk for infection related to inadequate secondary defenses (impaired WBC functioning) secondary to reduced ATP

Desired outcome: Patient is free of infection as evidenced by normothermia and absence of erythema, swelling, warmth, and purulent drainage at invasive sites.

- Monitor temperature q4h for evidence of infection. Obtain cultures of wounds and drainage as prescribed if infection is suspected.
- Use meticulous aseptic technique when changing dressings or manipulating indwelling lines (e.g., TPN catheters, IV needles).
- Provide oral hygiene and skin care at regular intervals. Intact skin and membranes are the body's first line of defense against infection.

NIC Infection Protection

HYPERPHOSPHATEMIA (SERUM PHOSPHATE LEVEL>4.5 mg/dl OR >2.6 mEq/L)

Pathophysiology

Hyperphosphatemia is common in patients with renal insufficiency/failure whose kidneys are unable to effectively excrete excess phosphorus. Other causes of hyperphosphatemia include increased intake of phosphates, extracellular shifts (i.e., movement of phosphorus out of the cell and into the ECF), cellular destruction with concomitant release of intracellular phosphorus, and decreased urinary losses that are unrelated to decreased renal function. As serum phosphorus levels increase, serum calcium levels often decrease, leading to hypocalcemia. Hypocalcemia is most likely to occur in sudden, severe hyperphosphatemia (e.g., after IV administration of phosphates) or in patients prone to hypocalcemia (e.g., those with chronic renal failure).

The primary complication of hyperphosphatemia is metastatic calcification (i.e., the precipitation of calcium phosphate in the soft tissue, joints, and arteries). Chronic hyperphosphatemia in the patient with chronic renal failure may contribute to the development of renal osteodystrophy.

Precipitation of calcium phosphate occur when the product of the serum calcium and serum phosphorus (i.e., calcium × phosphorus) exceeds 70 mg/dl.

Assessment
History and risk factors
Renal failure: Acute and chronic. Hyperphosphatemia is an early feature of chronic renal failure secondary to declining glomerular filtration.
Increased intake: Excessive administration of phosphorus supplements; vitamin D excess with increased GI absorption; excessive use of phosphorus-containing laxatives or enemas; massive transfusion.
Extracellular shift: Respiratory acidosis; diabetic ketoacidosis (before treatment).
Cellular destruction: Neoplastic disease (e.g., leukemia, lymphoma) treated with cytotoxic agents; increased tissue catabolism (breakdown); rhabdomyolysis (breakdown of striated muscle).
Decreased urinary losses: Hypoparathyroidism; volume depletion.
Clinical presentation: Anorexia, nausea, vomiting, muscle weakness, hyperreflexia, tetany, tachycardia.

Note: Usually patients experience few symptoms with hyperphosphatemia. The majority of symptoms relate to development of hypocalcemia or soft tissue (metastatic) calcifications. Indicators of metastatic calcification include oliguria, corneal haziness, conjunctivitis, irregular heart rate, and papular eruptions.

Physical assessment: See "Hypocalcemia," p. 554. In addition, see preceding "Clinical Presentation" for indicators of metastatic calcifications.
ECG changes: See "Hypocalcemia," p. 554. Deposition of calcium phosphate in the heart may lead to dysrhythmias and conduction disturbances.

Diagnostic tests
Serum phosphate level: Will be >4.5 mg/dl (2.6 mEq/L).
X-ray: May show skeletal changes of osteodystrophy.
PTH level: Will be decreased in hypoparathyroidism.

Collaborative management
Identification and elimination of the cause.
Use of aluminum, magnesium, or calcium antacids: To bind phosphorus in the gut, thus increasing GI elimination of phosphorus. *Calcium carbonate and calcium acetate are the preferred preparations for the patient with chronic renal failure. Magnesium antacids are avoided in renal failure because of the risk of hypermagnesemia. Aluminum-containing antacids are contraindicated because they may lead to aluminum accumulation and contribute to the development of bone disease.* Serum phosphorus levels may be allowed to remain slightly elevated (4.5-6 mg/dl) in chronic renal failure to ensure adequate levels of 2,3-DPG. This helps to minimize the effects of chronic anemia on oxygen delivery to the tissues.
Hemodialysis: May be necessary for acute, severe hyperphosphatemia accompanied by symptoms of hypocalcemia. See "Renal Replacement Therapies," p. 334.

Nursing diagnoses and interventions
Knowledge deficit: purpose of phosphate binders and the importance of reducing GI absorption of phosphorus to control hyperphosphatemia and prevent long-term complications
Desired outcome: Within the 24-hr period before discharge from intensive care unit (ICU), patient describes the potential complications of uncontrolled hyperphosphatemia and preventive measures.

Note: Prevention of long-term complications relies primarily on adequate patient education, because symptoms of hyperphosphatemia may be minimal.

- Teach patients the purpose of phosphate binders. Stress the need to take binders as prescribed with or after meals to maximize effectiveness.
- Educate patients about possible constipation from phosphate binders. Encourage use of bulk-building supplements or stool softener if constipation occurs. *Phosphate-containing laxatives and enemas must be avoided (i.e., Fleets Phosphosoda products).*
- Phosphate binders are available in liquid, tablet, or capsule form. Confer with physician regarding an alternate form or brand for individuals who find binders unpalatable or difficult to take. Phosphate binders vary in aluminum, magnesium, or calcium content. One may not be exchanged for another without first ensuring that the patient is receiving the same amount of elemental aluminum, magnesium, or calcium.
- Discuss avoiding or limiting foods high in phosphorus (see Table 10-14).
- Review the importance of avoiding phosphorus-containing OTC medications: certain laxatives, enemas, and mixed vitamin-mineral supplements. Instruct the patient and significant others to read the label for the words "phosphorus" and "phosphate."

▌NIC   Teaching: Prescribed Medication; Electrolyte Management: Hyperphosphatemia

Risk for injury related to internal factors associated with precipitation of calcium phosphate in the soft tissue (e.g., corneas, lungs, kidneys, gastric mucosa, heart, blood vessels) and periarticular region of the large joints (e.g., hips, shoulders, elbows); development of hypocalcemic tetany

Desired outcome: Patient does not develop symptoms of physical injury caused by precipitation of calcium phosphate in the soft tissue or joints, or by hypocalcemic tetany.

- Monitor serum phosphorus and calcium levels. Calculate the calcium-phosphorus product (calcium × phosphorus). Values >70 mg/dl are associated with precipitation of calcium phosphate in the soft tissues. Consult physician for abnormal values. *Phosphorus values may be kept slightly higher (4-6 mg/dl) to ensure adequate levels of 2,3-DPG in chronic renal failure patients, to minimize effects of chronic anemia on oxygen delivery to the tissues.*
- Vitamin D products and calcium supplements (taken between meals) may be limited until the serum phosphorus approaches a normal level.
- Consult physician if patient develops indicators of metastatic calcification: oliguria, corneal haziness, conjunctivitis, irregular heart rate, and papular eruptions.
- Monitor patient for symptoms of increasing hypocalcemia that may precede overt tetany: numbness and tingling of the fingers and circumoral region, hyperactive reflexes, and muscle cramps. Positive Trousseau's or Chvostek's sign may signal latent tetany. Consult physician promptly if these symptoms develop. (For a discussion of these signs and for additional information regarding treatment and prevention of hypocalcemia, see p. 554.)
- Because hyperphosphatemia can impair renal function, monitor renal function carefully: urine output, BUN, and creatinine values.

▌NIC   Neurologic Monitoring; Electrolyte Management: Hyperphosphatemia

MAGNESIUM IMBALANCE (NORMAL SERUM MAGNESIUM LEVEL 1.5-2.5 mEq/L)

Approximately 60% of the body's magnesium is located in bone, and approximately 1% is located in the ECF. The remaining magnesium is contained within the cells. Mg^{++} is the second most abundant intracellular cation ($^+$ or positive ion) after potassium. Magnesium is regulated by a combination of factors, including vitamin D–regulated GI absorption and renal excretion.

Because magnesium is a major intracellular ion, it plays a vital role in normal cellular function. Specifically, it activates enzymes involved in the metabolism of carbohydrates and protein, and it triggers the sodium-potassium pump, thus affecting intracellular potassium levels. Magnesium also is important in the transmission of neuromuscular activity, neural transmission within the CNS, and myocardial functioning.

HYPOMAGNESEMIA (SERUM MAGNESIUM LEVEL <1.5 mEq/L)

Pathophysiology

Hypomagnesemia usually results from decreased GI absorption, increased urinary loss, or excessive GI loss (e.g., vomiting, diarrhea), and with prolonged administration of magnesium-free parenteral fluids. Chronic alcohol abusers (see "History and Risk Factors" that follows) and critically ill patients most commonly experience low Mg^{++}. Hypomagnesemia is associated with increased mortality in the critical care setting. Dysrhythmias and sudden death increase when decreased magnesium levels occur in combination with myocardial infarction, heart failure, or digitalis toxicity. Hypomagnesemia usually is associated with hypocalcemia and hypokalemia (see "Diagnostic Tests," p. 554, for additional information). Symptoms of hypomagnesemia tend to develop once the serum magnesium level drops below 1 mEq/L. Decreased magnesium intake has been identified as a risk factor for hypertension, cardiac dysrhythmias, ischemic heart disease, and sudden cardiac death.

Assessment
History and risk factors
Chronic alcoholism: The most common cause of hypomagnesemia is a combination of poor dietary intake, decreased GI absorption, and increased urinary excretion secondary to ethanol effect.
Decreased GI absorption: May occur with cancer, colitis, pancreatic insufficiency, surgical resection of the GI tract, use of laxatives, diarrhea.
Increased GI loss: Prolonged vomiting or gastric suction.
Administration of low-magnesium or magnesium-free parenteral solutions: Especially with refeeding after starvation.
Poorly controlled diabetes including DKA: A result of movement of magnesium out of the cell and loss in the urine because of osmotic diuresis.
Increased urinary excretion: Resulting from medications such as diuretics, amphotericin, tobramycin, gentamicin, cisplatin, cyclosporine, or digoxin, or from diuretic phase of ATN.
Protein-calorie malnutrition.
Cardiopulmonary bypass.
Clinical presentation: Lethargy, weakness, fatigue, mood changes, hallucinations, confusion, anorexia, nausea, vomiting, paresthesias.
Physical assessment: Increased reflexes, tremors, convulsions, tetany, and positive Chvostek's and Trousseau's signs (see p. 554), associated with hypocalcemia. Skeletal and respiratory muscle weakness, tachycardia, hypertension, and coronary spasm may be present.
ECG findings: PVCs and torsades de pointes may be seen. See "Hypokalemia," p. 549; and "Hypocalcemia," p. 554.

Diagnostic tests
Serum magnesium level: <1.5 mEq/L. Hypomagnesemia is the most frequently undiagnosed electrolyte imbalance in hospitalized patients.
Magnesium tolerance test: Used to identify individuals with, or at risk for, magnesium deficiency. Results are based on the amount of magnesium retained after an infusion of magnesium.
Serum potassium level: May be decreased because of failure of the cellular sodium-potassium pump to move potassium into the cell and the accompanying loss of potassium in the urine. This hypokalemia may be resistant to potassium replacement until the magnesium deficit has been corrected.
Serum calcium level: Hypomagnesemia may lead to hypocalcemia because of a reduction in the release and action of parathyroid hormone. Parathyroid hormone is the primary regulator of serum calcium levels.
ECG evaluations: May reflect magnesium, as well as calcium and potassium, deficiencies: tachyarrhythmias, prolonged PR and QT intervals, widening of the QRS complex, ST segment depression, and flattened T waves. Increased digitalis effect (as evidenced by multifocal or bigeminal PVCs, paroxysmal atrial tachycardia with varying AV block, and other heart blocks) also may occur. Dysrhythmias associated with hypomagnesemia include ventricular ectopy, torsades de pointes, and atrial fibrillation.

Collaborative management
Identification and elimination of the cause: For example, ensuring adequate replacement of magnesium in TPN solutions.
IV or IM magnesium sulfate ($MgSO_4$): For severe hypomagnesemia or its symptoms.
Oral magnesium: Chronic magnesium loss is treated with oral magnesium salts (oxide or chloride). Magnesium-containing antacids (e.g., Mylanta, Maalox, Gelusil, Milk of Magnesia) also may be used. Some foods high in magnesium are listed in Table 10-15.

Nursing diagnoses and interventions
Altered protection related to neurosensory alterations secondary to hypomagnesemia
Desired outcomes: Within 8 hr of initiation of treatment, patient verbalizes orientation to time, place, and person. Patient does not exhibit evidence of injury caused by complications of severe hypomagnesemia.
• Monitor serum magnesium levels in patients at risk for hypomagnesemia and its deleterious effects (e.g., those who are alcohol abusers or experiencing heart failure, cases of recent myocardial infarction

---

T A B L E   10 - 15   Foods High in Magnesium

Bananas	Molasses
Chocolate	Nuts and seeds
Coconuts	Oranges
Grapefruits	Refined sugar
Green, leafy vegetables (e.g., beet greens,	Seafood
collard greens)	Soy flour
Kelp	Wheat bran
Legumes	

---

or digitalis toxicity). Normal range for serum magnesium is 1.5-2.5 mEq/L. Consult physician for abnormal values.

Note: Symptoms of hypomagnesemia may be mistakenly attributed to delirium tremens of chronic alcoholism. Be alert to indicators of magnesium deficit in these patients.

- Administer IV MgSO$_4$ slowly. Refer to manufacturer's guidelines. Too-rapid administration may lead to dangerous hypermagnesemia, with cardiac or respiratory arrest. Patients receiving IV magnesium should be monitored for decreasing BP, labored respirations, and diminished patellar reflex (knee jerk). An absent patellar reflex signals hyporeflexia (seen with dangerous hypermagnesemia). Should any of these changes occur, stop the infusion and consult physician immediately (see "Hypermagnesemia," p. 565). Keep calcium gluconate at the bedside in the event of hypocalcemic tetany or sudden hypermagnesemia.
- For patients with chronic hypomagnesemia, administer oral magnesium supplements as prescribed. All magnesium supplements should be given with caution in patients with reduced renal function because of an increased risk of the development of hypermagnesemia. Caution patient that oral magnesium supplements may cause diarrhea. Administer antidiarrheal medications as needed.
- When it is appropriate, encourage intake of foods high in magnesium (see Table 10-15). For most patients, a normal diet is usually adequate.
- Maintain seizure precautions for patients with symptoms (i.e., those who have hyperreflexia). Decrease environmental stimuli (e.g., keep the room quiet; use subdued lighting).
- For patients in whom hypocalcemia is suspected, caution against hyperventilation. Metabolic alkalosis may precipitate tetany as a result of increased calcium binding.
- Dysphagia may occur in hypomagnesemia. Test the patient's ability to swallow water before giving food or medications.
- Assess and document LOC, orientation, and neurologic status with each VS check. Reorient patient as necessary. Notify physician for significant changes. Inform patient and significant others that altered mood and sensorium are temporary and will improve with treatment.
- See "Hypokalemia," p. 549; "Hypocalcemia," p. 554; and "Hypophosphatemia," p. 558; for nursing care of patients with these disorders.

Note: Because magnesium is necessary for the movement of potassium into the cell, intracellular potassium deficits cannot be corrected until hypomagnesemia has been treated.

NIC Neurologic Monitoring; Electrolyte Management: Hypomagnesemia; Electrolyte Management: Hypokalemia; Electrolyte Management: Hypocalcemia; Seizure Precautions; Medication Administration

Decreased cardiac output related to electrical alterations associated with tachyarrhythmias or digitalis toxicity secondary to hypomagnesemia

Desired outcomes: Within 24 hr of initiating treatment, patient's cardiac output is adequate as evidenced by CO ≥4 L/min; CI ≥2.5 L/min/m^2; normal configurations on ECG; and HR within patient's normal range. Patient exhibits brisk capillary refill (<2 sec) and urinary output ≥0.5 ml/kg/hr.
- Monitor heart rate and regularity with each VS check. Consult physician for changes. Be alert to decreased CO and CI.

- Assess ECG for evidence of hypomagnesemia. Consider hypomagnesemia as a possible cause if a patient develops sudden ventricular dysrhythmias.
- Because hypomagnesemia (and hypokalemia) potentiate the cardiac effects of digitalis, monitor for digitalis-induced dysrhythmias. ECG changes may include multifocal or bigeminal PVCs, paroxysmal atrial tachycardia with varying AV block, and other heart blocks.
- Monitor for and report decreased urinary output and delayed capillary refill.

NIC Cardiac Care; Dysrhythmia Management

Altered nutrition: less than body requirements of magnesium, related to history of poor intake or anorexia, nausea, and vomiting secondary to hypomagnesemia or starvation

Desired outcome: Within 24 hr of resumption of oral feedings, patient receives diet adequate in magnesium.

- Encourage intake of small, frequent meals.
- Teach patient about foods high in magnesium content (see Table 10-15), and encourage intake of these foods during meals.
- Administer antiemetics as prescribed.
- Include patient, significant others, and dietitian in meal planning as appropriate.
- Provide oral hygiene before meals to enhance appetite.
- As with the other major intracellular electrolyte levels, magnesium depletion may develop with refeeding after starvation. Anticipate hypomagnesemia with refeeding, and ensure increased dietary intake or supplementation.
- Consult physician for patients receiving magnesium-free solutions (e.g., TPN) for prolonged periods.

NIC Nutritional Monitoring; Nutrition Management; Nutrition Therapy; Nutritional Counseling

HYPERMAGNESEMIA (SERUM MAGNESIUM LEVELS >2.5 mEq/L)

Pathophysiology
Hypermagnesemia occurs almost exclusively in individuals with renal failure who have an increased intake of magnesium (e.g., those who use magnesium-containing medications). It also may occur in acute cases of adrenocortical insufficiency (Addison's disease) or in obstetric patients treated with parenteral magnesium for pregnancy-induced hypertension. In rare cases hypermagnesemia occurs because of excessive use of magnesium-containing medications (e.g., antacids, laxatives, enemas). The primary symptoms of hypermagnesemia are the result of depressed peripheral and central neuromuscular transmission. Symptoms usually do not occur until the magnesium level exceeds 4 mEq/L.

Assessment
History and risk factors
Decreased excretion of magnesium: Seen with renal failure or adrenocortical insufficiency.
Increased intake of magnesium: May include excessive use of magnesium-containing antacids, enemas, and laxatives or excessive administration of magnesium sulfate (such as in the treatment of hypomagnesemia or pregnancy-induced hypertension).
Clinical presentation: Nausea, vomiting, flushing, diaphoresis, sensation of heat, altered mental functioning, drowsiness, coma, and muscular weakness or paralysis. Paralysis of the respiratory muscles may occur when the magnesium level exceeds 10 mEq/L.
Physical assessment: Hypotension, soft tissue (metastatic) calcification (see description, p. 556), bradycardia, and decreased deep tendon reflexes (DTRs). The patellar (knee jerk) reflex is lost once the magnesium level exceeds 8 mEq/L.
Hemodynamic measurements: Decreased arterial pressure caused by peripheral vasodilation.

Diagnostic tests
Serum magnesium level: Will be >2.5 mEq/L.
ECG findings: Prolonged PR, QRS, and QT intervals occur with levels >5 mEq/L. Complete heart block and cardiac arrest may occur in severe hypermagnesemia (levels >15 mEq/L).

Collaborative management
Removal of cause: May include discontinuing or avoiding use of magnesium-containing medications (see Table 10-15) or supplements, especially in patients with decreased renal function.
Diuretics and 0.45% NaCl solution: To promote magnesium excretion in patients with adequate renal function.
IV calcium gluconate, 10 ml of a 10% solution: To antagonize the neuromuscular effects of magnesium for patients with potentially lethal hypermagnesemia.
Hemodialysis with magnesium-free dialysate: For patients with severely decreased renal function.

T A B L E 10 - 16   Magnesium-containing Medications

Antacids	Laxatives
Aludrox	Magnesium citrate
Camalox	Magnesium hydroxide (Milk of Magnesia, Haley's
Di-Gel	M-O)
Gaviscon	
Gelusil and Gelusil II	Magnesium sulfate (Epsom salts)
Maalox and Maalox Plus	Magnesium-containing mineral supplements
Mylanta and Mylanta-II	
Riopan	
Simeco	
Tempo	

Nursing diagnoses and interventions

Altered protection related to neurosensory alterations secondary to hypermagnesemia

Desired outcomes: Within 12 hr of initiation of treatment, patient verbalizes orientation to time, place, and person. Patient does not exhibit evidence of injury as a result of complications of hypermagnesemia. Patient has no symptoms of soft tissue (metastatic) calcifications: oliguria, corneal haziness, conjunctivitis, irregular heart rate, and papular eruptions.

- Monitor serum magnesium levels in the patient at risk for hypermagnesemia (e.g., those with chronic renal failure). Normal range for serum magnesium levels is 1.5-2.5 mEq/L.
- Assess and document LOC, orientation, and neurologic status (e.g., hand grasp) with each VS check. Assess patellar (knee jerk) reflex in patients with a moderately elevated magnesium level (>5 mEq/L). With patient lying flat, support the knee in a moderately fixed position and tap the patellar tendon firmly just below the patella. Normally the knee will extend. An absent reflex suggests a magnesium level of =7 mEq/L. Consult physician for significant changes.
- Reassure patient and significant others that altered mental functioning and muscle strength will improve with treatment.
- Keep side rails up and the bed in its lowest position with the wheels locked.
- Assess patient for the development of soft tissue calcification. Consult physician for significant findings.
- Monitor for cardiopulmonary effects of hypermagnesemia: hypotension, flushing, bradycardia, respiratory depression.

NIC Neurologic Monitoring; Electrolyte Management: Hypermagnesemia

Knowledge deficit: importance of avoiding excessive or inappropriate use of magnesium-containing medications, especially for patients with chronic renal failure

Desired outcome: Within the 24-hr period before discharge from ICU, patient verbalizes the importance of avoiding unusual magnesium intake and identifies potential sources of unwanted magnesium.

- Caution patients with chronic renal failure to review all OTC medications with physician before use.
- Provide a list of common magnesium-containing medications (Table 10-16).
- Caution patients to avoid combination vitamin-mineral supplements because they usually contain magnesium.

NIC Teaching: Prescribed Diet; Teaching: Prescribed Medication

Acid-Base Imbalances

A steady balance must be maintained between bodily acids and bases for optimal functioning of the cells. Respiratory and metabolic acids are generated as cells work and must be buffered or eliminated to maintain a neutral chemical environment. Hydrogen ions (H^+) build the acids in the system. *Arterial pH* is an indirect measurement of (H^+) concentration, which reflects the overall acid level and effectiveness of maintaining the balance. The balance largely depends on interaction of the respiratory acid carbon dioxide (CO_2), the gaseous component of carbonic acid (H_2CO_3) regulated by the lungs, and hydrogen ion (H^+), the nongaseous acid regulated by the kidneys. CO_2 cannot be buffered. CO_2 is the largest contributor of H^+ in its gaseous state.

When the acid level increases, the bicarbonate (HCO_3^-), a base/buffer regulated by the kidneys, is used to neutralize the acid to maintain the balance. The kidneys also excrete additional hydrogen ions in the urine to reduce the acid level. The normal acid-base ratio is 1:20; one part acid (CO_2, a component of H_2CO_3) to 20 parts base (HCO_3^-). If the balance is altered, the pH changes. If extra acids are present or base is lost from cells, there is *acidosis*; pH is <7.35. If extra base is present or acid is lost from cells, *alkalosis* is present; pH is >7.45.

When evaluating patients, it is essential to have a basic understanding of the acid-base balancing system. The main formula for maintenance of acid-base balance is the following:

$$CO_2 + H_2O \leftrightarrow \underset{\text{carbonic acid}}{H_2CO_3} \leftrightarrow \underset{\text{bicarb}}{HCO_3^-} \text{ and } H^+$$

The equation is constantly shifting from left to right and right to left to show how the body uses bicarbonate and carbonic acid to maintain acid-base balance.

Buffering occurs in three primary ways:
- Rapid buffering using bicarbonate, proteins, intracllular electrolytes and chloride.
- Respiratory compensation: the respiratory center immediately stimulates hyperventilation to compensate.
- Renal compensation: if capable, the kidneys increase the amount of bicarbonate reabsorbed and hydrogen ions excreted. This may take up to 24-48 hours to occur.

> **Note:** Note: As the nonvolatile acid H^+ increases, it will displace the intracellular potassium, resulting in a serum hyperkalemia but an intracellular hypokalemia.

Pathophysiology of acid-base regulation

When the plasma contains either too many hydrogen ions (*acidemia: pH <7.35*) or too few hydrogen ions (*alkalemia: pH >7.45*), the pH changes. A pH change is a symptom that a pH regulation problem has occurred. For example: If metabolic acids have accumulated (H^+ increases and HCO_3^- decreases), the lungs should respond with hyperventilation to excrete more CO_2. If respiratory acids accumulate because of respiratory insufficiency (i.e., CO_2 is retained or increased), the kidneys should respond by excreting more hydrogen ions and retaining bicarbonate. If either the kidneys or lungs do not respond to a pH change, or they provide an ineffective response, the patient will remain in acid-base imbalance; either *acidotic* or *alkalotic*.

Respiratory system (CO_2 management) The respiratory system provides a quick response to pH changes—within 1-2 min. The lungs either eliminate or retain CO_2 in direct relation to arterial pH. Although the compensatory effect of the respiratory system cannot correct imbalances completely, it is 50%-75% effective. The compensatory effects of the respiratory system occur in response to an increase in tissue or metabolic acids and require an optimally functional respiratory system.

Response to acidosis: When H^+ (acid) increases, pH decreases in the plasma. The central respiratory center in the brain responds by *increasing the rate and depth of ventilation* to 4-5 times the normal level to exhale additional CO_2.

Response to alkalosis: When H^+ (acid) decreases, pH increases in the plasma. The central respiratory center in the brain responds by *decreasing the rate and depth of ventilation* (in the normal lung) to 50%-75% of the normal level.

Renal system (H^+ and HCO_3^- management) Although the kidneys' response to an abnormal pH level is slow—several hours to days—they are able to facilitate a nearly normal pH level by excreting or retaining large quantities of HCO_3^- or H^+ from the body. Acid-base balance is regulated by increasing or decreasing H^+ and bicarbonate (HCO_3^-) concentration in body fluids. A series of complex reactions with H^+ secretion, sodium ion (Na^+) resorption, HCO_3^- retention, and ammonia synthesis (excretes H^+ in the urine) occurs.

Response to acidosis: H^+ secretion is regulated by the amount of carbon dioxide in extracellular fluid (ECF): the greater the concentration of CO_2, the greater the amount of H^+ (acid). If the kidneys are functional, there will be an increase in renal tubular H^+ secretion, resulting in excretion of acidic urine. When H^+ is secreted, HCO_3^- is generated and resorbed by the kidneys, helping to restore the 1:20 balance of acids and bases.

Response to alkalosis: When ECF is alkalotic, the kidneys conserve H^+ and eliminate HCO_3^-, resulting in excretion of alkalotic urine. Renal excretion of acid load and increase in circulating buffer is the major compensation for respiratory deficits and requires a normally functioning kidney.

Buffers: all buffers absorb acids (H^+), but do so with a varying affinity

Buffers are present in all body fluids acid cells and act within one second after acid accumulation begins. They combine with excess acid to form substances that may not greatly affect pH. Some buffers have a strong affinity to acid; others are weak. The three primary plasma buffers are bicarbonate (HCO_3^-), proteins, and chloride (Cl^-). All are negatively charged to facilitate attraction to positively charged hydrogen ions (H^+). Combining positively charged with negatively charged ions yields a neutral substance.

Bicarbonate (HCO_3^-): The primary buffer of acid; largest quantity present in the body fluids. If bicarbonate accumulates, this indicates a primary problem with HCO_3^- regulation by the kidneys, or that the kidneys are compensating for increased CO_2 (respiratory failure increases CO_2). The kidney is responsible for the regeneration of bicarbonate ions, as well as excretion of the hydrogen ions.

Proteins: Serum and intracellular proteins offer a significant contribution to buffering acids. Hemoglobin is not only used for oxygen transport, but provides a very strong buffer for hydrogen ions (H^+). Albumin is also a significant buffer.

Chloride (Cl^-): The number of positive and negative ions in the plasma must balance at all times. Aside from the plasma proteins, bicarbonate and chloride are the two most abundant negative ions (anions) in the plasma. To maintain electrical neutrality, any change in chloride must be accompanied by the opposite change in bicarbonate concentration. If chloride increases, bicarbonate decreases (hyperchloremic acidosis) and vice-versa. Chloride concentration may influence acid-base balance.

Other buffers: Other buffers, including phosphate and ammonium, are present in very limited quantities and have a lesser impact on to the regulation of acid.

Cellular electrolytes: The cells also offer protection in the metabolic acid environment. H^+ may exchange across the cell wall, attracted by negatively charged intracellular proteins. When this happens, K^+ shifts out of the cell, causing an excess of K^+ in the blood.

EVALUATING ACID-BASE BALANCE

In order to determine the effector (what caused the change in pH) and any compensation that occurs, arterial blood gas studies should be acquired.

ABG values: ABG analysis usually is based on arterial sampling. Venous values are given as a reference.

Arterial values	**Venous values**
pH: 7.35-7.45	pH: 7.32-7.38
$Paco_2$: 35-45 mm Hg	$Pvco_2$: 42-50 mm Hg
Pao_2: 80-95 mm Hg	Pvo_2: 40 mm Hg
Saturation: 95%-99%	Saturation: 60%-80%
Base excess: −2 to +2	
*Serum HCO_3^-: 22-26 mEq/L	Serum CO_2^-: 23-27 mEq/L

---

pH (normal value 7.35-7.45): Reflects the level respiratory and metabolic acid found in the blood: the continuous balancing act that regulates the acid environment. If this balance is altered, derangements in pH occur. When pH is <7.35 or >7.45, it will be considered acute, or uncompensated.

Acidosis: Extra acids are present or base is lost, with a pH <7.40.

Alkalosis: Extra base is present or there is loss of acid, with a pH >7.40.

Any alteration in gaseous acid (CO_2) or nongaseous acid (H^+) will affect the pH. Several factors that increase H^+ are lipolysis (results in ketosis), cellular hypoxia (results in lactic acidosis), and failure to excrete H^+ and/or generate buffer (often results from renal failure).

Neutral: The pH measured when there is a perfect balance of acid and buffer. *"Perfect pH"* occurs when the body preserves neutrality (pH 6.8) inside the cells, where most chemistry occurs, and maintains the blood at pH 7.40. For the purposes of learning, the perfect pH is where all measurement begins. When the body contains either too many hydrogen ions (acidemia) or too few hydrogen ions (alkalemia) the pH will reflect the change.

$$PaCO_2 + H_2O \leftarrow H_2CO_3 \rightarrow HCO_3^- \text{ and } H^+$$

equal dissociation in a neutral environment $Paco_2$ (normal value 35-45 mm Hg): Measures pressure (partial pressure) that the dissolved carbon dioxide exerts in the arterial blood. CO_2 is released during aerobic metabolism and is the main contributor to bodily acid. CO_2 is controlled through ventilation. In the normal lung, CO_2 is regulated by changes in the rate and depth of alveolar ventilation. Respiratory compensation occurs rapidly in metabolic acid-base disturbances with normal lungs. When a patient hyperventilates, level of $Paco_2$ decreases or is "blown off" by rapid exhalations. During hypoventilation (slow and/or shallow breathing), $Paco_2$ increases or is retained due to

---

*Although serum bicarbonate is a buffer, it is usually reported in the venous blood sample as "CO_2 content" or "total CO_2" or "CO_2," and not as bicarbonate. The serum HCO_3^- concentration is usually obtained separately from ABG analysis and is critical in the determination of acid-base status.

inefficient exhalation. Chemically, the CO_2 does not contain H^+, but when dissolved in water, CO_2 + H_2O yields H_2CO_3 (carbonic acid). The pH equation shifts to the right, as the H_2CO_3 *disassociates* into H^+ and HCO_3^-. Due to the *dissociation* process, CO_2 is the largest contributor of H^+, which should be eliminated so normal pH can be maintained.

Respiratory acidosis: Alveolar hypoventilation, which results in a decreased pH.

Hypercapnia (Paco$_2$ >45 mm Hg): Signals alveolar hypoventilation and respiratory acidosis. It must be determined if the acidosis is the problem or a compensatory mechanism for metabolic alkalosis.

When respiration is insufficient (CO_2 goes up and H_2CO_3 dissociation increases)

$$\uparrow CO_2 + H_2O \rightarrow H_2CO_3 \rightarrow \uparrow HCO_3^- \text{ and } \uparrow H^+$$

CO_2 cannot be buffered in its gaseous state; thus, when CO_2 increases, the equation shifts to the right. This contributes more H^+ to the system and creates an acidotic environment. The kidneys, within 4-48 hours, should retain bicarbonate and excrete additional H^+ in an attempt to compensate for the additional respiratory acid. This process of *compensation* increases the pH to help neutralize the environment in response to acidosis created by excess CO_2.

Respiratory alkalosis: Alveolar hyperventilation, which results in an increased pH.

Hypocapnia (Paco$_2$ <35 mm Hg): Signals alveolar hyperventilation and respiratory alkalosis. It must be determined if the alkalosis is the problem or a compensatory mechanism for metabolic acidosis.

When respiration is too fast (CO_2 goes down, and H_2CO_3 dissociation decreases)

$$\downarrow CO_2 + H_2O \rightarrow H_2CO_3 \rightarrow \downarrow HCO_3^- \text{ and } \downarrow H^+$$

The kidneys, within 4-48 hr, should excrete bicarbonate and retain additional H^+ in an attempt to compensate for the lack of respiratory acid.

Partial pressure of oxygen; Pao$_2$: **(normal value 80-100 mm Hg):** The Pao$_2$ is a measure of the dissolved (usable) gas in the arteries. The dissolved gas exerts the pressure of oxygen, enabling it to diffuse across the capillary and cell wall to oxygenate cells.

Hypoxemia (Pao$_2$ <80 mm Hg): Low partial pressure of oxygen impairs the ability of the cells to extract oxygen from the blood and can lead to anaerobic metabolism, resulting in lactic acid production and metabolic acidosis. Pao$_2$ normally declines in the older adult.

P/F ratio (>400): Pao$_2$ is evaluated in relationship to Fio$_2$; that is, the higher the oxygen pressure that is delivered to the lungs, the higher the oxygen in the blood should be.

$$\text{Pao}_2/\text{Fio}_2 \text{ (in the decimal)} = \text{the P/F ratio}$$
$$100/0.21 = 476$$
$$\text{Normal P/F} > 400$$

Oxygen saturation; Sao$_2$: (normal values 95%-100% or 0.95-1.00) Hemoglobin is the primary transporter of oxygen and supplies a reservoir (reserve) of oxygen for cellular use. Each hemoglobin (Hgb) molecule carries 1.36 ml of oxygen. Oxygen must be released from the Hgb, dissolve in blood, and exert pressure to diffuse across the cell wall. Saturation (Sao$_2$) reflects the loading of oxygen onto Hgb in the lungs. The uptake/use of oxygen by the tissues can only be measured by Svo$_2$ and/or Scvo$_2$ (mixed venous and central venous saturation of Hgb). Cellular metabolism and oxygen utilization is affected by changes in stress level, temperature, pH, blood flow, and Paco$_2$. When the Pao$_2$ falls to <60 mm Hg, there is a large drop in saturation, reflected by the oxyhemoglobin dissociation curve.

Pulse oximetry (Spo$_2$): Can be used to monitor arterial oxygen saturation and determine ventilation status (the loading of oxygen onto hemoglobin in the lungs). This noninvasive monitoring technique is frequently used in critical care areas for patients at high risk of ventilation problems, in operating rooms, and emergency departments. Spo$_2$ should be correlated with Sao$_2$ (or oxyhemoglobin) via ABG studies, with the initiation of oximetry to assess accuracy of Spo$_2$ readings. Pulse oximetry is a close correlate to Sao$_2$, but the measure of true oxyhemoglobin (saturation) requires an ABG analysis.

Mixed venous oxygen saturation (Svo$_2$: normal values 60%-80% or 0.60-0.80) or central venous (Scvo$_2$: normal values 65%-85% or 0.65-0.85) oxygen saturation: Mixed venous or central venous saturation of Hgb evaluates the tissue use of oxygen. The comparison of postcellular and precellular Hgb saturation is used to evaluate the tissue oxygen consumption compared to oxygen delivery. Mixed venous (Svo$_2$) or central venous oxygen saturation (Scvo$_2$) is measured by an indwelling oxygen probe/sensor in a central vein or pulmonary artery (on a PA catheter). Measurement may provide an early indication of perfusion failure or increased tissue demands for oxygen, reflected by a decreased mixed venous saturation of Hgb. If this saturation is normal or high but the patient has an increased lactate level, the cells may be unable to extract or use the oxygen. Mixed venous saturation values are always correlated with tissue indicators of hypoxia, base deficit, serum bicarbonate, and lactate levels.

Base excess or deficit (normal value -2 to +2): A calculated indicator of circulating buffer (or available base) which reflects the tissue and renal tubular presence (or absence) of acid. As the proportion of acid rises, the relative amount of base decreases (and vice versa). Abnormally high values (>+2) reflect alkalosis; low values (<−2) reflect acidosis.

Serum bicarbonate (normal value 22-26mEq/L): Serum HCO_3^- is the major renal component of acid-base regulation. It is generated or excreted by the kidneys in direct proportion to the amount of circulating acid to maintain a normal acid-base environment. When the bicarbonate level changes, acid level changes in the opposite direction. To determine the cause of bicarbonate changes (problem vs. compensation), the relationship to pH must be evaluated. The pH will respond to the presence or absence of acid, and the directional relationship reflects how the pH alteration was caused.

Metabolic acidosis: Decreased HCO_3^- levels (<22 mEq/L) signify an increase in circulating metabolic acid and are indicative of metabolic acidosis. Not often seen as a compensatory mechanism for respiratory alkalosis. Metabolic acids are bodily acids which cannot be exhaled. These acids should be neutralized by buffers, excreted by the kidneys, or metabolized. The end product of normal aerobic glucose metabolism (when oxygen enters the cell) is pyruvate, which must be metabolized into CO_2, H_2O, and a small amount of lactate. With anaerobic metabolism (oxygen is not entering the cell), production of lactate and pyruvate are increased, creating more metabolic acids (increased H^+). Abundant lactate and ketones cause lactic acidosis and ketoacidosis. When an increase in H^+ occurs, H^+ and HCO_3^- combine on the right side of the formula and shift the equation to the left. CO_2 is then created from the excess metabolic acids.

When metabolism is failing (H^+ goes up and H_2CO_3 dissociation increases)

$$\uparrow CO_2 + H_2O \leftarrow H_2CO_3 \leftarrow HCO_3^- \text{ and } \uparrow H^+$$

The lungs, if normal, can exhale CO_2 by hyperventilation. The process of exhaling CO_2 in response to excess metabolic acids is called *compensation.*

Metabolic alkalosis: Elevated HCO_3^- levels (>26 mEq/L) reflect decreasing circulating metabolic acids. Occurs either as a primary metabolic disorder or as a compensatory alteration in response to respiratory acidosis.

When metabolic acids are lost or bicarbonate is depleted, dissociation of H_2CO_3 decreases

$$\downarrow CO_2 + H_2O \leftarrow H_2CO_3 \leftarrow \downarrow HCO_3^- \text{ and } \downarrow H^+$$

The lungs should decrease the rate and depth of respirations to retain carbon dioxide, to compensate for the lack of metabolic acid or excess of bicarbonate, so the pH can return to normal range.

Step-by-step guide to ABG analysis

A systematic analysis is critical to the accurate interpretation of ABG values.

Step 1: Check the pH: Determine if pH is perfect (7.40). If it is not perfect, determine if the direction of the difference is above or below 7.40. Next, determine if it is in the range of normal (7.35 to 7.45). If it is abnormal, identify whether it is on the acidotic (<7.35) or alkalotic (>7.45) side of normal.

Step 2: Check the Paco$_2$: Check Paco$_2$ for perfect levels (40 mm Hg). If not perfect, determine if the direction of change is above or below 40 mm Hg. Next, determine if CO_2 is in the range of normal (35-45 mm Hg). If abnormal, identify whether it is on the acidotic (>45 mm Hg) or alkalotic (<35 mm Hg) side of normal. If Paco$_2$ has been retained as a result of hypoventilation or overly removed through hyperventilation, the change in pH will be in the opposite direction of the Paco$_2$. Elevated CO_2 lowers pH, while decreased CO_2 increases pH. If the change in pH is in normal range but not perfect, with a Paco$_2$ value which has traveled in the opposite direction, respiratory acid changes caused an imbalance that may be compensated by the kidneys. Using this technique helps determine whether the primary problem is respiratory (involving Paco$_2$) or metabolic (reflected by HCO_3^-).

Step 3: Check HCO$_3^-$ and base (deficit or excess): Check bicarbonate (24 mEq/L) and base (0) for perfect levels. If not perfect, determine if the direction of change is above or below perfect. Next, determine if HCO_3^- (22-26 mEq/L) and base (+2 to −2) are in the range of normal. If the values are abnormal, relate the two values to metabolic acid (H^+). If bicarbonate and base are decreased (a deficit), metabolic acid is increased. If bicarbonate and base are increased (in excess), metabolic acid is decreased. If changes in the metabolic acid (determined by the change in bicarbonate and base) caused a change from perfect pH, the change in pH will be in the same direction as the amount of buffer, which is the opposite direction of the amount of metabolic acids. Elevated bicarbonate or base cause increased pH (low H^+ level). Decreased levels of bicarbonate or base cause decreased pH (high H^+ level). If the change in pH is inside normal range but not perfect and the HCO_3^- or base has traveled in the same direction, metabolic acid (H^+) changes caused the problem, and the lungs may be attempting to compensate by regulating CO_2. Using this technique helps determine whether the primary problem is respiratory (involving $Paco_2$) or metabolic (reflected by bicarbonate).

Step 4: (Evaluate both CO2 and HCO$_3^-$): If both $Paco_2$ and HCO_3^- are abnormal, the value that deviates the most from normal suggests the primary disturbance responsible for the altered pH. A mixed metabolic-respiratory disturbance or compensatory elements may be present, as discussed in prior $Paco_2$ and HCO_3^- steps 2 and 3.

Step 5: Check Pao2 and Sao2: Check Pao_2 and oxygen saturation to determine whether they are decreased, normal, or increased. Decreased Pao_2 and O_2 saturation can lead to lactic acidosis and may signal the need for increased concentrations of oxygen. Conversely, high Pao_2 may indicate the need to decrease delivered concentrations of oxygen.

COMPENSATION

When evaluating the arterial blood gas, the pH change is what determines the problem. Anytime the pH deviates from perfect, an evaluation must be made to determine whether the opposing systems (on opposite sides of the acid-base equation; respiratory or metabolic) are contributing acid or providing compensatory regulation. Values indicate whether arterial pH is perfect (7.4), acidic (<7. 4), or alkalotic (>7.4). When pH is <7.35 or >7.45, it will be considered acute, or uncompensated. Even though perfection is difficult to achieve, pH must be first evaluated as being perfect or within the normal range. The effect on pH is always related to the acid (H^+) direction, for example:

Problem of respiratory acidosis: $Paco_2$ 60 mm Hg ($\uparrow$above normal range)
pH: 7.24 ($\downarrow$below normal range)
Renal compensation: $HCO_3^-\uparrow$ to 30 mEq/L and $H^+\downarrow$, so pH increases to 7.35
Full compensation: pH returns to normal range but on the acid side (7.35 is below 7.40)

$$\uparrow CO_2 + H_2O \rightarrow H_2CO_3 \rightarrow \uparrow HCO_3^- \text{ and } \downarrow H^+ \text{ in 4-48 hr}$$

Note: If renal compensation increased the HCO_3^- to 28 mEq/L and the pH increased to only 7.33, the patient achieves ***partial compensation***. Full compensation indicates the pH has returned to normal range.

When CO_2 goes up, there is a shift to the right, prompting increased excretion of H^+ of HCO_3^- by the kidneys.

Because of buffers and other compensatory mechanisms, a near-normal pH level does not exclude the possibility of an acid-base disturbance. However, it is rare to see a perfect pH with compensation for either a metabolic or respiratory deficit. Compensation will bring the pH into range but generally not back to perfect.

CARING FOR ADULTS WITH ACID-BASE IMBALANCES

ACUTE RESPIRATORY ACIDOSIS

Pathophysiology
Respiratory acidosis (hypercapnia) occurs secondary to alveolar hypoventilation and results in an elevated $Paco_2$. $Paco_2$ derangements are direct reflections of the degree of ventilatory function or dysfunction. The degree to which the increased $Paco_2$ alters the pH depends on the rapidity of onset and the body's ability to compensate through the blood buffer and renal systems. The pH may be profoundly affected initially because of the delay (hours to days) before renal compensation occurs. Acute rises in $Paco_2$ precipitate a rise in extracellular buffering systems (primarily hemoglobin and proteins) even before renal compensation occurs, but the extracellular rise is not sufficient to maintain a normal pH in the presence of an elevated $Paco_2$.

The most common cause of inadequate CO_2 excretion is inadequate alveolar ventilation and may be a symptom of poor ventilatory support.

$$\uparrow CO_2 + H_2O \rightarrow H_2CO_3 \rightarrow \uparrow HCO_3^- \text{ and } H^+ \text{ (not enough time for excretion)}$$

Too much acid!!

ACUTE RESPIRATORY ACIDOSIS (UNCOMPENSATED)

Clinical presentation: Dyspnea, tachypnea, nausea, vomiting, headache, fine tremors, asterixis, and restlessness and confusion leading to lethargy and coma. The restlessness and confusion are early signs that may be subtle but are very important indicators.

Physical assessment: Increased heart and respiratory rates, diminished or absent breath sound; patient may have asymmetric chest expansion, hypotension, and diaphoresis. Severe hypercapnia may cause cerebral vasodilation, resulting in increased intracranial pressure (IICP). Another finding may be dilated conjunctival and facial blood vessels.

Monitoring parameters: Presence of ventricular dysrhythmias; IICP.

Diagnostic tests

ABG analysis: Aids in diagnosis and determination of severity of respiratory acidosis. $Paco_2$ will be >45 mm Hg and pH will be <7.35 (if acute). If the patient is breathing room air, hypoxemia always will be present to some degree with increased $Paco_2$.

Serum bicarbonate: Initially, HCO_3^- values will be normal (22-26 mEq/L), unless a mixed disorder is present.

Serum electrolyte levels: Usually not altered; depend on cause of respiratory acidosis.

Chest x-ray: Determines presence of underlying respiratory disease.

Drug screen: Determines presence and quantity of drug if patient is suspected of taking an overdose.

Collaborative management

Restoration of effective alveolar ventilation: Support ventilation. If $Paco_2$ is >50-60 mm Hg, Pao_2 is ≤50 mm Hg, and clinical signs of ventilatory failure (e.g., confusion, lethargy) are present, the patient usually requires intubation and mechanical ventilation. The primary mechanism to treat respiratory acidosis is to increase the tidal volume (Vt) and/or the respiratory rate (F), to increase minute ventilation (Vt × F). Generally, use of bicarbonate is avoided because of the risk of alkalosis when the respiratory disturbance has been corrected. Although a life-threatening pH must be corrected to an acceptable level promptly, a normal pH is not the immediate goal.

Treatment of underlying disorder.

Nursing diagnoses and interventions

Nursing diagnoses and interventions are specific to the pathophysiologic process. See the "Respiratory" section, p. 175, for acute pneumonia (p. 180), acute lung injury and respiratory distress syndrome (p. 189), and acute respiratory failure (p. 201), along with mechanical ventilation (p. 14).

CHRONIC RESPIRATORY ACIDOSIS (COMPENSATED)

Pathophysiology

This disorder occurs in pulmonary diseases in which effective alveolar ventilation is decreased. For CO_2 to be removed from the blood, the partial pressure of CO_2 in the alveoli must be less than that in the blood. In air-trapping syndrome or profound hypoventilation states, the alveolar concentration of CO_2 will limit the removal of CO_2 from the blood. Over time, the amount of CO_2 eliminated is less than the amount generated and thus $Paco_2$ levels increase. Chronic hypercapnia occurs with chronic obstructive pulmonary disorders (e.g., chronic emphysema and bronchitis, cystic fibrosis), restrictive disorders (e.g., pneumothorax, hemothorax, pickwickian syndrome), neuromuscular abnormalities (e.g., myasthenia gravis, Guillain-Barré syndrome, amyotrophic lateral sclerosis), and respiratory center depression (e.g., brain tumor, stroke, bleed, head injury). In patients with a chronic lung disease, a near-normal pH can be seen if renal function is normal, even if the $Paco_2$ is as high as 60 mm Hg. Chronic compensation from the kidney (retention and generation of serum HCO_3^- >26 mEq/L and an increase in renal excretion of metabolic acid) occurs and maintains an acceptable acid-base environment, which results in a near-normal pH level. Patients with chronic lung disease can experience acute rises in $Paco_2$ or lose their metabolic compensation (increased production of metabolic acid or loss of renal function) secondary to superimposed disease states such as pneumonia, hypermetabolic cellular hypoxia, or renal dysfunction. If the chronic compensatory mechanisms in place (e.g., elevated HCO_3^-) are inadequate to meet the sudden increase in $Paco_2$, or if the circulation of metabolic acids increases, decompensation may occur with a resultant decrease in pH.

Carbon dioxide is the main contributor of H^+. As CO_2 increases, a shift to the right occurs over time.

$$\uparrow CO_2 + H_2O \rightarrow H_2CO_3 \rightarrow \uparrow HCO_3^- \text{ and } H^+ \textbf{ (excreted)}$$

Making room for acid!

Assessment
History and risk factors
Chronic obstructive pulmonary disease (COPD): Predominantly emphysema and bronchitis; cystic fibrosis.
Extreme obesity: Pickwickian syndrome.
Acute respiratory infection in a patient with COPD.
Exposure to pulmonary toxins: Occupational risk; pollution.
Clinical presentation: If the $Paco_2$ does not exceed the body's ability to compensate, no specific findings will be noted. If $Paco_2$ rises rapidly, the following may occur: dyspnea, asterixis, agitation, and insomnia progressing to somnolence, hypotension (vasodilating properties of CO_2), and coma. The progression of symptoms may be subtle. Thorough assessment and evaluation are important.
Physical assessment: Tachypnea, cyanosis (depending on the underlying disorder). Severe hypercapnia ($Paco_2$ >70 mm Hg) may cause cerebral vasodilation resulting in increased intracranial pressure (IICP), papilledema, and dilated conjunctival and facial blood vessels. Depending on the underlying pathophysiologic process, edema may be present secondary to right ventricular failure.
Monitoring parameters: Supraventricular tachycardia and ventricular tachycardia are common with an acute exacerbation.

Diagnostic tests
ABG values: These provide data necessary for determining the diagnosis and severity of respiratory acidosis. Although the $Paco_2$ will be elevated, the pH level will be near normal, although on the acidic (low) side of normal. Increased excretion of H^+ shifts the equation to the right except in patients who also have an acute pulmonary disorder or metabolic problem superimposed on chronic hypercapnia (e.g., pneumonia). If the $Paco_2$ has increased abruptly from baseline value, a pH value lower than normal may be seen.
Serum electrolyte levels: Serum HCO_3^- is especially helpful in determining the level of metabolic compensation that has occurred (e.g., HCO_3^- increased with a near-normal pH value if fully compensated). This information is particularly useful in identifying "mixed" acid-base disturbances, because the HCO_3^- is expected to be elevated in chronic respiratory acidosis. If the HCO_3^- is normal or low in a patient who has a history of chronic respiratory acidosis or who was previously compensated, the pH will be dropping and may signal a second pathologic process
Chest x-ray: Determines extent of underlying pulmonary disease and identifies further pathologic changes that may be responsible in acute exacerbation (e.g., pneumonia).
ECG: Isoelectric P wave and an isoelectric QRS complex in lead I in a middle-aged or older adult suggest chronic bronchitis or emphysema.
Sputum culture: Determines presence of pathogens causing an acute exacerbation of a chronic pulmonary disease (e.g., pneumonia) present in a patient with COPD.

Collaborative management
Oxygen therapy: Used cautiously in patients with chronic CO_2 retention for whom hypoxemia, rather than hypercapnia, stimulates ventilation. Patient may require intubation and mechanical ventilation for stupor and coma precipitated by oxygen, if the drive to breathe is eliminated by high concentrations of oxygen. Continuous pulse oximetry may be used for close monitoring of oxygen delivery and to help ensure maintenance of oxygen saturation within acceptable range (e.g., 90%-92%).
Pharmacotherapy: Bronchodilators and antibiotics as indicated. Narcotics and sedatives can depress the respiratory center and are avoided unless intubation and mechanical ventilation are in place.
IV fluids: Maintain adequate hydration for mobilizing pulmonary secretions.
Chest physiotherapy: Aids in expectoration of sputum. Includes postural drainage if hypersecretions are present. Assess patient closely during this procedure because it may be poorly tolerated, especially the postural drainage component.
Bronchoscopy: Visualizes the airways and secretions of the patient. Protected bronchoalveolar lavage (BAL) may be performed in order to fully appreciate the content and amount of secretions.

Nursing diagnoses and interventions
Impaired gas exchange related to alveolar-capillary membrane changes secondary to pulmonary tissue destruction
Desired outcome: Within 24 hr of initiation of treatment, patient has adequate gas exchange as evidenced by $Paco_2$, pH, and Sao_2 that are normal or within 10% of patient's baseline.

- Monitor serial ABG results to assess patient's response to therapy. Consult physician for significant findings: increasing $Paco_2$ with decreasing pH, Pao_2, and Sao_2 values.
- Monitor oxygen saturation via pulse oximetry (Spo_2). Compare Spo_2 with Sao_2 values to assess reliability. Watch Spo_2 closely, especially when changing Fio_2 or to evaluate patient's response to treatment (e.g., repositioning, chest physiotherapy).
- Assess and document patient's respiratory status: respiratory rate and rhythm, exertional effort, and breath sounds. Compare pretreatment findings with posttreatment findings (e.g., oxygen therapy, physiotherapy, medications) for evidence of improvement.
- Assess and document patient's LOC. If $Paco_2$ increases, be alert to subtle, progressive changes in mental status. A common progression is agitation/insomnia/somnolence/coma. To avoid a comatose state caused by rising CO_2 levels, always evaluate the arousability of a patient with elevated $Paco_2$ who appears to be sleeping. Consult physician if patient is difficult to arouse.
- Ensure appropriate delivery of prescribed oxygen therapy. Assess patient's respiratory status after every change in Fio_2. Patients with chronic CO_2 retention may be very sensitive to increases in Fio_2, resulting in depressed ventilatory drive. If patient requires mechanical ventilation, be aware of the importance of maintaining the compensated acid-base status. If the $Paco_2$ is rapidly decreased by excessive mechanical ventilation, a severe metabolic alkalosis (posthypercapnic metabolic alkalosis) could develop. The sudden onset of metabolic alkalosis may lead to hypocalcemia, which can result in tetany (see "Hypocalcemia," p. 554). Severe alkalosis also can precipitate cardiac dysrhythmias.
- Assess for presence of bowel sounds, and monitor for GI distention, which can impede movement of the diaphragm and restrict ventilatory effort further.
- Assess for presence of symmetric lung expansion and normal resonance of lung fields. Hyperresonance and asymmetry indicate pneumothorax; dullness and asymmetry indicate solid tissue or fluid occupation of lung or pleural space (e.g., hemothorax, pleural effusion, hyperplasia).
- In patient without intubation, encourage use of pursed-lip breathing (inhalation through nose, with slow exhalation through pursed lips), which helps airways to remain open and allows for better air excursion. Optimally, this technique will diminish air entrapment in the lungs and make respiratory effort more efficient.

ACUTE RESPIRATORY ALKALOSIS (HYPOCAPNIA)
Pathophysiology
Respiratory alkalosis occurs as a result of an increase in the rate of alveolar ventilation (alveolar hyperventilation). It is defined as $Paco_2$ <35 mm Hg. Acute alveolar hyperventilation results most frequently from anxiety and is commonly referred to as *hyperventilation syndrome*. In addition, numerous physiologic disorders that cause hypoxemia (e.g., early acute respiratory distress syndrome, pneumonia, pulmonary edema, pulmonary emboli) can cause acute hypocapnia. Hypocapnia causes increased pH and a fall in the alveolar (A-a) gradient of oxygen.

The rise in pH is modified to a small degree by intracellular buffering. To compensate for increased CO_2 loss and the resultant base excess, hydrogen ions are released from tissue buffers, which in turn lowers the plasma HCO_3^- concentration. Whenever hydrogen ions are released from tissue, potassium will enter the cell and the result may be hypokalemia. Renal compensation for the respiratory alkalosis is not clinically apparent for hours; maximal compensation is not seen for days. Acute respiratory alkalosis can progress to chronic respiratory alkalosis if it persists for >6 hr and renal compensation occurs.

$$\downarrow CO_2 + H_2O \rightarrow H_2CO_3 \rightarrow \text{ (not enough time for } H^+ \text{ resorption)}$$

No compensation: Not enough acid!!

Assessment
History and risk factors
Anxiety: Patient is often unaware of hyperventilation.
Acute hypoxemia: Pulmonary disorders (e.g., pneumonia, pulmonary edema, pulmonary thromboembolism) and extremely high altitudes (e.g., >6500 ft) may result in hypoxemia, which stimulates the ventilatory effort, causing respiratory alkalosis. Tissue acidosis (e.g., systemic inflammation, sepsis, DKA, lactic acidemia) will stimulate the respiratory effort, resulting in respiratory alkalosis.
Hypermetabolic states: Fever; sepsis, pain, agitation.
Salicylate intoxication.
Excessive mechanical ventilation: Increased tidal volume or RR.
CNS trauma: That which results in damage to respiratory center.

Clinical presentation: Lightheadedness, anxiety, paresthesias (especially of the fingers), circumoral numbness. In extreme alkalosis, confusion, tetany, syncope, and seizures may occur.
Physical assessment: Increased rate and depth of respirations (hyperventilation).
Monitoring parameters: Cardiac dysrhythmias.

Diagnostic tests

ABG values: $Paco_2$ <35 mm Hg and pH >7.45 will be present. A decreased Pao_2, along with the clinical picture (e.g., pneumonia, pulmonary edema, pulmonary embolism), may help diagnose cause of the respiratory alkalosis.
Serum electrolyte levels: HCO_3^- will be decreased 2 mEq/L for each 10 mm Hg drop in $Paco_2$ as a result of the release of H^+ release from nonbicarbonate buffers and tissues, the excretion of bicarbonate, and the shift to the left.

Caution: BE SURE that the respiratory alkalosis is NOT COMPENSATING FOR primary metabolic acidosis.

- *Sodium* and *potassium* may be decreased slightly (potassium will shift from the extra cellular space to the intracellular space in exchange for H^+).
- *Serum calcium* may be decreased because of increased calcium and bicarbonate binding. Signs of hypocalcemia include muscle cramps, hyperactive reflexes, carpal spasm, tetany, and convulsions.
- *Serum phosphorus* may decrease (<2.5 mg/dl), especially with salicylate intoxication and sepsis, because the alkalosis causes increased uptake of phosphorus by the cells. No symptoms occur, and treatment usually is not required unless a preexisting phosphorus deficit is present.

ECG: Detects cardiac dysrhythmias, which may occur with alkalosis.

Collaborative management
Treatment of underlying disorder.
Reassurance or sedation: If anxiety is the cause of decreased $Paco_2$. If symptoms are severe, it may be necessary for patient to rebreathe exhaled air via a paper bag. Not all care providers support this strategy.
Oxygen therapy: If hypoxemia is the causative factor, increase Fio_2. If increases in Fio_2 do not result in resolution of hypoxemia and the patient does not have acute restrictive disorders, increase PEEP with circuit PEEP (dialed at ventilator) or mechanical PEEP (prolonged inspiratory time, high frequency ventilation).
Adjustments to mechanical ventilators: Settings are checked and adjustments made to ventilatory parameters in response to ABG results that signal hypocapnia. Respiratory rate and/or volume are decreased, and dead space is added, if necessary, by attaching extra tubing to the mechanical ventilator circuitry.
Pharmacotherapy: Sedatives and tranquilizers may be given for anxiety-induced respiratory alkalosis.
Evaluate for tissue hypoxia: If tissue hypoxia is the problem and respiratory alkalosis is the compensation, see "Acute Metabolic Acidosis," p. 576.

Nursing diagnoses and interventions
Ineffective breathing pattern related to anxiety, tissue hypoxia, or work of breathing
Desired outcome: If the respiratory alkalosis is primary, within 4 hr of initiating treatment, patient's breathing pattern is effective as evidenced by a state of eupnea; $Paco_2$ ≥35 mm Hg; and pH =7.45.
- To help alleviate anxiety, reassure patient that a staff member will remain with him or her.
- Encourage patient to breathe slowly. Pace patient's breathing pattern by having him or her mimic your own breathing pattern.
- Monitor patient's cardiac rhythm. Consult physician for new or increased dysrhythmias. With acute respiratory alkalosis, even a modest alkalosis can precipitate dysrhythmias in a patient with a preexisting heart disease who is also taking inotropic drugs (see Appendix 7). In part, this is caused by the hypokalemia that occurs with alkalosis.
- Administer sedatives or tranquilizers as prescribed. Assess and document effectiveness.
- Have patient rebreathe into a paper bag as indicated (if practice is supported by institution).
- Ensure that patient rests undisturbed after his or her breathing pattern has stabilized. Hyperventilation can result in fatigue.

Note: Hyperventilation may lead to hypocalcemic tetany despite a normal or near-normal calcium level because of increased binding of calcium.

CHRONIC RESPIRATORY ALKALOSIS

Pathophysiology

Chronic respiratory alkalosis is a state of chronic hypocapnia caused by stimulation of the respiratory center. The decreased $Paco_2$ stimulates the renal compensatory response and results in a proportionate decrease in plasma bicarbonate (and retention of H^+) until a new, steady state is reached. Maximal renal compensatory response requires several days to occur and can result in a normal or near-normal pH. Chronic respiratory alkalosis is not commonly seen in acutely ill patients, but when present it can signal a poor prognosis.

$$\downarrow CO_2 + H_2O \rightarrow H_2CO_3 \rightarrow \downarrow HCO_3^- \text{ and } \uparrow H^+ \text{ (resorbed)}$$

Compensation attained: Retaining acid!!

Assessment

History and risk factors

Cerebral disease: Tumor, encephalitis, stroke.

Chronic hepatic insufficiency: A sustained respiratory alkalosis with this diagnosis has a poor prognosis.

Restrictive lung diseases: Interstitial pulmonary fibrosis. Respiratory alkalosis continues throughout the course of the disease. A normal $Paco_2$ followed by increased $Paco_2$ occurs in the terminal stage of the disease.

Pregnancy.

Chronic hypoxia: Adaptation to high altitude, cyanotic heart disease, lung disease resulting in decreased compliance (e.g., fibrosis).

Clinical presentation: Individuals with chronic respiratory alkalosis are usually free of symptoms.

Physical assessment: Increased respiratory rate and depth.

Diagnostic tests

ABG values: $Paco_2$ will be <35 mm Hg, with a near-normal or normal pH; Pao_2 may be decreased, and hypoxemia can either be the causative factor or a result of inadequate time/flow of oxygen.

Serum electrolyte levels: Probably will be normal, with the exception of plasma HCO_3^-, which will decrease as renal compensation occurs.

Phosphate levels: Hypophosphatemia (as low as 0.5 mg/dl) may be seen with intense hyperventilation. Alkalosis causes increased uptake of phosphate by the cells.

Collaborative management

Treatment of underlying cause.

Oxygen therapy: If hypoxemia is present and identified as causative factor in respiratory alkalosis.

Nursing diagnoses and interventions

Nursing diagnoses and interventions are specific to the pathophysiologic process. See appropriate medical disorders and nursing diagnoses in this and other chapters.

ACUTE METABOLIC ACIDOSIS

Pathophysiology

Metabolic acidosis occurs for a variety of reasons, so unlike simple respiratory alterations, metabolic acidosis (bicarbonate down and/or base in deficit and pH below 7.35) must be evaluated for a variety of problems.

Excess H+ production: The most common cause of metabolic acidosis is the excessive production of organic acids such as lactate in anaerobic metabolism (tissue hypoxia or extreme exercise). When tissues metabolize anaerobically, pyruvate fails to be fully converted to CO_2 and H_2O, instead increasing the yield of lactate and H^+. Another type of metabolic acidosis is caused by increased production of ketone bodies after metabolizing fats (diabetic ketoacidosis). This abnormal metabolic pathway produces H^+ in excess.

Loss of alkali: When patients have persistent diarrhea or loss of small bowel contents, they may have an excessive wasting of bicarbonate.

Decreased acid excretion by the kidneys (e.g., acute and chronic renal failure): When the renal tubules are dysfunctional (acute tubular necrosis or chronic renal failure), there is a concomitant failure to excrete H^+ and reabsorb bicarbonate.

The decrease in pH (high presence of H^+) stimulates respirations. Attempts to compensate occur rapidly, as manifested by lowering of the $Paco_2$, which may be reduced to as little as 10-15 mm Hg. The most important mechanism for ridding the body of excess H^+ is the increase in acid excretion through ventilation. In addition, if the kidney is functional, acid will be excreted and bicarbonate reabsorbed. Nonvolatile acids, however, may accumulate more rapidly than they can be neutralized by the body's buffers, compensated for by the respiratory system, or excreted by the kidneys.

$$\text{(slight)} \downarrow CO_2 + H_2O \leftarrow H_2CO_3 \leftarrow \downarrow HCO_3^- \text{ and } H^+ \uparrow$$

Not enough compensation: Too much acid!!

Measuring metabolic acidosis: In any patient whose condition arouses suspicion (e.g., with tachycardia, tachypnea, hyperventilation and/or hypotension), it is essential to directly measure acid. All patients who run the risk of cellular hypoxia must have a sample drawn for a lactate level. An arterial lactate sample should be placed on ice and taken as soon as possible to the lab. Any lactate >4 mMol/dL is indicative of severe tissue hypoxia and hypoperfusion. If the glucose is elevated a serum ketone level should also be drawn.

- Lactate and ketone measurements are a direct indicator of acid production.
- Total CO_2 (serum CO_2) is a direct measure of the reservoir for bicarbonate and reflects level of both bicarbonate and acidosis.
- Bicarbonate is a direct calculated measure of the content of buffer in the blood and indirectly reflects acid.
- Base is a calculation based on the bicarbonate.

Assessment
History and risk factors
Ketoacidosis: Diabetes mellitus, alcoholism, starvation.
Lactic acidosis: Respiratory or circulatory failure, drugs and toxins, hereditary disorders, septic shock, hypovolemia, and hemorrhage. Lactic acidosis can be associated with other disease states such as leukemia, pancreatitis, bacterial infection, and uncontrolled diabetes mellitus.
Renal disease: Acute renal failure, renal tubular acidosis.
Poisonings and drug toxicity: Salicylates, methanol, ethylene glycol, ammonium chloride.
Loss of alkali: Draining wounds (e.g., pancreatic fistulas), diarrhea, and ureterostomy.
Clinical presentation: Findings vary, depending on underlying disease states and the severity of the acid-base disturbance and the speed with which it developed. There may be changes in LOC that range from fatigue and confusion to stupor and coma.
Physical assessment: Tachycardia (until pH <7, then bradycardia), decreased BP, tachypnea leading to alveolar hyperventilation (Kussmaul respirations), dysrhythmias, and shock state. Depending on the type of shock and the vascular response, skin temperature and color will be affected. Mild metabolic acidosis (HCO_3^- 15-18 mEq/L) may result in no symptoms, whereas symptoms will develop with a pH <7.2.
Monitoring parameters: A waveform suggestive of hyperkalemia (prolonged PR interval, widened QRS, and peaked T waves) may occur. Persistent tachycardia may indicate tissue hypoperfusion.

Diagnostic tests
ABG values: Determine pH (usually <7.35) and degree of respiratory compensation as reflected by $Paco_2$, which is usually <35 mm Hg.
Serum bicarbonate: Determines presence of metabolic acidosis (HCO_3^- <22 mEq/L, signifying a significant increase in H^+).
Serum electrolyte levels: Elevated potassium (K^+ >5 mEq/L) may be present as the H^+ moves into the cells to be buffered and the K^+ moves out of the cells to maintain electroneutrality. Hyperkalemia related to metabolic acidosis occurs most frequently in renal failure and diabetic ketoacidosis. If the K^+ is normal or low in the presence of metabolic acidosis, this signals low body stores of K^+ or profound hypokalemia.

Anion gap
To help identify the cause of metabolic acidosis, an analysis of serum electrolytes to detect anion gap may be helpful. *Anion gap* reflects immeasurable anions (acids or H^+) present in plasma and is calculated by subtracting the sum of chloride (bases) and sodium bicarbonate (or total serum CO_2) from plasma sodium concentration.

$$\text{Anion gap} = Na^+ - (Cl^- + HCO_3^-) \text{*or replace } HCO_3^- \text{ with total } CO_2$$

Normal anion gap is 12 (±2) mEq/L. Normal anion gap acidosis results from direct loss of HCO_3^- (e.g., diarrhea, renal tubular acidosis, pancreatic fistulas) or the addition of chloride-containing acids (e.g., ammonium chloride, hydrochloric acid), some hyperalimentation fluids, and oral calcium chloride. "**Non–gap acidosis**" may occur with hyperchloremia. If the patient is in metabolic acidosis, an increased anion gap acidosis >20 mEq/L indicates an increase of nonvolatile acids (H^+: acids from lactic acidosis, DKA, renal failure, salicylate and methanol toxicity).

ECG: Detects dysrhythmias, which may be caused by metabolic acidosis or hyperkalemia. Changes seen with hyperkalemia include peaked T waves, depressed ST segment, decreased size of R waves, decreased or absent P waves, and widened QRS complex. Ventricular fibrillation may occur.

Collaborative management
Sodium bicarbonate (NaHCO₃): May be indicated when arterial pH is ≤7.15. The usual mode of delivery is IV drip: 2-3 ampules (44.5 mEq/ampule) in 1000 ml D_5W, although $NaHCO_3$ may be given by IV push in emergencies. Deficit should be calculated and replaced accordingly.

Total body weight × base deficit/4 = the amount of sodium bicarbonate that must be replaced

Concentration depends on severity of the acidosis and presence of any serum sodium disorders. $NaHCO_3$ must be given very cautiously to avoid metabolic alkalosis and pulmonary edema as a result of the sodium load.
Potassium replacement: Usually, serum hyperkalemia is present, but an intracellular potassium deficit may be present. If a potassium deficit exists (K^+ <3.5), it must be corrected before $NaHCO_3$ is administered, because when the acidosis is corrected, the potassium shifts back to intracellular spaces. This shift in K^+ could result in serum hypokalemia with serious consequences, such as cardiac irritability with fatal dysrhythmias and generalized muscle weakness. See "Hypokalemia," p. ###, for more information.
Mechanical ventilation: If mechanical ventilation is required on the basis of ABG results and clinical signs, it is important that the patient's compensatory hyperventilation be allowed to continue to prevent acidosis from becoming more severe. Therefore the respiratory rate on the ventilator should not be set lower than the rate at which patient has been breathing spontaneously, and the tidal volume should be large enough to maintain compensatory hyperventilation until the underlying disorder can be resolved.
Treatment of underlying disorder:
Diabetic ketoacidosis: Insulin and fluids. If acidosis is severe (with a pH of <7.15 or HCO_3^- 6-8 mEq/L), judicious administration of $NaHCO_3$ may be necessary.
Alcoholism-related ketoacidosis: Glucose and saline.
Diarrhea: Usually occurs in association with other fluid and electrolyte disturbances; correction addresses concurrent imbalances.
Acute renal failure: Hemodialysis or peritoneal dialysis to maintain an adequate level of plasma HCO_3^-.
Renal tubular acidosis: May require modest amounts (<100 mEq/day) of bicarbonate.
Poisoning and drug toxicity: Treatment depends on drug ingested or infused. Hemodialysis or peritoneal dialysis may be necessary.
Lactic acidosis: Correction of underlying disorder related to hypoxia and/or hypoperfusion. Mortality associated with lactic acidosis is high. Unless pH is life-threatening, treatment with $NaHCO_3$ is generally not indicated and may actually be harmful.

Nursing diagnoses and interventions
Nursing diagnoses and interventions are specific to the pathophysiologic process. See "Altered Oral Mucous Membrane" in other sections of this text. Also see nursing diagnoses and interventions in "Mechanical Ventilation," p. 14; "Psychosocial Support," p. 68; "Psychosocial Support for the Patient's Family and Significant Others," p. 78; "Acute Renal Failure," p. 315; and "Diabetic Ketoacidosis," p. 393.

CHRONIC METABOLIC ACIDOSIS
Pathophysiology
Most often, chronic metabolic acidosis is seen with chronic renal failure in which the kidneys' ability to excrete acids (endogenous and exogenous) are exceeded by acid production and ingestion. The acidosis is usually mild in the initial stage, with HCO_3^- 18-22 mEq/L and a pH of 7.35. Treatment is indicated when serum HCO_3^- levels reach 15 mEq/L. Respiratory compensation occurs but only to a limited degree. A modest decrease in $PaCO_2$ will be noted on ABG values. If the patient suffers a respiratory failure state, acidosis will become profound.

$$\text{(Hyperventilated)} \downarrow CO_2 + H_2O \leftarrow H_2CO_3 \leftarrow \downarrow HCO_3^- \text{ and } H^+\uparrow$$

Better compensation: Exhaling or "blowing off" acid!!

Assessment
History and risk factors: Chronic renal failure, renal tubular acidosis, loss of alkaline fluid (e.g., with diarrhea or pancreatic or biliary drainage) for >3-5 days.
Clinical presentation: Usually the process leading to chronic metabolic acidosis is gradual and the patient is symptom free until serum HCO_3^- is ≤15 mEq/L. Fatigue, malaise, and anorexia may be present in relation to the underlying disease.

Diagnostic tests
ABG values: $Paco_2$ will be <35 mm Hg; pH will be <7.35.
Serum bicarbonate: Will be <22 mEq/L (usually 18-21 mEq/L). With severe acidosis, it will be <15 mEq/L.
Serum electrolyte levels: Serum calcium level is checked before treatment of acidosis is initiated to prevent tetany induced by hypocalcemia (caused by a decrease in ionized calcium). Serum phosphorus level is evaluated to determine presence of hyperphosphatemia, a common complication of chronic renal failure. Serum potassium level should be monitored after acidosis has been corrected to detect hypokalemia, inasmuch as potassium shifts back into the cells after correction of the acidosis.

Collaborative management
Alkalizing agents: For serum HCO_3^- levels <15 mEq/L, oral alkalis are administered ($NaHCO_3$ tablets or sodium citrate and citric acid oral solution [Shohl solution]). They are used cautiously to prevent fluid overload and tetany caused by hypocalcemia.

Caution: Be alert to the possibility of pulmonary edema, if bicarbonate is administered parenterally to patients with renal insufficiency or cardiovascular disorders.

Oral phosphates: Given if hypophosphatemia is present (not common with chronic renal failure), but may result from overuse of phosphate binders given to treat hyperphosphatemia (very common with chronic renal failure).
Hemodialysis, CRRT, or peritoneal dialysis: Renal replacement therapies may be indicated for chronic renal failure or other disease processes (see p. 334).

Nursing diagnoses and interventions
Nursing diagnoses and interventions are specific to the underlying pathophysiologic process. See other sections of this text, particularly Chapter 5, p. 315.

ACUTE METABOLIC ALKALOSIS
Pathophysiology
Acute metabolic alkalosis reflects excessive loss of hydrogen ions, excessive resorption of bicarbonate, or ingestion of alkaline; evaluated by and elevated serum HCO_3^- (up to 45-50 mEq/L). The major causes of this disturbance are loss of gastric acid from vomiting or gastric suction, diuretic therapy, posthypercapnic alkalosis (which occurs when chronic CO_2 retention is corrected rapidly), and excessive $NaHCO_3$ administration (i.e., overcorrection of a metabolic acidosis). Even when the causative factors have been removed, the alkalosis will be maintained until volume and electrolyte disturbances that are contributing to the alkalosis have been corrected. Severe alkalosis (pH >7.6) is associated with high morbidity and mortality. The body can tolerate a greater degree of acidosis than alkalosis.

$$\text{Some hypoventilation}\uparrow CO_2 + H_2O \leftarrow H_2CO_3 \leftarrow \uparrow HCO_3^- \text{ and } H^+\downarrow$$

Not enough compensation: Decreased metabolic acids!!

Assessment
History and risk factors
Clinical circumstances associated with volume/chloride depletion: Vomiting or gastric drainage; cystic fibrosis in hot weather when excessive chloride and sodium losses are not replaced.
Diuretic use: Usually a mild metabolic alkalosis will occur with diuretic use. The alkalosis will be more severe if using a potent diuretic (i.e., furosemide), especially in patients on sodium-restricted diets.
Posthypercapnic alkalosis: May occur after rapid correction of chronic hypercapnia.

Excessive alkali intake.
Clinical presentation: Muscular weakness, neuromuscular instability, and hyporeflexia because of accompanying hypokalemia. Decrease in GI tract motility may result in an ileus. Severe alkalosis can result in apathy, confusion, and stupor. Seizures may occur.
Physical assessment: Decreased respiratory rate and depth, periods of apnea, tachycardia (atrial or ventricular).
Monitoring parameters: Atrial-ventricular dysrhythmias as a result of cardiac irritability secondary to hypokalemia; prolonged QT interval.

Diagnostic tests
ABG values: Determine severity of alkalosis and response to therapy.
Serum bicarbonate levels: Values will be elevated to >26 mEq/L.
Serum electrolyte levels: Usually, serum potassium will be low (<4 mEq/L) as will serum chloride (<95 mEq/L).
Urinalysis: Urine chloride levels can help identify the cause of the metabolic alkalosis. Urine chloride level will be <15 mEq/L if hypovolemia and hypochloremia are present, and >20 mEq/L with excess retained HCO_3^-. This test is not reliable if diuretics have been used within the previous 12 hr.
ECG findings: To assess for dysrhythmias, especially if profound hypokalemia or alkalosis is present.

Collaborative management
Management will depend on the underlying disorder. Mild or moderate metabolic alkalosis usually does not require specific therapeutic interventions.
Saline infusion: Normal saline infusion may correct volume (chloride) deficit in patients with gastric alkalosis because of gastric losses. Metabolic alkalosis is difficult to correct if hypovolemia and chloride deficit are not corrected.
Potassium chloride (KCl): Indicated for patients with low potassium levels. KCl is preferred over other potassium salts because chloride losses can be replaced simultaneously.
Sodium and potassium chloride: Effective for posthypercapnic alkalosis, which occurs when chronic CO_2 retention is corrected rapidly (e.g., via mechanical ventilation). If adequate amounts of chloride and potassium are not available, renal excretion of excess HCO_3^- is impaired and metabolic alkalosis continues.
Cautious IV administration of isotonic hydrochloride solution, ammonium chloride, or arginine hydrochloride: May be warranted if severe metabolic alkalosis (pH >7.6 and HCO_3^- >40-45 mEq/L) exists, especially if chloride or potassium salts are contraindicated. The medication is delivered via continuous IV infusion at a slow rate, with frequent monitoring of IV insertion site for signs of infiltration. Ammonium chloride and arginine hydrochloride may be dangerous to patients with renal or hepatic failure.

Nursing diagnoses and interventions
Nursing diagnoses and interventions are specific to the underlying pathophysiologic process. See Chapter 5, p. 315, particularly.

CHRONIC METABOLIC ALKALOSIS
Pathophysiology
Chronic metabolic alkalosis results in a pH >7.45 and HCO_3^- >26 mEq/L. $PaCO_2$ will be elevated (>45 mm Hg) to compensate for the loss of H^+ or excess serum HCO_3^-. The three clinical situations in which this can occur are the following: (1) abnormalities in the kidneys' excretion of HCO_3^- related to a mineralocorticoid effect; (2) loss of H^+ through the GI tract; and (3) long-term diuretic therapy, especially with the thiazides and furosemide. A compensatory increase in $PaCO_2$ (up to 50-60 mm Hg) maybe seen. Respiratory compensation is very limited because of the hypoxemia, which develops as a result of decreased alveolar ventilation.

$$\text{Retained } CO_2 + H_2O \leftarrow H_2CO_3 \leftarrow \uparrow HCO_3^- \text{ and } H^+ \downarrow$$

Better compensation: Increased acid!!

Assessment
History and risk factors
Diuretic use: Thiazide diuretics cause a loss of chloride, potassium, and hydrogen ions. Massive depletion of potassium stores with loss of up to 1000 mEq, which is one third of total body potassium, may occur, causing profound hypokalemia ($K^+ \leq 2.0$ mEq/L).

Hyperadrenocorticism: Cushing's syndrome, primary aldosteronism. This is not a chloride deficit but a chronic loss of potassium, which can lead to total body depletion of potassium with profound hypokalemia ($K^+ \leq 2.0$ mEq/L).

Chronic vomiting or chronic GI losses through GI suction.

Milk-alkali syndrome: An infrequent cause of metabolic alkalosis.

Hypercalcemic nephropathy and alkalosis: Develop as a result of excessive intake of absorbable alkali (antacids containing calcium carbonate).

Clinical presentation: Patient may be free of symptoms. With severe potassium depletion and profound alkalosis, patient may experience weakness, neuromuscular instability, and a decrease in GI tract motility, which can result in ileus.

Monitoring parameters: Frequent PVCs or U waves with hypokalemia and alkalosis.

Diagnostic tests

ABG values: Determine severity of acid-base imbalance. $Paco_2$ will be increased (>45 mm Hg), and pH will be >7.4.

Serum bicarbonate levels: Will be >26 mEq/L.

Serum electrolyte levels: Usually potassium will be profoundly low (may be ≤ 2 mEq/L) related to the exchange of H^+ and K^+. Chloride may be <95 mEq/L. Magnesium may be <1.5 mEq/L in both renal system abnormalities.

Collaborative management

The goal is to correct the underlying acid-base disorder via the following interventions.

Fluid management: If volume depletion exists, normal saline infusions are given.

Potassium replacement: If a chloride deficit also is present, KCl is the drug of choice. If a chloride deficit does not exist, other potassium salts are acceptable.

IV potassium: If the patient is undergoing cardiac monitoring, up to 20 mEq/hr of KCl is given for serious hypokalemia. Concentrated doses of KCl (>40 mEq/L) require administration through a central venous line because of blood vessel irritation.

Oral potassium: Tastes very unpleasant; 15 mEq/glass is all most patients can tolerate, with a maximum daily dose of 60-80 mEq. Slow-release potassium tablets are an acceptable form of KCl. All forms of KCl may be irritating to gastric mucosa.

Dietary: Normal diet contains 3 g or 75 mEq of potassium but not in the form of KCl. Dietary supplementation of potassium is not effective if a concurrent chloride deficit also is present.

Potassium-sparing diuretics: May be added to treatment if thiazide diuretics are the cause of hypokalemia and metabolic alkalosis.

Identify and correct cause of hyperadrenocorticism.

Nursing diagnoses and interventions

Nursing diagnoses and interventions are specific to the underlying pathophysiologic process. See Chapter 5, p. 315, for examples.

High-Risk Obstetrics

PATHOPHYSIOLOGY

Most pregnant patients are healthy women, rarely in need of critical care. Obstetric complications may arise during gestation, labor, delivery, and postpartum. Pregnancy-induced hypertension (PIH) is the most common obstetric complication requiring critical care. Approximately 7% of United States women develop pre-eclampsia-eclampsia. 5% of patients with preeclampsia will progress to eclampsia. Types of PIH are reflected in Table 10-17.

The etiology of *preeclampsia* is uncertain, but more recently it has been viewed as caused by a combination of vasospasms and damage to the vascular endothelium, which may prompt a cascade of events leading to multiple organ dysfunction. Patients sometimes have vague complaints common to patients in the third trimester and remain undiagnosed until severe preeclampsia develops. Hypertension, edema, and proteinuria are the three classic signs of preeclampsia. Slight hypertension that develops after 20 weeks' gestation (e.g., BP has increased from baseline 90/60 to 120/90) may signal preeclampsia, particularly if other symptoms are present. *HELLP syndrome* is an acronym for a condition including hemolysis, elevated liver enzymes, and low platelets; it involves hemolysis caused by RBCs circulating through damaged vascular endothelium, which narrows as fibrin is deposited over damaged areas. HELLP syndrome is found in 10% of patients with severe preeclampsia. The etiology

T A B L E 10 - 17   Classification of Hypertensive States of Pregnancy

Type	Description
Gestational	Mild hypertension that develops during pregnancy without addition PIH symptoms
Preeclampsia	Hypertension that develops during pregnancy after 20 weeks' gestation (except in molar pregnancies) with proteinuria
HELLP syndrome	Severe form of preeclampsia with hemolysis, elevated liver enzymes, and low platelets, which may lead to DIC. Rarely patients may be normotensive with HELLP.
Eclampsia	Preeclampsia complicated by seizures
Chronic hypertension	Hypertension that is present prior to pregnancy or develops before 20 weeks' gestation without a molar pregnancy
Chronic hypertension with PIH	Preeclampsia and/or eclampsia superimposed on chronic hypertension

DIC, Disseminated intravascular coagulation; *PIH,* pregnancy-induced hypertension.

of HELLP is uncertain. Microemboli produced lead to liver damage and rarely, a subcapsular hematoma. Vasospasms and endothelial damage lead to a cascade of disseminated intravascular coagulation (DIC), which initially consumes platelets, then clotting factors. DIC may also be caused by placental abruption (abruptio placentae), dead fetus syndrome, septic shock, transfusion reaction, and amniotic fluid embolism. Maternal complications from DIC lead to acute respiratory distress syndrome (ARDS) and acute renal failure. Hemodynamic monitoring may be required to manage patients with HELLP syndrome.

Numerous preexisting conditions lead to other obstetric complications (see "Assessment" section that follows). *Anaphylactoid syndrome of pregnancy (amniotic fluid embolism)* causes maternal mortality in up to 80% of affected patients and is not yet predictable; 50% of patients expire within the first hour following the event. The syndrome is a rare (1/20,000 to 1/80,000 pregnancies) and poorly understood condition that occurs during labor, vaginal or cesarean delivery, or immediately postpartum, seemingly after contact of maternal circulation with amniotic fluid. Amniotic fluid contains fetal cells, lanugo hairs, immunologic mediators, and waste products, which when introduced into the mother's bloodstream, may prompt a severe allergic or septic type of reaction with resultant shock. Rapid onset, severe hypoxia with bronchospasms leads to development of ARDS, left ventricular failure, lethal dysrhythmias, possibly seizures, cardiac arrest, and bleeding due to consumptive coagulopathy (likely DIC).

Collaboration between the critical care and obstetrics nurses is necessary in providing safe and comprehensive obstetric critical care. The knowledge of each specialty is needed to assess, diagnose, implement, and evaluate the responses of the patient. If the patient is pregnant when the need for critical care arises, the nurse is responsible for the care of both mother and child. Patients may expect the family-centered care rendered in obstetrics units. If the baby has been delivered, families may desire unrestricted visitation, or the mother may desire to have the baby remain in her ICU room. Feasibility and appropriateness of both family and "baby visits" to the critical care unit must be determined.

Obstetric patients may require hemodynamic monitoring if shock has ensued. Hypovolemic shock due to bleeding and septic shock are the most common causes of prolonged hypotension in obstetric patients. Incidence of septic shock is increasing and is most often caused by septic abortion, chorioamnionitis, pyelonephritis, and endometritis. Indications for hemodynamic monitoring include the following: pregnancy-induced hypertension with pulmonary edema or oliguria, refractory heart failure with pulmonary edema or oliguria, preexisting cardiovascular disease (e.g., valve disease, primary pulmonary hypertension), intraoperative or intrapartum cardiovascular decompensation, HELLP syndrome, postpartum hemorrhage or other massive blood or volume loss, development of ARDS, severe sepsis, or anaphylactoid syndrome of pregnancy. Recognition of expected, pregnancy-induced hemodynamic changes is needed for appropriate interpretation of hemodynamic profiles (Table 10-18).

T A B L E 10 - 18   Expected Hemodynamic Changes During Pregnancy, Labor, Delivery and Postpartum

Hemodynamic profile	Third trimester changes before labor	% Additional changes during active labor	Postpartal measurements	Normal values (before pregnancy)
Cardiac output (L/min)	↑25%-50% (~7.5 L/min)	↑~10%	To prelabor value in 1hr; normal in 10-14 days	5.0 L/min
Stroke volume (cc/beat)	↑20%-30% (~75-85 cc/beat)	↑~ 10%	To prelabor value in 24 hr; normal in 3-12 months	65 cc/beat
Central venous pressure (mm Hg)	Unchanged	Data unavailable	Data unavailable	2-6 mm Hg
Pulmonary artery pressures (mm Hg)				
PA systolic	Unchanged	Data unavailable	Unchanged	15-25 mm Hg
PA diastolic	Unchanged	Data unavailable	Unchanged	6-12 mm Hg
PA wedge	Unchanged	Data unavailable	Unchanged	4-12 mm Hg
Systemic vascular resistance (dynes)	May ↓ up to 20%	Unchanged	To normal in 3-12 months	800-1200 dynes/sec/cm^{-5}
Pulmonary vascular resistance (dynes)	May ↓ up to 25%	Data unavailable	Data unavailable	150-240 dynes/sec/cm^{-5}

ASSESSMENT

Risk factors for nonhypertensive obstetric complications: Many conditions may predispose women to developing complications including: diabetes mellitus, thyroid disease or other chronic endocrine disorders, asthma, bleeding or thromboembolic condition, chronic hypertension (present prior to 20 weeks' gestation), valvular or other heart disease, Marfan syndrome, anemia (i.e., sickle cell or folic acid or iron deficiency), rheumatologic or other autoimmune disease (e.g., lupus anticoagulant-anticardiolipin-antiphospholipid antibody syndrome), AIDS, carcinoma, substance abuse, prolonged or severe bacterial or viral infection (e.g., herpes genitalis, hepatitis, urinary tract infection), venereal disease (e.g., syphilis, gonorrhea, *Chlamydia)*, abnormal placenta, possible premature rupture of amniotic sac ("leaky water bag"), placental abruption, presence of an intrauterine catheter, and other conditions. The primary focus of the rest of the chapter is complications of pregnancy-induced hypertension.

Risk factors for development of pregnancy-induced hypertension: preeclampsia, eclampsia, and HELLP syndrome: Women with mild pregnancy-induced hypertension; especially those with extremes of age (preteenagers or women >40 years old).

Clinical presentation: preeclampsia, eclampsia, and HELLP syndrome: Preeclampsia is a progressive hypertension occurring 20 weeks into gestation and up to 6 weeks postpartum, with blood pressure at least 140/90 mm Hg with peripheral edema (i.e., lower extremities, hands, feet) and proteinuria. Eclampsia manifests in patients with symptoms of preeclampsia as seizures and/or coma in patients without neurologic or chemical predisposition for these problems. HELLP syndrome (hemolysis, elevated liver enzymes, and low platelet count) occurs in a subset of patients with severe PIH. It is difficult to predict which patients will progress from simple PIH into the more severe complications.

Physical assessment: The severity of preeclampsia-eclampsia can be assessed as follows:
Mild-to-moderate preeclampsia-eclampsia: Blood pressure <160 mm Hg systolic and 110 mm Hg diastolic, peripheral edema, arteriolar spasms of the retina, hyperreflexia, headache, low-to-normal urine output, and possibly oligohydramnios (reduced amount of amniotic fluid). The hemodynamic profile of patients with preeclampsia varies, so treatment must be individualized. Some patients experience marked reduction in cardiac output from early stages, while others remain normal.
Severe preeclampsia-eclampsia: Blood pressure >160 mm Hg systolic and 110 mm Hg diastolic, increasing peripheral edema, retinal hemorrhages, headache, blurred vision, irritability, scotomas, clonus, seizures, low urine output, epigastric pain, oligohydramnios, fetal growth retardation, and fetal distress.
HELLP syndrome: Symptoms of severe preeclampsia-eclampsia with added jaundice and epigastric or right upper quadrant pain. Jaundice that develops during pregnancy is due to HELLP syndrome 99.9% of the time. Rarely, patients can display jaundice prior to the onset of hypertension.

DIAGNOSTIC TESTS

Complete blood cell count (CBC): Hgb and Hct may be elevated (>35 Hct) and steadily rising with severe preeclampsia-eclampsia (Table 10-19).
Peripheral blood smear: Schistocytes or burr cells are present with HELLP syndrome.
Urinalysis: Positive for protein spillage.
24-hour urine collection for protein: Mild/moderate: 0.3-5 g protein with normal urine output. Severe preeclampsia-eclampsia: >5 g protein with low urine output.
Serum albumin: Decreases as urine protein spillage increases. Severe: <2.5 mg/dl.
Liver enzymes: Aspartate transaminase (AST), alanine amino transferase (ALT), and lactate dehydrogenase (LDH) are elevated with severe preeclampsia-eclampsia and HELLP syndrome. Bilirubin may be elevated with HELLP.
Renal serum chemistry: Mild-moderate: BUN, creatinine, and uric acid levels may be elevated. Severe preeclampsia-eclampsia: BUN, creatinine, and uric acid will be elevated.
Platelet count: Mild-moderate: >100,000/µL, Severe preeclampsia-eclampsia and HELLP syndrome: <100,000/µL
Bleeding time: Prolonged when platelet count is <100,000/mm^3.
Fibrinogen: Decreased (<300 mg/dl).
Screening coagulation tests (PT, PTT, thrombin time): Normal unless the patient develops HELLP syndrome that progresses to DIC, wherein all values are elevated.
Platelet antibody screen: May have positive findings with severe form.

COLLABORATIVE MANAGEMENT

Prenatal Care:
• Early recognition of preeclampsia during prenatal care is the most effective management strategy.
• Subtle changes in blood pressure and weight may signal the onset of pregnancy-induced hypertension.
• Once detected, all efforts to prolong the pregnancy should be implemented, to allow for maturation of the fetus, especially the lungs, without overly compromising the health of the mother.

T A B L E   10 - 19   Blood/Blood Volume/Circulatory Alterations Expected With Pregnancy

Parameter	Third trimester changes before labor	% Additional changes during active labor	Postpartal measurements
Blood volume	↑ by ~50%	Unchanged	↓0.5-1.0 L or ↓10%-20%
Plasma volume	↑ by 40%-50%	Unchanged	↓10% during 1st week to total 20% RBCs + plasma
Hematocrit	↓ by 10%-25%	Unchanged	Returns to normal
Hemoglobin	↓ by ~10%	Unchanged	Returns to normal
Blood pressure	↑5%-10% systolic ↑0%-10% diastolic	Increases Increases	Returns to normal
Heart rate	↑~15%-30%	↑0%-20%	Returns to normal

Considerations regarding gestational age:
• Preeclampsia arising at 34 weeks' (or more) gestation is generally managed by delivery. New hypertension may prompt delivery, to avoid progression to severe preeclampsia or eclampsia.
• Before 34 weeks, patients with severe preeclampsia-eclampsia require delivery unless the gestational age is <26 weeks, wherein attempts to prolong the pregnancy may be initiated. If the mother exhibits signs of HELLP syndrome such as thrombocytopenia, epigastric pain, or right upper quadrant pain or has visual disturbances, delivery should be strongly considered regardless of fetal age, since the mother is at risk of life-threatening illness if delivery is delayed.

Manage seizures: Once seizures begin, turn patient onto her side to prevent aspiration and to improve perfusion to the placenta. Magnesium sulfate 3-4 g is given in an IV bolus, or diazepam 5-10 mg IV push over 4 min is administered until the seizure stops. A continuous infusion of magnesium sulfate is given at 2-3 g/hr unless the patient has renal insufficiency, wherein the dose may be reduced. Therapeutic blood levels (4-6 mEq/L) are monitored for magnesium at least every 6 hr. Hourly urine output is monitored, as are signs of magnesium toxicity (i.e., decreased respiratory rate and depth, respiratory arrest, or loss of deep tendon reflexes). Magnesium toxicity is reversed with 1 g of 10% calcium gluconate IV.

Manage hypertension: If hypertension is present, with diastolic BP >110 mm Hg, antihypertensives should be given. Hydralazine 5-10 mg IV every 20 min or labetalol 10-20 mg IV every 20 min may be initiated.

Delivery: Delivery is mandated when eclampsia or severe HELLP manifests unless unusual circumstances prevail. Need for immediate delivery depends on both fetal and maternal status following seizures or any potentially life-threatening clinical event. If cesarean section is needed, either regional analgesia or general anesthesia may be implemented. Labor may be augmented or induced with oxytocin. If close to delivery (active labor with advanced dilation and effacement of the cervix), vaginal delivery may be attempted if the conditions of mother and fetus are stable and delivery seems imminent.

Hemodynamic Management:
See Table 10-20.

NURSING DIAGNOSES AND INTERVENTIONS

Protection, ineffective related to hemodynamic, hematologic, and neurologic changes associated with PIH
Desired outcomes: Within 1 hr of development of severe preeclampsia, eclampsia, or severe HELLP syndrome, the pregnant patient (mother and child) is monitored intensively and prepared for delivery, to avoid life-threatening complications of pregnancy-induced hypertension.
• Verify heart rates of mother and fetus prior to initiating electronic monitoring.
• Monitor blood pressure of mother at least every 5 min if severe hypertension or seizures have occurred. Monitor fetal heart rate for slowing, indicative of fetal distress.
• Initiate fetal resuscitation measures to treat abnormal fetal heart rhythms, as appropriate. Note response to all supportive interventions.
• Instruct woman and support person(s) about the need for monitoring and data to be obtained.
• Keep physician informed of significant changes in fetal heart rate, interventions for abnormal patterns, fetal response, labor progress, and maternal response to interventions.

T A B L E 10 - 20   Hemodynamic Profiles in Oliguric Patients With Preeclampsia

Probable etiology	Pulmonary artery wedge pressure	Systemic vascular resistance	Cardiac output	Treatment
Hypovolemia	Normal to decreased	Increased	Increased	Volume infusion
Spasm of renal arteries	Increased	Normal	Increased	Volume infusion Generalized vasodilation
Spasm of systemic arterial vessels	Increased	Increased	Decreased	Diuresis Arterial vasodilation

- Administer anticonvulsive medications as ordered to control seizures.
- Monitor magnesium levels, and be alert to hypermagnesemia: decreased respiratory rate and depth, loss of deep tendon reflexes.
- Assist with application of forceps or vacuum extractor, as needed, during delivery.
- Monitor the patient closely for hemorrhage if HELLP syndrome is present.
- Note Hgb and Hct levels before and after blood loss, as indicated.
- Monitor coagulation studies, including PT, PTT, fibrinogen, fibrin degradation products (FDP), fibrin split products (FSP), and platelet counts as appropriate.

▌NIC Electronic Fetal Monitoring: Intrapartum,; Surveillance: Late Pregnancy; Intrapartal Care: High Risk Delivery

Decreased adaptive capacity: related to potential for seizures and neurologic complications secondary to eclampsia or HELLP syndrome

Desired outcomes: Throughout the hospitalization, patient remains free of seizures and neurologic complications as evidenced by orientation to time, place, and person; normoreactive pupils and reflexes; patient's normal visual acuity, motor strength, and coordination; and absence of headache and other clinical indicators of increased intracranial pressure (IICP).

- Monitor for and document seizures. Protect patient from injury by initiating seizure precautions. When patient is seizing, turn her to the side to promote placental perfusion and prevent aspiration.
- Assess patient for initial signs of IICP, including diminished LOC, headaches, abnormal pupillary responses (i.e., unequal; sluggish/absent response to light), visual disturbances, weakness and paralysis, slow HR, and change in respiratory rate and pattern. Patient may be experiencing problems related to seizure management, or may experience intracranial bleeding if platelets are extremely low.
- Monitor trend of Glasgow Coma Scale if patient has difficulty awakening after seizures. If patient exhibits signs of magnesium toxicity, consult physician and consider calcium gluconate administration.
- Increase frequency of neurologic monitoring as appropriate.
- Assess the epidural site (as appropriate), if patient received epidural analgesia during labor and delivery. Patients with coagulopathy may develop an epidural hematoma, manifested by sensory or motor deficits, bowel or bladder dysfunction, or back pain. Report problems to the physician immediately. The epidural catheter should remain in place until coagulation studies normalize.
- Avoid activities that increase intracranial pressure.
- If initial signs of IICP are noted, consult physician immediately. Signs of impending herniation include unconsciousness, failure to respond to deeply painful stimuli, decorticate or decerebrate posturing, Cushing's triad (i.e., bradycardia, increased systolic BP, widening pulse pressure), nonreactive/fixed pupils, unequal pupils, or fixed and dilated pupils. See p. 100 for more information about herniation. For additional interventions for IICP, see Table 2-6.

▌NIC Cerebral Edema Management; Cerebral Perfusion Promotion; Neurologic Monitoring; Electrolyte Management; Fluid Management;

Risk for fluid volume deficit related to active loss secondary to antepartum, postpartum, intraabdominal, or other bleeding

Desired outcome: Patient remains normovolemic as evidenced by HR, RR, and BP within 10% of expected normal range; urinary output ≥0.5 ml/kg/hr; and absence of epigastric or abdominal pain or tenderness, and frank bleeding resulting from HELLP syndrome.

- Monitor fluid status, including I&O, signs of hypovolemia, including increases in HR and RR, decreases in BP and urinary output, restlessness, and VS.
- Initiate hemodynamic monitoring if necessary to assess shock state and/or manage hemodynamics.
- Monitor Hgb and Hct as ordered. Postpartum, the uterus contracts and blood is released into the central circulation as it decreases in size. With a normal 500-ml vaginal delivery blood loss, often the Hgb and Hct increase despite the blood loss.
- Inspect for bleeding from mucous membranes, bruising after minimal trauma, oozing from puncture sites, and presence of petechiae. Maintain patent IV access.
- Administer supplemental oxygen as necessary for active bleeding.
- Perform fundus checks and initiate gentle fundal massage to help the uterus remain firm and promote hemostasis.
- Initiate bleeding control therapy as ordered. Methylergonovine, ergonovine, and carboprost may be used to manage prolonged bleeding or hemorrhage.
- Replace lost volume with plasma expanders (e.g., albumin, hetastarch) and/or blood products as indicated. See Table 9-2 for information about blood products.

NIC Bleeding Precautions; Bleeding Reduction: Antepartum Uterus; Bleeding Reduction: Postpartum Uterus; Fluid Monitoring; Hypovolemia Management; Invasive Hemodynamic Monitoring; Intravenous (IV) Therapy; Shock Management: Volume; Blood Products Administration

Risk for infection related to inadequate secondary defenses (HELLP syndrome causes liver dysfunction, which may impair the reticuloendothelial system phagocytic activity and portal-systemic shunting); multiple invasive procedures; stress and risks associated with pregnancy, labor, and delivery

Desired outcome: Patient is free of infection as evidenced by normothermia; HR <100 beats/min; RR <20 breaths/min; negative culture results; WBC count <11,000/mm^3; clear urine; and clear, thin sputum.

- Monitor VS for evidence of infection (e.g., increases in heart and respiratory rates). Check rectal or core temperature q4h for increases.
- If temperature elevation is sudden, obtain specimens for blood, sputum, and urine cultures or from other sites as prescribed. Consult physician for positive culture results.
- Monitor CBC, and consult physician for significant increases in WBCs. Be aware that a normal or mildly elevated leukocyte count may signify infection in patients with liver dysfunction.
- Evaluate secretions and drainage for evidence of infection (e.g., sputum changes, cloudy urine).
- Evaluate IV, central line, and other site(s) for evidence of infection (i.e., erythema, warmth, unusual drainage).
- Provide routine episiotomy care by spraying the area with warm water at least every 4 hours. Sitz baths are usually not possible with critically ill patients. Ice packs and topical anesthetics may be used to enhance comfort.
- Provide daily breast care by cleansing the breasts with mild soap and water. Breast engorgement should be managed per physician's orders to help prevent infection and control pain. If left unrelieved, breast engorgement can result in stoppage of lactation. If breast-feeding is planned, breasts can be massaged and milk manually expressed or pumped.
- Prevent transmission of infectious agents by washing hands well before and after caring for patient and by wearing gloves when contact with blood or other body substances is possible. Dispose of all needles and other sharp instruments in puncture-resistant, rigid containers. Keep containers in each patient room and in other convenient locations. Avoid recapping and manipulating needles before disposal. Teach significant others and visitors proper hand-washing technique. Restrict visitors with evidence of communicable disease.
- Administer antibiotics as prescribed. Use caution and reduced dosage when administering antibiotics (especially aminoglycosides) to patients with low urinary output or renal insufficiency.

NIC Infection Protection; Surveillance; Breast-Feeding Assistance; Cesarean Section Care; Postpartal Care

Family coping: compromised related to abnormal circumstances surrounding labor, delivery, and postpartum; creating need for mother to be separated from infant and other family members.

Desired outcome: Patient and family demonstrate adequate coping behaviors and are facilitated in being together as soon as possible in the postpartal hospitalization.

- Provide regular updates to family members about the condition of both mother and infant.
- Invite family members to participate in care of the mother as possible.
- Promote infant-mother bonding by allowing baby visitations in the ICU as soon as the conditions of mother and infant stabilize. Allow mother to feed baby if possible. Maintain infant safety if mother's condition is marginally stable.
- Discuss feelings about labor, delivery, and complications with patient and family members. Relay information about the condition of the infant as often as possible, if mother is unable to visit with the baby.
- If the infant or mother expires, provide all possible support measures for the patient and significant others, including pastoral care and referrals to community support groups or professional counseling.

NIC Family Involvement Promotion; Family Mobilization; Family Presence Facilitation; Family Support; Grief Work Facilitation: Perinatal Death

ADDITIONAL NURSING DIAGNOSES

Uncontrolled bleeding and other complications can be terrifying for the patient and significant others, who may fear that the patient will die. Refer to nursing diagnoses in "Psychosocial Support," p. 68, and "Psychosocial Support for the Patient's Family and Significant Others," p. 78, for appropriate interventions. For pain management, refer to nursing diagnoses in "Pain," p. 51. See "Acute Respiratory Failure," p. 201, and "Mechanical Ventilation," p. 14, if the patient is unable to ventilate without mechanical assistance. See "Heart Failure," p. 220, if patient experiences cardiac decompensation. See "Hepatic Failure," p. 427, if patient has severe HELLP syndrome with liver decompensation. See

"Fluid and Electrolyte Disturbances," p. 538, if patient is being managed for eclampsia. See "Anaphylactic Shock," p. 513, if patient has anaphylactoid syndrome of pregnancy (amniotic fluid embolism.) See "Hemodynamic Monitoring," p. 23, if a Swan-Ganz catheter has been inserted.

Emerging Infections*

Emerging infectious diseases are a serious problem. Medicine and technology have moved forward to successfully overcome and prevent infections, yet new problems continue to emerge. The new infections are complex, and their evolution has been challenging for health care to recognize, understand, and treat. Many emerging infections originate from different species of animals and have spread to humans. Humans are vulnerable, without natural defenses against these infections. Researchers are hard-pressed to develop vaccines and cures. Regardless of sex, age, socioeconomic status, or ethnic background, infectious disease can strike at any time and may lead to death.

SEVERE ACUTE RESPIRATORY SYNDROME (SARS)

Severe acute respiratory syndrome (SARS) is a febrile respiratory infection that mimics many other respiratory illnesses and thus is difficult to diagnose. The virus may have originated from animals and spread to humans. SARS first emerged in the Guandong Province in China in 2002. A worldwide epidemic occurred when a SARS-infected physician contaminated several guests at a hotel in Hong Kong. The guests were the catalyst leading to large outbreaks of SARS in Hong Kong, Vietnam, Singapore, and Canada. Overall, 8000 probable SARS cases were identified during the outbreak, and 800 total deaths occurred from 29 different countries.

A novel coronavirus (CoV) has been identified as the cause of SARS and is now labeled SARS-associated coronavirus (SARS-CoV). Coronaviruses are enveloped RNA viruses that cause diseases in both humans and animals. In humans, this group of viruses is implicated in the causes of the common cold and pneumonia. The distinct microscopic appearance of a crown surrounding the viruses has led to its name. Research in China has detected several coronaviruses closely related to SARS-CoV in two animal species (masked palm civet cat and raccoon-dog). This provided the first link between human SARS-CoV and its presence in other animals. Both are considered delicacies in China and are consumed by humans. One theory states that this coronavirus mutated and was transmitted to humans through handling of these animals or contact with their saliva and feces.

PATHOPHYSIOLOGY

The pathophysiology of SARS is unclear. It begins much like the common flu, progressing to pneumonia and potentially to acute respiratory distress syndrome (ARDS) and death. Lymphopenia, thrombocytopenia, and leucopenia are noted. SARS-CoV may infect blood cells and/or induce autoantibodies to damage these cells, leading to immunological dysregulation in response to the SARS-CoV. Poor patient outcomes have been linked to advanced age and elevated total lactate dehydrogenase (LDH greater than 300 units/L). Increased LDH may reflect cell death or leakage of this enzyme from cells, possibly indicating cellular infection by SARS-CoV.

TRANSMISSION

The most common mode of transmission for SARS is close person-to-person contact: kissing, sharing eating or drinking utensils, close conversation (less than 3 feet), physical examination, and any other direct physical contact. Respiratory droplets are expelled by the infected person by a cough or sneeze into the air. Droplets then reach the mucosal membrane of the nose, mouth, or eyes of a nearby person, infecting him or her.

Surfaces contaminated with SARS droplets may serve as a reservoir for the virus. SARS droplets can remain viable up to several days according to the type of surface they are on. If a person contacts a contaminated surface and then touches the mouth, eyes, or nose, he or she may become infected with SARS-CoV. Contact with feces of an infected person has accounted for a few cases. Other modes of transmission are not yet clearly identified.

ASSESSMENT

SARS' initial presentation is similar to other lower respiratory tract infections. No specific clinical or laboratory findings are available to rapidly distinguish SARS from other respiratory illnesses.

---

*The comments and views expressed in this section on Emerging Infections do not represent the U.S. Army or Department of Defense.

Early recognition of SARS requires assessment of clinical and epidemiologic features. Incubation period is 2-10 days. Many early clinical manifestations are flu-like symptoms: fever, myalgias, headache, and rhinorrhea. Fever is a key component and occurs in most cases. As the disease progresses, more respiratory symptoms may arise. On the second day of the fever, a dry, nonproductive cough may develop, progressing to shortness of breath, hypoxemia, and ARDS. The Centers for Disease Control and Prevention (CDC) has delineated three different levels of how patients may clinically present with SARS:

Early illness
- Presence of two or more of the following: fever, chills, rigors, myalgia, headache, diarrhea, sore throat, rhinorrhea

Mild-to-moderate respiratory illness
- Temperature of greater than 100.4° F (greater than 38° C), and
- One or more of the clinical findings of lower respiratory illness (e.g., cough, shortness of breath, difficulty breathing)

Severe respiratory illness
- Meets clinical criteria for mild-to-moderate respiratory illness
- One or more of the following:
  ❑ Chest x-ray illustrating pneumonia
  ❑ ARDS (See "Acute Lung Injury Respiratory Distress Syndrome" section, p. 189)
  ❑ Autopsy findings of pneumonia or ARDS without an identifiable cause

The CDC-defined epidemiological criteria are the following:
- Possible exposure to SARS-CoV. One or more of the following exposures occurred within 10 days before onset of symptoms:
  ❑ Travel to a location with documented or suspected recent transmission of SARS-CoV
  ❑ Close contact with a person with respiratory illness and with a history of travel in 10 days before onset of symptoms to a location with documented or suspected, recent transmission of SARS-CoV
- Likely exposure to SARS-CoV. One or more of the following exposures in 10 days before onset of symptoms:
  ❑ Close contact with a confirmed case of SARS-CoV
  ❑ Close contact with a person with respiratory illness for whom chain of transmission can be linked to a confirmed case of SARS-CoV

DIAGNOSTIC TESTS

SARS-CoV reverse-transcription polymerase chain reaction (PT-PCR) test: Detects SARS-CoV viral RNA in respiratory samples, stool, and blood. Has not been licensed by the Food and Drug Administration (FDA). Currently approved as a FDA investigational device exemption (test). A signed consent should be completed prior to collection of a sample. The sample should be forwarded to a state or local public health laboratory for processing.

Enzyme immunoassay (EIA) test: Detects SARS-CoV antibodies in blood samples. Has not been licensed by the Food and Drug Administration (FDA). Has been allowed for use by the FDA as a result of the SARS outbreak. A signed consent should be completed before collection of the sample. The sample should be forwarded to a state or local public health laboratory for processing.

Specimen culture for SARS-CoV: Isolation of the SARS-CoV from a clinical specimen to confirm the virus.

Other tests: Other tests include the following: respiratory viral panels for influenza A and B, respiratory syncytial viruses, and specimens for legionella and pneumococcal urinary antigen. These tests aid in ruling out other potential sources of infection.

The following tests are influenced by the extent of the disease process and other underlying medical conditions:

Chest x-ray: Assists in identifying the progression of disease, and anatomic involvement.

CBC and clotting profile: Monitoring WBC counts to assist in evaluation of other bacterial infection. Evaluation for lymphopenia, thrombocytopenia, and leucopenia.

ABGs: Determination of patient oxygen saturation and acid-base balance.

Pulse oximetry: Used to measure patient oxygen saturation of arterial blood. Values >90% are normal.

COLLABORATIVE MANAGEMENT

Oxygen therapy: To support gas exchange and circumvent development of hypoxemia. Maintain pulse oximetry >90%.

Intubation and mechanical ventilation: To support gas exchange and help maintain acid-base balance.

Intravenous fluids: To prevent dehydration and maintain adequate circulatory volume.

Antibiotics: To prevent secondary infections. Empirical antibiotic therapy should be prescribed for typical and atypical community-acquired pneumonia. Therapy may include fluoroquinolone or macrolide.

Antiviral: Ribavirin is the antiviral of choice, but has had mixed results. Adverse side effects include hemolytic anemia and electrolyte imbalances (i.e., hypokalemia and hypomagnesemia). Patients must be monitored closely for significant side effects.

Corticosteroids: May be beneficial in patients with pulmonary infiltrates and hypoxemia. Methylprednisolone dosages range from 40 mg bid to 2 mg/kg daily.

Infection control: Patient is placed in a negative pressure room. Restricted visitation should be implemented and an ongoing log kept of all persons entering the patient's room. Minimize the number of health care personnel caring for the patient. A strict combination of contact precautions (i.e., eye protection, mask, gloves, and gown) and airborne precautions (e.g., N95 respirator) should be

---

Note: No noted vaccine has been developed for SARS.

---

used. All equipment and other items should remain in patient's room and should not be used with other patients or outside the isolation room.

NURSING DIAGNOSES AND INTERVENTIONS

See nursing diagnosis for "Acute Lung Injury and Respiratory Distress Syndrome," p. 189; "Acute Pneumonia," p. 180; "Acute Respiratory Failure," p. 201; "Mechanical Ventilation," p. 14; "Fluid and Electrolyte Disturbances," p. 538; "Psychosocial Support," p. 68; and "Psychosocial Support for the Patient's Family and Significant Others," p. 78.

CREUTZFELDT-JAKOB DISEASE (INCLUDES "MAD COW" DISEASE)

PATHOPHYSIOLOGY

Creutzfeldt-Jakob disease (CJD) is a rare, fatal, neurodegenerative disorder, believed to be caused by an abnormal isoform of a glycoprotein known as a *prion*, a proteinaceous infectious particle. The most common disorder is *bovine spongiform encephalopathy* or *"mad cow" disease*. Recently a new form of CJD has emerged, called *new variant CJD* (vCJD or nvCJD). This form of CJD is linked to consumption of cattle suffering from mad cow disease. Clinical and epidemiologic evidence supporting this link between "mad cow" disease and vCJD has become stronger. As of May 2004, a total of 153 cases of vCJD have been reported. vCJD generally affects younger people with a mean age of 29 years old, whereas CJD occurs in the age group between 65-69 years.

CJD is classified as a transmissible spongiform encephalopathy, a category which includes other diseases (e.g., Fatal Familial Insomnia, Gerstman-Sträussler-Scheinker syndromes). *Prion disease* occurs in animals, particularly cattle, sheep and goats. CJD is endemic around the world and its estimated incidence report is one case per million people. Three forms of "classic" CJD have been identified. *Sporadic CJD* affects the elderly with rapid onset dementia and neurologic symptoms of unknown cause. *Familial CJD* is an inherited disease and generally strikes younger individuals. It has a longer course in comparison to sporadic CJD. *Iatrogenic CJD* occurs through contact with infected tissue via medical procedures or treatments.

Prion proteins are normal proteins in the body and brain. In CJD, these proteins become abnormally shaped, as a result either of genetics or of contamination from an outside source. This leads to surrounding normal prion proteins taking on the abnormal shape. Central nervous system function is disrupted, leading to cognitive impairment and cerebellar dysfunction. As the process continues, the abnormal prions accumulate in the brain, causing neuronal dysfunction, neuron death, gliosis (proliferation of neuroglial tissue in the central nervous system), and ultimately death.

TRANSMISSION

CJD can spread either through infectious or hereditary means. Prion infections are transmitted by peripheral routes, either orally or transcutaneously. They may be introduced to lymphatic organs, particularly the spleen and lymph nodes, where initial replication of the infected prions occurs. Infections either enter the circulatory system and are hematogenously spread to the brain, or infected prions may travel via the vagus nerve to the brain. Genetic mutation of the human prion gene PrP on chromosome 20 leads to the dysfunction of the prion protein. More than 20 reported mutations of this chromosome have been reported. All mutations influence onset and duration of CJD. vCJD is theorized to be caused by the consumption of meat from cattle that is infected with bovine spongiform encephalopathy or mad cow disease (a prion disease). Once ingested the infected prions follow the same neuroinvasion route of CJD.

ASSESSMENT

"Classic" CJD: Median age at death is 68 years old in patients who are initially seen with dementia and neurologic deterioration. Course of illness is often 4 months. Early symptoms include memory loss, loss of interest, and mood changes with complaints of clumsiness, with jerky and stiff limbs. Blurred eyesight and incontinence follows. At end stage, patients are unable to move or speak and need 24-hour care. Death occurs approximately 6 months after the onset of the disease.
vCJD: The incubation period is unknown and may take up to several years before manifesting. Affects younger people with a mean age of 29 years old. Initial symptoms are more psychiatric than neurologic. Patients are anxious and depressed, and display withdrawal or other behavioral changes. Persistent pain and odd sensations in the face and extremities are common. As disease progresses, the patient develops ataxia, sudden erratic movements, and progressive dementia with marked memory loss. Ultimately, the patient will lose the ability to move or speak and will require 24-hour care. Death soon follows.

DIAGNOSTIC TESTS

CJD is diagnosis based on typical signs, symptoms, and progression of disease.
MRI: A T1, a T2, FLAIR, and diffusion weighted sequences should be ordered with the MRI test. Images will show abnormalities (hyperintensities and cortical ribboning) in specific areas of the brain (i.e., basal ganglia and medial and posterior thalamus).
EEG: For sporadic CJD cases. Will show a consistent slowing of brain waves and/or presence of periodic sharp wave complexes, generally late in the disease's course.
Cerebrospinal fluid examination: Usually normal with elevated CSF protein levels. A 14-3-3 CSF protein test should be highly sensitive and specific to CJD.
Brain biopsy: For cases where diagnosis is difficult. Biopsy the region of the brain that appears abnormal on MRI.
Autopsy: Mainly used to confirm CJD. vCJD is confirmed either through a brain biopsy or autopsy.

COLLABORATIVE MANAGEMENT

There is no known treatment or cure for CJD or vCJD. Management of these patients is supportive and palliative in nature.
Supportive care: Ventilatory support, pain management, patient safety, intensive skin care; and assessment, nutritional support, care for immobility, and treatment for secondary infections. Standard precautions should be taken at all times; follow organization's policy for appropriate personal protection category.

Note: No noted vaccine has been identified for CJD or vCJD.

NURSING DIAGNOSES AND INTERVENTIONS

See nursing diagnoses and interventions in "Nutritional Support," p. 1; "Mechanical Ventilation," p. 14; "Alteration in Consciousness," p.38; "Wound and Skin Care," p. 45; "Prolonged Immobility," p. 61; "Psychosocial Support," p. 68;"Psychosocial Support for the Patient's Family and Significant Others," p. 78; and "Ethical Considerations in Critical Care," p. 80.

WEST NILE VIRUS

PATHOPHYSIOLOGY

West Nile virus is a single-stranded positive RNA virus from the Japanese encephalitis virus serogroup of the genus *Flavivirus*, family Flaviviridae, which is known for Japanese encephalitis and St. Louis encephalitis. In rare cases, West Nile virus may lead to encephalitis or meningitis and death. West Nile virus has an incubation period of 3-14 days. It also can be divided into two lineages. Lineage I strains are more widely distributed and linked to human infections.

TRANSMISSION

West Nile virus is a disease that has spread worldwide. Initially, West Nile virus was a disease that only occurred in bird species. Approximately 146 different species of birds have been reported to acquire this disease. This disease is spread among the bird population by 29 different species of mosquitoes (vectors). The natural cycle is from bird 1 to mosquito 1 to bird 2 to mosquito 2, and so forth. Due to a complex intensification of this natural cycle, bridge vectors (mosquitoes that bite both birds and humans) became infected with the West Nile virus and spread the disease to humans. Only birds and humans in the United States and Israel have been known to die from West Nile virus.

ASSESSMENT

Patients are classified into two different stages of infections, mild infection or severe infection, based on their clinical signs and symptoms.

Mild infection: Symptoms last 3-6 days. Sudden onset of a fever with malaise, anorexia, nausea, vomiting, eye pain, headache, myalgia, rash, and lymphadenopathy.

Severe infection: Most significant risk factor is the patient's age. Older patients have a higher incidence of severe neurologic disease. Symptoms include fever, GI disturbances , change in mental status, and development of a maculopapular or morbilliform rash involving the neck, trunk, arms, or legs. Neurologic symptoms include seizures, myelitis, polyradiculitis, optic neuritis, cranial nerve abnormalities, severe weakness, flaccid paralysis, and ataxia/extrapyramidal signs.

> **Note:**   Myocarditis, pancreatitis, and fulminant hepatitis have been noted in outbreaks before 1990.

DIAGNOSTIC TESTS

Testing for West Nile virus can be obtained through local or state health departments. West Nile virus is on the list of designated nationally notifiable arboviral encephalitides, and the proper authorities should be informed. Check your local or state health department for guidance.

West Nile virus MAC-ELISA: The most efficient diagnostic test in detecting West Nile virus. Detects IgM antibodies to West Nile virus in serum or cerebrospinal fluid collected within 8 days of onset of illness. Patients who have been vaccinated or infected with other flaviviruses (e.g., Japanese encephalitis) may have a positive result.

CBC: Normal or elevated leukocyte counts with lymphocytopenia and anemia.

Serum chemistry: Hyponatremia may be present.

MRI: One third of patients may show enhancement of the leptomeninges and the periventricular areas.

COLLABORATIVE MANAGEMENT

Medication therapy: High-dose ribavirin and interferon alfa-2b have some activity against West Nile virus in vitro.

Supportive care: Intravenous fluids to prevent dehydration, antipyretics for fever management; oxygen therapy and ventilatory support, patient safety, nutritional support, treatment for secondary infections. Standard precautions should be taken at all times; follow organization's policy for appropriate personal protection category.

> **Note:**   No noted vaccine has been identified for West Nile virus.

NURSING DIAGNOSES AND INTERVENTIONS

See nursing diagnoses and interventions in "Nutritional Support," p. 1; "Mechanical Ventilation," p. 14; "Alteration in Consciousness," p. 38; "Wound and Skin Care," p. 45; "Prolonged Immobility," p. 61; "Psychosocial Support;" p. 68; "Psychosocial Support for the Patient's Family and Significant Others," p. 78; and "Ethical Considerations in Critical Care," p. 80.

AVIAN INFLUENZA ("BIRD FLU")

PATHOPHYSIOLOGY

Avian influenza or "bird flu" is an infectious disease of birds caused by the type A strain of the influenza virus. This virus is believed to affect all species of birds and some species of pigs. Fifteen subtypes of type A strain influenza have been identified based on their surface proteins. Two proteins, the hemagglutinin (H) and neuraminidase (N), are used to delineate the subtypes. All subtypes have been recognized in birds; only three subtypes of H (H1, H2, and H3) and two subtypes of N (N1 and N2) have been known to infect humans.

It is theorized that certain subtypes of avian influenza mutated, crossed species, and infected humans. Three subtypes of avian influenza are linked to human infections: H5N1, H7N7, and H9N2. The H5N1 subtype is of particular concern to humans because of its ability to mutate and its tendency to acquire genes from viruses from other animal species. It has demonstrated high pathogenicity and causes severe disease in humans.

TRANSMISSION

Avian influenza is seemingly spread from infected birds to humans, and does not appear to travel between humans. The virus is harbored in birds (in the intestine), which shed the virus through their saliva, nasal secretions, and feces. The most common means of transmission among birds is fecal to oral. Humans who come in direct contact with the contaminated shedding are susceptible to infection. Avian influenza survives on inanimate objects. Contaminated objects may transmit this virus from birds to humans.

ASSESSMENT

Clinical presentation of humans suffering from avian influenza is similar to the "common flu": fever, cough, sore throat, muscle aches, and eye infections. In more severe cases of avian influenza the patient may display signs and symptoms of pneumonia (see "Acute Pneumonia" for "Assessment" information, p. 180) and acute respiratory distress syndrome (see "Acute Respiratory Distress Syndrome" for "Assessment" information, p. 189).

DIAGNOSTIC TESTS

Viral tests: Respiratory viral panels for influenza A. Laboratories that participate in the World Health Organization's global influenza network have capabilities to conduct influenza test for birds and humans. Rapid bedside tests are available for humans, but are not as precise as laboratory testing.

The following tests are influenced by the extent of the disease process and other underlying medical conditions.

Chest x-ray: Assist in identifying the progression of disease, and anatomic involvement.

CBC: Monitoring WBC counts to assist in evaluation of other bacterial infections.

ABG: Determination of patient oxygen saturation and acid-base balance.

Pulse oximetry: Used to measure patient oxygen saturation of arterial blood. Values >90% are normal.

COLLABORATIVE MANAGEMENT

Medication therapy: Two classes of medications are available for treatment of avian influenza in humans. Neuraminidase inhibitors (oseltamivir and zanimivir) and M2 inhibitors (amantadine and rimantadine) have been licensed for prevention and treatment. (Note: Analysis of M2 inhibitors used in the recent outbreak in Viet Nam indicates that avian virus may be resistant. Further testing is needed to clarify this assessment.)

Supportive management: Intravenous fluids to prevent dehydration, antipyretics for fever management; oxygen therapy and ventilatory support, patient safety, nutritional support, treatment for secondary infections.

Infection control: Patient is placed in a negative pressure room. Restricted visitation should be implemented and an ongoing log kept of all persons entering the patient's room. Minimize the number of health care personnel caring for the patient. A strict combination of contact and droplet protection (i.e., eye protection, mask, gloves, and gown) and airborne (e.g., N95 respirator) precautions should be used. All equipment and other items should remain in patient's room and should not be used with other patients or outside the isolation room.

Note: No noted vaccine has been identified for avian influenza H5N1. Due to the rapid mutation rate of this virus, it has been difficult to develop a vaccine.

NURSING DIAGNOSES AND INTERVENTIONS

See nursing diagnoses for "Acute Lung Injury and Respiratory Distress Syndrome," p. 189; "Acute Pneumonia," p. 180; "Acute Respiratory Failure," p. 201; "Mechanical Ventilation," p. 14; "Psychosocial Support," p. 68; and "Psychosocial Support for the Patient's Family and Significant Others," p. 78.

Bioterrorism

Bioterrorism is the intentional release of a biologic agent, generally aimed at causing as great a number of people as possible to suffer illness and death. A bioterrorism event should be suspected when there is an unusual and unexplained increase in an illness. Bioterrorism should be suspected when the following situations are seen:

- An outbreak of an illness similar to one that happens in a healthy population, especially when there is no link to explain the transmission such as a similar food source
- An outbreak of an illness that happens at unusual time of year
- An outbreak with an unusual age distribution
- A cluster of patients is affected by an uncommon disease.

The Centers for Disease Control identified six biological agents of highest concern for use in terrorism: smallpox, anthrax, botulism, tularemia, hemorrhagic fever viruses, and plague. Several factors explain why these agents are more likely to be used:

1. Most people are susceptible to these organisms.
2. They can be aerosolized.
3. They are fairly stable in aerosolized form.
4. Because of point 3, they can cause disease in a large group of individuals.
5. Resultant diseases are difficult to diagnose and treat.
6. They have high morbidity and/or mortality rates.

SMALLPOX (VARIOLA)

PATHOPHYSIOLOGY

Smallpox is a serious, contagious, and sometimes fatal infectious disease. Smallpox is a member of the orthopoxvirus family, along with monkeypox, vaccinia, and cowpox. Though all of these can cause skin lesions, only smallpox is readily transmitted from person to person. There are two clinical forms of smallpox, variola major and variola minor. Variola major is the severe and most common form of smallpox, with a more extensive rash and higher fever. Historically, variola major had a 30% mortality rate. Variola minor was less common and much less severe. Smallpox was eradicated after a successful worldwide vaccination program. The last case of smallpox in the United States was in 1949. The last naturally occurring case in the world was in Somalia in 1977.

Smallpox virus enters the body through the mucosa in the oropharyngeal and respiratory tracts. The virus multiplies in the lymph nodes, the spleen, and the bone marrow. Eventually the virus, contained in lymphocytes, localizes in small blood vessels of the dermis and infects adjacent cells, causing the pustules to form.

TRANSMISSION

Smallpox is transmitted via droplet nuclei or aerosols expelled from an infected person's oropharynx. Usually direct and fairly prolonged face-to-face contact was required to spread smallpox from person to person. Smallpox can be spread through direct contact with infected bodily fluids or contaminated objects (e.g., bedding or clothing). Rarely, the virus spreads through the air in enclosed settings (e.g., buildings, buses, trains.) Humans are the only natural hosts of variola (no recorded transmissions from animals or insects.)

A person with smallpox is sometimes contagious with onset of fever (prodrome phase). Most infected persons become contagious with the onset of rash. At this stage, the person is usually very sick, unable to move around in the community. The person remains contagious until the last smallpox scab falls off.

ASSESSMENT

Clinical case definition: An illness with acute onset of fever $\geq 101°$ F (38.3° C), followed by a rash characterized by firm, deep-seated vesicles or pustules in the same stage of development without other apparent cause.

Incubation period: Usually 12-14 days, but can range from 7-17 days. During this time, the patient feels fine and is not contagious.

Prodromal period: Begins with a high fever (101°-104° F), malaise, headache and backache. May exhibit severe abdominal pains, vomiting, and delirium. This period lasts for 2-4 days before a rash develops. The rash begins with small red spots on the tongue and mouth. During this phase the person is most contagious.

Rash development: Progresses in the mouth and develops on the skin starting on the face, moves to the arms and legs, and then to the feet and hands. Usually spreads to all parts within 24 hr. When rash appears, the person's fever subsides and the person starts to feel better. On day 3, the rash is raised bumps. On day 4, the bumps fill with thick, cloudy fluid with possible indent in the center. Indentation is the classic sign of smallpox rash. The bumps become pustules and eventually scab over. During the pustule stage, the patient is again febrile. After 2 weeks, most of the sores have scabs, which begin to fall off, leaving marks that will become pitted scars on the skin.

DIAGNOSTIC TESTS

Laboratory diagnostic testing for variola should be done by a CDC Laboratory Response Network (LRN) laboratory utilizing LRN-approved polymerase chain reaction (PCR) tests and protocols for variola virus. **Initial confirmation of a smallpox outbreak requires additional testing at CDC.** Laboratory testing should be reserved for cases that meet the clinical case definition: thus classified as being a potential high risk for smallpox.

Laboratory criteria for confirmation of smallpox include the following:
- Polymerase chain reaction (PCR) identification of variola DNA in a clinical specimen, OR
- *Isolation* of smallpox (variola) virus from a clinical specimen (World Health Organization Smallpox Reference laboratory or laboratory with appropriate reference capabilities) with variola PCR confirmation.

COLLABORATIVE MANAGEMENT

There are no specific treatments for smallpox, only supportive care.

Vaccine: A key is to identify smallpox exposure and administer vaccine within 3 days, to prevent or significantly lessen the severity of the disease process. Vaccine administered within 4-7 days after exposure may provide some protection and lessen the disease severity.

Isolation: Patients presenting with symptoms should be isolated immediately in a negative pressure room. The door should be kept closed at all times. All health care workers entering the room should wear an N-95 respirator mask. Since smallpox is also transmitted via body fluids (contaminating the bedding), health care workers should use contact precautions (i.e., gown, gloves, and shoe covers) when entering the room. Other infection control practices, such as limiting patient transport, designating patient care equipment, and so forth, should follow the institution's policies.

SUPPORTIVE MANAGEMENT

Provide hydration: Intravenous fluids to prevent dehydration.
Control fever: Antipyretics to reduce body temperature if >103° F.
Reduce pain and anxiety: Analgesics and sedatives as indicated.

NURSING DIAGNOSES AND INTERVENTIONS

Alteration in comfort related to skin rash and fever
Desired outcome: Patient reports an increase in comfort.
- Keep room at a comfortable temperature for patient.
- Provide patient with distracting activities.
- Administer pain medications and antipyretics as indicated.

ADDITIONAL NURSING DIAGNOSES

Also see nursing diagnoses and interventions in "Psychosocial Support," p. 68; and "Psychosocial Support for the Patient's Family and Significant Others," p. 78.

ANTHRAX

PATHOPHYSIOLOGY

Anthrax is a serious disease caused by *Bacillus anthracis,* a spore-forming bacterium. A spore is a dormant (inactive) cell that activates under the right conditions. Anthrax spores, once inside the human body, are able to germinate. Once germinated, the replicating bacteria release endotoxins leading to hemorrhage, edema, and necrosis.

There are three types of anthrax: skin (*cutaneous*), lung (*inhalation*), and digestive (*gastrointestinal*). Hemorrhagic mediastinitis is present with the inhalation form, and bloody diarrhea in seen with the intestinal form. When enough endotoxin is released into the bloodstream, the disease can be fatal even if antibiotics eradicate the bacteria. Anthrax infections are usually very rare since it takes thousands of spores to cause an infection. *Inhalation anthrax* is usually fatal even with treatment. *Gastrointestinal anthrax* has a mortality rate of 25% to 60%, whereas 20% of those with *untreated cutaneous anthrax* die. Cutaneous anthrax is rarely fatal unless untreated.

TRANSMISSION

Anthrax has not been known to spread from one person to another. Humans may acquire anthrax by handling products from infected animals or inhaling anthrax spores from infected animal products (e.g., wool). People acquire gastrointestinal anthrax by eating undercooked meat from infected animals. Anthrax in soil may enter the body through open skin.

ASSESSMENT

The symptoms (warning signs) of anthrax differ depending on the type of the disease:

- *Inhalation*: the most serious form with the highest mortality rate. Begins 1-6 days after exposure with cold or flulike symptoms: sore throat, mild fever, and muscle aches. Later symptoms include cough, chest discomfort, shortness of breath, fatigue, and muscle aches. Inhalation anthrax quickly progresses to respiratory failure and shock. Chest x-ray reveals a widened mediastinum.
- *Cutaneous*: the first symptom is a raised, itchy bump that develops into a blister, seen 1-7 days after exposure. The blister progresses to a skin ulcer with a blackened center. The sore, the blister, and the ulcer are painless. Fever, headache, and swollen glands may occur.
- *Gastrointestinal*: Two to five days after exposure the person exhibits nausea, loss of appetite, bloody diarrhea, and fever, followed by bad stomach pain. If untreated, it can progress to generalized toxemia and sepsis.

DIAGNOSTIC TESTS

Diagnostic tests to isolate anthrax antigen are not widely available. Confirmation of the diagnosis is made by sending a specimen to a national reference laboratory *after the treatment begins*. Clinicians should begin treatment based on clinical signs and symptoms, since early treatment is imperative to enhance chances of survival from inhalation anthrax. Standard blood culture may be useful if the lab is told to look for bacillus species.

COLLABORATIVE MANAGEMENT

Antibiotics: Used to treat all three types of anthrax. The antibiotics of choice are penicillin, doxycycline, and ciprofloxacin. Early identification and treatment are crucial to minimize the amount of endotoxin released.

Intubation and mechanical ventilation (inhalation): To support gas exchange and help maintain acid-base balance.

Intravenous fluids (inhalation and gastrointestinal): To prevent dehydration and maintain adequate circulatory volume.

Prevention after exposure: Treatment differs when a person exposed to anthrax is not yet sick. Health care providers use antibiotics (e.g., ciprofloxacin, doxycycline, penicillin) combined with anthrax vaccine to prevent anthrax infection.

Treatment after infection: Treatment is usually a 60-day course of antibiotics. Success depends on the type of anthrax and how early treatment begins.

Vaccination: A vaccine to prevent anthrax exists, but it is not yet available to the general public. Anyone at risk for anthrax exposure, including certain members of the U.S. armed forces, laboratory workers, and workers who may enter or reenter contaminated areas, may be vaccinated. If anthrax is used as a weapon, a vaccination program will be initiated to vaccinate as many exposed people as possible.

NURSING DIAGNOSES AND INTERVENTIONS

See nursing diagnoses and interventions in "Mechanical Ventilation," p. 14; "Fluid and Electrolyte Disturbances," p. 538; "Psychosocial Support," p. 68; and "Psychosocial Support for the Patient's Family and Significant Others," p. 78.

BOTULISM

PATHOPHYSIOLOGY

Botulism is a muscle-paralyzing disease caused by a toxin produced from *Clostridium botulinum* bacteria. The toxin is the most potent lethal substance known to man. Man-made inhalational botulism is brought into being when aerosolized botulinum toxin is inhaled. The bacterium naturally lives for weeks in nonmoving water and food. There are three naturally acquired types of botulism:

- Foodborne: a person ingests toxin that leads to illness in a few hours to days.
- Infant: occurs in a small number of susceptible infants each year who harbor *C. botulinum* in their intestinal tracts.
- Wound: occurs when a wound is infected with *C. botulinum.*

Botulinum toxin, once absorbed into the bloodstream, is transported to the peripheral cholinergic synapses, where is binds irreversibly. The toxin then blocks the release of acetylcholine in the neuromuscular junctions, causing paralysis of the muscles.

TRANSMISSION

Botulism is not spread from person to person. Botulinum toxin is absorbed through lung or intestinal mucosa and nonintact skin. Foodborne botulism occurs in all age groups.

ASSESSMENT

Foodborne: Double vision, drooping eyelids, slurred speech, dysphagia, dry mouth, descending muscle weakness. Weakness starts in the shoulders and upper arms, descends to the lower arms and upper thighs and eventually down to the lower legs and feet. Paralysis of the respiratory muscles leads to respiratory failure unless ventilation is supported with mechanical ventilation. Patients are generally afebrile and alert.

DIAGNOSTIC TESTS

Currently, the CDC and less than 25 public health laboratories perform the diagnostic test for botulism. Diagnosis is made clinically, after ruling out other causes of paralysis. Classic botulism paralysis is descending in nature and involves the cranial nerves.

COLLABORATIVE MANAGEMENT

Antitoxin: Botulinum antitoxin is administered in a single 10 mL dose diluted 1:10 in 0.9% saline and given by slow intravenous infusion. Antitoxin helps prevent further nerve damage from the botulinum toxin but cannot reverse the existing paralysis.
Antibiotic: To treat wounds infected with *C. botulinum* and secondary infections. Antibiotics have no effect on botulinum toxin.
Vaccine: Investigational, not currently available.

SUPPORTIVE CARE:

Includes mechanical ventilation, nutritional support, care for immobility, and treatment for secondary infections.

NURSING DIAGNOSES AND INTERVENTIONS

See nursing diagnoses and interventions in "Mechanical Ventilation," p. 14; "Prolonged Immobility," p. 61; "Psychosocial Support," p. 68; and "Psychosocial Support for the Patient's Family and Significant Others," p. 78.

T̃ULAREMIA

PATHOPHYSIOLOGY

Tularemia is caused by a bacterial zoonosis called *Francisella tularensis.* One of the most infectious pathogenic bacteria known, it is found in infected water, soil, vegetation, small mammals, ticks, fleas, and mosquitoes. *F. tularensis* is a small, nonmotile, aerobic, gram-negative coccobacillus that targets the lymph nodes, the lungs, the pleura, the spleen, the liver, and the kidneys. Bacteria enter through skin, mucous membranes, gastrointestinal tract, and lungs to invade cells, causing inflammation and permanent damage if untreated.

TRANSMISSION

Tularemia is transmitted by bites from infected arthropods, handling infectious animal tissues or fluids, direct contact with or ingestion of contaminated water, food, or soil, and inhaling infected aerosols. There is no evidence of person-to-person transmission. Patient should be placed on standard precautions.

ASSESSMENT

Disease presentation: May vary depending on the infecting organism, dose, and site of inoculation. Usually starts abruptly with a fever 100. 1° to 104° F (38° to 40° C), headache, chills, generalized body aches, rhinitis, and a sore throat. Some patients have dry cough, substernal pain. *Illness progression*: progressive weakness, malaise, anorexia, and weight loss. If untreated, symptoms may persist for several weeks to months. Secondary sepsis, pleuropneumonia, and rarely meningitis may develop.

DIAGNOSTIC TESTS

Rapid diagnostic testing for *F. tularensis* is not widely available. If tularemia is suspected, specimens of respiratory secretions and blood should be collected and sent to a designated laboratory for microscopic identification using fluorescent-labeled antibodies.

COLLABORATIVE MANAGEMENT

Antibiotics: Antibiotic of choice is streptomycin, though gentamicin may be used. The patient should be placed on a 10-day course.
Vaccine: A vaccine is currently under review by the FDA.

NURSING DIAGNOSES AND INTERVENTIONS

See nursing diagnoses and interventions in "Nutritional Support," p. 1; "Psychosocial Support," p. 68, and "Psychosocial Support for the Patient's Family and Significant Others," p. 78.

PLAGUE

PATHOPHYSIOLOGY

Plague is an infectious disease caused by the bacterium *Yersinia pestis,* found in rodents and their fleas. Several forms of plague can occur individually or in combination: bubonic, pneumonic, and septicemic plague. *Bubonic plague* is the most common, occurring when an infected flea bites a human or when infectious materials enter through a break in the skin. *Pneumonic plague* occurs when *Y. pestis* infects lungs through direct or close contact with a person who has pneumonic plague, or in untreated patients with bubonic or septicemic plague, allowing bacterial spread to lungs. *Septicemic plague* can occur as a complication of either of the previous types of plague or alone. The bacteria enter the bloodstream and multiply, prompting the systemic effects of sepsis.

The *Y. pestis* bacteria travel to lymph nodes, where they resist defense mechanisms and rapidly multiply, causing destruction of lymph nodes. Bacteria enter the bloodstream and prompt sepsis, septic shock, disseminated intravascular coagulation (DIC), and coma.

TRANSMISSION

Pneumonic plague is spread through direct contact with an infected person. Neither bubonic nor septicemic plagues are transmitted by person-to-person contact.
Pneumonic plague: Droplet precautions until the patient receives antibiotics for 72 hours.
Bubonic or septicemic plague: Standard precautions.

ASSESSMENT

Pneumonic plague: Fever, headache, weakness, and rapidly developing pneumonia with shortness of breath, chest pain, cough, and sometimes bloody or watery sputum. The pneumonia progresses and in 2-4 days can cause respiratory failure and shock. Without treatment, patients with pneumonic plague will die.
Bubonic plague: Swollen, tender lymph glands (called buboes), fever, headache, chills, and weakness.
Septicemic plague: Fever and chills, abdominal pain, shock with bleeding (due to DIC).

DIAGNOSTIC TESTS

Gram's stain of sputum or blood: Reveals gram-negative bacilli. A laboratory may misidentify the bacteria unless notified that *Y. pestis* is suspected.

COLLABORATIVE MANAGEMENT

Antibiotics: Given within the first 24 hr of symptoms. Streptomycin, gentamycin, tetracyclines, and chloramphenicol are all effective in treating pneumonic plague
Vaccine: There currently is no vaccine available in the United States.

Supportive care: Ventilatory support, pain management, and treatment for shock, DIC and MODS, as appropriate.

NURSING DIAGNOSES AND INTERVENTIONS

See nursing diagnoses and interventions in "SIRS, Sepsio, and Septic Shock," p. 501; "Disseminated Intravascular Coagulation," p. 489; "Mechanical Ventilation," p. 14; and "Psychosocial Support for the Patient's Family and Significant Others," p. 78.

HEMORRHAGIC FEVER VIRUSES (HFVS)

PATHOPHYSIOLOGY

Hemorrhagic fever viruses (HFVs) include many diseases separated into four families of viruses; not all are viewed as risks for bioterrorism. Those felt to pose a significant risk include Ebola virus disease, Marburg virus disease, Lassa fever, New World Arenaviridae, Rift Valley fever, Yellow fever, Omsk hemorrhagic fever, and Kyasanur Forest disease. The pathophysiology of these diseases is not well understood. Outbreaks are sporadic and have occurred in areas with very limited health care. Infection with these viruses leads to thrombocytopenia and possibly platelet dysfunction. The effects of these viruses vary, but all lead to coagulation problems, hemorrhage, and shock. Mortality ranges range from <1 % with Rift Valley fever to 50%-90% with Ebola. Only one of the Arenaviridae viruses has been identified in the United States. Other HFVs have not emerged.

TRANSMISSION

HFVs reside in many animal hosts and arthropod vectors. Humans become infected when bitten by an infected arthropod, by inhaling aerosolized virus from infected rodent excreta, or from direct contact with infected animal carcasses. Humans infected with Ebola, Marburg, Lassa fever, and arenaviruses can spread the disease to close contacts.
Isolation: Strict airborne and contact isolation if a patient is suspected of infection.

ASSESSMENT

Clinical scenarios vary depending on the virus. *The most common symptom is a fever.*
Ebola and Marburg: Maculopapular rash, bleeding, disseminated intravascular coagulation.
Lassa fever and New World arenaviruses: Gradual onset of fever, nausea, abdominal pain, and conjunctivitis.
Rift Valley fever: Fever, headache, photophobia, and jaundice. .

DIAGNOSTIC TESTS

Only the CDC and U.S. Army Research Institute of Infectious Diseases laboratories have testing available.

COLLABORATIVE MANAGEMENT

Supportive care: Maintain fluid and electrolyte balances, treat hypotension with early use of vasopressors if fluid therapy is not effective, mechanical ventilation, renal dialysis, and anticonvulsive therapy.
Ribavirin: 10-day course if Lassa fever or New World arenavirus is confirmed.
   Intramuscular injections, aspirin, nonsteroidal antiinflammatory drugs, steroids, and anticoagulant therapies are contraindicated.

NURSING DIAGNOSES AND INTERVENTIONS

See nursing diagnoses and interventions in "Fluid and Electrolyte Disturbances," p. 538; "Mechanical Ventilation," p. 14, and "Psychosocial Support for the Patient's Family and Significant Others," p. 78.

Bibliography
Websites
Sepsis.com
www.sepsis.com
International Sepsis Forum
www.sepsisforum.org
Information on surviving sepsis
www.survivingsepsis.org

Information on Xigris (drotrecogin alfa) and sepsis
www.Xigris.com
Information on agents used in bioterrorism/Centers for Disease Control and Prevertion
http://www.bt.cdc.gov/agent/anthrax/index.asp
http://www.bt.cdc.gov/agent/botulism/index.asp
http://www.bt.cdc.gov/agent/plague/index.asp
http://www.bt.cdc.gov/agent/smallpox/disease/index.asp
http://www.bt.cdc.gov/agent/tularemia/index.asp
http://www.bt.cdc.gov/agent/vhf/index.asp

Literature

Ahrens T: Continuous mixed venous (Svo$_2$) monitoring: too expensive or indispensable? *Crit Care Nurs Clin North Am* 11(1):33-48, March 1999.

American College of Chest Physicians/Society of Critical Care Medicine Consensus Conference Committee: Definitions for sepsis and organ failure and guidelines for the use of innovative therapies in sepsis, *Crit Care Med* 20(6):864-874, 1992.

Angus DC et al: Epidemiology of severe sepsis in the United States: analysis of incidence, outcome and associated costs of care, *Crit Care Med* 29(7):1303-1310, 2001.

Arias B, Smith B: Deaths Preliminary Data for 2001, *Centers for Disease Control* 4, March 2003.

Arieff, AI: Acid-base, electrolyte and metabolic abnormalities. In Parrillo JE, Dellinger RP: *Critical care medicine: principles of diagnosis and management in the adult,* ed 2, St. Louis, 2002, Mosby.

Aron SS et al: Botulinum toxin as a biological weapon: medical and pubic health management, *JAMA* 285(8):1059-1070, 2001.

Baue AE et al: Systemic inflammatory response syndrome (SIRS), multiple organ dysfunction syndrome (MODS), multiple organ failure (MOF): are we winning the battle? *Shock* 10(2):79-89, 1998.

Belay ED, Schonberger LB: Variant Creutzfeldt-Jakob disease and bovine spongiform encephalopathy, *Clin Lab Med* 22:849-862, 2002.

Bernard GR et al: The effects of ibuprofen on the physiology and survival of patients with sepsis, *N Engl J Med*, 336:912-918, 1997.

Borio L et al: Hemorrhagic fever viruses as biological weapons: medical and public health management, *JAMA* 287(18):2391-2405, 2002.

Bridges EJ et al: Hemodynamic monitoring in high-risk obstetrics patients. I: Expected hemodynamic changes during pregnancy, *Crit Care Nurse* 23 (4):53-62, Aug 2003.

Bridges EJ et al: Hemodynamic monitoring in high-risk obstetrics patients. II: Pregnancy induced hypertension and preeclampsia, *Crit Care Nurse* 23 (5):52-56, Oct 2003.

Burns MJ, Schwartzstein RM: Decontamination of the poisoned adult, parts I and II, *Uptodate.com* 11(1):2002.

Burns MJ, Schwartzstein RM: Enhanced elimination of poisons, *Uptodate.com* 11(1), 2002.

Burns MJ et al: Alcohol withdrawal syndromes, *Uptodate.com* 11(1), 2002.

Cain AE, Khalil RA: Pathophysiology of essential hypertension: role of the pump, the vessel, and the kidney, Semin Nephrol 22(1):3-16, Jan 2002.

Carroll K et al: Nonpharmacologic approaches to substance abuse treatment, *Med Clin North Am* 81(4):927-944, 1997.

Centers for Disease Control and Prevention: Basic information about avian influenza, Jan 2004, retrieved May 3, 2004 from the World Wide Web http://www.cdc.gov/flu/avian/facts.htm.

Centers for Disease Control and Prevention: Bird flu fact sheet (n.d.), retrieved May 2004 from the World Wide Web http://www.cdc.gov/flu/avian/outbreak.htm.

Centers for Disease Control and Prevention: Clinical guidance on the identification and evaluation of possible SARS-CoV disease among persons presenting with community-acquired illness, Jan 2004, retrieved April 30, 2004 from the World Wide Web http://www.cdc.gov/ncidod/sars/clinicalguidance.htm.

Centers for Disease Control and Prevention: Consent form (SARS-CoV EIA laboratory testing), April 2004, retrieved April 30, 2004 from the World Wide Web http://www.cdc.gov/ncidod/sars/lab/eia/consent.htm.

Centers for Disease Control and Prevention: Fact sheet: new variant Creutzfeldt-Jakob disease, Jan 2004, retrieved May 2, 2004 from the World Wide Web http://www.cdc.gov/ncidod/diseases/cjd/cjd_fact_sheet.htm.

Centers for Disease Control and Prevention: Guidance for persons who may have been exposed to severe acute respiratory syndrome (SARS), Jan 2004, retrieved April 30, 2004 from the World Wide Web http://www.cdc.gov/ncidod/sars/exposuremanagement.htm.

Centers for Disease Control and Prevention: In the absence of SARS-CoV transmission worldwide: guidance for surveillance, clinical and laboratory evaluation, and reporting version 2, Jan 2004, retrieved April 30, 2004 from the World Wide Web http://www.cdc.gov/ncidod/sars/absenceofsars.htm.

Centers for Disease Control and Prevention: Questions and answers regarding bovine spongiform encephalopathy (BSE) and Creutzfeldt-Jakob disease (CJD), Dec 2003, retrieved May 2, 2004 from the World Wide Web http://www.cdc.gov/ncidod/diseases/cjd/bse_cjd_qa.htm.

Centers for Disease Control and Prevention: SARS-associated coronavirus (SARS-CoV) sequencing, March 2004, retrieved April 30, 2004 from the World Wide Web http://www.cdc.gov/ncidod/sars/sequence.htm.

Centers for Disease Control and Prevention: Severe acute respiratory syndrome (SARS), Jan 2004, retrieved April 30, 2004 from the World Wide Web http://www.cdc.gov/ncidod/sars/guidance/core/intro.htm.

Centers for Disease Control and Prevention: Severe acute respiratory syndrome (SARS); public health guidance for community-level preparedness and response to severe acute respiratory syndrome (SARS) version 2, Supplement B: SARS surveillance, Jan 2004, retrieved April 30, 2004 from the World Wide Web http://www.cdc.gov/ncidod/sars/guidance/B/index.htm.

Centers for Disease Control and Prevention: Severe acute respiratory syndrome (SARS); public health guidance for community-level preparedness and response to severe acute respiratory syndrome (SARS) version 2, Supplement F: Laboratory guidance, Jan 2004, retrieved April 30, 2004 from the World Wide Web http://www.cdc.gov/ncidod/sars/guidance/f/index.htm.

Centers for Disease Control and Prevention: Supplement I: Infection control in healthcare, home, and community settings. Jan 2004, retrieved April 30, 2004 from the World Wide Web http://www.cdc.gov/ncidod/sars/guidance/I/occupational.htm.

Centers for Disease Control and Prevention: West Nile virus (WNV) infection: information for clinicians, Sept 2003, retrieved May 2, 2004 from the World Wide Web http://www.cdc.gov/ncidod/dvbid/westnile/resources/fact_sheet_clinician.htm.

Chakraborti S: Protective role of magnesium in cardiovascular diseases: a review, *Mol Cell Biochem* 238(1-2):163-79, Sept 2002.

Chamberlain G, Steer P: ABC of labour care, *BMJ* 318:1342-1345, 1999.

Chan MH et al: Serum LD1 isoenzyme and blood lymphocyte subsets as prognostic indicators for severe acute respiratory syndrome, *J Intern Med* 255:512-518, 2004.

Chan L, Gaston R, Hariharan S: Evolution of immunosuppression and continued importance of acute rejection in renal transplantation, *Am J Kidney Dis* 38(6): S2-S9 2001.

CJD Support Network: Variant CJD, 2001, retrieved May 3, 2004 from the World Wide Web http://www.cjdsupport.net/pdf/c_variant.pdf.

CJD Support Network: What is CJD? (n.d.), retrieved May 3, 2004, from the World Wide Web http://www.cjdsupport.net/what_is.html.

Clark SL: Critical care obstetrics. In Scott JR et al: *Danforth's obstetrics and gynecology,* ed 9, Philadelphia, 2003, Lippincott Williams and Wilkins.

Costanzo MR: Severe heart failure. In Parrillo JE, Dellinger RP: *Critical care medicine: principles of diagnosis and management in the adult,* ed 2, St. Louis, 2002, Mosby.

Coupey S: Barbiturates, *Pediatr Rev* 18(8):260-264, 1997.

Crombleholme WR: Obstetrics. In Tierney LM, McPhee SJ, Papadakis MA: *CMDT 2004: current medical diagnosis and treatment,* ed 43, New York, 2004, Lange Medical Books/McGraw Hill.

Cunningham J: Ecstasy-induced rhabdomyolysis and its role in the development of acute renal failure, *Intens Care Nurs* 13(4):216-223, 1997.

Dahlen K et al: Acute lung failure induced by tricyclic antidepressants, *Toxicol Appl Pharmacol* 146(2):309-316, 1997.

Deftos LJ: Hypercalcemia: mechanism, differential diagnosis and remedies, *Postgrad Med* 100(6):119-126, 1996.

Dellinger RP et al: Surviving sepsis campaign guidelines for management of severe sepsis and septic shock, *Crit Care Med* 32(3):858-873, 2004.

DeJong MJ, Fausett MB: Anaphylactoid syndrome of pregnancy: a devastating complication requiring critical care, *Crit Care Nurse* 23(6):42-48, December, 2003.

DeJong MJ, Karch AM: *Critical Care Drug Guide,* Philadelphia, 2000, Lippincott.

Dennis DT et al: Tularemia as a biological weapon: medical and public health management, *JAMA* 285(21):2763-2773, 2001.

Diagnosis and management of preeclampsia and eclampsia, ACOG Practice Bulletin No. 33, *Int J Gynaecol Obstet* 77:67, 2002.

Dochterman JM, Bulechek GM: *Nursing interventions classification (NIC),* ed 4, St. Louis, 2004, Mosby.

Dreher HM et al: What you need to know about SARS, *Nursing* 34(1):59-63, 2004.

Dunne J et al: Practice parameter for the assessment and treatment of children and adolescents with substance use disorders, *J Am Acad Child Adolesc Psychiatry* 36(10):140S-156S, 1997.

Ely WE, Kleinpell RM, Goyette RE: Advances in the understanding of clinical manifestations and therapy of severe sepsis: an update for critical care nurses, *Am J Crit Care* 12(2):120-135, March 2003.

Erikson P: The role of acetaldehyde in the actions of alcohol, *Alcohol Clin Exp Res* 25(5):15s-32s, 2001.

Faist E, Kim C: Therapeutic immunomodulary approaches for the control of systemic inflammatory response syndrome and the prevention of sepsis, *New Horiz* 6(suppl 2):S97-S102, 1998.

Fencl V et al: Diagnosis of metabolic acid-base disturbances in critically ill patients, *Am J Respir Crit Care Med* 162:2246–2251, 2000.

Fraser CL, Arieff AI: Epidemiology, pathophysiology, and management of hyponatremic encephalopathy, *Am J Med* 102:67-77, 1997.

Freeman BD, Parrillo JE, Natanson C: Septic shock and multiple organ failure. In Parrillo JE, Dellinger RP: *Critical care medicine: principles of diagnosis and management in the adult,* ed 2, St. Louis, 2002, Mosby.

Fried LF, Palevsky PM: Hyponatremia and hypernatremia, *Med Clin North Am* 81(3):585-609, 1997.

Gorman M et al: What do you do when your patient uses illicit drugs? *Am J Nurs* 98(3):54, 1998.

Greenberg A: Hyperkalemia: treatment options, *Semin Nephrol* 18(1):46-57, 1998.

Greene K, Nierman D, Vallet B: Commentary and analysis on advances in the understanding and treatment of sepsis, *Adv Sepsis* 1(4):114-144, 2001.

Gross P et al: The treatment of severe hyponatremia, *Kidney Int* 53(64):S6-S11, 1998.

Halperin ML, Goldstein MB: *Fluid, electrolyte and acid-base physiology,* ed 3, Philadelphia, 1999, Saunders.

Harvey MA: Systemic inflammatory response syndrome and multiorgan dysfunction syndrome. In Kinney MR et al: *AACN clinical reference for critical care nursing,* ed 4, St Louis, 1998, Mosby.

Health Canada: Learning from SARS, Oct 2003, retrieved April 30, 2004, from the World Wide Web http://www.hc-sc.gc.ca/english/protection/warnings/sars/learning/EngSe30_ch1.htm.

Health Canada: Management of severe acute respiratory syndrome (SARS) in adults: interim guidance for health care providers, July 2003, retrieved April 30, 2004, from the World Wide Web http://www.hc-sc.gc.ca/pphb-dgspsp/sars-sras/pdf/sars-clin-guide-20030703_e.pdf

Henderson DA et al: Smallpox as a biological weapon: medical and public health management, *JAMA* 281(22):2127-2137, 1999.

Hodges B: Pharmacotherapy for alcohol withdrawal, *Hosp Pharmacy* 38(5):420-425, 2003.

Hoecker CC: Designer drugs in adults, *Uptodate.com* 11(1), 2002.

Hoffman R et al: Evaluation of the patient with chest pain after cocaine use, *Crit Care Clin* 13(4):809-828, 1997.

Hollander J et al: Predictors of coronary artery disease in patients with cocaine-associated myocardial infarction. Cocaine-Associated Myocardial Infarction (CAMI) Study Group, *Am J Med* 102(2):158-163, 1997.

Horne MM, Heitz UE, Swearingen PL: *Pocket guide to fluids and electrolytes,* ed 3, St Louis, 1997, Mosby.

Inglesby TV et al: Anthrax as a biological weapon: medical and public health management, *JAMA* 281(18):1735-1745, 1999.

Inglesby TV et al: Plague as a biological weapon: medical and public health management, *JAMA* 283(17):2281-2290, 2000.

Joint Council of Allergy, Asthma and Immunology: The diagnosis and management of anaphylaxis, *J Allergy Clin Immunol* 101(6 Pt 2):S465-S528, 1998.

Jones A: Recent advances in the management of poisoning, *Ther Drug Monit* 24(1)150-155, 2002.

Kalant H et al: Opium revisited: a brief review of its nature, composition, non-medical use and relative risk, *Addiction* 92(3):267-277, 1997.

Kokko JP, Tannen RL: *Fluids and electrolytes,* ed 3, Philadelphia, 1996, Saunders.

Kosten TR, O'Connor PG: Management of drug and alcohol withdrawal, *N Engl J Med* 348(18):1786-1795, 2003.

Krause RS: Anaphylaxis, *eMedicine Journal,* updated Dec 2001, retrieved May 1, 2003, from the World Wide Web http://www.emedicine.com/emerg/topic25.htm.

Lancaster L, editor: *Core curriculum for nephrology nursing,* ed 4, Pitman, NJ, 2001, Anthony J. Janetti.

Lauro R, Karp BI: Myelinolysis after correction of hyponatremia, *Ann Intern Med* 126(1):57-62, 1997.

Leung TF et al: Severe acute respiratory syndrome (SARS) in children: epidemiology, presentation and management, *Paediatr Respir Rev* 4:334-339, 2003.

Levraut J. Grimaud D: Treatment of metabolic acidosis, *Curr Opin Crit Care* 9(4):260-265, Aug 2003.

Levy MM, Vincent JL: *Sepsis: Insights and Current Management. Proceedings of the 2002 SCCM/ESICM Summer Conference,* Society of Critical Care Medicine 1-136, 2003.

Liebelt E et al: Serial electrocardiogram changes in acute tricyclic antidepressant overdose, *Crit Care Med* 25(10):1721-1726, 1997.

Lin RY et al: Histamine and tryptase levels in patients with acute allergic reactions: an emergency department-based study, *J Allergy Clin Immunol* 106(1Pt1):65-71, 2000.

Lundberg JS et al: Septic shock: an analysis of outcomes for patients with onset on hospital wards versus intensive care units, *Crit Care Med* 26(6):1020-1024, 1998.

Malek N: Acute salicylate overdose, *Hosp Pract (Off Ed)* 33(6):46, 1998.

Mandal AK: Hypokalemia and hyperkalemia, *Med Clin North Am* 81(3):611-639, 1997.

Marino PL: *The ICU book,* ed 2, Baltimore, 1998, Williams & Wilkins.

Mayo-Smith M et al: Pharmacological management of alcohol withdrawal: a meta-analysis and evidenced-based practice guideline, *JAMA* 278(2):144-151, 1997.

Mazur H: Critically ill immunosuppressed host. In Parrillo JE, Dellinger RP: *Critical care medicine: principles of diagnosis and management in the adult,* ed 2, St. Louis, 2002, Mosby.

McCance KL, Huether SE: *Pathophysiology: the biological basis for disease in adults and children,* ed 4, St. Louis, 2002, Mosby Year Book.

McCloskey JC, Bulechek GB, editors: *Nursing Interventions Classification* (NIC), ed 3, St. Louis, 2000, Mosby Year Book.

McDonough J: Emergency! Acetaminophen overdose, *Am J Nurs* 93(3):52, 1998.

McKinley BA, Butler BD: Comparison of skeletal muscle PO_2, PCO_2, and pH with gastric tonometric PCO_2 and pH in hemorrhagic shock, *Crit Care Med* 27(9):1869-1877, Sept 1999.

Miller PR et al: Systemic inflammatory response syndrome in the trauma intensive care unit: who is infected? *J Trauma* 47(6):1004-1008, 1999.

Mitchell I et al: Earlier identification of patients at risk from acetaminophen-induced acute liver failure, *Crit Care Med* 26(2):279-284, 1998.

Mokhlesi B: Adult toxicology in critical care part 1: general approach to the intoxicated patient, *Chest* 123(2):577-592, 2003.

Moldenhauer JS, Sibai BM: Hypertensive disorders of pregnancy. In Scott JR et al: *Danforth's obstetrics and gynecology,* ed 9, Philadelphia, 2003, Lippincott Williams and Wilkins.

Moriyama S et al: Evaluation of oxygen consumption and resting energy expenditure in critically ill patients with systemic inflammatory response syndrome, *Crit Care Med* 27(10):2133-2136, 1999.

Nowbal S, Anderson RJ: Chronic renal failure. In Parrillo JE, Dellinger RP: *Critical care medicine: principles of diagnosis and management in the adult,* ed 2, St. Louis, 2002, Mosby.

Nugent AI, Ghatak AT, Miller RL: Anaphylaxis in the United States: an investigation into its epidemiology, *Arch Intern Med* 161(1):15-21, 2001.

O'Connor P et al: Rapid and ultrarapid opioid detoxification techniques, *JAMA* 279(3):229-234, 1998.

Oh MS, Kim HJ: Basic rules of parenteral fluid therapy, *Nephron* 92(Suppl 1):56-59, 2002.

Osborn H et al: New-onset bronchospasm or recrudescence of asthma associated with cocaine abuse, *Acad Emerg Med* 4(7):689-692, 1997.

Palevsky PM: Hypernatremia, *Semin Nephrol* 18(1):20-30, 1998.

Perazella MA, Mahnessmith RL: Hyperkalemia in the elderly, *J Gen Intern Med* 12:646-656, 1997.

Petersen LR, Marfin AA: West Nile Virus: a primer for the clinician, *Ann Intern Med* 137(3):173-179, 2002.

Porche R, Brenner ZR: Allergy to protamine sulfate, *Heart Lung,* 28(6):418-428, 1999.

Preston RA: *Acid-base, fluids and electrolytes made ridiculously simple,* Miami, 1997, MedMaster.

Rauén C, Munro N: Shock. In Kinney MR et al: *AACN clinical reference for critical care nursing,* ed 4, St Louis, 1998, Mosby.

Sampathkumar P et al: SARS: Epidemiology, clinical presentation, management, and infection control measures, *Mayo Clin Proc* 78:882-890, 2003.

Sands KE et al: Epidemiology of sepsis syndrome in 8 academic medical centers, *JAMA* 278(3):234-240, 1997.

Schrier RW, editor: *Renal and electrolyte disorders,* ed 5, Philadelphia, 1997, Lippincott-Raven.

Shapiro M: Traumatic shock: non-surgical management. In Parrillo JE, Dellinger RP: *Critical care medicine: principles of diagnosis and management in the adult,* ed 2, St. Louis, 2002, Mosby.

Solomon T et al: West Nile encephalitis, *BMJ* 326:865-869, 2003.

Sporer K: Clinical course of crack cocaine body stuffers, *Ann Emerg Med* 29(5):596-601, 1997.

Stein M et al: Women and substance abuse, *Med Clin North Am* 81(4):979-998, 1997.

Sulkowski J et al: Acute mental status changes, *AACN Clin Issues* 8(3):319-334, 1997.

Talmor M, Hydo L, Barie PS: Relationship of systemic inflammatory response syndrome to organ dysfunction, length of stay, and mortality in critical surgical illness: effect of intensive care unit resuscitation, *Arch Surg* 134(1):81-87, 1999.

Trujillo M et al: Pharmacologic antidotes in critical care medicine: approach for drug administration, *Crit Care Med* 26(2):377-391, 1998.

Tsuneyoshi I et al: Hemodynamic and metabolic effects of low-dose vasopressin infusions in vasodilatory septic shock, *Crit Care Med* 29:487-493, 2001.

University of California, San Francisco, Memory and Aging Center: Creutzfeldt-Jakob Disease (CJD), (n.d.), retrieved May 2, 2003 from the World Wide Web http://memory.ucsf.edu/Education/education_cjd.html.

Vender JS, Franklin M: Hemodynamic assessment of the critically ill patient, *Int Anesthesiol Clin* 42(1):31-58, 2004.

Verbalis JG: Adaptation to acute and chronic hyponatremia: implications for symptomatology, diagnosis, and therapy, *Semin Nephrol* 18(1):3-19, 1998.

Weaver MF: Heroin and other opiates, *Uptodate.com* 11(1):2002.

Weaver MF: Sedative, stimulant, hallucinogen and inhalant abuse, *Uptodate.com* 11(1):2002.

Weinhous GL et al: Alcohol withdrawal syndromes, *Uptodate.com* 11(1):2002.

Whang R: Clinical disorders of magnesium metabolism, *Compre Ther* 23(3):168-173, 1997.

Wheeler AP, Bernard GR: Treating patients with severe sepsis, *N Engl J Med* 340:209, 1999.

White V: ActionStat. Aspirin overdose, *Nursing* 28(4):33, 1998.

World Health Organization: Avian influenza, Jan 2004, retrieved May 3, 2004 from the World Wide Web http://www.who.int/mediacentre/factsheets/avian_influenza/en/

World Health Organization: Avian influenza-fact sheet, Jan 2004, retrieved May 3, 2004 from the World Wide Web http://www.who.int/csr/don/2004_01_15/en/.

World Health Organization: Avian influenza frequently asked questions, Jan 2004, retrieved May 3, 2004 from the World Wide Web http://www.who.int/csr/disease/avian_influenza/avian_faqs/en/#drugs.

World Health Organization: Case definitions for surveillance of severe acute respiratory syndrome (SARS), May 2003, retrieved May 3, 2004, from the World Wide Web http://www.who.int/csr/sars/casedefinition/en/.

World Health Organization: Influenza A (H5N1): WHO interim infection control guide for health care facilities, March 2004, retrieved May 3, 2004 from the World Wide Web http://www.who.int/csr/disease/avian_influenza/guidelines/infectioncontrol1/en/.

World Health Organization: Preliminary clinical description of severe acute respiratory syndrome, (n.d.), retrieved May 3, 2004 from the World Wide Web http://www.who.int/csr/sars/clinical/en/.

Xigris ™ (drotrecogin alfa activated). Prescribing information, 2002.

Zafonte RD, Mann NR: Cerebral salt wasting syndrome in brain injury patients: a potential cause of hyponatremia, *Arch Phys Med Rehabil* 78:540-542, 1997.

ACLS Algorithms

T A B L E 1	**Primary ABCD Survey**

ASSESS RESPONSIVENESS

If responsive, ask patient questions to determine adequacy of airway and breathing

If unresponsive, call for help (9-1-1 "Phone first"), call for defibrillator

Continue Primary ABCD Survey

↓

AIRWAY

Open the airway

If the airway is open, evaluate breathing

If the airway is not open, assess for sounds of airway compromise and look in the mouth for blood, broken teeth, loose dentures, gastric contents, and foreign objects

Clear the airway and insert an airway adjunct as needed to maintain an open airway

↓

BREATHING

Look, listen, and feel for breathing

If the patient is responsive and breathing is adequate, evaluate circulation

If the unresponsive patient is breathing adequately, place in recovery position if no signs of trauma

If breathing is difficult and the rate is too slow or too fast, provide positive-pressure ventilation with 100% oxygen

If breathing is absent, insert an airway adjunct (if not previously done) and provide positive-pressure ventilation with a pocket mask or bag-valve-mask and 100% oxygen

Deliver two slow breaths and ensure the patient's chest rises with each breath

Administer oxygen as soon as it is available

Continue Primary ABCD Survey

↓

CIRCULATION

Assess for the presence of a pulse

If the patient is unresponsive, assess the carotid pulse on the side of the patient's neck nearest you

If the patient is responsive, assess the radial pulse. If a pulse is present, quickly estimate the rate and determine the quality of the pulse (e.g., fast/slow, regular/irregular, weak/strong), then perform the Secondary ABCD Survey

If there is no pulse, begin chest compressions until an AED or monitor/defibrillator is available

↓

DEFIBRILLATION

Attach AED or monitor/defibrillator when available

If cardiac rhythm is pulseless VT or VF:

Defibrillate up to 3 times in rapid succession pausing only to analyze/verify rhythm ("serial shocks")

Defibrillate with 200 J, 200 to 300 J, 360 J, or equivalent biphasic energy as necessary

If cardiac rhythm is not VT/VF, perform

Secondary ABCD Survey

From Aehlert B: *ACLS quick review study guide,* ed 2, St Louis, 2002, Mosby.

T A B L E 2   Pulseless Ventricular Tachycardia (VT)/Ventricular Fibrillation (VF)

Basic Life Support	**Perform Primary ABCD Survey**

(Correct critical problems IMMEDIATELY as they are identified)

Assess responsiveness

Call for help/call for defibrillator

Airway—open the airway

Breathing—deliver two slow breaths, administer oxygen as soon as it is available

Circulation—perform chest compressions

Ensure availability of monitor/Defibrillator

On arrival of AED/monitor/defibrillator, evaluate cardiac rhythm

▼

If PEA or asystole, continue CPR and go to appropriate algorithm.

If pulseless VT/VF, shock up to three times (200 J, 200 to 300 J, 360 J, or equivalent Biphasic energy).

▼

Reevaluate cardiac rhythm

• If persistent or recurrent pulseless VT/VF, continue CPR and perform secondary ABCD Survey	• If PEA or asystole, continue CPR and go to appropriate algorithm	If return of spontaneous circulation (ROSC): • Assess vital signs • Maintain open airway • Provide ventilation • Administer medications appropriate for rhythm, blood pressure, and heart rate

▼

Advanced Life Support	**Perform Secondary ABCD Survey** **(ADVANCED) AIRWAY**

Reassess effectiveness of initial airway maneuvers and interventions

Perform invasive airway management

▼

*B*REATHING

Assess ventilation

Confirm ET tube placement (or other airway device) by at least two methods

Provide positive-pressure ventilation/Evaluate effectiveness of ventilations

Secure airway device in place with commercial tube holder (preferred) or tape

▼

*C*IRCULATION

Establish IV access and administer appropriate medications

▼

*D*IFFERENTIAL DIAGNOSIS

Search for and treat reversible causes

▼

Epinephrine (Class indeterminate) 1 mg (1:10,000 solution) IV every 3 to 5 min (ET dose 2 to 2.5 mg diluted in 10-mL normal saline or distilled water)

or,

Pattern becomes CPR-drug-shock or CPR-drug-shock-shock-shock	**Vasopressin** (Class IIb) 40 U IV bolus (administer only once) (If no response to vasopressin, may resume epinephrine after 10 to 20 min; epi dose 1 mg every 3 to 5 min) Defibrillate with 360 J (or equivalent Biphasic energy) within 30 to 60 sec <div align="center">▼</div>

Continued

T A B L E 2   Pulseless Ventricular Tachycardia (VT)/Ventricular Fibrillation (VF)—cont'd

Consider antiarrhythmics (avoid use of multiple antiarrhythmics because of potential proarrhythmic effects)

- **Amiodarone** (Class IIb): Initial bolus: 300 mg IV bolus diluted in 20 to 30 mL of NS or D5W. Consider repeat dose (150 mg IV bolus) in 3 to 5 min. If debrillation successful, follow with 1 mg/min IV infusion for 6 hours (mix 900 mg in 500 mL NS), then decrease infusion rate to 0.5 mg/min IV infusion for 18 hours. Maximum daily dose 2.0 g IV/24 hours
- **Lidocaine** (Class indeterminate): 1 to 1.5 mg/kg IV bolus, consider repeat dose (0.5 to 0.75 mg/kg) in 5 min; maximum IV bolus dose 3 mg/kg. (The 1.5 mg/kg dose is recommended in cardiac arrest.) Endotracheal dose: 2 to 4 mg/kg. A single dose of 1.5 mg/kg is acceptable in cardiac arrest
- **Magnesium** (Class IIb if hypomagnesemia present): 1 to 2 g IV (2 to 4 mL of a 50% solution diluted in 10 mL of D5W if Torsades de Pointes or hypomagnesemia)
- **Procainamide** (Class IIb for recurrent pulseless VT/VF; Class indeterminate for persistent pulselsss [VT/VF]): 20 mg/min; maximum total dose 17 mg/kg
- Consider **sodium bicarbonate** 1 mEq/kg

From Aehlert B: *ACLS quick review study guide,* ed 2, St Louis, 2002, Mosby.

TABLE 3   Asystole

Basic Life Support

Perform Primary ABCD Survey
(Correct critical problems IMMEDIATELY as they are identified)
Assess responsiveness
Call for Help/Call for Defibrillator
Airway—open the airway
Breathing—deliver two slow breaths, administer oxygen as soon as
it is available
Circulation—perform chest compressions
Ensure availability of monitor/Defibrillator
On arrival of AED/monitor/defibrillator, perform secondary ABCD
Survey if rhythm is NOT pulseless VT/VF
▼

Scene Survey—Documentation or other evidence of
Do Not Attempt Resuscitation (DNAR)?
Obvious signs of death? If yes, do not start/attempt resuscitation
▼

Advanced Life Support

Perform Secondary ABCD Survey
(ADVANCED) *A*IRWAY
Reassess effectiveness of initial airway maneuvers and interventions
Perform invasive airway management
***B*REATHING**
Assess ventilation
Confirm ET tube placement (or other airway device) by at least two
methods
Provide positive-pressure ventilation/evaluate effectiveness of
ventilations
Secure airways device in place with commercial tube holder
(preferred) or tape
▼

Possible causes of
asystole:
PATCH-4-MD

***C*IRCULATION**
Confirm presence of asystole
(Check lead/cable connections, ensure power to monitor is on, correct
lead is selected, gain turned up, confirm asystole in second lead)
Establish IV access and administer appropriate medications
▼

Pulmonary embolism
Acidosis
Tension pneumothorax
Cardiac tamponade
Hypovolemia
Hypoxia
Heat/cold
  (hypo/hyperthermia)
Hypo-hyperkalemia (and
  other electrolytes)
Myocardial infarction
Drug overdose/accidents
  (cyclic antidepressants,
  calcium channel blockers,
  beta-blockers, digitalis)

***D*IFFERENTIAL DIAGNOSIS**
Search for and treat reversible causes **(PATCH-4-MD)**

Consider immediate transcutaneous pacing

Epinephrine 1 mg (1:10,000 solution) IV every 3 to 5 min
(ET dose 2 to 2.5 mg diluted in 10 mL normal saline or distilled
water)

Atropine 1 mg IV every 3 to 5 min to maximum 0.04 mg/kg
(Class IIb)
(ET dose 2 to 3 mg diluted in 10 mL normal saline or
distilled water)

Continued

T A B L E 3 Asystole—cont'd

Consider sodium bicarbonate 1 mEq/kg:
- Known preexisting hyperkalemia (Class I)
- Cyclic antidepressant overdose (IIa)
- To alkalinize urine in aspirin or other drug overdoses (IIa)
- Patient that has been intubated + long arrest interval (IIb)
- On return of spontaneous circulation if long arrest interval (IIb)

▼

Consider termination of efforts:
- Evaluate the quality of the resuscitation attempt
- Evaluate the resuscitation for atypical clinical features (e.g., hypothermia, reversible therapeutic or illicit drug use)
- Does support for cease-effort protocols exist?

From Aehlert B: *ACLS quick review study guide,* ed 2, St Louis, 2002, Mosby.

T A B L E 4   Pulseless Electrical Activity (PEA)

Basic Life Support

Perform Primary ABCD Survey
(Correct critical problems IMMEDIATELY as they are identified)
Assess responsiveness
Call for help/call for defibrillator
Airway—open the airway
Breathing—deliver two slow breaths, administer oxygen as soon as it is available
Circulation—perform chest compressions
Ensure availability of monitor/**D**efibrillator
On arrival of AED/monitor/defibrillator, perform secondary ABCD Survey if rhythm is NOT pulseless VT/VF
▼

Advanced Life Support

Possible causes of asystole:

Perform Secondary ABCD Survey
(ADVANCED) AIRWAY
Reassess effectiveness of initial airway maneuvers and interventions
Perform invasive airway management
***B*REATHING**
Assess ventilation
Confirm ET tube placement (or other airway device) by at least two methods
Provide positive-pressure ventilation/evaluate effectiveness of ventilations
Secure airways device in place with commercial tube holder (preferred) or tape
▼

PATCH-4-MD

Pulmonary embolism
Acidosis
Cardiac tamponade
Hypovolemia
Hypoxia
Heat/cold
  (hypo-/hyperthermia)
Hypo-hyperkalemia (and
  other electrolytes)
Myocardial infarction
Drug overdose/accidents
  (cyclic antidepressants,
  calcium channel
  blockers, beta-blockers,
  digitalis)

***C*IRCULATION**
Establish IV access
Assess blood flow with Doppler
(If blood flow detected with Doppler, treat using hypotension/shock algorithm)
Tension pneumothorax
Administer appropriate medications
▼

***D*IFFERENTIAL DIAGNOSIS**
Search for and treat reversible causes **(PATCH-4-MD)**
(Fast narrow-QRS—consider hypovolemia, tamponade, pulmonary embolism, tension pneumothorax; slow wide QRS—consider cyclic antidepressant overdose, calcium channel blocker, beta-blocker, or digitalis toxicity)
▼

Epinephrine 1 mg (1:10,000 solution) IV every 3 to 5 min
(ET dose 2 to 2.5 mg diluted in 10 mL normal saline or distilled water)
▼

If the rate is slow, atropine 1 mg IV every 3 to 5 min to max 0.04 mg/kg (Class IIb)
(ET dose 2 to 3 mg diluted in 10 mL normal saline or distilled water)
▼

Continued

T A B L E 4   Pulseless Electrical Activity (PEA)—cont'd

Consider sodium bicarbonate 1 mEq/kg:
- Known preexisting hyperkalemia (Class I)
- Cyclic antidepressant overdose (IIa)
- To alkalinize urine in aspirin or other drug overdoses (IIa)
- Patient that has been intubated + long arrest interval (IIb)
- On return of spontaneous circulation if long arrest interval (IIb)

▼

Consider termination of efforts

From Aehlert B: *ACLS quick review study guide,* ed 2, St Louis, 2002, Mosby.

TABLE 5 Pulseless Electrical Activity (PEA): Clinical Signs and Treatment

Cause	Typical ECG findings	History, physical findings	Management
Mechanical causes			
Tension pneumothorax	Narrow QRS complex, slow rate (because of hypoxia)	History (trauma, asthma, ventilator, COPD), unequal breath sounds, no pulse with CPR, neck vein distention, tracheal deviation, difficult to ventilate patient, hyperresonance to percussion on affect side	Needle decompression—second intercostal space, midclavicular line
Cardiac tamponade	Narrow QRS complex, rapid rate (impending tamponade)—deteriorating to sudden bradycardia as terminal event	History (trauma, renal failure, thoracic malignancy), no pulse with CPR, neck vein distention	Pericardiocentesis
Decreased preload			
Hypovolemia	Narrow QRS complex, rapid rate	History, flat neck veins	Volume replacement; find source (e.g., bleeding) and manage
Sepsis		History	Volume replacement, antibiotics
Massive pulmonary embolism	Narrow QRS complex, rapid rate	History, no pulse with CPR, neck vein distention, deep vein thrombosis in lower extremities	Pulmonary arteriogram, surgical embolectomy, fibrinolytics
Myocardial dysfunction			
Massive myocardial infarction	Q waves, ST segment changes, T wave inversion	History, ECG, enzyme levels	Emergency PTCA, if unavailable, fibrinolytics

Continued

T A B L E 5   Pulseless Electrical Activity (PEA): Clinical Signs and Treatment—cont'd

Cause	Typical ECG findings	History, physical findings	Management
Drug overdose			
Calcium channel blocker	Slow rate, prolonged PR interval, possible AV block	History of ingestion, empty bottles at the scene, check pupils, neurologic exam	Calcium IV, pacing
Beta-blocker	Slow rate, prolonged PR interval, possible AV block		Glucagon IV, pacing
Cyclic antidepressants	Rapid rate, prolonged QT interval, widening of QRS, ST segment changes		Sodium bicarbonate IV
Digoxin	Slow rate, prolonged PR interval, shortened QT interval, T wave inversion or flattening		Fab antibodies
Electrolytes			
Hypokalemia	ST segment depression, T waves flatten, prominent U waves, QRS widens (uncommon in adults)	Prolonged diuretic therapy; administration of K^+ deficient parenteral fluids; severe GI fluid losses from gastric suctioning or lavage; prolonged vomiting or diarrhea, or laxative abuse without K^+ replacement	Rapid, controlled potassium infusion
Hyperkalemia	Rapid rate; tall, narrow, peaked (tented) T waves; QRS widens; flattened or absent P waves; ST segment elevation	History of acute or chronic renal failure; diabetes; dialysis fistulas; medications; severe cell damage such as from burns, trauma, crush injuries	Calcium chloride IV push (immediate); then combination of insulin, glucose, sodium bicarbonate; then sodium polystyrene sulfonate/sorbitol; dialysis (long-term)

Hypocalcemia	Prolonged QT interval and ST segment; VT, TdP	Acute or chronic renal failure, acute pancreatitis	Calcium chloride IV
Hypercalcemia	Shortened QT interval	Excessive intake of Ca^{++} supplements, prolonged immobility, thiazide diuretics	Magnesium sulfate, potassium, diuretics
Hypomagnesemia	Flattened T waves, slightly widened QRS complex, diminished voltage of P waves and QRS complexes, prominent U waves	Severe GI fluid losses from gastric suctioning or lavage, prolonged vomiting or diarrhea, or laxative abuse; administration of IV fluids or TPN without magnesium replacement; cancer chemotherapy	Magnesium sulfate
Hypothermia			
Hypothermia	Initial tachycardia, then progressive bradycardia; J or Osborne waves	History of cold exposure, core body temperature	Rewarming guided by core temperature
Pulmonary causes			
Severe respiratory insufficiency/arrest resulting in hypoxia	Slow rate because of hypoxia	Cyanosis, blood gas results, airway obstruction	Ventilation
Post-defibrillation PEA			
After reversal of prolonged VF with electrical counter-shock			No specific intervention

From Aehlert B: *ACLS quick review study guide,* ed 2, St Louis, 2002, Mosby.

T A B L E 6 Symptomatic Bradycardia

Basic Life Support	**Perform Primary ABCD Survey** (Correct critical problems IMMEDIATELY as they are identified) Assess responsiveness, Airway, Breathing, Circulation, ensure availability of monitor/Defibrillator ▼
	Perform Secondary ABCD Survey Administer oxygen, establish IV access, attach cardiac monitor, administer fluids as needed (O_2, IV, monitor, fluids) ▼
Advanced Life Support	
	Assess vital signs, attach pulse oximeter, and monitor blood pressure Obtain and review 12-lead ECG, portable chest x-ray film Perform a focused history and physical exam ▼
	Identify the Patient's Cardiac Rhythm ▼
	Is the patient experiencing serious signs and symptoms because of the bradycardia?

Signs	Symptoms
Low blood pressure, shock, pulmonary congestion, congestive heart failure, angina, acute MI, ventricular ectopy	Chest pain, weakness, fatigue, dizziness, lightheadedness, shortness of breath, exercise intolerance, decreased level of responsiveness

- If no serious signs and symptoms, observe
- If serious signs and symptoms are present, further intervention depends on the cardiac rhythm identified

Is the QRS narrow or wide?	
Narrow QRS bradycardia	**Wide QRS bradycardia**
<ul><li>**Sinus bradycardia**</li><li>**Junctional rhythm**</li><li>**Second-degree AV block, type I or type 2**</li><li>**Third-degree (complete) AV block**</li><li>**Atropine 0.5 to 1.0 mg IV:** May repeat every 3 to 5 min to a total dose of 2.5 mg (0.03 to 0.04 mg/kg). Total cumulative dose should not exceed 2.5 mg over 2.5 hours</li><li>**Transcutaneous pacemaker (TCP):** Pacing should not be delayed while waiting for IV access or for atropine to take effect.</li><li>**Dopamine infusion:** 5 to 20 mcg/kg/min</li><li>**Epinephrine infusion:** 2 to 10 mcg/min</li><li>**Isoproterenol infusion:** 2 to 10 mcg/min (low doses)</li></ul>	<ul><li>**Second-degree AV block, type II**</li><li>**Third-degree (complete) AV block**</li><li>**Ventricular escape (idioventricular) rhythm**</li><li>**Transcutaneous pacemaker:** As an interim device until transvenous pacing can be accomplished</li><li>**Dopamine infusion:** 5 to 20 mcg/kg/min</li><li>**Epinephrine infusion:** 2 to 10 mcg/min</li><li>**Isoproterenol infusion:** 2 to 10 mcg/min (low doses)</li></ul>

From Aehlert B: *ACLS quick review study guide,* ed 2, St Louis, 2002, Mosby.

TABLE 7   Narrow QRS Tachycardia

Perform Primary ABCD Survey (Basic Life Support)
(Correct critical problems IMMEDIATELY as they are identified)
Assess responsiveness, **A**irway, **B**reathing, **C**irculation, ensure availability of monitor/**D**efibrillator
▼
Perform Secondary ABCD Survey (Advanced Life Support)
Administer oxygen, establish IV access, attach cardiac monitor, administer fluids as needed
(O_2, IV, monitor fluids)
Assess vital signs, attach pulse oximeter, and monitor blood pressure
Obtain and review 12-lead ECG, portable chest x-ray film
Perform a focused history and physical exam
▼
Is the patient stable or unstable?
Is the patient experiencing serious signs and symptoms because of the tachycardia?
▼
Attempt to identify patient's cardiac rhythm using:

- 12-lead ECG, clinical information
- Vagal maneuvers
- Adenosine 6 mg rapid IV bolus over 1 to 3 sec, if needed, administer adenosine 12 mg rapid IV bolus over 1 to 3 sec after 1 to 2 min. May repeat 12 mg dose in 1 to 2 min if needed. Follow each dose immediately with 20 mL IV flush of NS. Use of adenosine is relatively contraindicated in patients with asthma. Decrease dose in patients on dipyridamole (Persantine) or carbamazepine (Tegretol); consider increasing dose in patients taking theophylline or caffeine-containing preparations

▼
Identify the Patient's Cardiac Rhythm
▼

Junctional tachycardia		Paroxysmal supraventricular tachycardia (PSVT) (Includes AVNRT or AVRT)		Ectopic atrial tachycardia, multifocal atrial tachycardia (MAT)	
Stable patient		**Stable patient**		**Stable patient**	
Normal cardiac function	**Impaired cardiac function***	**Normal cardiac function**	**Impaired cardiac function***	**Normal cardiac function**	**Impaired cardiac function***
Amiodarone (IIb) **or** Beta-blocker *(Indeterminate)* or Ca++ channel blocker *(Indeterminate)*	Amiodarone (IIb)	*Priority order:* Ca++ channel blocker (Class I) Beta-blocker (Class I) Digoxin (IIb) Sync cardioversion	*Priority order:* Sync cardioversion Digoxin (IIb) Amiodarone (IIb) Diltiazem (IIb)	Ca++ channel blocker (IIb) **or** Beta blocker (IIb) **or** Amiodarone (IIb) **or** Flecainide (IIb) or Propafenone (IIb) **or** Digoxin *(Indeterminate)* **Cardioversion ineffective**	Amiodarone (IIb) **or** Diltiazem (IIb) **or** Digoxin *(Indeterminate)* **Cardioversion ineffective**

Continued

UNSTABLE PATIENT

If hemodynamically unstable PSVT, perform synchronized cardioversion: 50 J, 100 J, 200 J, 300 J, 360 J, (or equivalent Biphasic energy)

Medication dosing

Amiodarone—150 mg IV over 10, followed by an infusion of 1 mg/min for 6 hours and then a maintenance infusion of 0.5 mg/min. Repeat supplementary infusions of 150 mg as necessary for recurrent or resistant dysrhythmias. Maximum total daily dose 2.0 g

Beta-blockers—*Esmolol:* 0.5 mg/kg over 1 min, followed by a maintenance infusion at 50 mcg/kg/min for 4 min. If inadequate response, administer a second bolus of 0.5 mg/kg over 1 min and increase maintenance infusion to 100 mcg/kg/min. The bolus dose (0.5 mg/kg) and titration of the maintenance infusion (addition of 50 mcg/kg/min) can be repeated every 4 min to a maximum infusion of 300 mcg/kg/min. *Metoprolol:* 5 mg slow IV push over 5 min × 3 as **needed to a total dose of 15 mg over 15 min.**

Calcium channel blockers: *Diltiazem*—0.25 mg/kg over 2 min (e.g., 15 to 20 mg). If ineffective, 0.35 mg/kg over 2 min (e.g., 20 to 25 mg) in 15 min. Maintenance infusion 5 to 15 mg/hr, titrated to heart rate if chemical conversion successful. Calcium chloride (2 to 4 mg/kg) may be given slow IV push if borderline hypotension exists before diltiazem administration. *Verapamil*—2.5 to 5.0 mg slow IV push over 2 min. May repeat with 5 to 10 mg in 15 to 30 min. Maximum dose 20 mg

Digoxin—Loading dose 10 to 15 mcg/kg lean body weight

Flecainide, propafenone—IV form not currently approved for use in the United States

Type of countershock	Dysrhythmia	Recommended energy levels
Defibrillation	Pulseless VT/VF	200 J, 200-300 J, 360 J, or equivalent Biphasic energy
	Sustained polymorphic VT	200 J, 200-300 J, 360 J, or equivalent Biphasic energy
	VT with a pulse	100 J, 200 J, 300 J, 360 J, or equivalent Biphasic energy
	Undue delay in delivery of synchronized countershock	Depends on rhythm
Synchronized cardioversion	Paroxysmal supraventricular tachycardia (PSVT)	50 J, 100 J, 200 J, 300 J, 360 J, or equivalent Biphasic energy
	Atrial flutter	50 J, 100 J, 200 J, 300 J, 360 J, or equivalent Biphasic energy
	Atrial fibrillation	100 J, 200 J, 300 J, 360 J, or equivalent Biphasic energy
	VT with a pulse	100 J, 200 J, 300 J, 360 J, or equivalent Biphasic energy

From Aehlert B: *ACLS quick review study guide,* ed 2, St Louis, 2002, Mosby.
*Impaired cardiac function = ejection fraction <40% or CHF.

T A B L E 8   Atrial Fibrillation/Atrial Flutter Algorithm

Perform Primary ABCD Survey (Basic Life Support)
(Correct critical problems IMMEDIATELY as they are identified)
Assess responsiveness, **A**irway, **B**reathing, **C**irculation, ensure availability of monitor/**D**efibrillator

Perform Secondary ABCD Survey (Advanced Life Support)
Administer oxygen, establish IV access, attach cardiac monitor, administer fluids as needed
(O_2, IV, monitor, fluids)
Assess vital signs, attach pulse oximeter, and monitor blood pressure
Obtain and review 12-lead ECG, portable chest x-ray film, perform a focused history and physical exam

Is the patient stable or unstable?
Is the patient's cardiac function normal or impaired?
Is the patient experiencing serious signs and symptoms because of the tachycardia?
Attempt to identify patient's cardiac rhythm using 12-lead ECG, clinical information
Is Wolff-Parkinson-White syndrome (WPW) present? If yes, see WPW algorithm.
Has atrial fibrillation/atrial flutter been present for more or less than 48 hours?

STABLE PATIENT			
Normal cardiac function		**Impaired cardiac function***	
Onset <48 hours control rate	**Onset >48 hours control rate**	**Onset <48 hours control rate**	**Onset >48 hours control rate**
Calcium channel blocker (Class I) **or** Beta-blocker (Class I) **or** Digoxin (IIb)	Calcium channel blocker (Class I) **or** Beta-blocker (Class I) **or** Digoxin (IIb))	Diltiazem (IIb) **or** Amiodarone (IIb) **or** Digoxin (IIb)	Diltiazem (IIb) **or** Amiodarone (IIb) **or** Digoxin (IIb)
Convert rhythm	**Convert rhythm**	**Convert rhythm**	**Convert rhythm**
Cardioversion **or** Amiodarone (IIa) **or** Procainamide (IIa) **or** Ibutilide (IIa) **or** Flecainide (IIa) **or** Propafenone (IIa)	Delayed cardioversion **or** Early cardioversion	Cardioversion **or** amiodarone (IIb)	Delayed cardioversion **or** Early cardioversion

Delayed cardioversion: anticoagulation therapy for 3 weeks before cardioversion, for at least 48 hours in conjunction with cardioversion, and for at least 4 weeks after successful cardioversion.
Early cardioversion: IV heparin immediately, transesophageal echocardiography (TEE) to rule out atrial thrombus, cardioversion within 24 hr, anticoagulation × 4 wks

UNSTABLE PATIENT

If hemodynamically unstable, perform synchronized cardioversion: Atrial fibrillation: 100 J, 200 J, 300 J, 360 J, or equivalent Biphasic energy. Atrial flutter: 50 J, 100 J, 200 J, 300 J, 360 J, or equivalent Biphasic energy
Amiodarone—150 mg IV bolus over 10 min followed by an infusion of 1 mg/min for 6 hours and then a maintenance infusion of 0.5 mg/min. Repeat supplementary infusions of 150 mg as necessary for recurrent or resistant dysrhythmias. Maximum total daily dose 2.0 g

Continued

T A B L E 8   **Atrial Fibrillation/Atrial Flutter Algorithm—cont'd**

UNSTABLE PATIENT—cont'd

Beta-blockers—*Esmolol:* 0.5 mg/kg over 1 min followed by a maintenance infusion at 50 mcg/kg/min for 4 min. If inadequate response, administer a second bolus of 0.5 mg/kg over 1 min and increase maintenance infusion to 100 mcg/kg/min. The bolus dose (0.5 mg/kg) and titration of the maintenance infusion (addition of 50 mcg/kg/min) can be repeated every 4 min to a maximum infusion of 300 mcg/kg/min. *Metoprolol:* 5 mg slow IV push over 5 min × 3 as needed to a total dose of 15 mg over 15 min. *Propranolol:* 0.1 mg/kg slow IV push divided in 3 equal doses at 2 to 3 min intervals. Do not exceed 1 mg/min. Repeat after 2 min, if necessary. *Atenolol:* 5 mg slow IV (over 5 min). Wait 10 min, then give second dose of 5 mg slow IV (over 5 min)

Calcium channel blockers: *Diltiazem*—0.25 mg/kg over 2 min (e.g., 15 to 20 mg). If ineffective, 0.35 mg/kg over 2 min (e.g., 20 to 25 mg) in 15 min. Maintenance infusion 5 to 15 mg/hr, titrated to heart rate if chemical conversion successful. Calcium chloride (2 to 4 mg/kg) may be given **slow** IV push if borderline hypotension exists before diltiazem administration. *Verapamil*—2.5 to 5.0 mg slow IV push over 2 min. May repeat with 5 to 10 mg in 15 to 30 min. Maximum dose 20 mg

Ibutilide—Adults ≥ 60 kg: 1 mg (10 mL) over 10 min. May repeat × 1 in 10 min. Adults <60 kg: 0.01 mg/kg IV over 10 min

Procainamide: —100 mg over 5 min (20 mg/min). Maximum total dose 17 mg/kg. Maintenance infusion 1 to 4 mg/min. *Flecainide, propafenone*—IV form not currently approved for use in the United States

Sotalol—1 to 1.5 mg/kg IV slowly at a rate of 10 mg/min

From Aehlert B: *ACLS quick review study guide,* ed 2, St Louis, 2002, Mosby.
*Impaired cardiac function = ejection fraction <40% or CHF

T A B L E 9   Wolff-Parkinson-White (WPW) Syndrome Algorithm

Perform Primary ABCD Survey (Basic Life Support)
(Correct critical problems IMMEDIATELY as they are identified)
Assess responsiveness, **A**irway, **B**reathing, **C**irculation, ensure availability of monitor/**D**efibrillator

Perform Secondary ABCD Survey (Advanced Life Support)
Administer oxygen, establish IV access, attach cardiac monitor, administer fluids as needed
(O_2, IV, monitor, fluids)
Assess vital signs, attach pulse oximeter, and monitor blood pressure
Obtain and review 12-lead ECG, portable chest x-ray film, perform a focused history and physical exam

Is the patient stable or unstable?
Is the patient experiencing serious signs and symptoms because of the tachycardia?
Is the patient's cardiac function normal or impaired?
Attempt to identify patient's cardiac rhythm using 12-lead ECG, clinical information
Is Wolff-Parkinson-White syndrome (WPW) present? (e.g., young patient, HR >300, ECG: short PR interval, wide QRS, delta wave)
Has WPW been present for more or less than 48 hours?

Normal cardiac function		Impaired cardiac function*	
Onset <48 hours **Control rate**	**Onset >48 hours** **Control rate**	**Onset <48 hours** **Control rate**	**Onset >48 hours** **Control rate**
Cardioversion **or** Amiodarone (IIa) **or** Procainamide (IIa) **or** Flecainide (IIa) **or** Propafenone (IIa) **or** Sotalol (IIb)	Use antiarrhythmics with extreme caution because of embolic risk	Cardioversion **or** Amiodarone (IIb)	Use antiarrhythmics with extreme caution because of embolic risk
Convert rhythm	**Convert rhythm**	**Convert rhythm**	**Convert rhythm**
Cardioversion **or** Amiodarone (IIa) **or** Procainamide (IIa) **or** Flecainide (IIa) **or** Propafenone (IIa) **or** Sotalol (IIb)	Delayed cardioversion **or** Early cardioversion	Cardioversion	Delayed cardioversion **or** Early cardioversion

Delayed cardioversion: Anticoagulation therapy for 3 weeks before cardioversion for at least 48 hours in conjunction with cardioversion and for at least 4 weeks after successful cardioversion. *Early cardioversion:* IV heparin immediately, transesophageal echocardiography (TEE) to rule out atrial thrombus, cardioversion within 24 hr, anticoagulation × 4 weeks

Medication dosing

Amiodarone—150 mg IV bolus over 10 min followed by an infusion of 1 mg/min for 6 hours and then a maintenance infusion of 0.5 mg/min. Repeat supplementary infusions of 150 mg as necessary for recurrent or resistant dysrhythmias. Maximum total daily dose 2.0 g
Procainamide—100 mg over 5 min (20 mg/min). Maximum total dose 17 mg/kg. Maintenance infusion 1 to 4 mg/min
Flecainide, propafenone—IV form not currently approved for use in the United States
Sotalol—1 to 1.5 mg/kg IV slowly at a rate of 10 mg/min

From Aehlert B: *ACLS quick review study guide,* ed 2, St Louis, 2002, Mosby.
*Impaired cardiac function = ejection fraction <40% or CHF.

T A B L E 10   Sustained Monomorphic Ventricular Tachycardia

Perform Primary ABCD Survey (Basic Life Support)
(Correct critical problems IMMEDIATELY as they are identified)
Assess responsiveness, Airway, Breathing, Circulation, ensure availability of monitor/Defibrillator

Perform Secondary ABCD Survey (Advanced Life Support)
Administer oxygen, establish IV access, attach cardiac monitor, administer fluids as needed
(O_2, IV, monitor, fluids)
Assess vital signs, attach pulse oximeter, and monitor blood pressure
Obtain and review 12-lead ECG, portable chest x-ray film, perform a focused history and physical
exam

Is the patient stable or unstable?
Is the patient experiencing serious signs and symptoms because of the tachycardia?
Determine if the rhythm is monomorphic or polymorphic VT and determine patient's QT interval
▼

STABLE PATIENT	
Normal cardiac function	**Impaired cardiac function***

May proceed directly to synchronized cardioversion or use **one** of the following:

• Procainamide (IIa)	• Amiodarone (IIb)
• Sotalol (IIa)	• Lidocaine (*Indeterminate*)
• Amiodarone (IIb)	
• Lidocaine (IIb)	

If medication therapy ineffective, perform synchronized cardioversion

UNSTABLE VT WITH A PULSE

If hemodynamically unstable, sync 100 J, 200 J, 300 J, and 60 J, (or equivalent Biphasic energy)
If hypotensive (systolic BP <90), unresponsive, or if severe pulmonary edema exists, defibrillate with
same energy

Medication Dosing

Amiodarone: 150 mg IV bolus over 10 min. If chemical conversion successful, follow with IV
infusion of 1 mg/min for 6 hours and then a maintenance infusion of 0.5 mg/min. Repeat
supplementary infusions of 150 mg as necessary for recurrent or resistant dysrhythmias. Maximum
total daily dose 2.0 g.
Lidocaine: 1 to 1.5 mg/kg initial dose. Repeat dose is half the initial dose every 5 to 10 min.
Maximum total dose 3 mg/kg. If chemical conversion successful, maintenance infusion 1 to
4 mg/min. If impaired cardiac function, dose = 0.5-0.75 mg/kg IV push. May repeat every 5 to
10 min. Maximum total dose 3 mg/kg. If chemical conversion successful, maintenance infusion 1 to
4 mg/min.
Procainamide: 100 mg over 5 min (20 mg/min). Maximum total dose 17 mg/kg. If chemical
conversion successful, maintenance infusion 1 to 4 mg/min.
Sotalol: 1 to 1.5 mg/kg IV slowly at a rate of 10 mg/min.

From Aehlert B: *ACLS quick review study guide,* ed 2, St Louis, 2002, Mosby.
*Impaired cardiac function = ejection fraction <40% or CHF.

T A B L E 11   Polymorphic Ventricular Tachycardia

Perform Primary ABCD Survey (Basic Life Support)
(Correct critical problems IMMEDIATELY as they are identified)
Assess responsiveness, Airway, Breathing, Circulation, ensure availability of monitor/Defibrillator

Perform Secondary ABCD Survey (Advanced Life Support)
Administer oxygen, establish IV access, attach cardiac monitor, administer fluids as needed
(O_2, IV, monitor, fluids)
Assess vital signs, attach pulse oximeter, and monitor blood pressure
Obtain and review 12-lead ECG, portable chest x-ray film, perform a focused history and physical exam

Is the patient stable or unstable?
Is the patient experiencing serious signs and symptoms because of the tachycardia?
Determine if the rhythm is monomorphic or polymorphic VT and determine patient's QT interval

▼

Polymorphic VT Normal QT interval		Polymorphic VT Prolonged QT interval (suggests Torsades De Pointes)	
Normal cardiac function	**Impaired cardiac function***	**Normal cardiac function**	**Impaired cardiac function***
Treat ischemia if present	May proceed directly to electrical therapy or use **one** of the following:	DC meds that prolong QT	May proceed directly to electrical therapy or use **one** of the following:
Correct electrolyte abnormalities	Amiodarone (IIb)	Correct electrolyte abnormalities	Amiodarone (IIb)
May proceed directly to electrical therapy or use **one** of the following:	Lidocaine *(Indeterminate)*	May proceed directly to electrical therapy or use **one** of the following:	Lidocaine *(Indeterminate)*
Amiodarone (IIb)		Magnesium *(Indeterminate)*	
Lidocaine (IIb)		Overdrive pacing with or without beta-blocker *(Indeterminate)*	
Procainamide (IIb)		Isoproterenol *(Indeterminate)*	
Sotalol (IIb)		Phenytoin *(Indeterminate)*	
Beta-blockers *(Indeterminate)*		Lidocaine *(Indeterminate)*	

If medication therapy ineffective, use electrical therapy

UNSTABLE PATIENT

Sustained (>30 sec or causing hemodynamic collapse) polymorphic VT should be treated with an unsynchronized shock, using an initial energy of 200 J; if unsuccessful, a second shock of 200 to 300 J should be given and, if necessary, a third shock of 360 J

Continued

T A B L E 11 **Polymorphic Ventricular Tachycardia—cont'd**

Medication Dosing

Amiodarone—150 mg IV bolus over 10 min. If chemical conversion successful, follow with IV infusion of 1 mg/min for 6 hours and then a maintenance infusion of 0.5 mg/min. Repeat supplementary infusions of 150 mg as necessary for recurrent or resistant dysrhythmias. Maximum total daily dose 2.0 g

Beta-blockers—*Esmolol:* 0.5 mg/kg over 1 min followed by a maintenance infusion at 50 mcg/kg/min for 4 min. If inadequate response, administer a second bolus of 0.5 mg/kg over 1 min and increase maintenance infusion to 100 mcg/kg/min. The bolus dose (0.5 mg/kg) and titration of the maintenance infusion (addition of 50 mcg/kg/min) can be repeated every 4 min to a maximum infusion of 300 mcg/kg/min. *Metoprolol:* 5 mg slow IV push over 5 min × 3 as needed to a total dose of 15 mg over 15 min. *Atenolol:* 5 mg slow IV (over 5 min). Wait 10 min, then give second dose of 5 mg slow IV (over 5 min)

Isoproterenol—Can be used as a temporizing measure until overdrive pacing can be instituted if no evidence of coronary artery disease, ischemic syndromes, or other contraindications. 2 to 10 mcg/min. Mix 1 mg in 500 mL NS or D5W

Lidocaine—1 to 1.5 mg/kg initial dose. Repeat dose is half the initial dose every 5 to 10 min. Maximum total dose 3 mg/kg. If chemical conversion successful, maintenance infusion 1 to 4 mg/min. If impaired cardiac function, dose = 0.5 to 0.75 mg/kg IV push. May repeat every 5 to 10 min. Maximum total dose 3 mg/kg. If chemical conversion successful, maintenance infusion 1 to 4 mg/min

Magnesium—Loading dose of 1 to 2 g mixed in 50 to 100 mL over 5 to 60 min IV. If chemical conversion successful, follow with 0.5 to 1.0 g/hr IV infusion

Phenytoin—250 mg V at a rate of 25 to 50 mg/min in NS using a central vein

Procainamide—100 mg over 5 min (20 mg/min). Maximum total dose 17 mg/kg. If chemical conversion successful, maintenance infusion 1 to 4 mg/min

Sotalol—1 to 1.5 mg/kg IV slowly at a rate of 10 mg/min

From Aehlert B: *ACLS quick review study guide,* ed 2, St Louis, 2002, Mosby.

T A B L E 12   Wide QRS Tachycardia of Unknown Origin

Perform Primary ABCD Survey (Basic Life Support)
(Correct critical problems IMMEDIATELY as they are identified)
Assess responsiveness, Airway, Breathing, Circulation, ensure availability of monitor/Defibrillator

Perform Secondary ABCD Survey (Advanced Life Support)
Administer oxygen, establish IV access, attach cardiac monitor, administer fluids as needed
(O_2, IV, monitor, fluids)
Assess vital signs, attach pulse oximeter, and monitor blood pressure
Obtain and review 12-lead ECG, portable chest x-ray film, perform a focused history and physical
exam

Is the patient stable or unstable?
Is the patient experiencing serious signs and symptoms because of the tachycardia?
Use 12-lead ECG/clinical information to help clarify rhythm diagnosis

Rhythm confirmed as SVT (Go to narrow-QRS tachycardia algorithm)	Wide-complex tachycardia of unknown origin Stable patient	Rhythm confirmed as VT (Go to VT algorithm)
Normal cardiac function	**Impaired cardiac function***	
Sync cardioversion or Procainamide (IIb) or Amiodarone (IIb)	**Sync cardioversion or Amiodarone (IIb)**	

If medication therapy ineffective, perform synchronized cardioversion

UNSTABLE PATIENT

If hemodynamically unstable, sync 100 J, 200 J, 300 J, and 360 J, or equivalent Biphasic energy. If
hypotensive (systolic BP <90), unresponsive, or if severe pulmonary edema exists, defibrillate with
same energy

Medication Dosing

Amiodarone—150 mg IV bolus over 10 min. If chemical conversion successful, follow with IV
infusion of 1 mg/min for 6 hours and then a maintenance infusion of 0.5 mg/min. Repeat
supplementary infusions of 150 mg as necessary for recurrent or resistant dysrhythmias. Maximum
total daily dose 2 g
Procainamide—100 mg over 5 min (20 mg/min). Maximum total dose 17 mg/kg. If chemical
conversion successful, maintenance infusion 1 to 4 mg/min

From Aehlert B: *ACLS quick review study guide,* ed 2, St Louis, 2002, Mosby.
*Impaired cardiac function = ejection fraction <40% or CHF.

T A B L E 13   **Management of ST-Segment Elevation MI**

ST-segment elevation ≥1 mm in two or more anatomically contiguous leads or new, or presumably new, **LBBB**

▼

Confirm diagnosis by signs/symptoms, ECG, serum cardiac markers

▼

All patients with ST-segment elevation MI should receive (if no contraindications):

- **Antiplatelet therapy**—Aspirin 162 to 325 mg (chewed)
- **Anti-ischemia therapy** (Beta-blockers, nitroglycerin IV if ongoing ischemia or uncorrected hypertension)
- **Antithrombin therapy**—Heparin (if using fibrin-specific lytics)
- **ACE inhibitors** (after 6 hours or when stable)—Especially with large or anterior MI, heart failure without hypotension (SBP > 100 mm Hg), previous MI

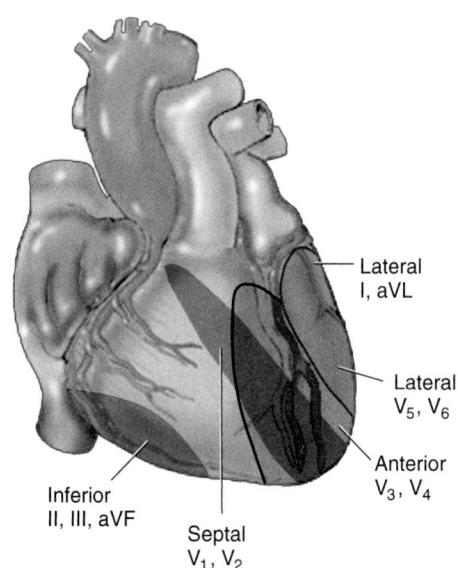

Lateral
I, aVL

Lateral
V_5, V_6

Anterior
V_3, V_4

Inferior
II, III, aVF

Septal
V_1, V_2

Symptom onset ≤12 hours?		Symptom onset =12 hours?
Patient Eligible for Reperfusion? Goals— • **Fibrinolytics:** Door-to-drug time < 30 min • **Primary PCI:** Door-to-dilation time 90 ± 30 min	Persistent symptoms	Resolution of symptoms

Continued

T A B L E 13   Management of ST-Segment Elevation MI—cont'd

Yes		No		Consider reperfusion	Medical management
Signs of cardiogenic shock or contraindications to fibrinolytics? changes?		Persistent or stuttering symptoms or ECG		Medical management	
Yes	**No**	**Yes**	**No**		
PCI, medical management	Can cath lab be mobilized within 60 min?	Cardiac cath, medical management	Medical management		
	Yes **No**				
	PCI | **Fibrinolysis** (alteplase, reteplase, streptokinase, anistreplase, **or** tenecteplase)				

From Aehlert B: *ACLS quick review study guide,* ed 2, St Louis, 2002, Mosby.
NOTE: *PCI,* Percutaneous coronary intervention (angioplasty ± stent).

T A B L E 14   Management of Unstable Angina/Non-ST-Segment Elevation MI

ECG changes in two or more automatically contiguous leads:
ST-segment depression > 1 mm or T wave inversion > 1 mm **or**
Transient (<30 min) ST-segment/T wave changes > 1 mm with discomfort
▼
Confirm diagnosis by signs/symptoms, ECG, serum cardiac markers
▼

- Aspirin: 162 to 325 mg (chewed) if not already administered (and no contraindications) (antiplatelet therapy)
- Heparin IV (antithrombin therapy)

▼

All patients with unstable angina/non-ST-segment elevation MI should receive
(if no contraindications)
▼

- Aspirin + glycoprotein IIb/IIa inhibitors (i.e., Integrilin, Aggrastat, ReoPro) + IV heparin or
- Aspirin + glycoprotein IIb/IIa inhibitors + SC low-molecular-weight heparin (i.e., enoxaparin [Lovenox], dalteparin [Fragmin])

HIGH-RISK CRITERIA

▼

- Persistent ("stuttering") symptoms/recurrent ischemia; left ventricular (LV) dysfunction, CHF; widespread ECG changes; prior MI, positive troponin or CK-MB

▼

Anti-ischemia therapy
- **Beta-blockers**—(e.g., metoprolol, atenolol, esmolol, propranolol) if patient not previously on beta-blockers or inadequately treated on current dose of beta-blocker (if no contraindications)
- **Nitroglycerin sublingual tablet or spray,** followed by IV nitroglycerin: If symptoms persist despite sublingual nitroglycerin therapy and initiation of beta-blocker therapy (and SBP >90 mm Hg), then administer:
- **Morphine:** 2 to 4 mg IV (if discomfort is not relieved or symptoms recur despite anti-ischemic therapy)—May repeat every 5 min (ensure SBP >90 mm Hg)

Assess clinical status: Is patient clinically stable?	
Yes	**No**

- Continue in-hospital observation
- Consider stress testing
	Cardiac cath:
	  - If anatomy suitable for revascularization: PCI, CABG
	  - If anatomy unsuitable: Medical management

From Aehlert B: *ACLS quick review study guide,* ed 2, St Louis, 2002, Mosby.

T A B L E 15   Management of Patient With a Suspected Acute Coronary Syndrome and Nondiagnostic or Normal ECG

Nondiagnostic or Normal ECG

▼

Evaluate signs/symptoms, serial ECGs, serum cardiac markers

▼

Aspirin + other therapy as appropriate

▼

- Assess patient's clinical risk of death/nonfatal MI
- History and physical exam
- Obtain follow-up serum cardiac marker levels, serial ECG monitoring
- Continue evaluation and treatment in Emergency Department, chest pain unit, or monitored bed
- Consider radionuclide, echocardiography

From Aehlert B: *ACLS quick review study guide,* ed 2, St Louis, 2002, Mosby.

T A B L E 16　　**Management of Acute Pulmonary Edema**

Perform Primary ABCD Survey (Basic Life Support)
(Correct critical problems IMMEDIATELY as they are identified)
Assess responsiveness, Airway, Breathing, Circulation, ensure availability of monitor/Defibrillator
▼
Perform Secondary ABCD Survey (Advanced Life Support)
(Obtain arterial blood gas before oxygen administration if possible)
Administer oxygen, establish IV access, attach cardiac monitor (O_2, IV, monitor)
Assess vital signs, attach pulse oximeter, and monitor blood pressure
Obtain and review 12-lead ECG, portable chest x-ray film
Perform a focused history and physical exam
▼
If feasible and BP permits, place patient in sitting position with feet dependent
• Increases lung volume and vital capacity
• Decreases work of respiration
• Decreases venous return, decreases preload
If systolic BP >100 mm Hg:
• **Sublingual nitroglycerin**—1 tablet or spray every 5 min (max 3 tablets) until IV nitroglycerin or nitroprusside can take effect
• **Furosemide IV:** 0.5 to 1.0 mg/kg (typically 20 to 40 mg) (can repeat in 30 minutes if symptoms persist and BP stable)
• **Consider morphine IV** 2 to 4 mg
Consider additional preload/afterload reduction—nitroglycerin or nitroprusside IV, ACE inhibitors (if SBP > 100 mm Hg)
• **Nitroglycerin IV**—Start at 5 mcg/min and increase gradually until mean systolic pressure falls by 10% to 15%, avoid hypotension (SBP <90 mm Hg) or
• **Nitroprusside IV**—0.1 to 5 mcg/kg/min
Evaluate early for:
• Readily reversible cause: Institute appropriate intervention (e.g., cardiac dysrhythmias, tamponade)
• Myocardial ischemia/infarction (Institute appropriate intervention—candidate for fibrinolytic therapy? PTCA?)
If patient is refractory to previous therapies, hypotensive, or in cardiogenic shock:
• Consider fluid or IV inotropic and/or vasopressor agents (e.g., dobutamine, dopamine, norepinephrine)
• Consider pulmonary and systemic arterial catheterization
• Obtain ECG to assist in diagnosis, evaluation, and reparability of culprit lesion or condition
• Consider need for mechanical circulatory assistance (balloon pump)

From Aehlert B: *ACLS quick review study guide,* ed 2, St Louis, 2002, Mosby.

T A B L E 17   Management of Hypotension/Shock: *Suspected Pump Problem*

Perform Primary ABCD Survey (Basic Life Support)
(Correct critical problems IMMEDIATELY as they are identified)
Assess responsiveness, Airway, Breathing, Circulation, ensure availability of monitor/Defibrillator
▼
Perform Secondary ABCD Survey (Advanced Life Support)
Administer oxygen, establish IV access, attach cardiac monitor, administer fluids as needed
(O_2, IV, monitor)
Assess vital signs, attach pulse oximeter, and monitor blood pressure
Obtain and review 12-lead ECG, portable chest x-ray film
Perform a focused history and physical exam
▼
Hypotension—Suspected Pump Problem
• If breath sounds are clear, consider fluid challenge of 250 to 500 mL NS to ensure adequate
  ventricular filling pressure before vasopressor administration
▼
Marked Hypotension (Systolic BP <70 mm Hg) Cardiogenic Shock
Pharmacologic management:
• **Norepinephrine** infusion: 0.5 to 30 mcg/min until SBP 80 mm Hg
• Then attempt to change to **dopamine:** 5 to 15 mcg/kg/min until SBP 90 mm Hg
• IV **dobutamine:** 2 to 20 mcg/kg/min can be given simultaneously in an attempt to reduce
  magnitude of **dopamine** infusion
Consider balloon pump or patient transfer to a cardiac interventional facility
Moderate Hypotension (Systolic BP 70 to 90 mm Hg)
• **Dopamine:** 5 to 15 mcg/kg/min
• If BP remains low despite dopamine doses >20 mcg/kg/min, may substitute **norepinephrine** in
  doses of 0.5 to 30 mcg/min
• Once SBP ≥90 with dopamine, add **dobutamine** 2 to 20 mcg/kg/min and attempt to taper off
  dopamine
Systolic BP ≥90 mm Hg
• **Dobutamine:** 2 to 20 mcg/kg/min

Medication dosing	
Norepinephrine IV	0.5 to 30 mcg/min
Dopamine IV	5 to 15 mcg/kg/min
Dobutamine IV	2 to 20 mcg/kg/min

From Aehlert B: *ACLS quick review study guide,* ed 2, St Louis, 2002, Mosby.

T A B L E 18   Management of Hypotension/Shock: *Suspected Volume Problem*
(Hypovolemia)

Perform Primary ABCD Survey (Basic Life Support)
(Correct critical problems IMMEDIATELY as they are identified)
Assess responsiveness, **A**irway, **B**reathing, **C**irculation, ensure availability of monitor/**D**efibrillator
▼
Perform Secondary ABCD Survey (Advanced Life Support)
Administer oxygen, establish IV access, attach cardiac monitor, administer fluids as needed
(O_2, IV, monitor, fluids)
Assess vital signs, attach pulse oximeter, and monitor blood pressure
Obtain and review 12-lead ECG, portable chest x-ray film
Perform a focused history and physical exam
▼
Hypotension: suspected volume (or vascular resistance) problem
▼

• Volume replacement
• Fluid challenge (250 to 500 mL IV boluses—reassess)
• Blood transfusion (if appropriate)
• If cause known, institute appropriate intervention (e.g., septic shock, anaphylaxis)
• Consider vasopressors, if indicated, to improve vascular tone if no response to fluid challenge(s)

From Aehlert B: *ACLS quick review study guide,* ed 2, St Louis, 2002, Mosby.

T A B L E 19   **Management of Hypotension/Shock:** *Suspected Rate Problem*
(Bradycardia, Tachycardia)

Perform Primary ABCD Survey (Basic Life Support)
(Correct critical problems IMMEDIATELY as they are identified)
Assess responsiveness, **A**irway, **B**reathing, **C**irculation, ensure availability of monitor/**D**efibrillator
▼
Perform Secondary ABCD Survey (Advanced Life Support)
Administer oxygen, establish IV access, attach cardiac monitor, administer fluids as needed
(O_2, IV, monitor, fluids)
Assess vital signs, attach pulse oximeter, and monitor blood pressure
Obtain and review 12-lead ECG, portable chest x-ray film
Perform a focused history and physical exam
▼
Hypotension: suspected rate problem
▼

* If rate too slow—bradycardia algorithm
* If rate too fast—determine width of QRS, then use appropriate tachycardia algorithm

From Aehlert B: *ACLS quick review study guide,* ed 2, St Louis, 2002, Mosby.

Heart and Breath Sounds

Assessing Heart Sounds

Sound	Auscultation site	Timing	Pitch	Clinical occurrence	End-piece/patient position
S_1 (M_1 T_1)	Apex	Beginning of systole	High	Closing of mitral and tricuspid valves; normal sound	Diaphragm/patient supine
S_1 split	Apex	Beginning of systole	High	Ventricles contracting at different times because of electrical or mechanical problems (e.g., longer time span between M_1 T_1 caused by right bundle-branch heart block, or reversal [T_1 M_1] caused by mitral stenosis)	Same as S_1
S_2 (A_2, P_2)	A_2 at second ICS, RSB; P_2 at second ICS, LSB	End of systole	High	Closing of aortic and pulmonic valves; normal sound	Diaphragm/patient supine
S_2 physiologic split	Second ICS, LSB	End of systole	High	Accentuated by inspiration; disappears on expiration. Sound that corresponds with the respiratory cycle because of normal delay in closure of pulmonic valve during inspiration. It is accentuated during exercise or in individuals with thin chest walls; heard most often in children and young adults	Same as S_2
S_2 persistent (wide) split	Second ICS, LSB	End of systole	High	Heard throughout the respiratory cycle; caused by late closure of pulmonic valve or early closure of aortic valve. Occurs in atrial septal defect, right ventricular failure, pulmonic stenosis, hypertension, or right bundle-branch heart block	Same as S_2

Sound	Location	Timing	Pitch	Description	Auscultation
S$_2$ paradoxic (reversed) split (P$_2$, A$_2$)	Second ICS, LSB	End of systole	High	Because of delayed left ventricular systole, the aortic valve closes after the pulmonic valve rather than before it (Normally during expiration the two sounds merge.) Causes may include left bundle-branch heart block, aortic stenosis, severe left ventricular failure, MI, and severe hypertension	Same as S$_2$
S$_2$ fixed split	Second ICS, LSB	End of systole	High	Heart with equal intensity during inspiration and expiration because of split of pulmonic and aortic components, which are unaffected by blood volume or respiratory changes. May be heard in pulmonary stenosis or atrial septal defect.	Same as S$_2$
S$_3$ (ventricular gallop)	Apex	Early in diastole just after S$_2$	Dull, low	Early and rapid filling of ventricle, as in early ventricular failure, heart failure. Common in children, during last trimester of pregnancy, and possibly in healthy adults >50 yr of age	Bell/patient in left lateral or supine position
S$_4$ (atrial gallop)	Apex	Late in diastole just before S$_1$	Low	Atrium filling against increased resistance of stiff ventricle, as in heart failure, coronary artery disease, cardiomyopathy, pulmonary artery hypertension, ventricular failure. May be normal in infants, children, and athletes	Same as S$_3$

ICS, Intercostal space; *LSB,* left sternal border; *MI,* myocardial infarction, *RSB,* right sternal border.

Commonly Occurring Heart Murmurs

Type	Timing	Pitch	Quality	Auscultation site	Radiation
Pulmonic stenosis	Systolic ejection	Medium-high	Harsh	Second, ICS, LSB	Toward left shoulder, back
Aortic stenosis	Midsystolic	Medium-high	Harsh	Second, ICS, RSB	Toward carotid arteries
Ventricular septal defect	Late systolic	High	Blowing	Fourth ICS, LSB	Toward RSB
Mitral insufficiency	Holosystolic	High	Blowing	Fifth-sixth ICS, left MCL	Toward left axilla
Tricuspid insufficiency	Holosystolic	High	Blowing	Fourth ICS, LSB	Toward apex
Aortic insufficiency	Early diastolic	High	Blowing	Second, ICS, RSB	Toward sternum
Pulmonary insufficiency	Early diastolic	High	Blowing	Second, ICS, LSB	Toward sternum
Mitral stenosis	Mid-late diastolic	Low	Rumbling	Fifth ICS, left MCL	Usually none
Tricuspid stenosis	Mid-late diastolic	Low	Rumbling	Fourth ICS, LSB	Usually none

ICS, Intercostal space; *LSB*, left sternal border; *MCL*, midclavicular line; *RSB*, right sternal border.

Assessing Normal Breath Sounds

Type	Normal site	Duration	Characteristics
Vesicular	Peripheral lung	I > E	Soft and swishing sounds. Abnormal when heard over the large airways
Bronchial	Trachea and bronchi	E > I	Louder, coarser, and of longer duration than vesicular. Abnormal if heard over peripheral lung
Bronchovesicular	Sternal border of major bronchi	E = I	Moderate in pitch and intensity. Abnormal if heard over peripheral lung

I, Inspiration; *E*, expiration.

Assessing Adventitious Breath Sounds

Type	Waveform	Characteristics	Possible clinical condition
Coarse crackle		Discontinuous, explosive, interrupted. Loud; low in pitch	Pulmonary edema, pneumonia in resolution stage
Fine crackle		Discontinuous, explosive, interrupted. Less loud than coarse crackles, lower in pitch, and of shorter duration	Interstitial lung disease; heart failure; atelectasis
Wheeze		Continuous, of long duration, high-pitched, musical, hissing	Narrowing of airway; bronchial asthma; COPD
Rhonchus		Continuous, of long duration, low-pitched, snoring	Production of sputum (usually cleared or lessened by coughing or suctioning)
Pleural friction rub		Grating, rasping noise	Rubbing together of inflamed parietal linings; loss of normal pleural lubrication

COPD, Chronic obstructive pulmonary disease.

Assessing Respiratory Patterns

Type	Waveform	Characteristics	Possible clinical condition
Eupnea		Normal rate and rhythm for adults and teenagers (12-20 breaths/min)	Normal pattern while awake
Bradypnea		Decreased rate (<12 breaths/min); regular rhythm	Normal sleep pattern; opiate or alcohol use; tumor; metabolic disorder
Tachypnea		Rapid rate (>20 breaths/min); hypoventilation or hyperventilation	Fever; restrictive respiratory disorders; pulmonary emboli
Hyperpnea		Depth of respirations greater than normal	Meeting increased metabolic demand (e.g., sepsis, MODS, SIRS, and exercise)
Apnea		Cessation of breathing; may be intermittent	Intermittent with CNS disturbances or drug intoxication; obstructed airway; respiratory arrest if it persists
Kussmaul		Deep, rapid (>20 breaths/min), sighing, labored	Renal failure, DKA, sepsis, shock

Continued

Assessing Respiratory Patterns—cont'd

Type	Waveform	Characteristics	Possible clinical condition
Cheyne-Stokes		Alternating patterns of apnea (10-20 sec) with periods of deep and rapid breathing. Lesions located bilaterally and deep within cerebral hemispheres	Heart failure, opiate or hypnotic overdose, thyrotoxicosis, dissecting aneurysm, subarachnoid hemorrhage, IICP, aortic valve disorders; may be normal in older adults during sleep
Central neurogenic hyperventilation		Rapid (>20 breaths/min), deep, regular. Lesions of midbrain or upper pons thought to be source of pattern	Primary injury (ischemia, infarction, space-occupying lesion); secondary injury (IICP, metabolic disorders, drug overdose)
Apneustic		Deep, prolonged inspiration, followed by 20-30 sec pause and short expiration. Lesion located in lower pons	Anoxia, meningitis, basilar artery occlusion
Cluster		Irregular breaths occurring in clusters with periods of apnea. Overall pattern irregular. Lesion located in lower pons or upper medulla	Primary and secondary neurologic injury may produce this respiratory pattern
Ataxic (Biot)		Irregular deep or shallow breaths. No discernible pattern. Lesion located in medulla	Primary and secondary neurologic injury may produce this respiratory pattern

CNS, Central nervous system; *DKA*, diabetic ketoacidosis; *IICP*, increased intracranial pressure; *MODS*, multiple organ dysfunction syndrome; *SIRS*, systemic inflammatory response syndrome.

Glasgow Coma Scale

Parameter	Patient Response	Score
Best eye opening response (record "C" if eyes closed due to swelling)	Spontaneously	4
	To speech	3
	To pain	2
	No response	1
Best motor response (record best upper limb response to painful stimuli)	Obeys verbal command	6
	Localizes pain	5
	Flexion—withdrawal	4
	Flexion—abnormal	3
	Extension—abnormal	2
	No response	1
Best verbal response (record "E" if endotracheal tube is in place or "T" if tracheostomy tube is in place)	Conversation—oriented × 3	5
	Conversation—confused	4
	Speech—inappropriate	3
	Sounds—incomprehensible	2
	No response	1

Total score	Interpretation
15	Normal
13-15	Minor head injury
9-12	Moderate head injury
3-8	Severe head injury
−7	Coma
3	Deep coma or brain death

Cranial Nerves: Functions and Dysfunctions

Cranial Nerve	Type	Functions	Dysfunctions
I Olfactory	Sensory	Smell	Anosmia
II Optic	Sensory	Sight	Blindness
		Visual acuity	
		Visual fields	
		Fundus	
III Oculomotor	Motor	Papillary constriction	Ptosis, diplopia, pupillary dilation, strabismus
		Elevation of upper eyelid	
		Extraocular movements	
IV Trochlear	Motor	Downward and inward movement of eye	Diplopia, visual disturbances with downward gaze
V Trigeminal	Sensory and motor	*Sensory:* Facial, scalp, anterior two thirds of tongue, lips, teeth, proprioception for mastication, corneal reflex	Loss of corneal reflex
		Motor: Temporal and masseter muscles (jaw clenching and lateral movement for mastication)	Paresis or paralysis of muscles of mastication, decreased facial sensation
VI Abducens	Motor	Lateral eye movement	Eye will not move laterally
VII Facial	Sensory and motor	*Sensory:* Taste in anterior two thirds of tongue, proprioception for face and scalp	Loss of taste in anterior two thirds of tongue
		Motor: Facial expression, lacrimal and salivary glands	Paresis or paralysis of facial muscles, facial droop, loss of glandular secretions
VIII Acoustic	Sensory	*Cochlear division:* Hearing	Tinnitus, deafness
		Vestibular division: Balance	Vertigo, nystagmus

Nerve	Type	Function	Dysfunction
IX Glossopharyngeal	Sensory and motor	*Sensory:* Taste in posterior one third of tongue; pain, touch, heat, cold in tongue, tonsils, soft palate, and pharynx *Motor:* Elevation of the soft palate, movement of pharynx, secretion and vasodilation of parotid glands for saliva; gag reflex	Loss of taste, pain, touch, heat, and cold in posterior one third of tongue, tonsils, and soft palate Paresis or paralysis of soft palate and pharynx, dysphagia, dysarthria, hoarseness, loss of gag reflex
X Vagus	Sensory and motor	*Sensory:* Muscles of pharynx, larynx, esophagus, thoracic and abdominal viscera; external ear, mucous membranes of larynx, trachea, esophagus, thoracic and abdominal viscera; lungs (stretch receptors), aortic bodies (chemoreceptors), respiratory/GI tract (pain receptors) *Motor:* Muscles of pharynx, larynx, esophagus, thoracic and abdominal viscera; respiratory/GI tract (smooth muscle), pacemaker and cardiac atrial muscle	Similar to dysfunction of glossopharyngeal Loss of gag reflex and difficulty swallowing
XI Spinal accessory	Motor	Sternocleidomastoid and trapezius muscles	Paresis of paralysis of sternocleidomastoid and trapezius muscles Inability to turn head or shrug shoulders
XII Hypoglossal	Motor	Tongue movement	Paresis or paralysis of the tongue

Major Deep Tendon (Muscle-Stretch) Reflexes

Reflex	Innervations	Examination technique	Normal response
Biceps	C5, C6	Arm partially flexed at elbow, palm down. Place thumb or finger on biceps tendon. Strike finger with reflex hammer	Contraction of biceps muscle Flexion at elbow
Triceps	C6, C7	Arm flexed at elbow, palm toward body, arm pulled slightly across body. Strike triceps tendon with reflex hammer above elbow	Contraction of triceps muscle Extension of arm at elbow
Brachioradialis	C5, C6	Hand resting on abdomen, palm slightly pronated. Strike radius with reflex hammer 3-5 cm above wrist	Contraction of brachioradialis muscle Flexion and supination of forearm
Achilles (ankle jerk)	S1, S2	Leg flexed at knee, dorsiflex the foot. Strike Achilles tendon with reflex hammer	Plantar flexion of foot
Quadriceps (knee jerk)	L3, L4	Leg flexed at knee. Strike patellar tendon with reflex hammer	Contraction of quadriceps muscle Extension of knee

Grading of Deep Tendon Reflexes

Scale (0 to 4+)	Interpretation
4+	Very brisk, hyperactive, repetitive, rhythmic flexion and extension (clonus); indicative of disease
3+	Brisker than average; may be normal for certain individuals or may indicate disease
2+	Average/normal
1+	Diminished response or low normal
0	No response

Major Superficial (Cutaneous) Reflexes

Reflex	Innervation	Examination technique	Normal response
Abdominals Above/upper Below/lower	T8, T9, T10 T10, T11, T12	Using tongue blade or wooden end of cotton-tipped applicator, lightly stroke abdomen in each quadrant, outer-to-inner direction, toward umbilicus	Contraction of abdominal muscles Umbilicus deviates (pulls) toward the stimulus
Bulbocavernous (male)	S3, S4	Pinch glans penis or apply pressure over bulbocavernous muscle behind scrotum	Scrotum will elevate toward the body
Corneal	Cranial nerves V and VII	Using wisp of cotton, lightly touch cornea	Eyelids will quickly close
Cremasteric (male)	L1, L2	Lightly stroke inner aspect of thigh	Testicle on side stroked will elevate
Gag	Cranial nerves IX and X	Using tongue blade, lightly touch posterior pharynx	Gagging or retching
Perianal	S3, S4, S5	Stroke tissue surrounding anus with blunt instrument, or examine rectum by gently inserting gloved finger	Anal puckering with external stimuli. Tightening of anal sphincter with internal examination

Inotropic and Vasoactive Agents

Inotropics/vasoactives

Agent	Effects (Preload) HR	(Preload) PAWP	(Afterload) SVR	(Afterload) Contractility	Dosage	Nursing implications
Dopamine hydrochloride (Intropin)	—↑	—	—	—↑	Low dose 1-2 mcg/kg/min; Moderate dose 2-10 mcg/kg/min; High dose >10 mcg/kg/min	Affect cardiac contractility and vascular resistance; Major effect may be to increase urine output; may potentiate effect of diuretics; Major effect is to increase contractility
Dobutamine (Dobutrex)	—↑	—↓	—↓	↑↑	2.5-10 mcg/kg/min	Can cause tissue necrosis and sloughing if infiltration occurs
Isoproterenol (Isuprel)	↑↑	—↓	↓↓	↑↑	2-10 mcg/min	Overall effect is improved CO; may cause tachycardia and dysrhythmias as side effects; Significant increase in myocardial oxygen consumption; can produce ventricular tachycardia and fibrillation
Epinephrine	↑↑	↑	↓↑	↑↑	0.5-1 mg for cardiac arrest; 1-4 mcg/min for inotropic support	May induce ventricular ectopy
Amrinone lactate (Inocor)	—↑	↓	↓	↑	2-20 mcg/kg/min	Can exacerbate myocardial ischemia
Milrinone lactate (Primacor)	—↑	↓	↓	↑	50 mcg/kg given over 10 min; start infusion of 0.375-0.75 mcg/kg/min	Can prompt supraventricular and ventricular dysrhythmias

Agent	HR	CO	SVR	PAWP	Dose	Comments
Vasopressors						Main effect is vasoconstriction of peripheral blood vessels
Methoxamine hydrochloride (Vasoxyl)	—	↑	↑↑↑	—	3-5 mg	Used rarely; may increase myocardial oxygen demand
Norepinephrine (Levophed)	↓↑	↑	↑↑↑	↑	2-12 mcg/min	Contraindicated when hypotension occurs secondary to hypovolemia. Can cause tissue necrosis and sloughing if infiltration occurs. Increased myocardial oxygen demand without increased coronary artery flow can cause myocardial ischemia and infarction
Phenylephrine (Neo-Synephrine)	—	↑	↑↑↑	—	0.1-0.5 mg	May cause dysrhythmias or trigger reflex bradycardia
Vasopressin	↑	—	↑↑	—	0.02-0.1 units/min	Higher doses cause marked splanchnic vasoconstriction
Vasodilators						Main effect is dilation of arterial and/or venous beds
Sodium nitroprusside (Nipride)	—↑	→	↓↓	—	Starting dose of 0.5-0.8 mcg/kg/min; titrate up to 10 mcg/kg/min	Drug is photosensitive; keep infusion container protected from light. Thiocyanate (a metabolite of nitroprusside) toxicity can occur after 72 hr. Monitor thiocyanate levels daily, being alert to levels >10 mg/dl and or signs of metabolic acidosis (see p. 576)
Nitroglycerin (Tridil, Nitrostat)	—↑	↓↓	→	—	Starting dose of 0.5 mcg/min; titrate up to 200 mcg/min	Absorbed by standard plastic IV tubing. Use special polyvinyl chloride tubing. Ensure that the drug is diluted for IV use

—, No effect; ↑, minimal effect; ↑↑, moderate effect; ↑↑↑, major effect; *CO*, cardiac output; *HR*, heart rate; *IV*, intravenous *PAWP*, pulmonary artery wedge pressure; *SVR*, systemic vascular resistance.

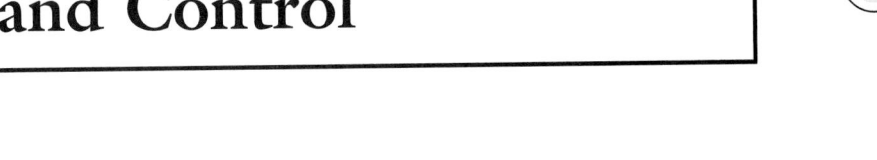

APPENDIX 8

Infection Prevention and Control

For several decades, infection prevention and control have focused on the use of barriers (e.g., gloves, gowns, masks) to interrupt transmission of organisms among and between patients and health care workers. These barriers are a major component of various systems of transmission precautions.

SYSTEMS OF TRANSMISSION PRECAUTIONS

Many different systems of transmission precautions have been used in hospitals over the years and were called *isolation precautions* until the most recent revision (2004) by the Centers for Disease Control and Prevention (CDC). The change in wording is to reflect clearly the purpose of these techniques and procedures, which is to interrupt transmission of organisms. The revised guideline adheres to four guiding principles: (1) to respond to challenges and needs not identified in previous guidelines, (2) to emphasize standard precautions as the essential foundation for preventing transmission of infectious agents in all health care settings, (3) to be epidemiologically sound and, whenever possible, evidence-based, and (4) to be useful to persons delivering care in a variety of health care settings. The 2004 guideline contains two tiers of precautions (Table 1): **Standard Precautions,** which are designed for the care of all patients in any health care setting, regardless of diagnosis or presumed infection status, and **Expanded Precautions,** which are used for patients known to be or suspected of being infected or colonized with epidemiologically important pathogens that can be transmitted by airborne or droplet transmission or by contact with dry skin or contaminated surfaces. A new type of Enhanced Precautions has also been added, the Protective Environment, which is specifically for patients receiving hematopoietic stem cell transplantation (HSCT) who are at particular risk for infections with airborne fungi.

The 2004 guideline replaces the 1996 guideline for isolation precautions in hospitals. The 1996 Standard Precautions system synthesized the major features of Universal Precautions and Body Substance Isolation and applied to (1) blood, (2) all body fluids, secretions, and excretions, except sweat, regardless of whether they contain visible blood, (3) nonintact skin, and (4) mucous membranes. In addition, Standard Precautions were designed to reduce risks of transmission of microorganisms from both recognized and unrecognized sources of infectious agents. The 2004 guideline continues these same principles of Standard Precautions and applies them to a broader range of situations and care settings. The 1996 Transmission-Based Precautions were designed for patients documented to be or suspected of being infected or colonized with organisms transmitted by the airborne route, by droplets, and by contact where extra precautions were necessary to interrupt transmission. The term *Expanded Precautions* replaces the term *Transmission-Based Precautions* and modifies the 1996 guideline consistent with new information about mechanisms of transmission of epidemiologically important organisms. As always, the CDC offers hospitals and other types of health care settings the option of modifying the recommendations according to their needs and circumstances and as directed by federal, state, or local regulations. For example, the Occupational Safety and Health Administration's (OSHA's) Bloodborne Pathogens Standard (1991) is still operable, and all facilities are required to comply with its provisions. The CDC's 2004 Standard Precautions incorporate all requirements of the OSHA Bloodborne Pathogens Standard.

EXPANDED PRECAUTIONS FOR PATIENTS WITH PULMONARY OR LARYNGEAL TUBERCULOSIS

Airborne Infection Isolation Precautions are for persons diagnosed with or suspected of having pulmonary or laryngeal tuberculosis (TB) that can be transmitted to others via the airborne route. These

Text continued on p. 666.

TABLE 1 Recommendations for Transmission Precautions in Healthcare Settings, 2004

	Standard Precautions	Expanded precautions: airborne infection isolation	Expanded precautions: droplet	Expanded precautions: contact	Expanded precautions: protective environment
When to use	For the care of all patients in all health care settings.	For patients known or suspected to be infected with microorganisms transmitted person-to-person by airborne droplet nuclei that remain suspended in the air and that can be dispersed widely by air currents.	For patients known or suspected to be infected with microorganisms transmitted by droplets that can be generated by the patient during coughing, sneezing, talking, or the performance of procedures.	For patients known of suspected of being infected or colonized with specific epidemiologically important organisms that can be transmitted by direct or indirect contact when there is evidence that standard precautions and hand hygiene are not effective in preventing health care associated transmission (see Guideline for specific organisms to which Contact Precautions apply).	For allogenic hematopoietic stem cell transplantation (HSCT) patients to minimize fungal spore counts in the air.

Hand hygiene:

1. If hands are not visibly soiled, use an alcohol-based waterless antiseptic agent

2. When hands are dirty or contaminated with proteinaceous material, wash with soap and water

Practice hand hygiene after touching blood, body fluids, secretions, excretions, and contaminated items, whether or not gloves are worn.

Use hand hygiene immediately after gloves are removed, between patient contacts, and when otherwise indicated in *Hand Hygiene Guideline* (2002). Decontaminate hands after contact with inanimate objects (including medical equipment) in the immediate vicinity of the patient.

Continued

TABLE 1 Recommendations for Transmission Precautions in Healthcare Settings, 2004—cont'd

	Standard Precautions	Expanded precautions: airborne infection isolation	Expanded precautions: droplet	Expanded precautions: contact	Expanded precautions: protective environment
Gloves	Wear gloves when it can be reasonably anticipated that contact with blood or other potentially infectious materials, mucous membranes, non-intact skin, or potentially colonized intact skin will occur. For purposes of preventing transmission of infectious agents, the choice of glove type (e.g., latex, vinyl, nitrile) is determined by permeability factors. Remove gloves after caring for patient. Do not wear the same pair of gloves for the care of more			Wear gloves as indicated according to Standard Precautions and whenever touching the patient's intact skin and the patient's environment and articles including medical equipment, computer keyboards, bed rails, etc. Remove gloves before leaving the patient's room and practice hand hygiene immediately. After glove removal and hand hygiene, ensure that hands do not touch surfaces or items in the patient's room to avoid transfer of microorganisms to other patients or surfaces or articles.	

	than one patient, and do not wash gloves between patients. Change gloves during patient care if moving from a contaminated body site to a clean body site.			
Mask, eye protection, face shield	Wear a mask and eye protection or a face shield to protect mucous membranes of the eyes, nose, and mouth during procedures that are likely to generate splashes or sprays.	Wear respiratory protection (N95 respirator) when entering the room or home of a patient with known or suspected infectious pulmonary tuberculosis. Persons susceptible to measles (rubeola), varicella (chickenpox), or smallpox should not enter the room of these patients if other immune caregivers are available. If susceptible persons must enter these rooms, respiratory protection should be used.	Wear a mask and eye protection when working within 3 feet of the patient.	Place a mask on patients when they leave the protective environment for diagnostic tests or treatments elsewhere in the facility to prevent inhalation of respirable particles and reaerosolization of exhaled particles. Consult infection control professional for appropriate type of mask.

Continued

TABLE 1 Recommendations for Transmission Precautions in Healthcare Settings, 2004—cont'd

	Standard Precautions	Expanded precautions: airborne infection isolation	Expanded precautions: droplet	Expanded precautions: contact	Expanded precautions: protective environment
Gowns	Wear a gown to protect skin and prevent soiling of clothing during procedures and patient-care activities that are likely to generate splashes or sprays of blood, body fluids, secretions, or excretions. Wear a gown for direct patient contact if patient has uncontained secretions, excretions, or wound drainage and contamination is likely to occur. Remove gown before leaving patient's environment.			Wear gowns as indicated according to Standard Precautions and whenever anticipating that the caregiver's clothing will have direct contact with the patient, environmental surfaces, or items in the patient's room. Remove gown before leaving patient's environment. After gown removal, ensure that clothing does not contact environmental surfaces.	
Patient placement	Consider potential for transmission of infectious agents when making patient placement decisions.	Inpatient or residential setting: Place patient in a private room that has monitored negative pressure ventilation,	Maintain spatial separation of at least 3 ft between the infected patient and other patients and visitors. This may be more easily	Place the patient in a private room to reduce the risk of transmission of epidemiologically important organisms.	Place allogenic HSCT patients in a protective environment that includes appropriate environmental controls

	adequate numbers of air changes, and appropriate discharge of air outdoors or filtered before recirculation. Keep the door closed and the patient in the room. If an appropriate private room is not available, consult infection control professional for alternatives.	achieved using a private room. When a private room is not available, patients with the same active infection may be in the same room (cohorting). Special air handling and ventilation are not necessary, and the room may remain open.	When a private room is not available, place the patient in a room with a patient(s) colonized or infected with the same organism. When these options are not available, consult infection control professional for alternatives.	to reduce the risk of transmission of environmental fungi. Consult infection control professional for details.
Patient transport	Limit movement and transport of the patient to essential purposes only. If transport or movement is necessary, minimize patient dispersal of droplet nuclei by placing a surgical mask on the patient. If patient has a viral infection that can be transmitted via the airborne route, cover patient to prevent aerosolization of virus from skin lesions that are not crusted.	Limit movement and transport of the patient to essential purposes only.	Limit movement and transport of the patient from the room to essential purposes only. If the patient is transported out of the room, ensure that precautions are maintained to minimize the risk of transmission of microorganisms to other patients and contamination of environmental surfaces or equipment.	

Continued

TABLE 1 Recommendations for Transmission Precautions in Healthcare Settings, 2004—cont'd

	Standard Precautions	Expanded precautions: airborne infection isolation	Expanded precautions: droplet	Expanded precautions: contact	Expanded precautions: protective environment
Patient care equipment	Handle used patient-care equipment in a manner that prevents skin and mucous membrane exposures, contamination of clothing, and transfer of microorganisms to other patients and environments.			Manage patient care equipment according to Standard Precautions. Note: Additional procedures may be indicated in outbreak situations.	
Care of the environment	Keep environmental surfaces visibly clean on a regular basis and as spills occur.			Clean the environment according to Standard Precautions. Note: Additional	

procedures may be indicated in outbreak situations.

| Textiles, laundry | Handle, transport, and process used linen in a manner that prevents skin and mucous membrane exposures and contamination of clothing, and that avoids transfer to microorganisms to other patients and environments. |

Modified from Strausbaugh L, Jackson M. Rhinehart E. Siegel J, and the Healthcare Infection Control Practices Advisory Committee (HICPAC): *Guideline to prevent transmission of infectious agents in healthcare settings.* To be published by the Centers for Disease Control and Prevention early 2004. **NOTE:** *This table was developed when this publication was in DRAFT form; therefore the final version may differ slightly from what is published here.*

guidelines focus on early identification and treatment of persons with a diagnosis or suspected diagnosis of active TB. In addition, the CDC defined requirements for special ventilation and use of respiratory protection masks that provide better filtration and a tighter fit than standard surgical masks. Masks of this type are called *particulate respirators (PRs)*, and the specific type of PR for TB protection is called an N95 respirator. This type of respiratory protection is also appropriate for susceptible persons caring for patients known or suspected of having measles (rubeola), varicella (chickenpox), or smallpox. Of course, the best protection for any of the vaccine-preventable infectious diseases is for all caregivers to be immunized, then respiratory protection masks are not necessary.

MANAGEMENT OF DEVICES AND PROCEDURES TO REDUCE RISK OF NOSOCOMIAL INFECTION

Use of barriers is but one of many strategies that can reduce the risk of nosocomial infection among patients and personnel. In fact, studies from the CDC show that significant gains can be made in reducing infection risks by focusing on the management of devices and procedures commonly used in patient care. For example, many patients need intravascular devices that deliver therapeutic medications, but they are put at risk for site infections and bacteremias when these devices are used. It is well known that rotating the access site at appropriate intervals reduces these risks to the patient, and catheter materials that are more "vein friendly" also reduce trauma to the vascular system. In addition, use of needles to deliver medications and fluids to patients through these intravascular devices can put the health care worker at risk for puncture injury. Needleless or needle-free IV access devices are used to access line ports so that it is not necessary to use needles once the intravascular catheter has entered the vascular system. Thus the use of newer and safer intravascular devices and procedures can benefit both the patient and health care worker by reducing their risk of nosocomial infection. Research studies of interventions to reduce nosocomial infection risks are published in general and specialty journals and presented at professional meetings each year. Infection control practitioners and hospital epidemiologists use these studies to make recommendations about changes in nursing and medical practice. The Joint Commission on Accreditation of Healthcare Organizations (JCAHO) requires that all accredited facilities have a person qualified to provide infection surveillance, prevention, and control services. The national associations for these professionals are the Association for Professionals in Infection Control and Epidemiology, Inc. (APIC), which publishes the *American Journal of Infection Control*, and the Society for Healthcare Epidemiology of America (SHEA), which publishes the journal *Infection Control and Hospital Epidemiology*.

Bibliography

Boyce JM, Pittet D: *Guideline for hand hygiene in health-care settings*: recommendations of the Healthcare Infection Control Practices Advisory Committee HICPAC/SHEA/APIC/IDSA Hand Hygiene Task Force 23 (12 Suppl):S3-40, 2002.

Department of Labor, Occupational Safety and Health Administration: *Occupational exposure to bloodborne pathogens*: final rule, 29 CRF, part 1910:1030, Federal Register 56:64003-64182, December 6, 1991.

Garner JS and the Hospital Infection Control Practices Advisory Committee (HICPAC), Centers for Disease Control Practices and Prevention: Guidelines for isolation precautions in hospitals, *Infect Control Hosp Epidemiol* 17 (1):53-80, 1996.

Strausbaugh L, Jackson M, Rhinehart E, Siegel J, and the Healthcare Infection Control Practices Advisory Committee (HICPAC): *Guideline to prevent transmission of infectious agents in health-care settings* (In press.)

Sample Relaxation Technique

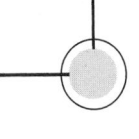

Give the patient the following instructions:

1. Sit quietly in a comfortable position. Close your eyes.
2. Relax all your muscles, starting at your feet and progressing to your facial muscles. Focus your attention on one body area at a time while you relax the muscles in that area.
3. Breathe through your nose. As you breathe out, say the word "one" silently to yourself. Become aware of your breathing. Continue this process for about 20 minutes.
4. Do not worry whether you are achieving deep relaxation. Maintain a passive attitude and permit relaxation to occur at its own pace. If distractions interfere, see your thoughts floating away like clouds. Continue breathing and repeating the word "one."

Abbreviations Used in this Manual

AACN: American Association of Critical Care Nurses
AAL: anterior axillary line
ABA: American Burn Association
ABG: arterial blood gas
ACC: American College of Cardiology
ACCP: American College of Chest Physicians
ACE: angiotensin-converting enzyme
ACh: acetylcholine
AChR: acetylcholine receptors
ACLS: advanced cardiac life support
ACS: abdominal compartment syndrome
ACT: activated clotting time
AD: autonomic dysreflexia
ADA: American Diabetes Association
ADH: antidiuretic hormone
ADL: activity of daily living
AED: automatic external defibrillator
AEG: atrial electrogram
AF: atrial fibrillation
AHA: American Heart Association
AIDS: acquired immunodeficiency syndrome
AIS: acute ischemic stroke
ALI: acute lung injury
ALP: alkaline phosphatase
ALT: alanine aminotransferase
AM: akinetic mutism
AMA: American Medical Association
AMI: acute myocardial infarct
ANA: American Nurses Association
ANP: atrial natriuretic peptide
APAS: antiphospholipid antibody syndrome
APSAC: anisoylated plasminogen streptokinase activator complex
aPTT: activated partial thromboplastin time
ARDS: acute respiratory distress syndrome
ARF: acute respiratory failure; acute renal failure
ARS: adjective rating scale
ASA: acetylsalicylic acid (aspirin)
ASO: antistreptolysin O
AST: aspartate aminotransferase
AT: antithrombin
AT$_1$: receptor antagonist
ATGAM: antithymocyte gamma globulin
atm: atmosphere (standard)

ATN: acute tubular necrosis
ATP: adenosine triphosphate
AV: atrioventricular; arteriovenous
AVM: arteriovenous malformation
AVNRT: atrial-ventricular non-reciprocating tachycardia
AVRT: atrial-ventricular reciprocating tachycardia
BAL: bronchoalveolar lavage
BEE: basal energy expenditure
BMI: body mass index
BP: blood pressure
bpm: beats per minute
BS: bowel sounds
BSA: body surface area
BUN: blood urea nitrogen
C: centigrade
Ca$^+$: calcium
CABG: coronary artery bypass grafting
CAD: coronary artery disease
CAPD: continuous ambulatory peritoneal dialysis
CASHD: coronary atherosclerotic heart disease
CAVH: continuous arteriovenous hemofiltration
CBC: complete blood cell count
CBF: cerebral blood flow
CD: Cotrel-Dubousset
CDC: Centers for Disease Control and Prevention
CDI: central diabetes insipidus
CHF: congestive heart failure
CI: cardiac index
CIE: counterimmunoelectrophoresis
CJD: Creutzfeldt-Jakob disease
CK: creatine kinase
Cl$^-$: chloride
CK-MB: creatine kinase-myocardial band
CM: cardiomyopathy
CMV: cytomegalovirus; controlled mechanical ventilation
CNS: central nervous system
CO: cardiac output; carbon monoxide
CO$_2$: carbon dioxide
COPD: chronic obstructive pulmonary disease
CPAP: continuous positive airway pressure
CPK: creatine phosphokinase
CPP: cerebral perfusion pressure; coronary perfusion pressure
C&S: culture and sensitivities
CSF: cerebrospinal fluid
CT: computed tomography
cTnI: cardiac troponin I
CVA: cerebrovascular accident; costovertebral angle
CVC: central venous catheter
CVP: central venous pressure
CVVH: continuous venovenous hemofiltration
CVVHD: continuous venovenous hemofiltration with dialysis
CVVHDF: continuous venovenous hemodiafiltration
CXR: chest x-ray
CyA: cyclosporine
DAI: diffuse axonal injury
DCM: dilated cardiomyopathy
DFI: diffusion weighted imaging (or DWI)
DI: diabetes insipidus
DIC: disseminated intravascular coagulation
DKA: diabetic ketoacidosis
DM: diabetes mellitus

DNR: do not resuscitate
Do$_2$: oxygen delivery
DOE: dyspnea on exertion
DPAHC: durable power of attorney for health care
DPL: diagnostic peritoneal lavage
DTR: deep tendon reflex
DVT: deep vein thrombosis
EACA: epsilon-(ε-) aminocaproic acid
EBV: Epstein-Barr virus
ECG: electrocardiogram
ECHO: electrocardiography
EEG: electroencephalogram
EFA: Epilepsy Foundation of America
ELISA: enzyme-linked immunosorbent assay
EMI: electromagnetic interference
EPS: electrophysiologic studies
ESR: erythrocyte sedimentation rate
ET: endotracheal
ETCO$_2$: end-tidal carbon dioxide
ETOH: alcohol
ETT: endotracheal tube
F: Fahrenheit
FAST: focused assessment with sonography for trauma
FDP: fibrin degradation product
FEF: forced expiratory flow
FEV: forced expiratory volume
FHF: fulminant hepatic failure
fr: French
Fio$_2$: fraction of inspired oxygen
FRC: functional residual capacity
FSP: fibrin split product
FVC: forced vital capacity
GABA: gamma-(γ-) aminobutyric
GBS: Guillain-Barré syndrome
GCS: Glasgow coma scale
GERD: gastroesophageal reflux disease
GI: gastrointestinal
GKI: glucose-potassium-insulin
G6PD: glucose-6-phosphate dehydrogenase
GU: genitourinary
H$_2$O: water
HAT: heparin-associated thrombocytopenia
HCM: hypertrophic cardiomyopathy
HCO$_3^-$: bicarbonate
Hct: hematocrit
HDL: high-density lipoprotein
HELLP: hemolysis, elevated liver enzymes, low platelet count
Hgb: hemoglobin
HHNS: hyperglycemic hyperosmolar nonketotic syndrome
HITT: heparin-induced thrombocytopenia thrombosis
HIV: human immunodeficiency virus
HOB: head of bed
HPO$_4$: phosphate
HR: heart rate
HRS: hepatorenal syndrome
HSV: herpes simplex virus
HUS: hemolytic-uremic syndrome
HVPG: hepatic venous pressure gradient
HVWP: hepatic vein wedge pressure
IABP: intraaortic balloon pump
IAP: intraabdominal pressure

ICA: internal cerebral artery
ICD: implantable cardioverter-defibrillator
ICH: intracerebral hematoma
ICP: intracranial pressure
ICS: intercostal space
ICU: intensive care unit
IE: infective endocarditis
I/E: inspiration/expiration
IER: in expected range
IgG: immunoglobulin G
IHSS: idiopathic hypertrophic subaortic stenosis
IICP: increased intracranial pressure
IM: intramuscular
INR: international normalized ratio
I&O: intake and output
IPD: intermittent peritoneal dialysis; intracranial pressure dynamics
IPPB: intermittent positive-pressure breathing
IRV: inverse ratio ventilation
ITP: idiopathic thrombocytopenic purpura
IV: intravenous
IVP: intravenous pyelogram
JNC VII: Joint National Committee VII
JT: junctional tachycardia
JVD: jugular vein distention
K$^+$: potassium
kcal: kilocalorie
KCl: potassium (K$^+$) chloride (Cl$^-$)
kg: kilogram
KUB: kidney, ureter, bladder
L: liter; lumbar
LAD: left anterior descending (coronary artery)
LAP: left atrial pressure
LDH: lactate dehydrogenase; also abbreviated LD
LDL: low-density lipoprotein
LIS: locked-in-syndrome
LMW: low molecular weight
LOC: level of consciousness
LOS: length of stay
LP: lumbar puncture
LR: lactated Ringer's
LUQ: left upper quadrant
LUT: lower urinary tract
LV: left ventricular
LVEDP: left ventricular end-diastolic pressure
LVH: left ventricular hypertrophy
m: meter
MAP: mean arterial pressure
MCA: middle cerebral artery
MCL: modified chest lead; midclavicular line
MCS: minimally conscious state
MCT: medium-chain triglycerides
MCV: mean corpuscular volume
Mg: magnesium
MG: myasthenia gravis
mg: milligram
MI: myocardial infarction
MODS: multiple organ dysfunction syndrome
mOsm: milliosmole
MPAP: mean pulmonary artery pressure; also abbreviated PAM
MRA: magnetic resonance arteriogram
MRI: magnetic resonance imaging

MS: multiple sclerosis
MSO$_4$: morphine sulfate
MUGA scan: multiple-gated acquisition scan
Na/Na$^+$: sodium
NaCl: sodium chloride/saline
NCV: nerve conduction velocity
NDI: nephrogenic diabetes insipidus
NG: nasogastric
NHO: National Hospice Organization
nl: normal
NMBA: neuromuscular blocking agent(s)
NPO: nothing by mouth
NRS: numeric rating scale
NSAID: nonsteroidal antiinflammatory drug
NSTEMI: non-ST segment elevation myocardial infarction
NTG: nitroglycerin
nvCJD: new variant Creutzfeld-Jakob disease
OT: occupational therapist
OTC: over the counter
PA: pulmonary artery
PAC: premature atrial complexes
PaCO$_2$: carbon dioxide (arterial pressure)
PAD: pulmonary artery diastolic
PaO$_2$: oxygen (arterial pressure)
PAP: pulmonary artery pressure/positive airway pressure
PASG: pneumatic antishock garment
PAT: paroxysmal atrial tachycardia
PAW: pulmonary artery wedge
PAWP: pulmonary artery wedge pressure
PBV: percutaneous balloon valvuloplasty
PCA: patient-controlled analgesia
PE: pulmonary embolus
PEEP: positive end-expiratory pressure
PEG: percutaneous endoscopic gastrostomy
PET: positron emission tomography
PIH: pregnancy-induced hypertension
PJC: premature junctional complexes
PK: pyruvate kinase
PMI: point of maximal impulse
PN: parenteral nutrition
PND: paroxysmal nocturnal dsypnea
PO: by mouth
PO$_4$: phosphates
PPF: plasma protein fraction
PRA: panel-reactive antibody
PRBCs: packed red blood cells
PSB: protected specimen brush
PSV: pressure support ventilation
PSVT: paroxysmal supraventricular tachycardia
PT: physical therapy; physical therapist; prothrombin time
PTCA: percutaneous transluminal coronary angioplasty
PTH: parathyroid hormone
PTT: partial thromboplastin time
PVC: premature ventricular complex; peripheral venous catheter
PVR: pulmonary vascular resistance
PWI: perfusion weighted imaging
RAP: right atrial pressure
RBC: red blood cell
RCM: restrictive cardiomyopathy
RDA: Recommended Daily Allowance; Recommended Dietary Allowance
rHuEPO: recombinant human erythropoietin

RLA: Rancho Los Amigos
ROM: range of motion
RPE: rate perceived exertion
RR: respiratory rate
rt-PA: recombinant tissue plasminogen activator
RV: right ventricle
RVP: right ventricular pressure
SA: status asthmaticus
SAH: subarachnoid hemorrhage
SAS: subarachnoid space
SBP: systolic blood pressure
SCCM: Society of Critical Care Medicine
SCI: spinal cord injury
Scvo$_2$: central venous oxygen saturation
SGOT: serum glutamic oxaloacetic acid transaminase
SGPT: serum glutamic pyruvic transaminase
SIADH: syndrome of inappropriate antidiuretic hormone
SIMV: synchronized intermittent mandatory ventilation
SIRS: systemic inflammatory response syndrome
Sjo$_2$: jugular venous oxygen saturation
SOB: shortness of breath
Spo$_2$: pulse oximetry oxygen saturation
SQ: subcutaneous; also abbreviated *SC*
SS: sensory stimulation
STEMI: ST segment elevation myocardial infarction
STSG: split-thickness skin graft
SV: stroke volume
Svo$_2$: mixed venous oxygen saturation
SVR: systemic vascular resistance
TBSA: total body surface area
TCD: transcranial Doppler
TdP: Torsades de Pointe
TE: thrombotic emboli
TEA: tranexamic acid
TEC: transluminal extraction catheterization
TEE: total energy expenditure; transesophageal echocardiography
TENS: transcutaneous electrical nerve stimulation
TIA: transient ischemic attack
TIBC: total iron-binding capacity
TIPS/TIPSS: transjugular intrahepatic portal-systemic shunt
TMP: transmembrane pressure
TNA: total nutrient admixtures
TNF: tumor necrosis factor
TOF: train-of-four
TPA: tissue plasminogen activator
TPN: total parenteral nutrition
TSF: triceps skinfold thickness
UF: ultrafiltration
URI: upper respiratory infection
UTI: urinary tract infection
VAD: venous access device; ventricular assist device
VAS: visual analog scale
VC: vital capacity
VCJD: variant (new) Creutzfeld-Jakob disease
VEDP: ventricular end-diastolic pressure
VF: ventricular fibrillation
VLDL: very-low-density lipoprotein
VMA: vanillylmandelic acid
Vo$_2$: oxygen consumption
VS: vital signs/vegetative state

VSD: ventricular septal defect
VT: ventricular tachycardia
Vt: tidal volume
WBC: white blood cell
WNL: within normal limits
WPW: Wolff-Parkinson-White syndrome

Index

Protease inhibitors in DIC, 493
Protection, altered
  in ARF, 328
  in DIC, 494
  in heparin-induced thrombocytopenia, 485
  in hepatic failure, 444-445
  in high-risk obstetric conditions, 585-586
  in hypercalcemia, 557
  in hypermagnesemia, 566
  in hypernatremia, 548
  in hypocalcemia, 555
  in hypomagnesemia, 563-564
  in hyponatremia, 547
  in hypophosphatemia, 559
  in immune thrombocytopenic purpura, 487-488
  with intraaortic balloon pump procedure, 297
  in myxedema coma, 413
  during renal replacement therapies, 343
  with SAH/cerebral aneurysm, 364
  during thrombolytic therapy, 308-309
  in thyroid crisis, 410
  in valvular heart disease, 265-266, 268
  with ventricular assist devices, 297
Protein
  buffering function of, 568
  in calorie count for parenteral nutrition, 4
  enteral formulas for, 7
  parenteral formulas for, 8
Protein requirements, estimating, 4
Proteus pneumonia, risk groups, onset, characteristics, complications, 182t
Pseudohyponatremia, 546
Pseudomonas pneumonia, risk groups, onset, characteristics, complications, 182t
Psychosocial support, 68-80
  for anticipatory grieving, 73
  for anxiety, 69
  for body image disturbance, 75-76
  for dysfunctional grieving, 73-74
  for fear, 71
  for hopelessness, 76-78
  for impaired communication, 69-70
  for ineffective coping/denial, 71-73
  in knowledge deficit, 68-69
  nursing diagnoses/interventions in, 68-78
  for patient's family/significant others, 78-80
  for powerlessness, 74
  in risk for violence, 76, 77t
  for sensory/perceptual alterations, 70-71
  for sleep pattern disturbance, 71, 72t
  for social isolation, 75
  for spiritual distress, 74
PTCA. See Percutaneous transluminal coronary angioplasty
PTH. See Parathyroid hormone
Pulmonary artery diastolic pressure, 24
  normal values for, 25t
Pulmonary artery pressure
  abnormal, 27t
  increased, 187
  normal values for, 27, 28
Pulmonary artery systolic pressure, normal values for, 25t
Pulmonary artery wedge pressure, 24
  normal values for, 25t, 28
Pulmonary care in spinal cord injuries, 139

Pulmonary disorders. *See also* Acute lung injury; Lung disease
  alterations in consciousness due to, 39
Pulmonary edema, 220-226
  acute, management of, 630t
  assessment of, 221
  diagnostic tests for, 221-222
  management of, 222-223
  nursing diagnoses/interventions for, 223-225
  pathophysiology of, 220-221
  from salicylate overdose, 536
Pulmonary embolism, 192-198
  after intracranial surgery, 367
  assessment of, 193-194
  diagnostic tests for, 194-195
  management of, 195-196
  nursing diagnoses/interventions for, 196-198
  pathophysiology of, 192-193
  PEA due to, 613t
Pulmonary function
  in acute lung injury/ARDS, 190
  in Guillain-Barré syndrome, 354
  in pulmonary hypertension, 188
  and weaning from mechanical ventilation, 19t
Pulmonary hypertension, 187-189
  assessment of, 188
  defined, 187
  diagnostic tests for, 188
  management of, 188-189
  nursing diagnoses/interventions for, 189
  pathophysiology of, 187, 188t
Pulmonary vascular resistance, 24
  calculation/normal values, 28
  increased, 187
Pulse oximetry
  in acid-base disturbances, 569
  in acute lung injury/ARDS, 190
  in acute pneumonia, 184
  in burn patient, 164
  in compartment syndrome, 134
Pulse pressure in abdominal trauma, 152
Pulseless electrical activity
  advanced cardiac life support for, 611t-612t
  clinical signs and treatment, 613t-615t
Pulseless ventricular tachycardia, assessment of, 607t-608t
Pulsus paradoxus
  in cardiac tamponade, 119t
  measuring, 121t
  in pericarditis, 275
Purpura fulminans, 493

Q

Q waves in myocardial infarction, 207
QS/QT ratio in acute lung injury/ARDS, 190
Quality of life, ethical considerations in, 82

R

Radioactive iodine for thyrotoxic crisis, 409
Radionuclide studies in cardiomyopathy, 227
Rancho Los Amigos cognitive functioning scale, 41
Range-of-motion exercises
  for activity intolerance, 61-62
  modifications of, 63
  in pain management, 58t